Advanced Nursing Practice

Advanced Nursing Practice

An Integrative Approach

Second Edition

ANN B. HAMRIC, PhD, RN, FAAN

Associate Professor and Master's Program Director
University of Virginia School of Nursing
Charlottesville, Virginia

JUDITH A. SPROSS, PhD, RN, AOCN, FAAN

Senior Scientist
Center for Applied Ethics and Professional Practice at
Education Development Center, Inc.
Newton, Massachusetts

CHARLENE M. HANSON, EdD, RN, CS, FNP, FAAN

Professor
Georgia Southern University
Statesboro, Georgia and
Family Nurse Practitioner
Family Health and Birth Center
Rincon, Georgia

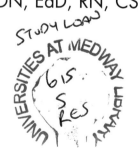

W.B. SAUNDERS COMPANY
An Imprint of Elsevier Science
Philadelphia • London • New York • St. Louis • Sydney • Toronto

W.B. SAUNDERS COMPANY
An Imprint of Elsevier Science

The Curtis Center
Independence Square West
Philadelphia, Pennsylvania 19106

Library of Congress Cataloging-in-Publication Data

Hamric, Ann B.

   Advanced nursing practice : an integrative approach / Ann B. Hamric, Judith A. Spross,
Charlene M. Hanson.—2nd ed.

       p. ; cm.

   Rev. ed. of: Advanced nursing practice : an integrative approach / [edited by] Ann B.
Hamric, Judith A. Spross, Charlene M. Hanson. c1996.

   Includes bibliographical references and index.

   ISBN 0–7216–8632–X

   1. Nurse practitioners.   2. Midwives.   3. Nurse anesthetists.   I. Spross, Judith A.   II.
Hanson, Charlene M.   III. Title.
     [DNLM: 1. Specialties, Nursing—methods.   2. Nurse Anesthetists.   3. Nurse Clinicians.
4. Nurse Midwives.   5. Nurse Practitioners. WY 101 H232a 2001]

RT82.8 .A384 2001
610.73—dc21

                                                                                    00–038806

Vice President and Nursing Editorial Director: Sally Schrefer

Editorial Manager: Thomas Eoyang

Editorial Assistant: Adrienne Simon

Production Manager: Donna L. Morrissey

ADVANCED NURSING PRACTICE   ISBN 0–7216–8632–X

Printed in the United States of America

Last digit is the print number: 9   8   7   6   5   4

To Mom and Dad and to my sisters and brothers, Carolyn, Betsy, John, and Jim, for their unfailing support and love during difficult times.

ABH

To my first teachers—my parents, Anne and Jerry Spross and to my aunt and godmother, Mary D. McVeigh (deceased 1999)—with love and gratitude.

JAS

To my husband, Dick, who makes all things possible for me.

CMH

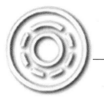

Contributors

AARA AMIDI-NOURI, BSN, RN
Graduate Student, Samuel Merritt
College; Staff Nurse II, Children's
Hospital Oakland, Oakland,
California
*History and Evolution of Advanced
Nursing Practice*

ANNE-MARIE BARRON, MS, RN,
CS
Instructor, Department of Nursing,
Simmons College, Boston; Doctoral
Candidate in Nursing, Boston College,
Chestnut Hill, Massachusetts
Consultation

JAMES BEAUREGARD, PhD
Clinical Neuropsychologist,
Generations Geriatric Mental Health,
Manchester, New Hampshire
Expert Coaching and Guidance

JERI L. BIGBEE, PhD, RN, CS, FNP,
FAAN
Adjunct Professor, California State
University, Stanislaus, Turlock,
California
*History and Evolution of Advanced
Nursing Practice*

ROBERT J. BOYLE, MD
Associate Professor of Pediatrics and
Attending Neonatologist; Faculty
Associate, Center for Biomedical
Ethics and Director, Ethics

Consultation Service, University of
Virginia Health System, Charlottesville,
Virginia
Ethical Decision-Making Skills

SARAH JO BROWN, PhD, RN
Research Consultant,
Practice-Research Integrations,
Norwich, Vermont
Direct Clinical Practice

KAREN A. BRYKCZYNSKI, DNSc,
RN, CS, FNP
Associate Professor, University of
Texas at Galveston School of Nursing,
Galveston, Texas
*Role Development of the Advanced
Practice Nurse*

DANIEL B. CARR, MD, FABPM
Saltonstall Professor of Pain Research
and Vice Chair for Research,
Department of Anesthesia, New
England Medical Center; Professor of
Anesthesia and Medicine, Tufts
University School of Medicine, Boston,
Massachusetts
Collaboration

ELLEN B. CLARKE, EdD, RN
Bioethics/Critical Care Graduate
Nursing Educator, Cohasset,
Massachusetts; Research Associate,
Education Development Center, Inc.,
Newton, Massachusetts
Expert Coaching and Guidance

MARGARET W. DORROH, MN, RN, CNM, FNPC
Clinician, Family Health and Birth Center, Rincon, Georgia
The Certified Nurse-Midwife

SUSAN E. DAVIS DOUGHTY, MSN, RN, CS
Adjunct Faculty, Simmons College, Boston, Massachusetts, Westbrook College, Portland, and University of Southern Maine, Portland; Nurse Practitioner, Co-owner, and Co-founder, New England Womencenter, Portland, Maine
Marketing and Contracting Considerations

MARGARET FAUT-CALLAHAN, DNSc, CRNA, FAAN
Professor and Chair, Adult Health Nursing, and Director, Nurse Anesthesia Program, Rush University College of Nursing, Chicago, Illinois
The Certified Registered Nurse Anesthetist

SHIRLEY A. GIROUARD, PhD, RN, FAAN
Consultant, Washington, D.C.
New Directions for the Advanced Practice Nurse in Health Care Quality: Performance and Outcome Improvement

ANN B. HAMRIC, PhD, RN, FAAN
Associate Professor and Master's Program Director, University of Virginia School of Nursing, Charlottesville, Virginia
A Definition of Advanced Nursing Practice; The Blended Role of the Clinical Nurse Specialist and the Nurse Practitioner

DIANE L. HANNA, MS, RNC, FNP
Nurse Practitioner and Clinical Instructor, Virginia Commonwealth University, Richmond, Virginia
The Primary Care Nurse Practitioner

CHARLENE M. HANSON, EdD, RN, CS, FNP, FAAN
Professor, Georgia Southern University, Statesboro and Family Nurse Practitioner, Family Health and Birth Center, Rincon, Georgia
Leadership: Empowerment, Change Agency, and Activism; Collaboration; Understanding the Regulatory and Credentialing Requirements for Advanced Practice Nursing

DOREEN C. HARPER, PhD, RN, CS, ANP, FAAN
Dean and Professor, University of Massachusetts Medical School Graduate School of Nursing, Worcester, Massachusetts; Formerly Associate Professor, George Mason University College of Nursing and Health Science, Fairfax, Virginia
Education for Advanced Nursing Practice

KERRY V. HARWOOD, MSN, RN
Director, Cancer Patient Education Program, Duke University Medical Center, Durham, North Carolina
Research

JEAN JOHNSON, PhD, RN, FAAN
Associate Dean and Professor, George Washington University School of Medicine and Health Sciences, Washington, D.C.
Health Policy Issues in a Changing Environment: An Interdisciplinary Perspective

JENNIFER M. KELLER, MSN, RNC
Women's Health Nurse Practitioner, East Boston Neighborhood Health Center, East Boston, Massachusetts
Marketing and Contracting Considerations

MAUREEN A. KELLEY, PhD, RN, CNM
Interim Coordinator, MSN Program, Emory University, Nell Hodgson Woodruff School of Nursing; Director,

Nurse-Midwifery Practice, Emory
Women's Care, Crawford Long
Hospital, Atlanta, Georgia
  The Certified Nurse-Midwife

CHRISTINA C. KING, MSN, RN,
CS, FNP
Family Nurse Practitioner and
Administrator, Mercy Maritime Family
Practice, Peaks Island, Maine
  *Managing Advanced Nursing
  Practice: Business Planning and
  Reimbursement Mechanisms*

MICHAEL J. KREMER, DNSc, CRNA
Assistant Professor, Adult Health
Nursing, and Assistant Director,
Nurse Anesthesia Program, Rush
University College of Nursing,
Chicago, Illinois
  *The Certified Registered Nurse
  Anesthetist*

CAROLYN K. LEWIS, PhD, RN, FAAN
Executive Director, American Nurses
Credentialing Center, Washington,
D.C.; Adjunct Faculty, George Mason
University, Fairfax, Virginia
  *Conceptualizations of Advanced
  Nursing Practice*

KATHY S. MAGDIC, MSN, RN,
ACNP-CS
Instructor, Acute Care Nurse
Practitioner Program, and Manager,
Cardiopulmonary Clinical Emphasis,
University of Pittsburgh School of
Nursing; University of Pittsburgh
Medical Center Cardiac Pavilion
Service, Pittsburgh, Pennsylvania
  The Acute Care Nurse Practitioner

VICKY A. MAHN, MS, RN
Director of Outcomes Management,
MIDS, Inc., Tucson, Arizona; Adjunct
Faculty, University of Arizona College
of Nursing, Tucson, AZ; Faculty, The
Institute for Johns Hopkins Nursing

Case Management Academy,
Baltimore, Maryland
  *The Advanced Practice Nurse Case
  Manager*

BEVERLY L. MALONE, PhD, RN, FAAN
Deputy Assistant Secretary for Health,
Department of Health and Human
Services Office of Public Health and
Science, Washington, D.C.
  *Leadership: Empowerment, Change
  Agency, and Activism*

LUCY MARION, PhD, RN
Head, Department of Public Health,
Mental Health, and Administrative
Nursing, and Associate Dean,
Community Practice, University of
Illinois, Chicago, College of Nursing;
Clinical Chief, Ambulatory Care,
University of Illinois, Chicago, Medical
Center, Chicago, Illinois
  *Innovative Practice Models:
  Uniting Advanced Nursing Practice
  and Education*

DEBORAH B. McGUIRE, PhD, RN,
FAAN
Associate Professor, University of
Pennsylvania School of Nursing;
Member, University of Pennsylvania
Cancer Center, Philadelphia, Pennsylvania
  Research

BRENDA M. NEVIDJON, MSN, RN
Chief Operating Officer, Duke
University Hospital; Clinical Associate,
Duke University School of Nursing,
Durham, North Carolina
  *Strengthening Advanced Nursing
  Practice in Organizational
  Structures and Cultures:
  Administrative Considerations*

L. GREGORY PAWLSON, MD, MPH
Adjunct Professor, George Washington
University; Executive Vice President,

National Committee for Quality Assurance, Washington, D.C.
Health Policy Issues in a Changing Environment: An Interdisciplinary Perspective

JUANITA REIGLE, MSN, RN, ACNP-CS
Associate Professor of Nursing, University of Virginia School of Nursing; Acute Care Nurse Practitioner for Heart Failure, University of Virginia Health System, Charlottesville, Virginia
Ethical Decision-Making Skills

DEBORAH M. RUST, MSN, RN, CRNP, AOCN
Coordinator, Acute Care Nurse Practitioner Program, and Manager, Oncology Clinical Emphasis, University of Pittsburgh School of Nursing; Nurse Practitioner, Adult Bone Marrow Transplant Program, University of Pittsburgh Medical Center, Pittsburgh Cancer Institute, Pittsburgh, Pennsylvania
The Acute Care Nurse Practitioner

KAREN SKALLA, MSN, ARNP
Palliative Care Coordinator, Dartmouth Hitchcock Medical Center, Lebanon; Instructor in Medicine, Hematology/Oncology, Dartmouth Medical School, Hanover, New Hampshire
The Blended Role of the Clinical Nurse Specialist and the Nurse Practitioner

PATRICIA S. A. SPARACINO, MS, RN, FAAN
Clinical Professor, University of California-San Francisco, School of Nursing; Clinical Nurse Specialist, Quality Improvement Clinical Coordinator, University of California Home Care Center; San Francisco, California
The Clinical Nurse Specialist

JUDITH A. SPROSS, PhD, RN, AOCN, FAAN
Senior Scientist, Center for Applied Ethics and Professional Practice at Education Development Center, Inc., Newton, Massachusetts
Expert Coaching and Guidance; Collaboration

MARGRETTA MADDEN STYLES, EdD, RN, FAAN
Professor Emerita, University of California, San Francisco, San Francisco, California; Consultant, American Nurses Credentialing Center, Washington, D.C.
Conceptualizations of Advanced Nursing Practice

DIANA TAYLOR, PhD, RN, FAAN
Associate Professor, School of Nursing-Department of Family Health Care Nursing, and Co-Director, Center for Collaborative Primary Care, University of California, San Francisco, California
Innovative Practice Models: Uniting Advanced Nursing Practice and Education

PATRICIA A. WHITE, MS, RN, CS
Assistant Professor, Graduate School for Health Studies, Graduate Program in Primary Health Care Nursing, Simmons College, Boston; Adult Nurse Practitioner, Hingham Weymouth Family Medical Associates, North Weymouth, Massachusetts; Doctoral Student, University of Rhode Island, Kingston, Rhode Island
Consultation

DONNA J. ZAZWORSKY, MS, RN, CCM
Adjunct Clinical Assistant Professor, University of Arizona; Program Director, Home Health/Outreach, St. Elizabeth of Hungary Clinic, Tucson, Arizona
The Advanced Practice Nurse Case Manager

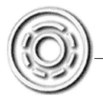

Preface

Since the first edition of this book was published, change in the health care system has continued to race ahead. In times that remain uncertain for nursing and health care at large, advanced nursing practice continues to grow, as evidence accumulates of its substantive benefits to patients/consumers. The reforms of the last decade included major growth in managed care, new configurations of providers and settings for health care delivery, the increased use of information and other technologies, and organizational redesign and restructuring initiatives. Continuing concerns regarding cost containment have led to an increased focus on evidence-based practice, a proliferation of quality initiatives at federal and state levels, and increased competition among providers—notably physicians and advanced practice nurses (APNs).

The swiftness with which these developments have occurred and the resultant uncertainty have heightened the need for clarity about advanced nursing practice and standards to ensure the competence of all APN providers. Increasingly, APNs must be able to deal with competitive and environmental forces within the health care marketplace to ensure that their practices survive this turbulent era. The nursing profession has rapidly increased the number of APN programs, particularly for nurse practitioners (NPs). This proliferation has raised questions about program quality, faculty preparation and practice, and standardization. All of these changes required us to re-envision this book and deepen our conceptual understanding of the core of advanced nursing practice.

PURPOSE

Among the seismic transformations of the United States' health care system and its associated provider disciplines, there are clear signals that new specialty roles for APNs are emerging. At the same time, the gains APNs have made in providing primary care services must be sustained. Our goal, for both specialty and primary care roles, is to propose a standardized, clear, and structured understanding of advanced nursing practice for both students and practicing APNs, and to ensure their abilities to manage proactively the environments in which they practice.

This new edition explores advanced nursing practice, its definition, competencies, roles, and the issues facing APNs with more clarity and authority than our first effort. To understand fully the meaning of advanced practice nursing and its potential contributions to shaping the future of health care, the contributions of all APN roles, whether established or evolving, must be considered. It is gratifying to see the growing agreement to embrace certified registered nurse anesthetists and certified nurse-midwives as advanced practice nursing groups. In addition, the debate has shifted away from the NP versus clinical nurse specialist (CNS) tensions so evident at the time of the first edition. There is now a clearer understanding that both roles, as well as the blended CNS/NP, are valuable. There is encouraging evidence of strong alliances developing among the professional groups and leaders that guide advanced nursing practice. These are clear signs of progress toward a unified understanding of advanced nursing practice.

For certain patient populations, APNs are the best providers for delivering quality care at a reasonable cost. It is essential to identify the opportunities for advanced practice that can be envisioned in a future health care system, where APNs and all nurses participate more fully, visibly, and equitably with their medical and other colleagues. In this revision we have identified these potential opportunities, and have focused much of this text on strategies to assist APNs to take advantage of the environment's uncertainty and complexity.

UNDERLYING PREMISES

This book is grounded in the conviction that advanced nursing practice must have a definable and describable core that provides a framework for standardizing the profession's understanding of this level of practice. At the same time, the core must be flexible enough to accommodate the differing roles necessary to enact the varied practices of all APNs. Several premises underlie this conviction:

- A uniform definition of advanced nursing practice and standards for educating and credentialing that are consistent across APN groups are essential for continued legitimacy of APN roles and regulatory parity with other providers. In the absence of a consistent definition, both the instability of the health care system and the increased competition among providers will threaten the legitimacy of all APNs as providers; such threats may lead to the loss of hard-won legal and regulatory battles.
- A consistent definition of core competencies for APNs is essential in order to standardize APN education and evaluate outcomes of APN care across roles. It is also imperative that APNs practice these competencies in order to demonstrate the value-added component they bring to care delivery, so that advanced nursing practice is not confused with physician substitution.
- A consistent definition is essential for interdisciplinary teamwork. Administrators and other providers must be able to rely on a core set of role expectations to design and implement cost-effective health care delivery systems that fully utilize all APN practices.
- We remain convinced that advanced nursing practice is good for patients, but a higher level of standardization must be attained for the larger health care establishment to agree with this claim.

ORGANIZATION

As noted, the second edition of *Advanced Nursing Practice: An Integrative Approach* has been extensively updated and revised to reflect current literature and trends. In

Part I, "Historical and Developmental Aspects of Advanced Nursing Practice," the history of case management has been incorporated into the first chapter's discussion of the origins of the four earlier APN roles (nurse anesthetist, nurse-midwife, CNS, and NP). Chapter 2 adds newer conceptual work such as that of the National Association of Clinical Nurse Specialists to the analysis of conceptualizations of advanced nursing practice. In Chapter 3, the core definition and conceptual model of advanced nursing practice have been modified to make explicit the centrality of direct clinical practice to advanced nursing practice. While APNs perform many activities in addition to direct clinical practice, their practice expertise is central to and informs all of these other activities. Developing and maintaining a cutting-edge clinical expertise in their specialty area must be expected of every APN. Additionally, the model and discussion have been expanded to address critical factors in practice environments that must be managed to benefit patients and enable APNs to succeed. Readers will see clear evidence that this reconceptualization is reflected throughout the book. Chapter 4 proposes changes in APN education consistent with this new definition. The chapter provides a prototype for the standardization of APN education and curricula that can support both existing and newly developing APN roles. In addition, policy making as an imperative shaping APN education and articulated models for interdisciplinary education are discussed. The discussion of role development in Chapter 5 has been extensively updated to incorporate recent research and new understandings of role acquisition and transition.

In Part II, "Competencies of Advanced Nursing Practice," the seven core competencies are examined. Important changes have been made to this section. As noted, direct clinical practice is described as the central and overriding competency that informs and shapes all of the other competencies. Chapter 6 expands and elaborates the key characteristics of APN direct practice: use of a holistic perspective, formation of partnerships with patients, expert clinical reasoning and skillful performance, use of research evidence in practice, and use of diverse health and illness management approaches.

Health care that is affordable, accessible, and of high quality requires well-prepared clinical leaders who can collaborate across disciplines. Effective care delivery increasingly depends on interdisciplinary thinking, communication, and practice. Consequently, chapters on expert coaching and guidance, collaboration, and ethical decision making (Chapters 7, 11, and 12) include the perspectives of interdisciplinary colleagues of the APN authors. In Chapter 8, nursing and medical literature have been synthesized to provide a model and an algorithm for APN consultation. Chapter 9 incorporates the current emphasis on evidence-based practice in discussing the research competency of the APN.

In Chapter 10, change agency and political activism have been incorporated with empowerment as fundamental elements of APN leadership. This new understanding of APN leadership resulted from our recognition that contemporary leadership requires change agent skills: one can no longer be an effective leader without being an effective change agent. Advanced nursing practice is evolving in a context of continuous change, and APNs must be prepared to respond, manage, and lead in the midst of change. The instability and uncertainty of the current health care system will require APNs to provide effective clinical leadership if a transformation to delivery models that are more consistent with nursing's vision of equitable, accessible health care is to be realized.

The chapters in Part III, "Advanced Practice Roles: The Operational Definitions of Advanced Nursing Practice," have been revised to reflect the current practices of each APN role. Each chapter explicitly incorporates the core competencies and demonstrates how these competencies are played out in specific APN roles. Features unique to each APN role are also described, and exemplars are used to help students understand how to implement the particular APN role. Chapters describing the three newest APN roles—the acute care nurse practitioner (ACNP), the blended clinical nurse specialist/nurse practitioner (CNS/NP), and the APN case manager—have been extensively reworked to reflect their current state of practice. The ACNP chapter reflects the rapid and dramatic evolution of this role in acute care in general and critical care in particular. The blended CNS/NP role chapter clarifies this evolving practice through a model that incorporates key CNS and NP competencies as well as features unique to the blended role. The APN case manager is another example of a rapid and dramatic APN role evolution. The revision of the APN case manager chapter strengthens the advocacy for APN-directed case management and demonstrates the need for the nursing profession to differentiate case coordination from case management. The unique competency of data management that is practiced by APN case managers is clearly described.

Part IV, "Critical Elements in Managing Advanced Nursing Practice Environments," has been reframed to explore key environmental factors. Chapter 20 helps the reader understand the complexities of reimbursement and practice management, using the direct and indirect processes of care delivery as a framework for understanding business planning. This chapter gives readers practical strategies for running an APN practice whether one is an independent provider (entrepreneur) or an employee in an established practice organization (intrapreneur). Information on job hunting, contracting, and marketing for both novice and experienced APNs is provided in Chapter 21. Health policy content has been substantially expanded and includes an examination of both micro and macro health policy environments. Chapter 22 helps students understand the regulatory and credentialing mechanisms that govern advanced nursing practice. Chapter 23 provides an overview of national health policies and traces the historical development of health care financing. Together these two chapters allow students and practicing APNs to gain a fuller understanding of the policy landscape as it affects APN scope-of-practice issues. Chapter 24 discusses the critical issue of administrative support for APNs given the context of managed care changes and innovative health care delivery systems. Both administrators and APNs will find strategies for collaborating to improve patient care and strengthen advanced nursing practice. Chapter 25 has been expanded to focus on the health care quality movement in addition to classic structure, process, and outcome evaluation. Resources for developing quality indicators are provided, and recent research, particularly in relation to outcomes and costs, is reviewed. Chapter 26 documents rich examples of the ways in which APN practice-education models have increased health care access to vulnerable populations and created innovative partnerships among institutions, communities, and providers to improve patient care. These models provide a fitting conclusion that illustrates the opportunities and challenges of making advanced nursing practice more visible in the new century's health care delivery system.

AUDIENCE

This book is intended for graduate students, practicing APNs in all roles, educators, administrators, and leaders in the nursing profession. For graduate students in any

APN graduate program, the book provides a comprehensive resource useful throughout their program of study. Initial clarity and understanding about the definition and competencies of advanced practice nursing can guide students as they enter their clinical coursework, and we strongly recommend the book's use early in the program of study. The text is useful throughout clinical courses as students see the various APN roles and related competencies in action, and as they begin practicing their chosen APN role. Students nearing graduation in role transition or capstone courses will appreciate the role development chapter and the content in Part IV that explores issues that they must be prepared to manage in the workplace.

For practicing APNs, the book contains both theoretical and practical content to guide role implementation. Individuals interested in strengthening or changing their roles will find many strategies for accomplishing these changes. The new edition's expansion to explore critical issues in the environment makes the book particularly useful to practicing clinicians who face issues within a marketplace that changes daily. The addition of interdisciplinary collaborative authors broadens the audience to include other clinicians and educators. For example, interdisciplinary teams could benefit from discussions of such chapters as expert coaching and guidance, collaboration, ethical decision-making skills and health care policy.

For educators, the book will serve as a comprehensive curricular resource in preparing APNs for practice. It also serves as a guide to standardize core education for advanced practice. Extensive current references and additional reading lists can assist educators to design relevant course content on all the facets of advanced nursing practice. Nursing administrators will appreciate the descriptions of various APN roles and the strategies for justifying and supporting APN positions. Clarity regarding advanced practice nursing is a professional imperative. For nursing leaders, this book is a clarion call to reach greater consensus regarding our understanding of and preparation for advanced nursing practice and the roles APNs assume, so that we speak with increasing authority and consistency to policy makers, to other disciplines, and to one another.

APPROACH

Time and a serious commitment by the APN community at large have softened the early disparate and conflicting stances of the various APN groups. This emerging consensus has enabled us to craft a more definitive and authoritative understanding of advanced nursing practice. Workforce dynamics, health policy issues, and system changes further influenced this revision. We have sought to describe advanced nursing practice at its best, as it is being enacted by APNs throughout the country. There is still much work to be done: not all APN students are educated to practice with the competencies described here; too many nurses are in advanced nursing practice roles without the necessary credentials or competencies, so that true advanced practice is not demonstrated; and there is still too much "alphabet soup" in role titles (for example, the APN case manager is variously called outcomes manager, clinical outcomes consultant, disease management specialist, and so on and so on).

There is no doubt that roles will continue to evolve as nursing matures in its understanding and enactment of advanced nursing practice. But advanced nursing practice must be distinct, recognizable, and describable if it is to continue to flourish. It will be clear to the reader that the diverse roles described in Part III, while they share the core criteria and competencies of advanced nursing practice, are different and distinct from one another in their role enactment. This should be a cause for celebration, as nursing recognizes its strength and range in meeting client needs.

We owe a special debt of gratitude to Thomas Eoyang of W.B. Saunders for his support and advocacy of our work. Thomas has shepherded this book and the prior edition with characteristic grace, humor, and wisdom. His understanding of this integrated vision and his commitment to advanced nursing practice have been invaluable in bringing both books from idea to reality.

We acknowledge the hard work of our contributors who substantially revised their chapters to portray this leading-edge understanding of advanced practice nursing. We are privileged to participate with them in shaping this important arena of nursing practice. Creating this new edition has been as challenging an undertaking as was the first edition. Advanced practice nursing is a relatively young idea in the profession's evolution. We continued to see how difficult it is to integrate and incorporate the perspectives of all APN specialties. The literature from the various advanced practice specialty groups remains unfortunately separated, and clinicians and educators tend to read and cite only their own group's literature. In addition, not all groups have addressed the core concept of advanced practice or the competencies of APNs in a complete or consistent manner. One of the major contributions of this second edition is the effort to solidify our understanding of advanced nursing practice. Adopting this integrative approach, as challenging as it continues to be, has in our view immeasurably enriched this work.

We remain convinced that advanced nursing practice is absolutely essential to improving the health and well-being of the citizens of this nation. As a critical component of present and future health care delivery systems, APNs are and must continue to be active participants in solving some of the pressing problems in health care delivery being experienced as we enter the 21st century.

Ann B. Hamric
Judith A. Spross
Charlene M. Hanson

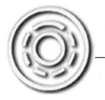

Contents

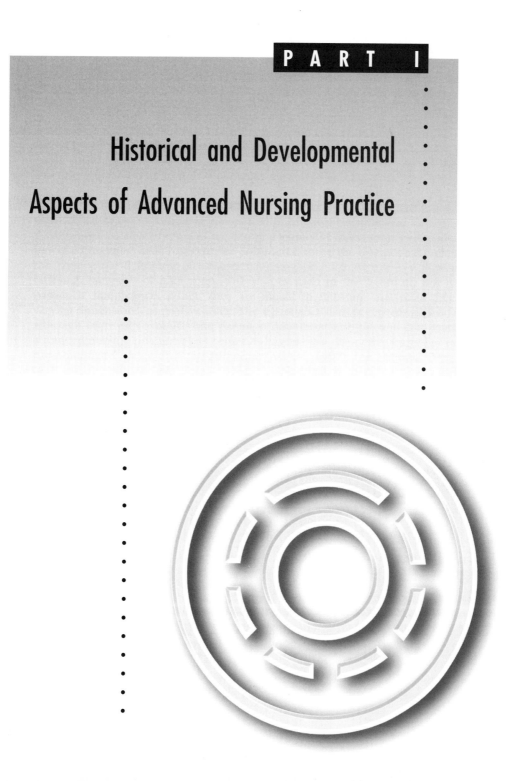

PART I

Historical and Developmental Aspects of Advanced Nursing Practice

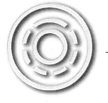

History and Evolution of Advanced Nursing Practice

• J E R I   L.   B I G B E E
• A A R A   A M I D I - N O U R I

INTRODUCTION

NURSE ANESTHETISTS
   Historical Review
   Organizational Development
   Educational Development
   Inter- and Intraprofessional Dynamics

NURSE-MIDWIVES
   Historical Review
   Organizational Development
   Educational Development
   Inter- and Intraprofessional Dynamics

CLINICAL NURSE SPECIALISTS
   Historical Review
   Organizational Development
   Educational Development
   Inter- and Intraprofessional Dynamics

NURSE PRACTITIONERS
   Historical Review
   Organizational Development
   Educational Development
   Inter- and Intraprofessional Dynamics

ADVANCED PRACTICE NURSE CASE MANAGERS
   Historical Review
   Organizational Development
   Educational Development
   Inter- and Intraprofessional Dynamics

SUMMARY AND CONCLUSIONS

INTRODUCTION

This chapter focuses on the historical development of one evolving and four established advanced practice roles, specifically certified registered nurse anesthetists (CRNAs), certified nurse-midwives (CNMs), clinical nurse specialists (CNSs), nurse practitioners (NPs), and advanced practice nurse case managers (APNCMs). It is acknowledged that other advanced nursing roles exist and are evolving. However, these five major roles were selected for review because of the depth of the historical information available. The history of each of the five advanced nursing practice roles is examined, including significant professional and educational developments, inter- and intraprofessional struggles, and legal and legislative advances. In addition, the broader historical context that has shaped the nursing profession, including gender, health manpower, and other sociopolitical issues, is discussed.

The evolution of the term "advanced" in relation to nursing practice is unclear. The use of the related term "specialist" in nursing can be traced back to the turn of the century, when postgraduate courses were offered by hospitals. Using an apprenticeship model, these courses were offered in a variety of specialty areas, including anesthesia, tuberculosis, operating room, laboratory, and dietetics. Some of these areas of specialization, such as dietetics, actually broke off to form new professions (Bullough, 1992). In the first issue of the *American Journal of Nursing,* an article by Dewitt (1900) entitled "Specialties in Nursing" addressed the development of specialized clinical practice within the profession. At that time the term "specialist" was used to designate a nurse who had completed a postgraduate course in a clinical specialty area or who had extensive experience and expertise in a particular clinical area. With the increasing complexity of health care knowledge and technology and enhanced professional sophistication, specialization became a force in the 20th century. By 1980, the American Nurses Association (ANA) declared that "specialization in nursing is now clearly established" and contended that "specialization is a mark of the advancement of the nursing profession" (p. 22). Early in the evolution of the NP role during the 1960s and 1970s, the term "expanded" or "extended" role was used throughout the literature, implying a horizontal movement to encompass expertise from medicine and other disciplines. The more contemporary term, "advanced," suggests a more hierarchical movement encompassing increasing expertise and graduate education within nursing rather than expansion into other disciplines. Several progressive state nursing practice acts, such as the one in Washington, included the term "advanced practice nurse" (APN) in the 1970s and 1980s to delineate CRNAs, CNMs, CNSs, and NPs. This regulatory influence promoted the contemporary use of the term "advanced" and served to demonstrate the commonalities of the various advanced practice specialties.

NURSE ANESTHETISTS

Historical Review

Nurse anesthesia is the oldest advanced nursing specialty. Since the mid-1800s, with the advent and development of anesthesia agents and care, nurses have been involved in administering anesthesia. Major advances in anesthesia science paved the way for the development of the CRNA role. Nitrous oxide was the first anesthesia agent identified in the mid-1800s. This anesthetic agent was adopted initially by American dentists. About the same time, ether and chloroform were widely used as anesthesia agents for surgical procedures. The concurrent advancement in antiseptic surgery and anesthesia promoted the growth of hospitals, because surgeries were becoming too complex to be conducted in the home.

Diers (1991) noted that "anesthesizers" were originally often unpaid or minimally paid surgeons in training who were logically most interested in the surgical procedure and not the anesthesia care. Under this system there was no incentive for physicians to become full-time anesthetists. So, in order to provide surgeons with the anesthesia care needed, nurses were recruited and trained. These early nurse anesthetists were readily accepted, because the nurse offered more stability over time and would solely concentrate on the anesthesia process versus the medical intern, who would tend to focus more on the surgical procedure. These first nurse anesthetists were religious sisters who did not expect any remuneration, which contributed to their early acceptance. Gender was also an issue that promoted early female nurse anesthetists, whose practice was justified because of their "gentle touch" (Olsen, 1940).

The first nurse anesthetist was Sister Mary Bernard at St. Vincent's Hospital in Erie, Pennsylvania, in 1877 (Bankert, 1989). In the late 1800s the Sisters of the Third Order of St. Francis established a network of hospitals throughout the Midwest through contracts with the Missouri Pacific Railroad. One of these hospitals was the Mayo Clinic, where all anesthesia was administered by nurses. The "mother of anesthesia," Alice Magaw, was an early nurse anesthetist at Mayo who reported and published an accounting of her work. By 1906, she had participated in over 14,000 surgical cases without one anesthesia-attributable death (Thatcher, 1953). Her visionary evaluative research is paralleled by the early work of nurse-midwife Mary Breckinridge and speaks to the importance of evaluative research in the early development of the advanced specialties. Magaw contended that hospital-based anesthesia services, which at the time included only nurse anesthetists, should remain separate from nursing service administrative structures, because anesthesia was a specialized field requiring education and recognition not possible under a nursing department (Thatcher, 1953). This early move away from nursing service reflects the alienation of nurse anesthesia from mainstream nursing still somewhat seen today.

Historically, nurse anesthesia has been greatly influenced by and involved with the American military and major wars because of the need for accessible anesthesia care for combat trauma victims. Nurses administered anesthesia during the American Civil War and the Franco-Prussian War (Garde, 1988). During World War I, hospital-sponsored medical units provided anesthesia care on the battlefield, resulting in reduced mortality. Nurse anesthetist Sophie Winton provided battlefront anesthesia care in France during World War I and received the Croix de Guerre in recognition for her service (Faut-Callahan & Kremer, 1996). World War I thus served to greatly enhance the visibility and public enthusiasm for nurse anesthetists. However, this growing acceptance of nurse anesthetists became an increasing concern for physician anesthetists.

Physicians began specializing in anesthesia practice around the turn of the century. Interestingly, female physicians were the initiators, because the low pay and status of anesthesia practice made it unattractive to male physicians. These women were active in the establishment of the Association of Anesthetists of the United States and Canada in the early 1920s (Bankert, 1989). Although they shared a great deal with nurse anesthetists in terms of gender discrimination and stereotyping, the early women physician anesthetists unfortunately were actively opposed to nurse anesthetists. The medical journal *Anesthesiology* was established in 1940, further strengthening medicine's claim to anesthesia practice. By the 1950s, increasing numbers of male physicians specialized in anesthesiology, and women's leadership in the field declined.

World War II served to institutionalize the nurse anesthetist role even further, with the military clarifying the position and elevating the status of the nurse anesthetist. Nurse anesthesia was declared a clinical nursing specialty within the military nursing structure with unique pay and assignments (Bankert, 1989). Immediately after the end of the war in 1945, the American Association of Nurse Anesthetists (AANA) initiated their certification program. This formal credentialing of CRNAs was far ahead of the other nursing specialties, and was a significant benchmark in the history of advanced practice.

In the postwar period, the close association of nurse anesthesia with the military continued. The Army established nurse anesthesia educational programs, including one at Walter Reed General Hospital, which graduated its first class in 1961. This class consisted of only men. Soon after, the Letterman General Hospital School of Anesthesia in San Francisco also graduated an all-male class. This significant movement of males into nurse anesthesia is unparalleled in any of the other advanced nursing specialties. Not surprisingly, nurse anesthetists played an active role in the Vietnam War, providing vital services in the prompt surgical treatment of the wounded. Of the 10 nurses killed in Vietnam, two were male nurse anesthetists (Bankert, 1989).

The number of CRNAs nationally has grown consistently over time. The AANA estimated that, as of 1999, the total number of CRNAs in the United States was approximately 28,000 (AANA Executive Office, personal communication, September 1999).

Organizational Development

The nurse anesthesia specialty was highly successful in building a strong national presence early in its history. The AANA was established in 1931 by Agatha Hodgins, who served as the organization's first president. At the first meeting of the association, the group voted to affiliate with the ANA, but were rebuffed. Thatcher (1953) contended that the ANA's refusal was based on its fear of assuming legal responsibility for a group that could be charged with practicing medicine. Nurse anesthesia's early organizational development also resulted in mandatory certification, which was instituted in 1945 by the AANA. As of 1996, 84.4% of CRNAs were nationally certified (Table 1-1) (U.S. Department of Health and Human Services, 1996). Men were first admitted to the AANA in 1947, reflecting the growing role and acceptance of men in the specialty. This opening of the professional organization to men was followed by special efforts of the American military to increase the number of male nurse anesthetists. Nurse anesthesia remains unique among the advanced nursing specialties in its success in attracting a significant percentage of males (approximately 42% of practicing CRNAs are male). This success has been influenced by historical efforts to recruit males, the close relationship with the American military, the relatively high salaries available to nurse anesthetists, and strong leadership among men in the specialty. The total membership of the AANA as of 1999 was 27,912, which represents the largest advanced practice nursing specialty organization in the United States (AANA Executive Office, personal communication, September 1999).

TABLE 1-1	NUMBER OF ADVANCED PRACTICE NURSES IN THE UNITED STATES AS OF MARCH 1996		
TITLE	TOTAL NUMBER	% CURRENTLY IN NURSING	% NATIONALLY CERTIFIED
CRNAs	30,386	86.7	84.4
CNMs	6,534	81.7	87.9
CNSs	53,799	90.5	23.6
NPs	63,191	88.2	63.5
CNS/NPs*	7,802	100	70.9
NCMs	No data available	No data available	No data available

* CNS/NPs are individuals who are prepared as both CNSs and NPs.
Taken from the U.S. Department of Health and Human Services, Division of Nursing. (1996). *The registered nurse population March 1996: Findings from the National Sample Survey of Registered Nurses.* Washington, DC: Author.

Educational Development

Educationally, nurse anesthesia training initially involved informal apprenticeship programs operated within hospitals. The first official postgraduate course was offered at St. Vincent's Hospital in Portland, Oregon, in 1909, consisting of 6 months of instruction under the direction of Agnes McGee (Thatcher, 1953). Subsequently, a postgraduate course in anesthesia for Sisters only was established at one of the Sisters' hospitals, St. John's Hospital in Springfield, Illinois, in 1912, admitting the first secular nurse in 1924. By the onset of World War I, there were five postgraduate schools of nurse anesthesia in the United States. At the well-established Lakeside Hospital program in Cleveland, critical experimentation with combined nitrous oxide–oxygen administration, as well as the first use of morphine and scopolamines as adjuncts to anesthesia, was conducted with the participation of nurse anesthetist Agatha Hodgins. In 1952 an accreditation program to monitor the quality of anesthesia programs was established under the AANA. By 1972, there were 208 schools of anesthesia, most of which were small, graduating approximately 800 nurse anesthetists each year (Bullough, 1992).

Despite early advances in credentialing, nurse anesthesia education has only recently joined mainstream graduate nursing education. Because of their historical "stepchild" relationship with nursing, nurse anesthesia programs, if they were associated with educational institutions, were often housed in schools of medicine or allied health, similar to some early NP programs. During the mid-1970s through mid-1980s the number of nurse anesthesia educational programs declined significantly, largely because of the closure of many small certificate programs. Physician pressure, inadequate financial support, limited clinical facilities, and lack of accessible universities for affiliation contributed to these closures (Faut-Callahan & Kremer, 1996). The first master's degree nurse anesthesia program was established at the University of Hawaii in 1973. By 1980, there were four master's programs in nurse anesthesia, growing to 17 in 1990 and 82 in 1999 (AANA Executive Office, personal communication, September 1999). The AANA mandated a baccalaureate degree for certification in 1987, and as of 1998 all accredited programs were required to be at the master's level. Currently CRNA master's programs are housed in a variety of disciplines, including schools of nursing, medicine, allied health, and basic science.

Inter- and Intraprofessional Dynamics

Interprofessional conflict has been an ever-present dynamic for CRNAs, intensifying as medical anesthesiologists increased their control over anesthesia practice. These struggles were often played out in the courts and state legislatures in the early 1900s and ultimately served to establish the legal basis of the practice of nurse anesthesia. In 1911, the New York State Medical Society unsuccessfully declared that the administration of an anesthetic by a nurse violated state law (Thatcher, 1953). The Ohio State Medical Board passed a resolution in 1912 specifying that only physicians could administer anesthesia, which culminated in action taken against the Lakeside Hospital program as the "chief source of the nurse-anesthetist abuse." This action was also unsuccessful but resulted in nurse anesthetists amending the Ohio Medical Practice Act, protecting the practice of nurse anesthesia. Shortly after, the Kentucky attorney general ruled that the administration of anesthesia fell within the practice of medicine, resulting in the first landmark court case. A suit was filed against the State Board of Health by a Louisville surgeon and nurse anesthetist team, Louis Frank and Margaret Hayfield. Initially the court ruled in favor of the State Board; however, on appeal the decision was reversed, and the appeals court ruled in 1917 that nurse anesthesia was not the practice of medicine. Legal challenge then moved to California, where nurse anesthetist Dagmar Nelson was sued by the Anesthesia Section of the Los Angeles County Medical Association for practicing medicine without a license. Nelson argued successfully that the Medical Association had no standing to sue. In response, a physician, William Chalmers-Frances, filed a similar suit against Nelson in 1936, which again resulted in a judgment for Nelson. The ruling was appealed, and in 1938 the California Supreme Court supported the decision, stating that Nelson was not practicing medicine because she was supervised by the operating surgeon (Thatcher, 1953). Thus the *Frank et al. v. South et al.* (1917) and *Chalmers-Frances v. Nelson* (1936) cases provide the critical legal basis of nurse anesthesia practice.

The relationship between organized nurse anesthesia and anesthesiology has reflected these historical interprofessional struggles. Between 1947 and 1963, there was no official communication between the AANA and the American Society of Anesthesiologists (ASA), because of the ASA's stand that only physicians could be involved in anesthesia education (Bankert, 1989). In 1972, after years of negotiation, the AANA and the ASA issued the "Joint Statement on Anesthesia Practice," which promoted the concept of the anesthesia team. However, in 1976 the ASA Board of Directors voted to withdraw support from the 1972 statement, preferring one that explicitly maintained physician control and leadership.

Over the years, legal tension with physician anesthesia groups has continued, particularly in relation to malpractice policies and most recently in relation to antitrust and restraint of trade issues, similar to those experienced by CNMs. *Oltz v. St. Peter's Community Hospital* (1986) established the standing of CRNAs to sue for anticompetitive damages when anesthesiologists conspire to restrict practice privileges. A second case (*Bhan v. NME Hospitals, Inc., et al.,* 1985) established the right of CRNAs to be awarded damages as a result of exclusive contracts.

Legislatively, beginning in 1977, the AANA led a long and complex effort to secure third-party reimbursement under Medicare. They were finally successful in 1989. In relation to modification of state nursing practice acts to reflect nurse anesthesia practice, historical activity has been limited. This may be explained by the legal view of nurse anesthesia as performing a dependent function under physicians in the administration of anesthesia. In 1972, over a century after the inception of nurse anesthetists, only four state practice acts specifically mentioned them. By 1999, that number had grown to 48 (AANA Executive Office, personal communication, September 1999).

NURSE-MIDWIVES

Historical Review

Nurse-midwifery was the second major advanced nursing specialty to develop histori-cally, but its history is commingled with the ancient practice of midwifery. In the United States, as in most other parts of the world, deliveries were assisted by traditional (lay) midwives until the turn of the century. Midwives were imported to the United States with the slave trade in 1619 (Robinson, 1984) and later with waves of European immigration. Midwives were respected and rewarded community members in early Native American, colonial, and pioneer communities. However, by the early 1900s, midwives in America were discredited because of religious attitudes, economic de-mands, replacement by physicians, inadequate education, lack of organization, influx of immigrants, and the low status of women (Varney, 1987). Most early midwives were educated in England, where midwifery was controlled by the Church of England, which placed moralistic and church doctrine restrictions on practice. In early Puritan communities, midwives were suspected of witchcraft, especially if birth defects oc-curred.

During the 1700s and 1800s, major advancement in nursing and medical science greatly enhanced the scholarly basis of obstetrical practice. Improved technology produced improved outcomes related to cesarean sections, obstetric anesthesia, and puerperal fever. These scientific advancements excluded the midwife because of her limited education and lack of professional organization. Immigration patterns, which peaked in the late 1800s, produced culturally isolated ethnic communities in urban areas that used "old country midwives" who were untrained, similar to "granny midwives" in the South whose practice was passed on through generations of women within families. Their practice focused on home remedies, prayer, and patience (Varney, 1987). By the late 1800s, European obstetrical trends had changed, making it fashionable to use male midwives (physicians), and soon this trend was reflected in the United States. At that time physicians made a concerted effort to gain control over birthing as a means of recruiting patients and increasing income (Fox, 1969). Concurrently, the status of women was an increasingly volatile issue in turn-of-the-century America. Swenson (1968) contended that the status of women was at a "low ebb," with women seen as economically exploitable but socially and politically incompetent. These negative views particularly undermined the status of American midwives, as well as the profession of nursing.

Between 1900 and 1920, the health status of the American population, particularly with regard to perinatal health indicators, was poor. Midwives were falsely blamed for the poor maternal-child health outcomes of the period. Maternal and infant mortality rates were high because of inadequate hospital resources for the treatment of complicated deliveries, the inadequate preparation of physicians related to obstet-rics, the lack of attention to prenatal care, and the inadequate education, regulation, and supervision of midwives. A 1906 study conducted by the New York City Health Department indicated that 40% of the births in the city were attended by 3,000 untrained midwives (Varney, 1987). In response, the Children's Bureau and the

Maternity Center Association were established to promote improved maternal and child health and welfare. The Children's Bureau, established in 1912 and spearheaded by nursing leader Lillian Wald, conducted studies of infant and maternal mortality, which demonstrated the importance of early and continuous prenatal care. In 1921 the Sheppard-Towner Act was passed, allocating federal funds to be administered by the Children's Bureau to provide improved maternal-child care. The impetus behind the increasing attention to public health and the passage of the Sheppard-Towner Act of 1921 was based on national security concerns. In the post–World War I sociopolitical climate, supporting the health of women and children was viewed as essential to maintain national security, particularly in ensuring an adequate supply of healthy soldiers (Tom, 1982). Interestingly, over time organized medicine withdrew its support of this legislation because programs were not under physician control, and the legislation lapsed (Diers, 1991).

Negative attitudes related to traditional midwives peaked around 1912, with heated debates surrounding issues of midwife licensing and control. Concurrently, medicine was assuming ever-increasing control of obstetrical care with a mass movement away from home births. Several states passed laws granting legal recognition of midwives with regulatory controls, resulting in the establishment of midwifery schools. Public health nurses were involved as instructors in these midwifery schools.

A landmark in nurse-midwifery history was the establishment of the Maternity Center Association (MCA) in 1918 in response to a study conducted by the New York City health commissioner, which indicated the need for comprehensive prenatal care. The MCA served as the central organization for a network of community-based maternity centers throughout the city, providing education and administrative support to the centers. In 1921 their efforts narrowed, demonstrating the provision of comprehensive maternity care in just one district. The MCA also collaborated with the Henry Street Visiting Nurse Association, identifying the need to prepare nurses to provide maternity services. These groups proposed the establishment of a school of nurse-midwifery, which was tabled because of strong opposition from medicine, nursing, and city officials. This opposition was related to professional turf issues as well as the increasingly discredited public view of traditional midwifery.

Meanwhile, in England, traditional midwives were being replaced by nurse-midwives with the emergence of nursing education. In the United States, in 1925 Mary Breckinridge, a registered nurse and British-trained nurse-midwife, established the Frontier Nursing Service (FNS), which would serve as a futuristic model of advanced nursing practice in nurse-midwifery as well as later for NPs. In an economically depressed rural mountain area of Kentucky, Breckinridge established a network of clinics to serve Appalachian women and children, using imported British midwives traveling on horseback (Breckenridge, 1952). Outstanding evaluation data were maintained from the outset. When analyzed by the Metropolitan Life Insurance Company in 1951, findings indicated that 8,596 births were attended, 6,533 in the home, since 1925 (Varney, 1987). The FNS maternal mortality rate of 1.2 per 1,000 was significantly lower than the national average of 3.4 per 1,000 over the same period. General primary health care and dental services were also provided to the population.

Early nurse-midwifery graduates either practiced with the MCA or the FNS or became involved in public health programs, which often included teaching and supervising indigenous midwives in rural areas. Many early graduates were not able to practice clinical nurse-midwifery because of limited opportunities, so they assumed roles in nursing education and administration. In the late 1950s and 1960s, nurse-midwives made efforts to practice in hospitals, where 70% of births took place,

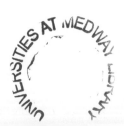

bringing with them models of family-centered maternity care that would revolutionize maternity care. However, barriers to practice were formidable. In 1963, only 11% of CNMs who responded to a national survey were practicing midwifery. This proportion increased to 23% by 1967; however, about one in four of these CNMs were practicing abroad through church and international health organizations. Within the United States, the proportion of CNMs actually practicing midwifery was highest in areas with strong educational programs, specifically New Mexico, Kentucky, and New York City (American College of Nurse-Midwives [ACNM], 1968).

In the late 1960s and early 1970s, nurse-midwifery finally turned the corner, experiencing rapidly increasing demand. This dramatic change was due in part to the increased visibility and involvement of the women's movement in birthing issues, which resulted in increased consumer recognition of and demand for nurse-midwifery services. In addition, sociopolitical developments, including the increased utilization of CNMs in federally funded health projects, the official recognition of CNMs by the American College of Obstetricians and Gynecologists in 1971, and the increased birth rate resulting from baby boomers reaching adulthood coupled with inadequate supplies of obstetricians, served to foster the rapid blossoming of CNM practice (Varney, 1987). Although in 1971 only 36.9% of CNMs who responded to an ACNM survey were in clinical midwifery practice, by 1977 this percentage had increased to 50.7%, with the majority practicing in the Southwest, Southeast, and Southern Appalachia, often in rural areas. Also in the early 1970s, the first nurse-midwifery private practice was instituted, leading to the rapid "discovery" of midwifery services by middle- and upper-income families. By 1977, approximately 26% of all practicing CNMs were engaged in private practices.

The more recent expansion of nurse-midwifery practice and education has been influenced by factors similar to those affecting the other advanced specialties, including the shortage of physicians, the availability of federal funding, and changes in nurse practice acts. In addition, the women's movement, including the demands for sensitive and caring approaches to women's health care, has fueled the success of nurse-midwifery in the United States. By mid-1982 there were almost 2,600 CNMs, with the majority located on the East Coast. The percentage of nurse-midwives in midwifery practice increased to 67% in 1982. As Varney (1987) stated, "Nurse-midwifery had become not only acceptable but also desirable and demanded. Now the problem was that, after years during which nurse-midwives struggled for existence there was nowhere near the supply to meet the demand" (p. 31). This pattern is also seen within the evolution of other advanced practice nursing specialties. As shown in Table 1–1, as of 1996, of the 6,534 CNMs nationally, 81.7% were employed in nursing, including 70.7% practicing as CNMs (U.S. Department of Health and Human Services, 1996). The 1996 National Sample Survey of RNs also indicated that 87.9% of CNMs were nationally certified. The ACNM estimated that, as of 1999, there were approximately 6,600 CNMs nationally (ACNM Executive Office, personal communication, September 1999).

Organizational Development

Historically, nurse-midwives have been highly active and well organized since the 1920s. The American Association of Nurse-Midwives (AANM) was founded in 1928, originally as the Kentucky State Association of Midwives, an outgrowth of the FNS. Nationally, nurse-midwives first organized as a section within the National Organization of Public Health Nurses in the mid-1940s. When that organization was subsumed within the ANA and the National League for Nursing (NLN), the maintenance of a distinct section to address the needs of nurse-midwives was not possible. As a result, the American College of Nurse Midwifery was incorporated in 1955 as an independent specialty nursing organization. In 1956, the AANM merged with the College, forming the American College of Nurse-Midwives. Beginning with a charter membership of 124, the College grew to 860 members in 1975, 2,434 in 1984, and 6,995 in 1999 (ACNM Executive Office, personal communication, September 1999). This relatively young organization made major progress in a relatively short time, including the establishment of an accreditation process in 1962, implementation of a certification examination and process in 1971, and the publication of a professional journal (*Journal of Nurse-Midwifery,* formerly the *Bulletin of the American College of Nurse Midwifery*) begun in 1955. In recent decades some have argued that nurse-midwifery has moved away from nursing and attempted to establish itself as a separate profession (Diers, 1991). Since certification was begun in 1971, approximately 4,000 nurse-midwives have been certified by the ACNM. The ACNM also currently certifies non-nurses as certified midwives (CMs). The same certification examination is used for CNMs and CMs, with both types of midwives defined as primary care providers and case managers for women and newborns (ACNM, 1997).

In 1962, the ACNM established the definitions of the nurse-midwife and nurse-midwifery. These definitions clearly emphasized that the role was an "extension" of nursing practice (ACNM, 1962). These definitions of practice and philosophy were revised in 1978, reflecting more of an emphasis on the distinct midwifery and nursing origins of the role (ACNM, 1978a, 1978b). Thus, CNMs are unique from other APNs in that they conceptualize their role as the combination of two disciplines, nursing and midwifery. That conceptualization has resulted in CNMs aligning with professional midwives, who are not nurses, organizationally and politically (see Chapter 17 for more discussion of this issue).

The ACNM has been active historically in policy formation related to some controversial areas. In 1971, the College approved a statement prohibiting CNMs from performing abortions. The College also issued a statement in 1980 allowing CNMs to practice in a variety of settings, including hospitals, homes, and birthing centers.

Educational Development

Educationally, the first nurse-midwifery training program was established in 1932 in connection with the Maternity Center of New York City. Named the School of the Association for the Promotion and Standardization of Midwifery, this program was also known as the Lobenstine Midwifery School. The impetus for creating this program was to prepare public health nurses to work as instructors and supervisors of traditional midwives as well as nurses with limited obstetrical training. The school was operated in connection with the Lobenstine Midwifery Clinic, and its students attended 7,099 deliveries between 1932 and 1958, producing a maternal mortality rate of 0.9 per 1,000 births as compared with a rate of 10.4 per 1,000 for the same geographic area (Varney, 1987). Between 1933 and 1959, the Maternity Center Association School of Nurse-Midwifery graduated 320 students.

The second formal nurse-midwifery training program was established by the FNS in 1939. With the advent of World War II, the FNS faced a crisis when many of the British nurse-midwives returned to their homeland. As a result, the Frontier Graduate

School of Midwifery was established in 1939. This historic school graduated 460 nurse-midwives by 1976 and continues today as the Frontier School of Midwifery and Family Nursing. In the 1930s through 1960s, several nurse-midwifery educational programs were established throughout the country, including Tuskegee, Philadelphia, and New Mexico, although some operated only briefly. In 1955 there were three certificate and two master's degree programs; by mid-1982 there were 11 certificate and 14 master's degree programs, consistent with the trend toward master's preparation reflected in the other advanced practice specialties (Adams, 1983). As of 1999, there were a total of 47 CNM educational programs (ACNM Executive Office, personal communication, September 1999). As of 1999, all nurse midwifery programs are required to award a minimum of a bachelor's degree to be eligible for ACNM accreditation. This requirement is divergent from the trend among the other APN specialties that have moved to requiring master's preparation. According to the American Association of Colleges of Nursing (AACN) (1999), based on data supplied by 30 graduate-level CNM programs, as of the fall of 1998 there were a total of 738 students enrolled and 395 graduates. This represented 3.7% of all master's enrollees.

Inter- and Intraprofessional Dynamics

Like nurse anesthesia, nurse-midwifery has been highly active in the legal and legislative arenas, often related to interprofessional struggles. As nurse-midwives reached increasing levels of acceptance and demand, interprofessional conflicts increased, with medicine perceiving CNMs as a competitive threat. This conflict was manifested by state legislative battles over statutory recognition of CNMs, denial of hospital privileges, attempts to deny third-party reimbursement, and malpractice insurance struggles. As a result, in 1980 an investigative congressional hearing was conducted regarding the problems of CNMs, specifically restraint-of-trade issues, involving the Federal Trade Commission. In two cases, one in Tennessee and one in Georgia, the Federal Trade Commission obtained consent orders against hospitals and insurance companies that attempted to limit the practice of CNMs (Diers, 1991). Third-party reimbursement was first approved in 1980 for CNMs in the Civilian Health and Medical Program of the Uniformed Services (CHAMPUS) for military dependents and in Medicaid. From a state regulatory perspective, as late as 1963 only three states and New York City legally authorized CNM practice. By 1984 all states had recognized nurse-midwifery within state laws or regulations (Varney, 1987).

One unique legal issue relates to the contention of CNMs that they represent the combination of two disciplines, nursing and midwifery. Legally, this has resulted in several interesting cases involving nurses practicing midwifery who were not educated as nurse-midwives (*Leggett v. Tennessee Board of Nursing,* 1980; *Leigh v. Board of Registration in Nursing,* 1984; *Smith v. State of Indiana ex rel. Medical Licensing Board of Indiana,* 1984). In all cases midwifery and nursing were found to be separate disciplines. However, there has never been a case of a CNM being sued for practicing medicine without a license, a legal challenge that both CRNAs and NPs have been forced to confront (Diers, 1991).

The history of nurse-midwifery in America certainly reflects significant interprofessional struggle and some intraprofessional tension as evidenced by early organizational efforts. CNMs, however, have consistently promoted an interdisciplinary perspective as reflected in a 1971 joint statement of the ACNM, the American College of Obstetricians and Gynecologists, and the Nurses' Association of the American College of

Obstetricians and Gynecologists. In this statement, the three groups supported the development and utilization of CNMs in obstetrical teams "directed by a physician." This dated concept of physician-directed teams will certainly be challenged as CNMs develop increasingly independent practice models.

CLINICAL NURSE SPECIALISTS

Historical Review

The historical development of CNSs has followed quite a different pattern from other advanced nursing specialties. According to Hamric (1989), the role of the CNS "originated for the purpose of improving the quality of nursing care provided to patients" (p. 3). Historically there is disagreement as to the origin of the CNS concept. According to Peplau (1965), the title originated in 1938. In 1943, Reiter (1966) first coined the term "nurse clinician" to designate a nurse with advanced clinical competence and recommended the preparation of such clinicians in graduate educational programs. Norris (1977) contended that the CNS concept was first introduced in 1944 in connection with the Committee to Study Postgraduate Clinical Nursing Courses of the National League for Nursing Education. Smoyak (1976) traced the origin of the concept to a national conference of directors of graduate programs that was held in 1949 at the University of Minnesota. During this period, the dominant view of nursing education was that the diploma was the preferred basic preparation for professional nursing, a stance that greatly limited the growth of graduate programs. Thus, until the second half of the 20th century, graduate nursing education focused primarily on functional rather than clinical specialization, with students concentrating on administration, education, or supervision. According to Sills (1983), this trend was influenced by the following factors: the orientation of nursing's early leaders in graduate nursing education at Teachers College, Columbia University; the increased emphasis on inpatient hospital care in the post–World War II era; and the resultant shift in the delivery of nursing care from a private-duty to a supervisory model within the hospital administrative structure. The conservative gender attitudes related to the roles of women that predominated during the midcentury period also served to inhibit the emergence of innovative and autonomous leadership roles in clinical nursing.

The evolution of the CNS role is expansive because of the multiple specialties represented. The historical development of psychiatric CNSs is presented as an example, because theirs is the oldest and one of the most highly developed CNS specialties. Peplau (1965) contended that the development of areas of specialization is preceded by three social forces: (1) an increase in specialty-related information, (2) new technological advances, and (3) response to public need and interests. All of these forces clearly helped shape the development of the psychiatric CNS role. The first American training program for psychiatric nurses was opened in 1880 at McLean Hospital in Massachusetts (Critchley, 1985). Nursing's role in mental health care at the time was basically providing custodial care and supervision of ancillary physical care providers under the direction of physicians (Goodnow, 1938). In the early 1900s, the specialty area of psychiatric nursing emerged, largely because of the leadership of Linda Richards. Between 1900 and 1930, psychiatry changed dramatically as a result of increasing scholarship, including the influence of Freud and Sullivan. It was in this period that the first psychiatric nursing text, *Nursing Mental and Nervous Diseases,* was published in 1920 by Harriet Bailey and served as the primary resource in the field for over 30 years. Sullivan's classic writings in psychiatry beginning in the 1930s had a dramatic effect on psychiatric nursing. The emphasis on interpersonal interaction with patients and milieu treatment supported the movement of nurses into a more direct role in the psychiatric care of hospitalized patients. Technological advances during this period, including insulin, chemotherapy, and electroshock therapies, supported the growing emphasis on interpersonal therapy, with nurses serving a direct, active role in treatment.

Sociopolitically, World Wars I and II produced increased public recognition of mental health concerns because of war-related psychiatric problems in returning soldiers (Critchley, 1985). Thus the stage was set in the late 1930s and 1940s for psychiatric nursing to make major strides in developing a specialized direct-care role. By 1943, three postgraduate programs in psychiatric nursing were established, but more developed soon, including the first master's program at Rutgers in 1954. The National Mental Health Act of 1946 designated psychiatric nursing as a core discipline; as a result, funding for graduate and undergraduate educational programs and research became available. During the late 1940s and 1950s, the scholarship in psychiatric nursing blossomed, including the classic writings of Peplau, who proposed the first conceptual framework for psychiatric nursing. This growth in the psychiatric nursing body of knowledge provided the support for psychiatric nurses to begin exploring new leadership roles in the care of mental health clients in both inpatient and outpatient settings. The expansion of the psychiatric CNS role in outpatient mental health was greatly enhanced by the Community Mental Health Centers Act of 1963 as well as the growing interest in child and adolescent mental health care during the 1960s. By 1970, a cadre of graduate-prepared psychiatric CNSs assumed roles as individual, group, family, and milieu therapists and obtained direct third-party reimbursement for their services. Soon after, psychiatric nurses led the way in identifying minimal educational and clinical criteria for CNSs and the establishment of national specialty certification through the ANA (Critchley, 1985).

The impressive development of the psychiatric CNS role helped initiate the growth of other CNS specialty areas. Following the enactment of the Nurse Training Act (Title VIII of the Public Health Service Act) in 1965, attention to clinical specialization in graduate education increased, in contrast to the prior emphasis on education and administration. The Nurse Training Act was instrumental in the development of master's programs emphasizing clinical specialization in schools of nursing. In the development of these new clinically focused graduate programs, nursing faculty members were instrumental in further developing and defining the role of the CNS. This specialist would provide a high level of specialized nursing care as well as serve as a change agent in hospital settings through role modeling and consultation with other providers (Christman, 1991).

As with the other advanced nursing specialties, the development of the CNS role included early evaluation research that served to validate and promote the innovation. Landmark studies by Georgopoulos and his colleagues (Georgopoulos & Christman, 1970; Georgopoulos & Jackson, 1970; Georgopoulos & Sana, 1971) evaluated the effect of CNS practice on nursing process and outcomes in inpatient adult health care settings. These and other evaluative studies (Ayers, 1971; Girouard, 1978; Little & Carnevali, 1967) demonstrated the positive effect of the introduction of the CNS in relation to nursing care improvements and functioning. More recently, McBride and her associates (1987) similarly demonstrated that nursing practice, particularly in relation to documentation, improved as a result of the introduction of a CNS in an inpatient psychiatric setting. Increasingly, evaluation of the CNS role has also focused on client outcomes (e.g., Barnason, Merboth, Pozehl, & Tietjen, 1998; Brooten et al., 1986; McCorkle, Robinson, Nuamah, Lev, & Benoliel, 1998; Wammack & Mabrey, 1998), which provide even stronger data supporting the contribution of the CNS role.

Employment opportunities for CNSs, particularly in nonpsychiatric specialties, were initially limited, so like CNMs, many early CNS graduates assumed roles in administration or education. Over time, the role became more institutionalized, especially in large health care institutions and in the professional and educational communities. As a result, the CNS role became accepted by and included in the practice arena relatively rapidly and without significant controversy, as noted by the National Commission on Nursing (1983) and the Task Force on Nursing Practice in Hospitals (McClure, Poulin, Sovie, & Wandelt, 1983). However, by the mid-1980s, concerns related to the future of the CNS role were surfacing in light of the increasing concern with health care cost containment (Hamric, 1989). In spite of these concerns, CNSs made impressive gains in the 1990s at the state and national levels, including being specifically defined and specified for Medicare reimbursement eligibility in the Balanced Budget Act of 1997 (Safriet, 1998).

As of 1996, there were 61,601 CNSs in the United States. These numbers reflected little change since 1992. Almost 91% of these CNSs were employed in nursing; however, only 23% were practicing in CNS-specific positions (U.S. Department of Health and Human Services, 1996) (see Table 1-1). This low percentage may reflect the variety of positions that CNSs assume in nursing, along with the decline of CNS positions in the mid-1990s. The 1996 Sample Survey of Registered Nurses also revealed that a significant number (7,802) of CNSs were prepared also as NPs. These dual-role-prepared APNs were more likely to function in the NP role and are discussed in more depth in the following section on NPs. It is difficult to obtain an accurate estimate of the number of CNSs nationally because CNSs are members of a variety of specialty organizations. A rough estimate as to the total number of CNSs in the United States ranges from 30,000 to 60,000 (National Association of Clinical Nurse Specialists Executive Office, personal communication, September 1999).

Organizational Development

Organizationally, CNSs have actively participated in independent specialty nursing organizations as well as councils within the ANA that reflect their particular clinical area of interest. The National Association of Clinical Nurse Specialists (NACNS) was established in 1995, which represented a major step in the organizational development of this specialty. As of 1999, membership within this organization totaled 830 (NACNS Executive Office, personal communication, September 1999). Certification of CNSs began in the mid-1970s under the ANA and has increased in specialty organizations over time. This process has been somewhat slow because of the multiple specialties of CNSs. Complicating the situation is the fact that certification in many specialty areas has been available primarily at the basic specialty level, rather than the advanced level. For example, in oncology, basic certification has been available for several years through the Oncology Nursing Society (ONS). In 1995, the first certification examination for advanced practice in oncology nursing was administered by the ONS. For some specialties no certification at either the basic or the advanced level is available. This may explain why a minority of CNSs (23.6%) are nationally certified (U.S. Department of Health and Human Services, 1996) (see Table 1-1).

Historically, legislative or regulatory turmoil relative to the CNS has been limited, although psychiatric CNSs were early leaders in seeking third-party reimbursement and changes in state nursing practice acts to recognize APNs. Currently, not all state nursing practice acts specifically recognize the CNS role.

Educational Development

As previously discussed, psychiatric nursing was the first nursing specialty to initiate clinical preparation at the master's level. According to Critchley (1985), this emergence was directly influenced by the effect of nurses returning from World War II, who were eligible to pursue advanced education under the GI Bill. Early educational programs were developed in psychiatric nursing and other specialties, often in connection with universities, although graduate degrees were not conferred. As noted earlier, Peplau established the first master's program in psychiatric nursing at Rutgers University in 1954. This is considered the first CNS educational program. The expansion of the Professional Nurse Traineeship Program to include CNS students in 1963 served as a major impetus for the development and expansion of graduate programs preparing CNSs. By 1984, the NLN accredited 129 programs for preparing CNSs (NLN, 1984). In the early 1990s, CNS programs were the most numerous of all the master's nursing programs nationally, serving over 11,000 students (NLN, 1994). The largest area of specialization was adult health/medical-surgical. However, with the increasing emphasis on primary care in the mid-1990s and the rapid growth of NP programs, there was a sharp decline in demand for and number of CNS educational programs. Between 1997 and 1998, enrollments and graduation in CNS programs fell by 19.4% and 11.7%, respectively (AACN, 1999). Many educational programs have responded by developing combined NP/CNS programs that prepare graduates for dual certification. As of 1998, CNS majors comprised 10.8% of master's enrollees and 13.6% of the graduates. In spite of the declines in CNS educational programs, the National Advisory Council on Nurse Education and Practice (1998) concluded that "the CNS provider is a viable member of the evolving health care delivery team, even as the direct and indirect roles of the CNS continue to change, adapting to changing population needs and the health care market place" (p. 26).

Inter- and Intraprofessional Dynamics

The relative ease with which the CNS was incorporated into the health care system contrasts with the experience of the other advanced nursing specialties. This could be because the CNS role did not represent a radical change in the organization or power dynamics of health care delivery patterns but was incorporated within existing nursing organizational structures. The CNS role was an innovation born out of mainstream nursing and enjoyed the strong support of nursing leaders. Territoriality struggles related to perceived turf encroachment with other disciplines, particularly medicine, were less public, occurring more quietly within institutions. The initial establishment of CNS preparation at the graduate level was also probably a positive factor in reducing controversy.

From an intraprofessional perspective, however, the CNS role produced some highly controversial dynamics. The introduction of a CNS may be interpreted by staff as a criticism of staff performance, resulting in suspicion and hostility toward the

CNS. Woodrow and Bell's (1971) experience confirmed the isolation and rejection encountered by many CNSs, especially initially. Christman (1991) wrote as follows:

> *For many years nurses received their advanced preparation under such rubrics as education, management, or supervision. This advanced preparation usually was devoid of clinical content . . . . This may be one of the reasons that nurse specialists threaten nurse managers, who do not have extensive clinical training, and why they are down played or underemployed by these administrators . . . . In breaking new ground at the graduate level, the nurse specialist was perceived as a threat to the status quo because she took as her model the full professional role in its broadest sense.*

(pp. 111–112)

Historically, these intraprofessional struggles were faced first by psychiatric CNSs, who were successful in delineating the differences between generalist and advanced practice within psychiatric nursing, thereby promoting collaborative intraprofessional practice. More recently, the intraprofessional tension of role ambiguity has emerged, particularly as the role boundaries between CNSs and NPs have become blurred (National Advisory Council on Nurse Education and Practice, 1998). In addition, the recent burgeoning of nurse case management has also served to raise intraprofessional issues regarding the current role of CNSs.

NURSE PRACTITIONERS

Historical Review

NPs developed somewhat later than CNSs, again with very different dynamics. In the late 1950s and early 1960s, discussion about the expansion of nursing functions increased, especially as related to domains of practice traditionally seen as "medical" (McGivern, 1986). Growing out of the role of the public health nurse as the closest example of a broad scope of practice with a relatively high degree of autonomy, examples of innovative practice emerged in settings such as rural nursing, occupational settings, and venereal disease clinics (Kalisch & Kalisch, 1986). Early experiments with role expansion in the United States and Canada also focused on chronic illness management, reflecting a physician extender perspective (Lewis & Resnick, 1967). A major impetus for NP development was the shortage of primary care physicians, which was acute in the 1960s and 1970s. The trend toward medical specialization drew increasing numbers of physicians away from primary care, leaving many areas underserved. Socially and politically, the United States was engaged in a period of rapid change related to the Vietnam War, domestic unrest, and movements promoting racial and gender equity. The consumer movement was at its height, demanding accessible, affordable, and sensitive health care. The women's movement also increased the awareness of nurses and of society that nurses were undervalued and underutilized. In health care delivery, costs were increasing at an annual rate of 10% to 14% (Jonas, 1981). One innovation growing out of the shortage of physicians and the Vietnam War was the introduction of the physician assistant role in the 1960s. Nursing leaders were not generally supportive of this new role, contending that nurses were more logical health professionals to assume a more direct role in primary health care. Thus the NP role emerged in a unique context in response to needs within the population, the nursing profession, and the health care delivery system. The development of the NP role was fueled by an increasing emphasis on primary health care in the 1970s and 1980s (McGivern, 1986). The focus was on ambulatory, interdisciplinary, and family-centered care as exemplified by demonstration projects such as the Yale Family Care Project and the Martin Luther King Health Care Center in New York.

Growing out of this period of social change, the NP role rapidly made a major impact on nursing and health care delivery. Loretta Ford (1991), one of the originators of the NP concept, wrote in retrospect, "The nurse practitioner movement is one of the finest demonstrations of how nurses exploited trends in the larger health care system to advance their own professional agenda and to realize their great potential to serve society" (p. 287). Ford contended that the NP concept initially took hold because of the political perception of the NP as a physician substitute in a climate of physician shortage. However, "the movement thrived because the foundation of the nurse practitioner was deeply rooted in the enduring values and goals of professional nursing" (Ford, 1991, p. 287).

The landmark event marking the birth of the NP role was the establishment of the first pediatric NP program by Loretta Ford and Henry Silver at the University of Colorado in 1965. This demonstration project, funded by the Commonwealth Foundation, was designed to prepare professional nurses to provide comprehensive well-child care as well as to manage common childhood health problems. Family dynamics and community cultural values were strongly emphasized. A study evaluating the project indicated that pediatric NPs were highly competent in assessing and managing 75% of well and ill children in community health stations. In addition, pediatric NPs increased the number of clients served in private pediatric practice by 33% (Ford & Silver, 1967). These strong evaluation data, similar to those collected by innovators in the other advanced practice specialties, demonstrate the importance of concurrent research activities with the development of new advanced nursing practice roles. This first pediatric NP program shifted the focus of NP practice from the care of medical illness to the strong family-oriented health promotive approach. The Colorado experience was a postbaccalaureate certificate program including a 4-month intensive educational and practical training period, followed by a 20-month period of concentrated training and practice in community-based health stations, often in rural areas. Interestingly, Ford (1991) saw the development of the pediatric NP as a reclaiming of the nurse's role in well-child care, which was lost in the 1930s when the American Academy of Pediatrics claimed that well-child care was the domain of pediatricians rather than public health nurses.

The emergence of the NP role attracted considerable attention from professional groups and policy makers. Health policy groups, such as the National Advisory Commission on Health Manpower, issued statements in support of the NP concept (Moxley, 1968). In the early 1970s, Health, Education and Welfare Secretary Elliott Richardson established the Committee to Study Extended Roles for Nurses. This group of health care leaders was charged with evaluating the feasibility of expanding nursing practice (Kalisch & Kalisch, 1986). They concluded that extending the scope of the nurse's role was essential to providing equal access to health care for all consumers. The committee urged establishment of innovative curricular designs in health science centers with increased financial support for nursing education. They also advocated commonality of nursing licensure and certification, including a model nursing practice law suitable for national application. In addition, the report called for further research related to cost-benefit analyses and attitudinal surveys to assess the impact of the new role. The report resulted in increased federal support through the Maternal and Child Health Service, Regional Medical Programs, and the Division of Nursing of the U.S. Public Health Service. This federal support, as well as support through private funding agencies, stimulated the rapid development of educational programs for family NPs, adult NPs, pediatric NPs, rural NPs, emergency NPs, and obstetrical/gynecological NPs. Numerous research studies that evaluated the role of the NP were conducted, both within nursing and outside the profession. These studies consistently demonstrated the efficacy and effectiveness of NPs in collaborative practice with physicians.

By 1984, approximately 20,000 graduates of NP programs were employed, for the most part in settings "that the founders envisioned" (Kalisch & Kalisch, 1986, p. 715): outpatient clinics, health maintenance organizations (HMOs), health departments, community health centers, rural clinics, schools, occupational health clinics, and private offices. However, only 12% of all NPs were employed in remote or satellite clinics, often because of problems securing physician collaboration (Kalisch & Kalisch, 1986).

During the 1990s, the number of NPs increased dramatically in response to increasing demand. An important innovation was the development of the acute care NP role, which emerged in the early 1990s. This new advanced practice role in inpatient settings grew out of an increasing need for "house officer" services in many large urban hospitals as a result of the declining number of medical residents. Advanced practice nursing responded quickly to this need, creating a role that promoted both quality patient care and nursing's leadership in health care delivery. Between 1992 and 1996, the total number of NPs increased 47%. As of 1996, there were 63,191 NPs nationally, representing the largest APN specialty. Of these NPs, 88.2% were currently employed in nursing; however, only 52% of NPs were practicing in specific NP positions. As noted earlier, the 1996 Sample Survey of Registered Nurses also revealed that there were 7,802 individuals prepared as both NPs and CNSs. Within this subgroup, 100% were employed in nursing, with most practicing as NPs (U.S. Department of Health and Human Services, 1996) (see Table 1–1).

Organizational Development

Organizationally the ANA Commission on Nursing Education functionally described the NP role in 1972. The NLN's Council of Baccalaureate and Higher Degree Programs immediately endorsed the NP role description. Nevertheless, considerable controversy regarding the educational preparation of NPs and their role within nursing versus medicine continued within the profession. Several independent NP organizations also developed in the 1970s and 1980s, including the National Association of Pediatric Nurse Associates and Practitioners and the American Academy of Nurse Practitioners. The Primary Health Care Nurse Practitioner Council was established within the ANA in the early 1980s. About the same time, the National Alliance of Nurse Practitioners was established as an umbrella organization of all the various NP associations. Those efforts at unifying the organizational voice of NPs further evolved in the mid-1990s with the establishment of the American College of Nurse Practitioners. Membership in this organization includes national organizational affiliates, state NP organizations, and individuals. The focus of the organization is addressing public policy related to all NPs as well as relevant clinical issues.

Since the 1970s, credentialing of NPs has also been evolving, with certification offered through multiple specialty organizations with varying requirements. As of 1996, 63.5% of NPs and 70.9% of CNS/NPs were nationally certified (U.S. Department of Health and Human Services, 1996) (see Table 1–1).

Educational Development

The development of NP education was controversial. As with nurse anesthesia and nurse-midwifery, early NP education did not develop for the most part within the mainstream of nursing education. Based on the Colorado project, new programs rapidly developed, including some "mutations" (Ford, 1991), that shifted from a nursing to a medical model with little consistency in academic standards. Over time, however, NP programs were increasingly institutionalized within major schools of nursing at the graduate level. By 1990, there were 135 master's degree and 40 certificate NP programs, and by 1998, there were over 750 master's and/or post-master's programs and only 12 post–basic RN certificate programs (AACN, 1999; Bullough, 1992). The majority of the certificate programs focus on women's health care. Most NP leaders support the master's degree as the educational requirement for NP practice. As noted earlier, in the mid-1990s, NP educational programs proliferated rapidly in response to increasing demand and national emphasis on primary care. Between 1992 and 1994, the number of institutions offering NP programs doubled from 78 to 158, doubling again to 325 by 1998. These institutions offered a total of 384 NP programs in 1994 and 769 programs in 1998 (AACN, 1999; National Organization of Nurse Practitioner Faculties, 1995). As of 1998, NP majors comprised the majority of master's enrollees and graduates (56.1% and 57.5%, respectively) (AACN, 1999). This rapid proliferation of programs raised serious concerns among NP leaders, educators, and state regulators and fueled the refinement of educational standards and discussions regarding program accreditation (Allan, 1998; Safriet, 1998). Currently, the growth of NP educational programs has leveled off, but they continue to produce the highest percentage of advanced practice nurses.

Inter- and Intraprofessional Dynamics

The legal and legislative history of NPs has been stormy. In 1971, Idaho became the first state to officially authorize an expanded role for nurses with a focus on NPs. The control and regulation of NP practice was often shared between state boards of nursing and medicine initially, moving to mainly nursing boards in the 1980s and 1990s. Prescriptive authority was and is a particularly volatile legislative issue. Most states that allow prescriptive authority specify it as a delegable function under the physician. A few states, including Oregon and Washington, have passed independent prescriptive authority statutes.

Inter- and intraprofessional relationships surrounding the NP role have also been controversial. Initially, there was considerable intraprofessional resistance from the nursing community, which viewed NPs as not practicing nursing (Ford, 1982). Martha Rogers (1972), one of the most outspoken opponents of the NP concept, argued that the development of the NP role was a ploy to lure nurses away from nursing to medicine and thereby undermine nursing's unique role in health care. This view divided nurse leaders and educators, resulting in barriers to the establishment of NP educational programs within mainstream nursing education. NPs were increasingly accepted by nursing over time as they proved to provide a high quality of care using a nursing approach. The increasing move toward NP educational standardization at the master's level has also served to reduce intraprofessional tension.

Interprofessional conflicts with organized medicine and to a lesser extent with pharmacy have centered on control issues and the degree of independence the NP is allowed. These conflicts have intensified as NPs have moved beyond the "physician extender" model to a more autonomous one. In 1980, a landmark case, *Sermchief v. Gonzales* (1983), was brought against two women's health care NPs charged with practicing medicine without a license by the Missouri medical board (Doyle & Meurer, 1983). The initial ruling was against the NPs, but on appeal the Missouri Supreme Court overturned the decision, concluding that advanced nursing functions may evolve without statutory constraints (Wolff, 1984). This case supported the development of liberalized state nursing practice acts that addressed advanced practice in generalized wording. Such practice acts are important in promoting future development of APN roles and functions.

Over time, the territorial and legal struggles faced by NPs have changed, similar to the experience of other advanced practice specialties. Most recently, legislative efforts to secure third-party reimbursement and maintain nursing's control over NP practice have been active areas. In addition, restraint-of-trade issues are being addressed as NPs are increasingly viewed as a competitive threat by other providers, particularly physicians.

ADVANCED PRACTICE NURSE CASE MANAGERS

Historical Review

The historical development of APNCMs as the newest advanced practice specialty has been quite different than that of the other specialties. It must be noted that there is not universal agreement that nurse case managers (NCMs) should be defined and prepared as APNs. Some argue that case management is a role within administrative or community health nursing and therefore not a distinct advanced practice role. However, as NCMs have increasingly defined their unique area of practice, it is clear that they represent an emerging advanced practice specialty with many common characteristics and struggles with the more established advanced practice roles. Case management is also unique in that, since its inception, it has represented a multidisciplinary practice activity that involves providers from varying professional disciplines, with nursing and social work being the most common. This presents challenges as well as opportunities as this area of specialty in nursing develops.

Although the term "case management" is often equated with the recent emergence of managed care, its history dates back well into the 1800s. This first phase of case management history reflects the case coordination activities of various disciplines, including nursing. Two powerful social factors in the 19th century contributed to the early development of case management: rapid urbanization and the influx of immigrant populations. These social phenomena, resulting largely from the shift from an agrarian to industrialized economy, produced social service and public health concerns related to densely populated, low-income communities. By 1860, case management strategies were used by early settlement houses serving new immigrants and the poor. In 1863, the first Board of Charities was established in Massachusetts to coordinate public services and conserve public funds, and by 1877, the Charity Organization Societies became the dominant force in providing cost-effective and efficient services to the poor through interagency cooperation and coordination (Tahan, 1998). In 1901, Mary Richmond, a social services pioneer, published a model of case coordination in which social workers played the role of mediator between those who needed services and the service providers. Social planning agencies were established in the 1920s with the emergence of child guidance centers. These centers were the result of the Community Chest Movement that garnered donations to support human services agencies and coordinate services for abused children and families in distress.

During these early years, nursing played a major role in the development of case management. In the 1890s, Lillian Wald established the role of the public health nurse who practiced autonomously to organize and mobilize families and community resources while providing direct nursing care (Kersbergen, 1996). At the turn of the century, Annie W. Goodrich, superintendent of the Yale University School of Nursing, developed the first visiting nurse service. Wald persuaded the Metropolitan Life Insurance Company to fund visiting nursing services, resulting in an estimated $43 million savings for the company (Kersbergen, 1996). Wald also founded the first nursing settlement house, Henry Street Settlement House, in 1938 in New York, which provided comprehensive health and social services for the urban poor.

World War II served as a catalyst for the further development of nurse case management, similar to other specialties. After the war, the need for affordable and comprehensive health care services for returning veterans with complex needs became apparent. In response to this need, particularly for community services for psychiatric patients, including mentally disabled or emotionally disturbed veterans and their families, the concept of "continuum care" developed in the 1950s. The need for coordinated community-based care was further reinforced by the deinstitutionalization of chronically mentally ill and developmentally disabled individuals beginning in the 1960s. In 1962, the President's Commission on Mental Retardation recommended the use of a "program coordinator" to help patients stay in the community and to improve accessibility to health care services. This coordinator role was fulfilled by the community mental health nurse, who ensured availability of services and expedited the delivery and responsiveness of care (Tahan, 1998). It is interesting to note that these early advances in psychiatric nursing served as a common base for the development of both the CNS and the APNCM role. Another significant event during this period in the evolution of case management was the passage in 1965 of the Medicare bill, which provided health coverage to the elderly, including home health services.

The term "case management" appeared first in social welfare literature in the 1970s, but soon also emerged in public health nursing journals. It was also during this time that case management services became increasingly available, particularly for elderly and disabled people, as mandated by federal legislation. The Allied Services Act of 1972 resulted in a series of demonstration projects creating the role of "systems agents." These agents coordinated resources for clients with complex health and social services needs, because many programs had become so fragmented and complex that it was difficult for clients to seek appropriate services independently. Several long-term demonstration projects were established that provided case management services funded by both Medicaid and Medicare. These case management services were provided by registered nurses, physicians, social workers, physical and occupational therapists, or dietitians (Tahan, 1998). The Older Americans Act of 1973, which led to the development of the Area Agencies on Aging (AAAs) throughout the country, also served as a powerful impetus in the development and dissemination of case management services. AAAs provide comprehensive services for the elderly to enable them to remain independent as long as possible (Gerber, 1994). They use case management teams, composed of registered nurses and social workers, to assess for, develop, implement, and evaluate needed services, and serve as brokers to obtain appropriate community resources for the client. In addition, the Education for All Handicapped Children Act of 1975 brought case management into the nation's school systems, with nurses and social workers coordinating services with educators. Similarly, the Developmental Disabilities Assistance and Bill of Rights Act of 1975 stipulated that each client be assigned a program coordinator for comprehensive services for deinstitutionalized mentally disabled persons. The President's Commission on Mental Health in 1978 identified case management as the keystone to integration of services for deinstitutionalized clients (Kersbergen, 1996).

In the 1980s a new emphasis on cost containment emerged, producing legislative and economic changes that continued to promote case management. The Omnibus Budget Reconciliation Act of 1981 enabled state Medicaid programs to implement case management systems and required documentation of cost-effectiveness (Conti, 1996). A landmark development in case management history occurred in 1983 with the establishment of prospective payment systems using diagnosis-related groups (DRGs) for hospitalized Medicare recipients. This major change was an effort to control rising costs and reimbursement to hospitals by shifting reimbursement from payment for services provided to payment by case (capitation). This shift created pressure to decrease length of inpatient stays to save funds in all hospital settings.

It was at this point that the second major phase in APN case management history emerged, with case management becoming distinguished as a specialized nursing role, but not yet an advanced practice specialty. Karen Zander (1988) developed the acute care nurse case management model in 1985 at New England Medical Center Hospital in Boston. She envisioned this model as an evolution and further development of primary nursing. Zander's model used clinical pathways that focused on prospective planning of nursing care and on measuring outcomes. These critical paths also led to the development of case management tools using a multidisciplinary approach that was not limited to nursing outcomes. The critical pathway is now one of the most widely used tools by case managers to enhance outcomes and contain costs within a constrained length of stay (Tahan, 1998). It has also been used in evaluative research studies that have demonstrated the benefits of NCMs (Rudisil, 1993). A community-based nursing case management model was developed at Carondelet Saint Mary's Hospital in Tucson, Arizona (Ethridge, 1991). This model established a nursing HMO with an NCM at the hub, and showed effective cost savings without compromising quality of care.

In the 1990s, the development of nurse case management accelerated significantly as a result of the rapid proliferation of managed care. In 1985, only 19% of the U.S. population received care through HMOs, as compared to 56% in 1995 (Fox, 1997). This major shift in health care financing has resulted in a dramatic increase in the use of case managers by both health care institutions and insurers. As a result, case management heads the list of the Bureau of Labor Statistics' projections of growth in health care professions, with a greater than 250% projected increase in case manager positions by the year 2003 (Conti, 1996). Currently there are no published estimates of the number of NCMs nationally.

The current emergence of APNCMs represents the third phase in this historical process. In the early 1990s, a variety of nursing leaders contended that case management was best done by APNs (Connors, 1993; Fralic, 1992; Hamric, 1992). Mahn and Spross (1996) differentiated the basic NCM from the APNCM. They proposed that the APNCM was a graduate-prepared advanced practice nurse who, like NCMs, maintains a direct clinical relationship with clients and families, but also assesses the need for system or process improvements (see also Chapter 19). Because APNCMs must attend to both complex clinical and system/fiscal outcomes, Mahn and Spross contended that APNCMs "might be more likely than other APNs to perform more detailed assessment of environmental, organizational, and contextual factors that affect *individual* patients" (p. 454). Within the emerging APNCM role there exists considerable overlap with other APN specialities, particularly CNSs. However, in light of the increasing complexities of managed care systems, it seems doubtful that CRNAs, CNMs, CNSs, and NPs will be adequately prepared to "do it all," including case management. The evolution of the APNCM as a distinct advanced practice role appears to be near the point of acceptance in the professional, educational, and practice communities. Solidification and institutionalization of this new advanced practice role will occur in the coming decade, along with advances in the organizational and educational development of this emerging APN specialty.

Organizational Development

The organizational development history related to nurse case management is quite recent and reflects the multidisciplinary history of the specialty. The Case Management Society of America (CMSA), founded in 1990, is currently the sole professional organization for case managers. In 1996 it consolidated with the Individual Case Management Association and currently has a membership of approximately 7,500 (CMSA Executive Office, personal communication, September 1999). It is an international nonprofit organization with about 100 affiliated chapters, including ones in Australia, Hong Kong, and London. Members must be in the field of case management and possess a health professional degree or current license or national certification in a health or human services profession. In 1995, the CSMA developed the "Standards of Practice for Case Management" and the "Ethics Statement on Case Management Practice." The Center for Case Management Accountability, a division of CSMA, provides evidence-based standards of practice to help members achieve such standards through the measurement, evaluation, and reporting of outcomes. There is currently no organization exclusively for NCMs or APNCMs, although the ANA has recognized this area of practice and offers a specific discussion forum for NCMs on their website.

Educational Development

NCMs currently have a variety of educational backgrounds, varying from diploma to master's preparation. The only standard for case managers in general is voluntary certification, which was first established by the Commission for Case Manager Certification (CCMC) in 1995. The certification is designed to serve as an adjunct to another professional credential in a health or human services profession. The minimum educational requirement for certification eligibility is a postsecondary degree in a field that promotes physical, psychosocial, or vocational well-being of the people being served. Furthermore, the applicant must have the ability to legally and independently practice without the supervision of another licensed professional, and to perform the six essential activities of case management: assessment, planning, implementation, coordination, monitoring, and evaluation (CCMC, 1999). The American Nurses Credentialing Center (ANCC) has recently established the first certification program specifically for NCMs. Eligibility requirements for the ANCC examination include a bachelor's degree in nursing and 2,000 hours of experience in nurse case management within the last 2 years (ANCC Executive Office, personal communication, September 1999). These requirements are not consistent with those for advanced practice specialty certification through the ANCC.

The ANA set initial educational guidelines specifically for the NCM in 1988 (ANA, 1988; Bower, 1992). The minimum recommended education is a baccalaureate in nursing with 3 years of appropriate clinical experience. In keeping with the more recent development of APNCMs, Newman (1990) and others have proposed that the education needed for the case management position is a postbaccalaureate professional degree. Cronin and Maklebust (1989) studied case-managed care at Harper Hospital and found that bachelor's-prepared nurses were frustrated with their inability to case manage effectively while delivering patient care. When master's-prepared case managers were used, improvements were noted for clients and the hospital. Advanced clinicians saved time and money by using early interventions based on in-depth clinical expertise. Master's-prepared nurses are better able to focus on managing system issues because of their preparation in developing critical pathways and staff development programs (Nolan, Harris, Kufta, Opfer, & Turner, 1998). Berger and her associates (1996) also maintained that competencies in the research process, communication, informatics, diversity, total quality management, and health policy are essential for case managers to function in the ever-changing health care delivery system. However, no curriculum standards or accreditation mechanisms for nurse case management or for APNCMs have yet been developed. As of the fall of 1998, there were 16 graduate nursing programs in case management, with an enrollment of 334 students and 50 graduates (AACN Executive Office, personal communication, September 1999). This was the first year that program data for nurse case management education programs were specifically reported; however, the number of case management students and graduates has reportedly increased since 1997.

Inter- and Intraprofessional Dynamics

The relatively recent entry of NCMs in health care delivery has produced a limited amount of inter- and intraprofessional conflict. The major question from an intraprofessional perspective has been, who should be a case manager? This discussion centers on the educational and practice preparation necessary to function as NCMs and APNCMs. Some authors argue that all professional nurses are NCMs (Conti, 1996). Others argue that CNSs or NPs are best prepared to provide case management services (Schroer, 1991; Trinidad, 1993; Wagner & Menke, 1992). The case manager must be an expert clinician and facilitator, promoting multidisciplinary collaboration while continuously evaluating clinical and financial outcomes based on standards of care (Lynn-McHale, Fitzpatrick, & Shaffer, 1993). This debate as to preparation and overlapping functions of NCMs, APNCMs, and other APNs will not be resolved until clear educational and credentialing standards for APNCMs are established that are consistent with the other advanced practice specialties.

From an interprofessional perspective, again the question of who should be a case manager has emerged because of the multiple disciplines who currently practice case management. This has created conflict as to who is best prepared to provide case management services, particularly between nurses, social workers, and to some extent physicians. Mundinger (1984) contended that nurses can provide the majority of services that social workers offer clients, but the reverse does not hold true, since social workers lack the physical assessment and illness detection skills of the nurse. The social work community, however, emphasizes their contribution to case management, particularly in the areas of social and economic assistance to clients, including housing, economic support, transportation, education, and recreation (Spitler, 1996). These services are needed especially among elderly, homeless, chronically mentally ill, developmentally disabled, and chemically dependent client populations. This conflict among the disciplines can result in larger case management teams because everyone feels his or her role is vital. This practice can become costly, negating the reason for establishing such programs in the first place. This professional posturing, similar to that which has historically occurred between medicine and CRNAs, CNMs, and NPs, approaches the issue from a competitive rather than collaborative perspective. It seems doubtful that the activities of case management will or should ever become the domain of only one discipline. In arguing that nursing is the preferred discipline to provide case management, it could be argued that nursing may be reflecting a somewhat narrow view. Certainly clients with complex health challenges benefit from APN case management, while clients with complex social and economic needs may require social work case management. Ideally case managers work collaboratively and focus on individual clients, addressing all the client's needs. Promoting collegiality and collaboration among all case management providers appears to be the wisest and most futuristic approach. With that said, however, if APNCMs are to become established, clarity regarding their distinct activities as APNs must be articulated (see Chapter 19).

A somewhat more volatile interprofessional issue has surfaced in response to case managers' decision-making and review powers within institutions and managed care systems. Some direct care providers, particularly physicians, have voiced strident opposition to perceived intrusions into the patient-provider relationship by case managers. Case managers are often negatively viewed by some providers as uninvolved "bean counters" who should not be given the power to limit services or "second guess" the judgment of direct providers. As a licensed health care provider, this tension places the NCM in a sensitive position as an advocate for quality client care as well as cost-effectiveness and institutional efficiency. This tension again demonstrates the need for APNCMs, who are best prepared to deal with these complexities by fully utilizing their high-level clinical and systems management competencies.

SUMMARY AND CONCLUSIONS

The preceding historical review of the development and evolution of advanced nursing practice makes it clear that the various specialties have areas of commonality. Recurrent themes and dynamics are apparent, including the impact of societal forces, dynamic inter- and intraprofessional struggles, and the importance of organizational, educational, and research development.

Societal forces have clearly influenced the development of advanced nursing practice. Gender issues have affected all the specialties to some degree because of the unique position of nursing as a female-dominated profession. In nurse anesthesia, the increasing acceptance of males in the specialty has been a challenge. Within nurse-midwifery, the status of women and their health was a powerful force in the establishment and development of the specialty. Gender biases have impeded attempts by CNSs and NPs to assume an autonomous role in the male-dominated health care system. Changing societal attitudes toward women have promoted advanced nursing practice; however, gender-related conflicts have also contributed to intra- and interprofessional tensions. A second powerful societal influence is the impact of wars and the relationship between advanced nursing practice and the American military. Each of the five nursing specialties reviewed was influenced in some significant way by the major wars of the 20th century. Historians have noted that major social changes often follow periods of war, and this phenomenon is certainly demonstrated in the history of advanced nursing practice. In general, wars have served as catalysts to promote the development of advanced nursing practice, education, and professional organization. Finally, economic changes, particularly in relation to health care financing, have had a powerful effect on the development of advanced nursing practice. The dramatic growth of managed care systems in the last decade in particular has presented new challenges and opportunities for APNs related to reimbursement, scope of practice, and autonomy (Safriet, 1998). The recent growth of the APNCM role is largely a result of the economic restructuring of health care in the 1990s.

The powerful influence of interprofessional struggles is also apparent in all the advanced specialties, with the possible exception of CNSs. The historical struggles between nursing and medicine are longstanding, particularly in relation to nurse anesthesia and nurse-midwifery. Most of these tensions revolve around issues of control, autonomy, and economic competition. The resulting legal and legislative battles for the most part have proven to be positive for nursing and have helped to institutionalize APN roles.

Similarly, struggles within the nursing community have been characteristic of the evolution of all the advanced practice specialties. CRNAs, CNMs, and to some extent NPs and NCMs have developed parallel to mainstream nursing, with CNSs developing more within the mainstream. Regardless, each specialty has had to deal with resistance from other nurses. These intraprofessional struggles are understandable in relation to the fact that each of the advanced nursing specialties represented innovations that shook the status quo of the nursing establishment as well as the health care system. CRNAs, CNMs, and NPs perhaps presented the most unsettling innovations for some because they challenged the boundaries between nursing and medical practice. However, each specialty has struggled for acceptance and recognition with nursing colleagues at individual practice, institutional, and larger professional levels. These territorial struggles will continue, particularly as the health care delivery system changes. History teaches us that these issues must be assertively confronted through strong and proactive organizational efforts. Organizational unity and consensus among all the advanced nursing specialties should be a goal to enhance political and legislative effectiveness. Fortunately, over time, the intraprofessional tensions seem to be lessening for all the advanced practice specialties, perhaps as the interprofessional struggles intensify.

Within the development of each of the advanced nursing specialties, several common themes emerge. Strong national organizational leadership has been clearly demonstrated to be of critical importance in enhancing the growth and protection of the specialty. Based on the experience of the two oldest specialties, nurse anesthesia and nurse-midwifery, the process of establishing an effective national organization has taken a minimum of three decades. The newest advanced practice specialties, NPs, CNSs, and APNCMs, are still struggling with their organizational development. The specialty organizations have also historically played a critical role in the credentialing process for individuals within the specialty, with nurse anesthesia and nurse-midwifery being most developed. The strength, unity, and depth of the organizational development of the two oldest advanced nursing specialties should serve as a model for the younger developing specialties.

Along with organizational development, the establishment of credible and stable educational programs is a crucial step in the evolution of advanced nursing specialties. Historically, educational programs have moved from informal, institutionally based models with a strong apprenticeship approach to more formalized graduate education models housed in nursing units within institutions of higher education. This movement from informal specialty preparation to advanced practice education in formal graduate programs can be seen in the newest role examined, the APNCM. It is a clear trend in the evolution of advanced practice. Clearly, the national commitment among nursing leaders and educators is that preparation for advanced nursing practice should be at the master's level. If current trends continue, this commitment will soon be realized. Ensuring consistency and quality across programs, a process that is complemented by strong specialty organizations and clear-cut curricular standards, is a related vital issue for all the advanced practice specialties.

The history and evolution of advanced nursing practice has also demonstrated the importance of evaluative research to document the contribution of the specialty to health care and client well-being. The early APNs were particularly visionary in their inclusion of evaluative studies within their development processes. This research clearly served to promote the growth and acceptance of the specialties using facts and measurable outcomes.

With the rapid changes in nursing and health care, it is apparent that the advanced nursing practice specialties will continue to evolve and diversify. Current examples of these newly evolving roles include the parish nurse and the acute care NP. The beauty of the concept of advanced nursing practice is the inherent flexibility and creativity to quickly adapt to changing health care needs. As new advanced practice roles emerge, the historical trends and struggles of the "older siblings" can certainly provide guidance and support in terms of current and future strategies. Close collaboration and support among all the advanced practice specialties are necessary to promote the dynamic evolution of all the roles.

In summary, the history and evolution of advanced nursing practice indicate that the leaders in these nursing specialties were clearly the vanguard of the development of modern nursing. Their position as trailblazers was neither safe nor comfortable in terms of attacks from within and beyond. As a result of their concerted and dedicated "pushing of the limits" through strong collective action, the profession of nursing and health care as a whole have benefited immeasurably.

ACKNOWLEDGMENT

The authors thank Rhonda Ramirez, RN, MSN, for her assistance in the preparation of this chapter.

REFERENCES

Adams, C. J. (1983). *Nurse-midwifery: Health care for women and newborns.* New York: Grune & Stratton.

Allan, J. D. (1998). Striving for quality in advanced practice nursing education. *Advanced Practice Nursing Quarterly, 4*(3), 6-14.

American Association of Colleges of Nursing. (1999). *Enrollment and graduations in baccalaureate and graduate programs in nursing.* Washington, DC: Author.

American College of Nurse-Midwives. (1962). *Definition of a certified nurse-midwife.* Washington, DC: Author.

American College of Nurse-Midwives. (1968). *Descriptive data, nurse-midwives—U.S.A.* Washington, DC: Author.

American College of Nurse-Midwives. (1978a). *Definition of a certified nurse-midwife.* Washington, DC: Author.

American College of Nurse-Midwives. (1978b). *Philosophy.* Washington, DC: Author.

American College of Nurse-Midwives. (1997). *Position statement.* Washington, DC: Author.

American Nurses Association. (1980). *Nursing: A social policy statement.* Kansas City, MO: Author.

American Nurses Association. (1988). *Nursing case management.* Kansas City, MO: Author.

Ayers, R. (1971). Effects and development of the role of the clinical nurse specialist. In R. Ayers (Ed.), *The clinical nurse specialist: An experiment in role effectiveness and role development* (pp. 32-49). Duarte, CA: City of Hope National Medical Center.

Bankert, M. (1989). *Watchful care: A history of America's nurse anesthetists.* New York: Continuum.

Barnason, S., Merboth, M., Pozehl, B., & Tietjen, M. J. (1998). Utilizing an outcome approach to improve pain management by nurses: A pilot study. *Clinical Nurse Specialist, 12*(1), 28-36.

Berger, A. M., Eilers, J. G., Pattrin, L., Rolf-Eixley, M., Pfeifer, B. A., Rogge, J. A., Wheeler, L. M., Bergstrom, N. I., & Heck, C. S. (1996). Advanced practice roles for nurses in tomorrow's health-care systems. *Clinical Nurse Specialist, 10*(5), 250-255.

Bhan v. NME Hospitals, Inc., et al. (1985). 772 F.2d 1467 (9th Cir.).

Bower, K. A. (1992). *Case management by nurses.* Kansas City, MO: American Nurses Publishing.

Breckenridge, M. (1952). *Wide neighborhoods: A study of the Frontier Nursing Service.* New York: Harper.

Brooten, D., Kumar, S., Brown, L. P., Butts, P., Finkler, S. A., Bakewell-Sachs, S., Gibbons, A., & Delivoria-Papadopoulos, M. (1986). A randomized clinical trial of early hospital discharge and home follow-up of very-low-birth-weight infants. *New England Journal of Medicine, 315,* 934-939.

Bullough, B. (1992). Alternative models for specialty nursing practice. *Nursing and Health Care, 13*(5), 254-259.

Case Management Society of America. (1995). *Standards of practice.* Little Rock, AR: Author.

Chalmers-Frances v. Nelson. (1936). 6 Cal.2d 402.

Christman, L. (1991). Advanced nursing practice: Future of clinical nurse specialists. In L. H. Aiken & C. M. Fagin (Eds.), *Charting nursing's future: Agenda for the 1990s* (pp. 108-120). New York: J. B. Lippincott.

Commission for Case Manager Certification. (1999). *CCM certification guide.* Rolling Meadows, IL: Author.

Connors, H. (1993). Impact of care management modalities on curricula. In K. Kelly & M. Maas (Eds.), *Managing nursing care: Promise and pitfalls* (pp. 190-207). St. Louis: Mosby.

Conti, R. M. (1996). Nurse case manager roles: Implications for practice and education. *Nursing Administration Quarterly, 21*(1), 67-80.

Critchley, D. L. (1985). Evolution of the role. In D. L. Critchley & J. T. Maurin (Eds.), *The clinical specialist in psychiatric mental health nursing* (pp. 5-22). New York: John Wiley & Sons.

Cronin, C. J., & Maklebust, J. (1989). Case-managed care: Capitalizing on the CNS. *Nursing Management, 20*(3), 38-47.

Dewitt, K. (1900). Specialties in nursing. *American Journal of Nursing, 1,* 14-17.

Diers, D. (1991). Nurse-midwives and nurse anesthetists: The cutting edge in specialist practice. In L. H. Aiken & C. M. Fagin (Eds.), *Charting nursing's future: Agenda for the 1990s* (pp. 159-180). New York: J. B. Lippincott.

Doyle, E., & Meurer, J. (1983). Missouri legislation and litigation: Practicing medicine without a license. *Nurse Practitioner, 8,* 41-44.

Ethridge, P. (1991). A nursing HMO: Carondelet St. Mary's experience. *Nursing Management, 22,* 222-227.

Faut-Callahan, M., & Kremer, M. (1996). The certified registered nurse anesthetist. In A. B. Hamric, J. A. Spross, & C. M. Hanson (Eds.), *Advanced nursing practice: An integrative approach* (pp. 421-444). Philadelphia: W. B. Saunders.

Ford, L. C. (1982). Nurse practitioners: History of a new idea and predictions for the future. In L. H. Aiken (Ed.), *Nursing in the 80s* (pp. 231-248). Philadelphia: J. B. Lippincott.

Ford, L. C. (1991). Advanced nursing practice: Future of the nurse practitioner. In L. H. Aiken & C. M. Fagin (Eds.), *Charting nursing's future: Agenda for the 1990s* (pp. 287-299). New York: J. B. Lippincott.

Ford, L. C., & Silver, H. K. (1967). The expanded role of the nurse in child care. *Nursing Outlook, 15*(8), 43–45.

Fox, C. G. (1969). Toward a sound historical basis for nurse-midwifery. *Bulletin of the American College of Nurse-Midwives, 14,* 76.

Fox, P. D. (1997). An overview of managed care. In P. R. Kongstvedt (Ed.), *Essentials of managed health care* (pp. 3–16). Gaithersburg, MD: Aspen.

Fralic, M. (1992). The nurse case manager: Focus, selection, preparation, and measurement. *Journal of Nursing Administration, 22*(11), 13–14, 46.

Frank et al. v. South et al. (1917). 175 Ky. 416–428.

Garde, J. (1988). Preface. In W. Waugaman, S. Foster, & B. Rigor (Eds.), *Principles and practice of nurse anesthesia* (pp. xiii). Norwalk, CT: Appleton & Lange.

Georgopoulos, B. S., & Christman, L. (1970). The clinical nurse specialist: A role model. *American Journal of Nursing, 70,* 1030–1039.

Georgopoulos, B. S., & Jackson, M. M. (1970). Nursing Kardex behavior in an experimental study of patient units with and without clinical specialists. *Nursing Research, 19,* 196–218.

Georgopoulos, B. S., & Sana, M. (1971). Clinical nursing specialization and intershift report behavior. *American Journal of Nursing, 71,* 538–545.

Gerber, L. S. (1994). Case management models. *Journal of Gerontological Nursing, 20*(7), 18–24.

Girouard, S. (1978). The role of the clinical nurse specialist as change agent: An experiment in preoperative teaching. *International Journal of Nursing Studies, 15,* 57–65.

Goodnow, M. (1938). *Outline of nursing history* (6th ed.). Philadelphia: W. B. Saunders.

Hamric, A. B. (1989). History and overview of the CNS role. In A. B. Hamric & J. A. Spross (Eds.), *The clinical nurse specialist in theory and practice* (2nd ed., pp. 3–18). Philadelphia: W. B. Saunders.

Hamric, A. B. (1992). Creating our future: Challenges and opportunities for the clinical nurse specialist. *Oncology Nursing Forum, 19*(1, Suppl.), 11–15.

Jonas, S. (1981). *Health care delivery in the United States.* New York: Springer.

Kalisch, P. A., & Kalisch, B. J. (1986). *The advance of American nursing* (2nd ed.). Boston: Little, Brown and Company.

Kersbergen, A. L. (1996). Case management: A rich history of coordinating care to control costs. *Nursing Outlook, 44,* 169–172.

Leggett v. Tennessee Board of Nursing. (1980). 612 S. W. 2nd 476.

Leigh v. Board of Registration in Nursing. (1984). 481 N.E.2d 401 (Ind. App.).

Lewis, C. E., & Resnick, B. A. (1967). Nurse clinics and progressive ambulatory patient care. *New England Journal of Medicine, 277*(3), 1236–1241.

Little, D. E., & Carnevali, D. (1967). Nurse specialist effect on tuberculosis. *Nursing Research, 16,* 321–326.

Lynn-McHale, D. J., Fitzpatrick, E. R., & Shaffer, R. B. (1993). Case management: Development of a model. *Clinical Nurse Specialist, 7*(6), 299–307.

Mahn, V. A., & Spross, J. A. (1996). Nurse case management as an advanced practice role. In A. B. Hamric, J. A. Spross, & C. M. Hanson (Eds.), *Advanced nursing practice: An integrative approach* (pp. 445–465). Philadelphia: W. B. Saunders.

McBride, A. B., Austin, J. K., Chesnut, E. E., Main, C. S., Richards, B. S., & Roy, B. A. (1987). Evaluation of the impact of the clinical nurse specialist in a state psychiatric hospital. *Archives of Psychiatric Nursing, 1,* 55–61.

McClure, M. L., Poulin, M. A., Sovie, M. D., & Wandelt, M. A. (1983). *Magnet hospitals.* Kansas City, MO: American Nurses Association.

McCorkle, R., Robinson, L., Nuamah, I., Lev, E., & Benoliel, J. Q. (1998). The effects of home nursing care for patients during terminal illness on the bereaved's psychological distress. *Nursing Research, 47*(1), 2–10.

McGivern, D. (1986). The evolution of primary care nursing. In M. Mezey & D. McGivern (Eds.), *Nurses, nurse practitioners: The evolution of primary care* (pp. 3–14). Boston: Little, Brown and Company.

Moxley, J. (1968). The predicament in health manpower. *American Journal of Nursing, 68,* 1490.

Mundinger, M. O. (1984). Community based care: Who will be the case managers? *Nursing Outlook, 32*(6), 294–295.

National Advisory Council on Nurse Education and Practice. (1998). *Report to the Secretary of Health and Human Services: Federal support for the preparation of the clinical nurse specialist workforce through Title VIII.* Washington, DC: U.S. Department of Health and Human Services.

National Commission on Nursing. (1983). *Summary report and recommendations.* Chicago: The Hospital Research and Educational Trust.

National League for Nursing. (1984). *Master's education in nursing: Route to opportunities in contemporary nursing, 1984–1985.* New York: Author.

National League for Nursing. (1994). *Nursing Datasource 1994: Vol. XX. Graduate education in nursing, advanced practice nursing.* New York: Author.

National Organization of Nurse Practitioner Faculties. (1995). *Nurse practitioner program number of institutions and specialty tracks by state: New York.* Washington, DC: Author.

Newman, M. A. (1990). Toward an integrative model of professional practice. *Journal of Professional Nursing, 6*(3), 167–173.

Nolan, M. T., Harris, A., Kufta, A., Opfer, N., & Turner, H. (1998). Preparing nurses for the acute care case manager role: Educational needs identified by existing case managers. *Journal of Continuing Education in Nursing, 29*(3), 130–134.

Norris, D. M. (1977). One perspective on the nurse practitioner movement. In A. Jacox & C. Norris (Eds.), *Organizing for independent nursing practice* (pp. 21–33). New York: Appleton-Century-Crofts.

Olsen, G. W. (1940). The nurse anesthetists: Past, present and future. *Bulletin of the American Association of Nurse Anesthetists, 8*(4), 298.

Oltz v. St. Peter's Community Hospital. (1986). CV 81-271-H-Res (D. Montana).

Peplau, H. E. (1965). Specialization in professional nursing. *Nursing Science, 3*, 268–287.

Reiter, F. (1966). The nurse-clinician. *American Journal of Nursing, 66*, 274–280.

Robinson, S. (1984). A historical development of midwifery in the black community: 1600–1940. *Journal of Nurse-Midwifery, 29*(4), 247–250.

Rogers, M. E. (1972). Nursing: To be or not to be. *Nursing Outlook, 20*, 42–46.

Rudisil, P. (1993). Clinical paths for cardiac surgery patients: A multidisciplinary approach to quality improvement outcomes. *Journal of Nursing Care Quality, 8*(3), 27–33.

Safriet, B. J. (1998). Still spending dollars, still searching for sense: Advanced practice nursing in an era of regulatory and economic turmoil. *Advanced Practice Nursing Quarterly, 4*(3), 24–33.

Schroer, K. (1991). Case management: Clinical nurse specialist and nurse practitioner, converging roles. *Clinical Nurse Specialist, 5*(4), 190–194.

Sermchief v. Gonzales. (1983). 660 S.W.2d 683.

Sills, G. M. (1983). The role and function of the clinical nurse specialist. In N. L. Chaska (Ed.), *The nursing profession: A time to speak* (pp. 563–579). New York: McGraw-Hill.

Smith v. State of Indiana ex rel. Medical Licensing Board of Indiana. (1984). 459 N.E.2d 401 (In. App. 2 Dist.).

Smoyak, S. A. (1976). Specialization in nursing: From then to now. *Nursing Outlook, 24*, 676–681.

Spitler, B. (1996). A social work perspective of care management. In D. L. Flarey & S. S. Blancett (Eds.), *Handbook of nursing case management: Health care delivery in a world of managed care* (pp. 169–179). Gaithersburg, MD: Aspen.

Swenson, N. (1968). The role of the nurse-midwife on the health team as viewed by the family. *Bulletin of the American College of Nurse-Midwives, 13*, 125.

Tahan, H. A. (1998). Case management: A heritage more than a century old. *Nursing Case Management 3*(2), 55–60.

Thatcher, V. S. (1953). *A history of anesthesia: With emphasis on the nurse specialist.* Philadelphia: J. B. Lippincott.

Tom, S. A. (1982). Nurse-midwifery: A developing profession. *Law, Medicine and Health Care, 10*, 262–266.

Trinidad, E. A. (1993). Case management: A model of CNS practice. *Clinical Nurse Specialist, 7*(4), 221–223.

U.S. Department of Health and Human Services. (1996). *The registered nurse population March 1996: Findings from the National Sample Survey of Registered Nurses.* Washington, DC: Author.

Varney, H. (1987). *Nurse-midwifery* (2nd ed.). Boston: Blackwell Scientific Publishing.

Wagner, J. D., & Menke, E. M. (1992). Case management of homeless families. *Clinical Nurse Specialist, 6*(2), 65–71.

Wammack, L., & Mabrey, J. D. (1998). Outcomes assessment of total hip and total knee arthroplasty: Critical pathways, variance analysis, and continuous quality improvement. *Clinical Nurse Specialist, 12*(3), 122–131.

Wolff, M. A. (1984). Court upholds expanded practice roles for nurses. *Law, Medicine and Health Care, 12*, 26–29.

Woodrow, M., & Bell, J. (1971). Clinical specialization: Conflict between reality and theory. *Journal of Nursing Administration, 1*, 23–27.

Zander, K. (1988). Nurse case management: Resolving the DRG paradox. *Nursing Clinics of North America, 23*(3), 503–520.

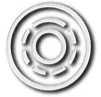

Conceptualizations of Advanced
Nursing Practice

- M A R G R E T T A   M A D D E N   S T Y L E S
- C A R O L Y N   K.   L E W I S

INTRODUCTION

Fundamental to the sound progress of any practice field is the development of a common language and conceptual framework for communication and for guiding and evaluating practice, policy, theory, research, and teaching. Such a foundation is particularly crucial at this stage in the development of advanced practice nursing. In this chapter, some of the conceptual impediments to developing a shared understanding of advanced practice nursing are identified; working definitions and conceptual models to serve the previously noted purposes are explored.

THE NATURE, PURPOSES, AND COMPONENTS OF CONCEPTUAL MODELS

What is a conceptual model? What purposes does it serve? What are its components? There are a number of answers to these questions in the nursing literature. In describing nurse-midwifery, Carveth (1987) drew heavily from various expert sources to arrive at a clear, comprehensive explanation of a conceptual model, paraphrased as follows.

A conceptual model is that which orders, clarifies, and systematizes selected components of the phenomenon/a (e.g., nursing) it serves to depict. The model then becomes a tool for interrelating concepts in a way in which the concepts can be better understood and explained. The term "conceptual framework" is often used synonymously with "conceptual model," as is the case in this chapter. Conceptual models are abstract and untestable, unlike theories, which are less abstract and able to be tested.

Conceptual frameworks serve many purposes. In professional role identity and function, such models help practitioners organize their beliefs and knowledge about their professional roles and practice and provide a sound base for further development of knowledge. In research, the conceptual model provides structure to the development of theory in relation to the concepts being studied. In education, conceptual models help in curriculum planning in the identification of important concepts and the relationships among them and in the selection of experiences to enhance student learning and their application of these relationships. In clinical practice, conceptual models allow practitioners to see the bigger picture so that holistic, comprehensive care is provided.

The components of conceptual frameworks are concepts and relationships (i.e., concepts in meaningful configuration) serving as building blocks that reflect assumptions about the philosphy, values, and practices of a profession. Carveth (1987) identified three schools of conceptual models in nursing, which she classified according to their foci and their derivation from other disciplines. *Interactionist* models are derived from social psychology and focus on the gestalt of the individual. *Developmental* models are derived from developmental psychology and focus on concepts of change and growth and levels of development. *Systems* models are derived from physics and sociology and focus on the integrity of the system through structure and organization. The conceptual frameworks reviewed in this chapter are variously derived from these three schools and are identified as such.

Holt (1984) defined a conceptual framework as "a network or an interrelationship of concepts that provides a rationale for action" (p. 446). She posited that conceptual frameworks encompass several types of concepts:

- Concepts that explain the nature of the unit (whether that unit be a cell, a person, a community, or a world)

- Concepts that identify the goal of the unit
- Concepts that describe the "normal" sequential growth and development of the unit
- Concepts that explore the deviation from the expected developmental pattern
- Concepts that describe other units in the universe and the environment in which the units exist
- Concepts that address relationships—internal and external

As previously stated, conceptual models reflect assumptions about the philosophy, values, and practices of the profession. Two key *assumptions* guide the present discussion of conceptualizations of advanced practice nursing. The first is that advanced practice nursing will reach its full potential to the extent that identified conceptual components are appropriately addressed. The second assumption is that the development and strengthening of the field of advanced practice nursing will lead to two *goals:*

1. A maximum social contribution in health care
2. The actualization of practitioners of advanced practice nursing

PROBLEMS AND PITFALLS IN CONCEPTUALIZATIONS OF ADVANCED NURSING PRACTICE

Currently there appear to be two general areas of conceptual confusion or uncertainty in the evolution of advanced practice nursing. The first is the shunned, but essential, distinction between *advanced practice nursing* and *advanced nursing practice.* The second conceptual hazard is a quagmire filled with ill-defined and inconsistently applied terms of reference. A core, stable vocabulary, a *lingua franca,* is needed for definition and model building. These two conceptual problems are briefly described below.

Advanced Practice Nursing and Advanced Nursing Practice

In the view of these authors, advanced practice nursing includes but is not synonymous with nor limited to advanced nursing practice, just as the nursing profession is not limited to direct practice. Nursing, and similarly advanced practice nursing, is the whole field, the profession—its members, its institutions, its values, and all that define and enable its practice; the practice is the vital function of the profession. If one envisions *advanced practice nursing* as a pyramid, at the base are foundational or support factors; at the apex is *advanced nursing practice.*

When these terms are used interchangeably, when conceptual confusion exists, the purposes for which conceptual models are developed (theory building, knowledge development, educational scope and definition, clinical practice) are in jeopardy. Moreover, there is great potential for neglecting the key components underpinning advanced nursing practice. For example, if the education of advanced practice nurses (APNs) follows a narrow practice model ignoring the social, economic, and political elements underlying and enabling that practice, practitioners may just as narrowly perceive their roles in furthering their profession. The same could be said in defining appropriate areas of research, confining it largely to clinical practice and excluding study of those financial, structural, and regulatory elements impinging on that practice (see later section on "Research Paradigms"). In examining a range of conceptual frameworks today, some deal with the profession, some deal with the practice, and some focus upon selected aspects of both, rendering the titling and organization of this chapter on conceptualization exceedingly difficult.

Only Brown (1998) has explicitly acknowledged the distinction between advanced practice nursing and advanced nursing practice and boldly developed an overarching framework encompassing the former, and accordingly including the clinical practice dimension (see "Conceptualizations of Advanced Practice Nursing"). Most of the existing frameworks deal with advanced nursing practice, which is the major focus of the remainder of this chapter.

Lack of a Core Vocabulary for Conceptual Frameworks

As to the second conceptual problem, lack of a consistent, stable vocabulary, it can be seen that the basic elements or building blocks of conceptual models within the advanced practice nursing literature are variously domains, theories, roles, subroles, competencies, functions, activities, skills, abilities, and others. The problem in comparing, refining, or developing models is that these terms are used with no universal meaning or frame of reference; occasionally no definition is offered at all or the meaning seems uncertain or inconstant. Shuler and Davis (1993), in introducing their nurse practitioner (NP) model, stated that "one of the greatest barriers to using nursing models in practice relates to vocabulary and communication within the models" (p. 11). This instability and inconsistency in terminology are pointed out as various models are cited in this chapter. It is rightly anticipated that conceptual models of the field and its practice change over time. However, it would assist such evolution and its comprehension if scholars and practitioners in the field could agree on the use and definition of fundamental terms of reference.

It should also be noted that some conceptual models, as reviewed, are more narrowly focused than others. Holt (1984) has identified a range of foci from cells to the universe. Some advanced nursing practice models are more homogeneous and some are mixed with respect to the phenomenon/a studied. Some could be seen as micromodels in terms of the unit of analysis, and others could be seen as metamodels, incorporating a number of conceptual frameworks. Some seek to explain systems; others look to explain relationships between systems.

All foci are important depending upon the purposes to be served. However, in developing conceptual models, it is essential that the phenomenon to be modeled is carefully defined. For example, is the model encompassing the entire field of advanced practice nursing or confined to distinctive concepts in collaborative practice between physicians and nurses? When dimensions are not clearly delimited, there is the possibility of being so inconsistent or mixed or far-reaching as to be confusing or to dilute or lose the impact of the seminal contribution.

FOUNDATIONAL FACTORS THAT SUPPORT ADVANCED NURSING PRACTICE

When the field of advanced practice nursing is conceptualized as a pyramid, what are the foundational factors supporting and enabling the practice at the apex? And why do we use the term *factor*?

The term *factor* does not customarily appear in any formal sense as a concept or building block in conceptual models. *Factor* is a nonesoteric term appearing widely throughout the public discourse; it is not the proprietary claim of a particular discipline or family of conceptual models within the Carveth classification (1987). The dictionary defines factors as conditions bringing about a result; in mathematics, factors are quantities that form a product when multiplied together. As the term is used herein, *factors are conditions that in combination lead to a result.* The result is the fullest development of advanced practice nursing, as put forth in the aforementioned assumptions and goals. The term *factor* is generous, permitting conditions or qualities of a different nature to be clustered.

There are several types of conditions that form the essential platform that supports a profession or occupational field. Herein are identified 13 foundational factors, both internal and external to the field, as categorized by Roy and Martinez (1983) in their systems framework for clinical nurse specialist (CNS) practice.

Within the external environment, there are four factors creating the opportunity for the field to exist and flourish:

1. The health needs of the people
2. New administrative structures of the health delivery system and the openness to innovation
3. The health policy of the government
4. The status of and fluidity within the health workforce situation

The history of the field of advanced practice nursing discloses many of these "opportunity factors." Ford (1982; cited in Mezey & McGivern, 1993) noted that society's needs and nursing's potential led to the development of the first NP program in 1965. The shortage of primary care physicians, described in some areas as a contributing factor, was seen by Ford as the opportunity, and not the reason, for the new role.

Within the environment of the greater nursing profession, some significant factors that have contributed to the development of advanced practice nursing are

5. The strength of the profession to advocate and advance a new area of practice
6. The profession's sanction and support for the development of advanced specialties, manifested, for example, in lobbying for favorable governmental laws and policies
7. Nursing's willingness to grant a special status and privilege to a segment of its members and to delegate certain powers of self-determination to the group, as reflected, for instance, in credentialing policies

Within the environment of advanced practice nursing are various factors that have, in particular, contributed to the quality of advanced nursing practice and enabled its growth. Principal among them are conditions relating to the characteristics of the practitioners themselves. Within this category are such factors as the practitioners'

8. Proper role identity and understanding of the field
9. Positive values and attitudes
10. Advanced education
11. Substantial experience

A very useful developmental framework for analyzing the role and attitude transformation that occurs as a practice field develops has been provided by Thibodeau and Hawkins (1994). They administered two instruments to NPs to determine correlations among (1) role attitudes and values, (2) confidence about practice knowledge and skills, and (3) orientation to a medical or nursing model to guide practice. A direct positive correlation was found between level of confidence and degree of nursing orientation.

Role theory provided the framework for articulating the research questions and analyzing the results of the Thibodeau and Hawkins (1994) study. Specifically, Oda (1977) identified three phases for specialized nursing role development: role identification, role transition, and role confirmation. (See Chapter 5 for discussion of role development models.) The practitioners studied appeared to have reached the stage of role confirmation.

A recent contribution to the understanding of the role transition process undergone by NPs is the theoretical model developed by Brown and Olshansky (1997). Using grounded theory methodology, they determined that, during the first 12 months after graduation, novice NPs progressed from limbo to legitimacy. Four nonlinear, not mutually exclusive categories of experiences, each with subcategories, were identified: (1) laying the foundation, (2) launching, (3) meeting the challenge, and (4) broadening the perspective. (See Chapter 5 for more discussion of this research.) Role development frameworks should be extremely useful in efforts to trace over time the role identity of nurses in advanced practice, a critical enabling factor in the continuing evolution of advanced nursing practice. These frameworks largely fall within the category of developmental models, focusing on concepts of change and growth and levels of progress, as defined by Carveth (1987). The focus or unit of analysis is essentially the attitudinal development of the individual APN.

Two final factors are essential to the ongoing progress of advanced nursing practice:

12. The development and dissemination of a significant research base for the practice
13. The existence of an organization to mobilize the practitioners and enable them to exert control over the standards and influence of the field, promote the development of a literature and sound educational programs, and represent the field within the external environment

These thirteen foundational factors are essential conditions to be addressed if the overall field of advanced practice nursing is to develop to its fullest and if advanced nursing practice is to rise to its pinnacle.

CONCEPTUALIZATIONS OF ADVANCED NURSING PRACTICE

As explained earlier, practice conditions are supported by environmental opportunities and internal and external professional advocacy. They further are derived from the expertise of practitioners and from research in the field. *Practice is the central, the clinical work of the field.* Practice is the reason for which the field was created. Maximizing that work in terms of its development and impact is the reason why the factors discussed previously are so important.

What are the characteristics of that advanced nursing practice? How does it differ from other nursing practice? What is its scope and purpose? What knowledge and skills are required? Within what roles does this practice occur? Scores of writers have written on this subject from a variety of different angles. As mentioned earlier, comparisons are difficult because terms of reference and their meanings vary according to the type of framework used and the level of anlaysis performed.

The American Nurses Association's (ANA's) *Nursing's Social Policy Statement* (ANA, 1995) identifies and defines three concepts to differentiate advanced nursing practice from basic nursing practice:

- *Specialization* is concentrating or delimiting one's focus to part of the whole field of nursing.
- *Expansion* refers to the acquisition of new practice knowledge and skills, including knowledge and skill legitimizing role autonomy within areas of practice that overlap traditional boundaries of medical practice.
- *Advancement* involves both specialization and expansion and is characterized by the integration of theoretical, research-based, and practical knowledge that occurs as part of graduate education in nursing. (p. 14)

Practitioners must be highly educated and experienced to practice within a field so characterized. Although they may practice in a variety of roles—CNS, NP, certified nurse-midwife (CNM), certified registered nurse anesthetist (CRNA), and others—what characterizes the practice is knowledge and expertise, clinical judgment, skilled and self-initiated care, and scholarly inquiry, not job description, title, or setting (Diers, 1985; see also Chapter 6).

In the conceptual frameworks reviewed in this section, the term *role* is used loosely and variably, sometimes seemingly describing *functions,* such as management or teaching or research or consultation, and sometimes taking a psychological or sociological perspective on developing social roles or selves in relation to environment. Dictionaries, adding to the confusion, use the terms *role, function, occupation,* and *duties* to define one another. In this discussion, *role* is used only in a concrete sense to refer to titles appearing in legal documents, certification programs, or job descriptions. For example, from this perspective the CNS, NP, CNM, and CRNA designations represent advanced practice roles.

Turning now from consideration of who engages in advanced nursing practice and in what capacity to consideration of models depicting the practice itself, one sees that such practice models could serve a variety of purposes. They could serve as a template against which (1) levels of practice can be distinguished, (2) educational programs can be developed and evaluated, (3) knowledge and behaviors can be measured for certification purposes, (4) practitioners can understand, examine, and improve their own practice, (5) job descriptions can be developed, and (6) progress in a field can be traced for historical purposes. Models can also be used in the identification of and as a context for researchable questions, and for theory development.

In the following discussion, the ultimate usefulness of particular practice models is assessed according to the extent they serve one or more of these purposes and to the degree that they provide some clarity about and direction to the field. Also, the purposes served are determined by the concepts explicated within the framework. For example, frameworks that depict configurations of knowledge are applicable to test construction and curriculum content. Frameworks that depict configurations of competencies are useful in examining behavior and in role development.

From the present review of a number of frameworks, it can be seen that *competency* may be the most commonly used concept in explaining nursing practice and advanced nursing practice. Again, meanings are not consistent.

Benner's Model of Expert Practice

Many of the models use, adapt, and refine Benner's (1984) seminal work, *From Novice to Expert.* It is important to note that Benner did not study advanced practice nurses; her research describes the expert-by-experience. In using an interpretive approach to identifying and describing clinical knowledge, Benner defined two key terms (pp. 292–293):

> *Competency:* An interpretively defined area of skilled performance identified and described by its intent, function, and meanings
> *Domain:* A cluster of competencies that have similar intents, functions, and meanings

Through the analysis of clinical exemplars discussed in the interviews, Benner derived a group of competencies. Clustering the competencies resulted in further identification of seven domains of expert nursing practice. Within her lexicon, these domains are a combination of roles, functions, and competencies, although the three have not been precisely differentiated. The seven domains are

1. The helping role
2. Administering and monitoring therapeutic interventions and regimens
3. Effective management of rapidly changing situations
4. The diagnostic and monitoring function
5. The teaching-coaching function
6. Monitoring and ensuring the quality of health care practices
7. Organizational and work-role competencies (Benner, 1984)

In a later work, Benner (1985) more directly described advanced nursing practice expertise in discussing the CNS. She saw CNS expertise as a hybrid of practical knowledge gained from frontline clinical practice and sophisticated skills of knowledge utilization. The CNS has in-depth knowledge of a particular clinical population and grasps in theory and practice the illness and disease trajectory of that patient population.

Fenton's and Brykczynski's Expert Practice Domains of the CNS and NP

Fenton (1985) and Brykczynski (1989) each independently applied Benner's model of expertise at the advanced nursing practice level in examining the practice of CNSs and NPs, respectively. In a later publication, Fenton and Brykczynski (1993) compared their earlier research findings to identify similarities and differences between CNSs and NPs. They used Benner's understanding of the concepts of domains, competencies, roles, and functions. Fenton and Brykczynski verified that nurses in advanced practice were indeed experts, as defined by Benner, and identified some additional domains and competencies as outlined in Figure 2-1.

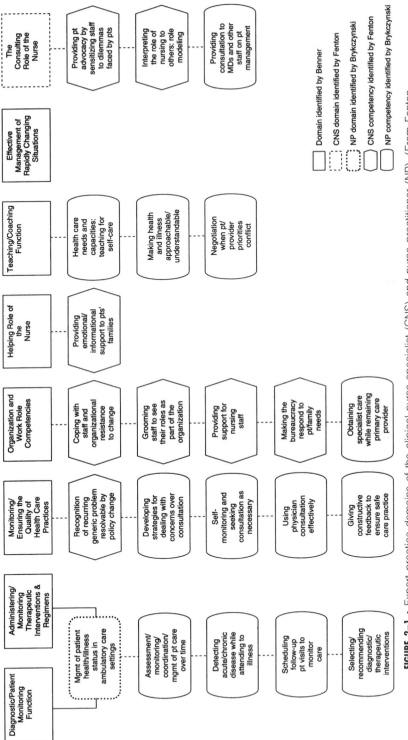

FIGURE 2–1 • Expert practice domains of the clinical nurse specialist (CNS) and nurse practitioner (NP). (From Fenton, M. V., & Brykczynski, K. A. [1993]. Qualitative distinctions and similarities in the practice of clinical nurse specialists and nurse practitioners. *Journal of Professional Nursing, 9*, 313–326; reprinted with permission.)

In considering the applications of the Benner model and the Fenton refinements to CNS practice, Spross and Baggerly (1989) made recommendations for further development. With some modification, their recommendations apply to advanced nursing practice in general. Needed are (1) further application of the model to advanced nursing practice, (2) extension of the teaching/coaching domain to teaching nurses, (3) comparison of the non-master's-prepared clinician's competencies and the APN's competencies to further elucidate components of expert versus advanced practice; and (4) student experience with ethnographic methods to enable graduates to address Benner's challenge to uncover knowledge embedded in practice (Spross & Baggerly, 1989).

In an examination of the domains of advanced nursing practice conducted for the National Organization of Nurse Practitioner Faculties (Zimmer et al., 1990), a further reworking occurred to facilitate use of the domains as a framework for primary care NP curricula. The original six domains were collapsed to five:

1. Management of client health/illness status in ambulatory care settings
2. Monitoring and ensuring the quality of health care practices
3. Organizational and work role competencies
4. Helping role
5. Teaching-coaching function

These domains were seen as a beneficial organizing framework for NP curricula development because they described the lived experience of NP practice, offered a way to organize a large amount of content while retaining a primary health care focus, and allowed for individual NP faculties to overlay other nursing frameworks as desired (Price et al., 1992).

Calkin's Model of Advanced Nursing Practice

Benner and her colleagues derived their framework from the data upward. They began by collecting samples of nursing practice, to which they applied their interpretive expertise. Others have taken a more deductive approach, first developing a theoretical rationale to explain particular phenomena. In this manner, Calkin (1984) developed a model for nurse administrators to use in determining how to differentiate advanced nursing practice in personnel policies. She proposed this be accomplished by matching (1) patient responses to health problems (as nursing was defined in the ANA 1980 Social Policy Statement) to (2) the skill level and (3) the knowledge level of nursing personnel. Three curves were overlaid on a normal distribution chart. Calkin depicted the skills and knowledge of novices, experts-by-experience, and advanced practitioners (APNs) in relation to knowledge required in caring for a range of patients (see Figure 2–2).

FIGURE 2–2 • Patient responses correlated with the knowledge and skill of beginning practitioners, experienced nurses, and advanced practice nurses. (From Calkin, J. D. [1984]. A model for advanced nursing practice. *Journal of Nursing Administration, 14*[1], 25–27; reprinted with permission.)

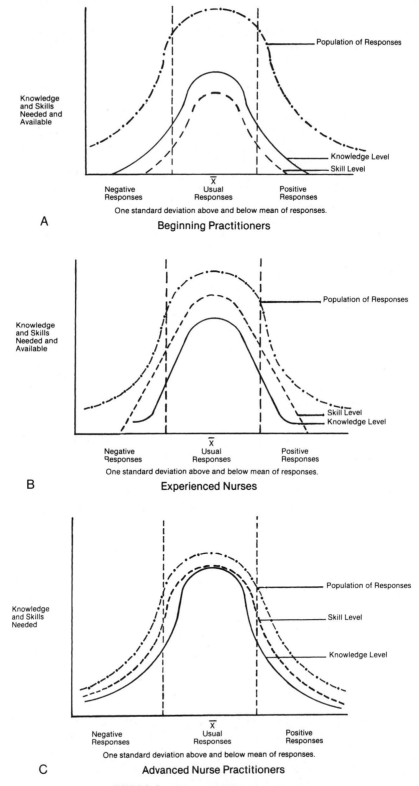

Knowledge and Skills Needed and Available

Population of Responses

Knowledge Level

Skill Level

Negative Responses

X̄ Usual Responses

Positive Responses

One standard deviation above and below mean of responses.

A

Beginning Practitioners

Knowledge and Skills Needed and Available

Population of Responses

Skill Level

Knowledge Level

Negative Responses

X̄ Usual Responses

Positive Responses

One standard deviation above and below mean of responses.

B

Experienced Nurses

Knowledge and Skills Needed

Population of Responses

Skill Level

Knowledge Level

Negative Responses

X̄ Usual Responses

Positive Responses

One standard deviation above and below mean of responses.

C

Advanced Nurse Practitioners

FIGURE 2–2 • See legend on opposite page

Calkin illustrated the application of this framework in explaining how APNs perform under different sets of circumstances: when there is a high degree of unpredictability; when there are new conditions or a new patient population or new sets of problems; and when there are a wide variety of health problems, requiring the services of "specialist generalists," as she called them. She defined what NPs do in terms of functions. For example, when patients' health problems may elicit a wide range of human responses with continuing and substantial unpredictable elements, the APN functions are to

- Identify and develop interventions for the unusual by providing direct care
- Transmit this knowledge to nurses and in some settings to students
- Identify and communicate needs for, or carry out research related to human responses to these health problems
- Anticipate factors that may lead to the presence of unfamiliar responses
- Provide anticipatory guidance to nurse administrators when the changes in the diagnosis and treatment of these responses may require altered levels or types of resources (Calkin, 1984, p. 28)

A principal advantage to Calkin's model is that the skills and knowledge of the practitioner are placed in the direct context of patient needs. The model, however, has been left for others to test. It does provide a framework for scholars to use in studying the function of APNs in a variety of work situations. It should be a useful conceptualization for administrators who must maximize a multilevel nursing workforce and thus need to rationalize the use of APNs.

Shuler's Model of NP Practice

Shuler's NP practice model is a systems model that is wellness oriented and definitive in terms of how the NP-patient interaction, patient assessment, intervention, and evaluation should occur (Shuler & Davis, 1993). It was derived from a number of disciplines and is most ambitious in embracing myriad theoretical constructs within an internal-external–input-throughput-output systems framework. The elements include (1) the four concepts of nursing's metaparadigm (person, health, nursing, and environment), (2) nursing process, (3) a table of humanistically based assumptions about patients and students, and (4) a table of theoretical concepts underlying practice model constructs. The model appears to be, in fact, a network or system of frameworks.

Shuler's model is intended "to impact the NP domain at four levels: theoretical, clinical, educational, and research" (Shuler & Davis, 1993, p. 17). Its scope and intent are enormous; the model is perhaps best utilized when single constructs are isolated and addressed although visualized within the larger whole. The most helpful subframework for identifying elements of practice may be the model constructs and underlying theoretical concepts depicted in Table 2-1.

Model of the National Association of Clinical Nurse Specialists

The National Association of Clinical Nurse Specialists (NACNS) published a *Statement on Clinical Nurse Specialist Practice and Education* in 1998. They moved from an earlier conceptualization of subroles to a complex of

TABLE 2-1	MODEL CONSTRUCTS AND UNDERLYING THEORY CONCEPTS INCLUDED IN SHULER'S MODEL OF NURSE PRACTITIONER (NP) PRACTICE					
THEORETICAL PRACTICE MODEL CONSTRUCTS	WHOLISTIC PATIENT NEEDS	NP-PATIENT INTERACTION	SELF-CARE	HEALTH PREVENTION	HEALTH PROMOTION	WELLNESS
Underlying Theory Concepts	Basic needs Wellness activities Health/illness Psychological health Family Culture Social support Environmental health Spirituality	Contracting Role-modeling Self-care activities Teaching/ learning Communication Problem-solving Decision-making	Wellness activities Preventive health activities Health promotion activities Compliance Problem-solving Teaching/ learning Contracting Culture Family Social support Environmental health	Primary prevention Secondary prevention Tertiary prevention Preventive health behavior Family Culture Environmental health	Health promotion behavior Wellness Family Culture Environmental health Social support	Self-care activities Wellness activities Disease prevention activities Health promotion activities Family Culture Social support Environmental health Spirituality Contracting Teaching/ learning

From Shuler, P. A., & Davis, J. E. (1993). The Shuler nurse practitioner practice model: A theoretical framework for nurse practitioner clinicians, educators, and researchers, Part I. *Journal of the American Academy of Nurse Practitioners, 5*(1), 11–18; reprinted with permission.

1. Essential characteristics—a combination of leadership, collaboration, and consultation skills and professional attributes
2. Spheres of influence—patients/clients, nursing personnel, and organizational/network—with outcomes and competencies for each sphere
3. Content areas for the competencies (NACNS, 1998)

Thus a virtual matrix was created to serve purposes ranging from making explicit the contributions of CNSs to providing a basis for curricula and certification examinations.

Models for Midwifery and Nurse Anesthesia Practice

Models of the CNM and CRNA roles are available to amplify and clarify the picture of advanced nursing practice; their scopes are delimited and specific to these two advanced roles. Official statements of CNM and CRNA organizations describe these practices.

The model of the American College of Nurse-Midwives (1997), *The Core Competencies for Basic Midwifery Practice* includes 14 *hallmarks* characterizing the art and science of midwifery and *components* of midwifery care within which are prescribed competencies. Competencies are defined as the knowledge, skills, and attitudes expected of a new practitioner. The components and associated competencies are identified as follows:

• Professional responsibilities of CNMs (certified nurse-midwives) and CMs (certified midwives)

- Midwifery management process
- The childbearing family
    Preconception care
    Care of the childbearing woman
    Newborn care
- The primary care of women
    Health promotion and disease prevention
    Management of common health problems
    Family planning gynecologic care
    Perimenopause and postmenopause

These components and related core competencies are said to comprise the foundation upon which practice guidelines and curricula are built.

The American Association of Nurse Anesthetists (1996) has published *Scope and Standards for Nurse Anesthesia Practice*. The scope is defined in terms of 17 acts described in one instance as *responsibilities* and in another as *functions*. The 11 *standards* that ensue are intended to fulfill four purposes relating to (1) evaluating care, (2) providing a common base for practitioners, (3) informing the public as to what to expect from practitioners, and (4) preserving the basic rights of patients. A statement of interpretation is attached to each standard.

FUTURE DEVELOPMENT

Further work is needed to clarify and harmonize the conceptual basis of advanced nursing practice. This review of models of advanced practice points out at least five striking areas for future work in model development and testing.

Consensus Building Around NP and CNS Roles

For some time, cross-matching of frameworks has been going on to contrast, compare, and combine the role of CNS and NP. Now is the time for the focus to shift toward bringing the practice of all APNs, including CNMs and CRNAs, into conceptual unity. This is not to suggest that the practice is identical for all, but that the common elements should be identified and differences noted. (See Chapter 3 for further discussion of this important recommendation.) The melange of terms, constructs, concepts, and levels of abstraction, as mentioned before, makes this an imposing challenge.

Fortunately, a process of consensus building is underway. In an excellent article on comparing practice domains, Lindeke, Canedy, and Kay (1997) summarized the evolution of advanced practice domains and the efforts of a number of organizations to reach agreement about advanced practice education, roles, and competencies. Additionally, these authors reported their own research on comparing and contrasting the practices of CNSs and NPs. Rasch and Frauman (1996) identified the conceptual and practical issues in guiding the possible merger of the two roles and recommended further dialogue. Both of these writings should assist in the multiple efforts to find common ground.

Consensus Building Around Specialty Scopes

Attention should be directed to the "scope" dimension of advanced nursing practice. Among its other characteristics, advanced nursing practice is specialized. Most of nursing's specialties have statements of scope, often with associated competencies or functions. At this stage in the evolution of advanced nursing, it would be helpful to devise, test, and utilize a conceptual framework for comparing and contrasting respective scopes of practice for advanced practice specialties. This is being done at the higher level of analysis, that of the NP and CNS (Fenton & Brykszynski, 1993; Williams & Valdivieso, 1994). Sometime soon, the respective scopes of practice in various specialties within advanced practice roles must be addressed and a rationale articulated for further development and refinement. The ANA's work in developing uniform formats and scopes and standards in cooperation with various specialty organizations should serve as a good platform for launching the project (ANA, 1996).

Conceptualization of Collaborative Practice

The relationship of advanced nursing practice to medical practice is either a theme or an undercurrent throughout most models (Thibodeau & Hawkins' [1994] role delineation; Ford's [1982] explanation of the origins of the NP role; and multidisciplinary partnerships and collaborative practice models [Brown, 1983; Walton, Jakobowski, & Barnsteiner, 1993]). Furthermore, it is an issue in the contemporary debates about autonomy, direct reimbursement, and "junior doctors." The relationship of advanced nursing practice to medical practice must be identified as a significant practice factor requiring ongoing attention.

A recent conceptual contribution to explain and promote medical-nursing collaboration and introduce a more active nursing component to the current dominant medical model is that of Dunphy and Winland-Brown (1998). The Circle of Caring model is said to incorporate the strengths of medicine and nursing in a transforming way. The conceptual elements are the *processes* of assessment, planning, intervention, and evaluation and a feedback loop. Each of these processes is greatly enriched by a multiparadigmatic perspective. By superimposing a nursing-based template upon a traditional medical model,

- The database in assessment and evaluation is contextualized, incorporating subjective and environmental elements.
- The approach to therapeutics is broadened to include holistic approaches to healing and makes nursing more visible.
- Measured outcomes include patients' perceptions.

The assessment-planning-intervention-evaluation processes in linear configuration are "encircled by caring," described as interpersonal processes occurring between caregiver and patient/family. These interpersonal or caring processes, drawn from Mayerhoff and Boykin and Schoenhofer, are patience, courage, advocacy, authentic presence, commitment, and knowing (Dunphy & Winland-Brown, 1998, p. 246). The authors intend that the model be applied on both the micro level of one-to-one relationships in acute care and the macro level of caring for communities and populations, although the feasibility and desirability of the latter are not specifically addressed.

The model undoubtedly serves well in addressing the interrelationship between the medical and nursing paradigms, thus fostering collaborative practice. Moreover, it does have the potential for rendering nursing's contribution more visible, and for increasing its presence in health care guidelines and reimbursement policies. The conceptual significance of encircling the four practice processes with the six caring processes may be questioned. Practically, one would expect the caring processes, which appear to be attitudes and values, to be integrated throughout each practice step in a value-added collaborative model.

The related issue of authority for practice deserves mention. Many in nursing would prefer the word *autonomy* instead of *authority*. The authors, however, prefer *authority* as the broader and more descriptive term. *Authority is the right to act, to take action, to make decisions, even to command.* The higher authority of those nurses in advanced practice derives from the recognition of their expertise by the public, regulatory bodies, the health policy arena, the health care system, and the greater profession—foundational factors supporting advanced nursing practice. Authority is not just received; it must also be asserted. APNs must themselves have confidence in the power of their expert knowledge and service and their right and responsibility to use it fully in the public's behalf.

Two milestones in establishing APNs' authority have been recognition of APNs for reimbursement by the government and other payers and the National Council of State Boards of Nursing's (NCSBN's) *Position Paper on the Regulation of Advanced Nursing Practice* (1993). In the NCSBN document, the state regulatory bodies are encouraged to recognize APNs by conferring an expanded legal scope of practice. The central thrust is to authorize, through the jurisdiction of states, greater autonomy in decision making for the highly educated, expert APN (NCSBN, 1993).

Research Paradigms

Research on patient outcomes and cost-effectiveness that leads to increased knowledge about advanced nursing practice is critical. The worth of any service depends on the extent to which practice meets the needs and priorities of the society, health care systems, and the public policy arena. These needs are, by and large, for appropriate services at a reasonable cost. Critical challenges to APNs are to demonstrate enhanced effectiveness in meeting social needs and to increase the public's awareness of the benefit or desirability of those services. APNs must communicate within the nursing profession, to other health care providers, and to society as a whole, in clear and powerful language, the difference advanced nursing practice makes. Styles (1990) identified five principles of knowledge empowerment, two of which have implications for this discussion:

• Appropriate paradigms or theoretical frameworks must be used to elicit politically powerful knowledge (i.e., knowledge significant to decisions about the allocation of resources). As Harrington (1988) wrote,

> *The new imperative for nursing is to move beyond its heavy reliance on individualist frameworks and to include theoretical frameworks that examine health care systems, organizations, professionals and the society as a whole. Only with a basic understanding of the larger issues drawn from*

the fields of sociology, political science, public policy and economics, can nursing become a full-fledged player in the political arena.

(p. 121)

• To have political impact, knowledge must be packaged and presented in such a manner that its meaning and relevance are unmistakable and widely disseminated.

Naylor and Brooten (1993) reviewed research literature demonstrating the differences that CNSs make in health outcomes, and the NACNS included a very helpful "Summary of Research on the Effects of Clinical Nurse Specialist Practice" in their position paper (1998). These works could serve as a model for other researchers seeking to strengthen the value attributed to advanced nursing practice. Specifically, Naylor and Brooten (1993) recommended that additional studies be done on patient and family outcomes, that the next phase of studies relate to unique functions, and that research be conducted to compare the practice patterns and outcomes of CNSs with those of physicians and other health providers. (See Chapter 25 for further discussion of strengthening APN evaluation.)

Conceptualizations of Advanced Practice Nursing

The observation was made earlier that conceptual frameworks tend to address advanced nursing practice and seldom the broader field of advanced practice nursing, and that inattention to foundational, enabling factors could inhibit the practice dimension from reaching its potential. What are the possibilities for widening the perspective?

Brown (1998) responded to the challenge to provide a framework for the entire field of advanced practice nursing, encompassing advanced nursing practice and the environments that surround and impact upon that practice. In addition to *environments* (society, health care economy, local conditions, nursing, advanced practice community), Brown has included the concepts of *role legitimacy* (graduate education, certification, licensure); *advanced practice nursing* (scope, clinical practice, competencies); and *outcomes* (patient, health care, nursing, individual). This comprehensive model will be useful to the extent that it calls attention to external factors impinging upon advanced clinical practice and the relationship of those factors to health care and professional outcomes (see Figure 2–3).

The ANA *Scope and Standards of Advanced Practice Registered Nursing* (1996) is a helpful document in striving for consensus among advanced practice roles and specialities. Within that framework, the generic scope and standards deal with the broader field of advanced practice nursing, as the title of the document makes clear, and standards of care have been differentiated from standards of professional performance. Although the professional performance standards focus upon the individual practitioner, they do refer to the individual as a member of the collective profession and open the door to consideration of all that is implied in the professional role relative to foundational factors.

SUMMARY

Conceptual models serve many purposes for the fields they seek to describe. Importantly, they are useful for guiding and evaluating the evolution of advanced nursing

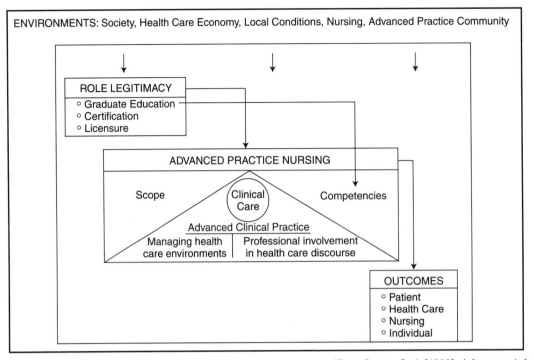

FIGURE 2–3 • Framework of advanced practice nursing. (From Brown, S. J. [1998]. A framework for advanced practice nursing. *Journal of Professional Nursing, 14*[3], 160; reprinted with permission.)

practice. Such progress is dependent upon the extent to which practice meets the needs and priorities of the society, health care systems, and the public policy arena. This chapter has identified pitfalls in conceptualizing advanced nursing practice, has reviewed a number of frameworks, and has traced recent progress in addressing some prior limitations. Continued model development and testing can enable the realization of the two goals of maximum social contribution of the APN to the health needs of society and the actualization of advanced practitioners.

REFERENCES

American Association of Nurse Anesthetists. (1996). *Scope and standards for nurse anesthesia practice.* Park Ridge, IL: Author.

American College of Nurse-Midwives. (1997). *The core competencies for basic midwifery practice.* Washington, DC: Author.

American Nurses Association. (1980). *Nursing: A social policy statement.* Kansas City, MO: Author.

American Nurses Association. (1995). *Nursing's social policy statement.* Washington, DC: Author.

American Nurses Association. (1996). *Scope and standards of advanced practice registered nursing.* Washington, DC: Author.

Benner, P. (1984). *From novice to expert.* Menlo Park, CA: Addison-Wesley.

Benner, P. (1985). The oncology clinical nurse specialist as expert coach. *Oncology Nursing Forum, 12*(2), 40–44.

Brown, M. A., & Olshansky, E. F. (1997). From limbo to legitimacy: A theoretical model of the transition to the primary care nurse practitioner role. *Nursing Research, 46*, 46–51.

Brown, S. J. (1983). The clinical nurse specialist in a multidisciplinary partnership. *Nursing Administration Quarterly, 8,* 36–46.

Brown, S. J. (1998). A framework for advanced practice nursing. *Journal of Professional Nursing, 14,* 157–164.

Brykczynski, K. A. (1989). An interpretive study describing the clinical judgment of nurse practitioners. *Scholarly Inquiry for Nursing Practice, 3,* 75–104.

Calkin, J. D. (1984). A model for advanced nursing practice. *Journal of Nursing Administration, 14*(1), 24–30.

Carveth, J. A. (1987). Conceptual models in nurse-midwifery. *Journal of Nurse-Midwifery, 32,* 20–25.

Diers, D. (1985). Preparation of practitioners, clinical specialists, and clinicians. *Journal of Professional Nursing, 1,* 41–47.

Dunphy, L. M., & Winland-Brown, J. E. (1998). The circle of caring: A transformative model of advanced practice nursing. *Clinical Excellence for Nurse Practitioners, 2,* 241–247.

Fenton, M. V. (1985). Identifying competencies of clinical nurse specialists. *Journal of Nursing Administration, 15*(12), 31–37.

Fenton, M. V., & Brykczynski, K. A. (1993). Qualitative distinctions and similarities in the practice of clinical nurse specialists and nurse practitioners. *Journal of Professional Nursing, 9,* 313–326.

Ford, L. C. (1982). Nurse practitioners: History of a new idea and predictions for the future. In L. H. Aiken & S. R. Gortner (Eds.), *Nursing in the 1980's: Crises, opportunities, challenges* (pp. 231–247). Philadelphia: J. B. Lippincott.

Harrington, C. (1988). The political economy of health: A new imperative for nursing. *Nursing and Health Care, 9,* 121.

Holt, F. M. (1984). A theoretical model for clinical specialist practice. *Nursing and Health Care, 5,* 445–449.

Lindeke, L. L., Canedy, B. H., & Kay, M. M. (1997). A comparison of practice domains of clinical nurse specialists and nurse practitioners. *Journal of Professional Nursing, 13,* 281–287.

Mezey, M. D., & McGivern, D. O. (Eds.). (1993). *Nurses, nurse practitioners: Evolution to advanced practice.* New York: Springer-Verlag.

National Association of Clinical Nurse Specialists. (1998). *Statement on clinical nurse specialist practice and education.* Glenview, IL: Author.

National Council of State Boards of Nursing. (1993). *Position paper on the regulation of advanced nursing practice.* Chicago: Author.

Naylor, M. D., & Brooten, D. (1993). The roles and functions of clinical nurse specialists. *Image: The Journal of Nursing Scholarship, 25,* 73–78.

Oda, D. (1977). Specialized role development: A three-phase process. *Nursing Outlook, 25,* 374–377.

Price, M. J., Martin, A. C., Newberry, Y. G., Zimmer, P. A., Brykczynski, K. A., & Warren, B. (1992). Developing national guidelines for nurse practitioner education: An overview of the product and the process. *Journal of Nursing Education, 31,* 10–15.

Rasch, R. F. R., & Frauman, A. C. (1996). Advanced practice in nursing: Conceptual issues. *Journal of Professional Nursing, 12,* 141–146.

Roy, C., & Martinez, C. (1983). A conceptual framework for CNS practice. In A. B. Hamric & J. A. Spross (Eds.), *The clinical nurse specialist in theory and practice* (pp. 3–20). New York: Grune & Stratton.

Shuler, P. A., & Davis, J. E. (1993). The Shuler nurse practitioner practice model: A theoretical framework for nurse practitioner clinicians, educators, and researchers, Part I. *Journal of the American Academy of Nurse Practitioners, 5,* 11–18.

Spross, J. A., & Baggerly, J. (1989). Models of advanced nursing practice. In A. B. Hamric & J. A. Spross (Eds.), *The clinical nurse specialist in theory and practice* (2nd ed., pp. 19–40). Philadelphia: W. B. Saunders.

Styles, M. M. (1990). A common sense approach to nursing research. *International Nursing Review, 37,* 203–218.

Thibodeau, J. A., & Hawkins, J. W. (1994). Moving toward a nursing model in advanced practice. *Western Journal of Nursing Research, 16,* 205–218.

Walton, M. K., Jakobowski, D. S., & Barnsteiner, J. H. (1993). A collaborative practice model for the clinical nurse specialist. *Journal of Nursing Administration, 23,* 55–59.

Williams, C. A., & Valdivieso, G. C. (1994). Advanced practice models. A clinical comparison of clinical nurse specialist and nurse practitioner activities. *Clinical Nurse Specialist, 8,* 311–318.

Zimmer, P., Brykczynski, K. A., Martin, A. C., Newberry, Y. G., Price, M. J., & Warren, B. (1990). *Advanced nursing practice: Nurse practitioner curriculum guidelines* (Final Report: NONPF Education Committee). Washington, DC: National Organization of Nurse Practitioner Faculties.

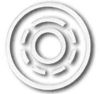

A Definition of Advanced Nursing Practice

• A N N B. H A M R I C

INTRODUCTION

The advanced practice of nursing builds upon the foundation and core values of the nursing discipline. According to the American Nurses Association (ANA, 1995), contemporary nursing practice has four essential features: (1) inclusion of the full range of human experiences and responses to health and illness without restriction to a problem-focused orientation; (2) practice based on the integration of objective and subjective experience; (3) the ability to apply scientific knowledge to diagnostic and treatment processes; and (4) the ability to provide a caring relationship that facilitates health and healing. These four characteristics are equally essential for advanced nursing practice. Core values that guide nurses in practice include advocating for patients; respecting patient and family values and informed choices; viewing individuals holistically within their environments and cultural traditions; and maintaining a focus on disease prevention, health restoration, and health promotion (Creasia & Parker, 1996; Leddy, 1998). These core professional values also inform the central perspective of advanced practice. As Smith (1995) stated, ''The core of advanced practice nursing lies within nursing's disciplinary perspective on human-environment and caring interrelationships that facilitate health and healing. This core is delineated specifically in the philosophic and theoretic foundations of nursing'' (p. 3).

Advanced nursing practice is a dynamic and evolving entity. Differing interpretations are evident at this stage of its development as compared to the first edition of this text. In this chapter, advanced nursing practice is defined and the scope of practice of advanced practice nurses (APNs) is discussed. Various APN roles are differentiated and key factors in advanced nursing practice environments are identified.

DISTINGUISHING BETWEEN SPECIALIZATION AND ADVANCED NURSING PRACTICE

Before exploring the definition of advanced nursing practice, it is important to distinguish between specialization in nursing and advanced nursing practice. Specialization involves concentration in a selected clinical area within the field of nursing. All nurses with extensive experience in a particular area of practice (e.g., pediatric nursing or trauma nursing) are specialized in this sense. As the profession has advanced and responded to changes in health care, specialization and the need for specialty knowledge have increased. Although family nurse practitioners (NPs) classically see themselves as generalists, they are also specialists in the sense being discussed here, because they have specialized in one of the many facets of health care, namely primary care. Thus there are few nurses who are generalists in the true sense of the word (Kitzman, 1989). As Bigbee and Amidi-Nouri note in Chapter 1, early specialization involved primarily on-the-job training or hospital-based training courses; many nurses continue to develop specialty skills through practice experiences and continuing education. Examples of such currently evolving specialties include parish nursing and holistic nursing practitioners. As specialties mature, they may develop graduate-level clinical preparation and incorporate the competencies of advanced practice nursing as the concept is defined below. This progression is clearly seen in the APN roles of certified registered nurse anesthetist (CRNA) and NP.

The nursing profession has responded in a variety of ways to the increasing need for specialization in both clinical and clinical support arenas. The creation of specialty organizations, such as the American Association of Critical-Care Nurses and the Oncology Nursing Society (ONS), has been one response. The creation of advanced clinical practice roles—the CRNA and certified nurse-midwife (CNM) roles early in nursing's evolution and the clinical nurse specialist (CNS) and NP roles more recently—has been another response. The development of specialized faculty, such as pediatric and obstetric faculty; researchers who focus on particular phenomena, such as nursing ethics or the care of dying patients; and nursing administrators who direct clinical nursing services has been a third response. Nurses in all of these roles can be considered specialists in an area of nursing; some of these roles may involve advanced education in a clinical specialty as well. They are not necessarily advanced nursing practice roles, however.

Advanced nursing practice includes specialization but goes beyond it. Advanced nursing practice involves expansion, advancement (ANA, 1995; Cronenwett, 1995), and other characteristics in addition to specialization. *Nursing's Social Policy Statement* (ANA, 1995) defined these elements:

> *Expansion refers to the acquisition of new practice knowledge and skills, including the knowledge and skills that legitimize role autonomy within areas of practice that overlap traditional boundaries of medical practice. Advancement involves both specialization and expansion and is characterized by the integration of a broad range of theoretical, research-based, and practical knowledge that occurs as a part of graduate education in nursing.*

(p. 14)

APNs are further characterized by their autonomy to practice at the edges of the expanding boundaries of nursing, their predominantly self-initiated treatment regimens rather than dependent functions, and the greater complexity of their clinical decision making and skill in managing organizations and environments than is seen in basic nursing practice (ANA, 1995).

DEFINING ADVANCED NURSING PRACTICE

As recently as 1996, O'Malley, Cummings, and King wrote, "In most settings, the role of APNs has not been fully understood . . . APNs are still not identified by the public as primary care providers, partially due to misunderstanding of their roles" (p. 63). The concept of advanced nursing practice continues to be defined in various ways in the nursing literature. The *Cumulative Index to Nursing and Allied Health Literature* defined advanced practice broadly as anything beyond the staff nurse role: "The performance of additional acts by registered nurses who have gained added knowledge and skills through post-basic education and clinical experience" ("Advanced nursing," 1999, p. 10). A definition this broad incorporates many nursing roles, not all of which should be considered advanced practice. For example, some authors have proposed the "health policy analyst" as an advanced practice role (Stimpson & Hanley, 1991). This role contains no direct practice component, focusing as it does on consultation to decision makers regarding health policy. As the ANA (1995) noted, "The term advanced practice is used to refer exclusively to advanced *clinical* practice" (p. 15). In the understanding being developed here, the health policy analyst is a specialized nursing role but not an advanced practice role.

Advanced nursing practice is most often defined as a constellation of four roles: the NP, CNS, CNM, and CRNA (ANA, 1992; Donley, 1995; Ray & Hardin, 1995). Some authors, although they explicitly state that they are addressing advanced practice, discuss only NP and CNS roles (Lindeke, Canedy, & Kay, 1997; Rasch & Frauman, 1996). Others have focused exclusively on the NP role (Hickey, Ouimette, & Venegoni, 1996; Thibodeau & Hawkins, 1994). Snyder and Mirr (1995) defined advanced nursing practice as the merged roles of the CNS and NP. These definitions of advanced practice in terms of particular roles limit the concept and deny the reality that nurses practicing in other roles are also APNs. These definitions are also limiting because they do not incorporate evolving APN roles, such as the APN case manager. It thus seems preferable to define advanced nursing practice in a way other than referring to particular roles.

It is also important to advance a definition that clarifies the critical point that advanced nursing practice involves advanced *nursing* skills; it is not a *medical* practice, although APNs perform expanded medical therapeutics in many roles. In addition, advanced nursing practice needs to be understood in a conceptually clear fashion that recognizes the core competencies that all APNs share.

CORE DEFINITION OF ADVANCED NURSING PRACTICE

As can be seen from this brief review, advanced nursing practice is defined in differing and sometimes contradictory ways. A central and agreed upon definition of advanced nursing practice and clarity regarding how it is enacted in various health care settings are critical to the continued development of advanced practice and, indeed, the nursing profession itself.

The definition proposed in this chapter builds on and extends the understanding of advanced practice proposed in the first edition of this book. In this section, a core definition of advanced nursing practice is proposed; the differences among the advanced practice roles are described in the following section. Important assertions of this discussion are as follows:

- Advanced nursing practice is a function of educational and practice preparation *and* a constellation of primary criteria and core competencies.
- Direct clinical practice is the central competency of any APN role.
- All APNs share the same core criteria and competencies, though the actual clinical skill set varies depending upon the needs of their patient population.
- Actual practices differ significantly based on the needs of the specialty patient population served and the organizational framework within which the role is performed. Particular APN roles have different "shapes" and include additional competencies specific to them. This is most clearly exemplified in the CRNA and CNM roles, but it is true for all the roles. Consequently, it is both necessary and preferable to retain varied job titles that reflect these actual practices, rather than reduce all APNs to one title.

In spite of the need to keep job descriptions and job titles distinct in practice settings, it is critical that the public's confusion about advanced practice be decreased and its acceptance of advanced nursing practice be enhanced. As Safriet (1993) noted, nursing's future depends on reaching consensus on titles and consistent preparation for these title holders. The burden is clearly on the nursing profession and its APNs to be clear, concrete, and consistent about APN titles and their functions in discussions with nursing's larger constituencies: consumers, other health care professionals, health care administrators, and health care policymakers.

Conceptual Definition

Davies and Hughes (1995) noted, "The term advanced nursing practice extends beyond roles. It is a way of thinking and viewing the world based on clinical knowledge, rather than a composition of roles" (p. 157). The ANA's *Scope and Standards of Advanced Practice Registered Nursing* (1996) defines the central activities of APNs as follows:

> *Advanced practice registered nurses manifest a high level of expertise in the assessment, diagnosis, and treatment of the complex responses of individuals, families, or communities to actual or potential health problems, prevention of illness and injury, maintenance of wellness, and provision of comfort. The advanced practice registered nurse has a master's or doctoral education concentrating in a specific area of advanced nursing practice, had supervised practice during graduate education, and has ongoing clinical experiences. Advanced practice registered nurses continue to perform many of the same interventions used in basic nursing practice. The difference in this practice relates to a greater depth and breadth of knowledge, a greater degree of synthesis of data, and complexity of skills and interventions.*
>
> (p. 2)

Integrating this understanding with the ANA's (1995) components of advanced practice, the author conceptualized advanced nursing practice as follows:

> **Advanced nursing practice is the application of an expanded range of practical, theoretical, and research-based therapeutics to phenomena experienced by patients within a specialized clinical area of the larger discipline of nursing (Hamric, 1996, p. 47).**[1]

The term "therapeutics" refers to any of the activities undertaken as part of delivering care, and includes assessment, diagnosis, planning, intervention/treatment, and evaluation. Through graduate education and practice experiences, APNs acquire expanded capabilities in providing care, some of which involve traditionally medical therapeutics. Although certain activities may also be performed by physicians and other health care professionals, the experiential, theoretical, and philosophical perspectives of nursing make these activities advanced *nursing* practice when they are enacted by an APN. In addition, advanced practice nursing involves highly developed nursing skills as well as performance of selected medical therapeutics, as the defining characteristics will clarify. The nursing profession needs to be clear on this point, for *the advanced practice of nursing is not the junior practice of medicine.*

The definition recognizes that not all nursing therapeutics are research based at this point in nursing's evolution. Theoretical understandings and practice expertise are also key adjuncts to advanced practice therapeutics. The definition acknowledges the strong experiential component necessary to develop the competencies of advanced nursing practice. Although graduate education in nursing provides a critical foundation for the expanded knowledge and theory base necessary to support advanced practice, in-depth clinical experiences are equally critical. Indeed, graduate

---

[1] The term "patient" is intended to be used interchangeably with "individual" and "client."

education and clinical practice experience work synergistically to develop the APN. The definition also emphasizes the patient-focused and specialized nature of advanced practice. Finally, the critical importance of ensuring that any type of advanced nursing practice is grounded within the larger discipline of nursing is made explicit.

Advanced nursing practice is further defined by three primary criteria, a central competency, and six core competencies. This discussion and the chapters in Part II will isolate each of these core competencies to clarify them. It is important for the reader to recognize that this is only a cognitive device for clarifying the conceptualization of advanced nursing practice used in this book. In reality, these elements are integrated in an APN's practice; they are not separate and distinct features. The concentric circles in Figures 3–1 through 3–3 represent the seamless nature of this interweaving of elements. In addition, the APN's skills function synergistically to produce a whole that is greater than the sum of its parts. The essence of advanced nursing practice is found not only in the primary criteria and competencies demonstrated, but also in the synthesis of these elements, along with individual nurse characteristics, into a unified composite practice (Davies & Hughes, 1995) that conforms to the conceptual definition presented earlier.

Primary Criteria

Certain criteria (or qualifications) must be met before one can be considered an APN. Although these baseline criteria are not *sufficient* in and of themselves, they are *necessary* core elements of advanced nursing practice. The three primary criteria for advanced practice are diagrammed in Figure 3–1 and include: an earned graduate degree with a concentration in an advanced nursing practice category, professional certification of practice at an advanced level within a given specialty, and a practice that is focused on patients/clients and their families. These criteria are most often the ones used by states to regulate APN practice, because they are objective and easily measured.

First, the APN must possess an *earned graduate (master's or doctoral) degree with a concentration in an APN specialty.* Advanced practice students acquire specialized knowledge and skills through study and supervised practice at either the master's or the doctoral level. The content of study includes theories and research findings relevant to the core of the given nursing specialty. The expansion of practice

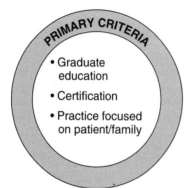

FIGURE 3–1 • Primary criteria of advanced nursing practice.

skills is acquired through clinical experience in addition to faculty-supervised practice (ANA, 1995). As noted previously in the ANA's definition, there is consensus that master's education in nursing is a requirement for advanced nursing practice.

Why is graduate educational preparation necessary for advanced nursing practice? Some of the differences between basic and advanced nursing practice are apparent in the range and depth of APNs' clinical knowledge; in APNs' ability to anticipate patient responses to health, illness, and nursing interventions; in their ability to analyze clinical situations and produce explicit clinical judgments (Calkin, 1984) and to explain why a phenomenon has occurred or why a particular intervention has been chosen; and in their skill in assessing and addressing nonclinical variables that influence patient care. Because of the interaction and integration of graduate education in nursing and extensive clinical experience, the APN is able to exercise a level of discrimination in clinical judgment that is unavailable to other experienced clinicians (Spross & Baggerly, 1989). Professionally, requiring graduate preparation is important to create parity among all APN roles, so that all can move forward together in addressing policy-making and regulatory issues. This parity advances the profession's standards and ensures more uniform credentialing mechanisms. Creating a normative educational expectation enhances nursing's image and credibility with other disciplines, especially medicine. Finally, the research and theory base required for advanced nursing practice mandates education at the graduate level.

Second, APNs must have *professional certification for practice at an advanced level within a specialty.* The continuing growth of specialization has dramatically increased the amount of knowledge and experience required to practice safely in modern health care settings. National certification examinations have been developed by specialty organizations and are used to determine whether nurses meet standards for practice in a particular clinical specialty. By and large, these examinations have tested the specialty knowledge of experienced nurses and not knowledge at the advanced level of practice. Two notable exceptions are CNM and CRNA certifying examinations (see Chapter 1). NPs have developed a number of certification options for both primary care and acute care practices. Although the American Nurses Credentialing Center (ANCC) has sponsored CNS certification examinations in medical-surgical and psychiatric areas for years, advanced practice certification examinations in particular specialties such as maternal-child health have been slow to develop. The number of examination options for CNSs are increasing. For example, the ONS began administering an advanced practice certification examination in 1995, and the ANCC is working with a number of specialty organizations to develop examinations for advanced-level practitioners in particular specialties. If no certification examination exists for the advanced practice level of a particular specialty, the APN should be certified at the highest level available. The ANA and various specialty organizations should continue to develop certification for advanced nursing practice based on graduate education so that, ultimately, all APN certifications will be at the graduate level.

Third, the APN engages in a *practice focused on patients and their families.* It is critical to promoting clarity about advanced nursing practice that the term be used to describe advanced *clinical* practice (ANA, 1995), and refer to roles that have direct clinical practice as their central focus. This does not imply that direct practice is the only activity that APNs undertake. APNs also educate others, participate in and conduct research, and serve as consultants, among other activities (Brown, 1998). However, to be considered an APN role, the patient/family direct practice focus must be primary. As noted earlier, there are other important specialized roles in the profession, notably, educators, administrators, and researchers. These roles are valuable and vital to the profession's continued development. They are "critical to the preparation of nurses for practice, the provision of environments that are conducive to nursing practice, and the continued development of the knowledge base that nurses use in practice" (ANA, 1995, p. 15). Some of the nurses in these roles possess advanced practice knowledge and skills as well. However, if they do not have a patient/family-focused clinical practice, they are not considered APNs by this definition.

This requirement puts some community health nurses in a gray area between advanced nursing practice and specialized practices of program development or consultation. There are APNs in community practices who take a community view of their practice and indeed consider the community to be their patient/client. Certainly the broad perspective of the APN encompasses the community and society in which care is provided (Davies & Hughes, 1995); effecting positive outcomes for populations of patients is an important expectation for the APN. However, advanced nursing practice as it is conceptualized by the profession is focused on and realized at the level of clinical practice with patients and families. So long as APNs in community health practices maintain a direct clinical practice focused on patients and their families in addition to programmatic or consultative responsibilities, they are APNs in this definition. Community health nurses who do not have a patient-focused practice have specialty skills in community assessment and program planning, and would be more appropriately considered specialty nurses rather than APNs.

Why limit the definition of advanced nursing practice to roles focused on clinical practice to patients and families? There are many reasons. Nursing is a practice profession. The nurse-patient interface is at the core of nursing practice; in the final analysis, the reason the profession exists is to render nursing services to individuals in need of them. Clinical practice expertise in a given specialty develops from these nurse-patient encounters and lies at the heart of advanced nursing practice. In addition, ongoing direct clinical practice is necessary to maintain and develop an APN's expertise. Without regular immersion in practice, the cutting-edge clinical practice expertise found in APN practices cannot be sustained.

The focus of all the APN roles discussed in this book is the patient/family. Newly emerging roles must be similarly focused on direct clinical practice to be considered advanced practice. If every specialized role in nursing were considered advanced nursing practice, the term would become so broad as to lack meaning and explanatory value (see also Cronenwett, 1995). For example, a nurse administrator functions very differently than does a CNM. Distinguishing between APN roles and other specialized roles in nursing can help clarify the concept of advanced nursing practice to consumers, to other health care providers, and even to other nurses. In addition, the monitoring and regulation of advanced nursing practice are increasingly important issues as APNs work toward more authority for their practices (see Chapter 22). If the definition of advanced nursing practice included nurses in nonclinical roles, developing sound regulatory mechanisms would be impossible.

Some nurses with specialized skills in administration, research, and community health have viewed this direct practice requirement as a devaluing of their contributions to the nursing profession. Some faculty who teach clinical nursing but do not themselves maintain an advanced clinical practice have also felt "disenfranchised" because they are not considered APNs by virtue of this primary criterion. Perhaps this problem has been exacerbated by using the term "advanced" to apply to this practice, because this term can inadvertently imply that other nurses not fitting into the APN definition are not "advanced." It is critical to understand that this definition is not a value statement, but a differentiation of one group of nurses from other groups for the sake of clarity within and outside of the profession. As the ANA noted, *all* nurses, whether their focus is clinical practice, educating students, conducting research, planning community programs, or leading nursing service organizations, are valuable and necessary to the integrity and growth of the larger profession. However, all nurses, particularly those with advanced degrees, are *not the same,* nor are they necessarily APNs. Historically, the profession has had difficulty differentiating itself and has struggled with the prevailing lay notion that "a nurse is a nurse is a nurse." This view does not match the reality of the health care arena, nor does it celebrate the diverse contributions of all the various nursing specialties.

Direct Clinical Practice: The Central Competency

As noted earlier, the primary criteria are necessary but insufficient elements of the definition of advanced nursing practice. Advanced practice is further defined by a set of core competencies that are enacted in each APN role. The term "competency" is used here to refer to a defined area of skilled performance. As noted previously, the first core competency of direct clinical practice is central to and informs all of the others (see Figure 3-2). Advanced nursing practice is first and foremost characterized by excellence in direct clinical practice.

However, clinical expertise alone should not be equated with advanced nursing practice. The work of Patricia Benner and her colleagues (Benner, 1984; Benner, Hooper-Kyriakidis, & Stannard, 1999; Benner, Tanner, & Chesla, 1996) is a major contribution to understanding clinically expert nursing practice. The reader will see this important work reflected in various ways throughout the chapters of this book. These researchers have studied expert nurses in acute care clinical settings exten-

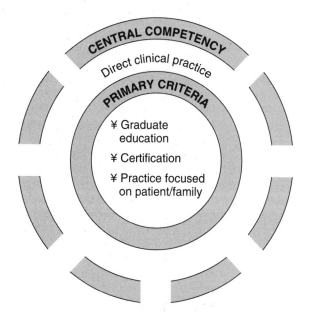

FIGURE 3-2 • The central competency of advanced nursing practice.

sively, and have described the engaged clinical reasoning and domains of practice seen in clinically expert nurses. Although some of the participants in this research were APNs (in the most recent report [Benner et al., 1999], 16% of the nurse participants were APNs), the majority were nurses with extensive clinical experience who did not have APN preparation. Calkin (1984) characterized these latter nurses as "experts by experience." (See Chapter 2 for a discussion of her conceptual differentiation between these levels of nursing practice.) Benner and her colleagues have not discussed differences in the practices of APNs as compared to other nurses they have studied. In fact, they stated, " 'Expert' is not used to refer to a specific role such as an advanced practice nurse. Expertise is found in the practice of experienced clinicians and advanced practice nurses" (Benner et al., 1999, p. 9).

Although clinical expertise is certainly a central ingredient of the direct practice competency that defines advanced nursing practice, it is not the only or complete understanding of the clinical practice of APNs. As noted in Chapter 6, advanced direct care practice includes five characteristics: (1) use of a holistic perspective, (2) formation of partnerships with patients, (3) use of expert clinical reasoning, (4) reliance on research evidence as a guide to practice, and (5) use of diverse health and illness management approaches. These characteristics help to distinguish the practice of the expert-by-experience from that of the APN. As previously noted, experiential knowledge and graduate education work synergistically to develop these characteristics in an APN's clinical practice.

The specific content of the direct practice competency differs significantly by specialty. For example, the clinical practice of a CNS dealing with critically ill children differs from the expertise of an NP managing the health maintenance needs of elderly people or a CRNA administering anesthesia in an outpatient surgical clinic.

Core Competencies

Six core competencies further define advanced nursing practice regardless of role function or setting. These competencies have repeatedly been identified as essential features of advanced practice (American Association of Colleges of Nursing, 1995; ANA, 1995; Davies & Hughes, 1995; National Association of Clinical Nurse Specialists, 1998; National Council of State Boards of Nursing, 1993; National Organization of Nurse Practitioner Faculties, 1995; Spross & Baggerly, 1989). As depicted in Figure 3-3, they are

1. Expert guidance and coaching of patients, families, and other care providers
2. Consultation
3. Research skills, including utilization, evaluation, and conduct
4. Clinical and professional leadership, which includes competence as a change agent
5. Collaboration
6. Ethical decision-making skills

These competencies are similarly learned by all APNs, who then apply them to specific patient populations and settings. In Figure 3-3, the openings between the central practice competency and these additional competencies represent the fact that the APN's direct practice skill interacts with and informs all the other competencies. For example, APNs consult with other providers who seek their practice expertise to plan care for specialty patients. They are able to provide expert guidance and

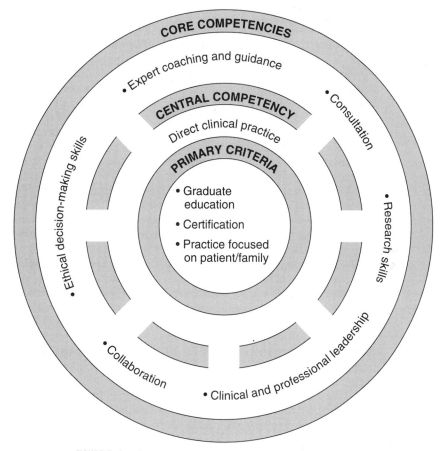

FIGURE 3–3 • Core competencies of advanced nursing practice.

coaching for patients going through health and illness transitions because of their direct practice experience and insight.

It is important to emphasize that these complex competencies develop over time. No APN emerges from a graduate program fully prepared to enact them all. However, it is critical that graduate programs provide exposure to each competency in the form of didactic content as well as practical experience, so that new graduates can be tested for initial credentialing and be given a base on which to build their practices. These key competencies are described in detail in subsequent chapters and so are not further elaborated here.

Scope of Practice

The term ''scope of practice'' refers to the legal authority granted to a professional to provide and be reimbursed for health care services. This authority for practice emanates from many sources, such as state and federal laws and regulations, the profession's code of ethics, and professional practice standards. For all health care professionals, scope of practice is most closely tied to state statutes; for nursing, these statutes are the Nurse Practice Acts of the various states. As previously discussed, an APN's scope of practice is characterized by specialization; expansion of services provided, including diagnosing and prescribing; and autonomy to practice (ANA, 1996). There are differences in the scopes of practice among the various APN roles; various specialty organizations have provided detailed and specific descriptions for their specialties. Carving out an adequate scope of APN practice authority has been a historic struggle for most of the advanced practice specialties (see Chapter 1), and this continues to be a hotly debated issue among and within the professions. Significant variability in state practice acts continues such that APNs can perform certain activities, notably prescribing medications and practicing without physician supervision, in some states but may be constrained from performing these same activities if they move to another state (Safriet, 1992, 1994). Safriet (1998) noted that, in the last few years, regulatory challenges have been compounded by changes in the financial restructuring of the health care delivery system. APNs now face new nongovernmental, market-based barriers to their practices. "These impediments, combined with the remaining restrictions embedded in state licensure laws and state and federal payment schemes, will define nursing's agenda in the next few years" (1998, p. 25).

The Pew Commission's Taskforce on Health Care Workforce Regulation (Finocchio et al., 1998) noted the tension and turf battles between professions and the increased legislative activities in this area that "clog legislative agendas across the country" (p. ii). These battles are costly and time-consuming, and lawmakers' decisions related to scope of practice are too often distorted by campaign contributions, lobbying efforts, and political power struggles rather than being based on empirical evidence. The Pew Commission Taskforce Report contains a number of recommendations that directly address scope of practice concerns, including the need for a national policy advisory body to research, develop, and publish national scopes of practice and continuing competency standards. They noted that this body should develop and press the states to enact model legislative language for uniform scopes of practice authority for the health professions, based on evidence of competence (see Chapter 22 for further discussion).

DIFFERENTIATING ADVANCED PRACTICE ROLES: OPERATIONAL DEFINITIONS OF ADVANCED NURSING PRACTICE

As noted earlier, it is critical to the public's understanding of advanced nursing practice that APN roles and resulting job titles reflect actual practices. Because actual practices differ, job titles should differ. (The corollary is also true: If the actual practices do not differ, the job titles should not differ.) These differences among roles must be clarified in ways that promote understanding of advanced practice, rather than divide the profession (Davies & Hughes, 1995). It is this spirit of promoting understanding and clarity that informs the ensuing discussion. A key assumption is that *all of these APN roles are valuable* in meeting the needs of patients in current and evolving health care settings.

The National Council of State Boards of Nursing (NCSBN, 1993) noted the differences in scopes of practice in each of the advanced roles. Although the NCSBN recognized overlapping activities within the four APN roles of CNS, NP, CNM, and CRNA, there were activities unique to each role. In addition to each role's unique competencies, differentiation between APNs occurs along a number of dimensions. The nature of the patient population receiving APN care, organizational expectations, emphasis given to specific competencies, and practice characteristics unique to each role also serve to distinguish the practice of one APN group from others. It is important to note at the outset of this discussion that these differences between ANP roles are not rigid demarcations. Nursing's scope of practice is dynamic and continually evolving, and this is especially true at the boundaries of the discipline, where advanced practice occurs (ANA, 1995). "Differences among nurses in their scopes of practice can be characterized as intraprofessional intersections across which collegial, collaborative practice occurs" (ANA, 1995, p. 12). These intersections are not rigid lines, but rather are fluid and involve overlapping areas. The intent of this discussion is not to create stereotypical divisions or to deny the dynamic and evolving nature of advanced nursing practice, but rather to describe key differences that are evident in actual practices at this stage in the evolution of advanced practice.

Advanced nursing practice is applied in a variety of roles, some established, some newly emerging. These roles can be considered to be the operational definitions of the conceptual definition of advanced nursing practice. Figure 3-4 illustrates the differing "shapes" of ANP roles. The shapes used in the figure do not have any particular significance; rather, they are meant to illustrate that roles differ along varying dimensions, as noted earlier. The figure also visually represents the fact that, although each APN role has the common definition, criteria, and competencies of advanced nursing practice at its center, it has its own distinctive form. For example, the American College of Nurse-Midwives (ACNM, 1997), the National Organization of Nurse Practitioner Faculties (1995), the National Association of Clinical Nurse Specialists (NACNS, 1998), and the American Association of Nurse Anesthetists (1992) have identified additional core competencies for the CNM, NP, CNS, and CRNA roles,

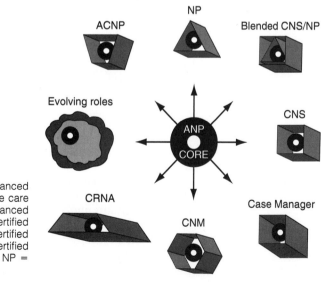

FIGURE   3–4 • Different advanced practice roles. ACNP = acute care nurse practitioner; ANP = advanced nursing practice; CNM = certified nurse-midwife; CNS = certified nurse specialist; CRNA = certified registered nurse anesthetist; NP = nurse practitioner.

respectively. Some of these distinctive features of the various roles are listed here. Differences and similarities between roles are further explored in Part III.

The CNS role has been distinguished by the expectation of practice in four subroles: clinical expert, consultant, educator, and researcher (Hamric & Spross, 1989; see also Chapter 13). CNSs are first and foremost clinical experts, who provide direct care to patients with complex health problems. CNSs not only learn consultation processes as do other APNs, but also function as formal consultants within their organizations. Their multifocal practice in these different subroles means that CNS practice is fluid and changeable. Developing, supporting, and educating nursing staff; managing system change in complex organizations to build teams and improve nursing practices; and "massaging the system" (Fenton, 1985) to advocate for patients are unique role expectations of the CNS. Expectations regarding research activities have been central to this role since its inception. More recently, the NACNS (1998) has distinguished CNS practice by characterizing "spheres of influence" in which the CNS develops competencies. These include the patient/client sphere, the nursing personnel sphere, and the organization/network sphere.

NPs, whether in primary care or acute care, possess advanced health assessment, diagnostic, and clinical management skills that include pharmacology management (see Chapters 14 and 15). Their focus is expert direct care, managing the health needs of individuals and their families. Incumbents in the classic NP role provide primary health care focused on wellness and prevention; NP practice also includes caring for patients with minor, common, acute conditions and stable chronic conditions. The newer acute care NP (ACNP) brings practitioner skills to a specialized patient population within the acute care setting. The ACNP's focus is the diagnosis and clinical management of acutely or critically ill patient populations in a particular specialized setting. Acquiring additional medical diagnostic and management skills, such as interpreting computerized tomography and magnetic resonance imaging scans, inserting chest tubes, or performing lumbar punctures, also characterize this role.

The blended CNS/NP role (see Chapter 16) combines the CNS's in-depth specialized knowledge of a particular patient population with the NP's primary health care expertise. It is important to clarify that CNSs who obtain NP skills are not necessarily functioning in a blended role. Many work as NPs in either primary care NP or ACNP roles as described earlier. The CNS/NP provides primary and specialty care, including clinical management, to a complex patient population, such as children with diabetes. A unique feature of this role is the provision of primary and specialized care such that the blended CNS/NP crosses setting boundaries to provide continuity of care. An additional characteristic that distinguishes this role from that of the ACNP is the expectation for CNS competencies in the three spheres of influence noted earlier. For example, this role combines individual patient management with expectations to develop nursing staff as well as effect change in complex organizational practices. In addition to learning the core advanced practice competencies, education for this role must include functional role preparation for both the CNS and the NP roles. Blended-role APNs also must ensure that their roles are carefully structured to allow time and emphasis in the three spheres of influence.

The CNM (see Chapter 17) has advanced health assessment and intervention skills focused on women's health and childbearing. CNM practice involves independent management of women's health care. CNMs focus particularly on pregnancy, childbirth, the postpartum period, and care of the newborn, but their practices also include family planning, gynecological care, and primary health care for women (ACNM, 1997). The CNM's focus is on direct practice to a select patient population.

CRNA practice (see Chapter 18) is distinguished by advanced procedural and pharmacological management of patients undergoing anesthesia. CRNAs practice independently, in collaboration with physicians, or as employees of a health care institution. Like CNMs, their focus is on direct practice to a select patient population. Both CNM and CRNA practices are also distinguished by well-established national standards, national examinations, and certification for practice at the advanced specialty level.

APN case managers (see Chapter 19) provide complex patient management of high-risk or resource-intensive patients. They identify patient needs for interdisciplinary care and develop and coordinate an integrated plan of care. In addition to direct clinical practice, APN case managers develop interdisciplinary clinical guidelines that support quality and cost outcomes for individual patients and patient populations. Patient management across delivery networks is an expectation of some of these roles. APN case managers are responsible for patient outcome identification and evaluation and share the risk for accomplishing or not accomplishing outcomes with other team members, and the institution as well. It is important to note that many APN roles, particularly the CNS and ACNP, may have case management as a part of their expectations in managing complex patient problems. However, their roles are not structured solely around case management practice, as is the role of the APN case manager.

These differing roles and their similarities and distinctions are explored in detail in subsequent chapters. This brief discussion underscores the rich and varied nature of advanced nursing practice and the necessity for retaining and supporting different APN roles and titles in the health care marketplace. At the same time, a consistent definition of advanced practice undergirds each of these roles.

CRITICAL ELEMENTS IN MANAGING ADVANCED NURSING PRACTICE ENVIRONMENTS

The health care arena is increasingly fluid and changeable—some would even say it is chaotic. Advanced nursing practice does not exist in a vacuum or a singular environment. Rather, the practice is imbedded in an increasing variety of health care delivery contexts. These diverse environments are complex admixtures of interdependent elements that mutually affect one another. There are certain core features of these environments that dramatically shape advanced practice, and must be managed by APNs for their practices to survive and thrive (see Figure 3-5). Although not technically part of the core definition of advanced practice, they are included here to frame the growing understanding that APNs must be aware of these key elements in any practice setting. Furthermore, APNs must be prepared to contend with and shape these aspects of their practice environment to be able to fully enact advanced practice.

Part IV of this book explores these elements in depth. They include managing reimbursement and business aspects of the practice, dealing with marketing and contracting considerations, understanding regulatory and credentialing requirements, understanding and shaping health policy considerations, strengthening organizational structures and cultures to support advanced nursing practice, and enabling outcome evaluation and performance improvement. Managing the business and legal aspects of practice is increasingly critical to survival as a primary care provider in the competitive

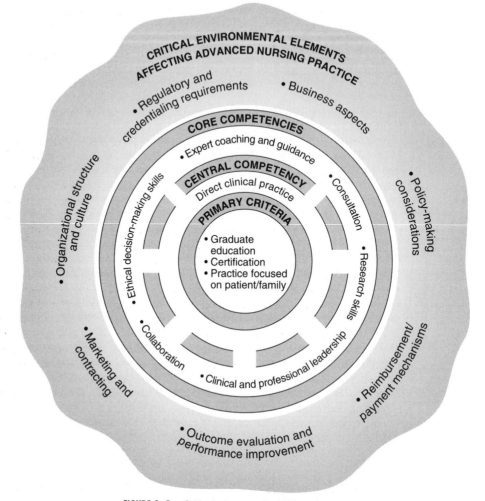

FIGURE 3–5 • Critical elements in APN environments.

health care marketplace. However, APN roles that exist primarily in tertiary settings also must understand the reimbursement issues and legal constraints within their organizations. Given the increasingly competitive environment between physicians, APNs, and nonphysician providers, APNs must be prepared to assertively and knowledgeably market their services. Often, they must be prepared to advocate for and actively create positions that do not currently exist. Contracting considerations are much more complex at the APN level, and all APNs, whether newly graduated or experienced, must be prepared to enter into contract negotiations. Health policy at state and federal levels is an increasingly potent force shaping advanced nursing practice; regulations and policies that flow from legislative actions can enable or constrain APN practices. Variations in the strength and number of APNs in various states attest to the power of this environmental factor. Organizational structures and cultures are also important facilitators or barriers to advanced practice; APN students must learn to assess and intervene to build organizations that strengthen APN practice. Finally, APNs are accountable for both patient and system outcomes. Measuring the favorable impact of advanced practice nursing on these outcomes and effecting performance improvements are essential activities all APNs must be prepared to undertake.

IMPLICATIONS OF THIS DEFINITION OF ADVANCED NURSING PRACTICE

Many of the implications of the definition of advanced nursing practice presented here have been noted throughout the chapter, such as the necessity for graduate preparation for APN roles and the need for an individual nurse to meet the core definition, criteria, and competencies to be considered an APN. Because of the centrality of direct clinical practice, it is essential that APNs hold onto and make explicit their direct patient care activities. In addition, there are other implications for education, practice, and research that flow from this understanding of advanced practice.

Implications for APN Education

APN roles involve many components and competencies. As a result, APNs require a considerable period of role development to implement fully the varied aspects of their practice (see Chapter 5). Graduate programs should provide anticipatory socialization experiences to prepare students for their chosen role. It is important that graduate experiences include practice in all the competencies of advanced practice, not just clinical practice expertise. For example, students who have no theoretical base or guided practice experiences in consultative skills or clinical leadership will be ill-equipped to enact these competencies upon entering a new APN role. However, even with the best graduate education, no APN new to practice can be expected to perform all the role components and competencies with equal skill.

Two other implications concern the education of APNs, which is discussed in more detail in Chapter 4. It is critical that universities (1) develop articulation programs to help certificate-prepared nurses currently functioning in APN roles obtain master's preparation and (2) transition certificate programs to the master's level. Graduate educators need to support these articulation programs and develop curricula to enable this education. The profession has embraced a wide variety of graduate educational models for preparing APNs, including direct-entry programs for non-nurse college graduates and RN-to-MSN programs. These programs have differing experience and academic requirements. Assuring quality and standardization of APN education in the various specialties is a professional imperative. Research is needed on the outcomes of these different APN master's educational programs in terms of APN graduate experiences and patient outcomes. Such data would be invaluable in continuing to refine advanced practice education.

Schools of nursing must not completely homogenize the preparation for advanced practice. Certainly, all students need exposure to the core definition and competencies of advanced practice described here. However, APNs enact these competencies in widely varying ways in differentiated positions. It is essential that schools provide sufficient functional role preparation that students are prepared to enter a specific work role. This point seems obvious when discussing CNMs and CRNAs, but it is equally important for CNSs and NPs as well. In a study of NPs who had previously practiced as CNSs, Lindeke and colleagues (1997) found distinct practices between the roles, which demonstrated that different knowledge and skills were needed to adequately enact each role. They stated, "Master's-level educational programs in nursing that combine NP and CNS roles into a single advanced practice role face the danger of diluting the strong competencies of each role" (p. 287). Educational standards developed by national specialty organizations for particular APN roles are assuming increasing importance in guiding curricular decisions. These standards have significant differences among them, particularly in the skill set expected for each role. Programs that prepare only a generic APN who has no preparation for the reality of assuming one of the ANP roles (or more, in the case of the blended CNS/NP) are doing their students, prospective employers of APNs, and the nursing profession a disservice. This role preparation is difficult to ensure when the content is not explicitly addressed but rather "integrated" in clinical coursework. In clinical courses, students are understandably focused on gaining the clinical knowledge base needed for their APN role, and often do not concentrate on the other core APN competencies and particular competencies unique to their chosen APN role. Role courses are also extremely helpful in enabling students to differentiate themselves from other APNs and other providers (such as physician assistants), and to explore the many issues surrounding advanced nursing practice.

A final educational implication relates to the need for APN students to understand the critical elements in health care environments that must be managed if their practices are to survive and grow. It is this author's experience that beginning graduate students are frequently unaware of the issues involved in enabling advanced practice, particularly the larger policy and regulatory issues. They have often come from clinical environments where their roles were standardized and focused solely on patient care. Graduate education exposes them to a broader field of vision, and exposure to the issues is invaluable. However, graduate programs must go beyond discussion of issues and trends to give students strategies for managing these issues. Many promising APNs have been unprepared to handle the rough-and-tumble practice environments they entered after graduation, and as a result their practices have not survived. In some cases, influential leaders in a particular environment have interpreted an individual APN's difficulties to mean that advanced practice was not necessary to achieve desirable patient outcomes and to improve system practices. Such experiences devalue advanced practice and are harmful for individual APNs and the profession. Developing clinically active and astute faculty who understand practice realities and can provide tools for dealing with them is one strategy that graduate programs can use to help students. Clinical practice experiences that include guided reflection on these key elements is another. Projects designed to focus on the critical elements, such as analyzing regulatory requirements for particular roles, developing an outcome management plan for a complex patient problem, and designing a marketing portfolio, can give students a significant advantage as they enter the marketplace in search of APN positions.

Clearly, graduate program length is an issue with many of these recommendations. Programs that endeavor to shorten clinical practice time or course requirements must balance their desires to be "user friendly" and competitive with other programs with their obligation to prepare APN students who are equipped to enter challenging practice roles in complex settings. As the knowledge base grows and the profession's understanding of advanced practice increases, curricula of necessity must also grow. Finding a balance remains an ongoing challenge. However, adequate graduate preparation is the necessary foundation for advanced practice nursing to survive and reach its full potential in the new millennium.

Implications for Practice Environments

The fact that new APNs need a period of role development before they can master all of the components and competencies of their chosen role has important implications for employers of new APNs. These include the need to provide experienced preceptors, the provision of some structure for the new APN, and ongoing support for role development (see Chapter 5 for further recommendations).

"Each individual who practices nursing at an advanced level does so with substantial autonomy and independence requiring a high level of accountability" (NCSBN, 1993, p. 3). Advanced practice roles require considerable autonomy and authority to be fully enacted. Practice settings have not always structured APN roles to allow sufficient autonomy or accountability to achieve the patient and system outcomes that are expected of advanced practitioners. Federal and state regulations have further limited the potential of APN roles by not recognizing advanced practice or by placing APNs in dependent positions with respect to their physician colleagues. Although encouraging progress has been made, APNs and their advocates must continue to work actively for removal of these barriers if advanced nursing practice is to flourish.

It is equally important to emphasize that APNs have direct and expanded responsibilities to patients. Expanded authority for practice requires expanded responsibility for practice. It is crucial for APNs to demonstrate a higher level of responsibility and accountability if they are to be seen as legitimate providers of care and full partners on provider teams responsible for patient populations. This willingness to be accountable for one's practice will also further consumers' and policy makers' perceptions of the APN as a credible provider in line with physicians.

The APN leadership competency mandates that APNs serve as visible role models and mentors for other nurses (Cronenwett, 1995; also see Chapter 10). Practice environments need to structure the roles to allow time and opportunities for this mentoring activity.

Finally, APN roles must be structured and understood as providing advanced nursing skills rather than as simply substituting for physicians. This is particularly an issue for CRNA, NP, and ACNP roles, which involve additional medical therapeutics in their practices. As physician numbers increase, particularly physicians prepared in family practice and the new "hospitalist" practices, this distinction must be clear in the minds of employers and insurers. Indeed, it needs to be equally clear in the minds of APNs' staff nurse and physician colleagues. As noted earlier, the advanced practice of nursing is not the junior practice of medicine. Advanced nursing practice provides a value-added service to patients that involves all of the differing perspectives and elements discussed in this chapter. In most cases, advanced nursing practice needs to be understood as complementary to, rather than competing with, medical practice. APNs must be able to clearly and forcefully articulate this critical point if their practices are to survive continued cost cutting in the health care sector.

Implications for Research

As noted in Chapter 9, there are different levels of research involvement for the APN. However, being actively involved in research related to patient care at whatever level the APN is comfortable is a crucial ingredient of advanced nursing practice. If research is to be relevant to care delivery and to nursing practice at all levels, APNs must be involved. APNs need to recognize the importance of advancing both the profession's and the health care system's knowledge about effective patient care practices, and that they are a vital link in building this knowledge. APNs are in a key position to uncover the knowledge imbedded in clinical practice (Benner, 1984).

Related to this research involvement is the necessity for more research differentiating basic and advanced nursing practice, and identifying the patient populations that most benefit from APN intervention. Increasing research evidence that APNs affect or improve outcomes of care is presented in each of the chapters of Part III and in Chapter 25. However, linking advanced nursing practice to specific patient outcomes remains a major research imperative for this new century.

CONCLUSION

Today's APNs, future APNs, educators, administrators, and other nursing leaders need to be clear and consistent about the definition of advanced nursing practice so that the profession speaks with one voice. For a profession to succeed, it must have internal cohesion and external legitimacy, at the same time (Safriet, 1993). Clarity about the core definition of advanced nursing practice and recognition of the primary criteria and competencies necessary for all APNs will enhance nursing's external legitimacy. At the same time, recognizing the differences among, and the legitimacy of different, advanced practice roles will enhance nursing's internal cohesion.

REFERENCES

Advanced nursing practice. (1999). *Cumulative Index to Nursing and Allied Health Literature, 44,* 10.

American Association of Colleges of Nursing. (1995). *The essentials of master's education for advanced practice nursing.* Washington, DC: Author.

American Association of Nurse Anesthetists. (1992). *Guidelines and standards for nurse anesthesia practice.* Park Ridge, IL: Author.

American College of Nurse-Midwives. (1997). *Core competencies for basic nurse-midwifery practice.* Washington, DC: Author.

American Nurses Association. (1992). *Nursing facts.* Washington, DC: Author.

American Nurses Association. (1995). *Nursing's social policy statement.* Washington, DC: Author.

American Nurses Association. (1996). *Scope and standards of advanced practice registered nursing.* Washington, DC: Author.

Benner, P. (1984). *From novice to expert.* Menlo Park, CA: Addison-Wesley Publishing.

Benner, P., Hooper-Kyriakidis, P., & Stannard, D. (1999). *Clinical wisdom and interventions in critical care.* Philadelphia: W. B. Saunders.

Benner, P., Tanner, C. A., & Chesla, C. A. (1996). *Expertise in nursing practice: Caring, clinical judgment, and ethics.* New York: Springer.

Brown, S. J. (1998). A framework for advanced practice nursing. *Journal of Professional Nursing, 14,* 157–164.

Calkin, J. D. (1984). A model for advanced nursing practice. *Journal of Nursing Administration, 14*(1), 24–30.

Creasia, J. L., & Parker, B. (1996). *Conceptual foundations of professional nursing practice* (2nd ed.). St. Louis: Mosby–Year Book.

Cronenwett, L. R. (1995). Modeling the future of advanced practice nursing. *Nursing Outlook, 43,* 112–118.

Davies, B., & Hughes, A. M. (1995). Clarification of advanced nursing practice: Characteristics and competencies. *Clinical Nurse Specialist, 9,* 156–160.

Donley, S. R. (1995). Advanced practice nursing

after health care reform. *Nursing Economics,* *13*(2), 84–88.

Fenton, M. V. (1985). Identifying competencies of clinical nurse specialists. *Journal of Nursing Administration, 15*(12), 31–37.

Finocchio, L. J., Dower, C. M., Blick, N. T., Gragnola, C. M., & the Taskforce on Health Care Workforce Regulation. (1998). *Strengthening consumer protection: Priorities for health care workforce regulation.* San Francisco: Pew Health Professions Commission.

Hamric, A. B., & Spross, J. A. (Eds.). (1989). *The clinical nurse specialist in theory and practice* (2nd ed.). Philadelphia: W. B. Saunders.

Hickey, J. V., Ouimette, R. V., Venegoni, S. L. (1996). *Advance practice nursing: Changing roles and clinical applications.* Philadelphia: J. B. Lippincott.

Kitzman, H. (1989). The CNS and the nurse practitioner. In A. B. Hamric & J. A. Spross (Eds.), *The clinical nurse specialist in theory and practice* (2nd ed., pp. 379–394). Philadelphia: W. B. Saunders.

Leddy, S. K. (1998). *Conceptual bases of professional nursing* (4th ed.). Philadelphia: J. B. Lippincott.

Lindeke, L. L., Canedy, B. H., & Kay, M. M. (1997). A comparison of practice domains of clinical nurse specialists and nurse practitioners. *Journal of Professional Nursing, 13*(5), 281–287.

National Association of Clinical Nurse Specialists. (1998). *Statement on clinical nurse specialist practice and education.* Glenview, IL: Author.

National Council of State Boards of Nursing. (1993). *Position paper on the regulation of advanced nursing practice.* Chicago: Author.

National Organization of Nurse Practitioner Faculties. (1995). *Advanced nursing practice: Curriculum guidelines and program standards for nurse practitioner education.* Washington, DC: Author.

O'Malley, J., Cummings, S., & King, C. S. (1996). The politics of advanced practice. *Nursing Administration Quarterly, 20*(3), 62–72.

Rasch, R. F. R., & Frauman, A. C. (1996). Advanced practice in nursing: Conceptual issues. *Journal of Professional Nursing, 12*(3), 141–146.

Ray, G. L., & Hardin, S. (1995). Advanced practice nursing: Playing a vital role. *Nursing Management, 26*(2), 45–47.

Safriet, B. J. (1992). Health care dollars and regulatory sense: The role of advanced practice nursing. *Yale Journal of Regulation, 9*(2), 417–487.

Safriet, B. J. (1993, February). *Keynote address— one strong voice.* Paper presented at the National Nurse Practitioner Leadership Summit, Washington, DC.

Safriet, B. J. (1994). Impediments to progress in health care workforce policy: License and practice laws. *Inquiry, 31*(3), 310–317.

Safriet, B. J. (1998). Still spending dollars, still searching for sense: Advanced practice nursing in an era of regulatory and economic turmoil. *Advanced Practice Nursing Quarterly, 4*(3), 24–33.

Smith, M. C. (1995). The core of advanced practice nursing. *Nursing Science Quarterly, 8,* 2–3.

Snyder, M., & Mirr, M. P. (1995). *Advanced practice nursing: A guide to professional development.* New York: Springer.

Spross, J. A., & Baggerly, J. (1989). Models of advanced practice. In A. B. Hamric & J. A. Spross (Eds.), *The clinical nurse specialist in theory and practice* (2nd ed., pp. 19–40). Philadelphia: W. B. Saunders.

Stimpson, M., & Hanley, B. (1991). Nurse policy analyst: Advanced practice role. *Nursing and Health Care, 12,* 10–15.

Thibodeau, J. A., & Hawkins, J. W. (1994). Moving toward a nursing model in advanced practice. *Western Journal of Nursing Research, 16,* 205–218.

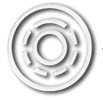

Education for Advanced Nursing Practice

• D O R E E N   C.   H A R P E R

INTRODUCTION

Education for advanced practice nurses (APNs) has progressed rapidly over the past 35 years as the roles of APNs have become more clearly defined regarding the provision of direct clinical care and the management of health care environments. APN role legitimacy has been established through graduate education, certification, and licensure (Brown, 1998). Recognition by policy makers at federal and state levels, consumers, foundations, health systems, and communities in the areas of scope of practice, prescriptive authority, and reimbursement have also served to legitimate these roles (Donaldson, Yordy, Lohr, & Vanselow, 1996; Gelmon et al., 1999; Kellogg Foundation, 1999; Mundinger et al., 2000; O'Neil et al., 1998; Robert Wood Johnson Foundation, 1999). The interactions between the nursing profession's values, direct clinical care, and the management of the health care environment continue to drive the core values defining APNs' roles, specialty knowledge, and clinical competencies. Grounded in theory and nursing practice, the elements of graduate, advanced practice *and* specialty knowledge and skill have led to competency-based advanced clinical practice. During the past decade, advanced practice nursing has begun to differentiate its contribution from that of other health care providers. This differentiation and legitimacy has influenced graduate nursing educators and APNs to analyze, communicate, and modify curricula and practice within the context of health care needs and the legal parameters of APN practice. Professional and educational organizations have been instrumental in leading these efforts, building on the broad repertoire of APN knowledge and skills while continuing to negotiate the larger health care system where APNs practice (Bellak, Graber, O'Neil, Musham, & Lancaster, 1999).

Advanced practice nursing educators have built on these developments in synergy with a dynamic health care environment. Consequently, core graduate, APN, and specialty knowledge, skills, and competencies aimed at improving practice have evolved. As the demands for health care shift, new and existing educational programs for APNs have continued to thrive because of APNs' adaptability and flexibility. Education for advanced nursing practice over the past decade has been standardized and expanded through formal guidelines for curriculum, program standards, evaluation criteria, and program review. Although educational programs have moved toward standardization, evaluation criteria are far from proscriptive, allowing graduate nursing education to remain open to the creation of leading-edge APN roles.

The general goals of APN education programs are

- To continue to prepare competent APNs as leaders and members of the nursing profession and the future health care workforce
- To prepare APNs as cost-effective, competent health care providers, based on supply-and-demand needs
- To maintain flexibility in educating APNs for innovative roles in a dynamic health care system
- To improve health care through the education of APNs

Preparation for advanced nursing practice has moved well beyond its early beginnings toward meeting these ambitious goals. This chapter discusses the definition and context of APN education and the environmental elements affecting it, proposes a model for APN curriculum and education, describes teaching and learning strategies in APN education; and raises challenges for the future.

DEFINING APN EDUCATION

Definition

Chapter 3 states that the APN applies "an expanded range of practical, theoretical, and research-based therapeutics to phenomena experienced by patients within a specialized clinical area of the larger discipline of nursing" (p. 56). This statement addresses the centrality of direct clinical practice in advanced nursing practice and the integration of specialization, expansion, and advancement in a clinical field. As Hamric explains, this description of the APN role recognizes the primary criteria and competency-based features of advanced nursing practice. APNs share the same primary criteria and core competencies, although actual clinical practice skills vary depending on the needs of the patient population and the corresponding environment (see Chapter 3 and the chapters in Part IV for discussion of important environmental elements).

The primary criteria for advanced practice incorporate several elements, including (1) an earned graduate degree in nursing at either the master's, post-master's, or doctoral level; (2) the integration of theory, research, and APN role function into practice; (3) the expansion of specialized knowledge and skills relevant to the core competencies of the particular nursing specialty; and (4) sufficient faculty-supervised clinical practice in the appropriate specialty. The specialized clinical knowledge and skill base, essential to the provision of care, allows the APN to exercise highly refined clinical judgment in a given specialty within the context of the patient-provider relationship and the health care environment.

Core competencies are the performance-based features of APN graduate educational programs. Direct clinical practice, the central competency, is characterized by a holistic and optimistic perspective, partnerships with patients and communities, clinical reasoning, and diverse management approaches (see Chapter 6). Because nursing education programs are derived from society's fundamental needs for health care, the curricular content, skills, and competencies needed by APNs are constantly evaluated for their practice-based relevance within the larger context of a dynamic health care environment. The demand for APN roles continues to evolve as the characteristics of advanced nursing practice environments change in conjunction with the organizational, business, regulatory, policy, reimbursement, population, and health workforce elements in health care (see Part IV).

Domains of Practice

APN educators are essential in defining the specialized knowledge and skills needed in the advanced roles of nurse practitioner (NP), certified nurse-midwife (CNM), clinical nurse specialist (CNS), and certified registered nurse anesthetist (CRNA). In addition to constantly monitoring existing APN roles, APN educators should be at the forefront of clarifying evolving roles such as the APN case manager and the blended CNS/NP role. Some authors have organized the knowledge and skills needed for advanced nursing practice according to domains and competencies derived from qualitative analysis of expert nurses in practice (Benner, 1984; Boodley et al., 1995; Fenton & Brykczynski, 1993). Benner (1984) defined "domain" as a cluster of competencies with similar intentions, functions, and meanings. Graduate nursing educators have used domains to identify and cluster curriculum knowledge and skills needed for the education of APNs. These practice domains have provided a potential curriculum infrastructure (Boodley et al., 1995; Fenton & Brykczynski, 1993) for APN clinical education, particularly for NPs and CNSs. More recently, the National Association of Clinical Nurse Specialists (NACNS) (1998) has developed a statement on CNS education that provides a beginning framework for the progression and evolution of CNS education at the graduate level. The roles chapters in Part III further describe these frameworks for the various APN specialties. The domains and competencies converge in APN educational programs through curriculum guidelines, evaluation criteria, and/ or the identification of competency behaviors needed for graduation from APN programs.

APN CRITERIA WITHIN THE CONTEXT OF GRADUATE NURSING EDUCATION

As is evident, advanced nursing practice curricula and competencies are not stagnant but evolve in response to numerous forces. New models of clinical practice, new therapies in disease and prevention management, and new roles emerge and lead to further revision and development of curricula. The interface between the spheres of advanced clinical practice, research, and education orbits in an upward spiral synergistically, building on the knowledge embedded in theory and practice. Hence the APN curriculum develops through this relationship between theory and practice, testing existing roles and initiating new APN roles and competencies (Brown, 1998).

Curricular depth and breadth matured with the growth and development of each of the APN roles. Because each role originated at different points in time over the past 60 years, the educational programs for NPs, CNSs, CRNAs, and CNMs were formed originally as separate entities, rather than in one unified educational framework in graduate nursing (see Chapter 1). However, during the past 10 years, the core nursing, core APN, and core specialty content has created a unifying curricular framework for graduate nursing and associated specialty education. This section describes this framework within the context of graduate nursing education: its models for articulation, accreditation standards, credentialing, regulation, and program review.

Graduate Nursing Education

APNs are prepared at the graduate level in master's, post-master's, or doctoral educational programs. Typically, these graduate programs are 1 to 2 years of full-time study or 2 to 4 years of part-time study. The 1-year programs typically involve intensive coursework and practica experiences to meet the competency requirements. Clinical practica in which students provide direct clinical care and negotiate various aspects of health care systems are an essential part of the educational program. APN graduate programs prepare students to engage in advanced clinical decision making both for professional nursing functions and, in selected roles, for medical functions traditionally performed by physicians and other health professionals.

The educational requirements for each APN role shifted toward graduate nursing education as the nursing profession recognized the need for the master's degree to be the educational standard for advanced practice (see Chapter 1). Although variation once existed in the level of preparation for the NP, CNM, and CRNA roles, from master's to post-master's to postbasic (certificate), the graduate degree in nursing is now viewed as the minimum standard for APN practice. There are exceptions, however. For example, the American Association of Nurse Anesthetists (AANA) (see Chapter 18) has required a master's- or higher level degree effective 1998, but the master's degree is not required to be in the nursing discipline (AANA, 1999). Although past variation in educational level has been a longstanding issue for graduate nursing education, APN programs are currently offered in all graduate nursing schools with the exception of less than 1% of postbasic certificate NP programs (American Association of Colleges of Nursing [AACN], 1999a). These few remaining certificate programs are affiliated with master's nursing programs for core master's and APN coursework is readily available through electronic coursework and/or teaching strategies among schools of nursing throughout the country. An excellent example is the distance education offered for CNMs through the Frontier Nursing Service (AACN, 1996b). The trend toward graduate preparation of APN roles arose in the 1980s and accelerated in the 1990s, as the norm for new APN programs became graduate nursing or postbasic certification programs affiliated with graduate schools of nursing.

CNSs have traditionally been graduates of master's-level nursing programs. The CNS role consistently established its roots in and has been supported by the nursing education community. Since the early 1990s, the trend to offer dual-track CNS/NP role preparation has increased based on the demand for subspecialty APN practice (see Chapter 16). Also, in response to the perceived demand, programs were offered to prepare nurses (usually CNSs) with graduate degrees (master's and doctoral) as NPs, CNMs, or CRNAs through post-master's graduate nursing coursework. The growth in merged CNS/NP roles and the tremendous movement of CNSs toward post-master's NP programs has offered the potential for expansion of APN roles into new practice areas. Graduate educational programs for the APN case manager role are being developed as the new health system creates opportunities for this role in response to society's need for health care.

Articulated APN Educational Models

APN education has moved well beyond its origins of continuing education in postbasic (registered nurse [RN] certificate) programs in affiliated schools of medicine to graduate-level preparation in schools of nursing at master's, post-master's and doctoral levels. Differing educational preparation has been a prevailing issue for nurses, including APNs, and continues to be an issue. For example, an estimated 66% of practicing NPs, CNMs, and CRNAs were not educated in master's-level nursing programs as recently as 5 years ago (Aiken, Gwyther, & Whelan, 1994). Hence, there remains an apparent need for a process through which individuals practicing in APN roles progress to higher levels of education with minimal barriers and minimal duplication of knowledge and skills (AACN, 1993). Educational mobility is an issue for all APNs given the redesign of the health system and emergence of new roles. In the past two decades, nursing education has had great success in developing articulated educational models in its RN-to–bachelor's of science in nursing (BSN) and RN to master's in nursing programs. Similar principles of educational mobility have been applied to nurses needing either undergraduate or graduate coursework for APN preparation, such as seen with post-master's NP programs.

There are five general types of students who need articulated educational programs:

1. Certificate-prepared NPs, CNMs, and CRNAs with a baccalaureate degree: master's of science in nursing (MSN) pathway
2. RNs without BSN preparation seeking accelerated master's preparation as an APN: RN to MSN pathway
3. Students who have a baccalaureate degree other than nursing and are seeking APN preparation at the master's level: generic master's pathway
4. Students with BSN degrees seeking a clinical doctoral degree as APNs: BSN to doctorate pathway
5. Master's prepared APNs seeking post-master's preparation as an NP: post-master's certificate pathway

Students in these various pathways, such as those students pursuing the clinical doctorate for APNs at the University of Tennessee at Memphis, have unique needs based on their personal and educational characteristics. Numerous programs have been tailored to the specific needs of each of these student groups. The common denominators in these programs are flexibility, acceleration and consolidation of content to avoid repetition, identification of a common core of content at either the graduate or undergraduate level, and an established programmatic competency-based curriculum model for articulation. These characteristics define the type of articulation model based on the unique needs and past experiences of the group of students being served.

An articulated curriculum model for RNs seeking master's preparation as APNs frequently includes advanced placement credit for undergraduate nursing coursework through examination, an accelerated curriculum that consolidates core graduate coursework with undergraduate coursework, and specially tailored clinical practice experiences. An articulated curriculum model for a certificate-prepared NP, CNM, or CRNA who does not have a baccalaureate degree often incorporates baccalaureate content for nursing and general education courses. Advanced placement exams are used in both undergraduate and graduate nursing courses, with standard APN core courses identified to prevent duplication of content. Graduate nursing coursework is tailored to incorporate a stronger emphasis on theory and research application. These programs need to explicitly address the APN core competencies identified early in the program, so graduates are prepared to function at an advanced level.

Two nontraditional educational pathways need further scrutiny by nurse educators seeking to build flexible APN pathway programs: the generic master's and the RN-to-MSN APN programs. The generic master's program builds on a bachelor's degree in a non-nursing field and incorporates the curriculum in the first professional nursing degree with the advanced practice curriculum to prepare an APN. These programs usually incorporate accelerated content for undergraduate and graduate knowledge, skills, and competencies. They are typically offered over a 2- to 3-year period, with intensive curricular content and clinical practicum experiences incorporating both undergraduate- and graduate-level APN clinical experiences.

The RN-to-MSN articulated pathway builds on professional nursing preparation at the associate degree or diploma level and incorporates the bachelor's and master's in nursing curricula to prepare an APN. Given that advanced nursing practice is built on the foundation of professional nursing practice and is competency based, each of these nontraditional pathways requires additional curricular content and clinical practicum experiences with faculty supervision. The direct practice component is enhanced in these programs in several ways: (1) the inexperienced graduate learner receives direct faculty supervision; (2) faculty supervision is conducted by clinically practicing faculty; and (3) additional clinical time is constructed through internship, residency, and/or mentoring experiences. Accelerated programs for students seeking a second degree are relatively expensive, because of the faculty resources needed to prepare these students both as competent RNs and as APNs. Students selected for these programs need to be highly motivated and willing to commit to full-time study and, particularly for the generic master's student, to clinical practice in order to be able to synthesize the broad-based content needed in these programs. Nontraditional graduate learners can be successful at achieving APN competencies through programs designed to provide additional clinical faculty resources and more concentrated faculty-supervised clinical practicum experiences.

In addition to the generic master's and RN-to-MSN programs, attention must be directed to clinical doctoral programs (Vesser, Stegbauer, & Russel, 1999) as well as professional development for lifelong learning. The ongoing advancements in clinical knowledge and technology development will demand new professional skills and competencies by all types of health care providers. Further testing must be conducted to determine the advanced clinical knowledge, skills, and competencies needed for future APN roles. Finally, the need for continuing professional development for APNs continues to offer leadership opportunities for graduate nursing educators to reinvent and realign continuing professional development through postgraduate programs and/or professional organizations. Given that change is a constant in health care and the knowledge age, informatics and electronic communications will open up new fields of learning in the new century. Furthermore, as the environment becomes more integrated, continuing professional education will become more interdisciplinary for all health care providers as health systems more clearly define a collaborative paradigm for health care.

Educational Standards for APN Programs

Leadership in promoting quality APN educational programs at the graduate level remains paramount, given the increased use of APNs in the health care workforce and the growing momentum for public accountability (Gelmon et al., 1999). Initially, APN educators were particularly successful in safeguarding the quality of educational programs through careful attention to educational program outcomes using a peer process of program review associated with federal funding of APN programs. Among the educational strategies used to safeguard the quality of program outcomes were selective admission to APN programs, limited numbers of APN students, low faculty-to-student ratios, and systematic evaluation of clinical knowledge and skills. These professional self-regulation strategies are implicit in program review and accreditation. The federal review process for APN education is currently being revised to reflect the most recent standards and regulations for APN credentialing and practice.

Quality control was furthered by ensuring that program graduates met established competency levels for designated clinical practice areas. For example, the American College of Nurse-Midwives (ACNM) (1992) and AANA Council on Accreditation (1994, 1998) were pioneers in delineating the fundamental knowledge, skills, and behaviors expected of new CNMs and CRNAs. The National Organization of Nurse Practitioner Faculties (NONPF; Boodley et al., 1995) delineated practice domains and competencies expected of new graduates. Likewise, the NACNS (1998) developed curriculum guidelines for CNSs. Because of the distinctive nature of specialty content in APN programs, professional associations define their own specialty content through standards of practice and competencies. As examples of this, the Oncology Nursing Society, the National Association of Pediatric Nurse Associates and Practitioners, and the National Association of Nurse Practitioners in Reproductive Health all stipulate specialty content, standards, and competencies for graduates of these respective programs. Because no specialty organizations stipulate adult, family, or gerontological NP competencies, the NONPF has begun to develop competencies for each of these specialized clinical areas (NONPF, 1999).

Other organizational statements and positions have contributed to more uniform standards for APN education. *Nursing's Social Policy Statement* (American Nurses Association [ANA], 1995) and *Scope and Standards of Advanced Practice Nursing* (ANA, 1996) provide a strong philosophical foundation for educating nurses in advanced practice roles. The AACN (1996, 1998) developed consensus statements on the essentials of master's and baccalaureate nursing education. In response to the growing debate over the education of APN clinicians, the AACN master's essentials document (1996) identified the core elements of master's program curricula for nurses, establishing a unified framework through the identification of a "common educational core." This important work led toward the standardization of a common core curriculum in programs for NPs, CNSs, CNMs, and CRNAs as well as other evolving roles. In addition, this project has been instrumental in distinguishing the common features of APN graduate education. These features include (1) the graduate core generic to all master's nursing degrees, (2) the advanced practice core generic to all advanced nursing practice, and (3) the specialty role core specific to each APN role (Figure 4–1). The "essential" curriculum elements identified through consensus among graduate nursing educators include (1) a common graduate core curriculum

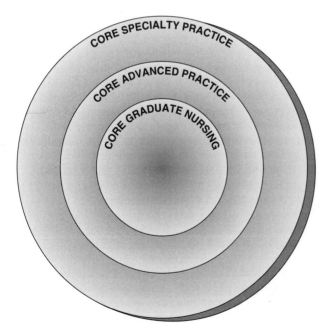

FIGURE 4–1 · Core advanced nursing practice curriculum.

for all master's degree nursing students and (2) the core curriculum content for APNs. In the AACN project, the graduate core curriculum for all master's students identified the common content areas of research and outcome evaluation, role theory, economics, ethical/decision-making issues, health policy, integrated health systems, informatics, managed care, business, reimbursement, regulatory and marketing principles, nursing theory, and cultural diversity. The APN core curriculum identified advanced health assessment, pathophysiology and/or related science, advanced pharmacology (AACN, 1995), population-based care, health promotion, and disease prevention as common to all APN roles.

Figure 4–2 visually combines the conceptual model and competencies defined by Hamric in Chapter 3 with the educational process for APN education. The core APN competencies of leadership, collaboration, coaching and teaching, consultation, research, and ethical decision-making skills are superimposed on the three levels of APN education—core graduate nursing, core advanced practice nursing, and core specialty practice nursing. The central competency, direct clinical practice, drives the process and is key to both education and practice for APNs. All levels of the

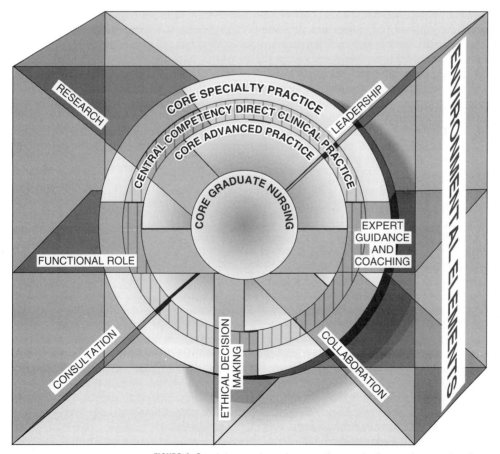

FIGURE 4–2 • Advanced nursing practice curriculum and competencies.

curriculum are taught within the context of the dynamic elements within the practice and educational environments.

The analysis of core components of APN education has been a progressive process, building on organizational and individual linkages and contributions. The most efficient mechanism for developing consistency in the education of nurses for advanced practice is to identify the common graduate educational requirements for each of these roles and to compare and contrast the differences and similarities in these requirements and the specific content among the roles and specialties. Future work needs to be done to analyze the content of specific APN roles, including their associated competencies within the standardized core APN curriculum.

The NONPF, in collaboration with the National Council of State Boards of Nursing, published a report on *Curriculum Guidelines and Regulatory Criteria for Family Nurse Practitioners Seeking Prescriptive Authority to Manage Pharmacotherapeutics in Primary Care* (Yocum, Busby, Conway-Welch, & Viens, 1999). This project contributes to improving standardization among pharmacology/pharmacotherapeutics curricula that prepare family NPs for prescriptive privileges. It also can assist state-level regulatory boards to develop criteria for determining eligibility for prescriptive authority (Yocum et al., 1999).

With the exception of well-developed specialties such as oncology and critical care nursing, standards for the CNS role have been highly variable because of the lack of core APN requirements. Graduate educators must define the specialty knowledge, skills, and competencies needed for CNS practice in conjunction with the standards of various specialty organizations and collaborate on developing a system to administer those standards if this APN role is to survive. The NACNS has begun this important work through its position statement (1998).

APN programs have demonstrated their willingness to develop program accountability through educational standards. This is most clearly seen in the case of CRNA and CNM standards and programs. Yet the process of accountability needs further development through ongoing program review and evaluation (NONPF, 1999) for all APN roles.

Graduate Nursing Accreditation

The major accrediting bodies for undergraduate and master's level nursing education are the National League for Nursing Accreditation Council (NLNAC) and the Commission of Collegiate Nursing Education (CCNE). The NLNAC accreditation process uses 20 outcome-based criteria as essential components for achieving positive graduate and program outcomes. These 20 outcome-based criteria are categorized according to (1) structure and governance, (2) material resources, (3) students, (4) faculty, (5) curriculum, and (6) required outcome criteria for the program. In addition to the outcome-based criteria, other specific areas must be demonstrated as part of the evaluation for accreditation. These areas include critical thinking, communication, therapeutic nursing interventions, graduation rates, and patterns of employment. This approach is particularly relevant for the preparation of APNs because graduate nursing educators must validate educational outcomes for the production of skilled, competent providers. Hence, the current NLNAC accreditation process enables graduate educators to move toward this goal.

The CCNE (1998) based its accreditation process on compliance with standards, their key elements, and examples of evidence used for baccalaureate and/or graduate nursing education programs. Among the standards used to evaluate the quality of educational programs and institutional performance are mission and governance, institutional commitment and resources, curriculum and teaching-learning practices, student performance, and faculty achievements. Of particular relevance to graduate nursing education is the program quality standard on curriculum and teaching-learning practices (CCNE, 1998). This standard describes key elements of APN curricula:

III-B. The master's curriculum builds on the competencies of baccalaureate graduates and focuses on advanced nursing roles.
III-C. The curriculum, teaching-learning practices and teaching environments foster behaviors *consistent with professional nursing standards and guidelines.*
III-Fb. The master's nursing curriculum incorporates content and learning experiences essential to performance in advanced nursing roles (CCNE, 1998; emphasis added).

These selected curriculum areas reinforce the performance- (read competency-) based nature of advanced practice nursing consistent with professional nursing guidelines and standards. Among the professional standards identified in CCNE's accreditation standards are *The Essentials of Master's Education for Advanced Practice Nursing* (AACN, 1996), *Criteria for Evaluation of Nurse Practitioner Programs* (National Task Force on Quality Nurse Practitioner Education, 1997), and various professional practice standards of the American Nurses Association. The AANA Council on Accreditation (1999) and the ACNM (1993) provide companion accreditation processes that are administered in concert with graduate accreditation procedures. Both CNM and CNRA educational programs must receive preapproval before they offer a program or admit students (AANA, 1992; ACNM, 1993).

APN Regulation, Credentialing, and Program Review

Given the abilities of specific schools, state regulatory agencies, accrediting bodies, and credentialing centers to independently establish differing standards, it is incumbent upon APN educators to exercise leadership in promoting the maintenance of quality APN programs through consistent curriculum standards and program review. External processes intrinsic to the regulation of APNs include national and state certification, state credentialing processes, and program review and accreditation. Each of these external processes supports mechanisms for validating knowledge and competencies for graduates of APN programs. These external processes have had a major influence on APN education, linking educational preparation to professional competency and accountability. Each of the advanced practice roles has its own distinct procedures for obtaining certification and credentialing.

As for NP educational programs, the NONPF has established minimum standards for NP programs in its *Advanced Nursing Practice: Curriculum Guidelines and Program Standards for Nurse Practitioner Education* (Boodley et al., 1995). Furthermore, the National Task Force on Quality Nurse Practitioner Education (1997) advocates a voluntary program review process in relation to these standards. Beyond these program standards, selected evaluation criteria have been addressed for specific groups (AANA, 1999; ACNM, 1993; National Task Force on Quality Nurse Practitioner Education, 1997). These evaluation criteria establish the minimum requirements for the designated roles without being highly proscriptive, thereby maintaining a degree of flexibility to accommodate emerging APN roles. The National Task Force on Quality Nurse Practitioner Education (1997), convened by the NONPF, is representative of 11 advanced nursing practice educational and credentialing organizations that endorse a criteria-based framework of evaluation for NP programs.

In addition, depending on the NP specialty (i.e., obstetrical/gynecological, pediatric, family, adult, women's health, or neonatal), several mechanisms for certification and credentialing are available. Each of these respective NP specialties has separate credentialing bodies, such as the National Certification Center, the American Nurses Credentialing Center, the National Certification Board for Pediatric Nursing Specialties, and the American Academy of Nurse Practitioners. Similarly, each credentialing body has its own distinct criteria to allow graduates of NP programs to sit for their respective national certification exams. Among the criteria are

- The type of educational degrees or certificates awarded (i.e., graduate nursing credit)
- The number of didactic and faculty-supervised clinical hours in the educational program
- The type of curriculum offered in the program, including core master's, advanced practice, and specialty
- Whether the curriculum matches the standards of practice or competencies for each particular specialty

Likewise, the ACNM and the AANA allow only those graduates of approved programs to sit for the national certification exams. CNSs are able to receive national certification through the American Nurses Credentialing Center and a variety of other specialty organizations, but frequently national and/or state certification is not a requirement for CNSs to practice in their role (see Chapter 22). Through these credentialing centers and certification bodies, the APN community has strengthened its linkages among educational, accrediting, and regulatory bodies, as well as other APN organizations. However, much work remains to develop common standards among national and state regulatory bodies, credentialing processes, and accreditation if APNs are to demonstrate accountability for continued improvement in health care.

APN Educators

Within the context outlined earlier, APN educators must be responsive and resilient in their orientation toward curriculum development, implementation, and evaluation. This orientation requires that APN educators maintain current and timely knowledge and competency in their clinical fields associated with trends in the health care marketplace, flexibility in curriculum adaptation and revision, and a willingness to restructure as needed. In fact, these requisite skills are contingent upon current clinical knowledge and faculty practice (see Chapter 26) for the integration of the academic mission.

Advanced practice nursing's strength lies in its ability to span nursing as well as selected interdisciplinary boundaries while concurrently enhancing the student's depth and breadth of knowledge in an APN specialty area. These areas include but are not limited to medicine and its specialties, including managed care configurations, alternative health practices, public health, psychology, sociology, anthropology, informatics, and a host of other fields integrally related to specialty practice.

ENVIRONMENTAL ELEMENTS AFFECTING APN EDUCATION

Environmental elements have created educational challenges for the preparation of APNs. Advanced nursing practice has been particularly responsive to society's needs by developing the leading-edge roles described throughout this book. Several categories emerge as priorities among environmental elements influencing health care delivery and APN education in the 21st century. Foremost among these are policy-making considerations driven by population-based and health care trends, such as the rapid increase in culturally and ethnically diverse populations, and the financing of graduate nursing education. A second priority is reimbursement and payment mechanisms driven by the increasing numbers of aging and medically underserved populations in the United States. Another key environmental element is organizational structure and culture, which are being influenced by managed care and changing health workforce requirements. Following is a discussion of these environmental forces and their potential impact on future APN education.

Policy-Making Considerations

CULTURAL DIVERSITY

The growing number of diverse populations is creating new demands for a diverse workforce prepared to deliver culturally sensitive health care in the United States and globally. Yet the growing ethnic diversity associated with this cultural shift is not reflected in the health workforce of today or the foreseeable future. An estimated 28% of this country's population represents racially and/or ethnically diverse groups, with an anticipated growth to 40% by 2010 (O'Neil et al., 1998). However, the supply pipeline continues to have relatively low numbers of ethnically diverse and/or culturally disadvantaged faculty or students in APN programs. In the most recent survey of master's and NP programs (Berlin, Bednash, and Hosier, 1999), less than 11% of all NP students represented ethnic minorities. These diversity trends have significant implications for APN education and the preparation of a culturally competent workforce. Improvement in the recruitment, retention, and graduation of ethnic minorities in APN roles is critical if the workforce is to be representative of the population it serves. Relative to the development of a culturally competent APN workforce, APNs will also need to expand their language skills to accommodate and meet the health needs of populations who have English as a second language. These relatively new phenomena call for APN programs to address both the cultural components of care and language capabilities among faculty and students.

FINANCING APN EDUCATION

One of the most significant influences in developing educational programs for NPs, CNMs, CNSs, and CRNAs in the past 20 years has been the Title VIII funding for advanced education of professional nurses provided by the Division of Nursing of the U.S. Department of Health and Human Services. From the perspective of the federal government, APN programs are an innovative way both to prepare new types of advanced nurses with an emphasis on delivering care and to expand access to care for medically underserved populations. For this reason, some of the Title VIII monies were originally designated to provide line-item funding for CNS, NP, CNM, and CRNA educational programs. This legislation provided the stimulus to support faculty and operational costs for many of the APN programs in the United States. The legislative mandate primarily supported new APN programs targeted to vulnerable populations and APN programs in remote geographic locations. The Nursing Education Act (Title VIII of the Public Health Service Act, 42 U.S.C. § 296 et seq.) was enacted 30 years ago and is reauthorized every 2 years through the federal legislature; the reauthorization in 1998 occurred through the Health Professions Education Partnerships Act of 1998. The fiscal year 1998 programs for APN education entitlements were as follows: advanced nursing education program grants, $12.5 million; NP and CNM program grants, $17.64 million: CRNA program grants, $2.77 million; traineeships for advanced education of professional nurses, $15.99 million; and Nursing Special Projects, $10.6 million (Nurse Education and Practice Improvement Amendments of 1992). Other federal initiatives that support APN preparation are the National Health Service Corps scholarships, the Area Health Education Centers, and the Office of Rural Health. As is evident from the fiscal year 1998 appropriations, federal funding for APN programs has had a significant impact on the maturation of APN roles through the nursing educational environment.

Another potential source of subsidy funding for APN education exists in the Medicare subsidy for Graduate Medical Education (GME) written into legislation in 1965. An estimated $200 million annually supports hospitals with diploma nursing programs in existence prior to 1985. These revenues need to be redirected to accountable funding for graduate nursing education instead of being used to support hospitals with pre-existing diploma nursing programs. By redirecting these GME dollars to clinical sites serving graduate APN programs, a clinical training infrastructure for *all* of nursing education could be developed (Pew Commission Federal Policy Task Force, 1998).

Policy Makers Influencing APN Education

Health policy centers, expert panels, and several foundations have had significant external influence in promoting advanced practice and its educational agenda as part of the future health system. Among the foundations are the Pew Charitable Trusts, the W. K. Kellogg Foundation, and the Robert Wood Johnson Foundation. For the past 10 years, the Pew Health Professions Commission has focused its efforts on restructuring health professions education. Among these efforts, the Commission's landmark report on schools in service to the nation (O'Neil et al., 1993) and its recent report on *Recreating Health Professional Practice for a New Century* (O'Neil et al., 1998) have exerted a direct impact on APN and other health professional education. The most recent recommendations and competencies needed by all health professional groups are listed in Tables 4–1 and 4–2. Specific recommendations for APNs are listed in Table 4–3.

In concurrent projects, both the Kellogg Foundation (1999) and the Robert Wood Johnson Foundation (1999) have focused initiatives on the development and training of interdisciplinary community-based primary care providers. Through its academic-

TABLE 4-1 RECOMMENDATIONS FOR ALL HEALTH PROFESSIONAL GROUPS

- Professional school faculties and administration should evaluate their current course of study to determine whether or not they are adequately preparing students to meet the challenges set forth in the competencies.
- Professional associations should integrate the competencies into their accreditation and licensing processes, benchmarks for graduation, entry into professional practice, and continuing competence.
- Students should assess the quality of educational programs based on how well they will prepare them to apply the competencies in their careers.
- Hospitals and other institutional providers should prefer partnerships with academic institutions that continuously revise their curricula to reflect changing market dynamics and those that embody the competencies.

Adapted from O'Neil, E. H., and the Pew Health Professions Commission. (1998). *Recreating health professional practice for a new century*. San Francisco: Pew Health Professions Commission, Pew Charitable Trust Foundation; reprinted with permission.

community partnership initiatives, the Kellogg Foundation has invested more than $61 million to craft new community-based, academic-service consortia to improve primary care education and delivery. These partnerships involve schools of medicine, schools of nursing, and communities as equity partners in attempts to shift the graduate and undergraduate education and clinical training of nurses, APNs, and physicians from traditional medical centers and ambulatory care centers to community-based centers. Likewise, the Robert Wood Johnson Foundation (1999) has provided significant support to reinvent primary care education and service

TABLE 4-2 COMPETENCIES FOR THE 21ST CENTURY

1. Embrace a personal ethic of social responsibility and service.
2. Exhibit ethical behavior in all professional activities.
3. Provide evidence-based, clinically competent care.
4. Incorporate the multiple determinants of health in clinical care.
5. Apply knowledge of the new sciences.
6. Demonstrate critical thinking, reflection, and problem-solving skills.
7. Understand the role of primary care.
8. Rigorously practice preventive health care.
9. Integrate population-based care and services into practice.
10. Improve access to health care for those with unmet health needs.
11. Practice relationship-centered care with individuals and families.
12. Provide culturally sensitive care to diverse society.
13. Partner with communities in health care decisions.
14. Use communication and information technology effectively and appropriately.
15. Work in interdisciplinary teams.
16. Ensure care that balances individual, professional, system, and societal needs.
17. Practice leadership.
18. Take responsibility for quality of care and health outcomes at all levels.
19. Contribute to continuous improvement of the health care system.
20. Advocate for public policy that promotes and protects the health of the public.
21. Continue to learn and help others learn.

Adapted from O'Neil, E. H., and the Pew Health Professions Commission. (1998). *Recreating health professional practice for a new century*. San Francisco: Pew Health Professions Commission, Pew Charitable Trust Foundation; reprinted with permission.

TABLE 4–3 RECOMMENDATIONS FOR ADVANCED PRACTICE NURSING

1. Reorient advanced practice nursing education programs to prepare APNs for the changing situations and settings in which they are likely to practice.
   • Prepare APNs to translate a core set of skills across institutions and settings, managing persons with health care problems regardless of their location.
   • Expand the proportion of advanced practice nurse training sites in ambulatory and long-term care settings favored by managed care systems.
2. Regardless of payer source (Health Care Financing Administration or an all-payer pool), federal funding for graduate medical education should be made available to support the training of advanced practice nurses and other nonphysician providers in clinical settings.
   • Pay funds directly to the clinical service site providing APN training and not to the educational programs that are responsible for planning education.
   • Develop a mechanism to ensure that this funding does not create an unwarranted expansion of the total number of training positions for APNs.
3. Develop standard guidelines for advanced nursing practice and reinforce them with curriculum guidelines, examination requirements, and accreditation regulations.
   • Establish standards for interdependent versus autonomous practice, prescriptive authority, hospital admitting privileges, civil liability, and other critical areas.
   • Gather input from a broad set of health disciplines to ensure that guidelines reflect the diversity of APN practice in the delivery system.
4. Emphasize the practice styles that are a critical part of advanced practice nursing, including the emphasis on preventive and health-promoting interventions and attention to psychosocial, environmental, and resource factors.
   • Support research to examine the effect of these practice characteristics on outcomes in the populations served by emerging health care networks.
   • Enhance the research training of APN students to ensure that future APNs have the background to evaluate and advocate for effective practice styles.

Adapted from O'Neil, E. H., and the Pew Health Professions Commission. (1998). *Recreating health professional practice for a new century.* San Francisco: Pew Health Professions Commission, Pew Charitable Trust Foundation; reprinted with permission.

delivery among interdisciplinary groups of primary care providers. These initiatives have been successful in increasing the supply and distribution of generalist physicians as well as NPs, physician assistants (PAs), and CNMs. They have also shaped health professions education to manage care more effectively. Each of these interdisciplinary primary care initiatives designates APNs as bona fide providers and essential members of the health care team. Common elements of interdisciplinary education for graduate medicine and nursing are discussed later in this chapter.

Other external forces have guided the development of population-based health competencies in APN curricula. *Healthy People 2010: National Health Promotion and Disease Prevention Objectives* is currently under revision by the Office of Disease Prevention and Health Promotion (ODPHP) of the U.S. Department of Health and Human Services (U.S. Public Health Service, 2000). With the health policy emphasis on effective, economical quality care, the ODPHP developed national clinical prevention guidelines and benchmarks to improve the consistent, systematic delivery of clinical preventive services. Population-based approaches to health care and education have gained recognition as the overarching concept to assess the health of a population and the capacity to develop outcomes for health-adjusted life expectancy (American Association of Colleges of Medicine, 1998; Kindig, 1999). APNs are key members of provider teams capable of designing and implementing these approaches (Wagner, 1998). Working from the historical context of nursing, APN faculty and students provide leadership in communities applying health promotion, systems care, disease prevention, and behavioral change across integrated health systems. However, population-based approaches to health require APN educators to expand content on community-based care, informatics, managed care, and health system competencies.

Reimbursement/Payment Mechanisms

MEDICARE AND AGING POPULATIONS

The demographic shift toward an aging population calls for a highly skilled health workforce that can address the health care needs of the skyrocketing elderly population in the United States. Currently, the elderly consume the vast majority of health resources, often during their last year of life. Considering current Medicare policy, chronic, case management, and preventive care will demand innovative strategies in providing care for the elderly in the next millenium. The complex health care needs of this population create demands in services across primary, secondary, and tertiary care settings, requiring knowledge and clinical decision-making, and continuity skills for rapidly changing, unpredictable situations—skills common among APNs. The advent of Medicare reimbursement for APNs and the prospect of dramatic changes in existing Medicare legislation will influence the APN's ways of learning, knowing, and practicing in the future (Buerhaus, 1998). The regulations governing Medicare require variation in clinical decision making that must be considered by APN educators as they construct curricula about clinical decision making for elderly persons. Likewise, Medicare regulations and payment policies for elder populations must be integrated into practice management, clinical decision making, and a research agenda, so APNs can be successful at rendering clinical services.

MEDICALLY UNDERSERVED POPULATIONS

The increasing proportion of medically underserved and vulnerable populations in the United States creates a tension and pressure on the existing health care system. Employers and managed care plans include approximately one third of all Medicaid recipients but continue to exclude segments of the working poor population in this country. An estimated 45 million people are categorized as being without health coverage or insurance (O'Neil et al., 1998). These access issues underscore the need for communities as partners and an accountable health system for all. APN programs, their faculty, and students have provided leadership in this area through the development of nursing centers in communities of need (National Health Policy Forum, 1999; see Chapter 26). These nursing centers serve as intermediary health resources for communities with limited access to health care, bridging the barriers associated with access-to-health-care issues. This type of educational environment mandates that APN programs provide curriculum and health system experiences in federal and state policy, regulations, and reimbursement for their graduate learners. Similarly, if APNs are to develop opportunities associated with negotiating Medicaid and Medicare managed care contracts for these underserved populations, they need to understand the legal context of federal and state requirements as well as qualifications for contractors within the context of the communities being served.

Marketing and Contracting in a Managed Care Environment

Managed care, with the focus on quality and cost, continues to be one of the major driving forces in the health care system. More than one half of the total U.S. population is covered under some type of managed care program. As managed care organizations have taken the lead as the major payer in health systems (Center for Health Policy and Research, 1999), so must the elements of managed care be incorporated into graduate nursing education with specific application for advanced practice nursing. These elements include, but are not limited to, epidemiology, business and partnership models, human and organizational behavior, information systems, quality measurement and improvement, health care financing and delivery, and systems-based care (Lurie, 1996). Other areas frequently cited (Yedidia & Gillespie, 1999) include practice guidelines, utilization management, evidence-based practice, disease management and preventive services, economics of managed care, and ethical and cost-effective decision making. The Partnerships for Quality Education (PQE) projects for medical residents and NPs are based on the integration of key managed care concepts into APN and medical curricula at both didactic and clinical levels (Robert Wood Johnson Foundation, 1999).

An APN needs to have the conceptual ability to move seamlessly through the health system. To navigate managed care and integrate care across systems requires boundary-spanning skills. Boundary-spanning skills include (but are not limited to) the following areas:

- The ability to practice in a variety of peer-unobserved settings and obtain consultation through the use of remote or technologically linked resources
- The ability to integrate care across settings with other providers (Mundinger & Gilliss, 1998)
- The ability to conduct "knowledge work" to analyze information and apply specialized expertise to solve problems, generate ideas, teach others, or create new products or services using information from a variety of disciplines
- The development of the "knowledge work team" based on particular knowledge and clinical skills, such as a palliative care, primary care, or geriatric care (Sorrells-Jones, 1999).

These essential skills for managed care practice are necessary if APNs are to move patients toward high-quality, cost-effective care. The information age emphasizes knowledge work and interdisciplinary collaboration for boundary spanning across systems to create innovative models of care. These areas need further development, integration, and testing within APN programs. Future attention must focus on faculty development and curriculum revision to include evidence-based practice and outcomes, population-based care, evaluation and research networks to promote "best/ innovative practices" in managed care environments, and the balance between costs of care and quality improvement to determine the value of care (see Chapter 25).

Organizational Structure and Culture

DEMOGRAPHICS OF THE NURSING WORKFORCE

While the demographics of the country are undergoing aging and cultural changes, similar issues are reflected among nursing professionals and faculty in schools of nursing. Many APNs are aging, with a concurrent "graying of the faculty." The mean age of RNs (44 years) has risen steadily over the past 10 years, and the average age of graduation from basic nursing education programs has also risen to 31.7 years (Moses, 1997). The average age of nursing faculty is estimated at 48 years (AACN, 1999a). The development and evolution of APN roles, particularly the NP and CNS roles, over the past 35 to 45 years has resulted in the convergence of natural retirement for APN educators with the national phenomenon of aging demographics in this country. As an example, in the past decade the original cohort of NP leaders and faculty have reached retirement age. Transferring the leadership for the profession to a new generation requires careful mentoring, executive leadership development, policy skills, and a population- and relationship-centered approach to people and health care.

According to the 1996 National Sample Survey of Registered Nurses, the proportion of racially/ethnically diverse members of the nursing workforce is estimated at almost 10% of the 2,559,000 nurses in the United States (Moses, 1997). However, estimates of minority populations approach 28% of the total population (Moses, 1997). Similarly, the ethnic diversity of advanced practice nursing faculty is not reflective of these shifts in population (AACN, 1999a). Attention must be directed toward recruiting, retaining, and developing qualified racial/ethnic minorities in the APN profession. Faculty development programs for ethnically diverse APNs need to be sustained to cultivate these individuals for leadership roles.

MULTIDISCIPLINARY HEALTH WORKFORCE TRENDS

During the past 8 years, tremendous growth has occurred in the supply of nonphysician clinicians such as APNs (NPs, CNMs, CRNAs and PAs) (Cooper, Laud, & Dietrich, 1998). The full impact of this increase has yet to be determined but bears watching. Combining this growth of APNs and PAs with the existing physician workforce has heightened the competition among clinicians. Health workforce requisites for primary and specialty care providers have begun to show clinician surplus in selected geographic regions. Yet provider preference, market forces, and federal and state funding continue to be the major predictors of the size, composition, and distribution of the clinician workforce (Harper & Johnson, 1998). Recommendations by the Council on Graduate Medical Education (COGME) (1999) call for the COGME and the National Advisory Council on Nurse Education and Practice to begin collaborative health workforce policy planning. This collaboration at a federal level has the potential to provide direction in nursing, medicine, and other health professions for the delivery of primary, specialty, and population-based care. APN educators need strong representation at such policy-making deliberations.

Outcome Evaluation and Performance Improvement

RESEARCH ON APN EDUCATION

Several studies have been conducted on curriculum trends in APN programs, particularly NP and CNS programs. Burns and colleagues (1993) analyzed the curricula of 176 NLN-accredited nursing master's programs, including the descriptive variables of length of program, credit requirements, academic degree offered, number and area of major and subspecialties, curricular organizing framework, and curricular organization of courses. Results showed that the semester-hour credits varied from 29 to 54, with 36 credits the mode; nine different categories of courses were identified. The most commonly cited course categories were core courses, APN courses, research, and theory. These findings, now approaching 10 years old, showed considerable variation in curricula, courses, credit structure, and titling for majors, subspecialties, and role functions. Further study and analyses of APN curriculum are needed for future curriculum standardization.

APN DATA TRENDS

Two nursing education associations (the AACN and the NONPF) partner to collect data annually about APN education. The latest enrollment and graduation data, collected from graduate nursing programs for 1997–1998 (AACN, 1999a) were based on an overall response rate of 88.5% among schools of nursing with master's and/or post-master's programs. The following findings are based on the statistical samples of the AACN data. Within master's programs, APN clinical tracks accounted for more than 56% of all types of graduate nursing programs. Among the APN programs, NP and CNS/NP (blended role) students accounted for 79% of enrolled master's-level APN students, while CNS students accounted for 14%, CRNA students for 4%, and CNM students for 3% of all APN students enrolled. These advanced practice clinical tracks accounted for more than 77% (25,161 students) of total master's enrollments in 1997–1998 and for 81% (8,728 graduates) of total master's level graduates from these graduate nursing programs. In the same year, an additional 2,233 post-master's students were enrolled in APN programs and 1,492 post-master's students completed APN programs. The predominant number of these students were enrolled in post-master's NP programs. The master's and post-master's APN enrollment and graduations for 1997–1998 were 27,394 and 10,220, respectively. Although there has been a steady increase in the number of APNs prepared at the graduate level, enrollments and graduations for all types of master's nursing programs have remained relatively stable or have decreased from the previous AACN 1996–1997 sample.

These findings about APN enrollment and graduation offer compelling evidence of the prevalence of graduate nursing students preparing for APN roles. Furthermore, they highlight the unrealized potential in APNs to positively influence care in a variety of settings. Likewise, with APN students comprising more than three quarters of all graduate nursing students, the emphasis on knowledge development and clinical competence in advanced nursing practice needs continued assessment and evaluation.

Looking to the future, there is an immediate need for health workforce data analyzing APN graduate and practice patterns and health improvement outcomes associated with the growth in advanced practice nursing. Two other factors contributing to changing demand or requirements of the health workforce should be integrated into forecasting models for health workforce requirements. These include monitoring existing and beginning APN educational programs for quality, and collecting and analyzing specific data for CNS practice and education. Likewise, APN workforce data need to be compared with national and state-wide health workforce requirements.

Each of these environmental forces has significant implications for graduate APN education. External forces create new demands and opportunities for the APN workforce and other health care providers in the areas of cultural competency, health workforce planning, interdisciplinary health professional team training, and community partnership development. These provocative issues have caused graduate educators to re-evaluate the primary criteria and generic and particular characteristics expected of their APN graduates.

CORE ADVANCED PRACTICE CURRICULUM

APN Curriculum Framework

The environmental forces that influence graduate nursing education stimulate questions about master's preparation for APNs given the primary definition and competencies of advanced practice. What is the core curriculum needed to prepare competent APNs? Does direct clinical practice within graduate nursing programs provide the knowledge and skills needed to develop APN core competencies for all roles and/or specialty practice? Do the core competencies build on advanced nursing and specialty practice? Identifying relationships among these concentric competency levels through the revision of standards of APN and specialty curricula is an ongoing process that can potentially strengthen the future of APN education. With the preparation for APN roles offered primarily in graduate nursing programs, graduate nursing educators are keenly aware of the need to delineate and standardize theory, direct clinical practice, and functional role content for each of the APN roles. Concurrently, graduate nursing educators recognize the intersection of the critical environmental elements described earlier (see also Chapter 3) and how they affect advanced nursing practice. Graduate nursing content, advanced practice nursing content, and specialty role practice content must be identified to delineate APN knowledge, skills, and competencies (see Figure 4-1). This process will permit refinement of the graduate curriculum and its framework, resulting in improved educational outcomes for the preparation of APNs.

The framework that illustrates the components of the APN core curriculum is analogous to a wheel with concentric circular layers rotating around an axis (see Figure 4-2). In this concentric layer framework, the substantive curriculum components are, in order, the graduate nursing core, the advanced practice core, and the specialty practice core. Superimposed over these core components are the environmental elements that must be managed by APNs. The components of this framework provide the foundation for central and core competencies (see Chapter 3), including specialization and expansion of direct clinical practice competencies at an advanced practice level. This curriculum process is developed and implemented within a dynamic environment interacting with advanced nursing practice (see Figure 4-2).

CORE GRADUATE NURSING CONTENT

The commonly occurring core graduate nursing content consists of research, evidence-based outcomes, health policy, nursing and health-related theory, organizational/leadership theory, environmental health, ethical/legal issues, multicultural care, economics and business theory, community partnerships, managed care, and health care delivery systems. This content is generic to all master's-level nursing programs, be they APN or other types of advanced nursing programs, such as administration or informatics. This content has clearly expanded with the growing complexity of health systems.

ADVANCED PRACTICE CORE CONTENT

The second curriculum layer, APN core content, is foundational to the development of depth in the clinical specialty and differentiates advanced *clinical* nursing roles from other advanced roles, such as administration and education. Among the components common to all APN curricula are advanced health assessment; pharmacology; physiology; advanced pathophysiology or other related sciences (depending on the APN specialty); the process of clinical decision making; using complex or advanced nursing interventions/therapeutics; health promotion/disease prevention/population-based care; role functions and differentiation; and interpersonal and family theory.

Advanced assessment incorporates health assessment and risk appraisal for individuals and populations; physical and mental status assessment; interpretation of diagnostic studies; and psychosocial, family, and/or community assessment. Advanced pathophysiology consists of the study of disease and provides an important basis for medical and nursing clinical decision making. Advanced nursing therapeutics consists of the study of patient responses and related nursing interventions for special patient populations. These may be instituted as distinct interventions but are most often combined with medical or alternative therapeutics. Pharmacology includes pharmacokinetics, pharmacodynamics, drug therapies and their appropriate selection, and particular legal issues associated with prescriptive authority defined according to regulatory statutes (Yocum et al., 1999). Depending on the specialty role content, other related sciences may be necessary, such as human genetics, which is typically required for pediatric nurse practitioners and nurse-midwifery students; chemistry and physics, required for nurse anesthetist students; and immunology, required for oncology CNS students and others.

APN CORE COMPETENCIES

APN role content includes the competencies of ethical decision making, consultation, expert guidance and coaching, research, clinical and professional leadership, and collaboration (see Chapter 3 and specific chapters in Part II). Functional role content, such as the NP, CNM, CRNA, and CNS scopes of practice, is also important for students to be able to competently practice. The content is woven through each of the concentric layers and interfaces with the environment affecting advanced nursing practice (Fig. 4–2). This content moves, rotating around the axis from the graduate core. It is this dynamic state that propels learning and the acquisition of knowledge, skills, and central and core competencies essential for advanced nursing practice. Graduate APN students acquire beginning ability and skills through learning and integrating their knowledge and relevant experiences. The foundation for the acquisition of these competencies is laid in the graduate program, but the APN central and core competencies continue to develop and change after graduation through practice and interaction with the environment affecting practice.

APN SPECIALTY CORE

The specialty-related core content is unique to each type of APN role (NP, CRNA, CNS, CNM, APN case manager, or CNS/NP) as well as the health care needs of the respective specialty population (e.g., oncology, adult health, acute care, women's health, family, or pediatric). The specialty core content frequently must match standards and competencies established by professional specialty organizations, such as the Oncology Nursing Society; the NONPF (draft guidelines for adult, family, and gynecological NP competencies; see Boodley et al., 1995; NONPF, 1999); the ACNM (*Core Competencies;* see ACNM, 1992); and the AANA's Council on Accreditation (1994, 1999). The specialty content core is developed in depth as students learn clinical decision making applied to specialty practice based on the setting and patient population served. Courses in advanced therapeutics include pharmacological and nonpharmacological interventions used in changing health status and frequently combine nursing and medical interventions. Faculty-supervised clinical practice is essential for the expansion of central competencies in both the advanced practice and specialty-related core.

The hallmark of the APN curriculum model is the rotation of the graduate nursing, advanced practice, and specialty practice core on the axis of the central and core competencies that are acquired through the practice of direct clinical care (see Figure 4–2). These competencies must be explicitly addressed in all courses if students are to internalize the APN role. The central competencies are enhanced by each of the concentric layers as they are integrated through the various core courses.

The integration of curriculum content and competency-based practice needs to be achieved if nurses are to function as APNs. If the merger of the central and core competency content fails to occur, nurses educated as CNMs, NPs, CNSs, and CRNAs function in specialty practice roles rather than APN roles. The major curriculum components of this layered concentric framework define the generic educational requisites essential for advanced direct *clinical* practice, as distinguished from other types of graduate nursing preparation (AACN, 1996).

The educational challenge is to standardize and unify these core elements of the APN curriculum and competencies, providing a model for graduate-level APN preparation while maintaining the unique specialty focus of each APN role. The integration of curriculum and competencies is foundational to professional growth and positions APNs to be key providers in the emerging health care system. The core curriculum components and the APN competencies are embedded in a dynamic relationship with the environmental field, as indicated in Figure 4–2. The elements in this environmental field are in a state of constant flux.

A Generic APN Curriculum

On the basis of these core curriculum components, a generic curriculum for APN education may be proposed. It should be noted that this generic curriculum is not proscriptive, but rather serves as an example to identify the content in each of the core areas. A sample generic curriculum for APN master's-level preparation is presented in Table 4–4.

The sample curriculum and credit structure varies according to the type of APN specialty being prepared. For example, didactic content and clinical practica for the CNM must integrate perinatal physiology; neonatal, prenatal, intrapartum, and postpartum care; family planning; and well-woman gynecological care. Likewise, acute care NP and CRNA coursework is oriented toward acquisition of the knowledge and competencies needed to care for in-hospital critical care and surgical patient populations. Conversely, specialty didactic and clinical practicum content for the family NP incorporates a generalist approach to obstetrical, gynecological, pediatric, adult, and geriatric primary care. Distinguished from these other roles is the CNS. Although many CNS programs do not require the pharmacology and medical clinical

TABLE 4–4 SAMPLE GENERIC APN CURRICULUM FOR GRADUATE-LEVEL PREPARATION

Core Graduate Nursing Content (9–12 credits)
Research and outcome evaluation: 4–6 credits
Theoretical perspectives: 3 credits
  Nursing and health-related theory, role theory, ethical decision making, environmental theory
  Organization/policy perspectives: 3 credits
  Organizational/leadership theory, health policy, community-based care, epidemiology, integrated
    health systems, informatics, managed care, business, reimbursement, regulatory, marketing
Core Advanced Practice Content (12–18 credits)
Pharmacotherapeutics: 3 credits
Advanced health assessment: 3 credits
Pathophysiology, genetics, related science: 3 credits
APN role development: 3 credits
Core Specialty Practice Content (12–18 credits)
Specialties I, II, III
Clinical practica:
  Clinical decision-making, advanced therapeutics, health promotion and disease prevention,
    primary care and population-based health

management components required by the programs for other APN roles, the curriculum for this APN role substitutes significant content and skill development in formal consultation and educator subroles, in advanced nursing interventions for patients, and in system influence (NACNS, 1998; Naylor & Brooten, 1993). As is evident from these examples, the specialty content for each particular APN role is unique to the characteristics of the role, the patient population served, and the clinical environment. In addition, APN curricula for the APN case manager role must be responsive to the unique educational needs of this evolving role. Clear role development and specific specialty core content based on the central core competency of direct clinical practice is needed for APN case manager preparation.

The relatively new development of post-master's graduate nursing programs to prepare nurses with master's or doctoral degrees in other areas of nursing to become NPs in a designated specialty track (adult, family, gerontological, women's health care, and others) also builds on this generic APN curriculum. Because post-master's students have taken prior core master's-level coursework as part of their original graduate degree, they are not required to repeat to this core as part of their post-master's certificate. Instead, they take graduate-level coursework in the APN core and specialty content and complete adequate clinical hours in the new APN specialty, which often leads to a postgraduate certificate with preparation in the specialty areas. Also, non–MSN-prepared NPs, CNMs, and CRNAs need access to APN core coursework in order to fully actualize advanced practice or to prepare for blended role practice. This phenomenon demonstrates the utility of having a generic APN curriculum.

TEACHING/LEARNING STRATEGIES FOR APN EDUCATION

APN educators use several strategies in the process of teaching students to integrate APN core content, role functions, and competencies. Among them are the processes of clinical decision making, critical thinking, and clinical practicum experiences.

Clinical Decision Making

Clinical decision making is the interaction of knowledge and reasoning skills blending ethics with scientific knowledge and evidence-based practice for a humane approach to care (NONPF, 1999). This complex process is discussed extensively in Chapter 6. Graduate educators thread critical-thinking teaching strategies throughout APN master's programs. Core courses develop clinical decision making through the presentation of content and skills that are logically clustered to enhance diagnostic reasoning in simulated and clinical practice situations. Clinical decision making is fully developed throughout the specialty coursework and in clinical practicum experiences for each APN role. In the specialty core, students expand their specialized clinical decision-making knowledge and skills in classroom settings through the analysis of paradigm clinical cases and in clinical practice supervised by graduate faculty and preceptors.

Typically, a faculty-supervised clinical practicum consists of both direct and indirect supervision. In direct supervision, faculty provide students with on-site clinical supervision. Faculty who provide direct supervision usually bring students to ongoing faculty practice sites, where the faculty serve as role models and direct supervisors. Indirect supervision involves faculty supplementation of a preceptor's clinical teaching. It has three components: Faculty serve as student mentors, act as community liaisons, and evaluate student progress (Boodley et al., 1995).

Teaching strategies that serve to guide APN students through the process of clinical decision making include analysis of case studies; critique of research findings and scholarly literature as applied to the diagnosis and management of conditions or problems for individuals, families, or communities; case presentations; oral presentations; class discussions; seminars; clinical journals; preceptor and self-evaluation and written and performance examinations differentiating medical and nursing diagnosis; and peer reviewed decision making (Boodley et al., 1995; see Chapter 6).

Clinical Resources

Clinical practicum experiences are a central component of all APN programs. In addition to giving graduate students practice in the direct caregiver role, the clinical practica allow students to integrate core APN competencies into their practice, to learn particular aspects of their chosen APN role, to make clinical decisions, to function as members of an interdisciplinary team, and to begin to negotiate and manage health systems.

Accordingly, these direct care experiences depend on site-based learning through direct "hands-on" patient care experiences. A recent publication identified essential clinical resources for undergraduate and graduate nursing education (AACN, 1999a) (see Table 4–5). Within this report, some of the barriers to clinical resource development are identified as system and organizational issues, educational competition, and costs of clinical education. The report focused on these barriers and resources with a call to redefine three key areas:

- The relationship between education and practice
- The nature of educational/clinical partnerships
- The shared mission of nursing education and practice

TABLE 4–5	ESSENTIAL CLINICAL RESOURCES FOR NURSING EDUCATION

Essential Clinical Resources for Undergraduate and Graduate Education
1. Provide care along a continuum.
2. Work with interdisciplinary and intradisciplinary teams.
3. Work within and across diverse health care delivery environments and communities.
4. Provide care for diverse populations, including diverse ages, gender, ethnicity, healthy-ill populations, and acute-chronic health states.
5. Exercise delegation/management skills.
6. Practice case management.
7. Manage health-related data.
8. Use information technologies to provide nursing care.
9. Participate in nursing research.
10. Deal with the allocation and management of fiscal and human resources.
11. Work with role models and preceptors.

Additional Essential Clinical Resources for Graduate Education
1. Practice in the advanced practice nursing role.
2. Work with an agency staff committed to the advanced practice nursing role.
3. Engage in nursing research.

Adapted from American Association of Colleges of Nursing. (1999). *Essential clinical resources for nursing's academic mission.* Washington, DC: Author; reprinted with permission.

Within this context, APN education must continue to explore and analyze the costs and value-added benefits of faculty and student practice to clinical sites. A study of faculty practice with graduate APN learners (Kellogg Foundation, 1999) has shown the benefits to communities associated with community partnership educational models as APN students deliver a significant component of clinical services across a number of clinical sites. Similarly, the development of nursing centers by schools of nursing is dependent on APN faculty to practice with graduate learners for the delivery of primary care and population-based services with vulnerable populations (see Chapter 26).

Multidisciplinary Health Professions Education

Multidisciplinary education has emerged as a potential solution for the integration of services in the increasingly complex health system of the future. Yet multidisciplinary and/or interdisciplinary education, practice, and research have not been operationalized to their full extent within APN education over the years. Collaborative learning activities over the past 5 years have just begun to develop as a part of the formal educational process of APNs or in other health professions programs. Such activities have been developed at the behest of educational policy and foundation initiatives that include the Interdisciplinary Health Initiative (IHI), Interdisciplinary Professional Education Collaborative (Headrick et al., 1996), the W. K. Kellogg Community Partnerships and Health Professions Education Initiative (Harris, Starnaman, Henry & Bland, 1998), the PQE program (Robert Wood Johnson Foundation, 1999), Partnerships for Training (1997), and the Program for Health Profession's Schools in Service to the Nation (HPSISN) (Community-Campus Partnership for Health, 1998). These multidisciplinary educational models have built upon interdisciplinary team practice that frequently occurs through on-the-job training with little formal technical assistance or support from health professional educational programs. This type of educational model involves moving each discipline beyond its discipline-specific "silo" to foster interprofessional interactions that enhance the practice of each discipline (AACN, 1996).

Because collaboration is an expected competency of APNs (see Chapter 11), educators develop and improve interdisciplinary teaching/learning strategies for shared experiences that foster working together around common goals. Within the funded interdisciplinary initiatives referenced earlier in this chapter, APNs function as the continuity in these team models, despite numerous barriers (Minnick, 1997). The continuous presence of APNs on these teams is an indication of their value and reinforces the interdisciplinary imperative for graduate nursing.

An example of the interest in interdisciplinary models is the Institute of Medicine's report on *Primary Care* (Donaldson et al., 1996), which focuses on developing the interdisciplinary team as the provider unit of care. The "Partnerships in Training" initiative (Robert Wood Johnson Foundation, 1995) seeks to develop primary care interdisciplinary training models for physicians, NPs, CNMs, and PAs. Among the areas identified as core interdisciplinary content are health assessment, pharmacology, pathophysiology, health promotion and disease prevention, and selected aspects of specialty content. Likewise, the Partnerships in Quality Management II initiative (Robert Wood Johnson Foundation, 1999) aims to improve health through better interdisciplinary education of physicians, PAs, and APNs in managed care settings by incorporating content on collaboration, continuous quality improvement, interdisciplinary team building, and community-oriented primary care. Finally, the Community Partnership in Graduate Medical and Nursing Education initiative (Kellogg Foundation, 1999) established its community partnership multidisciplinary health professions education model as a means of providing high-quality community-based graduate medical and nursing education while improving access to care for vulnerable populations.

These foundation initiatives have challenged educators to expand their ways of thinking and being. The challenge inherent in health care interdisciplinary education is to create innovative, cutting-edge models for practice while maintaining equity among the disciplines and balancing the integrity of each discipline's philosophy and practice style. Shared interdisciplinary instruction has multiple benefits. Among them are the conservation of curriculum, instructional resources, and faculty (Johnson-Pawlson & Harper, 1993; Larson, 1995) and the opportunity to develop and test models of team learning, as well as educational and clinical outcomes with faculty and students that extend to clinical agencies.

DISTANCE EDUCATION TECHNOLOGY

Advances in technology have led to dramatic changes in APN education (AACN, 1999b). Distance technology has led to substantial positive changes in the delivery of and access to APN education while also contributing to concerns about standardization of curricula and oversight of APN students. Distance education has been defined (Reinert & Fryback, 1997) as a set of teaching and/or learning strategies to meet the learning needs of students separate from the traditional classroom setting and sometimes the traditional roles of faculty. Distance learning strategies are offered predominantly through interactive television and synchronous and asynchronous web-based modalities. According to the AACN (1999b), several factors need to be considered when opting to select distance education modalities in APN education:

1. Substantial institutional financial resources are required in the areas of faculty development, equipment, and infrastructure to design, implement, evaluate, and continuously improve distance education programs.
2. Technology-mediated teaching strategies are needed that can dramatically change the teaching-learning relationship and the traditional infrastructure components for educational offerings and related counseling, library access, health services, and the like.
3. New methods are needed for recruiting students and improving access for disadvantaged and culturally diverse students.

Distance education models have been federally supported and documented for the past several years through the Division of Nursing, Bureau of Health Professions, Nursing Grant Programs. Among the programs that have supported these educational innovations are those in Section 820: Nursing Special Projects; Section 821: Advanced Nurse Education; Section 822: Nurse Practitioner/Nurse Midwifery Programs; and Section 830: Nurse Anesthetists. However, because of the competency-based nature of advanced practice nursing education, distance education technology must be balanced with the evaluation of the central and core competencies implicit in the APN role.

Distance education for APNs offers excellent opportunities for nursing to prepare students who live in remote areas for APN practice with rural, inner-city, and underserved populations. Distance education provides unique opportunities for educational partners to match strengths with other programs to enhance the quality of APN education by matching APN faculty and enhancing clinical opportunities. As well, the Internet is a rich resource to augment educational experiences worldwide. Although these factors speak to the need to develop distance modalities, it is imperative that standards, program review, and accreditation processes require that distance programs preparing APNs adhere to the same rigor as face-to-face programs. This means that both didactic and clinical components must offer sound experiences that assure beginning competence in the APN specialty and that there is appropriate and adequate student oversight and evaluation. It also requires sufficient numbers of faculty who are skilled both clinically and in distance learning teaching techniques to oversee APN student learners. Current standards for NP programs require that faculty-supervised performance evaluation be documented (Boodley et al., 1995). To date, APN distance education programs continue to monitor and supervise student clinical experiences through faculty site visits. It is anticipated that more sophisticated forms of video teleconferencing may enhance this faculty clinical supervision capacity in the next century.

CONCLUSION

APN educators have moved toward standardizing graduate-level educational preparation to strengthen internal professional cohesion and extend external professional validity within the health care system. Continued progress toward standardizing the curricula of graduate nursing programs is necessary to strengthen APN credibility among nurses, other health care providers, consumers, and policy makers. APN educators are poised to focus on several challenges for the future:

- Maintaining educational flexibility while continuing to improve standardization of APN programs.
- Developing a new generation of APN faculty for teaching, practice, and scholarship.
- Increasing access for and retention of under-represented minority APN students and faculty reflective of the nation's populations.
- Developing a national APN database to monitor education and practice outcomes.
- Providing leadership for multidisciplinary health professions education for the discovery of knowledge, best practices, and improved health care outcomes.
- Developing distance education programs for education and professional development that meet quality standards for APN education.

APN educators have a mandate for the 21st century: to integrate the central and core APN competencies within the matrix of the health care workforce and environment. To fulfill this mandate, APN educators cannot afford to stand still. Instead, they must continue to design and refine outcomes-oriented educational programs that are responsive to society's needs and those of the existing and future health care system.

REFERENCES

Aiken, L., Gwyther, M., & Whelan, E. (1994). *Advanced practice nursing education: Allocation of the proposed graduate nursing education account* (Report submitted under contract to the Office of the Assistant Secretary of Health, U.S. Department of Health and Human Services). Philadelphia, PA: Center for Health Policy Research, University of Pennsylvania School of Nursing.

American Association of Colleges of Medicine. (1998). *Report II: Contemporary issues in medicine: Medical informatics and population health.* Washington, DC: Author.

American Association of Colleges of Nursing. (1993). *Position statement on educational mobility.* Washington, DC: Author.

American Association of Colleges of Nursing. (1995). *Position statement: Interdisciplinary education and practice.* Washington, DC: Author.

American Association of Colleges of Nursing. (1996). *The essentials of master's education for advanced practice nursing.* Washington, DC: Author.

American Association of Colleges of Nursing. (1998). *The essentials of baccalaureate nursing education.* Washington, DC: Author.

American Association of Colleges of Nursing. (1999a). *Essential clinical resources for nursing's academic mission.* Washington, DC: Author.

American Association of Colleges of Nursing. (1999b). *White paper. Distance technology in nursing education: Assessing a new frontier.* Available: http://www.aacn.nche.edu./publications/positions/White Paper.html

American Association of Nurse Anesthetists. (1992). *Guidelines and standards for nurse anesthesia practice.* Park Ridge, IL: Author.

American Association of Nurse Anesthetists. (1999). *Standards for accreditation of nurse anesthesia educational programs.* Park Ridge, IL: Author.

American Association of Nurse Anesthetists Council on Accreditation. (1994). *Standards and guidelines for programs of nurse anesthesia.* Park Ridge, IL: American Association of Nurse Anesthetists.

American Association of Nurse Anesthetists Council on Accreditation. (1999). *Standards and guidelines for programs of nurse anesthesia.* Park Ridge, IL: American Association of Nurse Anesthetists.

American College of Nurse-Midwives. (1992). *Core competencies in nurse-midwifery.* Washington, DC: Author.

American College of Nurse-Midwives. (1993). *Criteria for accreditation of basic certificate, graduate, and pre-certification nurse-midwifery programs.* Washington, DC: Author.

American Nurses' Association. (1995). *Nursing's social policy statement.* Washington, DC: Author.

American Nurses' Association. (1996). *Scope and standards of advanced practice nursing.* Washington, DC: Author.

Bellak, J., Graber, D., O'Neil, E., Musham, C., & Lancaster, C. (1999). Curriculum trends in nurse practitioner programs: Current and ideal. *Journal of Professional Nursing, 15,* 15–27.

Benner, P. (1984). *From novice to expert: Excellence and power in clinical nursing practice.* Menlo Park, CA: Addison Wesley.

Berlin, L., Bednash, P., & Hosier, K. (1999). *American Association of Colleges of Nursing: 1998–1999 enrollments and graduations in baccalaureate and graduate programs in nursing.* Washington, DC: American Association of Colleges of Nursing.

Boodley, C. A., Harper, D. C., Hanson, C. M., Jackson, P., Russell, D. D., Taylor, D., & Zimmer, P. (Eds.). (1995). *Advanced nursing practice: Curriculum guidelines and program standards for nurse practitioner education.* Washington, DC: National Organization of Nurse Practitioner Faculties.

Brown, S. (1998). A framework for advanced practice nursing. *Journal of Professional Nursing, 14,* 157–164.

Buerhaus, P. (1998). Medicare payment for advanced practice nurses: What are the research questions? *Nursing Outlook, 46*(4), 151–154.

Burns, P., Nishikawa, H., Weatherby, F., Forni, P., Moran, M., Allen, M., Baker, C., & Booten, D. (1993). Master's degree nursing education: State of the art. *Journal of Professional Nursing, 9,* 267–276.

Center for Health Policy and Research. (1999). *Negotiating the new health system: A nationwide study of Medicaid managed care contracts* (2nd ed.). Washington, DC: Author.

Commission on Collegiate Nursing Education. (1998). *CCNE standards for accreditation of baccalaureate and graduate nursing programs.* Available: www.aacn.nche.edu/Accreditation/standrds.htm

Community-Campus Partnerships for Health. (1998). An overview: The Health Professions Schools in Service to the Nation program and community-campus partnerships for health. San Francisco, CA: *Community-Campus Partnerships for Health, 1*(1), 77–79.

Cooper, R., Laud, P., & Dietrich, C. (1998). Current and projected workforce of nonphysician clinicians. *JAMA, 280,* 794.

Council on Graduate Medical Education. (1999). *Fourteenth report: COGME physician workforce policies: Recent developments and remaining challenges in meeting national goals.* Rockville, MD: U.S. Department of Health and Human Resources.

Donaldson, M., Yordy, K., Lohr, K., & Vanselow, N. (Eds.). (1996). *Primary care: America's health in a new era.* Washington, DC: National Academy Press.

Fenton, M., & Brykczynski, K. (1993). Qualitative distinctions and similarities in the practice of clinical nurse specialists and nurse practitioners. *Journal of Professional Nursing, 9,* 313–326.

Gelmon, S., O'Neil, E., Kimmey, J., and the National Task Force on Accreditation of Health Professions Education. (1999). *Strategies for change and improvement: The report of the National Task Force on Accreditation of Health Professions Education.* San Francisco: University of California–San Francisco, Center for the Health Professions.

Hamric, A. B., Spross, J. A., & Hanson, C. M. (1996). *Advanced nursing practice: An integrative approach.* Philadelphia: W. B. Saunders.

Harper, D., & Johnson, J. (1998). The new generation of nurse practitioners: Is more enough? *Health Affairs, 17*(5), 158–164.

Harris, D. L., Starnaman, S. M., Henry, R. C., & Bland, C. J. (1998). Multidisciplinary educational outcomes of the W. K. Kellogg Community Partnerships and Health Professions Education Initiative. *Academic Medicine, 73*(10, Suppl.), S13–S15.

Headrick, L. A., Knapp, M., Neuhauser, D., Gelmon, S., Norman, L., Quinn, D., & Baker, R. (1996). Working from upstream to improve health care: The IHI Interdisciplinary Professional Education Collaborative. *Joint Commission Journal on Quality Improvement, 22*(3), 149–164.

Health Professions Education Partnerships Act of 1998, Pub. L. 105–392 (1998).

Johnson-Pawlson, J., & Harper, D. (1993). An economic paradigm for NP education program development. *Journal of Professional Nursing, 9,* 148–152.

Kellogg Foundation. (1999). *Community partnerships in graduate medical and nursing education.* Battle Creek, MI: Author.

Kindig, D. (1999). Purchasing population health: Aligning financial incentives to improve health outcomes. *Nursing Outlook, 47*(1), 15–17.

Larson, E. (1995). New rules for the game: Interdisciplinary education for health professionals. *Nursing Outlook, 43*(4), 180–185.

Lurie, N. (1996). Preparing physicians for practice in managed care environments. *Academic Medicine, 71,* 1044–1049.

Minnick, A. (1997). Key issues in building a continuum of care. *Nursing Administration Quarterly, 21*(4), 41–46.

Moses, E. (1997). *The registered nurse population: March 1996. Findings from the National Sample Survey of Registered Nurses.* Rockville, MD: Health Resources Services Administration, Bureau of Health Professions, Division of Nursing.

Mundinger, M., & Gilliss, C. (1998). How is the role of the advanced practice nurse changing? In E. O'Neil & J. Coffman (Eds.), *Strategies for the future of nursing* (pp. 171–191). San Francisco: Jossey-Bass.

Mundinger, M., Kane, R., Lenz, E., Totten, A., Tsai, W. Y., Cleary, P., Friedewald, W., Siv, A., & Shelanski, M. (2000). Primary care outcomes in patients treated by nurse practitioners or physicians. *JAMA, 233,* 59–68.

National Association of Clinical Nurse Specialists. (1998). *Clinical nurse specialist practice and education.* Glenview, IL: Author.

National Health Policy Forum. (1999). *The nursing center in concept and practice: Delivery and financing issues in serving vulnerable populations* (Issue Brief No. 746, pp. 2-10). Washington, DC: George Washington University.

National Organization of Nurse Practitioner Faculties. (1999). *Assuring quality nurse practitioner education: A plan for action* (Working Paper). Available: www.nonpf.com/nped.htm.

National Task Force on Quality Nurse Practitioner Education. (1997). *Criteria for the evaluation of nurse practitioner programs.* Washington, DC: National Organization of Nurse Practitioner Faculties.

Naylor, M., & Brooten, D. (1993). The roles and functions of clinical nurse specialists. *Image: The Journal of Nursing Scholarship, 25,* 73-78.

Nurse Education and Practice Improvement Amendments of 1992, Pub. L. 105-78 (1997).

O'Neil, E., and the Pew Health Professions Commission. (1993). *Health professions education for the future: Schools in service to the nation.* San Francisco: Pew Health Professions Commission, Pew Charitable Trust Foundation.

O'Neil, E., and the Pew Health Professions Commission. (1998). *Recreating health professional practice for a new century.* San Francisco: Pew Health Professions Commission, Pew Charitable Trust Foundation.

Partnerships for Training. (1997). Available: www.ahcnet.org.

Pew Commission Federal Policy Task Force. (1998). *Beyond the Balanced Budget Act of 1997: Strengthening federal GME policy.* San Francisco: University of California-San Francisco, Center for the Health Professions.

Pew Health Professions Commission, Phase Two. (1995). *Shifting the supply of our health care workforce: A guide to redirecting federal subsidy of medical education.* San Francisco: Pew Charitable Trust Foundation.

Public Health Service. (2000). *Healthy People 2010: Understanding and improving health.* (DHHS Publication No. [PHS] 017001 00543-6). Washington, DC: U.S. Department of Health and Human Services.

Reinert, B., & Fryback, P. (1997). Distance learning and nursing education. *Journal of Nursing Education, 36,* 421.

Robert Wood Johnson Foundation. (1995). *Partnerships in training: Regional education systems for nurse practitioners, certified nurse midwives and physician assistants.* Washington, DC: Association of Academic Health Centers.

Robert Wood Johnson Foundation. (1999). *Partnerships for quality education.* Available: www.pqe.org.

Sorrells-Jones, J. (1999). The role of the chief nurse executive in the knowledge-intense organization of the future. *Nursing Administration Quarterly, 23*(3), 17-25.

Vesser, P., Stegbauer, C., & Russel, C. (1999). Doctoral education: Developing a clinical doctorate to prepare nurses for advanced practice at the University of Tennessee. Memphis. *Image: The Journal of Nursing Scholarship, 31*(1), 39-41.

Wagner, E. H. (1998). *Complementary patient care teams: Their contributions to patient outcomes and health systems.* Unpublished manuscript.

Yedidia, M., & Gillespie, C. (1999). Do PQE training programs make a difference? In *Partnerships for quality education: Learning together, shaping the future* (p. 5). Boston: Harvard Pilgrim.

Yocum, C., Busby, L., Conway-Welch, C., & Viens, D. (1999). *Curriculum guidelines and regulatory criteria for family nurse practitioners seeking prescriptive authority to manage pharmacotherapeutics in primary care.* Washington, DC: National Organization of Nurse Practitioner Faculties.

Additional Readings

Bullough, B. (1992). Alternative models for specialty nursing practice. *Nursing and Health Care, 13,* 254-259.

Grumbach, K., & Coffman, J. (1998). Physicians and nonphysician clinicians: Complements or competitors? *JAMA, 280,* 825-826.

Hamric, A., & Spross, J. (Eds.). (1989). *The clinical specialist in theory and practice* (2nd ed.). Philadelphia: W. B. Saunders.

Harper, D., & Johnson, J. (1996). *NONPF workforce policy technical report: Nurse practitioner programs 1988-1995.* Washington, DC: National Organization of Nurse Practitioner Faculties.

Huston, C., & Fox, S. (1998). The changing health care market: Implications for nursing education in the coming decade. *Nursing Outlook, 46*(3), 109-114.

Jordan, L. (1994). Qualifications and capabilities of the certified registered nurse anesthetist. In S. D. Foster & L. Jordan (Eds.), *Professional aspects of nurse anesthesia practice* (pp. 3-10). Philadelphia: F. A. Davis.

Lindeke, L., Canedy, B., & Kay, M. (1997). A comparison of practice domains of clinical nurse specialists and nurse practitioners. *Journal of Professional Nursing, 13,* 281-287.

McBride, A. (1999). Breakthroughs in nursing education: Looking back, looking forward. *Nursing Outlook, 47*(3), 114-119.

McCloskey, J. (1998). Interdisciplinary teams: The nursing perspective is essential. *Nursing Outlook, 46*(4), 157–163.

National Advisory Council on Nurse Education and Practice. (1996). *Report to the Secretary of the Department of Health and Human Services on the basic registered nurse workforce.* Rockville, MD: Health Resources and Services Administration.

National League for Nursing. (1994). *Nursing datasource, 1994, Vol. II: Graduate education in nursing, advanced practice nursing* (Publication No. 19-2643). New York: Author.

National League for Nursing Accreditation Committee, Council of Baccalaureate and Higher Degree Programs. (1992). *Criteria and guidelines for evaluation of baccalaureate and higher degree programs in nursing* (Publication No. 15-2474). New York: National League for Nursing Press.

Safriet, B. (1992). Health care dollars and regulatory sense: The role of advanced practice nursing. *Yale Journal on Regulation, 9,* 417–487.

Wakefield, M. (1997). Federal funding shapes nursing's future. *Nursing Economics, 15,* 110–111.

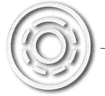

Role Development of the Advanced Practice Nurse

· K A R E N   A.   B R Y K C Z Y N S K I

INTRODUCTION

PERSPECTIVES ON APN ROLE DEVELOPMENT

NOVICE-TO-EXPERT SKILL ACQUISITION MODEL

ROLE CONCEPTS AND ROLE DEVELOPMENT ISSUES
Role Ambiguity
Role Incongruity
Interprofessional Role Conflict
Intraprofessional Role Conflict

ROLE TRANSITIONS
APN Role Acquisition (in school)
Strategies to Facilitate Role Acquisition
APN Role Implementation (at work)
Strategies to Facilitate Role Implementation
Facilitators and Barriers in the Work Setting
Evaluation of Role Development

CONCLUSION

INTRODUCTION

What is it like to become an advanced practice nurse (APN)? In the current managed care environment, the pressure to be cost-effective and to make an impact on outcomes is greater than ever. Yet literature indicates that the initial year of practice is one of transition (Brykczynski, 1996) and maximum potential is not reached until approximately 5 or more years in practice (Cooper & Sparacino, 1990). This chapter explores the complex processes of APN role development with the objectives of providing (1) anticipatory guidance for APN students, (2) concepts and strategies for faculty teaching APNs, and (3) role facilitation strategies for new APNs, APN preceptors, administrators, and interested colleagues.

This chapter also consolidates literature from all of the APN roles, including clinical nurse specialists (CNSs), nurse practitioners (NPs), nurse-midwives (CNMs), and nurse anesthetists (CRNAs), to present a generic process relevant to all APN roles. The discussion is separated into the educational component of APN *role acquisition* and the occupational or work component of *role implementation.* This division in the process of role development is intended to clarify and distinguish the changes occurring during role transitions experienced during the educational component of an APN role (role acquisition) and the changes occurring during the actual performance of the role following program completion (role implementation). Strategies for enhancing APN role development are described. The chapter concludes with summary comments and suggestions regarding facilitation of future APN role development.

PERSPECTIVES ON APN ROLE DEVELOPMENT

Professional role development is a dynamic, ongoing process that, once begun, spans a lifetime. The concept of graduation as commencement, whereby one's career begins upon degree completion, is central to understanding the evolving nature of professional roles over time in response to personal, professional, and societal demands (Gunn, 1998). Professional role development literature in nursing is abundant and complex, involving multiple component processes. These include (1) aspects of adult development, (2) development of clinical expertise, (3) modification of self-identity through initial socialization in school, (4) development and integration of professional subrole components, and (5) subsequent resocialization in the work setting. Like socialization for other professional roles, such as attorney, physician, teacher, and social worker, the process of becoming an APN involves aspects of adult socialization as well as occupational socialization.

NOVICE-TO-EXPERT SKILL ACQUISITION MODEL

Acquisition of knowledge and skill occurs in a progressive movement through stages of performance from novice to expert as depicted by Dreyfus and Dreyfus (1977, 1986) from their study of diverse groups, including pilots, chess players, and adult learners of second languages. This model of skill acquisition was applied to nursing and validated by Benner (1984) with neophyte and experienced hospital staff nurses. More recently, Benner has continued investigation of this skill model, specifically with critical care nurses (Benner, Hooper-Kyriakidis, & Stannard, 1999; Benner, Tanner, & Chesla, 1996).

A major implication of the novice-to-expert model for advanced practice nursing is the claim that even experts can be expected to perform at lower skill levels when they enter new situations or positions. Hamric and Taylor's (1989) report that experienced CNSs starting a new position experience the same role development phases as new graduates, only over a shorter period of time, supports this claim. Figure 5–1 depicts the multiple simultaneous processes expected during APN role development. For example, a professional nurse who functions as a mentor for new graduates may decide to pursue an advanced degree as an APN. As an APN graduate student, this nurse will experience the challenges of acquiring a new role, the anxiety of unfamiliar skills and practices, and the dependency of being a novice. At the same time, if this nurse continues to work as a registered nurse (RN), her or his functioning

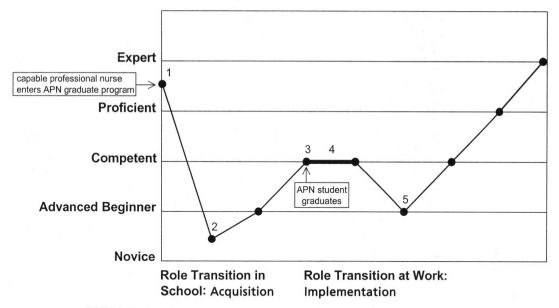

FIGURE 5–1 • Typical APN role development pattern:
1. APN students typically begin graduate school as proficient or expert nurses.
2. Depending on previous background, the new APN student will revert to novice or advanced-beginner level upon assuming the student role.
3. The graduate from an APN program is competent as an APN student but has no experience as a practicing APN.
4. A limbo or liminal period is experienced while the APN graduate searches for a position and becomes certified.
5. The newly employed APN reverts to advanced-beginner level in the new APN position as role trajectory begins again.

in this work role will be at the competent, proficient, or expert level (depending on experience and the situation). Upon graduation and taking a new APN position, this nurse will experience a return to the advanced-beginner stage as she or he proceeds through the phases of role implementation. Years later, the APN may decide to pursue yet another APN role. The processes of role acquisition, role implementation, and novice-to-expert skill development will again be experienced (although altered and informed by previous experiences) as the postgraduate student acquires additional skills and knowledge. Role development is thus pictured as multiple, dynamic, and situational processes with each new undertaking being characterized by passage through earlier transitional phases with some movement back and forth, horizontally and laterally, as different career options are pursued.

Another significant implication of the Dreyfus (1977, 1986) model for APNs is the observation that performance level also decreases when performers are subjected to intense scrutiny, whether it be their own or someone else's (Roberts, Tabloski, & Bova, 1997). The heightened anxiety of APN students during faculty on-site clinical evaluation visits or during videotaped testing of clinical performance in simulated situations can be understood as examples of such intense scrutiny. A third implication of this skill acquisition model for APNs is the need to accrue experience in actual situations over time, so that both practical and theoretical knowledge are refined, clarified, personalized, and embodied, forming an individualized repertoire of past experience that guides advanced practice performance.

According to this model, there is a generic process of skill acquisition through which humans proceed in stages from novice to expert as they acquire new psychomotor, perceptual, and judgment skills (see Table 5–1). The progression from novice level to advanced-beginner level and then to competent level is incremental. The competent level is a critical juncture in the development of expertise during which the crisis of confidence in others' abilities and the limits of available knowledge to ameliorate the health problems of real people occurs. There is a change from "acting like," sometimes referred to as "the imposter phenomenon" (Arena & Page, 1992; Brown & Olshansky, 1997, 1998), to individualized embodiment of the new role as the individual moves up to the proficient level. In other words, it takes time practicing new skills for them to become fully owned or embodied. Embodiment of a skill occurs after repeated experiences of performing the skill "as if" one actually could do it skillfully. It is a kind of "going through the motions" until over time the skill is transformed from the halting stepwise performance of the novice to the holistic fluid performance of the expert. It is important to note that the competent level is the one represented in computer processing and decision analysis models. Thus the Dreyfus model is inclusive of those models, but goes beyond them.

The proficient level represents a discontinuous, qualitative leap from the competent level whereby intuition, defined as "holistic situation recognition" (Dreyfus & Dreyfus, 1986, p. 28), replaces analytically reasoned responses. Expertise, according to this model, develops over time through direct personal encounters, which alter preconceptions and prior understanding developed from one's own background of particular experiences. The deep situational understanding associated with expertise involves holistic pattern recognition, described as "the intuitive ability to use patterns without decomposing them into component features" (Dreyfus & Dreyfus, 1986, p. 28). Decomposition of situations into abstract attributes is associated with earlier skill levels. The extent of an individual's involvement in a particular situation influences her or his decision-making ability (Benner et al., 1996). Deliberative rationality, a fine tuning of intuitions, takes place at the expert level, replacing the calculative rationality characteristic of other levels. Deliberative rationality is involved in distin-

TABLE 5–1	DREYFUS MODEL OF SKILL ACQUISITION			
SKILL LEVEL	COMPONENTS	PERSPECTIVE	DECISION	COMMITMENT
Novice	Context-free	None	Analytical	Detached
Advanced beginner	Context-free and situational	None	Analytical	Detached
Competent	Context-free and situational	Chosen	Analytical	Detached understanding and deciding; involved in outcome
Proficient	Context-free and situational	Experienced	Analytical	Involved understanding; detached deciding
Expert	Context-free and situational	Experienced	Intuitive	Involved

From Dreyfus, H. L., & Dreyfus, S. E. (1986). *Mind over machine: The power of human intuition and expertise in the era of the computer* (p. 28). New York: Free Press; reprinted by permission.

guishing a novel situation or a situation where there is an incorrect initial grasp from a situation in which experience can be trusted. Such personal expert knowledge is not totally idiosyncratic; it can be shared in ways described by Benner (1984), such as identifying maxims, common meanings, and exemplars that convey the contextual meanings of clinical situations. Narratives of situations from clinical practice can be studied to identify aspects of practical knowledge that enhance understanding of the knowledge embedded in practice.

ROLE CONCEPTS AND ROLE DEVELOPMENT ISSUES

This discussion of professional role issues incorporates role concepts from Hardy and Hardy (1988) along with the concept that different APN roles represent different subcultural groups within the broader nursing culture (Leininger, 1976). APNs can be described as tricultural and trilingual (Johnson, 1993). They share background knowledge, practices, and skills of three cultures: (1) biomedicine, (2) mainstream nursing, and (3) everyday life. They are fluent in the languages of biomedical science, nursing knowledge and skill, and everyday parlance. Some APNs—CNMs, for example—are socialized into a fourth culture as well, that of midwifery. Others are also fluent in more than one everyday language. Just as APN roles can be conceptualized as encompassing skills and knowledge from more than one culture, they can be seen as encompassing aspects of both male and female occupational sex roles. These ideas that APNs are multicultural, multilingual, and androgenous can be helpful for cultivating expertise in an increasingly diverse world.

The concepts of role stress and strain discussed by Hardy and Hardy (1988) are useful for understanding the dynamics of role transitions (see Table 5-2). They described role stress as a social structural condition in which role obligations are ambiguous, conflicting, incongruous, excessive, or unpredictable. Role strain is defined as the subjective feeling of frustration, tension, or anxiety experienced in response to role stress. It is believed that role strain can be minimized, although certainly not completely prevented, by the identification of potential role stressors, the development of strategies to cope with them, and rehearsal of situations designed to apply those strategies. It is acknowledged here that the difficulties experienced by neophytes in new positions can never be eliminated. As noted above, expertise is holistic, involving bodily perceptual skills and shared background knowledge as well as cognitive ability. A school-work, theory-practice, ideal-real gap will remain because of the nature of human skill acquisition.

Role Ambiguity

Role ambiguity (see Table 5-2) develops when there is a lack of clarity about expectations, a blurring of responsibilities, uncertainty regarding implementation of subroles, and the inherent uncertainty of the existent knowledge base of a discipline. According to Hardy and Hardy (1988), role ambiguity characterizes all professional positions. They pointed out that role ambiguity may be positive in that it offers opportunities for creative possibilities. It can be expected to be more prominent in professions undergoing change, such as those in the health care field. Role ambiguity has been widely discussed in relation to the CNS role (Chase et al., 1996; Payne & Baumgartner,

TABLE 5-2 SELECTED ROLE CONCEPTS		
CONCEPTS	DEFINITION	EXAMPLES
Role stress*	A situation of increased role performance demand	Learning a new role in school
Role strain*	Subjective feeling of frustration, tension, or anxiety in response to role stress	Feeling of decreased self-esteem when performance is below expectations of self or significant others
Role stressors*	Factors that produce role stress	Financial, personal, or academic demands and role expectations that are ambiguous, conflicting, excessive, or unpredictable
Role ambiguity*	Unclear expectations, diffuse responsibilities, uncertainty about subroles	All professional positions have some degree of ambuiguity because of the evolving nature of roles and expansion of skills and knowledge
Role incongruity*	A role with incompatibility between skills and abilities and role obligations or incompatibility between personal values, self-concept, and role obligations	A role requiring excellent therapeutic communication skills, but that also requires performing invasive procedures
Role conflict*	Occurs when role expectations are perceived to be mutually exclusive or contradictory	Interprofessional role conflict between APNs and physicians Intraprofessional role conflict between APNs and other nurses
Role transition*,†	A dynamic process of change over time as new roles are acquired	Changing from a staff nurse role to an APN role
Role insufficiency†	Feeling inadequate to meet role demands	New graduate
Role supplementation†	Anticipatory socialization	Role-specific educational components

* Developed from Hardy, M. E., & Hardy, W. L. (1988). Role stress and role strain. In M. E. Hardy & M. E. Conway (Eds.), *Role theory: Perspectives for health professionals* (2nd ed., pp. 159–239). Norwalk, CT: Appleton & Lange.
† Developed from Schumacher, K. L., & Meleis, A. I. (1994). Transitions: A central concept in nursing. *Image: The Journal of Nursing Scholarship, 26*(2), 119–127.

1993; Redekopp, 1997; see also Chapter 13), but it is a relevant issue for other APN roles as well.

Role Incongruity

Role incongruity is intrarole conflict, which Hardy and Hardy (1988) described as developing from two sources. Incompatibility between skills and abilities and role obligations is one source of role incongruity. An example might be an APN with excellent history-taking and therapeutic communication skills whose role requires performing invasive procedures, which may be experienced as more stressful and less satisfying. Another source of role incongruity is incompatibility between personal values, self-concept, and expected role behaviors. An APN who hoped for a position with 100% clinical practice may experience this incongruity if the position requires performing administrative functions. An example comes from Banda's (1985) study of psychiatric liaison CNSs in acute care hospitals and community health agencies. She reported that they viewed consultation and teaching as their major functions, while research and administrative activities were associated with role strain.

Interprofessional Role Conflict

Role conflict develops when role expectations are perceived to be contradictory or mutually exclusive. APNs may experience intrarole conflict as well as both inter- and intraprofessional role conflicts. Conflicts between physicians and APNs constitute the most common situations of interprofessional conflict of interest here. Major sources of conflict for physicians and APNs are the perceived economic threat of competition, limited resources in clinical training sites, and lack of experience working together.

The relationship between anesthesiologists and CRNAs provides a useful exemplar for considering the issues of interprofessional role conflict between physicians and APNs. The fact that nurse anesthetists predated the first physician anesthesiologists by 100 years (Aiken & Sage, 1992) perhaps partially explains why the relationship between anesthesiologists and CRNAs has historically been interpreted by anesthesiologists as one of direct competition, thus creating an adversarial stance. Their relationship over the years might be characterized as a cold war with overt offensives mounted periodically by anesthesiologists. Following World War II, anesthesiologists launched a major effort to eliminate nurses from the field of anesthesia (Gunn, 1991). In the mid-1980s, the concept of all-physician anesthesia was again promoted and many nurse anesthesia programs were closed (DePaolis-Lutzo, 1987). Recently another overt offensive has been advanced against CRNA autonomy in the operating room, with anesthesiologists calling for supervision of CRNAs by physicians (Federwisch, 1999; see also Chapter 18).

When APNs are viewed as direct competitors, it is understandable that some if not most physicians would be reluctant to be involved in assisting with APN education (National Commission on Nurse Anesthesia Education, 1990). In like manner, some nurse educators espouse the belief that physicians should not be involved in teaching and/or precepting APNs. Improved relationships between APNs and physicians will require redefinition of the situation by both groups. Fagin (1992) asserted that collaboration is imperative:

> *Comprehensive health care today requires the broad spectrum of knowledge that no one practitioner can provide. Costs of health and medical care have been shown to be reduced by the appropriate utilization of nurses working in teams or in consultative relationships with physicians. Nurses and physicians are not in competition for the patient. As physicians' work roles and autonomy change and more of them are salaried employees, the convergence of issues affecting nurses and doctors will benefit from collaboration.*

(pp. 357–358).

Redefinition of the situation between APNs and physicians may be facilitated by prioritizing public service over self-serving personal and professional interests. Collaboration between nurses and physicians is good for both groups as well as the public (see Chapter 11).

Rooks (1983) noted that "collegiality, cooperation, communication, and complementarity—not competition—should be the characteristics of nurse-midwives' relationships with physicians" (p. 3). King (1990) observed that "the collegial relationship is built on shared knowledge, confidence, and mutual trust in which an egalitarian working situation develops" (p. 172). Interprofessional role conflict results when there is a deficiency in any of these factors. Rooks and Haas (1986) discussed this problem in terms of nurse-midwifery and suggested that educating physicians about nurse-midwifery care, with emphasis on its complementary relationship to medical care, may decrease conflict. They also recommended CNM appointments on medical school faculties to increase awareness of nurse-midwifery and improve interprofessional communication. These recommendations are relevant for all APN groups.

However, the complementary nature of advanced nursing practice to medical care is a foreign concept for those physicians who view all health care as an extension of medical care and APNs as physician extenders. This misunderstanding of advanced nursing practice underlies their opposition to independent roles for nurses because they believe such nurses want to practice medicine without a license. The fact that nursing has its own knowledge and skills is a novel idea for physicians who see nursing as a subset of medicine. Thus an information campaign on individual, institutional, and national levels may be necessary to change such perceptions held by physicians and the general public.

More mundane matters also contribute to interprofessional role conflicts. The factors Long and Sharp (1982) identified nearly 20 years ago as contributing to conflictual relationships between CNMs and obstetrics (OB) residents still ring true today. Factors identified in their survey included residents' perceptions of CNMs having more favorable work schedules, working with a predominately low-risk patient population, and having positions somewhat separate from the OB faculty-resident hierarchy. These factors might be expected to be applicable to other APN-physician situations as well. Long and Sharp (1982) recommended using differences in practice between APNs and physicians as areas of inquiry rather than as targets of criticism. One way to promote positive interprofessional relationships is to structure education and practice experiences between APN and physician students and faculty to enhance mutual understanding. Developing such interdisciplinary experiences is difficult because of different academic calendars and clinical schedules. Such obstacles can be overcome if these interdisciplinary activities are considered essential for improved health care delivery.

Intraprofessional Role Conflict

APNs experience intraprofessional role conflict with other nurses and within the nursing profession for a variety of reasons. The historical development of APN roles has been fraught with conflict and controversy in nursing education and nursing organizations, particularly for CNMs (Varney, 1987), NPs (Ford, 1982), and CRNAs (Gunn, 1991; see also Chapter 1). Relationships between these APN groups and nursing as a discipline have improved markedly in recent years, yet difficulties remain to be surmounted. For example, the necessity of a nursing foundation for midwifery has been challenged (see Chapter 17). One would expect current discussions about broadening the scope of midwifery care to encompass primary care management of women's health to promote renewed interest in and commitment to maintaining a nursing foundation (American College of Nurse-Midwives, 1993).

Kimbro's (1978) description of communication difficulties between CNMs and staff RNs still seems relevant today for all APN roles. She noted a lack of communication between the two groups of nurses in three areas: (1) on an organizational level, (2) during educational programs, and (3) in the literature. She pointed out that value differences and structural role differences set up a situation for intraprofessional role conflict in that staff RNs were concerned with 24-hour coverage and smooth functioning of the unit as a whole while CNMs were more concerned with direct care of their individual patients.

Hazle's (1985) descriptive study of inter-role conflict between OB nurses and CNMs indicated that they generally viewed one another positively, but that conflicts did arise over intrapartum management. Lack of communication seemed to be a major source of conflict in the critical incidents reported (Hazle, 1985). She commented that when the OB nurse in the hospital setting encounters a CNM, it sets up a hierarchical relationship where another nurse (the CNM) performs functions usually within the purview of medicine and beyond the usual scope of nursing practice. If OB nurses are not adequately informed and oriented about CNM roles and functions, conflict may ensue. Familiarizing OB nurses with CNM job descriptions was recommended to decrease confusion about CNM role expectations.

Hamric and Taylor (1989) pointed out that staff resistance to change, complacency or apathy, and the fact that nurses are generally not accustomed to seeking consultation from other nurses as experts can impede CNS role development. Lurie (1981) and Brykczynski (1985) reported refusals by staff nurses to perform support functions, such as taking vital signs and drawing blood, for patients assigned to NPs, along with the absence of negative sanctions by their nursing supervisors for these behaviors. These behaviors are suggestive of horizontal violence commonly observed within oppressed groups (Roberts, 1983). Interpreting intraprofessional conflict as deriving from acting out hostility toward one's own less powerful group instead of toward the more powerful oppressors can be useful for increasing awareness of the need to develop strategies to overcome these difficulties. Such a perspective suggests that, by providing information and support, nurses can learn to value their own worth and significance, become empowered, and consequently practice supportive rather than destructive behaviors toward other nurses.

According to Curry (1994), important components of successfully integrating NP practice in an emergency room setting are thorough orientation of staff nurses to the APN role, including clear guidelines and policies regarding responsibility issues. Another significant strategy for minimizing intraprofessional role conflict is for the new APN (this holds true for APN students also) to spend time getting to know the nursing staff to establish rapport and learn as much as possible about the new setting from those who really know what is going on—the nurses. This affirms the value and significance of the nursing staff and sets up a positive atmosphere for collegiality and intraprofessional role cooperation and collaboration.

ROLE TRANSITIONS

Role transitions are defined here as dynamic processes of change that occur over time as new roles are acquired (see Table 5-2). Five essential factors found to influence role transitions were noted by Schumacher and Meleis (1994):

1. The personal meaning of the transition, which relates to the degree of identity crisis experienced
2. The degree of planning, which involves the time and energy devoted to anticipating the change
3. Environmental barriers and supports, which refer to family, peer, school, and other components
4. Level of knowledge and skill, which relates to prior experience and school experiences
5. Expectations, which are related to role models, literature, media, and the like

Role strain or role insufficiency accompanying the transition to APN roles can be minimized, although certainly not completely prevented, by (1) individualized assessment of these five essential factors, (2) development of strategies to cope with them, and (3) rehearsal of situations designed to apply those strategies.

APN Role Acquisition (in School)

The personal meaning of role transitions is a major focus of literature in nursing role development. In a review of APN role development literature from certificate and graduate nursing programs, alterations of self-identity and self-concept emerged as a consistent theme, with role acquisition experiences commonly depicted as identity crises (see Brykczynski, 1996, for a detailed discussion of this earlier work). It is important to note that literature on APN role transitions refers to individuals who are already nurses. The process of role transition for generic APN master's programs needs to be investigated. Because these individuals were not functioning as nurses prior to their APN educational program, one might speculate that their role transition experiences would be different from the more typical APN student with prior experience as a nurse.

Roberts and colleagues (1997) reported findings very similar to those observed more than 20 years previously by Anderson, Leonard, and Yates (1974). The earlier publication described the process of role development observed in three NP programs (a graduate program, a postbaccalaureate certificate program, and a continuing education program) while the later one refers to a current graduate NP program. Anderson and colleagues' (1974) description of NP students' progression from dependence to interdependence, accompanied by regression, anxiety, and conflict, was found to be similar to observations made by Roberts and associates (1997) with current graduate NP students over a period of 6 years (see Table 5–3). A similar role transition process has also been consistently observed by the author and her colleagues in teaching role and clinical courses for graduate NP students for the past 14 years.

Roberts and colleagues (1997) observed 100 NP graduate students and reviewed their student clinical journals. They identified three major areas of transition as students progressed from dependence to interdependence: (1) development of professional competence, (2) change in role identity, and (3) evolving relationships with preceptors and faculty. It is not surprising to note that the lowest level of competence coincided with the highest level of role confusion. This occurred at the end of the first semester and the beginning of the second semester in the three-semester program examined (Roberts et al., 1997). The author and her colleagues have observed that the most intense transition period comes at the end of the students' second semester (the first clinical preceptorship occurs during this semester) and continues through

TABLE 5-3	ROLE ACQUISITION PROCESS IN SCHOOL
STAGE	DESCRIPTIVE CHARACTERISTICS
I: Complete dependence	Immersion in learning medical components of care Role transition associated with role confusion and anxiety Decreased appreciation for psychosocial components of health and illness concerns Loss of confidence in clinical skills, feelings of incompetence
II: Developing competence	Ongoing clinical preceptorship experiences Didactic classes incorporate medical diagnostic and both nursing and medical therapeutic components along with personal experience of illness components Renewed sense of appreciation for the value of nursing knowledge and skills More realistic self-expectations of clinical performance, although still uncomfortable about accountability Increased confidence in ability to succeed in learning and making a valid contribution to care Begin forming own philosophy and standards of practice
III: Independence	Comfortable with ability to conduct holistic assessments (both physical and psychosocial) Concentrate on intervention and management options Conflicts with preceptors occur as student and preceptor challenge one another Conflicts with faculty relate to management options, clinical evaluations, exam questions, concern over not being taught all there is to know
IV: Interdependence	Renewed appreciation for the interdependence of nursing and medicine Each student develops her or his own individualized version of the advanced practice role

Developed from Anderson, E. M., Leonard, B. J., & Yates, J. A. (1974). Epigenesis of the nurse practitioner role. *American Journal of Nursing, 10*(18), 12–16; and Roberts, S. J., Tabloski, P., & Bova, C. (1997). Epigenesis of the nurse practitioner role revisited. *Journal of Nursing Education, 36*(2), 67–73.

half of the third semester in our four-semester graduate NP program. In other words, this phenomenon occurs after the first clinical immersion experience. It can be helpful for faculty to identify such periods of high stress in their particular program so that support can be built in during those periods.

Roberts and colleagues (1997) described the first transition as involving an initial feeling of loss of confidence and competence accompanied by anxiety (see Table 5–3, stage I). Initial clinical experiences were associated with the desire to observe rather than to provide care, the inability to recall simple facts, the omission of essential data from history taking, feelings of awkwardness with patients, and difficulty prioritizing. The students' focus at this time was almost exclusively on acquiring and refining assessment skills and continued development of physical examination techniques. By the end of the first semester, students reported returning feelings of confidence and the regaining of their former competence in interpersonal skills. Although still tentative about diagnostic and treatment decisions, they reported feeling more comfortable with patients as some of their ability to nurse began to return (see Table 5–3, stage II).

Transitions in nursing role identity occurring during the first two stages were associated with feelings of role confusion. Students were dismayed at how slow and inefficient they were clinically, and reported feelings of self-doubt and lack of confidence in their abilities to ever function in the "real world of health care." They sought short cuts to try to increase their efficiency. They reported profound feelings of responsibility regarding diagnostic and treatment decisions and at the same time increasingly realized the real limitations of clinical practice when confronted with the real-life situations of their patients. They recalled finding it easy to second guess physicians' decisions in their previous nursing roles, but now they found those decisions more problematic when they were responsible for making them. They joked about feeling like adolescents.

A blending of the new APN and the former nurse developed at this time as they renewed their appreciation for their previous interpersonal skills as teacher, supporter, and collaborator and again perceived their patients as unique individuals in the context of their life situations. Increased awareness of the uncertainty of the process of making definitive diagnostic and treatment decisions developed. Although these insights served to demystify the clinical diagnostic process, the students' anxiety about providing care increased. Learning about strategies to cope with clinical decision making in situations of uncertainty can lessen anxiety and promote increased confidence (Brykczynski, 1991).

The transition in the relationship between students and preceptors and students and faculty involved students feeling anxious that they were not learning enough and would never know enough to practice competently. They felt frustrated and perceived that faculty and preceptors were not providing them with all the information that they needed. As they felt more confident and competent, students began to question the clinical judgments of their preceptors and faculty. This process is thought to help students advance from independence to interdependence—the last stage of the transition process. Much of the conflict at this juncture appeared to derive from students' feelings of "ambivalence about giving up dependence on external authorities" such as preceptors and faculty and assuming responsibility for making independent judgments based on their own assessments from their clinical and educational experiences and the literature (Roberts et al., 1997, p. 71).

The relevance of these role acquisition processes for other APN roles has not been investigated. Several of the author's CNM faculty colleagues reported that these transition processes were congruent with the role transition experiences they observe with their students. CRNA faculty contacted by this author concurred that a similar process occurs with their students with the exception that their students seem more satisfied that they are being taught all they need to know.

Strategies To Facilitate Role Acquisition

The anticipatory socialization to APN roles that occurs in graduate education is analogous to immunization (Kramer, 1974). The overall objective is to expose role incumbents to as many real-life experiences as possible during the educational program to minimize their reality shock and role insufficiency upon graduation and initial role implementation. Role transition can be incorporated into APN curricula as: (1) the overall framework for designing an APN curriculum, (2) a specific role course, or (3) role seminars that span an entire curriculum. All APN programs today, regardless of specialty, should have requirements for basic content related to professional roles and issues. If there is not a separate role course, careful attention must be paid to this curriculum component so that it does not become integrated out of existence.

Specific strategies for facilitating role acquisition are presented here and categorized according to three major purposes: (1) role rehearsal (2) development of clinical knowledge and skills, and (3) creating a supportive network (see Table 5-4). For adequate role rehearsal, it is important that APN students experience all aspects of the core competencies (see Chapter 3) directly, while faculty and fellow students are readily available to help them process or debrief these experiences (Hamric & Taylor, 1989; Hupcey, 1990). APN students should be cautioned that other nurses, physicians, other providers, and administrators in the work setting may only value clinical expertise and not the other core competencies. Strategies for enhancing understanding of how the core competencies are embedded in each APN role include preparation of short- and long-term goals to use as guides in development of professional portfolios, analysis of existing position descriptions, and development of the ideal position description. These are also helpful for guiding students in their search for an initial APN position.

Portfolio materials (Hawkins & Thibodeau, 1993; see Chapter 21) can be used for learning assignments and seminar discussions by having APN students share drafts of their portfolio components with peers, faculty, and preceptors and then revise them based on the feedback received. These strategies contribute to refinement and modification of definitions and expectations for future APN roles and promote development of students as colleagues and peer evaluators. Learning experiences, such as role negotiation and identification with a role model, that offer students realistic opportunities for applying assessment, management, and role negotiation skills will enhance APN role acquisition (Hunter et al., 1996). Judith Spross (personal communication, 1995) recommended that beginning APN students conduct "burning question" interviews with experienced APNs to develop a realistic vision and to focus their role acquisition experiences.

A variety of panels can be convened during role seminars to stimulate exploration of issues and to promote greater role clarity. For example, a panel comprising various APNs is helpful for students to gain an appreciation of similarities as well as differences in available roles. Another useful panel is one composed of program graduates and potential employers that helps APN students target their résumés and position descriptions. An interdisciplinary panel comprising a nurse in an APN role and a physician in a complementary role can be beneficial for clarifying perceptions and discussing strategies for minimizing interprofessional role conflict. The impact and significance of students seeing successful APN graduates cannot be overstated.

Two popular role course activities are a discussion where students present critical incidents encountered while beginning to develop their roles and a social event, which includes faculty, graduates, APN students, preceptors, and administrators, specifically focused on describing the APN role in a social setting. Critical incident presentations require students to identify an actual role conflict situation from their clinical preceptorship experience. Students analyze these situations using the critical incident format adapted from Gordon and Benner (1980) and present them in small seminar groups for discussion. In the second activity, Diers' (1992) brief article, which reports reader responses to the questions "You're so smart, why are you just a nurse?" and "Why aren't you a doctor?" serves as a conversation starter at the social event. The purpose of this activity is to provide rehearsal for articulating responses to such questions in future social encounters.

The development of clinical knowledge and skills for APN role acquisition can be promoted by planning for realistic clinical experiences with the support of faculty and preceptors nearby. Clinical conferences can be conducted to share full details of clinical situations so that assessment and management decisions can be presented and refuted or defended in a supportive learning environment. Case studies can be

TABLE 5–4 STRATEGIES TO PROMOTE APN ROLE ACQUISITION IN SCHOOL

PURPOSE	STRATEGIES	IMPLEMENTATION
Role rehearsal	Directly experience all core skills	Faculty and students monitor experiences on all core competencies
	Professional marketing portfolio	Prepare a folder containing philosophy of care, résumé, ideal position description, salary data, certification details, APN brochures, etc.
	Lifelike role negotiation seminar	Invite interdisciplinary guests to participate
	Identify with a role model	Develop a mentee relationship with an APN and maintain contact throughout APN program
	Burning question interviews	Develop a list of questions of great importance to your future role satisfaction to ask APNs
	Panel discussions	Faculty and students can plan a variety of panels to increase understanding of positions available, practice settings, other health team members, etc.
	Critical incident presentations	Prepare an in-depth self-evaluation of a situation of role conflict you have experienced in learning the APN role and share this with peers and faculty
Develop clinical knowledge and skills	Realistic clinical immersion experiences	Clinical experiences need to reflect the real world of practice as much as possible
	Clinical conferences	Discussion of clinical experiences with faculty and peers promotes clinical understanding
	Clinical situation narrative seminars	Share full contextual details of situations to promote understanding of aspects of embedded clinical practice knowledge
	Case study analysis	Clinical examples make classroom learning more concrete and memorable
	Clinical logs	Maintain a listing of all patients seen, including pertinent details such as age, diagnosis, etc.
	Final clinical preceptorships	A final semester of clinical practice helps put it all together
	Faculty practice	Maintenance of faculty clinical competence enhances credibility of APN faculty
Create a support network	Establish peer support system	Join local, state, and national APN groups
	Share self and peer evaluations	Learn to be comfortable with giving and receiving feedback for improvement
	Faculty-student-preceptor social functions	Foster an APN supportive environment among faculty, clinicians, students, staff, and administrators
	Establish a pattern for continuing education	Subscribe to selected APN journals, participate in APN conferences, keep a record of continuing education hours
	Create a virtual community	Establish e-mail and Internet connections
	Establish a self-monitoring system	Select a framework for self-evaluating role enactment to keep track of progress in role transition over time

Adapted from Brykczynski, K. A. (2000). Chart 1–6: Strategies to promote NP role acquisition in school. In P. Meredith & N. M. Horan (Eds.), *Adult primary care* (p. 16). Philadelphia: W. B. Saunders; reprinted with permission.

incorporated into didactic classes, assignments, and exams to enhance their clinical relevance. Clinical logs were recommended by Hamric and Taylor (1989) to document experiences during the educational program for CNSs. Most current APN programs require that their students maintain clinical logs. Clinical logs provide a record of the variety and type of experiences students have had that can be useful for documenting their clinical hours to substantiate their qualification to sit for certification exams. They can also be useful for students in planning future clinical experiences and for graduates to describe their clinical experiences to potential employers. Final clinical preceptorships, sometimes called capstone experiences, are important for solidifying the acquisition of role components in actual practice.

Clinical experiences for APN students should emphasize realism and a holistic situational perspective to promote recognition that the complex clinical judgments involved in APN assessment and management of patient situations over time is not simply technical medical knowledge. Studies of APN practice demonstrate that advanced practice roles incorporate a holistic approach that blends elements of nursing and medicine (Brown, 1990; Brykczynski, 1989; Johnson, 1993; also see Chapter 6). Teaching and learning experiences for all of the APN role components should integrate elements of research, teaching, and theory and be incorporated into specialty APN courses to build on the knowledge gained in the traditional graduate core and clinical support courses in the curriculum.

Finally and perhaps most importantly, an overall strategy for enhancing APN clinical knowledge and skill is for faculty to maintain competency in clinical practice. Clinical competency enhances faculty ability to evaluate students clinically, to discuss clinically relevant examples in classes, to serve as a preceptor for students, and to evaluate the care provided in preceptorship sites. The clinical competence of faculty is important to prevent a wide gap between education and practice, to enhance faculty credibility, and to foster realistic expectations for new APN graduates.

The creation of a support network can be facilitated by establishing a peer support system, planning social functions with faculty and preceptors, and creating a virtual community (see Table 5–4). The establishment of a system for self-directed learning activities during the first few years following program completion forms the basis for maintaining competence throughout one's career (Gunn, 1998). The development of a system for lifelong learning should be initiated during the APN educational program as students create a self-monitoring system that includes clinical and role transition experiences over time to serve as a reality check or timetable. Upon graduation, continuing education program attendance could be incorporated into this monitoring system to facilitate compilation of necessary documentation for certification along with ongoing self-evaluation and role development.

APN Role Implementation (at Work)

After successfully emerging from the APN educational process, new APN graduates face yet another transition from the student role to the APN role (see Figure 5–1). APN graduates can be expected to experience attitudinal, behavioral, and value conflicts as they move from the academic world, where holistic care is highly valued, to the work world, where organizational efficiency is paramount. Anticipatory guidance is needed for role transition all over again. The process of APN role implementation is an example of a situational transition (Schumacher & Meleis, 1994), which has been described in the literature as a progressive movement through phases

(Baker, 1979; Hamric & Taylor, 1989; Oda, 1977; Page & Arena, 1991). There is general agreement that significant overlap and fluidity exist among the phases. However, for purposes of discussion the phases are considered sequentially. The two major research studies investigating APN role implementation processes that have been conducted include Hamric and Taylor's (1989) study of CNS role development and Brown and Olshansky's (1997, 1998) study of NP role transition.

Hamric and Taylor (1989) described seven phases of CNS role development along with associated characteristics and developmental tasks from analysis of questionnaires returned by 100 CNSs (see Table 5-5). All but 5% of the 42 CNSs in their first positions for 3 years or less experienced progression through the first three phases (identical to those phases identified by Baker [1979]). Most of the CNS respondents went through these three phases within 2 years. Phase one, orientation (see Table 5-5) is characterized by enthusiasm, optimism, and attention to mastery of clinical skills. The second phase, frustration is associated with feelings of conflict, inadequacy, frustration, and anxiety. The next phase, implementation is described as one of role modification in response to interactions with others. This phase is associated with a renewed or returning perspective.

Hamric and Taylor (1989) found that CNSs with more than 3 years' experience described their role development experiences in terms very different from Baker's (1979) phases. Content analysis of these data led to a description of four additional phases (see Table 5-5). They identified the integration phase (a new phase replacing Baker's [1979] reassessment phase), which was characterized by "self-confidence and assurance in the role, high job satisfaction, an advanced level of practice, and signs of recognition and respect for expertise within and outside the work setting" (Hamric & Taylor, 1989, p. 56). Only 10% of the CNSs with less than 5 years' experience in the role met the criteria for this phase, while 50% of those with more than 6 years' experience could be categorized as being in this phase. The integration phase was typically reached by 3 to 5 years in the CNS role. This fourth phase, integration (thought to be reached only after successful transition through the earlier phases) is characterized by refinement of clinical expertise and integration of role components appropriate for the particular situation.

Hamric and Taylor (1989) also described three negative phases not evident in previous literature. The frozen phase was described as being associated with frustration, anger, and lack of career satisfaction. The reorganization phase was characterized by the restructuring of role responsibilities and changing expectations. The complacent phase was characterized by comfort, stability, and maintenance of the status quo. Unlike the integration phase, these additional phases share a negative, nonproductive character. One might speculate that APNs experiencing these negative phases would be more vulnerable to position changes in response to health care reform.

The complexity of APN role development processes is further demonstrated by findings from Brown and Olshansky's (1997, 1998) grounded theory study of the role transition experiences of 35 novice NPs during their first year of practice. They described a four-stage process occurring during the first year of practice, which is depicted in Table 5-6 along with developmental tasks and strategies developed by the author. The first stage, an in-between or limbo stage, was not described in previous literature. During this stage, new graduates take certification examinations, obtain necessary recognition or licensure from state boards of nursing, and look for positions. This stage is influenced by the time required to obtain the necessary credentials for APN practice and may be shortened in the future by the availability of certification examinations by computer.

Phase	Characteristics	Strategies	
Integration	Self-confident and assured in role Rates self at advanced level of practice Activities reflect wide recognition, influence in area of specialty Continuously feels challenged; takes on new projects; expands practice Either moderately or very satisfied with present position Congruence between personal and organizational goals and expectations	Continued role evolution and skill development to strengthen subroles and competencies Share expertise and experience with others through publications, research, professional activities Maintain flexible approach Be alert for signs of complacency or boredom	Continue debriefing sessions Plan for role expansion and refinement Schedule performance and impact evaluations Develop broader professional interests Formulate short-term goals for further development
Frozen	Self-confident, assured in role Rates self at intermediate or advanced practice level Experiencing anger/frustration reflecting experience Conflict between self-goals and those of organization/supervisor Reports sense of being unable to move forward because of forces outside of self	Obtain feedback from supervisor and peers Re-evaluate self-goals in relation to CNS role and organization Objective assessment of organization: Is there potential for compatibility? Attempt to redesign or renegotiate the role If unsuccessful, consider change in position/career direction	Self-assessment and early recognition of problems Conflict resolution and role clarification discussions Appraisal of APN goals in relation to organizational goals Renegotiate role expectations Consider career move/change
Reorganization	Reports earlier experiences that represent integration Organization experiencing major changes Pressure to change role in ways that are incongruent with own concept of CNS role and/or self-goals	Open discussion with change agents Attempt compromise to preserve integrity of role and still meet needs of organization If unsuccessful, change position/title or negotiate job change	
Complacent	Experiences self in role as settled and comfortable Variable job satisfaction Questionable impact on organization	Need to re-energize Reconfigure role to allow growth by identifying new need of client population or institution	

Adapted from Hamric, A. B., & Taylor, J. W. (1989). Role development of the CNS. In A. B. Hamric & J. A. Spross (Eds.), *The clinical nurse specialist in theory and practice* (2nd ed., p. 48). Philadelphia: W. B. Saunders; reprinted with permission.

TABLE 5–6 TRANSITION STAGES IN FIRST YEAR OF PRIMARY CARE PRACTICE

STAGE*	CHARACTERISTICS*	DEVELOPMENTAL TASKS	FACILITATION STRATEGIES
Laying the foundation	Period of role identity confusion immediately postgraduation Not yet an NP, but no longer a student Feelings of worry, confusion, and insecurity about ability to practice successfully as an NP	Recuperate from school Initiate a job search and secure a position Obtain certification	Take time out to recuperate from the pressures of school Plan rewards for self Maintain peer support network Refine professional portfolio and use it to analyze available positions in terms of future goals
Launching	Discomfort of advanced-beginner level of knowledge and skills Feelings of unreality, insecurity—"the imposter phenomenon" Pervasive performance anxiety Daily stress Time pressure	Develop realistic expectations Incorporate feeling of legitimacy into NP role identity Cope with anxiety Mobilize problem-solving skills Work on time management and setting priorities† Develop support system†	Plan for longer appointments initially Anticipate need for time to feel comfortable in new role Realize that the transition process is time limited Schedule debriefing sessions with experienced MD or APN Seek peer and mentor support regularly Learn time-saving tips Clarify appropriate patient problems to work with initially Monitor internal self-talk—be positive

Meeting the challenge	Decreased anxiety Increased feeling of legitimacy Increased confidence develops along with increased competence Increased acceptance and comfort with the uncertainty inherent in primary care	Expand recognition of practice concerns to include the work environment Gain situated knowledge and skill in managing clinical problems Identify tangible accomplishments† Develop individualized style of approaching patients and organizing care Gain ability to handle uncertainty	Schedule a 6-month evaluation Sustain communication with peers, administrators, and others† Modify expectations to be more realistic Learn from repetitive practice Structure work situation so that resources are readily available Practice strategies to manage uncertainty
Broadening the perspective	Feeling of enhanced self-esteem Solid feeling of legitimacy and competence Realistic and positive feelings about future practice	Acknowledge strengths and identify ways to incorporate additional challenges Identify larger system problems and seek solutions (All the developmental tasks from the Integration phase of Table 5–5 would be appropriate here also†)	Schedule a 12-month evaluation to reflect on progress and accomplishments Continue to seek verification and feedback from colleagues Make changes in work situation to increase support and effectiveness Inform staff and colleagues about NP role Affirm self-worth (Facilitation strategies from the Integration phase of Table 5–5 would be useful here also†)

* Data from Brown, M. A., & Olshansky, E. (1997). From limbo to legitimacy: A theoretical model of the transition to the primary care nurse practitioner role. *Nursing Research, 46*(1), 46–51; and Brown, M. A., & Olshansky, E. (1998). Becoming a primary care nurse practitioner: Challenges of the initial year of practice. *The Nurse Practitioner, 23*(7), 46, 52, 58, 61–66.
† Developed from Hamric, A. B., & Taylor, J. W. (1989). Role development of the CNS. In A. B. Hamric & J. A. Spross (Eds.), *The clinical nurse specialist in theory and practice* (2nd ed., p. 48). Philadelphia: W. B. Saunders.

the clinical expert role. They also suggested making appointments with nursing leaders, physicians, and other health professionals during this phase to garner administrative support. They recommended distributing business cards and making their job description available for discussion. Strategies suggested for networking within the system include developing peer support groups, being accessible by beeper, and getting involved in interdisciplinary committees. They recommended withholding suggestions for change until the system is more fully assessed. Judith Spross (personal communication, 1995) suggested that, when a new APN joins the staff of an organization, the administrator should send a letter describing the APN's background experiences and new position to key people in the organization.

Hamric and Taylor (1989) observed that the frustration phase may come and go and may overlap other phases. They noted that painful affective responses are typical of this very difficult phase. They suggested that monthly sessions for sharing concerns with a group of peers and an administrator may facilitate movement through this phase. Strategies identified as helpful for energizing movement from the frustration phase to the implementation phase included assistance with time management, support groups to ameliorate feelings of inadequacy, conflict resolution and role clarification discussions, reassessing priorities and setting realistic expectations, and focusing on short-term, visible goals. Page and Arena (1991) recommended keeping a work portfolio to document activities so progress is more readily visible. This can be an expansion of the portfolio and self-monitoring system begun during the APN program. Brown and Olshansky (1997, 1998) pointed out that organized sources of support such as phone calls, seminars, planned meetings with mentors, and scheduled time for consultation can significantly decrease feelings of anxiety. They noted that recognition of the discomfort arising from moving from "expert back to novice" and realization that previous expertise can be valuable in the new role may help reduce feelings of inadequacy. They suggested that requesting reasonable time frames for initial patient visits, because novices take longer than experienced practitioners, is key to initial adjustment.

During the implementation phase, it is important for the APN to reassess demands to guard against feeling overwhelmed. Priorities may need to be readjusted, and short-term goals may be reformulated. Brown and Olshansky (1997, 1998) observed that competence and confidence are fostered through repetition. They also recommended scheduling a formal evaluation after approximately 6 months. Feedback about areas of strength and need for improvement should be sought as part of the evaluation process during this phase. Strategies mentioned as important during this time include seeking administrative support through involvement in meetings, maintaining visibility in clinical areas, and developing in-service programs with input from staff (Page & Arena, 1991). After some time in the implementation phase, APNs may plan and execute small-scale projects to demonstrate their effectiveness.

Hamric and Taylor's (1989) survey data indicated that it is during the integration phase that CNSs maximize their role potential. Satisfactory completion of the earlier phases appeared to be essential for passage into the integration phase. Strategies for enhancing and maintaining optimal role implementation during this phase include having a trusted colleague who can act as a safe sounding board for "feedback, constructive criticism, and advice" (Hamric & Taylor, 1989, p. 79). During this phase, it is important to have a plan to guide continued role expansion and refinement, such as the portfolio mentioned earlier. Seeking appointment to key committees is important to broaden organizational impact. Administrative support and constructive feedback from a trusted mentor continue to be important. Development of a promotional system that offers professional advancement in the APN practice role remains a challenge for practitioners and administrators. Page and Arena (1991) observed that less time is required for establishing relationships and assessing the system during this phase so more time can be devoted to areas of scholarly interests. Brown and Olshansky (1995) pointed out the importance of formulating short-term goals to further development.

Whether the frozen, reorganization, and complacent phases are distinct developmental phases or variations of the implementation and integration phases, they are clearly negative resolutions for APNs and their organizations. Strategies described by Hamric and Taylor (1989) for enhancing role development in these phases are included in Table 5–5. APNs should engage in periodic self-assessment so that they recognize beginning signs of characteristics associated with these phases, such as feelings of anger or dissatisfaction, conflict between self-goals and those of the organization or supervisor, feeling pressure to change one's APN role in ways that are incongruous with one's concept of the role, or feelings of complacency. Early problem recognition and taking proactive steps to deal with organizational changes can help prevent or ameliorate the negative feelings associated with these phases.

Hamric and Taylor (1989) stated that honest and open discussions with supervisors or individuals with whom the APN is experiencing conflict should be initiated to resolve conflicts and clarify role issues before they become serious problems. In situations of organizational turmoil that characterize the reorganization phase, APNs should evaluate their goals in relation to the organizational changes and renegotiate role expectations if necessary. Temporary role realignment may be negotiated to meet a short-term crisis, with explicit negotiated agreement that the APN would return to the original role after an agreed-upon time. Ann Hamric (personal communication, 1995) suggested that, in organizations increasingly concerned with fiscal efficiencies and patient outcomes, CNSs could negotiate to add a component of nurse case management to their practices for complex patients in their specialty. Wells, Erickson, and Spinella (1996) described their experience with developing a CNS role with a major focus on case management as one of role transition.

Ann Hamric (personal communication, 1995) asserted that APNs should not allow themselves, nor should administrators allow them, to remain in these negative phases. If discussion, compromise, and negotiations are unsuccessful, the APN should consider a career move, either to another position within the organization or to another organization. Career counseling may be a helpful strategy for the seriously disaffected APN.

Further analysis of the relationships between the stages described by Brown and Olshansky (1997, 1998) with NPs and the phases described by Hamric and Taylor (1989) with CNSs is needed. The relevance of these frameworks for transition processes experienced by other APNs, particularly CNMs and CRNAs, needs attention. Further refinement of these findings is needed for their incorporation into APN teaching, research, and practice. For example, two questions of interest are (1) Is the limbo stage common to other APN groups? and (2) Do the negative phases frozen, reorganization, and complacent appear after 3 years of practice in APN groups other than CNSs?

Facilitators and Barriers in the Work Setting

Aspects of the work setting exert a major influence on APN role definitions and expectations, thereby affecting role ambiguity, role incongruity and role conflict.

Findings from McFadden and Miller's (1994) survey of CNSs identified access to support services, such as computers, statistical consultation, and secretarial and library services, as facilitators to role development. Factors Lurie (1981) found to facilitate role development for NPs included being assigned their own caseload of patients and having access to their own exam room. Economic factors, such as pressure to manage large numbers of patients, impeded role development for the NPs studied. Lurie maintained that requirements to see 22 patients in one 8-hour day and physician evaluators' emphasis on assessment and management skills over counseling and patient education skills were two major factors that constrained NP teaching and counseling activities.

Lurie (1981) observed that, in spite of time pressures, some NPs managed to integrate counseling and teaching into the history and physical by performing these activities simultaneously. Research by Brykczynski (1985) and Johnson (1993) also reported that NPs incorporated counseling and teaching into the flow of patient visits — capturing the teachable moment without setting aside special time for it. The ability to incorporate teaching and counseling into the patient visit may be a factor of skill development gained with experience in the role. This observation may be used as a rationale for structuring longer time for visits and fewer total patients for new APNs, with gradual increases in caseloads as experience is accrued.

Administrative factors, including whether APNs are placed in line or staff positions, whether they are unit based, population based, or in some other arrangement, who evaluates them, and whether they report to administrative or clinical supervisors, are important to consider. Baird and Prouty (1989) maintained that the organizational design should have enough flexibility to change as the situation changes. The place-ments of various APN positions may differ even within one setting depending on size, complexity, and distribution of the patient population (Baird & Prouty, 1989; see also Chapters 20 and 24).

Issues of professional versus administrative authority underlie the importance of the structural placement of the APN within the organization. Effectiveness of the APN role is enhanced when there is a mutual fit between the goals and expectations of the individual and the organization (Cooper & Sparacino, 1990). Clarification of goals and expectations prior to employment and periodic reassessments can minimize conflict and enhance role development and effectiveness. One way to clarify goals and expectations, suggested by Cooper and Sparacino (1990), is to share one's position description with peers for critique and revise it based on their feedback before sharing it with one's supervisor or future employer and subsequently with other staff and colleagues.

Evaluation of Role Development

Evaluation is fundamental to enhancing role implementation. Evaluation of APNs should comprise both performance and impact (process and outcome) components (see Chapter 25). Development of a professional portfolio to document APN accom-plishments can be useful with both performance and impact evaluation. Performance evaluation for APNs should include self-evaluation, peer review, and administrative evaluation (Cooper & Sparacino, 1990; Hamric & Taylor, 1989). Use of a competency profile can be helpful for organizing evaluation in a dynamic way that allows for changes in subrole implementation over time as expertise, situations, and priorities change (Callahan & Bruton-Maree, 1994). The competency profile can be employed as an assessment of performance on each of the core APN skills.

Impact evaluation is important to demonstrate the effectiveness of each APN role. Ongoing development of appropriate impact evaluation measures, such as patient outcomes and patient satisfaction, are important. The existence of a reward system to provide for career advancement through a clinical ladder program and accrual of additional benefits is particularly important for retaining APNs in clinical roles. In less structured situations, APNs can negotiate for periodic reassessments and salary increases through options such as profit sharing.

The evaluation process expands to include interdisciplinary review when APN practice includes hospital privileges, prescriptive privileges, and third-party reimbursement. There are both positive and negative aspects to this expansion of the evaluation process. As Lurie (1981) noted, physicians may evaluate performance without recognizing the value of teaching and counseling, while a nursing supervisor may be more focused on general system components than individual patient care situations. Advantages to the review process associated with securing and maintaining hospital privileges include the multiple aspects that are considered in the evaluation, the variety of perspectives, and the visibility afforded APNs. In order to promote APN roles within organizations, it is important that APNs have key positions on hospital review committees. A major difficulty in implementing interdisciplinary peer review is lack of interaction between and among the incumbents of the various health professional groups during their formative educational programs (Brykczynski, 1989). The resurgence of interest in developing and implementing interdisciplinary educational experiences between nursing students and medical students is encouraging.

CONCLUSION

Role development experiences for APNs encompass role acquisition processes in school and role implementation processes after graduation. The limits of the educational process for preparing graduates for the realities of the work world need to be acknowledged. Students need to be informed about the human skill acquisition process and its stages, the processes of adult and professional socialization, identity transformation, role acquisition, role implementation, and overall career development. Knowing about (theoretical knowledge) and actually experiencing (practical knowledge) are very different phenomena, but at least students and new graduates can be forewarned. Anticipatory guidance can be provided through role rehearsal experiences, such as clinical preceptorships and role seminars. Students need to be encouraged to begin networking with practicing APNs through local, state, and national APN groups. This networking is especially important for APNs who will not be practicing in close proximity to other APNs. Experienced APNs and new APN graduates can form mutually beneficial relationships.

There needs to be open acknowledgment that anticipatory socialization experiences in school can facilitate role acquisition, but they cannot prevent the transition that occurs with movement into a new position and actual role implementation. It is essential that APN programs have a firm foundation in the real world. However, a certain degree of incongruence or conflict between academic ideals and work-world realities exists. It is important to guide and direct planned change and to guard against mere maintenance of the status quo. Support for the developmental phases of role implementation in the work setting needs to be developed and maintained. Support groups in local APN organizations are especially useful for enhancing both role acquisition (in school) and role implementation (at work).

APN role development has been described as dynamic, complex, and situational. It is influenced by many factors, such as experience, level of expertise, personal and professional values, setting, specialty, relationships with co-workers, aspects of role transition, and life transitions. Frameworks for understanding APN role development processes have been discussed. Strategies for facilitating role acquisition and role implementation, which have implications for students, educators, administrators, and APNs, have been presented. Future research studies to assess the applicability of this information for all APN specialty groups are needed to further the understanding of APN role development.

REFERENCES

Aiken, L. H., & Sage, W. H. (1992). Staffing national health reform: A role for advanced practice nurses. *Akron Law Review, 26,* 187–211.

American College of Nurse-Midwives. (1993). *Certified nurse-midwives as primary care providers.* Washington, DC: Author.

Anderson, E. M., Leonard, B. J., & Yates, J. A. (1974). Epigenesis of the nurse practitioner role. *American Journal of Nursing, 74*(10), 1812–1816.

Arena, D. M., & Page, N. E. (1992). The imposter phenomenon in the clinical nurse specialist role. *Image: The Journal of Nursing Scholarship, 24*(2), 121–125.

Baird, S. B., & Prouty, M. P. (1989). Administratively enhancing CNS contributions. In A. B. Hamric & J. A. Spross (Eds.), *The clinical nurse specialist in theory and practice* (2nd ed., pp. 261–283). Philadelphia: W. B. Saunders.

Baker, V. (1979). Retrospective explorations in role development. In G. V. Padilla (Ed.), *The clinical nurse specialist and improvement of nursing practice* (pp. 56–63). Wakefield, MA: Nursing Resources.

Banda, E. E. (1985). Role problems, role strain: Perception and experience of clinical nurse specialist. Unpublished master's thesis, Boston University School of Nursing, Boston, MA.

Benner, P., Hooper-Kyriakidis, P., & Stannard, D. (1999). *Clinical wisdom and interventions in critical care: A thinking-in-action approach.* Philadelphia: W. B. Saunders.

Benner, P., Tanner, C. A., & Chesla, C. A. (1996). *Expertise in nursing practice: Caring, clinical judgment and ethics.* New York: Springer-Verlag.

Benner, P. E. (1984). *From novice to expert. Excellence and power in clinical nursing practice.* Menlo Park, CA: Addison-Wesley.

Brown, M. A., & Olshansky, E. (1995, July). *Supporting novice nurse practitioners: The experience of the first year of NP practice.* Paper presented at the annual meeting of the National Organization of Nurse Practitioner Faculties, Keystone, CO.

Brown, M. A., & Olshansky, E. F. (1997). From limbo to legitimacy: A theoretical model of the transition to the primary care nurse practitioner role. *Nursing Research, 46*(1), 46–51.

Brown, M. A., & Olshansky, E. (1998). Becoming a primary care nurse practitioner: Challenges of the initial year of practice. *Nurse Practitioner, 23*(7), 46, 52–58, 61–66.

Brown, S. J. (1990). Tailoring nursing care to the individual client: An analysis of client-nurse dialogue. *Dissertation Abstracts International, 51*(10), 4774B. (University Microfilms No. 9106506)

Brykczynski, K. A. (1985). Exploring the clinical practice of nurse practitioners (Doctoral dissertation, University of California San Francisco, School of Nursing). *Dissertation Abstracts International, 46,* 3789B. (University Microfilms No. DA8600592)

Brykczynski, K. A. (1989). An interpretive study describing the clinical judgment of nurse practitioners. *Scholarly Inquiry for Nursing Practice: An International Journal, 3*(2), 75–104.

Brykczynski, K. A. (1991). Judgment strategies for coping with ambiguous clinical situations encountered in family primary care. *Journal of the Academy of Nurse Practitioners, 3*(2), 79–84.

Brykczynski, K. A. (1996). Role development of the advanced practice nurse. In A. B. Hamric, J. A. Spross, & C. M. Hanson (Eds.), *Advanced nursing practice: An integrative approach* (pp. 89–95). Philadelphia: W. B. Saunders.

Callahan, L., & Bruton-Maree, N. (1994). Establishing measures of competence. In S. D. Foster & L. M. Jordan (Eds.), *Professional aspects of nurse anesthesia practice* (pp. 275–290). Philadelphia: F. A. Davis.

Chase, L. K., Johnson, S. K., Laffoon, T. A., Jacobs, R. S., & Johnson, M. E. (1996). CNS role: An experience in retitling and role clarification. *Clinical Nurse Specialist, 10*(1), 41–45.

Cooper, D. M., & Sparacino, P. S. A. (1990). Acquiring, implementing, and evaluating the clinical nurse specialist role. In P. S. A. Sparacino, D. M. Cooper, & P. A. Minarik (Eds.), *The clinical nurse specialist: Implementation and impact* (pp. 41–75). Norwalk, CT: Appleton & Lange.

Curry, J. L. (1994). Nurse practitioners in the emergency department: Current issues. *Journal of Emergency Nursing, 20*(3), 207–215.

DePaolis-Lutzo, M. V. (1987). Factors influencing nurse anesthesia educational programs: 1982–1987. Unpublished doctoral dissertation, University of Pittsburgh.

Diers, D. (1992). One-liners. *Image: The Journal of Nursing Scholarship, 24*(1), 75–77.

Dreyfus, H. L., & Dreyfus, S. E. (1977). *Uses and abuses of multi-attribute and multi-aspect model of decision making.* Unpublished manuscript, Department of Industrial Engineering and Operations Research, University of California at Berkeley.

Dreyfus, H. L., & Dreyfus, S. E. (1986). *Mind over machine: The power of human intuition and expertise in the era of the computer.* New York: Free Press.

Fagin, C. M. (1992). Collaboration between nurses and physicians no longer a choice. *Nursing & Health Care, 13*(7), 354–363.

Federwisch, A. (1999). CRNA autonomy. Nurse anesthetists fight latest skirmish. *Health Week, 4*(1), 16.

Ford, L. C. (1982). Nurse practitioners: History of a new idea and predictions for the future. In L. H. Aiken (Ed.), *Nursing in the 1980s: Crises, opportunities, challenges* (pp. 231–247). Philadelphia: J. B. Lippincott.

Gordon, D., & Benner, P. E. (1980). Guidelines for recording critical incidents. In Benner, P. (1984). *From novice to expert. Excellence and power in clinical nursing practice* (pp. 299–302). Menlo Park, CA: Addison-Wesley.

Gunn, I. P. (1991). The history of nurse anesthesia education: Highlights and influences. Report of the National Commission on Nurse Anesthesia Education. *Journal of the American Association of Nurse Anesthestists, 59*(1), 53–61.

Gunn, I. P. (1998). Setting the record straight on nurse anesthesia and medical anesthesiology education. *CRNA: The Clinical Forum for Nurse Anesthetists, 9*(4), 163–171.

Hamric, A. B., & Taylor, J. W. (1989). Role development of the CNS. In A. B. Hamric & J. Spross (Eds.), *The clinical nurse specialist in theory and practice* (2nd ed., pp. 41–82). Philadelphia: W. B. Saunders.

Hardy, M. E., & Hardy, W. L. (1988). Role stress and role strain. In M. E. Hardy & M. E. Conway (Eds.), *Role theory: Perspectives for health professionals* (2nd ed., pp. 159–239). Norwalk, CT: Appleton & Lange.

Hawkins, J. W., & Thibodeau, J. A. (1993). Negotiating an employment contract. In J. W. Hawkins & J. A. Thibodeau (Eds.), *The practitioner* (3rd ed., pp. 130–140). New York: Tiresias Press.

Hazle, N. R. (1985). Perceptions of role conflict between obstetric nurses and nurse-midwives. *Journal of Nurse-Midwifery, 30*(3), 166–173.

Hunter, L. P., Bormann, J. E., & Lops, V. R. (1996). Student to nurse-midwife role transition process: Smoothing the way. *Journal of Nurse-Midwifery, 41*(4), 328–333.

Hupcey, J. E. (1990). The socialization process of master's level nurse practitioner students. *Journal of Nursing Education, 29*(5), 196–201.

Johnson, R. (1993). Nurse practitioner-patient discourse: Uncovering the voice of nursing in primary care practice. *Scholarly Inquiry for Nursing Practice: An International Journal, 7*(3), 143–157.

Kimbro, C. D. (1978). The relationship between nurses and nurse-midwives. *Journal of Nurse-Midwifery, 22*(4), 28–31.

King, M. B. (1990). Clinical nurse specialist collaboration with physicians. *Clinical Nurse Specialist, 4*(4), 172–177.

Kramer, M. (1974). *Reality shock.* St. Louis: Mosby.

Leininger, M. (1976). Two strange health tribes: The Gnisrun and the Enicidem in the United States. *Human Organization. Journal of the Society for Applied Anthropology, 35*(3), 253–261.

Long, W. N., & Sharp, E. S. (1982). Relationships between professions: From the viewpoint of the physician and nurse-midwife in a tertiary center. *Journal of Nurse Midwifery, 27*(4), 14–24.

Lurie, E. E. (1981). Nurse practitioners: Issues in professional socialization. *Journal of Health and Social Behavior, 22,* 31–48.

McFadden, E. A., & Miller, M. A. (1994). Clinical nurse specialist practice: Facilitators and barriers. *Clinical Nurse Specialist, 8*(1), 27–33.

National Commission on Nurse Anesthesia Education. (1990). Summary of Commission findings: Issues and review of supporting documents. *Journal of the American Association of Nurse Anesthetists, 58*(5), 394–398.

Oda, D. (1977). Specialized role development: A three phase process. *Nursing Outlook, 25,* 374–377.

Page, N. E., & Arena, D. M. (1991). Practical strategies for CNS role implementation. *Clinical Nurse Specialist, 5*(1), 43–48.

Payne, J. L., & Baumgartner, R. G. (1996). CNS role evolution. *Clinical Nurse Specialist, 10*(1), 46–48.

Redekopp, M. A. (1997). Clinical nurse specialist role confusion: The need for identity. *Clinical Nurse Specialist, 11*(2), 87–91.

Roberts, S. J. (1983). Oppressed group behavior: Implications for nursing. *Advances in Nursing Science, 5,* 21–30.

Roberts, S. J., Tabloski, P., & Bova, C. (1997). Epigenesis of the nurse practitioner role revisited. *Journal of Nursing Education, 36*(2), 67–73.

Rooks, J. P. (1983). The context of nurse midwifery in the 1980s: Our relationships with medicine, nursing, lay-midwives, consumers and health care economists. *Journal of Nurse-Midwifery, 26*(5), 3–8.

Rooks, J. P., & Haas, J. E. (Eds.). (1986). *Nurse midwifery in America.* Washington, DC: American College of Nurse-Midwives Foundation.

Schumacher, K. L., & Meleis, A. I. (1994). Transitions: A central concept in nursing. *Image: The Journal of Nursing Scholarship, 26*(2), 119–127.

Varney, H. (1987). *Nurse-midwifery* (2nd ed.). Boston: Blackwell Scientific.

Wells, N., Erickson, S., & Spinella, J. (1996). Role transition. From clinical nurse specialist to clinical nurse specialist/case manager. *Journal of Nursing Administration, 26*(11), 23–28.

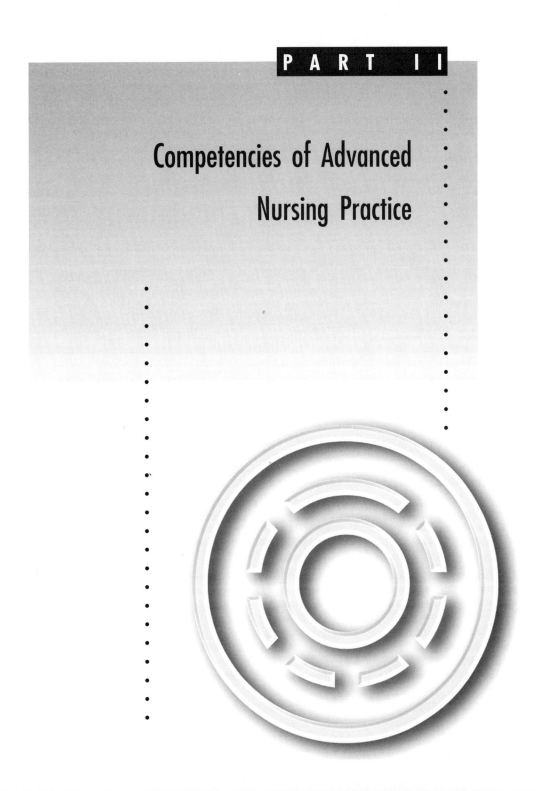

PART II

Competencies of Advanced Nursing Practice

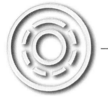

Direct Clinical Practice

• S A R A H   J O   B R O W N

INTRODUCTION

Few American advanced practice nurses (APNs) would dispute that their direct care activities have been affected by the financial restructuring of health care delivery that has occurred over the last half of the 1990s. Managed care, cost containment, prospective payment (e.g., capitation), integrated delivery systems, private contracting, and population-based management have changed the way APNs approach caregiving as well as the specifics of care provided to individual patients.

The dilemma many APNs face is how to maintain the characteristics of care that have helped patients achieve positive health outcomes and afforded APN care a unique niche in the health care marketplace. Characteristics such as use of a holistic perspective and the formation of partnerships with patients to co-produce individualized health care are threatened by the transition to managed care and capitation, in which the emphasis is on standardization of the processes of care to achieve population-based outcome targets. Conversely, characteristics of APN care such as health promotion, self-care, and low-technology modalities are valued by managed care and capitation systems because they result in low utilization of health care system resources. Their reasons are, of course, different from the reasons why APNs have valued, and continue to value, these components of care. Throughout the following discussion of the characteristics of APN care, observations are made regarding how each characteristic fits with managed care and capitation goals. Also, suggestions are offered regarding how to incorporate or defend the characteristics within the context of current delivery structures. To balance the picture, the special opportunities to improve care that exist within managed care are also noted.

Direct Care Activities

For the purposes of this chapter, the terms "direct care" and "direct clinical practice" will refer to the activities and functions APNs enact within the patient-nurse[1] interface. The activities that occur in this interface are unique because they are interpersonally and physically co-enacted with a particular patient for the purpose of promoting the patient's health or well-being. Many important processes transpire at this point of care, including formation and maintenance of an interpersonal relationship, creation of mutual understandings, definition of health problems, setting of health or recovery goals, and exploring and deciding on specific forms of management and treatment. In many APN-patient relationships, ministrations such as physical acts of treatment, therapy, comfort, and health monitoring also occur in this interface. The processes and activities that occur in the patient-nurse interface constitute the core of nursing practice and of advanced nursing practice (Hamric, 1996). Precise conceptualization of this core will help delineate the full range of clinical activities that contribute to patients' achieving desired health outcomes.

Although other APN activities occurring prior to and adjacent to the nurse-patient interface have a great influence on the direct care that occurs in the interface, they either are not co-enacted with an individual patient or their main purpose is something other than promoting the well-being of the individual patient. For instance, when an APN consults with another provider regarding the nature of a patient's condition or the care that should be recommended to a patient, the APN is engaging in advanced clinical practice, but not in direct care. Even though there may be adjunctive contact with the patient, the primary purpose of that contact is to acquire information and understandings to use in formulating recommendations for the patient's direct care provider. Another example is the APN who develops, conducts trials of, refines, and introduces a new assessment method or intervention for a population of patients. Even though this APN may assess patients using the new method or use the new interventions with several patients, the primary purpose of those contacts is to develop and refine a new method of care for the population of patients, not solely to promote the well-being of the individual patients. Thus, according to the definition of direct care used in this chapter, the APN is engaged in clinical practice but she or he is not providing direct care.

Although this delineation may seem too severely drawn to some people, the author believes restricting the use of the term "direct care" to what occurs in the patient-nurse interface serves heuristic and practical purposes. Importantly, this delineation is not intended to denigrate clinical activities that occur outside the nurse-patient interface—quite the contrary. The author believes these other clinical activities and functions should be recognized as influencing what happens in the interface and as having significant impact on patient outcomes. Because they so significantly affect patient outcomes, they should be valued by the nursing community and by health care systems. In the current environment of prospective payment, all activities that enhance patients' health, recovery, and adjustment should be valued regardless of whether they are antecedents of direct care, adjuncts to it, or actual direct care itself.

Many forms of clinical analysis, design, planning, and coordination are needed to develop and sustain the processes of direct care that help patients attain good health

[1] It is assumed in this definition that "the patient" may be an individual, a family, a community or community group, a workplace or school group, or a health interest group.

outcomes at reasonable cost. Too often these clinical activities and functions that improve patient care but occur outside the nurse-patient interface have been described using organizational terms. Referring to them as "indirect care," or even "clinical leadership," "consultation," or "planned change," assigns an organizational function to them but fails to recognize the impact they have on the clinical care individuals receive and on the clinical outcomes patients attain. Among domains of APN practice, (Fenton & Brykczynski, 1993), terms that describe the direct care activities of APNs would include: diagnostic/patient monitoring, administering/monitoring therapeutic interventions and regimens, helping patients and families during crisis, teaching/coaching, and effective management of rapidly changing situations. Activities and functions such as monitoring/ensuring the quality of health care practices, organization and work role competencies, and the consulting role would be recognized as domains of advanced nursing practice contiguous with direct care activities but do not define direct care.

Five Characteristics of the Direct Clinical Care of APNs

In this chapter the author proposes five characteristics of the direct clinical care provided by APNs as prevalent across health care settings, populations of patients, and advanced practice roles. They are

1. The use of a holistic perspective
2. The formation of partnerships with patients
3. Expert clinical thinking and skillful performance
4. Use of research evidence as a guide to practice
5. The use of diverse approaches to health and illness management

These characteristics have been widely present in APN practice for many years, and they constitute the themes one hears when APNs describe what they do. Moreover, there is accumulating research evidence supporting them as features of APN practice and as having positive influences on patient outcomes (Girouard, 1996). This evidence is cited throughout the chapter. These five characteristics of advanced direct care practice have their roots in the traditional values of the nursing profession. Nurses practicing in advanced practice roles often have a deep commitment to the values on which these characteristics rest, and are able to persuasively advocate these values in the discourse of daily practice. Importantly, the expanded scope of practice of APN roles has often enabled APNs to fully enact these characteristics in their daily interactions with patients. An overview of strategies for enacting these characteristics is provided in Table 6–1.

To maintain these characteristics in daily practice, as opposed to merely holding them as espoused values, APNs must be reflective practitioners. Reflection involves an intentional looking-back at situations to try to understand what happened and why it happened, and to speculate about how the situation might have been managed differently. The goal is to turn experience into personal knowledge by mining for insights that are not available with superficial recall (Atkins & Murphy, 1993; Rolfe, 1997a; Schön, 1991). Kim (1999) has described a method of reflective inquiry involving systematic analysis of situated or individual instances of nursing practice; this method could be used by individual APNs or groups to monitor and improve practice. Use of Kim's method of reflection also could help APNs detect assumptions and

TABLE 6–1 CHARACTERISTICS OF ADVANCED DIRECT CARE PRACTICE AND STRATEGIES FOR ENACTING THEM

Use of a Holistic Framework
- Take into account the complexity of human life
- Recognize and address how social, organizational, and physical environments affect people
- Consider the profound effects of illness, aging, hospitalization, and stress
- Focus on functional abilities and requirements
- Consider how symptoms, illness, and treatment affect quality of life

Formation of Partnership with Patients
- Use a conversational style to conduct health care encounters
- Encourage the patient to actively participate in decision making
- Listen to the indirect voices of patients who are noncommunicative
- Look for potential cultural influences on health care discourse
- Advocate the patient's perspective and concerns to others

Use of Expert Clinical Reasoning and Skillful Performance
- Acquire specialized knowledge and know-how
- Invest in deeply understanding the patient situations in which you are involved
- Generate and test alternative lines of reasoning
- Trust your hunches—check them out.
- Be aware of when you are time pressured and likely to make thinking errors.
- Consider multiple aspects of the patient's situation when deciding how to treat
- Make sure you know how to use technical equipment safely
- Make sure you know how to interpret the data produced by monitoring devices
- Pay attention to how you move and touch patients during care.
- Anticipate ethical conflicts.
- Acquire computer-related skills for accessing patient and best practice information

Use of Research Evidence
- Learn how to search health care databases for studies related to specific clinical topics
- Read research reports related to your field of practice
- Acquire skills in appraising the various forms of research evidence
- Work with colleagues to consider research-based improvements in care
- Be alert for midrange theories that are useful guides for practice

Use of Diverse, Direct Care Management and Treatment Approaches
- Use interpersonal interventions to influence patients
- Acquire proficiency in new ways of treating and helping patients
- Help patients maintain health and capitalize on their strengths and resources
- Provide preventive services appropriate to your field of practice
- Know what is allowed under managed care contracts
- Negotiate with managed care case managers for unallowed services when necessary
- Coordinate services among care sites and multiple providers

ineffective actions embedded in daily practice, as well as identify effective interpersonal strategies and behaviors that are enacted without much conscious awareness.

USE OF A HOLISTIC PERSPECTIVE

Holism Described

Holism has a variety of meanings, among which is the multifaceted view that it involves

- Viewing the patient as an integral part of larger social, physical, and energy environments

- Assuming that the mind, body, and spirit are closely related, so that one dimension should not be considered in isolation from the others
- Focusing on the meanings patients assign to health, illness experiences, and health care choices
- Viewing patients' current behaviors and responses as consistent with their life span patterns of response and choice (Hall & Allan, 1994; Kinney & Erickson, 1990; Newman, 1997)

This comprehensive and integrated view of human life and health becomes enacted as specific attention to the full range of factors influencing patients' experiences of health and illness. These factors include

- How patients view their health or illness situation
- Patterns of physical symptoms and amount of distress they cause
- How physical symptoms affect a patient's daily functioning and quality of life
- Symptom management approaches that are acceptable to the patient
- Life changes that could affect the patient's physical or psychological well-being (i.e., relationship breakup, job change, intrafamily conflict, retirement, death of a beloved person)
- The context of the patient's life, including the nuclear family unit, social support, job responsibilities, financial situation, health insurance coverage, responsibilities for the care of others (e.g., children, chronically ill spouse or partner, elderly parents)
- Spiritual and life values (e.g., independence, religion, beliefs about life, acceptance of fate)

Perhaps a shorter and more contemporary view of holism is that it involves a deep understanding of each patient as a complex and unique person who is embedded in a temporally unfolding life. This deep understanding enables the practitioner to view the patient as a sacred and unique person who is in the process of living life as best as she or he can within a particular context.

Holism and Health Assessment

Reaching a holistic understanding of the patient and his or her health-related situation is influenced by how the APN goes about acquiring information. Traditional disease-oriented, question-answer approaches clearly cannot lead to an understanding of the person who has specific health goals and/or problems. The interviewing approaches that foster holistic understanding are discussed in the next section, which is about the APN characteristic of forming partnerships with patients. However, the substance of interviewing (i.e., the content) is relevant to this discussion of holism.

When working with relatively healthy persons, the APN seeks to understand what the person's life goals, functional interests, and health risks are so as to preserve quality of life in the future. In contrast, when working with ill patients, the APN is interested in what they view as problems, how they are responding to problems, and what the problems and responses mean to them in terms of daily living and life goals. In a study of 199 primary care clinical situations, nurse practitioners (NPs) were found to engage in holistic assessment; they attended to the whole person and addressed both disease and illness experiences (Brykczynski, 1989).

The ability to function in daily activities and relationships is an important consideration for patients when they evaluate their health (Herth, 1989; Loomis & Conco, 1991), so it is an appropriate and essential focus for holistic, person-centered assessment of individuals. Many assessment formats focus on patients' functional health (Bates, 1987; Gordon, 1994; Richmond, McCorkle, Tulman, & Fawcett, 1997; Vallerand, 1998). Some of these formats are population specific (Dittmar & Gresham, 1997; Eisen, Wilcox, Leff, Schaefer, & Culhane, 1999; Neal, 1998), whereas others are more generic. The Short Form-36 Health Status Profile (SF-36) is a widely used tool for measuring general health, functional health status, and well-being in adults, and is available in several language versions. Most functional-abilities formats focus on (1) how patients view their health or quality of life; (2) how they accomplish self-care and household or job responsibilities; (3) the social, physical, financial, and environmental factors that augment or tax their functioning; and (4) the strategies they and their families use to cope with the stresses and problems in their lives.

An open-ended, screening functional health pattern assessment that can be used for outpatients or hospital inpatients is presented in Table 6–2. This form includes questions that allow the APN to identify problem areas efficiently. The questions can be asked conversationally in interviews with patients to ensure that all functional areas have been considered. Alternatively, patients can complete the questionnaire while waiting to be seen, or support staff can ask the questions of patients before the interview with the APN. The APN can use the answers to focus the visit/interview

---

TABLE 6–2 HEALTH SCREENING QUESTIONS

Your answers will help the advanced practice nurse in talking with you about your health and health problems.

1. How has your health been recently?
   Very good _____ Good _____ Fair _____ Poor _____
2. What "new" health problems do you have?
3. What "old" health problems still bother you?
4. Are you physically able to do the activities you would like to be able to do?
   Yes _____ No _____
5. Do you have pain, aches, or discomfort of any type?
   Yes _____ No _____ Not sure _____
6. Do you believe you eat well? Yes _____ No _____ Not sure _____
   Are you satisfied with your weight? Yes _____ No _____
7. Do you have any problems with your bowels or bladder?
   Yes _____ No _____ Maybe _____
8. Are you satisfied with the amount of sleep and rest you get?
   Yes _____ No _____ Not sure _____
9. Do you notice any problems with your vision, hearing, or feeling in your hands or feet?
   Yes _____ No _____ Maybe _____
10. Are you satisfied with how you handle the problems of daily life and with the decisions you make?
    Yes _____ No _____ Not sure _____
11. Do you generally feel good about yourself?
    Yes _____ No _____ Not sure _____
12. Are you generally satisfied with your relationships with others?
    Yes _____ No _____ Not sure _____
13. Are you satisfied with your sexuality and sexual relations?
    Yes _____ No _____ Not sure _____
14. Do you have beliefs about life that are very important to you and that you think we need to know to provide health care for you?
    Yes _____ No _____ Not sure _____

on problems or potential illness areas that need to be explored. The questions provide a time-efficient way of zeroing in on health issues that are of concern to patients while also broadly assessing their health status.

As APNs take on responsibilities that formerly were in the purview of physicians, concern has been expressed by some that APNs are being asked to function within a medical model of practice rather than within a holistic nursing model. This is particularly true in roles where APNs replace medical interns and/or residents (Ruth-Sanchez, Bosque, & Lee, 1996). There is, however, evidence to suggest that a nursing orientation is a strong component of APN practice. In a study of 10 collaborative pairs of physicians and NPs in primary care practices in Missouri, the NPs evidenced a holistic approach to care and conscious awareness of using both the medical model and a nursing model in their thinking (Flesner & Clawson, 1998). In addition, a national survey of 482 randomly selected NPs conducted in the early 1990s found that they are very confident about their practice skills and knowledge, and have a very strong nursing orientation (Thibodeau & Hawkins, 1994). The educational preparation of neonatal nurse practitioners (NNPs) has been found to influence their care orientation; certificate-prepared NNPs aligned themselves with a medical philosophy, whereas master's-prepared NNPs espoused a philosophy of nursing and a strong nursing identity (Beal, Maguire, & Carr, 1996). Another piece of evidence indicating that APNs do not abandon their nursing orientation is the fact that the standards and competencies issued by APN organizations and incorporated in the American Nurses Association's (ANA's) Social Policy Statement include strong endorsement of the nursing perspective (ANA, 1995; Manthey & Avery, 1996).

The Shuler Nurse Practitioner Practice Model is a theoretical and pragmatic tool for blending a nursing and medical orientation (Shuler & Huebscher, 1998). It has been proposed as a model that is holistic and wellness oriented, and emphasizes self-care while incorporating the role responsibilities involved in diagnosing and treating acute, episodic diseases and chronic illnesses.

Holism and Managed Care

The view of patients as unique, complex, and unitary persons is discordant with how managed care organizations (MCOs) view patients, that is, as a member of a "population" or "subpopulation" having in common a particular health problem. Typically, the health problem is a medical diagnosis. The processes of care and resources required by the majority of persons in the population to produce good health outcomes are of primary interest to health maintenance organizations (HMOs). When the care allowed for a certain population is prespecified by a health care system, the individuality of each patient is not factored in. As a result, there often is no provision for unique situations, needs, preferences, and beliefs. Increasingly, APNs find themselves in the position of having to contact case managers who represent the MCO to defend the need for reimbursement for treatment modalities, services, care products, or specific medications that are not paid for under the contract.

Although "there are compelling reasons to create systems of care to manage subpopulations of patients" (Britt, Schraeder, & Shelton, 1998, p. 20), it must be recognized that *only some* health care needs are predictable based on biostatistics, epidemiology, cost-benefit analysis, outcomes studies, resource utilization tracking, and variance reports. The APN must be ready to present a strong case for why resources not generally allowed for patients in the population are needed for a particular patient. This form of advocacy on behalf of patients is and will continue to be increasingly common in a financing environment that emphasizes cost containment through population-based management.

FORMATION OF PARTNERSHIPS WITH PATIENTS

APNs' person-centered, holistic perspective serves as the foundation for the kinds of relationships they co-create with patients. Research evidence reveals that APNs do indeed form collaborative relationships with patients (Brown, 1994; Brykczynski, 1989; Courtney & Rice, 1997; Flesner & Clawson, 1998; Grando, 1998; Johnson, 1993; Morten, Kohl, O'Mahoney, & Pelosi, 1991; Pearson, Borbasi, & Walsh, 1997). They do so by engaging in social story exchanges, expressing regard for patients, asking about patients' home lives, and helping patients plan how they can enact health and illness management recommendations. Taken together, these studies indicate that advanced nursing practice does embody the ideal of providing "skilled companionship" on illness "journeys" (Pearson et al., 1997).

In addition to eliciting disclosure that helps the APN understand the patient's illness experience, APNs also encourage patients to participate in decisions regarding how their disease and illness will be managed. There is substantial evidence from the field of cancer research to conclude that many patients want to participate in decisions about their illness management (Degner et al., 1997; Johnson et al., 1996; Petrisek, Laliberte, Allen, & Mor, 1997; Pyke-Grimm, Degner, Small, & Mueller, 1999). Because participatory decision making has been studied most extensively in decision making related to treatment for cancer, much less is known about what kind of decision making patients facing other kinds of decisions prefer (e.g., hormone replacement therapy or treatment of coronary heart disease). The cancer treatment studies clearly reveal considerable variation in preference for participation; therefore it is possible, even likely, that patients' decisions regarding other kinds of decisions and decisions made under less threatening conditions also vary widely. Also, it should be noted that the benefits of patient participation in treatment and management decisions have not been extensively studied (Guadagnoli & Ward, 1998).

Many conceptual models (e.g., Watson's Human Caring theory and the Modeling and Role-Modeling Theory of Erickson, Tomlin, and Swain) propose that forming partnerships with patients will result in improved health outcomes (Erickson, Tomlin, & Swain, 1983; Raudonis & Acton, 1997; Watson, 1997). Three middle-range theories address partnerships at a less abstract level (King, 1981; Powell-Cope, 1994; Swanson, 1991). The amount of research that has either tested or generated each of these theories is quite variable.

Based on current knowledge, providers should be reluctant to make any assumptions about an individual patient's preference for participation in clinical decisions regarding how to prevent and diagnose disease, or manage an illness. Instead, they should individually determine each patient's preference for participation in decision-making, and be sensitive to the fact that patients' preferences may change over time as they get to know the provider better and as different kinds of health problems arise. Once the patient's preference has been elicited, the provider should tailor his or her decision-making style to the patient's preference. The importance of this tailoring of care style was supported by a study of the decision-making preferences of ambulatory Veterans Affairs patients (Harvey, Kazis, & Lee, 1999). The veterans with a high preference for involvement in decision making and fewer provider-offered decision-making opportunities had significantly lower satisfaction with medical care than did the other three combinations of preference and offered opportunities.

Providers may find that, if they socialize patients to a more active role by discussing different ways of shaping the patient-provider relationship, many patients will opt for a collaborative relationship. Many patients have not had prior health care experiences in which shared decision making was even a possibility, but, when offered the idea, may come to view it as preferable after they have had a chance to discuss how it would work.

Cultural Influences on Partnerships

Another important factor affecting whether and how persons want to participate in health care decision making may be their cultural background. It is easy to forget that not all cultures value individual autonomy as much as young, Anglo-Saxon, North Americans do. Increasingly, recognizing and respecting the cultural identification of patients is being viewed as essential to building meaningful partnerships. Cultural groups form along lines of racial, national origin, religious, professional, organizational, sexual orientation, or age group identification. Some cultural groups are easier to identify than others. Physical differences in appearance among racial and ethnic groups often tip the provider off to the fact that she or he is dealing with a person of a different cultural orientation. Other cultural identifications are less obvious—for example, people with religious beliefs about fate, God-as-Healer, or treatment taboos.

Some of these groups have ways of thinking and communication expectations that are quite different from those of the health care provider, and possibly unfamiliar to her or him (Cooper-Patrick et al., 1999; Waite, Harker, & Messerman, 1994). These differences can cause confusion, misunderstandings, and even conflicts that disrupt the patient-provider relationship and discourse. Moreover, they often complicate attempts to resolve misunderstandings because different cultural groups approach conflict negotiation differently.

In every encounter, every provider needs to expect that the patient may hold values that are different in some ways from her or his own. Certainly, respect for diverse beliefs and soliciting patients' views will avoid some misunderstandings and conflicts, and may help in resolving others. However, when awkward communication, lack of interpersonal responsiveness, or hostility occurs, providers should suspect that a difference of cultural perspective is adversely affecting the relationship and communication. The obvious first step is to try respectfully to identify the problem by eliciting the patient's expectations, preferences, and goals. Once this is done, the provider most often should take the lead in trying to create mutually agreeable strategies to meet the goals of both parties. These strategies will be constrained by the need to not violate the fundamental personal values or ethical standards of both the patient and the provider (Jecker, Carrese, & Pearlman, 1995). Identifying and negotiating through and around cultural differences requires considerable sensitivity, self-awareness, and open-mindedness, but these skills are crucial to creating partnerships with patients who have value orientations different from those of the provider.

Partnerships with Noncommunicative Patients

Some patients are not able to enter fully into partnership with APNs because they are too young, have compromised cognitive capacity, or are unconscious. Clinical populations who may be unable to participate fully in shared decision making are listed in Table 6-3. Although these patients may be limited in their abilities to speak for themselves, they are not entirely without voice. Situations in which patients will experience temporary alterations in cognition or verbal abilities can often be anticipated (i.e., during general anesthesia and during intubation), and the APN can discuss their preferences for handling possible events and elicit their wishes.

In the absence of this kind of prior dialogue, experts who work with patients who cannot verbalize their concerns and preferences learn to pay close attention to how patients are responding to what happens to them; facial expressions, body movement, and physiological parameters are used to ascertain what causes the patient discomfort and what helps alleviate it (Benner, Tanner, & Chesla, 1996). Current practice in anesthesia is to rely on indirect hemodynamic measurements such as blood pressure and heart rate to monitor the sedative-hypnotic state of the patient's brain during general anesthesia; however, a new technology, a processed electroencephalographic recording, is in the development stages (Halliburton, 1998). This technology is expected to be valuable in detecting and preventing the possibility of awareness during general anesthesia, and hence, of recall after surgery.

In a study of persons who had experienced and recovered from unconsciousness (Lawrence, 1995), 27% of the patients reported being able to hear, understand, and respond emotionally while unconscious. These findings suggest that nurses should communicate with unconscious patients by providing them with interventions such as reassurance, bodily care, pain relief, explanations, and comforting touch. A naturalistic, interpretive study of critical care nurses revealed that recognizing subtle forms of communication requires expert perceptual acuity as well as interpersonal involvement with the patient (Benner, Hooper-Kyriakidis, & Stannard, 1999).

It is also important to identify alternative sources of information about patients who are unable to respond physically or to communicate. For example, siblings visiting an adolescent male with a major head injury would be able to tell you what kind of music he likes to listen to and would probably even bring you a tape or CD to play for the patient. His mother would know what has caused him to have skin reactions in the past. Responding to his father's off-handed comment that he can't stand to not have his glasses on when his contacts are out would most likely help both father and son. All of these are ways of building partnership with an unconscious teenager in an intensive care unit (ICU). In adults and adolescents, advance directives, heath care proxy documents, and organ donation cards represent another source of information regarding patients' wishes. Thus, noncommunicative patients are not without a voice, but hearing their voices does require presence, attentiveness, and relationship.

TABLE 6-3 PATIENT POPULATIONS UNABLE TO PARTICIPATE FULLY IN PARTNERSHIP
Infants and preverbal children
Anesthetized patients
Unconscious/comatose patients
People in severe pain
Patients receiving medications that impair cognition
People with dementia
People with psychiatric conditions that seriously impair rational thought
People with conditions that render them incapable of speech and conversation

EXPERT CLINICAL THINKING AND SKILLFUL PERFORMANCE

The public expects health care providers to be knowledgeable in their fields, to make recommendations that are appropriate to the patient's particular situation, and to administer treatments, therapies, interventions, procedures, and comfort care with skill. To meet these expectations, health care providers must

- Possess substantial domain-specific knowledge
- Be capable of acquiring a deep understanding of the patient's situation
- Be able to bring domain-specific knowledge to bear on understanding and managing the patient's situation
- Be able to safely and appropriately use technological equipment
- Possess skill in performing treatments, therapies, and comfort care

In brief, the provider must be a skilled clinical thinker and doer. Because skillful doing is specific to each clinical specialty and APN role, and because little is known about skilled performance of APN nursing functions, skilled performance is not extensively addressed in this chapter. However, there are commonalities of expert clinical reasoning that apply across specialties and roles, and expert clinical thinking has been studied extensively, hence a discussion of expert clinical thinking follows. It should be acknowledged, however, that although we know a great deal about expert clinical reasoning, and although there is considerable indirect evidence to support the proposition that APNs are expert clinical thinkers, the body of direct evidence establishing APNs as such is scant.

Two Schools of Thought

The research on how clinical experts think is less than cohesive. There are two main schools of thought about clinical reasoning, the information-processing school and the intuitive school; both are represented in the current research literature. The information-processing viewpoint is based on the assessment-diagnosis-treatment model of clinical practice and on an information-processing view of clinical judgment (Bulechek & McCloskey, 1999a; Gordon, Murphy, Candee, & Hiltunen, 1994; Narayan & Corcoran-Perry, 1997). Researchers in this tradition typically ask practitioners to think aloud as they make decisions in either hypothetical or real-time situations. Typically, these researchers are interested in the cognitive processes practitioners use in bringing clinical knowledge to bear on a particular situation. For instance, they look for evidence of cognitive strategies and processes such as the generation of diagnostic hypotheses, the search for patterns among the cues (i.e., data), and the deliberative search for data that will either support or disconfirm alternative hypotheses. Researchers may also look for evidence indicating that cues from the situation trigger the activation of domain-specific concepts from memory. These domain concepts then serve as lines of reasoning that can be used by clinicians to think about the particular situation (Narayan & Corcoran-Perry, 1997).

Thus, information-processing researchers focus on how discrete cognitive processes and the use of clinical knowledge help produce judgments about the particulars of a situation (Pesut & Herman, 1998). Although in the past these processes have been described as rule driven or as a prescribed series of steps (such as the nursing process), a more recent view is that the cognitive processes are data driven, that is, influenced by context and experiential knowledge (Fowler, 1997), and domain-specific knowledge structures and problem-solving strategies (Narayan & Corcoran-Perry, 1997).

Researchers in the intuitive, or thinking-in-action, tradition use naturalistic, descriptive, and interpretive methods to study clinical judgment. They employ observational interviews and clinical narratives to collect descriptions of actual episodes of clinical thinking. Clinical judgment is viewed as inextricably linked to knowing the particular patient and her or his unfolding clinical situation (Benner et al., 1996). Researchers in this tradition are interested in how clinicians think and reason about a particular patient across time. They document how the nurse's perceptual-recognition skills, grasp of the situation, clinical forethought, practical know-how, and emotional responses affect judgment and action (Benner et al., 1999).

Those who view clinical judgment through the intuitive lens focus on how the nurse comes to have a deep understanding of a particular patient's evolving situation or unfolding account. They seek to link the processes of perception and clinical reasoning to the specific content that is being reasoned about. They are interested in the nurse's recognition of qualitative distinctions in the patient's account or qualitative changes in the patient's condition, and how trends in the patient's condition are recognized. They pay close attention to the aspects of the situation that the nurse perceives, such as sequence, development and change over time, and nuance (Benner et al., 1999). They also look at reasoning processes such as how nurses' prior experiences create expectations for particular populations of patients; how they acquire a clinical grasp of a particular situation; how practitioners' notions of what is good and right influence what is noticed; and how they particularize actions to individual patients (Benner et al., 1996, 1999).

At this point, the two ways of thinking about clinical thinking do not share much common language, and articulation between their research findings is limited. Even though the two views of clinical reasoning are based on different epistemological assumptions, they are not inherently incompatible. It is possible that they focus on different aspects of clinical reasoning, judgment, and decision making. The two different ways of thinking they portray may operate together in ways that we as yet do not fully appreciate. For a nurse to acquire a deep and accurate understanding of a situation, these two ways of thinking may need to occur simultaneously and interactively. The intuitive view of clinical thinking may be most useful in portraying how clinicians perceive, make sense of what is occurring in, and come to deeply understand a situation in which they are embedded. The information-processing view may enlighten our understanding of the way clinicians activate theoretical, domain-specific knowledge to help make sense of a particular situation. This would mean that, to understand a patient situation, clinicians must simultaneously think deeply about the particulars of the situation while activating relevant concepts in memory to serve as lines of reasoning that help make sense of what is occurring or what could be done. When a problem-solver starts with insights or knowledge of a current situation and then activates knowledge stored in memory to better understand the situation at hand, the problem-solver is engaging in a form of reasoning called abduction (Rolfe, 1997b).

Currently, the reasoning strand highlighted in an account given by clinicians may depend on the clinical task at hand, on the procedures researchers use to identify episodes of clinical reasoning, and on what artifacts of thinking the researchers are interested in. The following discussion of clinical reasoning is eclectic in that it draws from both schools of thought.

An Eclectic Portrayal of Clinical Reasoning and Judgment

KNOWLEDGE

Specialized knowledge and accrued experience working with a population of patients lay the foundation for the expert clinical thinking that is associated with advanced direct care practice. Once an APN has been in practice for a while, formalized knowledge and experiential knowledge become so mixed together that they are no longer distinguishable. Importantly, the expert's clinical knowledge is characterized by the ability to make fine distinctions among common features of a particular condition that were not possible during beginning practice.

Illness trajectories and presentations of prior patients make an impression and come to mind when a patient with a similar problem is seen later (Benner, 1984). The expert also remembers what interventions worked and did not work in certain situations. Timetables that most patients attain in certain situations (e.g., the time after surgery when patients who have undergone general anesthesia are expected to begin to wake up) create expectations for patients who fit into that population (Benner et al., 1996). Eventually, the expert's clinical knowledge consists of a complex network of memorable cases, prototypic images, domain-relevant concepts, thinking strategies, moral values, maxims, probabilities, behavioral responses, associations, illness trajectories and timetables, research findings, and therapeutic information. Thus, experts have extensive, varied, and complex knowledge networks that can be activated to help understand clinical situations and events.

CLINICAL THINKING

Expertise involves more than accumulated stores of knowledge, however. Clinical reasoning brings together the clinical knowledge of the provider with specific observations, perceptions, events, and facts from the situation at hand to produce an understanding of what is occurring (O'Neill, 1995). Sometimes the understanding is arrived at using cognitive processes to logically consider evidence and alternative explanations. Other times the insight or understanding "arrives" intuitively, that is, via direct apprehension without recourse to deliberate reasoning (Benner et al., 1996).

Experts have the ability to rapidly scan a situation (e.g., past records, patient's appearance, and the patient's unexpressed concern or discomfort) and identify salient and relevant information. Relying heavily on their perceptions, observations, and physical assessment skills, experts quickly activate one or several lines of reasoning regarding what might be going on. They then conduct a more focused assessment to determine which one best explains the situation at hand. These lines of reasoning are really informal, personal theories about the specific patient situation; their formulation draws from personal knowledge of the particular patient, from personal knowledge acquired from past experiences, and from formalized domain-specific knowledge (Narayan & Corcoran-Perry, 1997; Rolfe, 1997a). Often these lines of reasoning can be tested by making a clinical intervention and noting how the patient responds. For example, the ventilator settings could be changed in ways suggested by the line of reasoning to see if the patient is better able to proceed with weaning (Narayan & Corcoran-Perry, 1997).

Most patient accounts unfold in a fairly predictable way, and the APN arrives at a diagnosis and/or intervention with considerable confidence in her or his clinical inferences. Other times, however, there is uncertainty and lack of understanding regarding the situation. The uncertainty may pertain to information the patient provides, to the diagnosis, to the best approach to management, or to how the patient is responding (Brykczynski, 1991). When there is ambiguity, experts often break into conscious problem solving or "detective-like thinking and questioning" (Benner et al., 1996, 1999) to try to figure out what is going on.

Knowing the patient as an individual person with certain patterns of responses enables experienced nurses to detect subtle changes in a patient's condition (Tanner, Benner, Chesla, & Gordon, 1993). In one study, experienced acute care nurses reported that they often sensed nonspecific changes in patients and experienced a gut feeling that the patient was in transition before they were able to detect significant objective changes (Smith, 1988). These subjective feelings led to "close searching" for confirmative evidence, which gradually led to detection and recognition of an objective pattern indicating a change in condition. Premonitory feelings were also reported by an NP who reported attending to her "feelings of lack of closure, of uneasiness, incompleteness, or discomfort" because they often indicated that something important was going to come up in the conversation (Brykczynski, 1989, p. 83).

Importantly, knowing the patient may be critical to the nursing functions of surveillance and rescuing (which are addressed more fully in the section on diverse management approaches). The extent to which a nurse knows the patient may be associated with that nurse's ability to

- Recognize that risk factors are present
- Detect early indicators of a problem (i.e., a slight change in pattern)
- Take timely preventive action

While looking for patterns, the expert nurse is alert to nonfitting data, that is, data that seem important but just do not fit into any of the clinician's explanations of the situation. Nonfitting data suggest to experts that they need to generate new, or additional, hypotheses because the current observations and parameters do not fully explain the clinical picture as it has been or as it should be. Two common types of alternative hypotheses pertain to the onset of a complication or to the worsening of the disease process.

THINKING ERRORS

The clinical acumen of APNs and the inferences/hypotheses/lines of reasoning they generate are highly dependable. However, as practice becomes repetitive, APNs may develop routine responses, and they then run the risk of making certain types of thinking errors (Schön, 1984). Errors of expectancy occur when the correct diagnosis is not generated as a hypothesis because there is a set of circumstances, in either the clinician's experience or the patient's circumstances, that predisposes the clinician to disregard it. For example, the NP who over several years has seen an elderly woman for problems associated with chronic pulmonary disease may fail to consider that the most recent onset of shortness of breath and fatigue could be related to worsening aortic stenosis; the NP has come to expect pulmonary pathology, not cardiac pathology.

Erroneous conclusions are also more likely when the situation is ambiguous, that is, when the meaning or reliability of the data is unclear, the interpretation of the data is not clear-cut, the best approach to treatment is debatable, or one cannot say for sure whether the patient is responding well to treatment (Brykczynski, 1991). To avoid errors in these kinds of situations, experts often revert to the use of maxims to guide their thinking (Brykczynski, 1989). One of the maxims that NPs use to deal with uncertain diagnoses is "Real disease will declare itself" (Brykczynski, 1989). This maxim recognizes that, with the passage of time, amorphous signs and symptoms may become more distinct, so that suspending judgment and monitoring the situation may be preferable to accepting a diagnosis that has a less than good fit with the data.

The maxim "When you hear hoofbeats in Kansas, think horses, not zebras," reminds clinicians who are about to make a diagnosis that occurs infrequently to consider the incidence of the condition in the population (i.e., the base rate information). Thus an elderly person with respiratory problems seen in a suburban office is unlikely to have tuberculosis; pneumonia is a more likely diagnosis. Because tuberculosis is rare in the population of which the elderly person is a member, the clinical data for tuberculosis should be quite convincing if one were to make that diagnosis.

To keep the use of axioms in perspective, the clinicians must be aware that over-reliance on a clinical axiom can be a source of error in clinical thinking (Kassirer & Kopelman, 1991). Poor judgment can also result from tunnel vision; overgeneralization; influence by a recent, dramatic experience; and fixation on certain problems to the exclusion of others (Benner et al., 1999). Faulty thinking is not the only source of error in clinical decision making. Other sources include inaccurate observations, misinterpretation of the meaning of data, a sketchy knowledge of the particular situation, and a faulty model of the disease/condition/response.

TIME PRESSURES

Many practitioners worry about the effect time pressures have on the accuracy and completeness of their clinical thinking and decision making. Surprisingly, in a MEDLINE search using various permutations of the terms "time," "accuracy," "error," "decision making," "adverse events," "clinical reasoning," and "role strain," no studies about the influence of time pressure on clinical reasoning were found. Thus the empirical evidence regarding the effects of time pressures and heavy workload on clinical reasoning, decision making, and performance is indirect, coming from studies of adverse events during hospitalization (Buerhaus, 1999; Kovner & Gergen, 1998). One study of the incidence of adverse events during hospitalization found that 4% of patients experienced an adverse event, and another study found that 18% of patients in a teaching hospital ICU had a serious adverse event (Buerhaus, 1999). Two thirds of the adverse events in the first study were determined to be preventable, that is, due to human error.

Being rushed, feeling time pressure, and feeling overworked are clearly among the reasons people make mistakes (Buerhaus, 1999). The curious thing is that investigators in this field of research discuss the need to reduce errors by improving work processes and designing systems of care, but there is little forthright discussion of the need to reduce the workload expectations of health care providers.

As lengths of visit/contact times are decreased or the number of visits/consultations practitioners are expected to make in a day is increased, it is logical to assume that the number of errors in clinical thinking will increase. Each contact requires the practitioner to "reset" her or his clinical reasoning process by closing out one thinking project and starting out on a whole new one. This resetting, which is done back-to-back many times during a day, is cognitively and physically demanding. We just do not know how these performance expectations affect clinical reasoning accuracy.

Moreover, time pressures often get compounded by hassles. Hassles come in the form of interruptions, noise in the environment, missing supplies, and system glitches that make clinical data or even whole charts unavailable to providers. It is probable that these hassles interfere with providers' ability to concentrate on what the patient is saying and disrupt their effort to make clinical sense of the patients' accounts. They also increase the likelihood of not completing tasks or of not proceeding through a task in an organized manner, both of which can contribute to erroneous thinking, omissions in care, or failure to respond to patients' requests for service.

Finally, we are naive if we think patients are unaffected by practitioners' heavy workloads or tight appointment schedules. Many patients are sensitive to the pace with which staff and providers greet them, talk with them, and do things, particularly those activities that involve verbal interaction and/or physical contact. Some patients respond to the fast-paced talk and hurried movements of providers by not bringing up some of the issues they had intended to ask about. Others may just get flustered and forget to mention important information; still others may become hostile and nondisclosing. Thus, error in the form of information omission by the patient enters the clinical reasoning and decision-making process. In summary, the lack of evidence regarding clinical reasoning accuracy and sources of error under conditions of hectic daily practice should be an issue of concern to APNs.

TREATMENT DECISIONS

The decision whether to treat or not can be complex, because the practitioner is faced with a string of probabilities that do not all point to the same decision. APNs consider four types of information when deciding whether and how to treat:

- The degree of certainty about the diagnosis/condition
- What is known about the effectiveness of the various treatment alternatives
- What is known about the risks of the treatment alternatives
- The clinician's comfort with a particular treatment or intervention

The most clear-cut situation is when the condition is assuredly present, a particular treatment is known to be highly effective, the treatment can be expected to be low in risk for the particular patient, and the clinician is comfortable with the treatment. Unfortunately, many (probably most) therapeutic decisions are not so clear-cut. Instead, the weight of factors in support of a particular treatment and the weight of those against treatment, or in support of another treatment, are close to equivalent.

One goal of treatment decision making is to choose from among several possible interventions the one that will have the highest probability of achieving the outcomes the patient most desires. However, another goal is to "particularize" the treatment or action to the individual patient (Benner et al., 1996). Particularizing requires that the final decision factor in

- The acceptability of the treatment to the patient
- What has worked for the patient in the past

- The patient's motivation and ability to use or follow the treatment
- The likelihood that the patient will continue to use the treatment even if side effects are experienced
- The financial burden of the treatment

Other investigative work has also delineated what is meant by individualized care. A discourse analysis study of an expert APN (Brown, 1992) revealed that a majority of the interventions she enacted were tailored to the individual client (91%, 77%, and 55% in three different encounters). Tailoring was defined as speech segments that were characterized by (1) discussing client singularity (Cox, 1982) and clinical issues in association with one another; and (2) proposing interventions and plans that are explicitly personalized to the individual. This definition of tailoring of care involves components similar to those identified by Radwin (1996) in a review of research on the concept of "knowing the patient": (1) the nurse's understanding of the patient, and (2) the selection of individualized interventions. Radwin concluded that knowing the patient may result in expert clinical decision making and positive patient outcomes.

ETHICAL REASONING

Clinical decision making is inextricably linked to ethical reasoning. Clinical reasoning generates possibilities of what *could* be done in a situation, whereas ethical reasoning adds the dimension of what *should* be done in the situation. (For a more extensive discussion of ethical decision making, see Chapter 12.) What is possible and what is appropriate in specific situations are furthest apart when dealing with decisions regarding the stopping or withholding of nutrition, hydration, or a treatment; when dealing with reproductive technology; and when cost must figure into clinical treatment decisions. These situations are at high risk for becoming ethically problematic.

The literature regarding how to resolve ethical dilemma issues is large, but an approach to incorporating ethical considerations into clinical thinking and decision making that makes a great deal of sense is preventive ethics (Forrow, Arnold, & Parker, 1993). This approach places an emphasis on preventing ethical conflicts from developing rather than waiting until a conflict arises; it does so by shaping the process of clinical care so that possible value conflicts are anticipated and discussed prior to outright conflict. In addition to emphasizing early communication between the patient and the provider(s) about values, preventive ethics requires explicit, critical reflection on the institutional factors that lead to conflict (Forrow et al., 1993). A third aspect of preventive ethics is an effort to create and preserve trust and understanding among providers as well as between patients (and their families) and providers. Thus preventive ethics is proactive in that it requires providers to consider how the routine processes of care either foster or prevent conflicts from occurring or at least being identified at an early stage.

In a study of 99 ICU patients who were treated with continuous mechanical ventilation, a proactive ethics consultation starting after approximately 96 hours of continuous mechanical ventilation resulted in improved communication and decision making (Dowdy, Robertson, & Bander, 1998). The quality of communication relevant to near-end-of-life decisions in their health care records was better than those of the two control groups. In addition, twice as many decisions to forgo life-sustaining treatment were documented and they had reduced lengths of stay in the ICU.

Many questions about preventive ethics remain (Dowdy et al., 1998, p. 293): When in a patient's illness should the values issues be discussed? How can they be raised without frightening patients? What information should be discussed? Is it better to discuss specific but hypothetical future clinical scenarios or to discuss a patient's more general goals and values? Even with these unanswered questions, the approach has the potential to avoid conflicts before they occur. It also has the potential to integrate ethical reasoning into clinical reasoning at an earlier point in time than it typically enters using a traditional conflict-based ethics approach.

Another approach to moral reasoning has been uncovered in the research of Benner and associates; in their work they have found that many nurses have a "disposition toward what is good and right" (Benner et al., 1996, p. 15). These notions of good arise from society, from the nursing profession, from personal and professional experience, and from the work setting. They include commitments to humanizing and personalizing care; promoting comfort and self-care; preventing needless suffering; maximizing patient participation in decision making; responding to the feelings and problems of families; and preventing the patient from experiencing hazards in the course of receiving health care (Benner et al., 1996, 1999). These notions of good guide the actions of nurses as well as influence how they see situations. When health care is in conflict with these values and commitments, practitioners experience moral conflict or anguish, and often take action to change these kinds of situations. This view of how nurses experience ethical dilemmas is very different from the kinds of ethical decisions that physicians face, and from the kinds of conflicts addressed by traditional biomedical ethics.

Liaschenko (1997) views knowing the significance of the person as critical when doing the moral work of nursing (i.e., acting for patients, helping them maintain the integrity of their lives or face physical deterioration or death). However, she also goes on to raise three reservations about this attention to the subjective experience of patient-persons: (1) it can be a form of intrusiveness into private lives; (2) it can immensely complicate nursing practice by raising dilemmas that would not exist for the nurse practicing in a less personally involved manner; and (3) it is a political viewpoint with implications about the kind of health care our society envisions and funds. Thus, the author calls us to an objective view of what is involved in basing care on knowledge of the patient as a unique person.

INFORMATION MANAGEMENT

A final aspect of APN clinical decision making is the increasingly important competency of managing the extensive data and knowledge that are required to base practice on available, current information (Kibbe, 1999; see also Chapters 9 and 19). In the shift to an electronic environment, APNs need to be able to use within-the-organization information systems and databases, connected-system databases, the Internet, and on-line libraries and journals to access the information they need to take care of patients (Brennan & Daly, 1996). These sources will have to be accessed to acquire clinical data about the patient as well as current information about best practice. Fortunately, computerized documentation systems will make clinical data more accessible to clinicians by facilitating the recording of patient data, obtaining prior authorizations, and arranging for specialty referrals. The completion of referral forms, reports, and discharge summaries will also be built into many clinical information systems (Yancey, Given, White, DeVoss, & Coyle, 1998). As is already happening, these information systems will serve clinical decision making and link it to the resource utilization management functions of managed care systems (Britt et al., 1998).

USE OF RESEARCH EVIDENCE

An important form of knowledge that must be brought to bear on clinical decision making, for individuals as well as for populations, is the ever-increasing volume of research findings. For the nursing profession, the use of research as a basis for practice is more than the latest trend. Our profession has been exploring and considering the issues of research utilization rather intensively since the early 1970s. Clinical nurse specialists (CNSs) have led efforts in many agencies to move toward research-based practice (Hanson & Ashley, 1994; Hickey, 1990; Mackay, 1998; Stetler, Bautista, Vernale-Hannon, & Foster, 1995). They have brought research findings to the attention of the nursing staff and interdisciplinary teams, and have worked to develop the research appraisal skills of nursing staffs (Stetler & DiMaggio, 1991). Recently, the expectation of the profession and of agencies for an APN's research competency has changed from that of conducting research to that of using research evidence as a guide and basis for practice (see Chapter 9).

The Research-Based Practice Process

Bringing research to bear on clinical practice requires systematic, precise analysis and careful consideration of whether and how credible findings should be incorporated into practice. The research-based practice process involves

- Formulation of a clinical question answerable by research findings
- Location of studies relevant to that question
- Appraisal of the credibility of the findings
- Deciding whether and/or how to change practice based on the evidence
- Subsequently evaluating whether the research-based change in practice has produced the benefits anticipated

Knowledge of one's clinical practice area and familiarity with its literature are essential to formulating a clinical question for which a body of research evidence can be found. Identifying the research reports that address the clinical question requires computer searching skills that are developed and honed with practice and with the assistance of a health science librarian (Pond, 1999).

Perhaps the most difficult step for most clinicians is appraising the research evidence, that is, deciding whether a study was well conducted and whether the results are clinically significant (Brown, 1999). Admittedly, appraising scientific soundness requires knowledge of research methods, standards of conduct, and statistics. For this reason, most clinician groups feel more comfortable embarking on a research-based practice project in collaboration with a doctorally prepared health science researcher. The inclusion of the researcher enhances the likelihood that the research-based practice group has the knowledge and skills required to evaluate the scientific soundness of a study.

Findings are judged to be credible if they were produced by a scientifically sound study and clinically significant if incorporating them into practice is likely to make a difference in patients' outcomes. For findings that pass these two screens, it is still necessary to think about what patients in one's own practice would benefit from the research-based change in practice being considered and whether the protocol or intervention would be feasible in your practice setting.

The decision to implement research findings in one's setting or with a subgroup of patients is a complex one that should take into account the setting's ability to safely, effectively, and consistently incorporate the change. Another consideration in deciding whether to make a change based on research evidence is the extent to which the patients involved in the studies are similar to the patients with whom the practice group is considering using the findings. Careful reading of research reports is required to ascertain if there is a similarity, and also to determine if there were subgroups of patients in the studies who did not respond well to the intervention even though on average the intervention was effective (Rolfe, 1998). For example, a study of people with human immunodeficiency virus infection found that guided imagery and progressive muscle relaxation on average improved participants' perceived health status. However, participants who were at midstage disease and those who used guided imagery less frequently had more benefit than those in the other two stages of disease or the other two frequency-of-usage groups (Eller, 1999). This particular study was designed to detect such differences in responses, but even studies looking for an overall effect of an intervention may report data suggesting that gender or age or some other factor influenced how individuals responded to the interventions.

Finally, a quality improvement project should be planned to evaluate whether the outcomes produced under research conditions have been realized in everyday practice. This evaluation should involve data collection and measurement, but it need not be a research study (Nelson, Splaine, Batalden, & Plume, 1998). Measuring results can lead to a better understanding of the extent to which general research knowledge works at the local level. By fine-tuning general knowledge to local conditions, improvement in care and patient outcomes can be realized and documented.

Forms of Research Evidence

The basic unit of evidence of research-based practice is a finding from a single study,[2] which may vary in design from a small observational study to a large randomized clinical trial. However, the findings of one study, even a well-conducted one, is a limited basis on which to design or change practice. Nevertheless, if one's current practice clearly is not working well, and if the approach supported by the study poses no risk to patients, a change should be considered.

The better strategy, however, is to review *all* the studies that have examined the clinical issue to determine what common findings have appeared in several settings and with different populations. The main obstacle to reviewing all the studies germane to a clinical question is obviously the time required to locate, read, critically appraise, and compare the findings of many studies (Stetler et al., 1998). When searching databases for studies relevant to a particular clinical question, several results are possible: too many studies are identified, too few are identified, or just the right

---

[2] Even though a study has more than one finding and even though clinicians are often interested in a set of findings, each finding must be appraised separately (Brown, 1999, p. 70).

number (4 to 10) are identified. It is important to remember that the studies identified in the search have not been screened for credibility. You may identify six studies but, after appraising them, end up with only three credible studies that you want to seriously consider. Finding too many studies is a problem because appraisal of them will tax the time and skills of those conducting the project. To keep a research-based practice project feasible, the number of studies included in the review should be limited by an objective method, rather than by arbitrarily ignoring study reports that are difficult to obtain or to read (Brown, 1999). The best way to limit the number of studies is to focus the clinical question of interest by being specific about what form of intervention or what outcomes you are interested in. Alternatively, you can decide to look only at studies that involved a certain population or phase of illness, or only those that randomly assigned patients to treatment groups.

If the search resulted in too few studies being identified, you may need to expand the search terms you employ, search other databases, or contact colleagues who might know of research being conducted but not yet published on the topic (Pond, 1999). Alternatively, you may need to settle for findings from related populations, similar but not identical interventions, or even basic research studies. Even though not directly addressing your question, these forms of indirect evidence can be informative and can provide some rationale for choosing one course of action over another.

Fortunately, summaries of many or all studies on clinically relevant topics are appearing in clinical journals with greater frequency. These summaries come in the forms of integrative research reviews, meta-analyses, and research-based clinical guidelines. These summaries, when throughly and systematically produced, provide a basis for assessing the scientific knowledge about a particular topic that is superior to only using the findings of one or a few studies. Clinical guidelines are also being produced with increased frequency by clinical specialty organizations as well as government agencies and evidence-based centers. Many of them are of excellent quality, but some are based on expert opinion rather than research evidence. The good ones communicate to the potential user the strength of the evidence for each recommendation (i.e., number and types of studies, expert consensus, logical reasoning).

In some cases the guidelines may be easy to implement, but in others the implementation may require resources or expertise not available in a particular agency or patient population. As a result, members of a particular practice may be able to implement some of the recommendations but not others. Implementing soundly produced clinical guidelines can bring great benefit to patients, but only if the guidelines are compatible with local philosophy of care, patient values, and resources.

Moving Toward Research-Based Practice

Research-based practice requires that some time be dedicated to its pursuit. This could take the form of time set aside to systematically scan clinical journals for reports relevant to one's clinical speciality. Alternatively, an APN could join or form a multidisciplinary group that meets monthly to discuss research reports on topics of mutual interest. Some APNs keep a small notebook to jot down clinical issues and questions about which they want to find research-based knowledge. Then once a month they use the 2 hours of library time that is built into their schedules to find studies about these issues. The recorded questions help them use the limited library time in the most efficient manner.

As the evidence-based movement has gained momentum across the health care disciplines, more research summaries, also called evidence reports, are being produced and made available in clinical journals, in government publications, and on Internet sites. The people who produced the summary report have done a great deal of the time-consuming work of evidence-based practice for clinicians. Such summaries will become increasingly important to busy clinicians who do not have the time to analyze the evidence firsthand themselves. Still, clinicians should be aware that these summary products will vary in quality depending on the process used to produce them. Thus, practitioners must be able to appraise the scientific soundness of these research summaries as well as the applicability of these summaries to their own practice (Brown, 1999).

Theory-Based Practice

The preceding discussion of research-based practice recognizes how research evidence informs practice but ignores the role of theory. APNs are getting quite comfortable with the idea of research evidence as a guide to practice, yet the idea of theory-based practice is less familiar. It should not be, because, contrary to common perception, theory can be a very practical tool. Theory often brings together research findings and concepts generated in practice in a way that helps practice be more purposeful, systematic, and comprehensive.

In the past, most references to theory-based practice referred to the use of a conceptual model of nursing to guide care (Bonamy, Schultz, Graham, & Hampton, 1995; Hawkins, Thibodeau, Utley-Smith, Igou, & Johnson, 1993; Laschinger & Duff, 1991; Sappington & Kelley, 1996). The use of conceptual models or theories (e.g., the models of Orem, Newman, and Roy) provide nurses with a broad perspective within which they can view client situations; this perspective helps them organize and make sense of the myriad of information relevant to each case. Conceptual models also help nurses plan and implement care in a purposeful, proactive, and comprehensive manner (Raudonis & Acton, 1997). Their value is enhanced if there is a natural fit between the model and the nature of the clinical issues of the patient population. For example, Orem's self-care model probably has a more natural fit with the care of a population of people with chronic mental illness than it does with a population of ICU patients. Most conceptual models require practitioners to spend some time considering how the abstract concepts of the model occur or are enacted with a particular patient population or in a particular setting. Some people enjoy and see benefit from engaging in this deductive operation, whereas other people find it contrived.

Theory-based practice is, however, more than the use of conceptual models as a guide to practice. More specific theories, called middle-range theories, guide practice in a different way. Middle-range theories address the experiences of particular patient populations or of a cohort of people who are dealing with a particular health or illness issue (e.g., changing a health-related behavior or coping with postpartum depression). Because middle-range theories are more specific in what they explain, practitioners often find them more directly applicable than the conceptual models.

A recent analysis of the nursing literature identified 22 middle range theories that met certain criteria (Liehr & Smith, 1999). The list of theories generated by that analysis is provided in Table 6-4. There are other middle-range theories that were not identified by the search methods and criteria used by these analysts; however,

TABLE 6–4 MIDDLE-RANGE THEORIES (LIEHR & SMITH, 1999)	
NAME OF THEORY	AUTHORS(S)
Uncertainty in illness	Mishel
Nurse-midwifery care	Thompson et al.
Facilitating growth and development	Kinney
Self-transcendence	Reed
Hazardous secrets and reluctantly taking charge	Burke et al.
Women's anger	Thomas
Caring	Swanson
Negotiating partnership	Powell-Cope
Unpleasant symptoms	Lenz et al.
Cultural brokering	Jezewski
Homelessness-hopelessness	Tollett & Thomas
Balance between analgesia and side effects	Good, Moore, & Good
Chronotherapeutic intervention for postsurgical pain	Auvil-Novak
Nurse-expressed empathy and patient distress	Olso & Hanchett
Interpersonal perceptual awareness	Brooks & Thomas
Resilience	Polk
Individualized music intervention for agitation	Gerdner
Affiliated individuation as a mediator for stress	Acton
Chronic sorrow	Eakes, Burke, & Hainsworth
Acute pain management	Huth & Moore
Psychological adaptation	Levesque et al.
Peaceful end of life	Ruland & Moore

the list provides a sampling of the middle-range theories currently available to practicing nurses.

In looking at this list, you can see that the topics of the theories are substantively specific, although some are more specific than others. "Balance between analgesia and side effects" is more specific and less abstract than "resilience." An APN in a particular practice field may find that only one or two of these theories is applicable to her or his area of practice. However, as middle-range theories are developed for other topics, APNs will be able to use several of these types of theories to guide different aspects of practice.

Knowledge-Based Practice

Beyond research-based practice and theory-based practice is the more essential issue of knowledge-based practice. Knowledge is the goal of both the conduct of research and the development of theory. Moreover, acquisition of useful and dependable knowledge requires both research work and theory work. Research findings are bits of knowledge, whereas theories are explanatory systems describing how some aspect of the world works. To be most useful, research findings must be brought together into an internally consistent explanatory description. The knowledge development process can, of course, work in reverse. A theory can be based on the experiences of practice; then that theory needs to be tested and refined through research. Research can be used to determine the extent to which a theory holds up across different groups of people and helps identify the circumstances in which it is applicable. The findings of theory-testing research may also reveal ways in which the theory should be modified.

Via either knowledge production pathway, the goal is meaningful and useful knowledge that has been tested using scientific methods and found to be an accurate and useful portrayal of certain realities. APNs have the educational background to appreciate how these two knowledge production pathways of science work together and separately to produce useful and dependable clinical knowledge.

DIVERSE APPROACHES TO DIRECT CARE: HEALTH AND ILLNESS MANAGEMENT

APNs' holistic approach to care and their commitment to using research evidence as a basis for care shape how they help patients. Generally, they use a variety of interventions to effect change in the health status or quality of life of an individual and/or family, including interpersonal interventions and discrete actions (Brykczynski, 1989). Interpersonal interventions are frequently referred to as "support," whereas discrete actions are those nonpharmacological and pharmacological interventions used to alleviate, prevent, or manage a specific physical symptom, condition, or problem.

Interpersonal Interventions

Support is not a discrete intervention; it is a composite of interpersonal interventions based on the patient's unique psychological and informational needs. Supportive interpersonal interventions include providing reassurance, giving information, affirming, providing anticipatory guidance, guiding decision making, listening actively, expressing understanding, and being available. Each of these interventions can be described in terms of the circumstances under which it is indicated; for example, reassurance is indicated when clients are experiencing uncertainty, distress, or lack of confidence (Boyd & Munhall, 1989), and active listening is indicated when patients have a strong need to tell their story. The actions that constitute these interventions are not mutually exclusive. Giving factual information can be reassuring, instructional, guiding, or all of these things at the same time.

In practice, these interpersonal interventions blend together, and APNs are not consciously aware of when they are doing one and when another. That is as it should be. There is no need to think "Now I'm doing active listening, now I'm going to do anticipatory guidance." Instead, APNs interact with patients in ways that intermingle the conceptually separate interventions. This crafting of support evolves as the APN talks with patients; infers their worries, fears, and concerns; and, without a great deal of conscious thought, acts to alleviate their distress. The patient may experience the interaction as just a good talk with the APN or as a feeling of being understood. However, support is a complex nursing intervention that is strategically crafted and purposefully administered and often makes a difference in how the patient feels and acts. Thus it is an intervention in the finest nursing tradition. Chapter 7 elaborates on the interpersonal interventions APNs use to teach and coach patients.

Discrete Management and Treatment Interventions

PREVENTIVE SERVICES IN PRIMARY CARE

Health promotion and disease prevention interventions are tools that APNs in primary care regularly use to help people achieve and/or maintain a high quality of life. These preventive services include (1) counseling regarding personal health practices that can protect a person from, or put her or him at risk for disability or disease, (2) screening for the presence of disease, and (3) immunization to prevent specific diseases. Discernment is needed in the use of these interventions because time and effort can be wasted if their use is not based on current scientific knowledge and tailored to the individual person or community. The U.S. Preventive Services Task Force's *Guide to Clinical Preventive Services* (1996) and the *Canadian Guide to Clinical Preventive Health Care* (Canadian Task Force on the Periodic Health Examination, 1994) provide specific preventive guidelines for many health conditions as well as valuable summaries for each that describe the state of the science regarding common preventive services.

An important point made in the *Guide to Clinical Preventive Services* (1996) is that primary prevention in the form of counseling aimed at changing health-related behavior may be more effective than diagnostic screening and testing. Many healthy people as well as people who have had a recent health scare are quite receptive to, even eager for, information and guidance about how to stay healthy and avoid age-related disabilities. However, other people who engage in one or several unhealthy behaviors can be quite defensive and resistant to talking about their risks and how behavior changes could reduce risks. Introducing behavior change issues with unreceptive people requires a high level of interpersonal skill and a good sense of timing. However, one has to also consider that it is likely that no health care provider has previously attempted to discuss the problem (e.g., smoking, lack of exercise, alcohol abuse) with the person even though signs of a problem have existed for quite a while (Stafford & Blumenthal, 1998). If this is the case, some of these people may even welcome the opportunity to be helped in facing the issue.

Talking about the risks of the current behavior and the benefits of the behavior change are not enough. To be effective, counseling regarding these issues most likely needs to also include a discussion of how the person perceives the burden of changing a personal behavior; that is, what would be lost and what would be required to make a change? The provider has to get in touch with how much effort will be required and what forms of self-help assistance are acceptable to the individual. Then and only then can a specific recommendation about a strategy or program be made.

For many risk-reduction behaviors, community-based interventions may be more effective than those delivered in a clinical setting. School-based education and media blitzes are being used to try to get through to children and adolescents regarding risky behaviors; however, the extent to which they are effective is not known. Small-group discussions with adolescents in church programs and community health centers about sexual behaviors have resulted in less intercourse, greater use of condoms, and less risky sexual behavior in some communities (Kirby et al., 1994; O'Donnell et al., 1999). And work-site health education is being used with increased frequency, particularly with regard to occupational risks such as back strain and eye injuries (Volinn, 1999), but also regarding cancer and heart disease prevention.

Clinicians also have at their disposal a wide array of screening tools, but some of these tools are better with certain populations than others. For example, electrocardiographic screening for heart disease yields little benefit in asymptomatic adults, or in asymptomatic children and adolescents prior to engaging in vigorous sports, but is clearly of value in symptomatic adults (U.S. Preventive Services Task Force, 1996). The clinical preventive guidelines cited earlier are invaluable for determining how much benefit can be realized with the screening tools available and in selecting the populations who would benefit most from their use.

PREVENTIVE SERVICES IN HOSPITALS AND HOME CARE

Although the nature of prevention in acute care is somewhat different from that provided in primary care, nurses working in hospitals, other inpatient settings, and home care also provide preventive services. Many of the actions and assessments performed on behalf of acutely ill patients are aimed at early detection and prevention of problems related to treatment, disease progression, self-care deficits, or the hospital environment itself. Nurses assist patients by *preventing* adverse events and complications, including medication interactions, physiological decline, poor communication, bedsores, and death. This function is also referred to as "rescuing," as in rescuing from a bad course of events and/or death (Aikens, Sochalski, & Lake, 1997).

One project aimed at identifying nursing-sensitive outcomes in hospitals identified four types of problems nurses frequently prevent: (1) complications related to treatment; (2) injuries/complications unrelated to treatment (e.g., falls); (3) extension of the disease process; and (4) complications related to a limited ability to engage in self-care activities at home (Stetler & DeZell, 1989). These problems typically result from a complex set of factors, some of which reside in inadequate delivery systems. They occur when health care professionals do not assess patients for risk of problems common to their condition and do not proactively enact interventions that would prevent the problem from developing (Harris, 1997).

THERAPEUTIC INTERVENTIONS

The treatment and management interventions that APNs use include a wide variety of self-care modalities and low-technology, nonpharmacological modalities (Avorn, Everitt, & Baker, 1991; Brown & Grimes, 1993; Brykczynski, 1989). However, even when technological and pharmacological modalities are used, they are used in combination with considerable discussion of why they are advantageous and how they will affect the patient (Flesner & Clawson, 1998). Information giving in the form of printed materials, small-group sessions, and personalized teaching to patients and their families are frequently used by APNs in all clinical settings. The following discussion provides examples and studies to support the general characterization just offered of ANP therapeutics.

APNs' consideration of many factors was evident in a study of 501 physicians and 298 NPs who were asked to describe how they would treat simulated cases involving patients with epigastric pain. The NPs were more likely than the physicians to recommend stopping aspirin; changing diet; reducing alcohol, caffeine, and tobacco intake; and obtaining counseling for stress (Avorn et al., 1991). They were also far less likely to recommend a prescription drug.

A slightly different result was found in another study of 10 collaborative pairs of physicians and NPs using a methodology similar to the Avorn et al. study: NPs and physicians were identical in their final recommendations related to medication management, although the processes used to reach decisions were different

(Flesner & Clawson, 1998). The NPs elicited more information about the context of the patients' lives and available resources, and collaborated with patients more frequently to work out the details of implementing the management plans.

When prescribing medications, APNs also consider many factors, including the patient's financial status, the patient's previous experience with similar medications, the ease of taking the medication, how many other medications the person is taking, how often it must be taken, the side effect profiles of the drugs being considered, and potential drug and disease interactions (Brown & Grimes, 1993). A descriptive study of the safety and effectiveness of APN prescriptive authority found that the 33 NPs in the project prescribed medications for 90% of 1,708 patients; 42% had one drug prescribed per visit, and 31% had two drugs prescribed per visit (Hamric, Worley, Lindebak, & Jaubert, 1998). This would seem to be a low number of prescribed medications, but further study of the extent to which APNs recommend prescription drugs vis-à-vis the extent to which other providers who care for similar patients do is needed before it can be established that a lower use of prescription drugs is characteristic of ANP.

In general, it can be said that there is evidence that APNs use a broad range of interventions, with substantial reliance on self-care and low-technology interventions. APNs in oncology settings report using nonpharmacological interventions such as cognitive activity; imagery; music; relaxation, breathing, and movement techniques; and cutaneous interventions (heat, cold, vibration, and transcutaneous electrical nerve stimulation) for symptom management (McMillan, Heusinkveld, & Spray, 1995; Spross & Wolff-Burke, 1996). Similarly, certified nurse-midwives (CNMs) report teaching perineal massage during late pregnancy (Labrecque et al., 1999) and recommending alternative birthing positions and styles of pushing to avoid having to perform episiotomies (Lydon-Rochelle, Albers, & Teaf, 1995; Sampselle & Hines, 1999). CNMs also use significantly less analgesia and anesthesia; perform less fetal monitoring, and fewer episiotomies, forceps deliveries, and amniotomies; use less intravenous fluids; and induce labor less frequently than do physicians (Brown & Grimes, 1993; Davis, Riedmann, Sapiro, Minogue, & Kazer, 1994). Another perspective on the use of nonpharmacological management by CNMs is added by a study comparing nurse-midwives' and obstetricians' processes of care; the CNMs emphasized educational/psychosocial care and restrained use of technology, whereas the obstetricians more routinely used state-of-the-art technology (Oakley et al., 1995). In a study of APNs' use of current procedural terminology (CPT) codes, family NPs and nurse-midwives used, on average, 30% to 33% of the codes, a relatively broad usage (Griffith & Robinson, 1993).

Acute care nurse practitioners (ACNPs), CNMs, certified registered nurse anesthetists (CRNAs), and CNSs clearly use different repertoires of therapeutic interventions than do APNs who provide primary care. For example, the therapeutic procedures used frequently by ACNPs include managing patients receiving ventilation, suturing lacerations, initiating and adjusting intravenous lines, performing cardioversion, and performing incision and drainage (Kleinpell, 1997).

The Nursing Interventions Classification Project (Bulechek & McCloskey, 1999b), the Omaha System, and the Home Health Care Classification are well along the road to capturing the full range of treatments/interventions nurses use, and are superior to the CPT system for categorizing nursing activities (Henry, Holzemer, Randell, Hsieh, & Miller, 1997). These discipline-specific classification systems have the potential to recognize nursing interventions that currently are not recognized by the CPT system as contributing to patients' outcomes. If these systems were linked with the

CPT classification system, a complete profile of the interventions patients receive from various health care providers in a variety of settings would be available.

The repertoire of interventions used by individual APNs clearly depends on the problems experienced by the population of patients with whom they work, but it also depends on the effort APNs have made to extend and refine their repertoire beyond the interventions they learned during graduate education and orientation to a position.

Management of Complex Situations

APNs' direct care often involves management and/or coordination of complex situations; many illustrations of this ANP characteristic may be found in the chapters on specific ANP roles (see Chapters 13 through 19). In some settings, APNs have been designated the providers responsible for coordinating discharge for patients with complex follow-up care or for conducting patient education with high-risk patients (Damato et al., 1993; Naylor et al., 1999). In other settings, APNs are assuming management responsibilities for discrete and complex aspects of care, such as care of elderly patients who become confused during hospitalization, pain management in patients who are chronically or terminally ill, skin care for patients at risk for skin breakdown or delayed healing, and aggressive management of complex cases (Urban, 1997). Daleiden (1993) described the role of the CNS as trauma case manager. The trauma CNS assessed each patient daily, did rounds with the medical director, made clinical nursing rounds on all trauma patients in the hospital, and met regularly with families. This coordination of care resulted in early identification of changes in patients' conditions and smooth transition of patients when transferred from one unit to another.

Many CNSs have had the experience of being called in on a consultation and finding that there is a need for skilled communication, advocacy, or coordination of the various providers' plans—or some combination thereof. The patient may not be progressing because wound care, pain management, and physical therapy have not been well thought out and coordinated. A family may be angry because plans keep changing and they are receiving conflicting information from various providers. Typically, the CNS talks with the patient and family to become familiar with their concerns and objectives, and then brokers a new plan of care that reflects the patient's and family's needs and preferences as well as the clinical objectives of the involved providers (Steele & Fenton, 1988). The agreed-upon plan must also be consistent with the care authorized by the third-party payers for the patient, or a special agreement must be negotiated. This brokering requires broad clinical knowledge regarding the objectives of various providers, interpersonal skill in calming the results of misunderstandings, diplomacy to get the stakeholders to see each other's points of view, and a commitment to keeping the patient's needs at the center of what is being done.

HELPING PATIENTS MANAGE CHRONIC ILLNESSES

Another type of complex situation that APNs manage effectively is chronic illness. Chronic diseases such as multiple sclerosis, arthritis, cognitive degeneration, psoriasis, congestive heart failure, chronic lung disease, cancer, acquired immunodeficiency syndrome, and organ failure with subsequent transplantation affect individuals and families in profound ways. The extent to which the disease can be altered significantly by treatment is often unknown. Individuals and their family members, however, develop perceptions about how the illness may unfold over time for them. The term "trajectory" has been used to describe the perceived illness course, because it conveys a sense of phases that unfold over time, each with different illness management issues and ways of intruding on life (Corbin & Strauss, 1992). Individual illness, however, is characterized by a great deal of uncertainty—uncertainty about the future life course, the effectiveness of treatment, the chances of leading a happy life, bodily functions, medical bills, and intimate relationships. Uncertainty is the single most stressful aspect of the illness experience (Mast, 1995) and APNs often take steps to help the patient and family overcome their powerlessness by helping them acquire a sense of control over their lives.

A study of families coping with breast cancer showed that the issues, problems, and challenges the families dealt with changed as the families moved through the year after diagnosis (Hilton, 1993). Facing the diagnosis, experiencing family communication problems, and dealing with the effects of tests and treatment were more prevalent during the diagnosis and treatment phases, whereas disruption of plans, household organization, and the health of other family members became issues later. However, for most of the families uncertainty remained a major issue throughout the course of the illness.

The spouses and significant others of people with chronic illness often bear considerable emotional and workload burdens (Gaynor, 1990; Laizner, Yost, Barg, & McCorkle, 1993; Northouse & Peters-Golden, 1993). One intervention approach is to enhance the couple's ability to work together. A study of 60 couples over a 2-year period showed that couples who worked together well had the following characteristics (Corbin & Strauss, 1984):

- Had come to terms with the illness and the reality that it would have major effects on their lives
- Were committed to the relationship and to the work that had to be done to manage the illness
- Were sensitive to cues indicating each other's moods, needs, and wants
- Recognized the need for self-renewal activities
- Were willing to negotiate and compromise
- Knew how to use resources
- Trusted that each was doing everything possible to make their shared and separate lives good

For a variety of reasons, APNs are successful in providing care to persons with chronic conditions, but an important one is that APNs are oriented toward patient self-care. One example of the value placed on self-care by APNs is found in the core competencies for nurse-midwifery. The American Association of Nurse Midwives (1997) specifies that one of the core competencies is "Providing information and support to enable women to make informed decisions and to assume primary responsibility for their own care" (p. 8). This focus on patients' self-management was also illustrated in a descriptive study of the meaning of advanced practice nursing for APNs (Grando, 1998). One subject, a family NP, believed that her emphasis on patient self-care was one of the biggest differences between her practice and that of a physician. Another subject, a CNM, communicated her support of patient autonomy when she described birthing: "the woman gives birth to the baby" rather than the provider "delivering the baby" (Grando, 1998, p. 507).

The benefits of emphasizing self-care are supported by research showing that, when patients are given information about illnesses and helped to manage their illnesses, the course of illnesses and quality of life are improved (Gifford, Laurent, Gonzales, Chesney, & Lorig, 1998; Lorig, Mazonson, & Holman, 1993; Von Korff et al., 1998). Moreover, the evidence suggests that health education for self-management works in part by building patients' self-confidence about controlling their lives in spite of the presence of disease (Sobel, 1995). Hence, many self-management, educational interventions for persons with chronic conditions are being designed to bolster the patients' sense of self-efficacy related to (1) coping with the associated disabilities and (2) gaining control over the impact of the disease on their lives.

APNs who see chronically ill patients either in a primary care setting or in a specialty setting improve care by coordinating the services patients receive from multiple providers. Chronic illnesses often affect several body systems or have numerous sequelae. Thus, persons who are chronically ill often receive care from a primary care provider and several other clinicians including physician and APN specialists, social workers, physical therapists, and dietitians. Some patients are receiving home care and family members, particularly children, may also need services such as supportive care. Insurance providers and HMOs are also stakeholders in the delivery of services to the chronically ill; they have the authority to allow or disallow services. Without coordination, families coping with chronic illness(es) can find themselves in an "agency maze" (Burton, 1995). This vivid phrase captures the confusing experiences that ensue when the agencies and providers rendering care to a family do not communicate with one another. Families do not know where to go for help and as a result many resort to a trial-and-error approach to getting what they need. They often suffer the negative effects of misinformation, repetitive intake interviews, being denied service, conflicting approaches, and unsolved problems. A resource-savvy APN can often assess such situations and intervene to reduce stress, improve communications, and benefit patients and families. By contacting other providers to develop a coordinated management plan and by linking patients with suitable agencies, the APN can do much to relieve the burdens of chronic illness on a family.

END-OF-LIFE CARE

End-of-life care is another realm requiring the expanded skills, attentive planning, and coordinating efforts of APNs (Weggel, 1997). When a person is nearing death, many decisions need to be coordinated to assure continuity of care and a peaceful death; these decisions involve issues such as pain control, plans for withholding or initiation of life support measures, where the patient will be cared for, the need for supportive services such as hospice care, and burden on the family. An APN's ability to smooth the patient's and family's experience often depends on knowing the resources of a particular community as well as how "to work" the patient's health care insurance system.

The Report of the National Task Force on End-of-Life Care in Managed Care (1999) described current end-of-life care in the United States as fragmented and inadequate, and pointed out that special tools and strategies are available within managed care to intervene at the system level to improve it. Examples of these tools include creative case management programs, financing of palliative care programs and referrals, clinical guidelines and education of staff regarding the management of pain at the end of life, collection of population-based data regarding the process of dying, and providing for bereavement counseling (National Task Force on End-of-Life Care in Managed

Care, 1999). Thus, APNs working within managed care need to consider whether the resources necessary to support patients at the end of life are available within their organization or from the payers with whom they contract. If they are not, an organized lobbying effort to secure palliative care benefits for subscribers should be embarked upon; the recommendations of national task forces, such as the one just cited, could be invoked as a standard for end-of-life care.

GAPS IN THE RESEARCH BASE PERTAINING TO APN CARE

The evidence cited previously establishes that the five characteristics of APN care result in better clinical outcomes at a reasonable cost and in a manner that is acceptable to patients. (The association between APN care and outcomes of care is discussed more fully in Chapter 25.) Unfortunately, there are important gaps in the research base regarding the impact of APN care on client health and illness outcomes.

   For instance, we know very little about how APNs form partnerships with patients and about how those partnerships develop and change over time. In addition, we do not know what the impact of partnerships is on patient outcomes or patients' feelings about the care they receive. The same is true of holistic care, expert clinical reasoning, and research-based practice. Practitioners everywhere are engaging in research-based practice projects, but there is little evidence that research-based practice produces better patient outcomes. It certainly makes sense that it should. If practitioners use approaches and interventions that were found to be effective in research studies, it is highly likely that, when used in practice, they will produce good patient outcomes. However, it is possible that the conditions that were present in the research study cannot be reproduced in real-world practice, hence the approach or intervention may not work, or may not work as well. Another reason why a research-based intervention might not work is that the population with whom it is being used is in some way different from the populations who participated in the research studies. For these reasons, quality improvement studies are needed to measure how well a research-based intervention is working when applied in practice. Measurement and data collection in clinical settings establish and document the extent to which the process of care is being implemented in accord with the research evidence and the degree to which the desired outcome targets are being achieved (Nelson et al., 1998). In short, there is respectable research evidence supporting the assertion that care from APNs results in good patient outcomes. However, we are not very knowledgeable about what actions, care strategies, and competencies of the APN produce those good outcomes. Such research is needed in order to design educational curricula that foster the acquisition of the efficacious competencies.

CONDITIONS CONDUCIVE TO APN PRACTICE

A Population Focus

It is no longer possible to serve patients well by providing only good clinical care (Britt et al., 1998). The reality is that, to serve patients well, clinical recommendations must be made within the financial structure of the patient's health care plan. This involves understanding how capitated health care delivery and financing work in general, as well as the terms of specific managed care plans.

Part of this understanding involves recognizing that MCOs approach health care using a population-based focus. They often use a combination of aggregated individual outcomes and/or population outcomes to demonstrate value for dollars spent on specified populations of patients (Britt et al., 1998; Grimes & Garcia, 1997). Evaluation of the degree to which desirable outcomes are attained enables an HMO to compare its effectiveness to that of a comparable system or to evaluate the relative effectiveness of a new program or new processes of care. These kinds of evaluations and comparisons can lead to the identification of best practice methods at the health care system level. Utilization of services, readmission rates, worked hours per patient day, and average total cost per case are examples of population outcomes used in these kinds of evaluations and comparisons.

Aggregated individual outcomes are useful in evaluation of program effectiveness. By requiring that care administered and individual outcomes be documented in standardized ways, the health care system can conduct programmatic evaluations of clinical outcomes. Population-based evaluations can also be used by APNs to evaluate and improve the care they provide. Such evaluations can help answer questions such as "Is the specific care I/we provide patients the best way of managing their health or illness?" and "Are my patients doing as well as similar patients who are cared for by other providers?" Conducting such an evaluation involves (1) identifying groups of patients (i.e., populations) who have high costs of care and/or less than optimal outcomes; (2) monitoring and analyzing variances in outcomes and costs; (3) examining processes of care to determine how management of the condition could be improved; and (4) incorporating management methods found to be effective in research or best practice networks.

Managed Care Contracts

As MCOs and capitation have evolved and taken on various organizational forms, the contractual arrangements APNs' practice groups are asked to enter with these organizations have become more complex. Although the specific nature of these contracts is beyond the scope of this chapter, it is important to realize that APNs' direct care can be affected through the terms of these contracts, MCOs acquire the ability to influence how providers clinically manage their patients. This is typically done by instituting contractual capitation agreements, monitoring service utilization, limiting diagnostic and treatment options, and assessing the efficiency and quality of individual provider groups (Britt et al., 1998). Providers are encouraged to practice preventive health care and constrain their use of costly services such as specialty referrals, hospitalization, and expensive technology. A stronger characterization of this constraint is "Every time the physician uses a resource, for example, consultation, diagnostic testing, or surgical procedures, he or she pays an economic penalty" (Chervenak, Laurence, McCullough, & Chez, 1996, p. 525). Financial incentives to avoid using resources create a conflict of interest for providers which may result in withholding of tests, treatments, and services from patients who really should have them. In addition, the contractual arrangements integrated MCOs form between care provider groups along the continuum from acute to long-term care influence what, where, and how illness is managed.

Learning About Managed Care Contracts

APNs should know who in their organizations negotiates and manages contracts with MCOs for the services the APN provides. An ongoing relationship and dialogue with this person (often called a contracting manager) is essential to assuring that APN services are fairly and fully represented in negotiations with MCOs (Adams, 1997). From the contracting manager the APN can learn who the top payers are for APN services; what managed care agreements have the most effect on the APN's service line; and how the rate of reimbursement relates to the cost of providing the service (e.g., what services/programs are operating within their reimbursement rate and which ones are not?). The APN should ask to be informed when new contracts are being negotiated and when changes in existing contracts are under discussion so problematic issues can be negotiated and new opportunities explored.

Clinical Guidelines

Clinical guidelines are often used by managed care plans to assure quality and limit resource utilization. Some guidelines have been developed in close association with providers, are based on research evidence, and have attained a balance between quality care and economic efficiency. Others, however, overly constrain clinical judgment and do not represent patients' interests well. Concern has also been expressed that clinical guidelines concentrate on common problems and on problems for which there are direct and immediate answers. This focus could result in failure to pursue less common and more poorly defined problems, which in turn would result in less complete care (Chervenak et al., 1996). Many MCOs clearly have quality care as their objective, and the introduction of capitation and managed care has introduced cost into the quality formula, which was surely needed. Inevitably, however, some providers will find themselves in the position of believing that the MCO's clinical guidelines are not in the best interest of a particular patient or more generally in the interests of a population of patients. Providers must be willing to take on the issue and be politically savvy about how to negotiate with managed care plans to secure changes that more optimally represent patients' interests.

For example, primary care providers and home health nurses are finding that, after elderly people have been hospitalized, the number of home visits allowed by MCOs is often inadequate for those who do not have family or social resources. A survey of home health nurses revealed that an immense amount of time is consumed in calls to MCOs in an attempt to obtain authorization for continued care that is needed by patients (Brennan & Cochran, 1998). Considerable work will be required to get the visit allotments changed so that obtaining more visits does not have to be negotiated so often.

Consultation, Collaboration, and Referral

Consultation, collaboration, and referral play out differently in various clinical settings. In primary care settings where the NP is viewed as an independent practitioner, collaboration takes the form of NP consulting with and referring to physicians for patient needs outside the NP's scope of practice. Conversely, the physician consults with and refers to NPs for patient needs that are outside the physician's scope of practice (King, Parrinello, & Baggs, 1996). It has been estimated that NPs can safely deliver up to 80% of the primary care needed by adults and 90% of that needed by children (Green & Conway Welch, 1995). This means that 10% to 20% of the patient care will need to be provided in consultation with or by the NP's primary care physician backup. Many contracts allow such consultation under a comprehensive patient case management agreement, but others view it as a referral.

In the past, primary care APNs have used referrals to specialists judiciously, and patients have valued APNs' ability to recognize when patients would most likely benefit from specialist care. A family NP was told by a patient that the fact that she called a dermatologist for advice on how to handle a persistent rash was one of the reasons he trusted her so much. He said, "You know what you know, and you know what you don't know. I like that." One gets the same sense from talking to patients who have received care from CNMs; one woman said, "She didn't take any chances with me or my baby. She just got on the phone and called the obstetrician—and she was right." CNMs and CRNAs have worked closely with physicians for years and are quite clear regarding what they can manage independently and when they need to consult, co-manage, or refer. Unfortunately, APNs must be more frugal about making referrals than they have in the past. At the same time, they must not hesitate to refer if the patient's condition is beyond their scope of practice or if the patient is not achieving good outcomes under APN management.

In the acute care setting, where any individual patient is assumed to require care from both disciplines, collaboration should be played out as interdependent, interdisciplinary practice (King et al., 1996). That is to say that the care provided by the different disciplines is complementary, and all patients benefit from ongoing collaboration between the disciplines. In settings where ANPs are employed, each patient should be assigned to a core team comprised of an ACNP and an attending physician who collaborate to provide the care required by the patient; trainees (i.e., NP students and residents) are then integrated into the team (King et al., 1996).

Experienced APNs who are in joint practices with physicians find them an important source of affirmation for the nursing perspective that APNs bring to care. APNs report that informal consultation is just as likely to consist of the physician's seeking the APN's opinion as it is the APN's seeking the physician's opinion. For the new APN, a carefully chosen joint practice provides ready informal consultation as well as opportunities for case review and discussions. Joint practice can make available to patients the benefits of different perspectives on care and can result in patients' being linked with the provider who has the interests and skills that correspond with their needs.

APNs who work in settings with APN peers report that relationships within the group are important sources of support and professional growth (Winch, 1989). Although many APNs work in geographical areas where peers are a considerable distance away, electronic communication has the potential to increase opportunities for dialogue and mutual support.

In a comprehensive book about collaboration among health care professionals, edited by Sullivan (1998), collaboration is viewed as "a health care imperative in the global information era of the next millennium" (p. xxv). At the societal level, collaboration is viewed as a value and an activity that transcends individual achievement and thereby contributes to harmony and a sense of community—experiences many people say are missing in their lives (Hobbs, 1998).

Others who also value interdisciplinary collaboration point out the potential constraints to it, including less than ideal communication, unequal power relationships, differing professional paradigms, and a dearth of shared time and space (Lindeke & Block, 1998). These authors describe the difficulty of maintaining professional identity and integrity while working toward shared goals. Along the same lines, McCloskey and Maas (1998) express a similar concern that "some nurses are abandoning discipline-specific successes because they have been led to believe that a disciplinary focus is not consistent with an interdisciplinary approach" (p. 157). They cite three examples as evidence of this concern: (1) nurse executives with titles that make nursing invisible in the organizational structure; (2) critical paths that focus on medical procedures and diagnoses; and (3) clinical documentation systems that exclude the use of nursing language. Few would disagree with the premise that interdisciplinary collaboration has great contributions to make to the improvement of health care, but it has to be thoughtfully undertaken if patients are to continue to benefit from the unique nursing perspective that has contributed to the health, comfort, recovery, and dignified death of individuals and populations since the profession's inception.

EDUCATIONAL STRATEGIES

The education of APNs should consider the health care problems and needs of the population the graduates of the program will serve, the expressed preferences of the public, the health care policy of the state and the nation, and the competencies set forth by professional nursing organizations and national commissions. In this brief discussion, selected issues that pertain directly to the five characteristics of APN practice discussed in this chapter are addressed.

Holistic Perspective

When student APNs begin to have learning experiences in the expanded domain of advanced practice (i.e., assessment and management of medical problems), they often experience a deterioration in their comfort level, motor skills, interviewing competency, and clinical problem-solving ability. As they become more competent in the new domain, they eventually emerge and recognize that they want to retain the holistic perspective from their basic nursing education and career experiences. They do not want to simply diagnose and treat disease; they want to continue to attend to how patients are responding to disease and to the effects patients' social and physical environments have on their illness, and they want to continue to be responsive to the health problems patients experience in their daily lives. Part of the solution may be to address the continued importance of a holistic perspective up front and to encourage students to evaluate the different perspectives they observe in their clinical placements.

Unfortunately, the theoretical, empirical, and educational literature are rather silent on how the medical and nursing perspectives can be brought together. What is needed is a way to unite cognitively the purposes of diagnosing and treating patients' disease-based problems with the purposes of helping patients adjust to and cope with their experiences of development, parenting, aging, and illness. However, union of the two perspectives on health and health care may not be possible, or even desirable, because the two perspectives have very different philosophical assumptions, traditions, and assessment interests that inform the design of medical and nursing curricula and affect role socialization. Each perspective has something unique to contribute to health care. Perhaps what should be pursued is facility with both perspectives and awareness of when to use one rather than the other. Although one cannot take the nursing perspective out of the APN, some issues patients raise during health care encounters may be better addressed by emphasizing the diagnostic processes and therapeutic approaches characteristic of the medical perspective. Other issues are likely to be better addressed by the holistic, functional perspective characterized by the nursing view of the patient. Until the blending of the two perspectives is better understood, the most effective strategy is to approach and think about patient care within a holistic framework but recognize that, when disease-related issues surface, it is necessary to think in a more causal way. The holistic framework is the most helpful for seeing issues from patients' perspectives and for seeing the relationship between disease and illness, but the linear cause-and-effect perspective may be necessary when underlying disease processes need to be considered. Dialogue on interdisciplinary education and demonstration projects that evaluate effects of interdisciplinary education of APNs and physicians are likely to illuminate this discussion (Larson, 1995).

Allan and Hall (1988) contrasted the technocratic framework of health care (i.e., the medical model) with the ecological framework of health care. The ecological model focuses on the interaction between the person and the environment and quality-of-life issues. The three major concepts that distinguish the ecological viewpoint are environment, holism, and process. Newman's (1994) conceptual model of health as expanding consciousness is one of several ecological theories in nursing. It provides a useful way of thinking about patients' experiences, about how people develop lifestyle patterns that affect their well-being, and about how people's choices can bring about expanding consciousness; it also suggests new ways of helping patients. However, this author does not find Newman's model particularly helpful for deliberating on how to join the medical and the holistic perspectives, because it places considerable emphasis on refraining from fixing things and letting go of personal control. It does not take into account the reality that many diseases are highly treatable using technological interventions. Yet the ecological paradigm has generated ideas that could eventually result in the evolution of a new holistic framework that brings together person-environment interaction care and disease-focused care.

Partnerships with Patients

Graduate programs should not assume that students have good communications skills and styles because they acquired them during undergraduate education. The reality is that some undergraduate students never acquired them, and some nurses who acquired them may have slipped into bad habits over the years in practice. In addition, return to graduate school often finds them willing to re-evaluate their communication skills and re-examine to what degree they are practicing their person-centered values.

Creating partnerships with patients, refraining from dominating patients, and helping patients be self-determining are some of the values that student APNs need to revisit. After a discussion of person-centered communication and conversational interviewing in one of this author's classes, students reflected on audiotapes of interviews they had held with patients, and several realized how controlling they had been. The assignment moved them to alter drastically their approaches to assessment interviewing.

Clinical Reasoning

There are learning strategies that can be used to assist students in becoming good clinical thinkers. First, it is important to recognize that expert clinical reasoning is more than arriving at a correct diagnosis, even though that is an important objective. Expert clinical reasoning also requires that the practitioner use communication competency as a medium of practice and be sensitive to the broader contexts in which disease, illness, and individual responses occur. To produce broad-based, discriminating, and proficient clinical thinkers, some combination of the learning experiences listed in Table 6–5 will be required.

One approach to bottom-up case analysis is problem-based learning (PBL), in which the student is guided through standardized cases by the tutor-teacher (Barrows & Pickell, 1991). The tutor is responsible for the process of learning, not for content. In PBL, the tutor guides students through analysis and synthesis by pushing them to identify what they know, what they do not know, and what resources they will have to use to acquire the information they need to manage a case. During the ensuing week, the students are expected to acquire the needed information so that they can continue analysis and synthesis at a more informed level. Evaluations of PBL indicate that it produces more self-motivated learners than do traditional learning methods and that students prefer it to traditional methods (Vernon & Blake, 1993; White, Amos, & Kouzekanani, 1999). The evidence regarding its effect on clinical performance suggests that PBL does result in a higher level of clinical functioning, although this is not a consistent finding across all applications of PBL (Doucer, Purdy, Kaufman, & Langille, 1998; Moore, Block, Style, & Mitchell, 1994; Vernon & Blake, 1993).

Like PBL, experiential learning requires students to be active learners, and it is also particularly useful in helping students approach care from an entirely new perspective. In this learning method, assignments require students to try an approach to care or intervention that they have not previously used and then to reflect on whether the approach has advantages over the method they are currently using (Jarvis, 1987). For example, an assignment might require students to conduct several health assessments to try out different interview formats: conversational assessment interviewing, functional health assessment, and a comprehensive health history. The reflection phase of experiential learning is crucial in helping students evaluate whether (and how) they should incorporate the method into their practices.

TABLE 6–5	LEARNING EXPERIENCES TO DEVELOP CLINICAL REASONING

Exposure to substantive clinical content
Practice using concepts and theories as thinking tools
Reflection on personal episodes of clinical practice (Kim, 1999; Rolfe, 1997a)
Tutored bottom-up case analysis
Experiential learning assignments
Self-directed study
Assignments in appraising research evidence and deciding how to use it in practice
Mentored clinical practice

Using Research Evidence

To prepare APNs to become consumers of research, their research course should focus on research-based practice, or the research utilization process, not on the research process. Research-based practice requires the clinician to appraise the scientific credibility, clinical significance, and readiness for practice of the best available research evidence. This threefold interest is broader than the in-depth focus on research methodology that is necessary to become a nurse researcher—although assuredly *basic* knowledge of research methodology is requisite to appraising the scientific credibility of findings.

During their program of study, APNs must be assisted in the activities involved in appraising the clinical significance of findings and their applicability for practice just as much as they are assisted in critiquing the scientific soundness of the study from which the findings came. Reading study reports and appraising findings must begin early in the program and be conveyed as a value throughout the program rather than "taught" within the confines of one or two research courses. From the beginning, the expectation should be that APN students will be discerning regarding the amount of research evidence on which an intervention or approach to care is based. The question "Is there any research to guide practice in this area?" should be asked over and over again throughout the program.

APN students will need help in appraising the research base germane to a clinical question or issue. This will be true particularly when the research base consists of many studies, some with different or even apparently contradictory findings. Also, help will be needed when appraising the summarized forms of research evidence (i.e., meta-analyses, integrative research reviews, and research-based clinical guidelines). If students are to have multiple opportunities to practice these appraisal skills, all faculty members must be committed to incorporating research reports and findings into their courses, and have the skills to assist students as they struggle to make sense of the research evidence.

Students should be required to base the care they are providing to patients on research findings. This requirement should be upheld when dealing with a patient who over time is not achieving desired outcomes, or when strategizing about how best to provide care to a population of patients with common experiences. No clinical course should be taught without reviewing the research that has been conducted on the important and recurring issues in that realm of practice. If students are repeatedly asked about the research base for practicing a certain way, and if faculty frequently refer to research studies, the students will acquire research-based practice as a value and they will become proficient in searching for research reports in the health care literature databases. Acquisition of this value and its associated skills increases the likelihood that graduates of the program have the necessary competencies to continue updating the scientific basis of their practices after graduation.

A more integrated approach to teaching research-based practice is to teach nursing theory and research utilization together in one course. Currently, theory and research are viewed as separate kinds of knowledge rather than as two approaches to nursing knowledge that must influence one another and be used together if meaningful and reliable knowledge for clinical practice is to be produced. With the current emphasis on evidence-based practice, there is a tendency to view empirical findings as the end product of science. This view does not recognize that the ultimate goal of science is to integrate empirical findings in ways that create explanations of how the world works (i.e., create theories). Another form of this integration is to test and/or explore how empirical findings support or refute existing theories. Creative educational strategies will be required to help students see how these various methods of knowledge production work together to provide knowledge that is useful to practitioners.

Diverse Approaches to Direct Care Management and Treatment

Graduate school should be a time when APN students expand their repertoire of therapeutic interventions. They should learn new skills and therapies and refine and expand existing ones. In a course taught by this author, students are required to use several interventions that are not in their current repertoires. They are also required to evaluate the research base regarding these interventions and to report back to the class on their experiences in learning and using the new interventions. One student tried foot reflexology, another used a transcutaneous nerve stimulation unit for a certain kind of pain, and another used guided imagery with adolescents in a psychiatric unit who were experiencing difficulty settling for sleep at bedtime. Students frequently expressed that the assignment forced them to try a new intervention and that the learning experience made them recognize the importance of continuing to expand their repertoire of interventions.

In summary, if graduate APN students are to begin to demonstrate the five process characteristics of direct care described in this chapter, they will require opportunities to think about how to incorporate the characteristics as well as opportunities to practice using them. Then these characteristics should be included as course and program competencies and evaluated either through multiple-station examinations using standardized patients or through video assessment and reflective analysis of actual patient-APN encounters (Kim, 1999; Ram, van der Vleuten, Rethans, Grol, & Aretz, 1999).

Interdisciplinary Education

Interdisciplinary educational experiences would seem to be ways of promoting comprehensive patient care and productive professional relationships in health care workplaces. Educational offerings could bring together students who subsequently will be working together (i.e., APNs, physicians, health care administrators, physical therapists, dietitians, occupational therapists, social workers, health policy specialists, and others) in ways that promote understandings of each other's views and contributions. Three models of interdisciplinary education have been explicated by Lindeke and Block (1998): (1) elective courses for health science students that are co-taught by teachers from several disciplines; (2) interdisciplinary clinical experiences; and (3) interdisciplinary project-based experiences. The authors of the article caution that, to truly succeed, all the involved faculty must be genuinely open to cross-disciplinary teaching and each discipline must deliberatively consider how such offerings fit into its curriculum. Issues such as deciding what discipline-specific learning experiences should precede involvement need to be thoughtfully planned. Thoughtful inclusion of interdisciplinary learning into curriculums should produce practitioners who bring to interdisciplinary teams strong disciplinary values, skills, and identity combined with a deep commitment to achieving high-quality health care through joint planning, cooperation, and coordination.

CONCLUSION

APNs are currently providing direct health care services that are

- Qualitatively different from those provided by other health care professionals
- Positively affecting patients' health care outcomes
- Cost-effective

There is research evidence to support each of these claims and hence to substantiate the nursing profession's and the public's confidence in the care provided by APNs. However, the impact of the full range of APN activities on individual and population outcomes will require ongoing documentation and examination. APN care should continue to incorporate: the holistic perspective, partnerships with patients, expert clinical reasoning and skilled performance, the use of research-based evidence, and the use of diverse management approaches. Together, these qualities form a solid foundation for providing scientifically based, person-centered, and population-validated health care.

R E F E R E N C E S

Adams, L. (1997). Perioperative managed care reimbursements. *Nursing Management, 28,* 32F, 32H.

Aikens, L., Sochalski, J., & Lake, E. (1997). Studying outcomes of organizational change in health services. *Medical Care, 35*(Suppl.), NS6–NS18.

Allan, J. D., & Hall, B. A. (1988). Challenging the focus on technology: A critique of the medical model in a changing health care system. *Advances in Nursing Science, 10*(3), 22–34.

American College of Nurse-Midwives. (1997). The core competencies for basic midwifery practice. *http://www.midwife.org/prof/corecomp.htm.*

American Nurses Association. (1995). *Nursing's social policy statement.* Washington, DC: American Nurses Publishing.

Atkins, S., & Murphy, K. (1993). Reflection: A review of the literature. *Journal of Advanced Nursing, 18,* 1188–1192.

Avorn, J., Everitt, D. E., & Baker, M. W. (1991). The neglected medical history and therapeutic choices for abdominal pain. *Archives of Internal Medicine, 151,* 694–698.

Barrows, H. S., & Pickell, G. C. (1991). *Developing clinical problem-solving skills.* New York: Norton.

Bates, B. (1987). *A guide to physical examination and history taking.* Philadelphia: J. B. Lippincott.

Beal, J. K., Maguire, D., & Carr, R. (1996). Neonatal nurse practitioners: Identity as advanced practice. *Journal of Obstetrical, Gynecological, and Neonatal Nursing, 25,* 401–406.

Benner, P. (1984). *From novice to expert: Excellence and power in clinical practice.* Menlo Park, CA: Addison-Wesley.

Benner, P., Hooper-Kyriakidis, P., & Stannard, D. (1999). *Clinical wisdom and interventions in critical care: A thinking-in-action approach.* Philadelphia: W. B. Saunders.

Benner, P. A., Tanner, C. A., & Chesla, C. A. (1996). *Expertise in nursing practice: Caring, clinical judgment, and ethics.* New York: Springer-Verlag.

Bonamy, C., Schultz, P., Graham, K., & Hampton, M. (1995). The use of theory-based practice in the Department of Veterans' Affairs Medical Centers. *Journal of Nursing Staff Development, 11,* 27–30.

Boyd, C. O., & Munhall, P. L. (1989). A qualitative investigation of reassurance. *Holistic Nursing Practice, 4*(1), 61–69.

Brennan, P. F., & Daly, B. J. (1996). Information requirements of advanced practice nurses. *Advanced Practice Nursing Quarterly, 2,* 54–57.

Brennan, S. J., & Cochran, M. (1998). Home healthcare nursing in the managed care environment. *Home Healthcare Nurse, 16,* 280–287.

Britt, T., Schraeder, C., & Shelton, P. (1998). *Managed care and capitation: Issues in nursing.* Washington, DC: American Nurses Publishing.

Brown, S. A., & Grimes, D. E. (1993). *Nurse practitioners and certified nurse-midwives: A meta-analysis of studies on nurses in primary care roles.* Washington, DC: American Nurses Publishing.

Brown, S. J. (1992). Tailoring nursing care to the individual client: Empirical challenge of a theoretical concept. *Research in Nursing and Health, 15,* 39–46.

Brown, S. J. (1994). Communication strategies used by an expert nurse. *Clinical Nursing Research, 3*(1), 43–56.

Brown, S. J. (1999). *Knowledge for health care practice: A guide to using research evidence.* Philadelphia: W. B. Saunders.

Brykczynski, K. A. (1989). An interpretive study describing the clinical judgment of nurse practitioners. *Scholarly Inquiry for Nursing Practice: An International Journal, 3,* 75–104.

Brykczynski, K. A. (1991). Judgment strategies for coping with ambiguous clinical situations encountered in primary family care. *Journal of the American Academy of Nurse Practitioners, 3*(2), 79–84.

Buerhaus, P. I. (1999). Lucian Leape on the causes and prevention of errors and adverse events in health care. *Image: The Journal of Nursing Scholarship, 31,* 281–286.

Bulechek, G. M., & McCloskey, J. C. (1999a). Nursing diagnoses, interventions, and outcomes in effectiveness research. In G. M. Bulechek & J. C. McCloskey (Eds.), *Nursing interventions classification: Effective nursing treatments* (3rd ed., pp. 1–26). Philadelphia: W. B. Saunders.

Bulechek, G. M., & McCloskey, J. C. (Eds.). (1999b). *Nursing interventions classification: Effective nursing treatments* (3rd ed.). Philadelphia: W. B. Saunders.

Burton, D. (1995). Agency maze. In I. M. Lubkin (Ed.), *Chronic illness: Impact and interventions* (3rd ed., pp. 457–480). Boston: Jones & Bartlett.

Canadian Task Force on the Periodic Health Examination. (1994). *The Canadian Guide to Clinical Preventive Health Care.* Ottawa: Health Canada.

Chervenak, F. A., McCullough, L. B., & Chez, R. A. (1996). Responding to the ethical challenges posed by the business tools of managed care in the practice of obstetrics and gynecology. *American Journal of Obstetrics and Gynecology, 175,* 523–527.

Cooper-Patrick, L., Gallo, J. J., Gonzales, J. J., Vu, H. T., Powe, N. R., & Ford, D. E. (1999). Race, gender, and partnership in the patient-physician relationship. *JAMA, 282,* 583–589.

Corbin, J. M., & Strauss, A. L. (1984). Collaboration: Couples working together to manage chronic illness. *Image: The Journal of Nursing Scholarship, 16,* 109–115.

Corbin, J. M., & Strauss, A. L. (1992). A nursing model for chronic illness management based upon the trajectory framework. In P. Woog (Ed.), *The chronic illness trajectory framework: The Corbin and Strauss nursing model* (pp. 9–28). New York: Springer-Verlag.

Courtney, R., & Rice, C. (1997). Investigation of nurse practitioner-patient interactions: Using the Nurse Practitioner Rating Form. *Nurse Practitioner, 22,* 46–48, 54–57, 60 passim.

Cox, C. L. (1982). An interaction model of client health behavior: Theoretical prescription for nursing. *Advances in Nursing Science, 5,* 41–56.

Daleiden, A. L. (1993). The CNS as trauma manager: A new frontier. *Clinical Nurse Specialist, 7,* 295–298.

Damato, E. G., Dill, P. Z., Gennaro, S., Brown, L. P., York, R., & Brooten, D. (1993). The association between CNS direct care time and total time and very low birth weight infant outcomes. *Clinical Nurse Specialist, 7,* 75–79.

Davis, L. G., Riedmann, G. L., Sapiro, M., Minogue, J. P., & Kazer, R. R. (1994). Cesarean section rates in low-risk private patients managed by certified nurse-midwives and obstetricians. *Journal of Nurse Midwifery, 39,* 91–97.

Degner, L. F., Kristjanson, L. J., Bowman, D., Sloan, J. A., Carriere, K. C., O'Neil, J., Bilodeau, B., Watson, P., & Mueller, B. (1997). Information needs and decisional preferences in women with breast cancer. *JAMA, 277,* 1485–1492.

Dittmar, S. S., & Gresham, G. E. (Eds.). (1997). *Functional assessment and outcome measures for the rehabilitation health professional.* Rockville, MD: Aspen Publishers.

Doucer, M. D., Purdy, R. A., Kaufman, D. M., & Langille, D. B. (1998). Comparison of problem-based learning and lecture format in continuing medical education on headache diagnosis and management. *Medical Education, 32,* 590–596.

Dowdy, M. D., Robertson, C., & Bander, J. A. (1998). A study of proactive ethics consultation for critically and terminally ill patients with extended lengths of stay. *Critical Care Medicine, 26,* 252–259.

Eisen, S. V., Wilcox, M., Leff, H. S., Schaefer, E., & Culhane, M. A. (1999). Assessing behavioral health outcomes in outpatient programs: Reliability and validity of the BASIS-32. *Journal of Behavioral Health Services and Research, 26,* 5–17.

Eller, L. S. (1999). Effects of cognitive-behavioral interventions on quality of life in persons with HIV. *International Journal of Nursing Studies, 36,* 223–233.

Erickson, H. C., Tomlin, E. M., & Swain, M. P. (1983). *Modeling and role-modeling: A theory and paradigm for nursing.* Englewood Cliffs, NJ: Prentice Hall.

Fenton, M. V., & Brykczynski, K. A. (1993). Qualitative distinctions and similarities in the practice of clinical nurse specialists and nurse practitioners. *Journal of Professional Nursing, 9,* 313–326.

Flesner, M., & Clawson, J. (1998). Clinical management by family nurse practitioners and physicians in collaborative practice: A comparative analysis. In T. J. Sullivan (Ed.), *Collaboration: A health care imperative* (pp. 207–224). New York: McGraw-Hill.

Forrow, L., Arnold, R. M., & Parker, L. A. (1993). Preventive ethics: Expanding the horizons of clinical ethics. *The Journal of Clinical Ethics, 4,* 287–294.

Fowler, L. P. (1997). Clinical reasoning strategies used during care planning. *Clinical Nursing Research, 6,* 349–361.

Gaynor, S. E. (1990). The long haul: The effect of home care on the caregiver. *Image: The Journal of Nursing Scholarship, 22,* 208–212.

Gifford, A. L., Laurent, D. D., Gonzales, V. M., Chesney, M. A., & Lorig, K. R. (1998). Pilot randomized trial of education to improve self-management skills of men with symptomatic HIV/AIDS. *Journal of Acquired Immune Deficiency Syndromes and Human Retrovirology, 18*(2), 136–144.

Girouard, S. A. (1996). Evaluating advanced nursing practice. In A. B. Hamric, J. A. Spross, & C. M. Hanson (Eds.), *Advanced nursing practice: An integrative approach* (pp. 569–600). Philadelphia: W. B. Saunders.

Gordon, M. (1994). *Nursing diagnosis: Process and application* (3rd ed.). St. Louis: Mosby.

Gordon, M., Murphy, C. P., Candee, D., & Hiltunen, E. (1994). Clinical judgment: An integrated model. *Advances in Nursing Science, 16,* 55–70.

Grando, V. T. (1998). Articulating nursing for advanced practice nursing. In T. J. Sullivan (Ed.), *Collaboration: A health care imperative* (pp. 499–514). New York: McGraw-Hill.

Green, A. H., & Conway-Welch, C. (1995). Negotiating capitated rates for nurse-managed clinics. *Nursing Economics, 13,* 105–107.

Griffith, H. M., & Robinson, K. R. (1993). Current procedural terminology (CPT) coded services provided by nurse specialists. *Image: The Journal of Nursing Scholarship, 25,* 178–186.

Grimes, D. E., & Garcia, M. K. (1997). Advanced practice nursing and work site primary care: Challenges for outcomes evaluation. *Advanced Practice Nursing Quarterly, 3*(2), 19–28.

Guadagnoli, E., & Ward, P. (1998). Patient participation in decision-making. *Social Science and Medicine, 47,* 329–339.

Hall, B. A., & Allan, J. D. (1994). Self in relation: A prolegomenon for holistic nursing. *Nursing Outlook, 2,* 162–170.

Halliburton, J. R. (1998). Awareness during general anesthesia: New technology for an old problem. *Certified Registered Nurse Anesthetist, 9,* 39–43.

Hamric, A. B. (1996). A definition of advanced nursing practice. In A. B. Hamric, J. A. Spross, & C. M. Hanson (Eds.), *Advanced nursing practice: An integrative approach* (pp. 42–56). Philadelphia: W. B. Saunders.

Hamric, A. B., Worley, D., Lindebak, S., & Jaubert, S. (1998). Outcomes associated with advanced nursing practice prescriptive authority. *Journal of the American Academy of Nurse Practitioners 10,* 113–118.

Hanson, J. L., & Ashley, B. (1994). Advanced practice nurses' application of the Stetler Model for Research Utilization: Improving bereavement care. *Oncology Nursing Forum, 21,* 720–724.

Harris, M. R. (1997). Reduced risk of complex response: An invisible outcome. *Nursing Administration Quarterly, 21*(4), 25–31.

Harvey, R. M., Kazis, L., & Lee, A. F. (1999). Decison-making preference and opportunity in VA ambulatory care patients: Association with patient satisfaction. *Research in Nursing and Health, 22,* 39–48.

Hawkins, J. W., Thibodeau, J. A., Utley-Smith, Q. E., Igou, J. F., & Johnson, E. E. (1993). Using a conceptual model for practice in nursing wellness centre for seniors. *Perspectives, 17,* 11–16.

Henry, S. B., Holzemer, W. L., Randell, C., Hsieh, S. F., & Miller, T. J. (1997). Comparison of nursing interventions classification and current procedural terminology codes for categorizing nursing activities. *Image: The Journal of Nursing Scholarship, 29,* 133–138.

Herth, K. A. (1989). The relationship between level of hope and level of coping response and other variables in patients with cancer. *Oncology Nursing Forum, 16,* 67–72.

Hickey, M. (1990). The role of the clinical nurse specialist in the research utilization process. *Clinical Nurse Specialist, 4,* 93–96.

Hilton, B. A. (1993). Issues, problems, and challenges for families coping with breast cancer. *Seminars in Oncology Nursing, 9,* 88–100.

Hobbs, D. (1998). Collaboration: More than a practice. In T. J. Sullivan (Ed.), *Collaboration: A health care imperative* (pp. 593–609). New York: McGraw-Hill.

Jarvis, P. (1987). Meaningful and meaningless experience: Towards an analysis of learning from life. *Adult Education Quarterly, 37,* 164–172.

Jecker, N. S., Carrese, J. A., & Pearlman, R. A. (1995). Caring for patients in cross-cultural settings. *Hastings Center Report, 25*(1), 6–14.

Johnson, J. D., Roberts, C. S., Cox, C. E., Reintgen, D. S., Levine, J. S., & Parsons, M. (1996). Breast cancer patients' personality style, age, and treatment decision making. *Journal of Surgical Oncology, 63,* 183–186.

Johnson, R. (1993). Nurse practitioner-patient discourse: Uncovering the voice of nursing in primary care practice. *Scholarly Inquiry for Nursing Practice: An International Journal, 7,* 143–163.

Kassirer, J. P., & Kopelman, R. I. (1991). *Learning clinical reasoning*. Baltimore: Williams & Wilkins.

Kibbe, D. C. (1999, March). Best practice interview: David C. Kibbe. *http://ww1.best4health.org/resources/interviews/interview-kibbe.cfm*

Kim, H. S. (1999). Critical reflective inquiry for knowledge development in nursing practice. *Journal of Advanced Nursing, 29,* 1205–1212.

King, I. M. (1981). *A theory for nursing: Systems, concepts, process.* New York: John Wiley & Sons.

King, K. B., Parrinello, K. M., & Baggs, J. G. (1996). Collaboration and advanced practice nursing. In J. V. Hickey, R. M. Ouimette, & S. L. Venegoni (Eds.), *Advanced practice nursing: Changing roles and clinical applications* (pp. 146–192). Philadelphia: J. B. Lippincott.

Kinney, C. K., & Erickson, H. C. (1990). Modeling the client's world: A way to holistic care. *Issues in Mental Health Nursing, 11,* 93–108.

Kirby, D., Short, L., Collins, J., Rugg, D., Kolbe, L., Howard, M., Miller, B., Sonenstein, F., & Zabin, L. S. (1994). School-based programs to reduce sexual risk behaviors: A review of effectiveness. *Public Health Reports, 109,* 339–360.

Kleinpell, R. M. (1997). Acute-care nurse practitioners: Roles and practice profiles. *AACN Clinical Issues, 8,* 156–162.

Kovner, C., & Gergen, P. (1998). The relationship between nurse staffing level and adverse events following surgery in acute care hospitals. *Image: The Journal of Nursing Scholarship, 30,* 315–321.

Labrecque, M., Eason, E., Marcoux, S., Lemieux, F., Pinault, J. J., Feldman, P., & Laperriere, L. (1999). Randomized controlled trial of prevention of perineal trauma by perineal massage during pregnancy. *American Journal of Obstetrics and Gynecology, 180* (3 Pt. 1), 593–600.

Laizner, A. M., Yost, L. M., Barg, F. K., & McCorkle, R. (1993). Needs of family caregivers of persons with cancer: A review. *Seminars in Oncology Nursing, 9,* 114–120.

Larson, E. L. (1995). New rules for the game: Interdisciplinary education for health professionals. *Nursing Outlook, 43,* 180–185.

Laschinger, H. K., & Duff, V. (1991). Attitudes of practicing nurses towards theory-based nursing practice. *Canadian Journal of Nursing Administration, 4,* 6–10.

Lawrence, M. (1995). The unconscious experience. *American Journal of Critical Care, 4,* 227–232.

Liaschenko, J. (1997). Knowing the patient? In S. E. Thorne & V. E. Hayes (Eds.), *Nursing praxis: Knowledge and action* (pp. 23–38). Thousand Oaks, CA: Sage Publications.

Liehr, P., & Smith, M. J. (1999). Middle range theory: Spinning research and practice to create knowledge for the new millennium. *Advances in Nursing Science, 21*(4), 81–91.

Lindeke, L. L., & Block, D. E. (1998). Maintaining professional integrity in the midst of interdisciplinary collaboration. *Nursing Outlook, 46,* 213–218.

Loomis, M. E., & Conco, D. (1991). Patients' perceptions of health, chronic illness, and nursing diagnoses. *Nursing Diagnosis, 2,* 162–170.

Lorig, K. R., Mazonson, P. D., & Holman, H. R. (1993). Evidence suggesting that health education for self-management in patients with chronic arthritis has sustained health benefits while reducing health care costs. *Arthritis and Rheumatism, 36,* 439–446.

Lorig, K., Gonzales, V. M., Laurent, D. D., Morgan, L., & Laris, B. A. (1998). Arthritis self-management program variations: Three studies. *Arthritis Care Research, 11,* 448–454.

Lyndon-Rochelle, M. T., Albers, L., & Teaf, D. (1995). Perineal outcomes and nurse-midwifery management. *Journal of Nurse Midwifery, 40,* 13–18.

Mackay, M. H. (1998). Research utilization and the CNS: Confronting the issues. *Clinical Nurse Specialist, 12,* 232–237.

Manthey, M., & Avery, M. D. (1996). Remembering the nurse in the business of advanced practice. *Advanced Practice Nursing Quarterly, 2,* 49–54.

Mast, M. E. (1995). Adult uncertainty in illness: A critical review of research. *Scholarly Inquiry for Nursing Practice: An International Journal, 9,* 3–24.

McCloskey, J. M., & Maas, M. (1998). Interdisciplinary team: The nursing perspective is essential. *Nursing Outlook, 46,* 57–163.

McMillan, S. C., Heusinkveld, K. B., & Spray, J. (1995). Advanced practice in oncology nursing: A role delineation study. *Oncology Nursing Forum, 22,* 41–50.

Moore, G. T., Block, S. D., Style, C. B., & Mitchell, R. (1994). The influence of the new pathway curriculum on Harvard medical students. *Academic Medicine, 69,* 983–989.

Morten, A., Kohl, D., O'Mahoney, P., & Pelosi, K. (1991). Certified nurse-midwifery care of the postpartum client: A descriptive study. *Journal of Nurse-Midwifery, 36,* 276–288.

Narayan, S. M., & Corcoran-Perry, S. (1997). Line of reasoning as a representation of nurses' clinical decision making. *Research in Nursing and Health, 20,* 353–364.

National Task Force on End-of-Life Care in Managed Care. (1999). *Meeting the challenge: Twelve recommendations for improving end-of-life care in managed care.* Newton, MA: Educational Development Center.

Naylor, M. D., Brooten, D., Campbell, R., Jacobsen, B. S., Mezey, M. D., Pauly, M. V., & Schwartz, J. S. (1999). Comprehensive discharge planning and home follow-up of hospitalized elders: A randomized clinical trial. *JAMA, 281,* 613–620.

Neal, L. J. (1998). Current functional assessment tools. *Home Healthcare Nurse, 16,* 766-772.

Nelson, E. C., Splaine, M. E., Batalden, P. B., & Plume, S. K. (1998). Building measurement and data collection into medical practice. *Annals of Internal Medicine, 128,* 460-466.

Newman, M. A. (1994). *Health as expanding consciousness* (2nd ed., Publication No. 14-2626). New York: National League for Nursing.

Newman, M. A. (1997). Experiencing the whole. *Advances in Nursing Science, 20,* 34-39.

Northouse, L. L., & Peters-Golden, H. (1993). Cancer and the family: Strategies to assist spouses. *Seminars in Oncology Nursing, 9,* 74-82.

Oakley, D., Martland, T., Mayes, F., Hayashi, R., Petersen, B. A., Rorie, C., & Andersen, F. (1995). Process of care. Comparisons of certified nurse-midwives and obstetricians. *Journal of Nurse Midwifery, 40,* 399-409.

O'Donnell, L., Stueve, A., San Doval, A., Duran, R., Haber, D., Atnafou, R., Johnson, N., Grant, U., Murray, H., Juhn, G., Tang, J., & Piessens, P. (1999). The effectiveness of the Reach for Health community youth service learning program in reducing early and unprotected sex among urban middle school students. *American Journal of Public Health, 89,* 176-181.

O'Neill, E. S. (1995). Heuristics reasoning in diagnostic judgment. *Journal of Professional Nursing, 11,* 239-245.

Pearson, A., Borbasi, S., & Walsh, K. (1997). Practicing nursing therapeutically through acting as a skilled companion on the illness journey. *Advanced Practice Nursing Quarterly, 3,* 46-52.

Pesut, D. J., & Herman, J. (1998). OPT: Transformation of nursing process for contemporary practice. *Nursing Outlook, 46,* 29-36.

Petrisek, A. C., Laliberte, L. L., Allen, S. M., & Mor, V. (1997). The treatment decision-making process: Age differences in a sample of women recently diagnosed with nonrecurrent, early-stage breast cancer. *Gerontologist, 37,* 598-608.

Pond, F. (1999). Searching for studies. In S. J. Brown (Ed.), *Knowledge for health care practice: A guide to using research evidence* (pp. 41-58). Philadelphia: W. B. Saunders.

Powell-Cope, G. M. (1994). Family caregivers of people with AIDS: Negotiating partnerships with professional health care providers. *Nursing Research, 43,* 324-330.

Pyke-Grimm, K. A., Degner, L., Small, A., & Mueller, B. (1999). Preferences for participation in treatment decision making and information needs of parents of children with cancer: A pilot study. *Journal of Pediatric Oncology Nursing, 16,* 13-24.

Radwin, L. E. (1996). 'Knowing the patient': A review of research on an emerging concept. *Journal of Advanced Nursing, 23,* 1142-1146.

Ram, P., van der Vleuten, C., Rethans, J. J., Grol, R., & Aretz, K. (1999). Assessment of practicing family physicians: Comparison of observation in a multiple-station examination using standardized patients with observation of consultations in daily practice. *Academic Medicine, 74,* 62-69.

Raudonis, B. M., & Acton, G. J. (1997). Theory-based nursing practice. *Journal of Advanced Nursing, 26,* 138-145.

Richmond, T., McCorkle, R., Tulman, L., & Fawcett, J. (1997). Measuring function. In M. Frank-Stromborg & S. J. Olsen (Eds.), *Instruments for clinical health-care research* (2nd ed., pp. 75-85). Boston: Jones & Bartlett.

Rolfe, G. (1997a). Beyond expertise: Theory, practice, and the reflexive practitioner. *Journal of Clinical Nursing, 6,* 93-97.

Rolfe, G. (1997b). Science, abduction, and the fuzzy nurse: An exploration of expertise. *Journal of Advanced Nursing, 25,* 1070-1075.

Rolfe, G. (1998). The theory-practice gap in nursing: From research-based practice to practitioner-based research. *Journal of Advanced Nursing, 28,* 672-679.

Ruth-Sanchez, V., Bosque, E. M., & Lee, K. A. (1996). Facilitators of and constraints to neonatal nurse practitioner practice: Comparing nursing and medical models. *Journal of the American Academy of Nurse Practitioners, 8,* 175-180.

Sampselle, C. M., & Hines, S. (1999). Spontaneous pushing during birth: Relationship to perineal outcomes. *Journal of Nurse Midwifery, 44,* 36-39.

Sappington, J., & Kelley, J. H. (1996). Modeling and role-modeling theory: A case study of holistic care. *Journal of Holistic Nursing, 14,* 130-141.

Schön, D. A. (1984). *The reflective practitioner: How professionals think in action* (2nd ed.). San Francisco: Jossey-Bass.

Shuler, P. A., & Huebscher, R. (1998). Clarifying nurse practitioners' unique contributions: Application of the Shuler Nurse Practitioner Practice Model. *Journal of the American Academy of Nurse Practitioners, 10,* 491-499.

Smith, S. (1988). An analysis of the phenomenon of deterioration in the critically ill. *Image: The Journal of Nursing Scholarship, 20,* 12-15.

Sobel, D. S. (1995). Rethinking medicine: Improving health outcomes with cost-effective psychosocial interventions. *Psychosomatic Medicine, 57,* 234-244.

Spross, J. A., & Wolff-Burke, M. (1996). Nonpharmacological management of cancer pain. In D. B. McGuire, C. H. Yarbro, & B. R. Ferrell (Eds.), *Cancer pain management* (2nd ed.; pp. 159-205). Boston: Jones & Bartlett.

Stafford, R. S., & Blumenthal, D. (1998). Specialty differences in cardiovascular disease prevention practices. *Journal of the American College of Cardiology, 32,* 1238-1243.

Steele, S., & Fenton, M. V. (1988). Expert practice of clinical nurse specialists. *Clinical Nurse Specialist, 2,* 45-52.

Stetler, C. B., Bautista, C., Vernale-Hannon, C., & Foster, J. (1995). Enhancing research utilization by clinical nurse specialists. *Nursing Clinics of North America, 30,* 457-473.

Stetler, C. B., Brunell, M., Giuliano, K. K., Morsi, D., Prince, L., & Newell-Stokes, V. (1998). Evidence-based practice and the role of nursing leadership. *Journal of Nursing Administration, 28*(7-8), 45-53.

Stetler, C. B., & DeZell, A. (1989). Implementing nursing case management. In M. L. Etheredge (Ed.), Collaborative care: Nursing case management (pp. 67-77). Chicago: American Hospital Publishing.

Stetler, C. B., & DiMaggio, G. (1991). Research utilization among clinical nurse specialists. *Clinical Nurse Specialist, 5,* 151-155.

Sullivan, T. J. (Ed.). (1998). *Collaboration: A health care imperative.* New York: McGraw-Hill.

Swanson, K. M. (1991). Empirical development of a middle range theory of caring. *Nursing Research, 40,* 161-166.

Tanner, C. A., Benner, P., Chesla, C., & Gordon, D. R. (1993). The phenomenology of knowing a patient. *Image: The Journal of Nursing Scholarship, 25,* 273-280.

Thibodeau, J. A., & Hawkins, J. W. (1994). Moving toward a nursing model in advanced practice. *Western Journal of Nursing Research, 16,* 205-218.

Urban, N. (1997). Managed care challenges and opportunities for cardiovascular advanced practice nurses. *AACN Clinical Issues, 8,* 78-89.

U.S. Preventive Services Task Force. (1996). *Guide to clinical preventive services: Report of the U.S. Preventive services Task Force* (2nd ed.). Baltimore: Williams & Wilkins.

Vallerand, A. H. (1998). Development and testing of the inventory of functional status—chronic pain. *Journal of Pain Symptom Management, 15,* 125-133.

Vernon, D. T., & Blake, R. L. (1993). Does problem-based learning work? A meta-analysis of evaluative research. *Academic Medicine, 68,* 550-563.

Volinn, E. (1999). Do workplace interventions prevent low-back disorders? If so why?: A methodological commentary. *Ergonomics, 42,* 258-272.

Von Korff, M., Moore, J. E., Lorig, K., Cherkin, D. C., Saunders, K., Gonzalez, V. M., Laurent, D., Rutter, C., & Comite, F. (1998). A randomized trial of a lay person-led self-management group intervention for back pain patients in primary care. *Spine, 23,* 2608-2615.

Waite, M. S., Harker, J. O., & Messerman, L. I. (1994). Interdisciplinary team training and diversity: Problems, concepts and strategies. In D. Wieland et al. (Eds.), *Cultural diversity and geriatric health care: Challenges to the health care professions* (pp. 65-82). New York: Haworth Press.

Watson, J. (1997). The theory of human caring: Retrospective and prospective. *Nursing Science Quarterly, 10,* 49-52.

Weggel, J. M. (1997). Palliative care: New challenges for advanced practice nursing. *Hospice Journal, 12,* 43-56.

White, M. J., Amos, E., & Kouzekanani, K. (1999). Problem-based learning. *Nurse Educator, 24*(2), 33-36.

Winch, A. E. (1989). Peer support and peer review. In A. B. Hamric & J. A. Spross (Eds.), *The clinical nurse specialist in theory and practice* (2nd ed., pp. 299-321). Philadelphia: W. B. Saunders.

Yancey, R., Given, B. A., White, N. J., DeVoss, D., & Coyle, B. (1998). Computerized documentation for a rural nursing intervention project. *Computers and Nursing, 16,* 275-284.

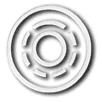

C H A P T E R   7

Expert Coaching and Guidance

• J U D I T H   A.   S P R O S S
• E L L E N   B.   C L A R K E
• J A M E S   B E A U R E G A R D

INTRODUCTION

EXEMPLAR   1

We were first-time parents and had gone through childbirth education. None of our prenatal care prepared us for the hour of intense pain and suffering my wife experienced. The day my daughter was born, my wife and I went to the hospital about 2 A.M. For the first few hours things went very well, but around 6 A.M. my wife began to experience unrelenting pain that she rated as 7/10. Our nurse-midwife had discussed with us the possibility of having epidural analgesia, to be determined during labor. As the pain intensified, my wife asked the staff for epidural analgesia. The midwife had not arrived yet; the nurse on duty said the midwife was on her way and we would have to wait for her arrival before anything could be done. Although the midwife had told the nurse she was on her way, she did not tell the nurse when she would arrive. The nurse may have been new and she may not have known what her alternatives were for contacting an anesthesiologist. The nurse didn't appreciate our distress or the significance of this information for us. In reflecting on the situation later, my wife said it was "not knowing how long she would have to endure the intense pain, waiting without any definite idea of when the pain she was feeling would end or at least diminish—that was the worst aspect of the morning." There was an hour (an eternity to my wife) of intense, untreated pain. When the nurse-midwife arrived some 45 minutes later, she agreed with initiating epidural analgesia and mobilized the resources needed. (JB).

Having worked in clinical settings, it seems to the authors there was a systems problem, a lack of communication between the midwife and the staff nurse, and a lack of empathy on the part of the staff. Where might coaching have made a difference? The nurse-midwife could have told the couple what the procedure was for being evaluated for an epidural if neither she nor the obstetrician was available. Staff could have been "coached" had there been a protocol available to them either for consulting with the obstetrics team caring for the couple or for paging the anesthesiologist. The staff themselves could have offered alternatives to comfort this wife and husband—coaching them through uncertainty, using nondrug methods when the husband's coaching efforts were no longer effective.

Patient education is a central and well-documented function of all nurses. Patient and other types of education provided by advanced practice nurses (APNs) are best conceptualized as interpersonal processes of coaching through transitions such as illness, childbearing, or bereavement. The authors synthesize their own practice and teaching experiences with theoretical, research, and clinical literature to develop a picture of coaching through transitions as the complex, interpersonal process APNs use to enlist clients' active and effective participation in their care. An interdisciplinary perspective informs the discussion of coaching. In this chapter the use of the terms "coach" and "coaching," rather than "education," is deliberate, because these terms imply the existence of a relationship that is fundamental to effective teaching. Coaching people through transitions is a relatively invisible, intangible, but complex process that must be made more explicit if APNs are to be seen by consumers and policy makers as a solution to health policy concerns such as access to and continuity of care, and if they are to secure reimbursement for their care. Because numerous resources exist to help APNs develop and implement educational programs for individuals and groups, this chapter describes the coaching competence of APNs and strategies for acquiring and using the skills needed to coach effectively. Although the focus is on coaching of patients and families, the processes of coaching can also be applied to student and staff education.

PATIENT EDUCATION AND COACHING BY APNs

Many studies document the content and amount of time APNs spend in teaching and counseling as well as the outcomes of these interventions (see Chapter 25 for more detail on outcome studies). Studies of nurse practitioners (NPs) indicate that they spend a significant proportion of their direct care time in teaching and counseling (Brown, 1995; Brown & Waybrant, 1988; Draye & Pesznecker, 1980; Mezey, Dougherty, Wade, & Mersmann, 1994). Health promotion topics covered by NPs include diet, exercise, smoking cessation, family planning, and stress management (Brown & Waybrant, 1988). Teaching and counseling are also significant clinical activities in nurse-midwifery (Scupholme, Paine, Lang, Kumar, & DeJoseph, 1994; Scupholme & Walsh, 1994) and clinical nurse specialist (CNS) (Scott, 1999) practices. In the Quality-Cost Model of Early Discharge and Nurse Specialist Transitional Care, teaching and counseling are provided during face-to-face contacts in the home as well as through regular telephone contact; these services are regarded as critical (Brooten et al., 1986). Analysis of CNSs' interventions revealed that 68% could be categorized as teaching. Other types of interventions were liaison, consultation, and referral; encouragement of self-care and infant care; and reassurance and reinforcement of client actions (Brooten et al., 1988, 1991).

Controlled trials of APN care that involved teaching and coaching activities have demonstrated statistically significant differences in patient outcomes and resource utilization for indigent, inner-city patients with asthma (George et al., 1999), low-birth-weight infants (Brooten et al., 1986), women undergoing unplanned cesarean births (Brooten et al., 1994), and hospitalized elders (Naylor et al., 1999). Interventions in these studies occurred in hospitals and during the postdischarge period. The range of interventions used by APNs in these studies indicate that APNs use a holistic focus that requires technical and interpersonal competence. In addition to these quantitative studies, qualitative studies and anecdotal reports suggest that coaching patients and staff through transitions is embedded in the practices of nurses, including APNs (Barnsteiner, Gillis-Donovan, Knox-Fischer, & McKlindon, 1994; Benner, Hooper-Kyriakidis, & Stannard, 1999).

Numerous factors in contemporary health care have increased the focus on patient education as a means of improving effectiveness and efficiency and achieving cost and quality outcomes. These include managed care and cost containment (Barger, 1997; Bauer, 1994; Cook, 1997; Spross & Heaney, 2000; Taylor, Resick, D'Antonio, & Carroll, 1997; Weiss, 1998); the evidence-based practice movement (Bero et al., 1998; Porter et al., 1997; Spross & Heaney, 2000; University of York NHS Centre for Reviews and Dissemination, 1999); the educational needs of informal caregivers (Kirk & Glendinning, 1998); efforts to develop interdisciplinary models of health care that are patient-centered (Pew-Fetzer Task Force on Advancing Psychosocial Health Education, 1994); and the widespread use of the World Wide Web for teaching and learning.

Given the research-based evidence of the effectiveness of nurses' and APNs' patient education, some investigators have questioned why the nature, process, and characteristics of nurse-client interactions have rarely been the focus of research on patient teaching and patient adherence to therapies (Kasch, 1983; Schwartz-Barcott et al., 1994; Squier, 1990). More needs to be understood about the process of patient teaching used by APNs and how it promotes adherence to therapies and self-care. That patient education generally improves outcomes and that telephone follow-up has been one of the important APN activities in studies of APN care and patient outcomes (George et al., 1999; Naylor et al., 1999) suggest several directions for research. Studies that identify the process and the "dose" of APN-delivered interventions, as well as the differential effects and costs of APN coaching, registered nurse coaching, and the coaching of other clinicians, are needed. The effects of World Wide Web–based information and education and the role of health professionals in helping patients use this information effectively should be studied. Finally, effective strategies for teaching clients who are functionally illiterate need to be identified.

Although more research is needed, the foregoing review supports the authors' premise that expert guidance and coaching are key foci of the APN's direct care role. APNs' coaching of clients, as it is described in this chapter, assumes an understanding of basic principles of education and an awareness of the research on which patient education is based. APNs are responsible for knowing the theoretical and scientific bases for patient teaching in their specialties and practice settings. Examples of the APN's integration of specialty knowledge with principles of patient education to operationalize the coaching competency are incorporated into the chapters on the different APN roles in Part III.

COACHING THROUGH TRANSITIONS: A SYNTHESIS OF THEORETICAL PERSPECTIVES

Coaching: An Interdisciplinary Perspective

The word "coach" is derived from the Middle English word, "coche," meaning "wagon or carriage, a means of conveyance from one destination to another." Modern usage of "coach" to mean a teacher is apt—a coach facilitates the safe passage of a person in transition from one situation to another. Coaching is complex interpersonal work that helps people who are facing equally complex personal transitions or journeys. These meanings of coaching can be applied to nurse-patient, faculty-student, preceptor-student, and mentor-protégé relationships.

Coaching has been used by several disciplines to describe interactions between experts and learners that focus on developing the learner's knowledge and skill in an area that is within the coach's expertise (Spross, 1994). The literature review supports the use of "coach" and "coaching" as terms that describe the teaching functions of APNs. The fact that "coach" and "coaching" are common terms may also make it easier for APNs to communicate with consumers and policy makers about what it is they do.

In cognitive psychology, social skills tutoring (Frisch, Elliott, Atsaides, Salva, & Denney, 1982) and interpersonal cognitive problem solving (Hops, 1983) are coaching techniques that have been used to improve individuals' social skills, language skills, and problem-solving abilities. Both techniques include direct verbal instructions in problem-solving principles. Interpersonal cognitive problem solving also emphasizes thinking processes such as identifying problems, generating alternative solutions, and anticipating the consequences of solutions (Pelligrini & Urbain, 1985).

In sports, coaches create and present complex challenges that develop athletes' physical and psychological capacities while providing support and motivation (Lombardo, 1987; Sullivan & Wilson, 1991). Coaches are expected to have technical competence, interpersonal skills, and leadership skills. Lombardo (1987) described humanistic coaches as those who can focus on strengthening the athlete's performance and self-concept because the coaches themselves are competent, secure in their self-concepts, and self-accepting. Such coaches help athletes believe in themselves; through coaching, athletes learn that they are trustworthy, responsible, capable of self-direction, and able to identify relevant goals.

Heifetz' (1994) work on leadership illuminates Lombardo's (1987) description of humanistic coaching. According to Heifetz, leadership is "mobilizing people to tackle tough problems" (p. 15). Situations that require leadership or expert coaching are those in which the problems are complex—a technical solution is unavailable, and would be inadequate anyway, and the problem demands adaptive work (Heifetz, 1994). Leaders identify the adaptive task. Leadership, as a type of coaching, can be viewed as helping people uncover opportunities for personal growth by helping them clarify their goals, decide what matters most to them, acknowledge trade-offs and losses, and develop coping strategies. Becoming a parent, losing a job, adjusting to and living with a chronic illness, and facing impending death are examples of transitions requiring complex, adaptive work that can be facilitated by APNs.

In a qualitative study of nurses' clinical experiences, Benner (1984) identified the teaching-coaching role as one of seven domains of nursing practice. Subsequent studies, based on Benner's work, have confirmed that APNs demonstrate this role as part of their practice (Benner et al., 1999; Fenton, 1984; Fenton & Brykczynski, 1993; Steele & Fenton, 1988). Benner (1985) elaborated on the teaching-coaching role of APNs who work with patients with chronic illness: "Coaches learn what the illness means to the individual, what the adaptive demands, tasks, and resources are for the patient at different stages in the illness" (p. 43). APNs use their knowledge of a patient as well as knowledge from past experiences with similar patients to craft patient-specific coaching interventions. Other nurses have used the term "coaching" to characterize the nature of nurses' relational, therapeutic interventions with patients.

In describing coaching as the interpersonal process nurses use to help those who suffer, Spross (1996) summarized the elements of the nurse-patient relationship connoted by the term "coaching":

> *Coaching captures the essence of the relationships nurses create with patients on which their effectiveness depends. . . . It is a term that permits the experience of intense emotions on both sides; it captures the temporal nature of the relationship (which may be brief or extended); it suggests both the one-sided aspect (the coach has information and expertise needed by the patient) and the mutuality (opportunities for personal growth) in the relationship; and it conveys the contractual or voluntary nature of the relationship (if the relationship is not working despite the best efforts of both, another coach may need to be found).*

(pp. 197–198)

Table 7–1 summarizes conceptualizations of coaching described by nurse clinicians and investigators. These descriptions of coaching by nurses are consistent with the

TABLE 7-1 NURSING CONCEPTUALIZATIONS OF COACHING

	BENNER (1985)	SPROSS (1994)	WILKIE ET AL. (1995)	CARRIER-KOHLMAN ET AL. (1996)	LEWIS & ZAHLIS (1997)	BENNER ET AL. (1999)
Purpose/focus	To teach and coach patients	To ameliorate suffering	To teach lung cancer patients to report pain perception and changes in pain perceptions to clinicians	To increase patients' self-efficacy in performing exercises and decrease anxiety in order to decrease dyspnea	To help clients (patients and significant others) process thoughts and feelings related to breast cancer experience; to enhance cognitive-behavioral management and self-care skills	An embodied clinical leadership skill in which relational skills are used to help others in their understanding, their judgment, their skilled know-how, and their openness to seeing new possibilities
Characteristics or elements of the coaching interaction or protocol	Capturing readiness to learn Assisting patients to integrate implications of illness and recovery Eliciting patient's understanding of situation Providing interpretation of the patient's condition and giving a rationale for procedures Making culturally avoided aspects of an illness approachable and understandable	Permits the experience of intense emotions on both sides Temporal aspects of the relationship (brief or extended) Relationship is both one sided (nurse has knowledge and skills needed by patient) and mutual (relationship is an opportunity for personal growth for nurse *and* patient) Relationship is, at least theoretically, voluntary and contractual	Encourages patients to mark a self-assessment tool to record pain intensity Encourages patients to report pain characteristics to clinicians Emphasizes and reinforces that pain characteristics reported by patient were important for clinicians' pain treatment decisions	Nurse coach teaches coping skills Nurse coach collaborates with patient to set goals for exercise session based on prior performance and clinical factors Nurse coach teaches relaxation and breathing exercises Nurse coach reinforces information given and encouraged patients	Attending to the story Encircling the experience Inviting the work Exploring solutions Anchoring the skill through feedback, self-monitoring, and homework Setting up success	Envisions realistic possibilities Makes excellent judgment Is able to balance patient's need for safety with team members' need to learn Is able to help others learn to interpret, forecast, and respond to patient transitions
Type of article/book	Qualitative research	Theoretical synthesis	Quantitative research (pilot study)	Quantitative research (experimental design)	Qualitative research	Qualitative research

concepts of coaching from other disciplines discussed previously. Thus coaching can be viewed as a relational, multidimensional process that involves all aspects of being human—cognitive, affective, behavioral, physical, social, and spiritual.

Transitions

The word "transition" comes from the Latin "transitus," meaning "to go across, to pass over or go through." Transitions—physiological, developmental, situational, and organizational—make up the natural course of human lives. Transitions are paradigms for life and living—"dangerous opportunities" in Chinese culture. Like life, they may be predictable or unpredictable, joyous or painful, obvious or barely perceptible, chosen and welcomed or unexpected and feared. Bridges (1980) described three phases of transition: an ending or leaving; a period of chaos, confusion, and distress; and a new beginning. Bridges indicated that, for some people, "transitionality" may be a semipermanent state. Schumacher and Meleis (1994) asserted that transition is a central concept in nursing, and Chick and Meleis (1986) offered a clinically useful definition of it:

> *Transition is a passage from one life phase, condition, or status to another. . . . Transition refers to both the process and outcome of complex person-environment interactions. It may involve more than one person and is embedded in the context and the situation.*

> (pp. 239–240)

Chick and Meleis (1986) also characterized the process of transition as having phases during which individuals experience (1) a disconnectedness from their usual social supports, (2) a loss of familiar reference points, (3) old needs that remain unmet, (4) new needs, and (5) old expectations that are no longer congruent with the changing situation. Becoming a parent, giving up cigarettes, learning how to cope with chronic illness, and dying in comfort and dignity are just a few examples of transitions. Transitions can also be characterized according to type, conditions, and universal properties. Schumacher and Meleis (1994) identified nursing therapeutics that support or facilitate transitions, and education was one of them.

Other models and concepts inform the conceptualization of APN coaching through transition (see Table 7-2). Themes that are common across models and studies of particular concepts include assessment, collaborating with patients, teaching, and mobilizing social support to accomplish health- and illness-related outcomes.

A TYPOLOGY OF TRANSITIONS

Schumacher and Meleis (1994) proposed that there are four categories of transitions in which nurses are involved: developmental, health/illness, situational, and organizational. Developmental transitions are those that reflect life cycle transitions, such as adolescence, parenthood, and aging. For the purposes of discussing APN coaching, the authors consider developmental transitions to include any intrapersonally focused transition, including changes in life cycle, self-perception, motivation, expectations, or meanings. Health/illness transitions were described by Schumacher and Meleis primarily as illness related, ranging from adapting to a chronic illness to being dis-

TABLE 7–2	MODELS AND CONCEPTS THAT INFORMED CONCEPTUALIZATION OF COACHING THROUGH TRANSITION	
MODEL OR CONCEPT	**AUTHOR(S)**	**COMMENTS**
Chronic illness trajectory framework	Corbin & Strauss (1992)	• Describes principles of framework: • Chronic illness has a course that varies over time • Nurses collaborate with patients to shape the trajectory
Self-help model	Braden (1990, 1993)	• Describes 5 stages of response to chronic illness • Notes that nursing interventions can facilitate the acquisition of self-help behaviors
Self-care in Chronic Illness Model	Connelly (1993)	• Is an extension of Health Belief Model
Transitional care	Lamm, Dungan, & Hiromoto (1991), Brooten et al. (1988)	• Describe discharge from hospital to home as a transition that can be shaped by nursing interventions
Self-efficacy	Bandura (1977), Carrieri-Kohlman et al. (1996), Clark & Dodge (1999), Lev (1997), McDougall (1999)	• Address interaction among factors that influence behavior change • Account for changes in motivation, self-confidence, and behavior that result from interventions
Patient-centered communication (PCC)	Squier (1990), Brown (1999)	• Describe empirical support for components of PCC (see Table 7–4)
Comforting-Interaction Relationship Model	Morse, Havens, & Wilson (1997)	• Addresses patient and nurse factors • Notes that comforting relationship is negotiated by means of nurse-patient interactions
Therapeutic relationships	Peplau (1952), Travelbee (1971)	• Address existential and spiritual aspects of relationship
Transition experiences	Schumacher & Meleis (1994), Chick & Meleis (1986), Benner et al. (1999)	• Delineate types and process of transitions

charged from the hospital to home. In this chapter, health/illness transitions are defined as transitions that are driven by an individual's experience of the body in a holistic sense. Such transitions can include modifying risk factors, adapting to a chronic illness, adapting to the physiological and psychological demands of pregnancy, and numerous other clinical phenomena. Some health/illness changes are self-limiting (e.g., the physiological changes of pregnancy), whereas others are long term or chronic, reversible or irreversible. Although Schumacher and Meleis excluded acute self-limiting illnesses (e.g., a cold) from the notion of transition, other variables are likely to influence whether a transition occurs as a result of self-limiting illnesses (e.g., if a cold prevents a person from attending an important event). Changes in educational, professional, or family roles were given as examples of situational transitions by Schumacher and Meleis. The authors also included situational transitions occurring as a result of changes in intangible or tangible structures or resources (e.g., role changes and financial reversals) that are specific to individuals and their relationships. Organizational transitions were defined as those that occur in the environment—within agencies, between agencies, or in society—and reflect changes in structures and resources at a system level.

The first three types of transitions are the ones most likely to lead to clinical encounters between APNs and patients in which expert coaching is required. However, APNs must also be skilled at dealing with organizational transitions, which tend to affect structural and contextual aspects of providing care (see Chapter 10). Barnsteiner and colleagues (1994) described an interesting project in which a standard for establishing therapeutic relationships in a pediatric setting was developed. As described, the process was an organizational transition implemented by staff who were coached by APNs. Wise APNs pay attention to all four types of transitions in their personal and professional lives, because transitions can affect the development and effectiveness of APNs' expert coaching.

In practice, the APN is also aware of the possibility of multiple transitions occurring as a result of one salient transition. While eliciting information on the primary transition that led the client to seek care, the APN is attending to verbal, nonverbal, and intuitive cues to identify other transitions and meanings associated with the primary one. Attending to the possibility of multiple transitions enables the APN to tailor coaching to the individual's particular needs and concerns. Table 7–3 lists some situations, based on this typology, that require APN coaching.

CHARACTERISTICS, CONDITIONS, AND OUTCOMES OF TRANSITIONS

Transitions can be characterized along the dimensions of time, the nature of the process that occurs, and the type of change that occurs (Schumacher & Meleis, 1994). All transitions seem to unfold over time, as opposed to being a one-time event. A single event may precipitate the transition, but the transition is experienced over some period of time. The process that occurs is directional, entailing movement from one state to another, and is often described as occurring in stages. The type of change tends to be substantive and internal, rather than incidental or superficial; transitions affect personal identities, roles, relationships, functional status, and behaviors (Schumacher & Meleis, 1994). The experience of transition can vary considerably from one individual, group, or organization to the next as a result of conditions affecting the transition (Corbin & Strauss, 1992; Schumacher & Meleis, 1994). Regardless of

TABLE 7–3 TRANSITION SITUATIONS THAT REQUIRE COACHING

HEALTH/ILLNESS	DEVELOPMENTAL	SITUATIONAL	ORGANIZATIONAL
Pregnancy/labor	Parenting	Job loss or change	Mergers
Hospitalization	Puberty	Divorce	Policy changes
Risk reduction	Suffering	Natural disasters	Change in leadership
Lifestyle changes	Loss of significant others	Quality of life	Change in organizational
Chronic illness	Caregiving for elderly	Change in social supports	structure
Disability	relatives	Social isolation	
Weight loss or gain	Changes in sexual function	Financial reversals or	
Symptoms	or activity	windfalls	
Violence		Change in living situations	

Note: The situations are categorized according, to the initiating change. Many of these transitions have reciprocal impacts across categories.

the type of change that occurs, similar conditions seem to influence transitions. These conditions include meanings, expectations, motivation, level of knowledge and skill, the environment, level of planning, and well-being.

Outcomes of transitions proposed by Schumacher and Meleis (1994) included subjective well-being, role mastery, and well-being of relationships. Quality-of-care outcomes could also be used as indicators of successful transitions. When one considers the direct, individual effects of APN coaching, the most relevant outcomes are those that are patient related. These could be traditional or emerging clinical outcomes, such as morbidity; mortality; medical complications; comfort; functional, physiological, or mental status; stress level; coping strategies; quality of life; patient satisfaction; and caregiver burden (Kolcaba, 1992; Lang & Marek, 1992; Naylor, Munro, & Brooten, 1991; Peplau, 1994). Although some researchers are beginning to study intrapersonal phenomena that might be considered outcomes of coaching, such as finding meaning and self-transcendence, more work is needed on how to assess such outcomes. Organizational or cost outcomes that might be affected by coaching processes include lengths of stay, costs of care, proportion of services that receive reimbursement, and use of health care services (Lang & Marek, 1992; Naylor et al., 1991). This description of transitions as a focus for APN coaching underscores the need for, and the importance of, a holistic orientation when helping individuals address their health and illness concerns.

THE FOUNDATIONS OF COACHING THROUGH TRANSITIONS

A Model of APNs' Expert Coaching and Guidance

APN coaching may be defined as a complex, dynamic, collaborative, and holistic interpersonal process that is mediated by the APN-patient relationship and the APN's self-reflective skills. APNs integrate self-reflection and the technical, clinical, and interpersonal competencies they have acquired through graduate education and experience with patients' understandings, experiences, and goals in order to shape transitional experiences and accomplish therapeutic and educational goals. Expert coaching by APNs depends on the interaction of four factors: clinical competence, technical competence, interpersonal competence, and self-reflection (Fig. 7–1). Graduate education is assumed. It is the interaction of self-reflection with these three areas of competence that drives the ongoing expansion and refinement of expertise in advanced nursing practice.

Several assumptions that underlie this model of APNs' coaching and guiding must be made explicit. First, the entire discussion of coaching assumes the integration of the client's significant other or the client's proxy as appropriate. Second, although technical competence and clinical competence may be sufficient to teach a task, they are insufficient to coach patients through transitions. For example, diabetic people may be taught how to monitor their blood sugar and administer insulin with technical accuracy, but, if the impact of the transition from health to chronic illness that requires major lifestyle changes is not evaluated, then coaching and guidance cannot occur. Failure to assess the need for coaching when teaching patients about health and illness may influence the outcomes of individual and group teaching approaches. Third, the APN's skill as an expert coach and guide depends on a combination of clinical experience with a particular population and graduate educa-

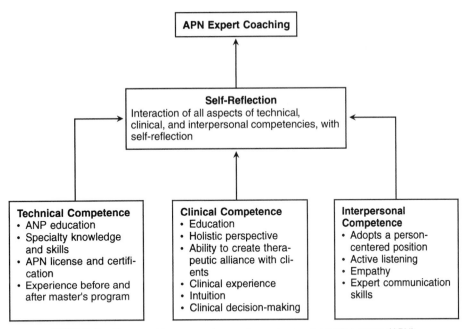

FIGURE 7–1 • The coaching competency of an advanced practice nurse (APN).

tion (see Chapter 3). The clinical and didactic content of graduate education extends the APN's repertoire of assessment skills, technical skills, interpersonal behaviors, and self-reflection abilities, enabling the APN to coach in situations that are broader in scope or more complex in nature. APNs are also able to be more explicit about the processes and outcomes of coaching.

Finally, the basis for expert APN coaching is the interaction of interpersonal, technical, and clinical competence with self-reflection. Expert coaching requires that APNs be self-aware and self-reflective as an interpersonal transaction is unfolding, so that they can shape communications and behaviors to maximize the therapeutic and educational goals of the clinical encounter. The ability to self-reflect and focus on the process of coaching as it is occurring implies that APNs are capable of the simultaneous execution of other skills. While interacting with a client, APNs integrate physical, cognitive, and intuitive skills such as physical examination, interviewing, attending to their own noncognitive reactions and those of the client, and interpreting these multiple sources of information. One might compare the process to simultaneous translation of a speech into several languages as it is being given. The difference is that the simultaneous translations are being carried out by one APN, not several translators. De la Cuesta (1994) characterized this as the "'product' [or outcome] taking shape or being 'manufactured' in the very process of the interaction" (p. 457).

Readers might be interested in comparing the model of APN expert coaching proposed here with two other models (Morse et al., 1997; Squier, 1990). Squier (1990) wondered why–if the goals of health care are preventing future illness, decreasing chronicity, limiting relapses or exacerbations of illnesses, alleviating suffering, and responding to crises–is the quality of provider-patient relationships not given more priority, at least as much as is given to technological treatments? To address his question, Squier analyzed existing literature including studies of physicians and APNs, and proposed a model linking a clinician's empathic understanding with a patient's adherence to therapeutic regimens. He hypothesized that empathic understanding has two components: cognitive and affective. Clinicians' cognitive ability to take accurately the perspective of the patient enables them to communicate effectively and reflect this understanding back to the patient. Patients are then more likely to elaborate their experiences of the concern that brought them to the clinician. Clinicians' emotional sensitivity to the patient's emotions and underlying concerns helps reduce the anxiety and stress that often affect the presenting health problem. Squier further described phases of the clinician-patient consultation and the client outcomes associated with each phase, the ultimate outcome being improved adherence to preventive and therapeutic strategies (self-care) and beneficial health outcomes.

Morse and colleagues (1997) synthesized research on patient interactions and nurse-patient relationships and proposed a model integrating these findings—the Comforting Interaction-Relationship Model. The components of the model include nursing actions that represent three interrelated levels—comforting strategies, styles of care, and patterns of relating. Nurses initiate these actions in response to patient actions—signals of distress, indices of discomfort, and patterns of relating. Nurse-patient interactions are the means by which the therapeutic relationship is negotiated and evolves.

Technical Competence and Clinical Competence

Technical and clinical competence are well-defined aspects of established APN roles, and their importance to coaching cannot be overestimated. However, these two factors are not addressed in detail in this chapter. The evolution of specialties in advanced nursing practice has focused on defining and describing the technical and clinical skills required for advanced practice with particular populations. Chapter 1 documents the evolution of these aspects of various APN roles. In addition, chapters on specific APN roles (e.g., Part III) illustrate the specific technical and clinical skills needed for a particular APN role.

An important part of clinical competence is clinical experience with the populations that are the APN's focus. Pregraduate school experiences, experiences within the clinical practica of graduate programs, and post-master's clinical experiences provide the grist for analyzing, developing, and making visible the coaching competency of APNs. Ongoing development of the APN's coaching competency depends on applying self-reflection to clinical experiences in order to acquire new coaching knowledge and skills that cannot be found in any textbook. Over the course of caring for patients, nurses learn the many ways people experience and manage health, birth, illness, pain, suffering, and death (Benner, 1985, 1991; Benner et al., 1999). These clinical experiences enable APNs to identify coaching alternatives that help other patients understand, learn, change, modulate, and control experiences of transitions.

Interpersonal Competence

Interpersonal competence encompasses the ability to communicate effectively and to establish therapeutic, caring relationships. These two components are briefly described and theoretical and research support for interpersonal competence as an integral part of coaching are provided. Interpersonal interactions can be characterized as position centered or person centered (Bernstein, 1974; Brown, 1999; Kasch & Dine, 1988; Kasch & Knutson, 1985). Position-centered interpersonal interactions are characterized by dependence on roles and rules and the use of power and authority. A person-centered encounter is characterized by an appreciation for the uniqueness of the individuals involved (the nurse and the patient) and attention to the patient's concerns. APNs do not assume they understand the patient's perspective (Kasch, 1983; Kasch & Dine, 1988; Squier, 1990); person-centered communication enables APNs to take accurately the patient's perspective and respond empathically (Squier, 1990). During patient encounters, APNs adopt an open, flexible, nonhierarchical stance with clients and communicate this verbally and behaviorally (Brown, 1995); they convey an attitude of openness, elicit and respond to feelings, express concern, confirm the patient's experience, and provide positive reinforcement (Quirk & Casey, 1995). APNs summarize, recap, and interpret as they coach. Verbal and nonverbal skills that characterize a person-centered approach to interviewing are listed in Table 7–4.

Establishing a caring, therapeutic relationship with a client demands that the APN be emotionally responsive, not distant. The nurse and patient enter the relationship as whole persons, complete with talents, goals, needs, and wishes, but the focus of the interpersonal process is on addressing the patient's potentials and goals (Martocchio, 1987; Montgomery, 1993). Nurses reveal themselves through their eyes, tone of voice, affect, body language, and silences. The APN "who withholds parts of herself [or himself] is unlikely to allow the patient to emerge as a whole, or to comprehend that wholeness if it does emerge" (Gadow, 1980, p. 87). Montgomery (1993) found that clinicians had predispositional qualities consistent with caring: a person orientation rather than role orientation, concern for the human element in care, person-centered intention, transcendence of judgment, hopeful orientation, lack of ego involvement, and expanded personal boundaries. She also described the properties of caring behaviors (Table 7–5). These properties are consistent with a person-centered style of communication. APNs who rely only on scientific and technical competencies in

TABLE 7–4	SKILLS ASSOCIATED WITH A PERSON-CENTERED STYLE OF COMMUNICATION

- Allowing patients to tell their stories using their own language and chronology
- Using a conversational style of interviewing
- Eliciting patients' thoughts, perspectives, expectations, values, and goals
- Asking about the contexts of patients' lives
- Encouraging self-disclosure
- Responding to patients' indirect and nonverbal clues regarding emotions and problems
- Providing patients with self-care information and enabling patients' participation in health care decision making
- Creating shared understandings with patients
- Developing health care plans collaboratively with patients
- Expressing concern for the patient's well-being
- Responding empathically
- Creating social connectedness with patients by humor, touch, and modest personal sharing
- Using open-ended questions and paraphrasing to elicit information and validate patients' communications
- Using a tone of voice and pace of speech appropriate to the topic being discussed
- Making eye contact and using a forward-leaning posture

Data from Brown (1999), Quirk and Casey (1995), and Montgomery (1993).

TABLE 7-5 PROPERTIES OF CARING EXPRESSED AS BEHAVIORS
• Empowerment through mobilization of resources
• Advocacy
• Authenticity
• Responsiveness
• Commitment
• Being present with
• Creating positive meaning and hope
• Competence

Data from Montgomery (1993).

their relationships with patients are unlikely to appreciate patients' holistic responses or enable patients to express themselves holistically (Gadow, 1980).

Studies of education done by nurses in basic and advanced practice suggest that a caring, person-centered relationship underlies successful educational interventions (Benner, 1984; Brown, 1999; Fenton, 1984; Lamb & Stempel, 1994; Morgan, 1994; Steele & Fenton, 1988). Selected findings to support the importance of interpersonal competence to APN coaching are summarized here.

In one study of nurses, nurse-patient interaction and the development of rapport were foundational in accomplishing patient education (Morgan, 1994). De la Cuesta (1994) affirmed that therapeutic alliances established by public health nurses with patients had an important enabling function—the relationship was seen as "a medium or vehicle for achieving goals" (p. 452) and as having a mediating function that allowed the nurse to adopt conflicting roles (e.g., being able to point out the patient's self-neglect behaviors while supporting the patient as a person or intervening to help the patient accomplish self-care goals).

Patients' experiences with nurse case management offer additional insight. Nurse case management seemed to help patients become "their own insider-experts" (Lamb & Stempel, 1994, p. 9). This process consisted of three phases: bonding, working, and changing. Lamb and Stempel noted that bonding or "the demonstration of concern [by nurses] appears to be a key factor in triggering cognitive change" (p. 10). Once the nurse was seen as both expert and insider, the working phase could begin. Patients were willing to examine relationships among their attitudes, behaviors, illness exacerbations, and use of health care resources. Patients began to see themselves differently and reported changes in self-image, changes in meaning, and mastery. Many patients became their own insider-experts, skilled at identifying changes in illness patterns, selecting effective self-care interventions, and using the health care system in a timely and appropriate way.

A caring, person-centered approach demands an involved, current, individualized, contextual understanding of the patient (Tanner, Benner, Chesla, & Gordon, 1993). This understanding serves to bridge the differences between APNs and their clients and enables clients to share power and collaborate with APNs to develop a realistic plan of care. If patients are to be coached effectively in making transitions that are genuinely their own, both the nurse and the patient must enter the relationship as whole persons.

Self-Reflection

The fourth component of the APN expert coaching model is self-reflection—the deliberate, internal examination of experience in order to learn from it. The

APN uses self-reflection during interactions with patients as well as retrospectively. Schön (1983) described these as "reflection-in-action" and "reflection-on-action." Reflection-in-action is the ability to pay attention to phenomena as they are occurring, giving free rein to one's intuitive understanding of the situation as it is unfolding. The APN is not restricted to using only familiar patterns of thought. APN coaching is analogous to the flexible and inventive playing of a jazz musician; APNs can attend to what is happening in the moment and respond with a varied repertoire of exploratory and transforming actions. The heart of reflective practice is action and paradox, not generalized scripts and certainty (Grimmett, 1988). In the APN-client relationship, it is simultaneously doing and learning and coming to know. Reflection-in-action can be compared to the Zen concept of mindfulness (Tremmel, 1993). Mindfulness means paying attention to "right here, right now" and investing the present moment with full concentration. Reflection-in-action, or mindfulness, involves awareness of the world and awareness of multiple aspects of consciousness—thoughts, feelings, behaviors.

Looking within involves listening to one's own thinking processes; it is part of preparing for and enacting reflective practice (Bartels, 1998; Pugach & Johnson, 1990). Extending the work done by Jackson (1986) on expert teaching, APN coaches might be characterized as those who "see more" than nonexperts do. "Seeing more" refers to the practice of "paying attention" (Jackson, 1986). APNs are sensitive to possibilities—within patients, within the processes of the clinical encounter, and within themselves. They anticipate what might happen during the encounter or after the patient leaves. They are sensitive to incipient difficulty: APNs' sensibilities, processes (including reflection), and skills interact to shape their encounters with patients, to support patients, and to enable patients to navigate transitions to achieve mutually determined goals. Action without reflection becomes automatic; there can be no transformation in the absence of action with reflection (Freire, 1970).

The capacity to reflect mindfully in action and on action is not readily mastered and requires continuous practice (Tremmel, 1993). However, certain qualities and characteristics can be developed to facilitate self-reflection. These include motivation, commitment, open-mindedness, self-awareness, the ability to describe phenomena or situations, critical analysis, and the ability to synthesize and evaluate (Atkins & Murphy, 1994). It is important to pay attention to both positive and negative experiences. What made this effective? Why didn't this work? APNs may be more likely to reflect on negative experiences than to reflect on positive experiences, because the feeling of failure is more uncomfortable than the feeling of satisfaction or success. However, reflecting on satisfying, successful experiences can provide clues to interventions that will be effective in future interactions. One of the key aspects of self-reflection is paying attention to feelings. Experienced nurses and APNs are more likely than inexperienced ones to pay attention to feelings or intuitions. However, novice APNs need to be taught to recognize that their affective responses to situations are clues to developing their expertise as clinicians and coaches.

COACHING ASSESSMENT, PROCESSES, AND OUTCOMES

Assessment

Patient assessment is the basis for determining which coaching interventions will be used. APNs use whatever physical and psychological assessment procedures, skills, or tools they need to evaluate the patient's presenting concerns. They understand that assessments have two purposes: (1) establishing and building a relationship and (2) collecting data. They make conscious efforts to build a relationship that will work by conveying caring and concern, being honest and dependable, and displaying professional knowledge and self-confidence. The person-centered approach adopted by nurses has been described by several researchers as "knowing the patient" (Jenny & Logan, 1992; Tanner et al., 1993). This entails getting to know the patient as a person and learning the patient's pattern of responses, including habits, practices, preferences, usual demeanor, and self-presentation (Jenny & Logan, 1992).

Assessment must extend beyond the individuals to consider the clients' communities and social milieu because social and contextual variables often influence the APN's ability to provide effective care. Thus a vital aspect of knowing the patient is what White (1995) calls "sociopolitical knowing." Sociopolitical knowing includes an understanding of the social and political context of the patient as well as the broader context in which nursing and health care take place. Both the APN's and the patient's cultural and political location powerfully influence their understandings of health, illness, language, identity, social roles, and historical issues. For example, domestic violence, child abuse, malnutrition, substance abuse, and stress-induced illnesses are responses to political, social, and personal problems. Both Steven (1989) and Chopoorian (1986) emphasized the need for nurses to provide a vocal critique of how domination, alienation, poverty, homelessness, and unemployment affect the health of persons and communities. APNs may find that coaching their clients requires that they expose, provoke, and problematize social and political inequities that affect people's health (Hagedorn, 1995; Kendall, 1992). Otherwise the core issues in many patients' transitions will be invisible and unidentified and the coaching strategies employed will be superficial, unfocused, and ineffective.

In addition to getting to know the patient and using strategic communication, APNs use their observations of themselves, the patients, and the interactive process to decode patients' behaviors and the content of their communications for significance (Kasch & Dine, 1988). They need to grasp the patient's perspective, including salient aspects of the patient's self-definition (Olesen, Schatzman, Droes, Hatton, & Chico, 1990). This understanding is critical for selecting coaching behaviors to help people who need to make lifestyle changes, reduce risk, or manage chronic illness.

Several conditions influence the experience of transition and its unfolding (Corbin & Strauss, 1992; Schumacher & Meleis, 1994) and should be assessed. Meaning and expectations are subjective phenomena that affect the anticipation and experience of transition (Schumacher & Meleis, 1994). Although many transition conditions can be affected by prior experience, meanings and expectations may be the ones most colored by memories and past experiences. Meanings may be positive, negative, or neutral. Regardless of whether the meaning is positive or negative, patients may experience uncertainty, grief, guilt, stress, or other emotional responses. Expectations may be accurate and realistic, or they may be unrealistic, even fantastic. Cognitive variables such as knowledge, self-care skills, motivation, coping style, habitual stressors, and personal preferences for control affect people's experience of and ability to accept, adjust to, or adapt to transitional experiences (Brooten et al., 1991; Corbin & Strauss, 1992; Jenny & Logan, 1992; Kasch & Dine, 1988; Schumacher & Meleis, 1994). The environment, including resources, relationships, social support, setting of care, and contextual variables, can mediate transitions (Brooten et al., 1991; Corbin & Strauss, 1992; Schumacher & Meleis, 1994). Role demands and responsibilities that may interfere with therapeutic self-care need to be identified (Connelly,

1993). Level of planning, including problem and need identification, organization of phase-related interventions, and communication, influences the success of the transition. Physical and emotional well-being also determine how the transition process is experienced (Schumacher & Meleis, 1994). The nature of the health concern; the degree of symptomatology, perceived vulnerability, and seriousness; and the degree of predictability or certainty about one's experience of the body can make for smooth or chaotic transitions.

APNs identify missing information that they might need for coaching and variables that might enhance or hinder coaching. Throughout the interaction, they try to regulate distress (Heifetz, 1994), respond to patients' needs for information, and create a physically and interpersonally comforting environment (Kasch & Lisnek, 1984). For example, the APN might observe that a patient is becoming fatigued during an examination. In addition to providing for rest and changing the pace of the examination, the causes, duration, and significance of the fatigue will be explored.

Several points can be made about the assessment aspects of coaching through transitions. First, not every encounter will involve a transition; many encounters will be self-limiting. Even in these more routine situations, the APN's coaching competence can result in efficient care delivery, improved patient satisfaction, and return business, all valued outcomes in managed care environments. Second, not every individual immersed in a transitional situation is interested in moving or adjusting; a person can become stuck or immobilized by the demands of the transition. APNs can often help patients who are immobilized. Indeed, these are often the patients for whom the help of an experienced APN is sought by physicians, staff nurses, or novice APNs. By working effectively with difficult cases, APNs expand their repertoire of coaching interventions. Some patients who are stuck simply need a new coach—someone with a different approach or personality. A smaller population may be help rejecters; in this case, coaching is unlikely to be effective and patients can only be "maintained." Third, whereas some conscious patients may reject help, noncommunicative patients can often be coached effectively. For example, the APN who is providing palliative care may talk to the dying person about letting go, review aspects of the patient's life, and provide comforting touch interventions. The APN observes responses that indicate relaxation and peace (e.g., less restlessness and moaning).

Processes and Outcomes

Coaching processes used by APNs focus on fostering involvement, choice, and independence. One study of patient education suggested that a continuum of nurse-patient interactions exists, from simple interactions to decrease anxiety to complex ones such as counseling to enhance problem-solving skills (Morgan, 1994). Intervention mapping, a strategy for tailoring educational interventions to the needs of the population, has been proposed as a strategy for planning health education initiatives (Bartholomew, Parcel, & Kok, 1998). The concept of intervention mapping may also be used to plan care for individuals; an individualized assessment often leads APNs to tailor the usual treatment to improve adherence and the likelihood of reaching a desired outcome.

Benner (1985) elaborated on APNs' coaching behaviors. In coaching a patient, APNs have four main tasks: interpreting unfamiliar diagnostic and treatment demands, coaching the patient through alienated stances (e.g., anger and hopelessness), identifying changing relevance as demands or symptoms of the illness change, and ensuring that cure is enhanced by care. These tasks can be accomplished through coaching processes. Both processes and outcomes can be categorized by focus: bodily or physical, affective/interpersonal/spiritual, cognitive/behavioral, and social. Processes and outcomes derived from the literature review presented earlier and references found in Spross (1996) are listed in Table 7-6.

APNs attend to issues of timing and sequencing in teaching and counseling patients. Thus they may need to coach the patient to become motivated before beginning to teach the patient a particular task. APNs integrate coaching into processes of consultation, collaboration, and referral. They use their knowledge of the patient to mobilize resources and interpret the patient's needs to team members, consultants, and family caregivers. Knowing the patient enables APNs to take risks, adopt stances that are unusual or unpopular, and make the system work in order to shape patients' transitional experiences, a quality of APN direct care that has been described as "fearlessness" (Koetters, 1989). Therefore, coaching is a holistic process, and, although there is a primary focus or target, coaching behaviors often have effects across all dimensions of the patient's experience.

EXEMPLAR 2

Drs. Spross and Beauregard collaborated on the care of a complex patient named Jack, who had been admitted to a rehabilitation hospital following a left hip arthroplasty and left tibial traction pin. His immediate postoperative course had been complicated by a staphylococcal infection at the surgical site, for which he was still receiving intravenous antibiotics. Jack had a history of substance abuse and has been on a methadone maintenance program. Jack was well known to the staff because he had been in the rehabilitation hospital 1 year earlier following a girdlestone surgical procedure on his right hip. During both admissions, pain management was a significant problem. He became easily frustrated and impatient, and expressed his anger verbally. These characteristics were heightened when he was in moderate to severe pain. For example, requests for pain medications were made in demanding and insistent tones. Jack currently reports pain in his left hip and left lower leg as well as some right shoulder and paralumbar pain. From the nursing assessment, his pain intensity data are as follows: worst pain is 10/10, least is 9/10, average is 9/10. Despite being on Percocet, 2 tabs every 6 hours, his pain is never below 9/10. He had not completed high school and was disabled. His parents were divorced. He has nieces and nephews he adored and was motivated to stay clean because he was not permitted to see them if he was abusing drugs.

The CNS (JAS) performed an initial, thorough assessment of Jack's pain. During this assessment, she initiated coaching by reviewing with him what they had learned during the prior admission about how to manage his pain using a combination of scheduled opioids and nondrug interventions. Jack expressed frustration that he wasn't as independent as he had been on the prior admission. JAS explained that, during the prior admission, he had had the use of his "good" leg to compensate for what the treated leg could not do. Although he had made a good recovery, the leg treated last year was not functional enough to support his weight and compensate for the temporary loss of function in the leg being treated during this admission. He acknowledged that this made sense. JAS knew from having reviewed the admission orders that she would need to talk to the physicians to get the analgesics changed to an around-the-clock schedule so Jack could participate effectively in therapies.

JAS and the psychologist (JB) conferred and agreed to share responsibility for coaching, with the CNS having a primary focus on the patient and the psychologist having a primary focus on the staff. JAS had been working with the staff for over a year to improve pain management practices on the unit. However, the staff would need coaching because they were being challenged to apply what they learned about pain management to a patient whose history they believed made use of opioids for pain risky. The psychologist would help the staff understand this patient and the reasons for treating pain with opioids in an addict who had had surgery, and, if needed, help staff see when attitudes and misbeliefs might be interfering with Jack's care. Jack needed coaching in communicating his pain and response to pain management interventions in order to avoid alienating staff and to maximize participation in therapy. In addition, the CNS would work with the nurses and physicians on titrating analgesia to effect. Given Jack's history, he was likely to need more analgesics, not less.

JB noticed during the course of working with Jack that staff often assumed that Jack was "drug seeking" if he requested medications for pain. Staff had other concerns that needed attention: fear of giving too much pain medication, getting Jack off analgesics as soon as possible (regardless of pain intensity level or impact of unrelieved pain on progress in rehabilitation), and concern that Jack would relapse with regard to substance abuse. JB listened to and acknowledged the staff's issues. He offered them new information to encourage them to modify their thinking about how pain in addicts should be managed. Both JB and JAS were able to show staff the effectiveness of their interventions—when Jack's pain was well managed, his participation in therapy was better. If someone had withheld or forgotten Jack's medication, it showed in a decreased level of activity during physical and occupational therapies.

JAS coached Jack in effective ways to communicate his frustration and explained why angry and blaming communications might make it harder for some staff to help him. Both JB and JAS used cognitive restructuring strategies to help Jack think differently about his problems and learn strategies to raise his threshold for frustration. For example, when Jack reported that nothing was going right or that he couldn't do anything, events of the day were reviewed for some evidence of some progress. The links between his thinking and behavior were identified. When Jack became an outpatient, JB and JAS praised his self-care and adherence to treatment plans. Jack was discharged 4 weeks after admission on an effective analgesic regimen so he could continue to make progress at home. Prior to his discharge JB and JAS collaborated with the social worker to find, and then coach, a primary care physician in the most effective strategies to help Jack because Jack was at high risk of being lost to follow-up. The staff also gained a better understanding of how to manage pain in a patient with a history of substance abuse.

This case illustrates the following aspects of coaching: recognizing the need for coaching early in a patient encounter and the risks of not coaching (poor pain management, poor rehabilitation outcome, alienation between staff and patient), identifying the multiple levels of coaching that were needed (patient, staff, postdischarge caregivers), and the use of relationships with patients and colleagues to shape a positive outcome in a complex situation.

DEVELOPMENT OF APNs' COACHING COMPETENCE

Becoming an expert coach requires a combination of education, experience, interpersonal competence, and self-reflection on one's practice. It is not a technical skill; technical skill is insufficient "in the swampy lowland [of clinical practice] where situations are confusing 'messes'" (Schön, 1983, p. 42). Although scientific and technical knowledge are essential for effective coaching, it is in the coaching of clients that the art of advanced nursing practice is fully expressed. APNs need a

TABLE 7-6 ADVANCED PRACTICE NURSES' COACHING PROCESSES AND POSSIBLE OUTCOMES

DOMINANT FOCUS	COACHING PROCESSES	POSSIBLE OUTCOMES*
Physical	Demonstrating self-care or self-monitoring skills	Effective self-care (e.g., fewer symptoms)
	Describing the likely physical trajectory of the health or illness concern, including physical and psychological demands, tasks, and resources	Improved functional status
		Improved mental status (e.g., as a result of decreased pain or normalized blood sugars)
	Describing the possibilities inherent in the physical transitions experienced	Increased physical comfort
	Identifying risk factors	
	Implementing pain and symptom management	
	Interpreting the person's experiences of the body	
	Offering alternative (e.g., more hopeful) interpretations of bodily sensations/functions	
	Offering strategies to modify risk factors	
	Providing hygiene and toileting and conducting invasive procedures and other physical interventions while preserving dignity	
	Using comforting touch	
Affective, interpersonal, spiritual	Accepting the person as he or she is	Acceptance of help from others
	Acknowledging the person's courage, strength, or other personal qualities	Decreased anxiety, stress, or uncertainty
		Decreased spiritual distress
	Acknowledging both expressed and possible fears and concerns	Finding meaning
		Hope
	Attuning oneself to client's needs and goals	Improved quality of life
	Being available/presencing	Increased ability to initiate self-care
	Being honest	Increased comfort, decreased suffering
	Bonding, establishing a therapeutic alliance	Revised future agendas
	Comforting through touch, behavior, and interactions	Self-acceptance
	Counseling	Self-report of satisfaction with decision making
	Eliciting expectations, fears, meanings, and values	Self-transcendence
	Enabling	
	Encouraging, praising	
	Ensuring safe passage	
	Expressing confidence in clients and their abilities	
	Inspiring/inspiriting	
	Listening	
	Keeping a vigil	
	Making a commitment to help	
	Offering hope	
	Reassuring	
	Supporting	
	Validating	

Category	Activities/Interventions	Outcomes
Cognitive, behavioral	Challenging Coaching in communication and technical skills Communicating strategically Confronting and identifying contradictions Dealing with conflict Demonstrating and role-modeling Explaining Guiding, offering a map Identifying adaptive tasks Identifying the goals of interventions Improving problem-solving skills Intervention mapping Mediating Monitoring Motivating Negotiating Offering options Organizing goals Presenting challenges Providing cognitive strategies to alter negative thought patterns Providing feedback Reframing expectations, goals, and meanings Setting tasks Using a variety of teaching strategies Using humor Effective use of cognitive coping strategies	Behavior change Change in beliefs or attitudes Decreased stress Effective self-care and problem solving related to clinical issues Improved functional status Improved quality of life Increased self-efficacy
Social	Advocating Bonding Collaborating with the client and with other providers Facilitating important relationships Interpreting patients' behaviors, needs, and goals to members of the health care team and patients' families Keeping tradition Mobilizing community, financial, and social resources Strengthening social supports through teaching, consultation, and referral	Affection Alienation and stigmatization averted or minimized Comfort Decreased caregiver burden Decreased costs of care Improved satisfaction with care Improved self-care Satisfaction with social support

Adapted from Spross, J. A. (1996). Coaching and suffering: The role of the nurse in helping people face illness. In B. R. Ferrell (Ed.), *The human dimensions of suffering* (Table 8.3, pp. 198–199). Boston: Jones & Bartlett; reprinted with permission. The reader is encouraged to refer to that publication for additional reference from which the coaching processes were derived.
* Although most outcomes are client/family related, some systems outcomes are included to help readers connect the individual coaching by advanced practice nurses with organization-level outcomes.

highly nuanced range of interpersonal skills to coach people through multifaceted transitions. The strategies used to develop coaching expertise are designed to groom reflective practice and a person-oriented interactive style. These are foundational abilities that APNs must develop to become skilled coaches.

Graduate Nursing Education: The Influence of Faculty and Preceptors

Graduate faculty and clinical preceptors are highly influential models for APN students seeking to develop coaching skills. A key step in assisting APN students to develop as coaches is for faculty to be reflective. In particular, faculty need to name and evaluate the processes and pedagogies to which they were exposed, distinguishing between effective, respectful experiences of being taught/coached and ineffective, disrespectful ones. Students who have been effectively coached by teachers and preceptors will know experientially what respectful coaching "feels like." They will be more likely to reproduce these behaviors with patients. Schön (1987) called this the "hall of mirrors" effect—the teacher, in the very process of supervising and coaching the student, exemplifies the coaching repertoire that the student is attempting to acquire. If ineffective, disrespectful teaching is recognized for what it is—a position-centered style—then students also learn how not to coach.

Clinical preceptors play a particularly salient role with APN students. In effect, there is a "double exposure" to coaching: the student experiences being coached and observes how patients are coached by the preceptor. Similarly, preceptors need to be able to coach students while coaching patients. The authors believe that a person-centered style of interaction on the part of the preceptor is just as important to developing the APN student's coaching skills as it is to helping clients accomplish their health goals. It is possible to have preceptors who use a person-centered style of interaction with clients yet, because of their own student experiences, adopt a position-centered style of interacting with students. Very experienced APNs can be novice preceptors (Meng & Morris, 1995), so that preceptors themselves may need coaching by faculty to develop in their preceptor roles. Davis, Sawin, and Dunn (1993) identified strategies preceptors should employ to create the best conditions for learning: using orientation strategies; managing the clinical environment to decrease student anxiety; and optimizing patient, student, and preceptor interactions. Just as APNs tailor their coaching to meet individual client needs, so APN preceptors need to tailor their coaching of students to the level of the student and the situation (Davis et al., 1993).

Faculty and APN preceptors need to be explicit with students in articulating the range of coaching strategies used in the classroom and the clinical area. In this way, the student learns the components of coaching. What was ineffable and undervalued in the process of coaching becomes defined, contextualized, reproducible, and valued (McKinnon & Erickson, 1988). Developing coaching competence requires attention to all ways of knowing, including personal knowing (Diemert Moch, 1990). Therefore, faculty and APN preceptors need to encourage students to pay close attention to their experiences. APN students should reflect on their past educational experiences, identifying and evaluating effective and ineffective coaching that they experienced. Bringing these educational moments to full consciousness and naming them is a key first step to envisioning coaching processes the students want to emulate or discard.

Strategies for Developing Coaching Competence

Coaching activities can be conceptualized along two dimensions: the degree of structure and the focus. Activities may be very structured (e.g., a lecture) or unstructured (e.g., storytelling). The focus of the APN's coaching may be individuals or groups. Table 7–7 organizes teaching activities and strategies along these dimensions. These strategies can be used to foster the development of coaching processes and can also be used to evaluate the APN's competence at coaching.

Less traditional teaching strategies must be used if one is to enlarge the APN student's interpersonal repertoire and self-reflective abilities. Expressive writing (Fulwiler, 1987; Sorrell, 1994; Van Manen, 1989) enables the student to recapture important experiences in nursing and reflect on them to arrive at new insights and interpretations. Keeping a journal and writing poetry are examples. Storytelling is another expressive strategy in which stories, the products of reflection, are relayed orally (Mattingly, 1998). Storytelling can build community and mutual respect among nurses (Lindesmith & McWeeny, 1994). Sharing stories from practice enables APN students to establish a shared history, and provides a means of offering and receiving support. The process promotes critical thinking, strengthens collegiality, and builds self-esteem and rapport (Lindesmith & McWeeny, 1994). One author (JAS) included journal writing as a teaching strategy in courses on role development. The journals were not graded. Through the students' writings and the instructor's responses, salient

TABLE 7–7	EDUCATIONAL STRATEGIES TO DEVELOP THE COACHING SKILLS OF THE ADVANCED PRACTICE NURSE
INDIVIDUAL	**GROUP**
Unstructured	
Coaching	Discussion group
Debriefing	Grand rounds
Discovery	Online chat rooms, listserve discussions
Experiential learning	Online communication
Expressive writing (e.g., poetry)	Storytelling
Use of humor	Support groups
Individual clinical supervision	Use of movies/media with a health care theme
Journal keeping	Walking rounds
Mentoring	
Peer coaching	
Reading about others' health-care experiences	
Support for risk taking	
Structured	
Chart review	Classroom-as-clinic (videotapes)
Critical incidents/exemplars	Continuing education programs
Demonstrations	Group patient education
Clear, immediate feedback on strengths *and* areas for growth	In-services
Competency-based instruction	Lecture
Computer-assisted learning	Orientation
Individualized media (e.g., patient education booklets and self-study programs)	Staff development
Intervention mapping	Standardized curricula
Objective tests	Standardized patient teaching plans
Practice laboratories	Virtual courses
Precepting	
Self-learning modules	

experiences were debriefed, a process described by Davies (1995). Sometimes debriefing consisted of the instructor's written response to the student's reflections. Other times, with the student's permission, the journal entries became the focus of a seminar discussion. Students' reflections on the experience of being new or uncertain of their skills led to discussions of developmental tasks such as embracing novicehood or learning to trust one's hands, heart, gut, and observations. Through journals and storytelling, cues and strategies for coaching used by different APN students and preceptors became available to a larger group of learners.

Aesthetic approaches to developing interpersonal competence can also develop APNs' coaching skills. The intense insights that can come from reading poetry and literature or watching a movie are often unexplored ways of knowing. Some of the most profound aesthetic experiences in which nurses are involved can never be known through scientific and transactional writing because of the limitations of these styles of writing. The acutely personal, reflective nature of poetry especially captures for nurses the person-oriented stance of interpersonal interaction that is required in APN coaching. Poetry and literature have been potent triggers for reflective practice. As a graduate student, one of the authors (EBC) had the experience of being invited to bring a short piece of prose, a poem, or a song that was meaningful to her. When she volunteered to share the piece with the class, the teacher coached her in the process of delivering the piece effectively by focusing and calming the student, demonstrating the process, standing close to the student, and offering encouragement. Similarly, movies with plots revolving around illness or disability, such as *Heartsounds, Passion Fish, Marvin's Room,* and *Regarding Henry,* can help APN students assess needs for coaching, evaluate clinicians' ineffective and effective interpersonal styles, and articulate the gaps in care that might require APN intervention.

Faculty should examine the curriculum for opportunities to incorporate aesthetic educational approaches into courses that tend to be structured. One of the authors (EBC) integrated aesthetics into a 3-credit graduate course on pathophysiology. The basic sciences and clinical features of various pathologies were presented to teach students "what disease is." Poetry and literature were used to help students understand the lived experience of illness—"what it is like for a person to have this disease." Patients' stories were integrated with scientific principles in the course activities and take-home tests. These strategies enabled students to acquire a holistic understanding of disease and illness as experienced by patients and families.

Harris (1997) asserted that APNs intervene to reduce the risk of complex responses to health problems, a practice outcome that tends to be invisible. Although not directly related to coaching, the suggested strategies for assessing risk in patient populations as a way to make the impact of APNs on patient outcomes visible can be applied to coaching. Assessing risk involves the following six steps:

1. Identify and describe the complex response.
2. Determine the group at risk.
3. Identify risk factors.
4. Assess the dose response.
5. Determine exposure to risk factors with and without APN intervention.
6. Characterize the risk by summarizing the information gathered in the previous steps.

To apply this strategy to the coaching competency, students might describe the observations made during the course of encounters, risk factors that were elicited as a result of intentionally shaping the interaction, and interpersonal or personality characteristics of the patient that might increase risk. Additional strategies and resources are available to APNs interested in refining their coaching skills: peer coaching (Aviram, Ophir, Raviv, & Shiloah, 1998; Robbins, 1991), thinking aloud (Corcoran & Moreland, 1988), teaching diagnostic reasoning using the classroom-as-clinic approach (Neistadt & Smith, 1996), and mentoring (Daloz, 1986).

PATIENT EDUCATION AND COACHING FOR APNs: ISSUES AND SELECTED LITERATURE REVIEW

Managed Care

Numerous factors in contemporary health care have increased the focus on patient education as a means of improving effectiveness and efficiency and achieving cost and quality outcomes. These include managed care (Cook, 1997; Spross & Heaney, 2000; Taylor et al., 1997); cost containment (Barger, 1997; Bauer, 1994; Smith, 1989; Weiss, 1998); the evidence-based practice movement (Bero et al., 1998; Porter et al., 1997; Spross & Heaney, 2000; University of York NHS Centre for Reviews and Dissemination, 1999); the educational needs of informal caregivers (Kirk & Glendinning, 1998); and the widespread use of the World Wide Web for teaching and learning. The emphasis in managed care on risk reduction (Harris, 1997), disease management (Weiss, 1998; see Chapter 19), and implementation of evidence-based practices requires that nurses establish partnerships with patients so that they can coach them in self-care and tailor interventions to the needs of the patient and the situational context. Although these trends underscore the importance of patient education, one writer expressed concern that the inability of APNs to participate in some managed care networks might limit patients' access to effective programs such as childbirth education (Cook, 1997).

Research Utilization and Research

Chapter 6 addresses the role of APNs in applying middle-range theories to practice, highlighting theories APNs are likely to use. Middle-range theories that have informed health education and counseling interventions for many clinical populations include self-efficacy (Bandura, 1977; Clark & Dodge, 1999; Lev, 1997) and the Health Belief Model (Becker, 1974; see Chapter 19). Given the importance of behavior change to improving health and coping with illness, applying these theories to better understand the expert coaching and guidance competency could yield important insights from both a nursing and an interdisciplinary perspective.

One of the problems in discerning the impact of APN education on patient care is the inconsistency with which the "nurse or APN dose" of the intervention is described. In updating the literature review for this chapter, it was difficult to know what the characteristics of the nurse delivering the intervention were. Of the dozen review articles or studies that examined teaching and coaching interventions (Brooten et al., 1994; Carrieri-Kohlman, Gormley, Douglas, Paul, & Stulbarg, 1996; Eller, 1999; Forshee et al., 1998; George et al., 1999; McDougall, 1999; Naylor et al., 1999;

Pettersson, Gardulf, Nordstrom, Svanberg-Johnsson, & Bylin, 1999; Ryan, 1999; Schwartz-Barcott et al., 1994; Taylor et al., 1997; Wilkie, Williams, Grevstad, & Mekwa, 1995), only those by Brooten et al. (1994), George et al. (1999), Naylor et al. (1999), and Taylor et al. (1997) specified that the nurse was an APN. It is important that APNs who participate in the design and execution of such studies ensure that the characteristics of the clinicians delivering the interventions be included in descriptions of intervention protocols and, where appropriate, that analyses account for clinician characteristics when evaluating the intervention. Such analyses are important for determining the most efficacious and cost-effective approaches to patient education and coaching. If patient education is effective and if efficient patient education is one of the solutions to reducing the costs of health care, more needs to be understood about the process of patient teaching used by APNs and how it promotes adherence to therapies and self-care.

Health Literacy

An important consideration in implementing the APN coaching and guidance competency is the extent of health illiteracy in the United States. Literacy is defined as "an individual's ability to read, write, and speak in English, and compute and solve problems at levels of proficiency necessary to function on the job and in society, to achieve one's goals, and develop one's knowledge and potential" (1991 National Literacy Act passed by the U. S. Congress and cited in Ad Hoc Committee on Health Literacy for the Council on Scientific Affairs, American Medical Association, 1999, p. 552). The National Adult Literacy Survey revealed that nearly one quarter of the U. S. population (40 to 44 million people) are functionally illiterate. The large number of individuals with marginal literacy skills (about 50 million) means that about one half of adults in this country have reading and computational skills that are inadequate to meet the demands of daily life (Kirsch, Jungeblut, Jenkins, & Kolstad, 1993). To further understand health literacy, investigators studied 3,260 Medicare enrollees over 65 years old to assess functional health literacy (Gazmararian et al., 1999). They found that one third of English-speaking ($N = 2,956$) and over one half of Spanish-speaking ($N = 304$) subjects had inadequate or marginal health literacy. Reading ability declined with age even when results were adjusted for variables such as cognitive impairment and years of school completed.

Assessing functional health literacy must be done sensitively. Years of education completed may not be an adequate indicator of reading and computational literacy (Davis, Michielutte, Askov, Williams, & Weiss, 1998). A variety of tools exist to assist clinicians in assessing patient literacy (Davis et al., 1998). APNs involved in developing programmatic approaches to patient education must ascertain that materials are appropriate to the literacy level of participants in educational programs.

Selected Literature Review on Patient Education

Redman (1988) described patient education as a complex set of interactions that include a diversity of subtasks and approaches. What and how to teach patients and how to help them cope with or master their health concerns have long been concerns of nurses in basic and advanced practice (Redman, 1997; Sparks, 1995; Walsh & Bernhard, 1998). Studies on client education were among the earliest types of clinical research performed by nurses. Much of what is considered standard practice in nursing, such as preparing patients for procedures and surgery by providing sensory, procedural, and other information, is based on a program of research initiated by Johnson and her colleagues (e.g., Johnson, Rice, Fuller, & Endress, 1978; Leventhal & Johnson, 1983) and replicated and extended by subsequent investigators (Hathaway, 1986).

Sufficient research on patient education exists to indicate how teaching should be done and that it influences outcomes. In an integrative review of research on patient education, Lindemann (1988) found that most teaching strategies are effective. Although this may be an artifact of various research designs, it may also underscore the strength of patient education as an intervention. A meta-analysis of patient teaching strategies revealed that nine strategies had small to moderate effect sizes (Theis & Johnson, 1995). The largest effect sizes were associated with structured approaches, reinforcement, independent study, and multiple strategies. Regardless of a strategy's effect size, all subjects in experimental groups had better outcomes than did those in control groups. In a meta-analysis of 84 experimental studies, Heater, Becker, and Olson (1988) evaluated the effectiveness of patient education for 4,000 subjects, including neonates, preterm infants, preschool children, grade school children, adolescents, new parents, parents and infants, adults, and elderly. They concluded that the average subject in an experimental group had a better outcome than did 72% of the subjects in comparison groups. Improved outcomes occurred in the cognitive (knowledge), behavioral, physiological, and psychosocial areas. A literature search for this revision using the keywords "patient education" and "advanced practice nurses," and specific advanced practice roles did not identify more recent meta-analyses.

An integrative review of 74 randomized, controlled trials of telephone-delivered interventions (TDIs) indicated that TDIs have been used to broaden the reach of health interventions, promote health behavior change, and increase the efficacy of health services delivery (McBride & Rimer, 1999). In 27 studies, interventions were delivered by nurses; of these, in only three could interventions be clearly identified as having been delivered by APNs. Table 7–8 lists the areas where TDIs have been associated with improvements in patient outcomes and better utilization of health services. This review article would be of interest to APNs who are interested in understanding the ways in which TDIs have been used effectively and who want to incorporate systematic use of TDIs in clinical programs. The review concluded with some of the unanswered questions about TDIs. For example, one of the research questions the authors posed was: What are the optimal characteristics of the interventions? These questions could be modified to guide research regarding the use of the World Wide Web for patient education.

CONCLUSION

APNs coach patients through transitions. In the APN, graduate education and technical, clinical, and interpersonal competence interact with self-reflection to produce a diverse set of coaching skills and the ability to invent new coaching processes in the midst of novel clinical encounters. This is an extremely complex skill that relies on APNs' human and professional qualities. Although coaching processes occur simultaneously, they are not automatic. APNs can usually describe the intent of coaching interventions and explain their selection of one approach over another.

TABLE 7–8	TYPES OF TELEPHONE-DELIVERED INTERVENTIONS	
GOAL	PURPOSES	TYPES OF TDIs
Reaching the underserved	• Smoking cessation • Pain management • Treatment adherence	• Hotline • Helpline • Callbacks • Counseling
Sustaining health behavior changes in populations with addictions, chronic diseases, or groups at risk for health problems	• Smoking cessation • Relapse prevention • Complication prevention (e.g., diabetics, asthmatics) • Cancer screening • Appropriate use of services	• Helpline • Counseling • Booster calls (reminders, encouragement)
Increasing the effectiveness of health care services	• Decrease system burdens • Decrease patient burdens • Increase/improve outpatient support for those with health problems • Improve treatment/medication adherence (e.g., hypertensives, elderly patients)	• Callbacks • Helpline

What may seem automatic is actually very deliberate; the APN has learned what has worked in similar encounters and uses it over and over. In using a person-centered style with a patient, the APN remains open to cues that the approach may not work in this particular encounter, thereby remaining flexible and aware of alternatives. An observer seeing the APN in action may think these processes are automatic because of how natural they seem. That such interactions appear to occur naturally arises from the APN's mindfulness of the encounter and the patient's and the APN's own responses.

In many arts and sports, coaches no longer perform the skill they coach and yet are still able to coach effectively. The nature of the health care environment and the delivery of clinical services are dynamic and complex. A nurse's coaching expertise can still develop when the nurse's primary responsibility shifts from direct care to another area within nursing, such as teaching or administration. However, the coaching processes that are developed will be related to the learners—students or staff. The ability to coach patients depends on direct care experiences in which new human responses, possibilities for growth, and new coaching strategies are revealed through APNs' encounters with patients and families as they experience health and illness and new technologies and therapies.

REFERENCES

Ad Hoc Committee on Health Literacy for the Council on Scientific Affairs, American Medical Association. (1999). Health literacy: Report of the Council on Scientific Affairs. *JAMA, 281,* 552–557.

Atkins, S., & Murphy, K. (1994). Reflective practice. *Nursing Standard, 8*(39), 49–54.

Aviram, M., Ophir, R., Raviv, D., & Shiloah, M. (1998). Experiential learning of clinical skills by beginning nursing students: "Coaching" project by fourth-year student interns. *J Nursing Education, 37,* 228–231.

Bandura, A. (1977). Self-efficacy: Toward a unifying theory of behavioral change. *Psychological Revue, 84*(2), 191–215.

Barger, S. (1997). Building healthier communities in a managed care environment: Opportunities for advanced practice nurses. *Advanced Practice Nursing Quarterly, 2*(4), 9–14.

Barnsteiner, J. H., Gillis-Donovan, J., Knox-

Fischer,C., & McKlindon, D. D. (1994). Defining and implementing a standard for therapeutic relationships. *Journal of Holistic Nursing, 12*(1), 35–49.

Bartels, J. E. (1998). Developing reflective learners—student self-assessment as learning. *J Professional Nursing, 14,* 135.

Bartholomew, L. K., Parcel, G. S., & Kok, G. (1998). Intervention mapping: A process for developing theory- and evidence-based health education programs. *Health Education & Behavior, 25,* 545–563.

Bauer, J. (1994). *Not what the doctor ordered: Reinventing medical care in America.* Chicago: Probus Publishing Company.

Becker, M. (1974). *The health belief model and personal health behavior.* Thorofare, NJ: Charles B. Slack.

Benner, P. (1984). *From novice to expert: Excellence and power in clinical nursing practice.* Menlo Park, CA: Addison-Wesley.

Benner, P. (1985). The oncology clinical nurse specialist as expert coach. *Oncology Nursing Forum, 12*(2), 40–44.

Benner, P. (1991). The role of experience, narrative, and community in skilled ethical comportment. *Advances in Nursing Science, 14*(2), 1–21.

Benner, P., Hooper-Kyriakidis, P., & Stannard, D. (1999). *Clinical wisdom and interventions in critical care: A thinking-in-action approach.* Philadelphia: W. B. Saunders.

Bernstein, B. (1974). *Class, codes, and control: Theoretical studies towards a sociology of language.* New York: Schocken Books.

Bero, L., Grilli, R., Grimshaw, I. M., Harvey, E., Oxman, A. D., & Thomson, M. A. (1998). Closing the gap between research and practice: An overview of systematic reviews of interventions to promote the implementation of research findings. *BMJ, 317,* 465–468.

Braden, C. (1990). Learned self-help response to chronic illness experience: A test of three alternative learning theories. *Scholarly Inquiry for Nursing Practice, 4*(1), 23–41.

Braden, C. (1993). Research program on learned response to chronic illness experience: Self-help model. *Holistic Nursing Practice, 8*(1), 38–44.

Bridges, W. (1980). *Transitions: Making sense of life's changes.* Reading, MA: Addison-Wesley.

Brooten, D., Brown, L., Hazard Munro, B., York, R., Cohen, S., Roncoli, M., & Hollingsworth, A. (1988). Early discharge and specialist transitional care. *Image: The Journal of Nursing Scholarship, 20*(2), 64–68.

Brooten, D., Gennaro, S., Knapp, H., Jovene, N., Brown, L., & York, R. (1991). Functions of the CNS in early discharge and home follow-up of very low birthweight infants. *Clinical Nurse Specialist, 5*(4), 196–201.

Brooten, D., Kumar, S., Brown, L., Butts, P., Finkler, S., Bakewell-Sachs, S., Gibbons, A., & Delivoria-Papadopoulos, M. (1986). A randomized clinical trial of early hospital discharge and home follow-up of very low birthweight infants. *New England Journal of Medicine, 315,* 934–939.

Brooten, D., Roncoli, M., Finkler, S., Arnold, L., Cohen, A., & Mennutti, M. (1994). A randomized clinical trial of hospital discharge and nurse specialist home follow-up of women with unplanned cesarean birth. *Obstetrics and Gynecology, 84,* 832–838.

Brown, M., & Waybrant, K. (1988). Health promotion, education, counseling, and coordination in primary health care nursing. *Public Health Nursing, 5*(1), 16–23.

Brown, S. (1995). An interviewing style for nursing assessment. *Journal of Advanced Nursing, 21,* 340–343.

Brown, S. (1999). Patient-centered communication. *Annual Review of Nursing Research, 17,* 85–104.

Carrieri-Kohlman, V., Gormley, J. M., Douglas, M. K., Paul, S. M., & Stulbarg, M. S. (1996). Exercise training decreases dyspnea and the distress and anxiety associated with it: Monitoring alone may be as effective as coaching. *Chest, 110,* 1526–1535.

Chick, N., & Meleis, A. (1986). Transitions: A nursing concern. In P. Chinn (Ed.), *Nursing research methodology: Issues and implementation* (pp. 237–258). Rockville, MD: Aspen Publishers.

Chopoorian, T. (1986). Reconceptualizing the environment. In P. Moccia (Ed.), *New approaches to theory development.* New York: National League for Nursing.

Clark, N. M., & Dodge, J. A. (1999). Exploring self-efficacy as a predictor of disease management. *Health Education & Behavior, 26*(1), 72–89.

Connelly, C. (1993). An empirical model of self-care in chronic illness. *Clinical Nurse Specialist, 7,* 247–253.

Cook, S. S. (1997). Configuring childbirth education to survive in managed care. *Advanced Practice Nursing Quarterly, 2*(4), 22–26.

Corbin, J., & Strauss, A. (1992). A nursing model for chronic illness management based upon the trajectory framework. In P. Woog (Ed.), *The chronic illness trajectory framework: The Corbin and Strauss model* (pp. 9–28). New York: Springer-Verlag.

Corcoran, S., & Moreland, H. (1988). "Thinking aloud" as a strategy to improve clinical decision making. *Heart & Lung, 17,* 463–468.

Daloz, L. (1986). *Effective teaching and mentoring: Realizing the transformational power of adult learning experiences.* San Francisco: Jossey-Bass.

Davies, E. (1995). Reflective practice: A focus for caring. *Journal of Nursing Education, 34,* 167–174.

Davis, M., Sawin, K., & Dunn, M. (1993). Teaching strategies used by expert nurse practitioner preceptors: A qualitative study. *Journal of the American Academy of Nurse Practitioners, 5,* 27–33.

Davis, T. C., Michielutte, R., Askov, E. N., Williams, M. V., & Weiss, B. D. (1998). Practical assessment of adult literacy in health care. *Health Education & Behavior, 25,* 613–624.

de La Cuesta, C. (1994). Relationships in health visiting: Enabling and mediating. *International Journal of Nursing Studies, 31,* 451–459.

Diemert Moch, S. (1990). Personal knowing: Evolving research and practice. *Scholarly Inquiry for Nursing Practice, 4,* 155–170.

Draye, M., & Pesznecker, B. (1980). Teaching activities of nurse practitioners. *Nurse Practitioner, 5,* 28–33.

Eller, L. S. (1999). Effects of cognitive-behavioral interventions on quality of life in persons with HIV. *International Journal of Nursing Studies, 36,* 223–233.

Fenton, M. (1984). Identification of the skilled performance of master's prepared nurses as a method of curriculum planning and evaluation. In P. Benner (Ed.), *From novice to expert* (pp. 262–274). Menlo Park, CA: Addison-Wesley.

Fenton, M., & Brykczynski, K. (1993). Qualitative distinctions and similarities in the practice of clinical nurse specialists and nurse practitioners. *Journal of Professional Nursing, 9,* 313–326.

Forshee, J. D., Whalen, E. B., Hackel, R., Butt, L. T., Smeltzer, P. A., Martin, J., Lavin, P. T., & Buchner, D. A. (1998). The effectiveness of one-on-one nurse education on the outcomes of high-risk adult and pediatric patients with asthma. *Managed Care Interface, 11*(12), 82–92.

Freire, P. (1970). *Pedagogy of the oppressed.* New York: Continuum Publishing.

Frisch, M., Elliott, C., Atsaides, J., Salva, D., & Denney, D. (1982). Social skills and stress management training to enhance patients' interpersonal competencies. *Psychotherapy Theory, Research and Practice, 19,* 349–358.

Fulwiler, T. (1987). *Teaching with writing.* Upper Montclair, NJ: Boynton/Cook.

Gadow, S. (1980). Existential advocacy: Philosophical foundations of nursing. In S. Spicker & S. Gadow (Eds.), *Nursing: Images and ideas* (pp. 79–101). New York: Springer-Verlag.

Gazmararian, J. A., Baker, D. W., Williams, M. V., Parker, R. M., Scott, T. L., Green, D. C., Fehrenbach, S. N., Ren, J., & Koplan, J. P. (1999). Health literacy among Medicare enrollees in a managed care organization. *JAMA, 281,* 545–551.

George, M. R., O'Dowd, L. C., Martin, I., Lindell, K. O., Whitney, F., Jones, M., Ramondo, T., Walsh, L., Grissinger, J., Hansen-Flashen, J., & Pannettieri, R. A. (1999). A comprehensive educational program improves clinical outcome measures in inner-city patients with asthma. *Archives of Internal Medicine, 159,* 1710–1716.

Grimmett, P. (1988). The nature of reflection and Schön's conception in perspective. In P. Grimmett & G. Erickson (Eds.), *Reflection in teacher education* (pp. 5–15). New York: Teacher's College Press.

Hagedorn, S. (1995). The politics of caring: The role of activism in primary care. *Advances in Nursing Science, 17*(4), 1–11.

Harris, M. (1997). Reduced risk of complex response: An invisible outcome. *Nursing Administration Quarterly, 21*(4), 25–31.

Hathway, D. (1986). Effect of preoperative instruction on postoperative outcomes: A meta-analysis. *Nursing Research, 35,* 260–275.

Heater, B., Becker, A., & Olson, R. (1988). Nursing interventions and patient outcomes: A meta-analysis of studies. *Nursing Research, 37,* 303–307.

Heifetz, R. (1994). *Leadership without easy answers.* Cambridge, MA: Belknap Press.

Hops, H. (1983). Children's social competence and skill: Current research, practices, and future directions. *Behavioral Therapy, 14,* 3–18.

Jackson, P. (1986). *The practice of teaching.* New York: Teacher's College Press.

Jenny, J., & Logan, J. (1992). Knowing the patient: One aspect of clinical knowledge. *Image: The Journal of Nursing Scholarship, 24,* 254–258.

Johnson, J., Rice, V., Fuller, S., & Endress, M. (1978). Sensory information, instruction in a coping strategy, and recovery from surgery. *Research in Nursing and Health, 1,* 4–17.

Kasch, C. (1983). Interpersonal competence and communication in the delivery of nursing care. *Advances in Nursing Science, 5*(1), 71–88.

Kasch, C., & Dine, J. (1988). Person-centered communication and social perspective taking. *Western Journal of Nursing Research, 10,* 317–326.

Kasch, C., & Knutson, K. (1985). Patient compliance and interpersonal style: Implications for practice and research. *Nurse Practitioner, 10*(3), 52–64.

Kasch, C., & Lisnek, P. (1984). Role of strategic communication in nursing theory and research. *Advances in Nursing Science, 6*(1), 56–71.

Kendall, J. (1992). Fighting back: Promoting emancipatory nursing actions. *Advances in Nursing Science, 15*(2), 1–15.

Kirk, S., & Glendinning, C. (1998). Trends in community care and patient participation: Implications for the roles of informal carers and community nurses in the United Kingdom. *Journal of Advanced Nursing, 28,* 370–381.

Kirsch, I., Jungeblut, A., Jenkins, L., & Kolstad, A. (1993). *Adult literacy in America: A first look at the findings of the National Adult Literacy Survey.* Washington, DC: U.S. Department of Education, National Center for Education Statistics.

Koetters, T. L. (1989). Clinical practice and direct patient care. In A. B. Hamric & J. A. Spross (Eds.), *The clinical nurse specialist in theory and practice* (2nd ed., pp. 107–124). Philadelphia: W. B. Saunders.

Kolcaba, K. (1992). Holistic comfort: Operationalizing the construct as a nurse-sensitive outcome. *Advances in Nursing Science, 15*(1), 1–10.

Lamb, G., & Stempel, J. (1994). Nurse case management from the client's view: Growing as insider-expert. *Nursing Outlook, 42*(1), 7–13.

Lamm, B., Dungan, J., & Hiromoto, B. (1991). Long-term lifestyle management. *Clinical Nurse Specialist, 5*(4), 182–188.

Lang, N., & Marek, K. (1992). Outcomes that reflect clinical practice. In *Patient outcomes research: Examining the effectiveness of nursing practice* (NIH Publication No. 93-3411) (pp. 27–38). Rockville, MD: National Institutes of Health.

Lev, E. (1997). Bandura's theory of self-efficacy: Applications to oncology. *Scholarly Inquiry for Nursing Practice, 11,* 21–37.

Leventhal, H., & Johnson, J. (1983). Laboratory and field experimentation: Development of a theory of self-regulation. In P. Woolridge, M. Schmitt, J. Skipper, & P. Leonard (Eds.), *Behavioral science and nursing theory* (pp. 189–262). St. Louis: C. V. Mosby.

Lewis, F. M., & Zahlis, E. (1997). The nurse as coach: A conceptual framework for clinical practice. *Oncology Nursing Forum, 24,* 1695–1702.

Lindemann, C. (1988). Nursing research in patient education. *Annual Review of Nursing Research, 6,* 29–60.

Lindesmith, K., & McWeeny, M. (1994). The power of storytelling. *Journal of Continuing Education in Nursing, 25,* 186–187.

Lombardo, B. (1987). *The humanistic coach: From theory to practice.* Springfield, IL: Charles C Thomas.

Martocchio, B. (1987). Authenticity, belonging, emotional closeness, and self representation. *Oncology Nursing Forum, 14*(4), 23–27.

Mattingly, C. (1998). Healing dramas and clinical plots: The narrative structure of experience. Cambridge, UK: Cambridge University Press.

McBride, C. M., & Rimer, B. K. (1999). Using the telephone to improve health behavior and health service delivery. *Patient Education & Counseling, 37,* 3–18.

McDougall, Jr., G. J. (1999). Cognitive interventions among older adults. *Annual Review of Nursing Research, 17,* 219–240.

McKinnon, A., & Erickson, G. (1988). Taking Schon's ideas to a science teaching practicum. In P. Grimmett & G. Erickson (Eds.), *Reflection in teacher education* (pp. 113–137). New York: Teacher's College Press.

Meng, A., & Morris, D. (1995). Continuing education for advanced nurse practitioners: Preparing nurse-midwives as clinical preceptors. *Journal of Continuing Education in Nursing, 26,* 180–184.

Mezey, M., Dougherty, M., Wade, P., & Mersmann, C. (1994). Nurse practitioners, certified nurse-midwives, and nurse anesthetists: Changing care in acute care hospitals in New York City. *Journal of the New York State Nurses' Association, 25*(4), 13–17.

Montgomery, C. L. (1993). *Healing through communication.* Newbury Park, CA: Sage Publications.

Morgan, A. (1994). Client education experiences in professional nursing practice—a phenomenological perspective. *Journal of Advanced Nursing, 19,* 792–801.

Morse, J. M., Havens, G. D., & Wilson, S. (1997). The comforting interaction: Developing a model of nurse-patient relationship. *Scholarly Inquiry for Nursing Practice, 11,* 321–343.

Naylor, M. D., Brooten, D., Campbell, R., Jacobsen, B. S., Mezey, M. D., Pauly, M. V., & Schwartz, J. S. (1999). Comprehensive discharge planning and home follow-up of hospitalized elders. *JAMA, 281,* 613–620.

Naylor, M., Munro, B., & Brooten, D. (1991). Measuring the effectiveness of nursing practice. *Clinical Nurse Specialist, 5,* 210–215.

Neistadt, M. E., & Smith, R. E. (1996). Teaching diagnostic reasoning: Using a classroom-as-clinic methodology with videotapes. *American Journal of Occupational Therapy, 51,* 361–368.

Olesen, V., Schatzman, L., Droes, N., Hatton, D., & Chico, N. (1990). The mundane ailment and the physical self: Analysis of the social psychology of health and illness. *Social Science and Medicine, 30,* 449–455.

Pelligrini, D., & Urbain, E. (1985). An evaluation of interpersonal cognitive problem solving training with children. *Journal of Psychology and Psychiatry, 26,* 17–41.

Peplau, H. (1952). *Interpersonal relations in nursing: A conceptual frame of reference.* New York: G. P. Putnam.

Peplau, H. (1994). Quality of life: An interpersonal perspective. *Nursing Science Quarterly, 7*(1), 10–15.

Pettersson, E., Gardulf, A., Nordstrom, G., Svanberg-Johnsson, C., & Bylin, G. (1999). Evaluation of a nurse-run asthma school. *International Journal of Nursing Studies, 36,* 145–151.

Pew-Fetzer Task Force on Advancing Psychosocial Health Education. (1994). *Health professions education and relationship-centered care.* San Francisco: Pew Health Professions Commission.

Porter, C. P., Pender, N. J., Hayman, L. L., Armstrong, M. L., Riesch, S. K., & Lewis, M. A. (1997). Educating APNs for implementing the guidelines for adolescents in Bright Futures: Guidelines of health supervision of infants, children, and adolescents. *Nursing Outlook, 45*(6), 252-257.

Pugach, M., & Johnson, L. (1990). Developing reflective practice through structured dialogue. In R. Clift, W. Houston, & M. Pugach (Eds.), *Encouraging reflective practice in teacher education* (pp. 186-207). New York: Teacher's College Press.

Quirk, M., & Casey, L. (1995). Primary care for women: The art of interviewing. *Journal of Nurse-Midwifery, 40*(2), 97-103.

Redman, B. (1988). *The process of patient education.* St. Louis: Mosby-Year Book.

Redman, B. K. (1997). *The practice of patient education* (ed. 8). St. Louis: Mosby Year Book, Inc.

Robbins, P. (1991). *How to plan and implement a peer coaching program.* Alexandria, VA: Association for Supervision and Curriculum Development.

Ryan, A. A. (1999). Medication compliance and older people: A review of the literature. *International Journal of Nursing Studies, 36,* 153-162.

Schön, D. (1983). *The reflective practitioner: How professionals think in action.* New York: Basic Books.

Schön, D. (1987). *Educating the reflective practitioner: Toward a new design for teaching and learning in the professions.* San Francisco: Jossey-Bass.

Schumacher, K., & Meleis, A. (1994). Transitions: A central concept in nursing. *Image: The Journal of Nursing Scholarship, 26,* 119-127.

Scupholme, A., Paine, L., Lang, J., Kumar, S., & DeJoseph, J. (1994). Time associated with components of clinical services rendered by nurse-midwives: Sample data from phase II of nurse-midwifery care to vulnerable populations in the United States. *Journal of Nurse-Midwifery, 39,* 5-12.

Scupholme, A., & Walsh, L. (1994). Home-based services by nurse-midwives: Sample data from phase II of nurse-midwifery care to vulnerable populations in the United States. *Journal of Nurse-Midwifery, 39,* 358-362.

Smith, C. (1989). Overview of patient education: Opportunities and challenges for the twenty-first century. *Nursing Clinics of North America, 24,* 583-587.

Sorrell, J. (1994). Remembrance of things past through writing: Esthetic patterns of knowing in nursing. *Advances in Nursing Science, 17*(1), 60-70.

Sparks, R. K. (1995). Client education. In M. Snyder & M. P. Mirr (Eds.), *Advanced practice nursing: A guide to professional development* (pp. 117-133). New York: Springer-Verlag.

Spross, J. (1994). *Coaching: An interdisciplinary perspective. Unpublished manuscript,* Doctoral Program in Nursing, Boston College.

Spross, J. (1996). Coaching and suffering: The role of the nurse in helping people face illness. In B. Ferrell (Ed.), *Suffering* (pp. 173-208). Boston: Jones & Bartlett.

Spross, J. A., & Heaney, C. A. (2000). Shaping advanced nursing practice roles in the new millennium. *Seminars in Oncology Nursing, 16,* 12-24.

Squier, R. (1990). A model of empathic understanding and adherence to treatment regimens in practitioner-patient relationships. *Social Science and Medicine, 30,* 325-339.

Steele, S., & Fenton, M. (1988). Expert practice of clinical nurse specialists. *Clinical Nurse Specialist, 2*(1), 45-52.

Steven, P. (1989). A critical social reconstruction of environment in nursing: Implications for methodology. *Advances in Nursing Science, 11*(4), 55-68.

Sullivan, P., & Wilson, D. (1991). The coach's role. In G. Cohen (Ed.), *Women in sport: Issues and controversies* (pp. 230-237). Newbury Park, CA: Sage.

Tanner, C., Benner, P., Chesla, C., & Gordon, D. (1993). The phenomenology of knowing the patient. *Image: The Journal of Nursing Scholarship, 25,* 273-280.

Taylor, C. A., Resick, L., D'Antonio, J. A., & Carroll, T. L. (1997). The advanced practice nurse role in implementing and evaluating two nurse-managed wellness clinics: Lessons learned about structure, process, and outcomes. *Advanced Practice Nursing Quarterly, 3*(2), 36-45.

Theis, S., & Johnson, J. (1995). Strategies for teaching patients: A meta-analysis. *Clinical Nurse Specialist, 9,* 100-105, 120.

Travelbee, J. (1971). *Interpersonal aspects of nursing.* Philadelphia: F. A. Davis.

Tremmel, R. (1993). Zen and the art of reflective practice in teacher education. *Harvard Educational Review, 63,* 434-458.

University of York NHS Centre for Reviews and Dissemination. (1999). Getting evidence into practice. *Effective Health Care, 5*(1), 1-16. Website: *http://www.york.ac.uk/inscr/crd/ehc51.hrm*

Van Manen, M. (1989). By the light of anecdote. *Phenomenological Pedagogy, 7,* 232-253.

Walsh, M., & Bernhard, L. A. (1998). Selected theories and models for advanced practice nursing. In C. M. Sheehy & M. McCarthy (Eds.), *Advanced practice nursing: emphasizing common roles* (pp. 88-113). Philadelphia: F. A. Davis.

Weiss, M. (1998). Case management as a tool for clinical integration. *Advanced Practice Nursing Quarterly, 4*(1), 9–15.

White, J. (1995). Patterns of knowing: Review, critique, and update. *Advances in Nursing Science, 17*(4), 73–86.

Wilkie, D. J., Williams, A. R., Grevstad, P., & Mekwa, J. (1995). Coaching persons with lung cancer to report sensory pain: Literature review and pilot study findings. *Cancer Nursing, 18,* 7–15.

Younger, J. (1995). The alienation of the sufferer. *Advances in Nursing Science, 17*(4), 53–72.

Additional Readings

Alexander, J., Younger, R., Cohen, R., & Crawford, L. (1988). Effectiveness of a nurse managed program for children with chronic asthma. *Journal of Pediatric Nursing, 3,* 312–317.

Beheshti, P., & Fonteyn, M. (1988). Role of the advanced practice nurse in continence care in the home. *AACN Clinical Issues, 9,* 389–395.

Brown, S. (1998). A framework for advanced practice nursing. *Journal of Professional Nursing, 14*(3), 157–164.

Brykczynski, K. (1989). An interpretive study describing the clinical judgment of nurse practitioners. *Scholarly Inquiry for Nursing Practice, 3*(2), 75–112.

Fenton, M. (1985). Identifying competencies of clinical nurse specialists. *Journal of Nursing Administration, 15*(12), 31–37.

Hodnett, E. (1999). *Continuity of caregivers for care during pregnancy and childbirth.* Available: *http://updateusa.com/CLIB/CLIBNET*

Leigh, S. (1998). The long-term cancer survivor: A challenge for nurse practitioners. *Nurse Practitioner Forum, 9*(3), 192–196.

Lipman, T. (1986). Length of hospitalization of children with diabetes: Effect of a clinical nurse specialist. *Diabetes Educator, 14*(1), 41–43.

Office of Technology Assessment. (1986). *Nurse practitioners, physician assistants, and certified nurse-midwives: A policy analysis* (Health Technology Case Study 37, No. OTA-HCS-37). Washington, DC: U. S. Congress.

Pozen, M., Stechmiller, J., Harris, W., Smith, S., Fred, D., & Voight, G. (1977). A nurse rehabilitator's impact on patients with myocardial infarction. *Medical Care, 15,* 830–837.

Priest, A. R. (1989). The CNS as educator. In A. B. Hamric & J. A. Spross (Eds.), *The clinical nurse specialist in theory and practice* (2nd ed., pp. 147–168). Philadelphia: W. B. Saunders.

Reiger, P. (1998). Overview of cancer and genetics: Implications for nurse practitioners. *Nurse Practitioner Forum, 9*(3), 122–133.

Schwartz-Barcott, D., Fortin, J., & Kim, H. (1994). Client-nurse interaction: Testing for its impact in preoperative instruction. *International Journal of Nursing Studies, 31*(1), 23–35.

Scott, R. A. (1999). A description of the roles, activities, and skills of clinical nurse specialists in the United States. *Clinical Nurse Specialist, 13,* 183–190.

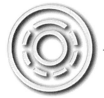

C H A P T E R   8

Consultation

- A N N E - M A R I E   B A R R O N
- P A T R I C I A   A.   W H I T E

INTRODUCTION

CONSULTATION AND ADVANCED NURSING PRACTICE

DEFINING CONSULTATION
Distinguishing Consultation from Co-management,
Referral, and Collaboration
Distinguishing Consultation from Clinical and
Administrative Supervision

BACKGROUND
Consultation in Mental Health Practice
Types of Consultation

A MODEL OF ADVANCED NURSING
PRACTICE CONSULTATION
Principles of Consultation
Description of the Model

COMMON APN CONSULTATION SITUATIONS
APN–APN Consultation
APN–Physician Consultation
APN–Staff Nurse Consultation

FORMAL AND INFORMAL CONSULTATION

MECHANISMS TO FACILITATE CONSULTATION

ISSUES IN ANP CONSULTATION
Developing Consultation Skills in APN Students
On-Line Consultation
Documentation and Legal Considerations
Stepping Out of the Consultation Process
Developing the Practice of Other Nurses
Consultation Practice over Time

EVALUATION OF THE CONSULTATION COMPETENCY

SUMMARY

INTRODUCTION

Consultation is an important aspect of advanced nursing practice. The nursing literature on consultation is largely focused on the clinical nurse specialist (CNS) role. Historically, CNS practice in the acute care setting has emphasized consultation as a critical role component, whereas other advanced practice nurses (APNs) have emphasized the direct care role. As the profession of nursing considers the educational and practice issues relevant to all advanced practice, it is important that consultation be considered an essential core competency of all advanced practice roles. Although CNSs have developed this aspect of their practice more completely, all APNs offer and receive consultation.

The authors are a psychiatric CNS with a background in psychiatric liaison nursing and a primary care nurse practitioner (NP) with a gerontology and adult health emphasis. Both are currently nursing faculty members. The synergy that developed from their collaboration and the sharing of experiences and perspectives was enriching and energizing and perhaps underscores the most fundamental points of this book—that there is much common ground across roles, that APNs have much to offer one another, and that together they can effect important changes.

This chapter has several goals. First, consultation is distinguished from supervision, collaboration, referral, and co-management. Of concern to the authors is the fact that these terms continue to be used interchangeably in practice without clear distinctions. Each term suggests very distinct relationships and responsibilities. For example, consultation is a role function utilized by APNs to offer their own clinical expertise to other colleagues or to seek additional information to enhance their own practice. Because consultation is often confused with co-management, supervision, and referral in practice settings, these terms are defined to distinguish them from consultation. The authors then describe their model of consultation in advanced practice, and the purposes and processes of consultation are discussed. Current realities of practice are considered and issues are explored. It is the authors' intent to provide more clarity regarding the nature of consultation because it has the potential to increase the APN's ability and skill in providing expert nursing care. APNs can also develop their own consultative skills in order to utilize their expertise to enhance their colleagues' nursing practice. The works of Caplan (1970), Caplan and Caplan (1993), and Lipowski (1974, 1981, 1983) are classic and continue to inform the thinking, writing, and practice of the authors. A number of the sources used to prepare this chapter are classic and currently relevant in spite of early publication dates.

CONSULTATION AND ADVANCED NURSING PRACTICE

Much of the recent literature related to consultation continues to be found in the CNS literature (Ingersoll & Jones, 1992; Norwood, 1998; Scott & Beare, 1993), with the notable exceptions of Monicken (1995) and Manley (1998). Although consultation is part of every APN's practice, the CNS and certified nurse-midwife (CNM) roles appear to address the competency most specifically (American College of Nurse Midwives [ACNM], 1992; Barron, 1983, 1989; Barron & White 1996). For other advanced nursing practice roles, consultation seems to have been less formally described. In CNS roles, consultation was primarily directed toward staff nurses as a way of directly or indirectly influencing patient care. Although CNSs might serve as consultants to physicians and other clinicians, staff nurses and their patients are the primary focus. The ACNM (1992) identifies consultation with physicians as one of several communicative/interactive processes used in providing well-woman care.

APNs should be aware that state laws and regulations may mandate a consulting physician as a requirement for advanced practice and prescriptive privileges. The wording of such mandates often directly states or implies a hierarchical relationship between APN and physician, which is contrary to the description of consultation being put forth here. Minarik and Price (1999) described the critical importance of conceptual clarity for legislative and regulatory reform. At the state and federal levels, medical societies are attempting to limit APN practice—the terminology included in the legislation describing the relationship between physicians and APNs is of enormous significance. They make the compelling argument that the practical effect of legislation related to financing of health care can be devastating to APN practice even though state boards of nursing are quite clear in their regulations about the appropriateness of the expanded scope of practice for APNs. Being sophisticated readers of legislative proposals that include mandated relationships between physicians and APNs is critical. As legislation is drafted regarding both scope of practice and direct reimbursement for practice, APNs need to be clear and articulate about the implications of such terms such as "collaboration," "supervision," "direction," and "consultation." Medical societies may use such terminology with a clear intent to mandate hierarchical relationships with physicians in order to limit APN practice. Because mandated relationships between APNs and physicians may constrain APN consultation, it is important that APNs be aware of the statutes and norms that regulate their practices.

The goals and outcomes of consultation are relevant to the current health care debate. APNs can help to bring about the national goal of high-quality, cost-effective health care for every American. Through consultation, APNs create networks with other APNs, physicians, and other colleagues, offering and receiving advice and information that can improve patient care and one's clinical knowledge and skills. Interacting with colleagues in other disciplines can enhance interdisciplinary collaboration (see Chapter 11). Consultation can also help to shape and develop the practices of consultees and protégés, thereby indirectly but significantly improving the quality, depth, and comprehensiveness of care available to populations of patients and families. Consultation offers APNs the opportunity to positively influence health care outcomes beyond the direct patient care encounter.

Given the importance of consultation for all APNs, it is surprising that so little emphasis is reflected in other APN nursing literature. Consultation within APN practice may be largely invisible (with the exception of CNS practice), but consultation activities may be an important variable in explaining the effectiveness of APNs. The authors urge all APNs to recognize the significance of consultation within their practices and to communicate the issues, concerns, and successes of this aspect of practice. It is also essential that APN researchers study the role that timely consultations play in the high-quality, cost-effective care delivered by APNs. Consultation is a variable that ought to be considered in health care outcomes research. Looking specifically at APN consultation in relation to outcomes may shed some light on the elusive phenomenon of nurse-sensitive outcomes in care.

DEFINING CONSULTATION

The term "consultation" is used in many ways. It is sometimes used to describe direct care: the practitioner is in consultation with the patient. It is also used interchangeably with "referral" or "collaboration." For example, a staff nurse might request consultation with the oncology CNS so that the CNS could assume management of the patient's pain. It is also used when there is a hierarchical or supervisory relationship and the person without decision-making authority presents an issue to the person with such authority for a decision. For example, a psychiatric CNS might consult with the psychiatrist regarding inpatient admission for a patient. Some consultants always see the patient being considered, and some consultants never see the patient being considered. It can be confusing, indeed, to know how the term is being used in any given situation and to therefore know exactly what is being requested and what is expected. The more precisely "consultation" is defined, the more likely consultation will be utilized well for its intended purposes. Because consultation is a core competency of advanced nursing practice, such precision is needed for communication within and outside the profession regarding APN roles and patient care. Although consultations can enhance patient care and promote positive professional relationships, it is important to understand the differences between consultation and other types of professional interactions. Table 8–1 summarizes these differences, which are further described in the remainder of this section.

Distinguishing Consultation from Co-management, Referral, and Collaboration

Providing direct care involves a variety of interactions with colleagues. "Consultation," "collaboration," "co-management," and "referral" are, at times, used interchangeably but should not be. Lack of clarity about the specific process being used for clinical problem solving leads to confusion about roles and clinical accountability. The primary characteristic that distinguishes consultation from co-management, referral, and supervision is the degree to which one assumes responsibility for the direct clinical management of a problem that falls within one's area of expertise. *Consultation* is an interaction between two professionals in which the consultant is recognized as having specialized expertise (Caplan, 1970; Caplan & Caplan, 1993). The consultee requests the assistance of that expert in the handling of a problem that she or he recognizes as falling within the expertise of the consultant. *Co-management* is the process whereby one professional manages some aspects of a patient's care while another professional manages other aspects of the same patient's care. Often, co-management takes place between professionals who consider themselves part of the same interdisciplinary team. Effective co-management requires excellent communication, coordination, and collaborative skills. *Referral,* another frequently encountered term, describes a situation in which the clinician making the referral relinquishes responsibility for care (or aspects of care), either temporarily or permanently.

Caplan and Caplan (1993), Spross (1989), and Hanson and Spross (1996) discussed collaboration in some depth. Collaboration is raised as an issue for consideration in relation to consultation because it has been the authors' experience that APNs are confused about the differences between collaboration and consultation. Hanson and

TABLE 8-1	CLARIFYING DEFINITIONS OF CLINICAL CONSULTATION, CO-MANAGEMENT, REFERRAL, AND SUPERVISION		
TYPE OF INTERACTION	GOALS	FOCUS	RESPONSIBILITY FOR CLINICAL OUTCOMES
Clinical consultation	To enhance patient care and/ or improve skills and confidence of consultee	Consultant may or may not see patient directly Degree of focus on consultee's skill is negotiated with consultee	Remains with consultee, who is free to accept or reject the advice of consultant
Co-management	To enhance patient care through availability of expertise of two (or more) professionals working together to optimize outcomes	Both professionals see patient directly and coordinate their care with one another (e.g., physician may monitor complex medication regimen while APN focuses on adaptation and human responses)	Shared
Referral	To enhance patient care by relinquishing care (or aspects of care) to another professional whose expertise is perceived to be more essential to care than is that of the professional who is referring	Establish connection between patient and professional who is accepting referral Negotiate responsibilities for outcomes	Negotiated, but responsibility is often assumed (at least for aspects of care) by professional accepting referral
Supervision	To enhance patient care by overseeing the work of a less senior professional	On developing the skill of the supervisee	Supervisor and supervisee

Spross (see Chapter 11) offer a thoughtful definition of *collaboration* slightly modified from the one they proposed in 1996:

> *A dynamic, interpersonal process in which two or more individuals make a commitment to each other to interact authentically and constructively to solve problems and to learn from each other in order to accomplish identified goals, purposes, or outcomes. The individuals recognize and articulate the shared values that make this commitment possible.*

(Chapter 11, p. 318)

This definition suggests that collaboration is a process that underlies the professional interactions involved in consultation, co-management, referral, and supervision. Therefore the discussion of consultation assumes collaboration as essential to the process. This differs from the definition of collaboration used in the chapter on consultation in the previous edition of this text (Barron & White, 1996), but offers conceptual clarity, which is very useful.

Distinguishing Consultation from Clinical and Administrative Supervision

Caplan and Caplan (1993), Critchley (1985), and Lewis and Levy (1982) described clinical supervision in mental health practice. The process of supervision can be helpful for enhancing the practice of clinicians, especially novice clinicians, regardless of specialty area. APNs can be competent supervisors. There are characteristics of supervision that distinguish it from consultation, and it is important that the supervisor and supervisee understand that supervision is different from consultation. The term "clinical supervision," as used in mental health, describes an ongoing supportive and educational process between a more senior and expert clinician and a less senior, more novice clinician. The goals of clinical supervision are to develop the knowledge, skills, self-esteem, and autonomy of the supervisee (Caplan & Caplan, 1993). Unlike the consultant, the supervisor generally is responsible for safeguarding the care of the supervisee's patients and is accountable in that respect for the work of the supervisee (Caplan & Caplan, 1993). Also unlike the consultant, who is often an outsider to the organization or unit where the consultation occurs, the supervisor and supervisee commonly are employed by the same organization and work together in the same clinical area. The supervisor and supervisee generally are in hierarchical positions, with the supervisor being in a higher position (Caplan & Caplan, 1993).

Although the ultimate goal of supervision and consultation are the same, namely, assisting another professional to enhance knowledge, skills, and abilities as they care for patients and families, the processes, relationships, and responsibilities are different. Administrative supervision (e.g., vice president for nursing of APNs) has much in common with clinical supervision (e.g., hierarchical relationship, responsibility for professional development of APNs). In administrative supervision, however, interactions are likely to focus on operations and the APN's ability to meet job responsibilities rather than the day-to-day clinical management of patients.

BACKGROUND

Consultation in Mental Health Practice

Gerald Caplan, the father of mental health consultation theory (Simmons, 1985), recognized that there were many more needs to be addressed in the Israeli community in which he worked than could possibly be met by available mental health professionals (Caplan & Caplan, 1993). In the late 1940s, Caplan and a small team of psychologists and social workers were expected to meet the mental health needs of 16,000 new immigrant children in Jerusalem. He developed his consultation model in response to these pressing needs. By consulting with other professionals, such as teachers and counselors, he found the recipients of consultation could effectively meet many of the mental health needs of the children. Both the need that gave rise to this model and the model itself are relevant to APNs, who must consider strategies that enable patients and families, beyond their direct practice reach, to benefit from APN knowledge and skills.

Lipowski (1981) also developed a model of mental health consultation for use in the general hospital setting. He stressed that it is essential for consultants to understand the context of the consultation situation. He recommended that consultation include an evaluation of the patient, the patient's interactions with the staff, and the specific needs of the consultee (the staff member). The family and social supports are considered as well. The consultant carefully communicates with the staff and provides regular follow-up of the patient for the course of the hospitalization. Although the Kaplan and Lipowski models were developed for application in mental health, they have informed the authors' evolving model of advanced nursing practice consultation.

Types of Consultation

There are four different types of consultation (Caplan, 1970). *Client-centered case consultation* is the most common type of consultation. The primary goal of this type of consultation is assisting the consultee to develop an effective plan of care for a patient who has a particularly difficult or complex problem. In client-centered case consultation, the consultant often sees the patient directly to complete an assessment of the patient and to make recommendations to the consultee for the consultee's management of the case. This is often a one-time evaluation. Follow-up by the consultant sometimes is needed. The primary goal is to assist the consultee in helping the patient. A positive experience with handling that specific case will enhance the consultee's ability so that future patients with similar problems can be managed more effectively.

In *consultee-centered case consultation,* improving patient care is important, but the emphasis is focused directly on the consultee's problem in handling the situation. Thus, the primary goal is to assist the consultee to acquire the knowledge, skill, confidence, or objectivity needed to address the problem effectively. In consultee-centered case consultation, the task for the consultant is to understand and remedy the problems of the consultee in managing a particular case. Usual problems, as noted, are lack of knowledge, skill, confidence, or objectivity. Thus the consultant may educate the consultee further on the issues presented by the patient or may suggest alternative strategies for dealing with the problem. This is probably the most common type of consultation sought by APNs. The consultant may seek to bolster the confidence of the consultee in handling the problem, if in the opinion of the consultant the consultee has the ability and potential to do so. If the problem presented by the consultee is a lack of professional objectivity, the consultant can help the consultee to identify the factors interfering with the consultee's ability to see the patient realistically. It may be that the consultee holds a stereotyped view of the patient, or perhaps the patient's difficulties in some way mirror or symbolize the consultee's personal difficulties and cloud the consultee's ability to see the reality of the situation. Effective consultation can foster orderly reflection and extend the frames of reference used by the consultee to solve clinical problems (Caplan & Caplan, 1993). Both client-centered and consultee-centered case consultations have been important activities in traditional CNS practice.

Program-centered administrative consultation focuses on the planning and administration of clinical services. *Consultee-centered administrative consultation* focuses on the consultee's (or group of consultees') difficulties as they interfere with the organization's objectives. APNs may be involved in all four types of consultation at various times. This chapter specifically considers client-centered case consultation and consultee-centered case consultation, because the focus of this chapter is the process of interacting with other professionals regarding the care of individual patients.

A MODEL OF ADVANCED NURSING PRACTICE CONSULTATION

Principles of Consultation

The model of advanced nursing practice consultation proposed by the authors is based on the following principles of consultation derived from the field of mental health (Caplan, 1970; Caplan & Caplan, 1993; Lipowski, 1981):

1. The consultation is usually initiated by the consultee.
2. The relationship between the consultant and consultee is nonhierarchical and collaborative.
3. The consultant always considers contextual factors when responding to the request for consultation.
4. The consultant has no direct authority for managing patient care.
5. The consultant does not prescribe but makes recommendations.
6. The consultee is free to accept or reject the recommendations of the consultant.
7. The consultation should be documented.

Description of the Model

Barron (1989) proposed a model of consultation for CNSs that was based on the nursing process and incorporated principles from Caplan's (1970; Caplan & Caplan, 1993) and Lipowski's (1974, 1981, 1983) work. This model, expanded by Barron and White (1996), has evolved into the model of advanced nursing practice consultation described in Figure 8-1. APNs tend to have a holistic orientation and an understanding of systems theory which will enable them to apply this consultation model in practice. At the center of the authors' proposed model are the purposes and outcomes of consultation which are essentially the same. Surrounding the center is the ecological field of the consultation. Consultations are embedded in the context of the specific circumstances surrounding the consultation request, so the ecological field in which the consultation takes place must be understood to provide effective consultation (Caplan & Caplan, 1993). This involves an appreciation for the interconnection and inter-relatedness of the systems and contexts influencing the consultation problem and process. Thus, the consultation process is an integral part of the ecological field. The process, in which the consultant evaluates the request, performs an assessment, determines the skills required to address the problem, intervenes, and evaluates the outcome, is further expanded in Figure 8-2. Other elements of the ecological field include the characteristics of the consultant, characteristics of the consultee, characteristics of the patient and family, and situational factors. The authors assume that there are reciprocal influences among the purposes, process, and contextual factors that can affect consultation processes and outcomes. Each component of the model is elaborated below.

PURPOSES AND OUTCOMES

The purpose of a consultation may be to improve patient outcomes, enhance health care delivery systems, extend the knowledge available to solve clinical problems,

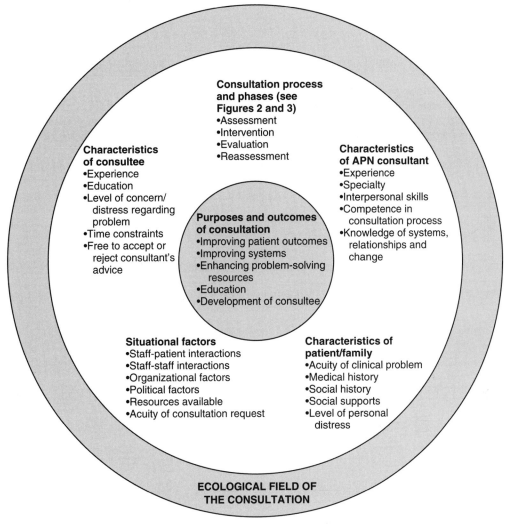

FIGURE 8-1 • A model of APN consultation.

and/or foster the ongoing professional development of the consultee. Consultants should be aware that the purposes for which they have been consulted may change or expand during the process of consulting. Often, APN consultants accomplish several purposes at once. If one uncovers additional purposes and possible outcomes during consultation, these should be made clear to the consultee. It may be that the consultee wants the consultant's assistance with a patient but does not have the time or interest to focus on her or his own development. It is also possible that patients reveal information that requires a shift in the consultation's focus, purpose, and outcome. Over the course of the consultation, being explicit about the goal or outcome of the consultation is essential if APNs are to evaluate the impact of consultation on practice.

THE CONSULTATION PROCESS

Figure 8-2 presents an algorithm of the consultation process. With experience and expertise, the process may occur fairly rapidly so that the expert consultant may not be aware of using these steps consciously. In addition, there are situations in which the problem for which help is sought is clear cut and the consultation is brief. These are discussed later in the chapter.

Assessment of the consultation problem begins with evaluation of the request itself. An important component of assessment is to confirm with the consultee that consultation is, in fact, the appropriate strategy for addressing the problem (rather than a referral, for example). At this stage, it is possible that the consultant and consultee decide that an alternative process is needed (e.g., shifting to co-management or referral). The consultant confirms that the problem has been accurately identified and falls within the realm of the consultant's expertise, and clarifies the nonhierarchical nature of the relationship between the consultant and consultee. The consultant also confirms that the consultee will remain clinically responsible for the patient who is the focus of the consultation. The consultant must remember that the consultee is ultimately free to accept or reject her or his recommendations. Once the request itself has been considered, the consultant gathers information from the consultee about the specific nature of the problem. The consultant tries to determine whether

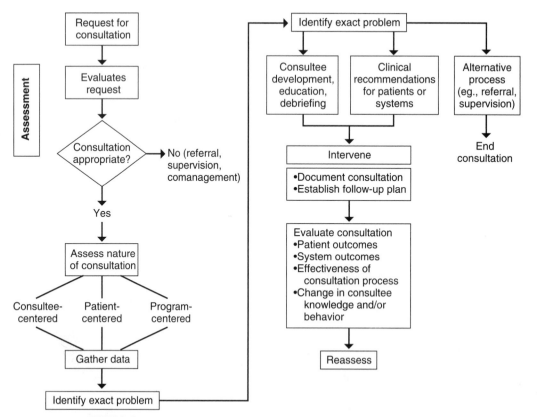

FIGURE 8-2 • Algorithm for consultation process.

the patient has unusually difficult and complex problems (patient-centered consultation) and whether the problem results from the consultee's lack of knowledge, skill, confidence, or objectivity (consultee-centered consultation). Once the request, the nature of the relationship, and appropriateness of consultation have been established, the consultant focuses on gathering data related to the consultation problem. This may include direct assessment of the patient. The consultant considers the ecological field of the consultation, which includes the systems and contexts that may influence the patient and family, the consultee and staff, and the setting in which the consultation takes place.

The consultant uses available resources such as patient records, direct assessment of the patient, and interviews with staff to *identify the exact problem* or problems that are to be the focus of consultation. This may or may not be the one for which help was sought. Some consultation problems are simple and do not require extensive data collection. Others are complex and may require extensive chart review for a longstanding problem or calls to referring clinicians when incomplete data have been provided. The consultant shares the identified problem with the consultee and validates this with the consultee. If the problem includes lack of expertise of the consultee, the consultant will want to use tact as the problem is identified and discussed. Interpersonal qualities of the consultant are crucial and are discussed later in this chapter.

Once the specific problem or problems have been identified, the consultant and consultee *consider interventions* that will address the problem(s). The consultant may intervene directly with the consultee using such approaches as education, assisting with reinterpretation of the problem, or identification of appropriate resources if the problem is the consultee's lack of experience with the consultation problem. If the problem results from a particularly difficult patient situation, the consultant may assist with the process of clinical decision making by providing alternative perspectives on the problem and recommending specific interventions. It may be that more data are needed to further analyze the situation and a decision needs to be made about whether the consultee or consultant will gather more data. If the consultee accepts the recommendations of the consultant, together they negotiate how the interventions will be carried out and by whom. If the consultant is to intervene directly with the patient, the consultee must understand her or his ongoing responsibility for the patient and agree to the consultant's interventions. Together they identify additional resources and determine the time frame for the consultation (one time or ongoing).

Following the intervention, the consultant and consultee engage in *evaluation*. Evaluating the success or lack of success of the intervention and the overall consultation is essential to the consultation process. If the problem is resolved, evaluation offers an opportunity for review, confirmation of the enhanced effectiveness of the consultee in managing the problem (underscoring the new skills and abilities or understanding of the situation by the consultee), and closure. If problems remain, reassessment offers the consultant and consultee another opportunity for problem solving.

ECOLOGICAL FIELD OF THE CONSULTATION PROCESS

Characteristics of the APN Consultant. In addition to theoretical understanding, self-awareness and interpersonal skills are essential for the consultant (Barron, 1989; Barron & White, 1996). For a model of consultative practice to be implemented, it is critical that APNs first value themselves and the specialized expertise they have developed. One must appreciate one's skills and knowledge before the possibilities for consultation can be envisioned (see Chapter 3). APNs have developed specialized expertise in the direct care of underserved populations, such as those who are homeless; the frail elderly; those who are chronically mentally ill, home-bound, or institutionalized; and patients with human immunodeficiency virus infection. The knowledge and skill developed by these APNs could serve to inform and expand the practices of staff nurses, other APNs, and health care professionals of various disciplines involved in the care of these populations of patients. The APNs must first appreciate that they have valuable understanding and knowledge to share, however.

Ideally, consultants know themselves well—they are aware of their own personal issues, strengths, weaknesses, and motives. A good consultant must be able to suspend judgment and avoid stereotyping. When consultation is sought, often what is needed is a fresh perspective. Self-understanding allows the consultant to see consultation issues realistically and without prejudice. It is not uncommon for a consultant to step into a highly emotionally charged situation. Self-awareness, understanding, and being able to remain centered and self-possessed are key to remaining objective and clear. It can be meaningful and helpful for the consultant to have a trusted colleague or supervisor with whom to share and review consultation situations. Such discussions can offer support and enhance one's understanding of personal and interpersonal responses to the consultation material.

It is also important that the consultant be able to establish warm, respectful, and accepting relationships with consultees. The initiation of a consultation request often is associated with a sense of vulnerability on the part of the consultee, who recognizes that assistance is required to help manage the situation at hand. The consultant must communicate (and sincerely believe) that the problem and the consultee are important and worthy of consideration. The consultant must also communicate confidence in the consultee's ability to overcome the difficulties resulting in the consultation request. When the consultant creates a climate of trust and acceptance, the consultee can then be willing to risk vulnerability and genuineness with the consultant. When a respectful, trusting connection is made between the consultant and consultee, a deep examination of the problem, implications, and solutions is possible.

It is important to understand that APNs are sometimes the consultee and often the consultation is made to a physician. As a consultee, the APN should be able to identify and articulate the nature of the problem for which help is being sought. It may be necessary to clarify the collegial, nonhierarchical nature of the consultation relationship. When consulting with an APN colleague or physician, APNs often have tried alternative plans or are thinking about possible directions to take based on their knowledge of the patient or clinical situation. Consultants find such information useful in planning their approaches to the consultation. Such dialogue can improve the effectiveness and efficiency of the consultation and can strengthen collaboration among colleagues.

In addition to their intrapersonal knowledge and interpersonal skills, APNs must be competent in the consultative process. To be an effective consultant, it is also important to be knowledgeable about systems, relationships, and change. While skill in consultation develops over time, the consultant attributes and consultation process described here can help novice APNs who are open to learning approach consultation with confidence (see "Developing Consultation Skills in APN Students" later in this chapter).

Characteristics of the Consultee. The consultee identifies a problem that exists in a clinical situation because of a lack of knowledge or uncertainty and believes that increased knowledge and assistance with clinical decision making would enhance practice. Depending on the consultee, there may be characteristics of the consultee to consider. Education, experience, level of distress (the consultee's) regarding the clinical problem for which help is sought, organizational skills, and availability to problem solve with the consultant are factors that can influence the consultation.

Patient and Family Factors. Among factors to consider are the acuity and complexity of the clinical problem, medical history, social history, social supports, and other resources. Depending on the nature of the problem, it may be important to consider concurrent stresses being experienced by the patient and family. An acute problem may demand the consultant's immediate assistance, requiring a shift in the consultant's priorities. A complex or unusual problem may take more time to solve.

Situational Factors. Numerous situational factors can affect the consultation process. The quality of relationships and interactions between staff and patients or among staff members themselves may be important issues. For example, a patient perceived as being nonadherent to some therapy may be responding to conflicts among team members the patient has inferred from clinicians' behaviors. A clinician may seek validation from a consultant as a way of getting support for an unpopular approach. Time pressures and lack of adequate resources can affect consultation. Organizational politics, power imbalances, and rapid or frequent systems changes are other things to consider. All of these factors can affect the consultee's view of the importance of the request.

For APNs, the status of advanced nursing practice and APNs in one's agency or state may influence consultation. For example, organizational policies and procedures regarding consultation, statutes regarding APN-physician "consulting" relationships, reimbursement policies, and degree of prescriptive authority may affect the consultation process.

COMMON APN CONSULTATION SITUATIONS

Depending on one's particular APN role, certain consultation situations may be more common than others. Patient- and consultee-centered case consultations are the most common requests APNs are likely to get. These types of consultations are described in this section. Experienced APNs may extend their consultative skills into other types of consultations, such as program centered. The exemplars included here vary in the complexity of consultations and the extent to which aspects of the consultation model are made explicit. Readers are encouraged to examine the ways in which the proposed model of ANP consultation is applied.

APN-APN Consultation

Within one's specialty or agency, APNs may take for granted the available APN consulting resources. They may not think of their interactions about patient care as consultation because they occur in the hallway or over coffee. Consultation among APNs may be more or less formal depending on the culture of the unit or clinic, the relationships among the APNs, and the specialty populations seen in the facility. Consultations are likely to involve specific patient issues—for example, "Could you look at this rash? I've never seen one quite like this before," or "I've done everything I can think of to try to make sure this pregnant teen comes to her prenatal visits and she still misses them. Here's what I've done . . . can you think of anything else before I get the City Department of Social Services involved?" An example of a formal APN-to-APN consultation follows.

Norwood (1998) discussed the importance of, and practicalities related to, APNs' seeking consultation from other APNs. She noted that APNs readily think of themselves as consultants but may overlook opportunities for seeking consultation. She outlined the following factors as relevant when considering the use of a consultant: cost savings, objectivity, politics, when not to seek consultation, and issues to consider when choosing a consultant.

In many settings, APNs may have some clinical as well as supervisory responsibilities. For example, a senior NP may supervise other APNs and staff as well as have a patient caseload. The supervisory relationship may constrain the consultation process as it is described here. An NP seeking consultation from a supervisor may worry that such a request reflects poorly on clinical competency. It is important to be aware that the nature of the relationship (i.e., whether it is with a colleague or a supervisor) can affect the consultation process. Given the authors' belief that a nonhierarchical relationship is essential for true consultation, it may be more accurate to refer to interactions with a supervisor as problem solving. Regardless of what the interaction is called, these types of interactions are important for professional development and optimal patient care. As APNs integrate consultation more explicitly into their practices and reflect on the process and outcomes of consultation, future discussions might illuminate this consultation dilemma.

EXEMPLAR   1

The medical-surgical CNS consulted the psychiatric liaison nurse regarding the care of a severely burned young man who had been transferred to the surgical service from the intensive care unit (ICU). An initial problem to be addressed was the frequent and painful dressing changes. The patient disliked the lingering effects of narcotic analgesia for the dressing changes, but clearly needed assistance with the pain during the dressing changes. The medical-surgical CNS asked if the psychiatric liaison nurse could teach the patient relaxation and imagery strategies for the dressing changes (and if the strategies proved to be helpful for the patient, also teach the staff to coach the patient with these tools). The medical-surgical CNS also recognized that there were many complex and difficult psychosocial issues to be confronted by the patient as he recovered. His hands and face were significantly burned. He would likely be permanently disfigured and disabled. She requested that the liaison nurse provide additional supportive care to the patient and be available to the staff as they planned for the psychosocial dimension of his care.

The patient and staff found relaxation and imagery techniques to be quite helpful for the dressing changes. The liaison nurse and staff planned his care together with the clear intention of providing a climate of trust, acceptance, and openness with the hope that the patient would experience himself as whole and respected and worthwhile in his relationships with them. In spite of his severe and disfiguring burns, the nurses could access the beauty of the patient's humanity as they established intentional relationships with him. They helped him to experience the depths of himself, which transcended the limits established by the burns. They helped him plan his first visit with his young child, preparing the patient for potential reactions and helping the patient to prepare his child for his first visit. Follow-up mental health care was arranged at discharge. (AMB).

Another example of APN-APN consultation is illustrated in the following scenario.

EXEMPLAR 2

A NP caring for an adolescent patient is concerned about the high-risk sexual practices her patient is reporting. Despite the rapport and longstanding nature of the relationship with her patient, the NP feels the need for additional expertise in order to facilitate caring for this patient. The APN sought the consultation of an NP colleague with clinical and research expertise in the area of adolescent health care. The APN caring for the patient incorporated her suggestions and advice into her plan of care for the patient. This APN-APN exchange depicts client-centered consultation. The expert provided important knowledge and suggestions, yet was not responsible for how the consulting APN utilized this information. The consultant provided important perspectives and input and indirectly affected the patient's care, yet was not responsible for the consultee's decision making or outcomes of care. (PAW).

APN-Physician Consultation

When consulting with other APNs or physicians, an APN is likely to be fairly far along in the problem-solving process. The need for consultation is often related to the consultee's level of diagnostic uncertainty (Colman, 1992). Experienced APNs often have a clear definition of the problem and a preliminary plan to address it that they wish to validate or reformulate, depending on the consultant's advice. APN-APN or APN-physician consultation is sophisticated and high level.

The need for statutory language that clearly describes the autonomous nature of APN practice has been addressed (Safriet, 1992; Birkholz & Walker, 1994) and continues. The ACNM (1992) was deliberate in describing the various kinds of interactions CNMs have, primarily with physicians. Unfortunately, as noted earlier, APN-physician consultative relationships have often been structured by laws and regulations that mandate or imply a supervisory relationship, which can reinforce stereotypical nurse-physician relationships. Many organizational cultures reinforce traditional nurse-physician relationships and the behavioral norms associated with them. One of the major challenges facing ANP educators is to explicitly address socialization to nurse-physician relationships that may undermine full expression of autonomous APN practice. When a hierarchical relationship exists between an APN and a physician, the APN who consults with a physician may defer to the physician's decisions, downplaying or ignoring first-hand knowledge of the patient. However, numerous descriptions of successful collaborative practices between physicians and APNs exist (Barron & White, 1996). Such practices embrace the nonhierarchical relationship we believe is key to effective consultation (see Chapter 11).

There are APN-physician exchanges where true consultation occurs; however, much of the language that defines relationships between APNs and physicians involve the terms "co-management," "referral," and "supervision." Physicians in primary care often seek the consultation of APNs regarding such issues as assisting clients in making lifestyle changes or in coping with the effects of chronic illness. Many APNs in primary care have special expertise in women's health care and are sought out by physicians for their consultation on such issues. Physicians might then choose to co-manage clients with APNs so that clients benefit from the expertise of both professionals. APNs in turn might seek the consultation of a physician regarding a medically unstable client, which evolves into co-management by the physician and APN each assuming responsibility for the outcomes of decision making. Consultation between APNs and physicians can highlight for each what APNs know—that is, a deep appreciation for the human responses related to health and illness—and what physicians know, a deep understanding of disease and treatment. When both areas of expertise are available to patients and their families, truly holistic, comprehensive, and individualized care is offered.

As APN knowledge evolves and deepens, an emerging issue in relation to APN-physician consultation is the crossover of traditional nurse-physician boundaries. As APNs become more and more specialized, the knowledge embedded in practice may be more closely related to what is generally thought of as medical practice. For example, an oncology CNS may have very highly developed skills in the area of pain management. As a physician consults with the CNS on an individual patient, the CNS may make recommendations for specific medications. Whether or not the APN has prescriptive authority, an appreciation for the inherent shifts in the usual "professional territories" of nurses and physicians and the need for flexibility are helpful. Tact and understanding of the longstanding boundaries that are being crossed can bring the consultation relationship to a new level.

APN–Staff Nurse Consultation

As CNSs implemented their consultative roles, it became apparent that the culture of nursing had not adopted consultation as an important strategy in providing patient care (Barron, 1983). Staff nurses were expected to take care of the patients themselves. A novice might consult a head nurse or more senior nurse, but staff were expected to know how to solve problems and use the policy and procedures manual. Part of implementing consultation meant teaching staff how and when to consult. In the early days, CNSs often engaged in active case-finding to identify the patients who needed the knowledge and skills they had, because CNSs were not "assigned" to patients and staff nurses. By building this kind of clinical caseload, they demonstrated to staff how consultation might be helpful. Of note, CNSs tended both to do direct consultation and to consult with other professionals to assist the staff with problem solving and enhancing patient care. For example, staff nurses might call the medical-surgical CNS regarding a patient with Guillain-Barré syndrome because they had had no previous experience caring for patients with this disorder. The CNS may have had little or no experience as well but would mobilize the resources needed, such as arranging in-services by the neuroscience or rehabilitation CNS, providing articles, being available to staff on all shifts as they implement unfamiliar assessments, and assisting with care plan development. The CNS would initiate processes (including additional consultation) and provide knowledge directly.

Once relationships are established and staff perceive that the APN consultant is approachable, respectful, and helpful, then staff will initiate contact with the consultant when complex clinical issues arise. The following example illustrates ICU nurses requesting a psychiatric liaison nursing consultation. The staff and consultant had a well-established relationship.

EXEMPLAR 3

A young adult male had been admitted to the ICU several hours before consultation was sought, following an overdose of acetaminophen. Unfortunately, a large quantity of acetaminophen had been ingested the night before and many hours had passed before he and his family sought medical assistance. His medical condition was grave. The psychiatric consultation service had been consulted to render an opinion about the current suicidal risk for the patient. The nurses were very concerned about the young man and his family. The patient was expressing regret about the overdose, saying he was no longer suicidal. He was terrified by the potential for slipping into liver failure and dying. His mother was beside herself with guilt. The patient had come home the night before intoxicated, telling his mother that he had taken the acetaminophen. She did not believe him—she thought he was looking for sympathy to avoid getting into trouble in relation to his drinking. She also reasoned that, if he had taken the acetaminophen, it was no big deal; after all, it was a relatively mild and safe drug. When he woke up in the morning very ill, she brought him to the local emergency room for care. He was treated initially and sent by ambulance to the medical center.

The gastroenterologist was not at all confident that liver failure could be prevented. The psychiatrists assessed the patient to no longer be at risk of suicide. Everyone involved was deeply moved and distressed by the tragedy they were witnessing. The nurses requested that the liaison nurse be available for additional supportive care for the patient, support and referral for the family, and assistance in planning nursing care for the patient.

After about a day and a half, the patient slipped into a coma. It became clear that he was dying. His mother had accepted referral to her local mental health center, which was arranged by the psychiatric consult service and liaison nurse. For the first 2 days the mother was in the unit most of the time. She spoke openly with staff and the liaison nurse about her guilt, regret, and pain. After her son became comatose, she did not spend much time in the unit. She said it was just too painful for her to see him deteriorate. Other family members and friends spent much time on the unit. The liaison nurse stopped by the unit frequently, talking with staff and with family members. Everyone (including the liaison nurse) had a great need to talk through the sorrow and sense of impotence in the situation. Everything that could be done was being done—but that was not enough to change the outcome.

The patient had lived for 5 days, but on Friday evening, when the liaison nurse was leaving for the weekend, it was clear that death was not far away. She invited the staff to call her if they needed her over the weekend. The nurses called her and asked her to come very late on Friday evening. They sensed that the patient would die within a matter of minutes or hours and they were concerned about how to respond to his mother when he actually died.

The liaison nurse came in and was present with the family and friends there to support the patient dying. His mother did not return to the hospital. Hands were held, songs chanted, and tears shed as the patient peacefully slipped into death. Unit nurses were in and out of the room also, being present as time allowed. After the emotionally tumultuous week with the young patient, there was some sense of satisfaction in knowing that, if his death could not be prevented, a peaceful death could be facilitated. The family and friends expressed their deep gratitude for that facilitation.

The client-centered consultation focused on the needs of the patient and family primarily. The consultant and staff regularly shared their own feelings of impotence and despair with one another as they discussed the care of the patient. That sharing and planning helped to shape the nursing perspective in the situation and clarify the goal of promoting a peaceful and comfortable death, once cure was no longer a viable goal. The consultation contributed to an active and compassionate nursing presence in the midst of tragedy and pain. (AMB).

FORMAL AND INFORMAL CONSULTATION

The process of consultation described previously is comprehensive and formal. The consultant brings clinical expertise as well as an understanding and appreciation of the process of consultation to the problem presented. According to the model, the consultant considers all elements of the nursing process in relation to the consultation problem. What about the quick questions to the consultant, when what is needed is a piece of information and a quick description of how to apply the information? Are these brief interactions related to a circumscribed problem true consultation? Absolutely, but the consultant needs to make a conscious decision about responding in a brief and simple way to the request and needs to consider with the consultee whether or not the quick response addresses the problem. There are times when the problem presented oversimplifies a complex concern requiring a more comprehensive approach. If the consultant and consultee consider the problem together, they can determine whether the quick response is adequate or whether consultation is needed. Conversely, there are times when what is truly needed is a short answer to a clinical question or validation that the approach to the problem is appropriate.

Staff nurses, at times, equate this brief type of consultation with consultation in general because they have experienced only this type of consultation with physicians, who quickly impart information and are then off to the next patient. The idea of the roving clinical expert dropping by with tidbits of expert advice is indeed the notion non-APNs can have of a consultant. That is another reason why it is important to make a conscious decision about responding in a brief way to the consultation request. In the informal situation, the consultee may not realize that a more comprehensive and thorough investigation of the problem and solutions with the consultant is possible. Also, there are clinical situations that require a more formal approach to the consultation problem. The authors suggest that APNs consider the kinds of problems in practice that require a formal approach and develop a system for integrating nurse-nurse and interdisciplinary consultations that make APN skills more visible and extend their knowledge and skills.

MECHANISMS TO FACILITATE CONSULTATION

Mechanisms to facilitate consultation need to be considered by all APNs regardless of setting. Traditionally, CNSs have offered consultation to staff in institutions where they are employed. Consultation is an explicit role expectation for CNSs and often a daily activity for these APNs. These services are rarely costed out or considered as directly reimbursable activities. As health care becomes more community focused and as APNs provide care to increasingly diverse and vulnerable populations, the breadth and depth of skills required for these newer roles are considerable. APN-APN consultation is an important way to develop these skills.

Current reimbursement mechanisms do not reimburse indirect patient care activities, as much as those activities may improve outcomes for patient care (Sebus, 1994). To the extent that APNs and other disciplines can demonstrate the benefits of consultation, this shortcoming of the current payment system for health care services should be addressed as part of reform efforts. With the current focus on reimbursement for direct care activities and capitation-based reimbursement, it seems unlikely that additional, specific funds will be available in the near future for consultative activities. Creative strategies for funding consultation need to be developed. For example, incorporating APN consultation into critical pathways for selected populations can be one strategy for ensuring the cost-effectiveness of capitation-based reimbursement and building in bottom-line consideration of consultation services.

Boyd and co-workers (1991) described CNS revenue-generating activities at their hospital in Columbia, South Carolina. They described relevant strategies for APNs as they creatively consider sources of funding for consultation services. They obtained third-party reimbursement for patient education and direct patient care. Funding was obtained by selling instructional and informational tapes and books written and produced by CNSs. Notably, they also received substantial funding from grants.

Another strategy is bartering of services among APN colleagues. Members of the Sara Beth Harris Clinical Nurse Specialist Group (A. Spang, personal communication, fall, 1994) described exchanging consultative services with a network of other providers. There was an informal understanding that consultation could be sought with reciprocal availability as consultant when the need arose in the future. APNs may also need to look to professional organizations for assistance in developing mechanisms to market and facilitate nursing consultation. Until the issues of financing and reimbursement in the health care delivery system are resolved and include mechanisms to reimburse consultative activities, creative strategies for this activity will be the responsibility of the profession.

In addition to funding considerations, it is important to consider new settings and potential beneficiaries of APN consultation (see Chapter 21). When the APN is involved in collaborative relationships, clarification of the possibilities for consultation could be discussed and negotiated. The consultant's services could be made available to interdisciplinary teams—even teams of which the APN is a member. Interdisciplinary teams exist in many settings. In addition to working collaboratively on such teams, APNs can offer valuable consultative services. Staff nurses in these settings may be without the benefit of abundant resources to enhance practice and professional development. APNs could offer such opportunities through consultation.

When APNs are the primary providers of care, such as in nursing homes and community health centers, opportunities for consultation may be missed because the most common interactions are collaborative or co-managerial or because of time constraints. Yet in these settings the outcome of consultation is often improved patient care. APNs should consider documenting their consultations in somewhat standard and easily retrievable forms. If such consultations were easy to access, their potential usefulness for research would be greatly enhanced and the effectiveness of consultation could be studied.

As APNs move into innovative practices, they should determine what consultative services they will market and what types of APNs and other consultants are available and will be needed. Consultation between APNs offers the additional benefit of collegial networking. Certified registered nurse anesthetists are establishing private independent practices (see Chapter 18). As independent practitioners, they are offering their services in home health (particularly to assist in the respiratory care of ventilator patients), in pain clinics, and in obstetrical care settings (M. Callahan, personal communication, June 14, 1995). Consultation with other APNs in those settings, in addition to the direct care they offer, has the potential to enhance the knowledge and practice of the APNs and creates co-management and collaborative possibilities for all of the APNs involved.

ISSUES IN ANP CONSULTATION

Developing Consultation Skills in APN Students

To learn the theoretical and practical issues involved with developing the abilities of the APN as consultant, it is important to include relevant content in graduate education curricula. Focusing on the theoretical issues in a seminar and engaging in a project as a clinical consultant was helpful for Barron in her graduate program and has been a strategy that some of her mental health CNS colleagues have described as part of their graduate programs. It is ideal to consider developing consultative skill during the educational process as role identity is beginning to be formed. Although this aspect of skill development may be more commonly part of CNS education, it is relevant for all APN graduate programs if APNs are to integrate the consultation competency into their practices.

Encouraging students to consider how the process of consultation differs from the direct care role and discussing the process and methods are easily accomplished in a professional seminar. The students complete assigned readings ahead of time and engage in a faculty-led discussion of the process and issues. Course requirements should include a clinical consultation project. Students could approach individuals or organizations that might benefit in some way from the sharing of their area of expertise. They would negotiate a consultation issue to focus on and engage in a consultation. In Barron's experience with this model, students were surprised by how well they were received and had a positive experience trying out these skills in a practical and real way. The entire focus on consultation was limited to two seminar discussions and the project, yet it was influential later in terms of position choice and role preparation. Judith Spross (personal communication, May 19, 1995) recommended having graduate APN students from different specialty areas consult one another. She devoted the first 20 minutes of the role seminar she facilitated for graduate APN students to consult with one another.

Students can also be asked to report on their observations of consultation in clinical settings. Students could reflect on the type of consultation offered, the skills demonstrated, the process engaged in, the problem focus, and the outcome. Considering real situations where consultation evolved into co-management or referral offers faculty an opportunity to explicate the differences in the terminology and implications of each type of interaction.

Graduate educators and APNs could collaborate on much-needed research to evaluate the effects of consultative activities on patient outcomes. Documentation of the value and cost-effectiveness of consultation could help to inform curricular decisions. It could also be presented by APNs to insurers and policy makers who determine policy and payment for health care services. Gurka (1991) suggested that some research questions could emerge from analyzing one's own consultations. In an analysis of her own practice, there were three major outcomes of CNS consultation. The first was prevention of complications. The CNS was able to identify high-risk situations and intervene to prevent complications. The second was the maintenance of standards of care and the development of new standards. The CNS's consultation activities assured that high-quality standards of care were consistently maintained. The third outcome she identified was improvement in staff nurses' clinical judgment skills. Students could be required to reflect on the outcomes of their consultation projects as an aspect of the assignment. Encouraging the process of reflection on practice, with a focus on outcomes of care, can help to build important practice "habits" with benefits to the students beyond acquiring consultation skills.

Developing comfort with seeking, providing, and evaluating consultation is an important goal of APN graduate education. APNs are expected to influence patients, other providers, and the systems within which they work. It is vital that they graduate equipped with knowledge, skill, and confidence in the consultation process. Effective consultation, whether seeking or providing it, enables APNs to establish credibility and build collaborative relationships with other members of the health care team.

On-Line Consultation

On-line consultation via the Internet is increasingly available. The legal questions regarding such consultations are complex. The authors suggest that APNs be cautious in relation to on-line consultation and keep abreast of legal challenges and precedents related to on-line health care. The potential benefits of on-line clinical consultation are considerable, but APNs must keep in mind that they may be getting inadequate or incomplete data regarding the patient care situation (see earlier discussion). The legal issues may vary from state to state in relation to on-line consultation. Given that list-serve discussions cross state and national boundaries with ease, APNs engaging in such consultation should seek clarification of legal considerations before offering consultation via the Internet. Also, APNs should keep in mind that few legal precedents have been established so far, because of the newness of the technology. Kuszler (1999) suggested that new technologies exponentially increase the opportunities for formal and informal medical consultations. Whereas the duty to care has been conferred by the courts on consulting physicians in formal rather than informal consultation encounters, the dividing line between the two is not always clear. Technology may further blur the distinctions between the two types of consultation. There is considerable promise in relation to on-line consultation possibilities, but also some peril.

Documentation and Legal Considerations

Although it has been stressed that the consultee remains clinically responsible for the patient who is the focus of the consultation, it is also critical to appreciate that APN consultants are also accountable for their practices relative to the consultation problem. Marie Snyder, RN, MS, JD (personal communication, June 14, 1995), described the overall responsibilities of the consultant as gathering accurate data about the consultation problem (or letting the consultee know that the data are incomplete), making reasonable recommendations, and giving good advice. She stressed that APN consultants who are working within the same organization as the consultees have a higher degree of accountability in relation to the patient care situations for which they are consulted than do consultants who come from outside the organization. APNs consulting within their own organizations would be expected to identify and follow through on urgent concerns and particularly problematic situations in ways that outside consultants would not be. APNs who are consulting should, therefore, know the organizational structure well and be certain that the APN consultation responsibilities are consistent with the overall job description of the APN. That is, if the job description required that APNs be in a line position of authority for a unit or a clinic (thereby being ultimately responsible for clinical care), for example, responsibility would constrain their ability to function as consultants as defined here. The hierarchical/supervisory relationship could interfere with the consultation process.

Kathleen Moore, RN, JD (personal communication, June 16, 1999) stressed that APNs be cognizant of their responsibility to adhere to the standard of practice for their specialty areas in all aspects of practice, including consultation. In terms of liability for consultation, Moore stated that an initial issue to be determined in the event of a suit would be: Does a nurse-patient relationship exist in the consultation situation, thereby invoking the duty of care? Although there are no clear-cut legal answers to the question of liability for consultation services, Moore emphasized the importance of the question as to whether or not a relationship exists between the clinician and the patient. In a court of law, whether or not a relationship exists would be a question of fact. If a relationship exists, then liability attaches. The likelihood of determining that there was a nurse-patient relationship increases when the consultant sees the patient directly, receives payment for the consultation, or becomes aware of gross negligence in clinical care.

When the APN consultant sees the patient directly, documentation of the consultation in the patient's record is appropriate and important. Ingersoll and Jones (1992) comprehensively described the elements of the consultation note. The consultant's assessment of the problem and recommendations for clinical problem solving should be clearly articulated in the documentation. When the patient is not seen directly, the consultant will want to decide whether or not it is appropriate to document the consultation in the patient's record. If the primary focus of the consultation is on education of the consultee in relation to the consultation problem, documentation in the patient's chart is not necessary. However, consultants should document all consultations in their own records, outlining the issues, the assessment data, and the recommendations (M. Snyder, personal communication, June 14, 1995). Such records provide important data. They enable APNs to make consultation visible and to analyze the nature, volume, and effects of consultation on patient care outcomes.

Snyder recommended documenting informal consultations (see ''Formal and Informal Consultation'' earlier in this chapter) only if they seem to raise particularly problematic situations (personal communication, June 14, 1995). The APN should keep in mind that an informal consultation may be inadequate in relation to the problem described. For example, there may not be enough assessment data to clearly identify the problem for the consultant, or the problem may be particularly complex or urgent. When that is the case, it is important to acknowledge the lack of sufficient information with the person seeking the informal consultation and recommend that a formal consultation be sought to comprehensively consider the problem. If the situation seems to be potentially urgent or emergent, the consultant should recommend the immediate initiation of an emergency consultation. The increased responsibilities inherent in advanced nursing practice expose APNs to increased liability (Poteet, 1989; Scott & Beare, 1993; Survillo & Levine, 1993). Specialists may be held to a higher standard than generalists (Survillo & Levine, 1993). Thus APNs should be cognizant of legal issues in all areas of advanced nursing practice, including consultation.

Stepping Out of the Consultation Process

The APN must recognize that unusual circumstances could necessitate abandoning the consultation process and assuming the stance of clinically responsible expert

(Barron, 1983, 1989). If the APN became aware that the patient being considered during the consultation was in a dangerous situation and the consultee was unable or unwilling to intervene on behalf of the patient, the consultant would then assume direct responsibility for assuring that safety needs were addressed. It is unusual that consultees, once aware of safety concerns, are unable or unwilling to address them, but it does happen. Barron described such a circumstance (1989). She was consulted by the coronary care unit (CCU) nursing staff because of a patient's unwillingness to adhere to the safety guidelines of his care protocol. The patient had had a myocardial infarction 2 days earlier. It became apparent during the consultant's psychosocial assessment of the patient that he was delirious. Recognizing the potentially dangerous implications of the delirium, the consultant went directly to the intern (having discussed her plan with the consultee, who fully supported her direct action) to share her concern and to recommend that the cause of the delirium be evaluated. The intern and then the resident minimized the delirium and attributed the patient's symptoms to psychological distress. The consultant then initiated a psychiatric consultation by discussing her concerns with one of the psychiatrists on the Consultation and Liaison Service and asked that he contact the attending CCU physician and offer psychiatric consultation. The psychiatrist consultant agreed with the liaison nurse consultant, and an investigation into the causes of the delirium revealed that the patient's digitalis level exceeded the therapeutic range. A potentially dangerous and correctable problem was identified.

Developing the Practice of Other Nurses

An outcome of nursing consultation, especially consultation over time, is to enhance the professional development and practice of nurse consultees. Consultation can clearly enhance the clinical knowledge and practice of nurses requesting consultation. One of the most satisfying aspects of the consultative process is to watch consultees master new skills and become more clinically expert.

A goal for consultation is to enable the consultee to manage future similar situations effectively. When the consultant and consultee evaluate the effectiveness of the consultation, they can recognize and reinforce helpful problem-solving strategies, which then can be applied in the future. As APNs engage in self-reflection and include staff in that reflection, they model a critical aspect of practice.

Evaluation of the consultation itself with the consultee is enormously important. It can enhance the learning and skill of both the consultee and the consultant. APNs can contribute to the development of other APNs in a meaningful way through the consultation process. APNs can also enhance their own professional development and practices by receiving nursing consultation.

Consultation Practice over Time

Initially, consultants must market their services to potential consultees. Setting, niche identification, workload, and experience are all issues that contribute to the time and focus an APN may have for consultation efforts. For novice APNs, the marketing may consist of demonstrating expertise and offering consultation services. Over time, staff and colleagues recognize the APN's skill, and the APN may need to develop strategies to deal with large numbers of requests. Setting priorities and identifying alternative resources when the consultant's caseload is full are important activities as the consultation practice becomes more and more recognized and valued. Identifying other APNs who can consult on similar issues may be a useful strategy for balancing requests with availability.

Clarifying availability and the timing of responses to requests is essential if consultees are to continue to consider consultation as a helpful, timely option for assistance with complex clinical situations. Negotiating directly with the consultee at the time of the request (or shortly thereafter) allows the consultant to express to the consultee the importance and worth of the request, even if the consultant cannot meet the need directly. It also provides the opportunity to consider appropriate alternative resources to assist the consultee in addressing the clinical problem. The consultant must have established backup resources who are available to handle emergencies when the consultant is not available. Establishing such resources at the beginning of the consultant's practice is essential. Consultees should always know who to contact in the event of a clinical emergency.

Over time the number of consultee-centered requests may increase. After trust has been established with the consultant, the consultee may feel more comfortable and able to focus on specific problems in handling the clinical situation. It may be more comfortable for the consultee, as the relationship is beginning with the consultant, to focus on the needs of the patient. Over time the consultee may be willing to examine lack of understanding, skill, or objectivity. Wonderful professional development can result from that level of self-examination, but trust usually needs to be firmly developed before such self-examination can take place with the consultant.

The consultant may find that the consultees' requests become more sophisticated over time. The consultee who often requested basic assistance with care may develop skill, understanding, and confidence with basic issues and move on to more expert levels of practice. Requests for consultation may reflect more expert levels of concern and understanding. Such requests can be catalysts for the consultant's ongoing professional growth. Experiencing the development of the consultee's professional practice is exciting.

Conversely, boredom with requests may be an issue for the established consultant. Particularly where there is high turnover of staff, the consultant may focus time and time again on the same clinical concerns. Seeking support from a trusted colleague may help the consultant cope with frustration and avoid sharing it with consultees. Communicating a lack of interest with concerns presented by consultees is a sure way to derail both the specific consultation and the use of consultation as a means to address clinical problems. The consultant may also consider developing an educational program to address, in a different way, the needs commonly being expressed in consultation requests. If the problem is common, the consultant may also want to develop written guidelines, protocols, or care plans to share with consultees.

As the APN's consultation skills become widely appreciated in the system and in the community, the nature and types of consultation requests may change. It can be stimulating to move into different types of consultation, such as programmatic or administrative consultation, and indeed APN consultants have much to contribute in these areas. APNs should be careful to consider the impact of such shifts, however, because such requests move them away from their original purposes. Such requests can lead to job restructuring or new positions, which may or may not be advanced practice roles. Initially, the request to move into new professional areas can be seductive. Furthermore, the shifts can be time- and energy-consuming, leading the APN away from direct practice and ultimately creating job dissatisfaction.

The message that skills and perspectives are valued and that new avenues are available for exploration is gratifying. Developing new ideas and plans also can be helpful to both the institution and the consultant. Recognizing the meaning that new directions have for consultees who have grown to rely on the consultant is critical. Planning with the consultees when such shifts occur can assure consultees that their concerns will continue to be considered even if the resource person changes temporarily or the response from the consultant is not going to be immediate.

EVALUATION OF THE CONSULTATION COMPETENCY

APNs evaluate individual consultations as the final step of the consultation process. Overall evaluation of the consultative process and skills is also important. Barron (1989) discussed both aspects of evaluation. APNs should consider strategies that will help them to determine their overall effectiveness (see Chapter 25) and their specific effectiveness in relation to consultation. Data may be obtained from consultees, peers, administrators, review of the APN's documentation of consults, and the APN's self-evaluation.

APN practices will vary considerably as to what questions and criteria are considered relevant to evaluation of consultation skills. (See Chapter 25 for a comprehensive discussion of evaluation of APN practice.) Some questions that may be useful in eliciting data regarding consultation have been suggested by Lewis and Levy (1982) and Barron (1989). Is the consultant recontacted after the initial consultation? Are consultation requests becoming more sophisticated over time (Lewis & Levy, 1982)? Was the APN able to respond to all requests for consultation? Do glaring issues or needs seem to be going unaddressed? Do there seem to be patterns in terms of either the theme, number, or location of consultations (Barron, 1989)?

The subjective experiences of the consultant are also important (Barron, 1989). Sensing openness and enthusiasm on the part of consultees can provide the APN with data. However, sensing resistance or unwillingness to implement consultation recommendations also can provide data. One would not want to rely solely on subjective data, but the feelings of the consultant can yield important information.

Clinical competency, competency in applying the consultation process, interpersonal skills, and professionalism are all areas to be considered in the evaluation process. Identifying the appropriate people to be involved in the evaluation and developing a systematic approach to data collection regarding the consultation aspects of an APN's practice are important. Evaluation can guide the APN's individual professional growth and can ultimately validate the need for the APN's service and skill in the specific work setting and beyond.

SUMMARY

APNs have had a long tradition in various aspects of direct and indirect patient care activities, including consultation. Consultation has the potential to influence patient care both directly and beyond the direct care encounter. The power of consultative activities to inform and advance practice compels all APNs to consider consultation as an integral aspect of role performance. Consultation offers APNs the opportunity to both share and receive the clinical expertise necessary to meet the increasingly challenging and diverse demands of patient care. This chapter has defined consultation, identified various types of consultation, and distinguished it from co-management, referral and supervision. The authors have offered a model of consultation for advanced nursing practice and have highlighted issues related to implementation of the consultative process. It remains imperative that the appropriate use of the term "consultation" be discussed and researched. The authors have attempted to clarify the concept of consultation because conceptual clarity will enhance its appropriate use in practice and in the literature.

The authors believe that APN consultation contributes to positive patient outcomes and may promote more appropriate use of scarce health care resources. These assumptions must be tested through quality improvement studies, cost-benefit studies, and research that examines the processes and outcomes of care. Outcomes of consultation activities can then be effectively measured. Ongoing discussion regarding this important topic will assist in the much needed clarification of the other terms utilized to characterize relationships with other professionals. APNs can contribute to this discussion as well as to the research by sharing their experiences as both recipients and providers of consultation. It is the authors' belief that consultation by and for APNs in all settings can enhance and extend quality nursing care and improve outcomes of care. Consultation can facilitate having comprehensive and specialty-related knowledge available to all patients who might need it, and therefore should be an expected and integral aspect of APN role performance.

REFERENCES

American College of Nurse-Midwives. (1992). *Clinical practice statement: collaborative management in nurse-midwifery practice for medical, gynecological and obstetrical conditions.* Washington, DC: Author.

Barron, A.-M. (1983). The clinical nurse specialist as consultant. In A. B. Hamric & J. A. Spross (Eds.), *The clinical nurse specialist in theory and practice* (pp. 91–113). New York: Grune & Stratton.

Barron A.-M. (1989). The clinical nurse specialist as consultant. In A. B. Hamric & J. A. Spross (Eds.), *The clinical nurse specialist in theory and practice* (2nd ed., pp. 125–146). Philadelphia: W. B. Saunders.

Barron, A.-M., & White, P. (1996). Consultation. In A. B. Hamric, J. A. Spross, & C. M. Hanson (Eds.), *Advanced nursing practice: An integrative approach* (pp. 165–183). Philadelphia: W. B. Saunders.

Birkholz, G., & Walker, D. (1994). Strategies for state statutory language changes granting fully independent nurse practitioner practice. *Nurse Practitioner, 19*(1), 54–58.

Boyd, J. N., Stasiowski, S. A., Catoe, P. T., Wells, P. R., Stahl, B. M., Judson, E., Hartman, A. L., & Lander, J. H. (1991). The merit and significance of clinical nurse specialists. *Journal of Nursing Administration, 21*(9), 35–43.

Caplan, G. (1970). *The theory and practice of mental health consultation.* New York: Basic Books.

Caplan, G., & Caplan, R. (1993). *Mental health consultation and collaboration.* San Francisco: Jossey-Bass.

Colman, N. S. (1992). Variability in consultation rates and practitioner level of diagnostic certainty. *Journal of Family Practice, 35*(1), 31–38.

Critchley, D. L. (1985). Clinical supervision. In D. L. Critchley & J. T. Maurin (Eds.), *The clinical specialist in psychiatric mental health nursing* (pp. 495–510). New York: John Wiley & Sons.

Gurka, A. M. (1991). Process and outcome components of clinical nurse specialist consultation. *Dimensions of Critical Care Nursing, 10*(3), 169–175.

Hanson, C. M., & Spross, J. A. (1996). Collaboration. In A. B. Hamric, J. A. Spross, & C. M. Hanson (Eds.), *Advanced practice nursing: An integrative approach* (pp. 229–248). Philadelphia: W. B. Saunders.

Ingersoll, G., & Jones, L. (1992). The art of the consultation note. *Clinical Nurse Specialist, 6,* 218–220.

Kuszler, P. (1999). Telemedicine and integrated health care delivery: Compounding malpractice liability. *American Journal of Law and Medicine, 25,* 297–326.

Lewis, A., & Levy, J. (1982). *Psychiatric liaison nursing: The theory and clinical practice.* Reston, VA: Reston Publishing Co.

Lipowski, Z. J. (1974). Consultation-liaison psychiatry: An overview. *American Journal of Psychiatry, 131,* 623-630.

Lipowski, Z. J. (1981). Liaison psychiatry, liaison nursing and behavioral medicine. *Comprehensive Psychiatry, 22,* 554-561.

Lipowski, Z. J. (1983). Current trends in consultation-liaison psychiatry. *Canadian Journal of Psychiatry, 28,* 329-338.

Manley, K. (1998). A conceptual framework for advanced practice: An action research project operationalizing an advanced practitioner/consultant role. In G. Rolfe & P. Fulbrook (Eds.), *Advanced nursing practice* (pp. 118-135). Boston: Butterworth Heinemann.

Minarik, P., & Price, L. (1999). Collaboration? Supervision? Direction? Independence? What is the relationship between the advanced practice nurse and the physician? States legislative and regulatory reform III. *Clinical Nurse Specialist, 13,* 34-37.

Monicken, D. R. (1995). Consultation in advanced practice nursing. In M. Snyder & M. Mirr (Eds.), *Advanced practice nursing* (pp. 183-195). New York: Springer-Verlag.

Norwood, S. L. (1998). When the CNS needs a consultant. *Clinical Nurse Specialist, 12,* 53-58.

Poteet, G. W. (1989). Consultation. *Clinical Nurse Specialist, 3*(1), 41.

Safriet, B. J. (1992). Health care dollars and regulatory sense: The role of advanced practice nursing (special issue). *Yale Journal on Regulation, 9*(2), 417-488.

Scott, L., & Beare, P. (1993). Nurse consultant and professional liability. *Clinical Nurse Specialist, 7,* 331-334.

Sebus, M. (1994). Developing a collaborative practice agreement for the primary care setting. *Nurse Practitioner, 19*(3), 44-51.

Simmons, M. K. (1985). Psychiatric consultation and liaison. In D. L. Critchley & J. T. Maurin (Eds.), *The clinical specialist in psychiatric mental health nursing* (pp. 362-381). New York: John Wiley & Sons.

Spross, J. A. (1989). The clinical nurse specialist as collaborator. In A. B. Hamric & J. A. Spross (Eds.), *The clinical nurse specialist in theory and practice* (2nd ed., pp. 205-226). Philadelphia: W. B. Saunders.

Survillo, A. I., & Levine, A. T. (1993). Strategies to limit CNS malpractice liability exposure. *Clinical Nurse Specialist, 7*(4), 215-220.

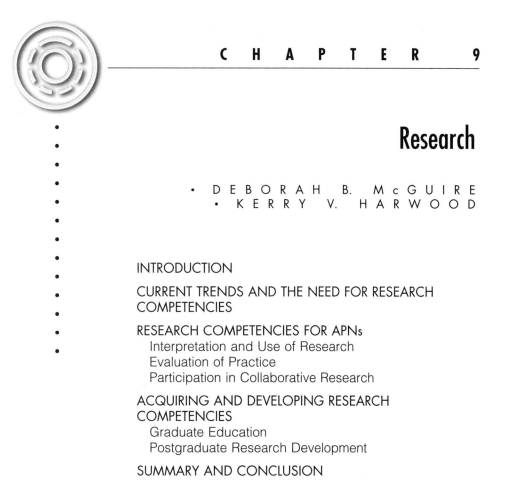

Research

· D E B O R A H   B.   M c G U I R E
· K E R R Y   V.   H A R W O O D

INTRODUCTION

The role of "researcher" has long been considered integral to the practice of clinical nurse specialists (CNSs) (Hodgman, 1983; McGuire & Harwood, 1989) and reflects the critical contribution they have made to nursing knowledge and to scientifically based practice. Research roles of other advanced practice nurses (APNs)—for example, certified nurse-midwives (CNMs), certified registered nurse anesthetists, and nurse practitioners (NPs)—typically have not been a major focus in education and practice, nor have they been well addressed in the professional literature.

With professional consensus on the definition, preparation, and practice of the APN (Cronenwett, 1995; American Association of Colleges of Nursing, 1999), it is essential that research be considered a "core competency" (see Chapter 3). This core competency, however, must be flexible enough to meet the needs of all types of APNs, who may choose or be requested to participate in a wide variety of research-related activities following graduate school. The academic and experiential preparation required for these competencies must be defined so that schools of nursing and clinicians both understand their respective responsibilities.

This chapter describes a set of research competencies for APNs ranging from basic activities (e.g., appraising scientific literature) that should be evident at graduation

245

from a master's degree program to advanced activities (e.g., developing institutional mechanisms for incorporating research into practice) that are developed through experience and individual initiative. Recommendations for academic curriculum content are presented, as are suggestions for how APNs may continue to expand their research competencies following graduate school.

In the health care environment of today and tomorrow, it is critical that research competencies of the APN, historically acknowledged as important yet never consistently embraced or enacted, now move to the forefront of advanced nursing practice. As Kachoyeanos stated,

> *Nurses can no longer rely on experience in making policy and patient care decisions. Accreditation bodies, such as the Joint Commission on Accreditation of Healthcare Organizations (JCAHO), want confirmation that patient care is based on research. Administrators and payers want evidence that the care delivery system will substantially affect patient care and contain cost*

(1995, p. 111)

The APN is a key link between research and patients when functioning as a direct care provider and is also a key link between research and other providers of care when functioning in a programmatic or leadership position. Thus research competencies are now not only a core competency for the APN, but also need to be internalized to the extent that they become part of the "infrastructure" (M. A. Whedon, personal communication, May 1999) for advanced practice nursing or become "embedded" in the APN's thinking process (see Chapter 6).

The foundation of APN research competencies consists in part of two related concepts: (1) research utilization (using research in practice) (Stetler, 1985), and (2) evidence-based medicine (basing practice on systematic scientific observation, with controlled randomized clinical trials providing the strongest levels of evidence) (Evidence-Based Working Group, 1992). Some authors prefer the term "evidence-based care" (Murphy, 1997), while others use terms such as "evidence-based practice" (Stetler, Brunell, et al., 1998) or "research-based care" (Brown, 1999), which suggest a blending of research utilization and evidence-based medicine. The terms "research utilization" (RU) and "evidence-based practice" (EBP) are used in this chapter and are described in more detail later. It is important to note here that both prescribe a relatively similar systematic process for reading, evaluating, and interpreting research literature to determine its applicability to practice. The desired outcome of this process is what the authors call research-based practice.

Three research competencies are described in this chapter: (1) interpretation and use of research, (2) evaluation of practice, and (3) participation in collaborative research. These research competencies must become a major focus in academic programs, individual APN practice, and administrative planning and implementation of APN positions across clinical settings. The skills embedded in these competencies will help guide the future utilization and scope of advanced nursing practice, as well as support standards of nursing practice that appropriately consider both cost and quality outcomes of care. In this chapter, current trends that build the case for the importance of research competencies are discussed; a flexible set of competencies, including specific knowledge and skills, is explicated; and recommendations are made for the responsibilities of both academic institutions and individual practitioners in preparing APNs for these research competencies.

CURRENT TRENDS AND THE NEED FOR RESEARCH COMPETENCIES

The research role for nurses with master's degree preparation initially focused on the conduct of research, exemplified by numerous graduate programs that taught the research process and required formal, original research theses for graduation. As doctoral education developed and the American Nurses' Association (ANA) (1981) recommended specific research roles for nurses prepared in various academic programs, the research role of the master's-prepared nurse focused on use of research findings in practice (McGuire & Harwood, 1989), commonly referred to as RU (Stetler, 1985). This evolution is demonstrated in part by elimination of the required master's thesis and inclusion of RU content in research courses. In the academic setting, many educators structure their curricula using *The Essentials of Master's Education for Advanced Practice Nursing* (American Association of Colleges of Nursing, 1996). Research is deemed part of the core of graduate education, necessary to "prepare a practitioner for the utilization of new knowledge to provide high quality health care, initiate change, and improve nursing practice" (p. 6). Inherent in this statement is use of research to improve outcomes. However, even in schools that incorporate RU content into formal coursework, the breadth and depth of its presentation and general integration into the graduate curriculum may be less than optimal (Firlit, Walsh, & Kemp, 1987; McGuire, 1992). In many APN programs today, important core content such as research receives minimal emphasis or time in a bulging curriculum that places a higher priority on clinical diagnosis and disease management independent of RU.

Current trends in health care delivery have dramatically affected how and where APNs practice, as well as the demands placed on them. In the health care environment of the 1990s, learning to provide care using new techniques, equipment, assistive personnel, and documentation systems was essential to survival. The external demands placed on the health care system by the effects of managed competition rapidly escalated the rate of change. In early managed care efforts, changes in the health care system were primarily driven by cost (i.e., reducing hospital stays, avoiding unnecessary tests). Later efforts exhibited a clear trend toward more emphasis on quality (albeit within the context of controlling costs) as managed care evolved into capitated care, although it is unclear whether quality improved significantly. These changes affected the research competencies needed by APNs, who play a significant role in defining research-based standards of care for specific patient populations, in evaluating the outcomes of such standards in individuals and groups, and in working with others on collaborative research to establish appropriate health care practices. Thus, changes in health care have provided an important impetus for renewing the focus on APN research competencies in the graduate programs of today and tomorrow. Such programs must find ways to build research competencies into the curriculum so that their graduates are adequately prepared for the challenges that await them in the workplace.

Primary cost-containment tools are differentiated practice and standardization of health care. Differentiated practice is a philosophy that structures roles and functions according to education, experience, and competence (Association of Nurse Executives, 1990). This trend is manifested both by APNs' performance of activities previously done by physicians and by unlicensed personnel's increasing performance of activities typically associated with licensed nurses. Many positions were restructured in the 1990s, resulting in both increased and innovative use of APNs as care providers (e.g., acute care NPs, blended role APNs) as well as decreased use of some traditional advanced practice roles (e.g., hospital-based CNSs) or evolution of APN roles into case managers or coordinators of managed care (McDermott-Blackburn, 1998). In these newer roles, APNs will need research competencies to help them determine the best care, appropriate resources, and feasible outcome evaluation mechanisms (Spross & Heaney, 2000; see Chapter 19). Through research competencies, APNs can demonstrate the value of their practice in producing better patient outcomes, be they quality of life, safety, satisfaction, or financial outcomes.

These trends suggest several possibilities for APN practice types in the future. Cooper, Laud, and Dietrich (1998) projected that nonphysician clinicians (including NPs and CNSs) would increase 20% by 2001. In addition, the increase of acutely ill patients in nonhospital settings, coupled with an impending shortage of registered nurses (RNs), portends a rapid growth in nonhospital sectors of care (Buerhaus, 1998), resulting in redefinition of APN roles (Whedon, 1996). Both individual APNs and health care administrators should give careful consideration to APN practice type possibilities, to ensure that the diverse competencies of the APN are fully utilized to the benefit of the health care system. The first possibility is independent practice, when APNs function in patient management roles previously performed by physicians. In nonhospital settings, NPs are increasingly utilized as primary care providers. In selected hospital settings, such as the newborn nursery, NPs are also assuming primary responsibility for patient management. These practices couple traditional medical management (assessment, diagnosis, treatment) with components inherent in advanced nursing practice, such as assisting patients and families to manage lifestyle choices and/or chronic illness. This type of practice necessitates that the APN assume responsibility for maintaining a research-based practice in both the nursing and medicine domains.

A second possibility is collaborative practice, in which physician and APN co-manage patients with some overlap in roles but more of a focus (for each practitioner) on one's traditional domain. Although this scenario is often the structure for CNS roles, other APNs, such as NPs and CNMs, may practice in this way as well. In a collaborative practice setting, the APN is ideally positioned to promote RU or EBP in areas that physicians have traditionally not addressed, such as symptom management or health promotion.

A third, less desirable, possibility is the utilization of APNs in physician surrogate roles. As pressures to cut costs have increased, and the labor pool of physicians-in-training has decreased, NPs (and physician assistants) have been used to stretch the ability of an individual physician or group of physicians to manage a group of patients. These roles tend to be narrow in their focus and activities commonly focus on one aspect of care, such as performing admission histories and physicals, performing procedures, or writing discharge prescriptions, historically all of which have been performed by residents in teaching hospitals. This type of APN utilization, while meeting immediate needs, does not fully use APNs' competencies and undermines APN autonomy.

Research suggests that there are many areas in which health care provided by APNs may result in *better* outcomes at lower cost than care provided by physicians (see Chapter 25) or, when APNS and physicians have the same authority and responsibilities, equivalent outcomes (Mundinger et al., 2000). The future of advanced nursing practice, in its preferred state of collaborative rather than supervised surrogate practice, hinges on research in all its manifestations—that is, interpretation and use of research (RU or EBP), evaluation of outcomes of advanced nursing practice, and knowledge building through participation in the conduct of theory-based research. Moreover, this future of advanced nursing practice also depends not only on demonstration of positive cost and quality outcomes for patients managed by APNs but on a definition of the specific components of nursing practice that lead to positive outcomes. The research competencies described in this chapter can provide APNs with skills in these important processes.

Current pressures to manage larger clinical caseloads may substantially decrease administrative support for research activities of APNs. Nevertheless, APNs are expected to integrate clinical expertise and specific research competencies to improve the care of their patients and to provide clinical leadership for other nurses (Cronenwett, 1995). Given the critical need for further studies of the short- and long-term outcomes of APN, RN, and specialty nursing care, a lack of administrative support for involvement in such research activities could adversely affect the future of APN roles and perhaps the nursing profession itself (see Chapter 24). When nursing administration provides departmental support for EBP, the outcome can be integration of scientific evidence into daily clinical practice through a process led by APNs, specifically CNSs in one example provided by Stetler, Brunell, and their colleagues (1998). Their work demonstrated the importance of the research competency "interpretation and use of research"—the APNs role-modeled the use of research language and behaviors to nursing staff and others as they increased the research foundation of clinical practice.

The trend toward differentiated practice within nursing, including the use of unlicensed personnel under the direction of RNs, further supports the need for clearly articulated standards of care, with more attention given to the translation/application component of the research utilization process (Stetler, 1994) and careful evaluation of the outcomes of research-based practice (McGuire et al., 1994). Clarifying both the rationale for and the details of differentiated practices for both licensed and unlicensed personnel is essential to achieve successful and appropriate practice changes. Such changes will also enhance the evaluation of nonfiscal outcomes, such as clinical variables and patient satisfaction.

An examination of current documents delineating the scope and standards of advanced practice in several specialties (American Association of Critical-Care Nurses and ANA, 1995; ANA, 1996; Oncology Nursing Society [ONS], 1997) is useful with respect to research and outcomes. These documents include research as a standard, most commonly defined as using research findings in practice, but only one organization (ONS, 1997) goes beyond use to indicating that research can improve outcomes.

Standards of practice for APNs thus do address the need for research to be integrated into care. However, the question that results, then, is who establishes the standards for delivering care? Several health maintenance organizations use guidelines (Doyle & Feren, 1992) that focus on care provided by physicians to determine standards of care for specific patient groups. The establishment of the World Wide Web–based National Guidelines Clearinghouse (NGC; *www.guideline.gov*) has provided a public repository for clinical practice guidelines. With over 600 guidelines currently included, the ability to compare guidelines on the same clinical topic, and topic-related e-mail groups, the NGC will undoubtedly speed the application of guideline-based practice in the future. Reimbursement for services will be based on such standards and guidelines; thus APNs must take an active role in their development. The development of appropriate clinical practice guidelines depends on a process of critically evaluating research findings and determining their applicability to practice, activities that are clearly within the scope of APNs' practice, skills, and qualifications (McGuire & Harwood, 1989, 1996; Stetler & DiMaggio, 1991). The research competency of "interpretation and use of research" helps the APN find, review, and judge the quality and appropriateness of clinical practice guidelines, and apply them in her or his setting.

An increasing emphasis on interdisciplinary approaches to care is also driving efforts to provide research-based practice. Tools used to manage patients include critical pathways, algorithms, and other structured approaches to managing specific patient populations or problems. These interdisciplinary plans of care incorporate mechanisms for care documentation and for tracking and analyzing outcome data. APNs often provide leadership in the development of these approaches (Lindeke & Block, 1998), particularly when they function as case managers (see Chapter 19). These activities provide opportunities to use nursing research, to incorporate the services and interventions of APNs into care delivery systems, and to advocate for holistic care of patients and families. Without adequate preparation in research competencies, APNs may find it difficult to assume these responsibilities.

Increased scrutiny of the APN role and associated outcomes vis-à-vis cost containment (with some APN positions eliminated) is another trend that supports the need for research competencies. Both RU and elements of the process of conducting research can be used in the development and evaluation of advanced nursing practice. The use and application of research can enhance the credibility of APNs and their interventions, because the research bases for advanced nursing practice are usually less familiar to physicians and interdisciplinary colleagues. For example, an APN may recommend the incorporation of structured decision support for a woman newly diagnosed with cancer based on data from a review of relevant studies indicating that this intervention can decrease depression at 6 and 12 months after surgery, regardless of the surgical option selected (Fallowfield, Hall, Maguire, & Baum, 1990). Similarly, an APN may recommend a structured support group intervention for newly diagnosed cancer patients based on data indicating that specific interventions for specific groups of patients are likely to be beneficial with regard to quantity and quality of life (Fawzy et al., 1993; Spiegel, Bloom, Kraemer, & Gottheil, 1989).

In addition to using research findings, there is a need to demonstrate through the research process that positive patient outcomes result from APNs' interventions (Brooten & Naylor, 1995). Chapter 25 addresses this issue in some detail. When APNs' interventions are judged effective through systematic research, there is no question but that they should be included in interdisciplinary and nursing standards of care. An increase in the visibility of such nursing research within the context of interdisciplinary publications or predominantly medical publications is an important advance in this regard (Mundinger et al., 2000; Naylor et al., 1999).

Another critical factor underlying many of the changes in the health care system and one which argues for the APNs research competencies put forth here, is access to information. The explosion in information technology demands that APNs be skilled in using it. Health care administrators are demanding not only clinical outcome data but "real-time" data access (i.e., immediate information that enables decision making for clinical problems as they occur, rather than monthly or quarterly reports that allow retrospective analyses and problem solving). As these information systems are developed, it is important that outcome parameters relevant to APN practice be incorporated into databases. In many instances, these parameters will be common variables such as length of stay, readmission rates, or morbidity and mortality, but it will be important to ensure that outcome variables typifying contributions of APN practice (e.g., patient satisfaction, functional status, symptom management) are included. Additionally, APNs should identify variables that will reflect the integration of specialty knowledge with a holistic nursing perspective (e.g., ability of Medicare patients with lymphoma to manage chemotherapy side effects at home; self-efficacy of a primary family caregiver to meet a patient's care needs; recurrent ear infection rates in a pediatric clinic serving a low-literacy population). The challenges inherent in identifying appropriate outcomes, interpreting outcome data, and attributing changes to specific variables within complex health care systems can be mitigated somewhat by knowledge of, and experience with, the research process. Inclusion of the areas discussed previously in graduate curricula appears mandatory. No longer is it acceptable to simply teach the "research process" as has been done traditionally, with students preparing hypothetical "research studies." Focused efforts are needed to integrate research competency content and exercises throughout the curricula, not just in research courses.

Increased emphasis in graduate programs on access to health and medical information is commensurate with the trend toward improved access not only within health care institutions or systems but in general. The capacity for biomedical literature searching is widely available, and abstracts or even full texts can often be printed out if journals are not immediately accessible. Multiple sources on the Internet and World Wide Web contain both peer-reviewed and non-peer-reviewed biomedical information. One new and challenging result of improved access to health and medical information is patients' access to and consumption of such information. Although this activity can have positive benefits with respect to education and making informed decisions, it can be negative when the information used is non-peer-reviewed and/or biased and misleading. A useful tactic might be the development of standards for information that is put on the Web.

Information overload can be minimized through the use of literature reviews completed by professional organizations and government agencies. These groups have already applied the RU or EBP process by analyzing existing knowledge to develop or validate practice standards (Mitchell, Armstrong, Simpson, & Lentz, 1989) as a means of supporting an organization's members or the health care and public community at large. One helpful resource is a bulletin published by the University of Kent [England] NHS Centre for Reviews and Dissemination (1999), *Effective Health Care,* which presents and discusses research evidence and mechanisms to initiate change in practice. Perhaps the most well-known efforts are those of the Agency for Healthcare Research and Quality (AHRQ), formerly the Agency for Health Care Policy and Research, which is responsible for developing clinical practice guidelines to assist practitioners in prevention, diagnosis, treatment, and management of clinical conditions (Carter, Moorhead, McCloskey, & Bulechek, 1995). Among the guidelines that have been released are those on acute pain management, urinary incontinence in adults, pressure ulcers in adults, sickle cell disease, early human immunodeficiency virus infection, unstable angina and cancer pain management. The Web-based NGC described earlier includes these AHRQ clinical practice guidelines in addition to many others. Other Web-based resources are described in Chapter 25 (see Table 25-4).

Nursing specialty organizations are also involved in efforts to promote practice standards that improve patient outcomes. For example, the Association of Women's

Health, Obstetric, and Neonatal Nurses published results of a research utilization project that tested a clinical protocol for the transition of the preterm infant to an open crib (Meier, 1994). In some cases, published practice standards are subsequently used to define and provide care in the managed environment. For example, one managed care company in Pennsylvania reported linking reimbursement for radiologists and diagnostic facilities to compliance with guidelines on fetal monitoring from the American Institute of Ultrasound in Medicine (Sandrick, 1993).

In summary, current trends in, and demands imposed by, the health care environment have direct implications for the research competencies of APNs. It is clear from the previous discussion that two major areas of research competency will be exceedingly important to APNs in defining, implementing, refining, validating, and evaluating advanced nursing practice: (1) critical appraisal of existing research to determine its suitability for use in practice, along with incorporation into practice of appropriate research findings including interdisciplinary or other clinical practice guidelines; and (2) evaluation studies to examine broad outcomes of nursing and interdisciplinary standards of care as well as more specific outcomes of the practice of individual APNs. Finally, a third research competency, less critical for the new APN, is collaborative participation in research studies to generate knowledge that defines optimal nursing interventions for particular populations and specific clinical problems (Brooten & Naylor, 1995).

RESEARCH COMPETENCIES FOR APNs

The authors previously described a *research role* for CNSs, developed from historical antecedents and clinical and scientific perspectives of the time (McGuire & Harwood, 1989). This role consisted of three levels of research involvement: (1) activities related to identifying researchable problems, enhancing the clinical relevance of research, and facilitating the use of research by nurses and others in the clinical setting; (2) activities using the research process to conduct quality improvement, replication, case study, and secondary analysis studies; and (3) activities related to conducting independent or collaborative research. When the notion of "competencies" for APNs was initially conceptualized by the editors of this text (Hamric, Spross, & Hanson, 1996), the levels of CNS research involvement evolved into three *research competencies* (McGuire & Harwood, 1996): (I) interpretation and use of research, (II) evaluation of practice, and (III) conducting research within a collaborative context. These new research competencies offered a realistic and feasible set of activities for APNs of any type and were conceptualized as consisting of basic and advanced activities. This chapter presents an updated version of the three research competencies (Table 9-1). APNs should be able to perform basic activities in competencies I and II upon completion of graduate school. They may then develop proficiency in the advanced activities of competencies I and II and in the activities of competency III (which does not have specific basic or advanced activities as discussed later) in their postgraduate work settings. In the sections that follow, necessary knowledge and skills for basic activities in competencies I and II and general activities for competency III (Table 9-1) are detailed. Advanced activities for the competencies are discussed briefly in the section on postgraduate education because they are envisioned to develop more fully following graduate school.

The research competencies discussed in this chapter are based not only on the concepts of RU and EBP (as mentioned previously) and the earlier work of the

TABLE 9-1	OVERVIEW OF RESEARCH COMPETENCIES AND LEVELS OF ACTIVITY	
COMPETENCY	BASIC LEVEL	ADVANCED LEVEL
I. Interpretation and use of research	• Incorporate relevant research findings appropriately into own practice • Assist others to incorporate research into individual or unit practice	• Develop programmatic and/or departmental research utilization process
II. Evaluation of practice	• Use existing data to evaluate nursing practice, individual and/or aggregate • Collaborate in conduct of evaluation studies	• Identify and/or develop practice-specific package of outcome criteria • Lead the conduct of evaluation studies
III. Participation in collaborative research	• Identify research problems • Develop study procedures • Assist with recruitment • Participate in interventions • Identify nurse-sensitive outcomes • Collect outcomes data	

authors, but also on the evolving work of Stetler and Grady, who have been developing and refining a model of RU competencies for several years (C. Stetler, personal communication, January 29, 2000). Although the model is not yet published in its entirety, several aspects might be helpful for readers. First, competencies are defined as a "set of knowledge-based abilities to perform behaviors related to using research in practice, as both a product and a process . . . and thus to integrating evidence into daily practice" (C. Stetler, unpublished materials, personal communication, October 1999). Stetler and her colleagues also described the importance of nursing leadership in developing a process for integrating EBP into a division of nursing (Stetler, Brunell, et al., 1998). Second, their RU competency model has three levels: basic, intermediate, and complex. Each level is characterized by certain expectations. For example, the intermediate level uses a beginning knowledge of research and statistics. The individual who is competent at the complex level is characterized by in-depth knowledge of a specialty area and its related literature, familiarity with theories of planned change, and advanced knowledge of research and statistics; this individual is likely to be an APN. Indeed, Stetler has long been an active proponent of APNs as the key players in RU (or EBP) activities (Stetler, Bautista, Vernale-Hannon, & Foster, 1995; Stetler, Corrigan, Sander-Buscemi, & Burns, 1999). The use of integrative reviews of research by APNs as a basis for making decisions about nursing actions and interventions is an example of the RU competencies for APNs and is a key component of EBP (Stetler, Morsi, et al., 1998). Information taken from such reviews can be combined with other data to develop effective protocols for integrating scientific evidence into clinical care and changing clinical outcomes in such important areas as fall prevention (Stetler et al., 1999).

Interpretation and Use of Research

Interpreting and using existing research in practice constitute the focal point of this competency, which is based on the concepts of RU and EBP. Both were defined earlier and noted to have similar systematic processes for reading and evaluating scientific literature for its applicability to practice. Key to both processes, and therefore at the heart of this research competency for APNs, is the critical appraisal of research for its scientific merit as well as its suitability/appropriateness for application to practice in a given setting. McGuire and Harwood (1996) described in some detail the importance of learning about RU, including its conceptual foundation (knowledge utilization), early and more contemporary nursing RU models, and how RU fits within nursing's "circle of knowledge" (a continuous interaction of theory, research, science, and practice) (National League for Nursing [NLN], 1987). Notable among the contemporary nursing RU models is the Stetler model for application of research findings to practice (Stetler, 1994). This model, based on the concepts of knowledge utilization (research knowledge and knowledge from other sources, such as clinical experience) and on systems theory, provides a six-phase process to help practitioners read and critique research studies, evaluate their clinical applicability, decide how to use relevant findings, and develop evaluation mechanisms. The model is heavily reliant on APNs' skills in these areas and is the foundation of Stetler's subsequent work on RU competencies (see earlier). Interested readers are referred to McGuire and Harwood's (1996) work for background reading to enhance their understanding of not only Stetler's model, but others as well.

Stetler and her colleagues (Stetler, Brunell, et al., 1998), as noted previously, have integrated RU with the concept of EBP. They developed a summary definition of EBP as it relates to nursing:

> *Evidence-based nursing deemphasizes ritual, isolated and unsystematic clinical experiences, ungrounded opinions and tradition as a basis for nursing practice . . . and stresses instead the use of research findings and, as appropriate, quality improvement data, other operational and evaluation data, the consensus of recognized experts and affirmed experience to substantiate practice.*

(pp. 48–49)

A key component of EBP is the notion of "levels" (or strength) of evidence, which emanated originally from the AHRQ clinical practice guidelines mentioned earlier (Stetler, Brunell, et al., 1998). Six levels were defined: (I) meta-analyses of multiple controlled studies: (II) individual controlled clinical trials: (III) quasi-experimental (nonrandomized) trials; (IV) nonexperimental studies using comparative and correlational techniques or qualitative methods: (V) program evaluation, RU, or quality improvement projects; and (VI) opinions of respected authorities. Studies are also rated on their overall basic quality or scientific credibility, on a scale of A (best) to D (seriously flawed). Additional discussion of levels of evidence used in evidence-based medicine can be found in Hadorn, Baker, Hodges, and Hicks (1996).

A more in-depth discussion of similarities and differences between RU and EBP is beyond the scope of this chapter. In essence, both RU and EBP are aimed at improving practice by combining research knowledge with clinical knowledge and experience, while also considering the perspectives of recipients of care. Thus, for the purposes of this research competency, they can be considered equivalent.

RU (and EBP) is one outcome, in a sense, of nursing and/or interdisciplinary research. Why? Because RU provides the means through which nursing or clinical science (the foundation of practice) is solidified, expanded, and actually used to guide or drive practice. That is, nurses read, evaluate, and use relevant research findings in order to improve the scope, content, and quality of their practice. These improved practices are then evaluated, and, if outcomes are positive, the value of the research they are based on is substantiated, and the scientific foundation (science) of nursing practice is strengthened.

RU (and EBP) must, however, be understood within the broader field of study called knowledge utilization, which was defined by Larsen (1980) as a process that uses specific information or knowledge accompanied by political, organization, socio-economic, and attitudinal aspects. Using research information within this broader context is appropriate for nurses, who rarely base their practice on research alone but tend to blend research-based information with information from clinical experience, expert judgment, professional standards, and other sources (Stetler, 1994). Although research-based information is recognized as the "first source of substantiation" in confirming research findings of a given study (Stetler, 1994, p. 21), the pressures of real clinical problems and the need for rapid decisions and solutions also necessitate the use of non-research-based information (hence "knowledge utilization") to deal with these problems (Stetler, 1994). This "real world" need also meshes nicely with the basic tenets of EBP (Stetler, Brunell, et al., 1998), which marries the best research evidence with clinical experience (Evidence-Based Working Group, 1992).

In an extensive review of RU literature, McGuire (1992) described RU as a complex process consisting of five essential components: (1) *dissemination/acquisition* of research findings to and by appropriate individuals and agencies, (2) *evaluation of merit and clinical applicability* of research findings, (3) *incorporation of research findings* into practice through various mechanisms, (4) *evaluation of research-based practice* through assessment of predetermined outcome parameters, and (5) *socialization* of nurses into the belief that research-based practice is not only desirable but necessary. This view of RU provides a useful conceptual framework for this competency and is used to organize the specific knowledge and skills that are required. In Table 9–2, each of these five components is briefly defined in column one; areas of related knowledge are presented in column two; and specific skills are listed in column three.

An example of how an APN (or faculty member in an APN program) might use this table is the following. The RU component of dissemination/acquisition requires that the APN understand not only theories of communication (as they relate to research findings) and RU, but also barriers and resources in applying research findings, and the relationships among these factors. This knowledge is critical in order for the APN to understand why nurses may or may not use research, how the use of research might be increased, and what their own roles might be. Thus the required knowledge can be used to fashion appropriate graduate school experiences and activities.

Skills needed for dissemination/acquisition include being able to identify literature databases and other resources and to find and retrieve literature. Of particular importance to APNs in all specialty areas is the ability to identify existing clinical guidelines based on research, such as those listed in the NCG mentioned earlier. The authors of such guidelines have already undertaken the task of identifying, retrieving, reviewing, and synthesizing available research and clinical information in order to apply it to practice. Additionally, dissemination and acquisition require that the APN have the ability to use a computer in order to identify and retrieve relevant literature, possess interpersonal and group process skills, write and speak effectively, and use appropriate audiovisual materials. Although some of these skills may seem only

TABLE 9–2 COMPETENCY 1: INTERPRETATION AND USE OF RESEARCH		
COMPONENT OF RU PROCESS*	KNOWLEDGE	SKILLS

Dissemination/Acquisition
Communication of research findings *and* research utilization outcomes to others
	• Theories of communication
	• Barriers to RU
	• Resources:
	  Media
	  Personnel
	  Institutions
		• Identification of relevant databases, literature, resources, and consultants
		• Literature searching and retrieval techniques
		• Computer skills
		• Interpersonal and group process skills
		• Effective written and oral presentation techniques
		• Audiovisual skills

Evaluation of Merit and Clinical Applicability Determination of scientific merit of research studies and their potential for clinical application	• Basic understanding of research paradigms, designs, sampling, instrumentation, procedures, analysis, and ethical aspects • Goals and process of a traditional research critique for scientific merit • Goals and process of a utilization critique for clinical applicability • Critique for use in practice • Awareness of specific critique tools • Relationship between type of research and potential type of use in practice	• Oral and written research critique • Oral and written utilization critique based on specific criteria defined by formal RU approaches (e.g., Stetler Model; Conduct and Utilization of Research in Nursing Model) • Ability to teach, guide, and mentor other nurses in research and utilization critiques
Incorporation of Findings into Practice Translation of research findings into practice through feasible and relevant application mechanisms that are commensurate with the clinical setting	• Goals, methods, and strategies of published approaches to RU • Clinical relevance of research-based practices to a given setting • Barriers and facilitators to RU • Goals, process, and outcomes of institutional quality management programs	• Assessment of institutions and individuals for readiness and receptivity to research-based practice • Development of policies, procedures, standards of care, and nursing protocols • Ability to identify and appropriately incorporate non-research-based knowledge • Negotiation with individuals and groups • Ability to teach, guide, and mentor other nurses
Evaluation of Research-Based Practice Determination of the value, efficacy, and cost-effectiveness of research-based practice	• Conceptual approaches to outcome evaluation • Relevant clinical and administrative outcomes • Methodologic approaches to outcome evaluation that are based on selected outcomes • Evaluation strategies of published RU approaches	• Design and conduct evaluation projects • Identification and development of tools to measure outcomes • Data collection procedures • Analysis techniques • Oral and written reports of evaluations

TABLE 9–2	COMPETENCY 1: INTERPRETATION AND USE OF RESEARCH *Continued*	
COMPONENT OF RU PROCESS*	KNOWLEDGE	SKILLS
Socialization Integration of the value and necessity of research utilization into the philosophy and practice of nursing at all levels	• Nursing's circle of knowledge • Contribution of RU to nursing knowledge • Roles of nurses in RU • Approaches for socializing nurses and changing the "research culture"	• Function as an RU role model for APNs and nursing staff • Teach, guide, and mentor other nurses in their RU roles • Provide leadership in RU-related activities • Negotiation with administrative and clinical leaders regarding incorporation of RU into institutional policy and practice

* The components of the RU process are from McGuire, D. B. (1992). The process of implementing research into clinical practice. *Proceedings of the Second National Conference on Cancer Nursing Research* (92-50M-No.3320.00-PE). Atlanta: American Cancer Society.

peripherally relevant to RU, on closer examination, they are important in both finding and communicating research results and thus are critical to this competency.

In summary, this research competency depends highly on both generic and specific knowledge and a set of specific skills that encompass literature retrieval, use of computer technology (including the World Wide Web), evaluation of research merit and clinical applicability, interpersonal communication, proficiency in group process, and understanding of political and organizational systems. Specific recommendations for how the requisite knowledge and skills can be taught in graduate programs, and acquired by APNs, are provided in the section of the chapter entitled "Acquiring and Developing Research Competencies." Two examplars of how APNs might use the knowledge and skills needed to engage in this research competency are presented next. These exemplars showcase two important areas of APN intervention—pain management and health promotion—that are cornerstones of advanced practice nursing across clinical specialties (McCloskey, Bulechek, & Donahue, 1998) and individual APN roles.

EXEMPLAR 1: PAIN MANAGEMENT

Managing pain is a key aspect of advanced nursing practice in a variety of clinical areas and settings, particularly as it relates to quality of life. An extensive body of research exists on assessment and management of pain, and has been used by experts to develop standards of practice and clinical practice guidelines. Such standards and guidelines are readily available to APNs, but need implementation in ways that capitalize on existing systems, personnel, and operating procedures.

Bookbinder and her colleagues (1995; 1996) described a continuous quality improvement (CQI) framework in their institution, a tertiary cancer hospital, that served as a foundation for a pain management project that was designed to improve institutional pain management practices. Existing practices were variable and did not result in uniform pain assessment and management across the institution. A complete discussion of the project is beyond the scope of this text, but interested readers are referred to Bookbinder and colleagues' (1995) detailed paper. Several specific aspects of the project, however, are relevant for this exemplar. First, the project was spearheaded by a group of APNs and a doctorally prepared expert in RU. Second, the underlying knowledge base was the American Pain Society's (APS's) quality assurance standards for pain management, derived from research and clinical experience (Max, 1990). Third, the group consisted of an interdisciplinary team, each with an important role to play in pain management within the institution. Fourth, the project capitalized on existing resources and processes such as internationally renowned pain experts, the CQI paradigm, and commitment from the nursing department. The implementation of this project included a systematic evaluation of the effects of the APS standards on nurses' knowledge about pain, their skills in managing it, and patients' pain relief. Evaluation of these outcomes is discussed in the section "Evaluation of Practice," where this exemplar is continued.

EXEMPLAR 2: HEALTH PROMOTION — SMOKING CESSATION

An important component of advanced nursing practice is health promotion, which is aimed at facilitating change in individual or community health-related behavior. It involves, first, identifying the behaviors that influence health outcomes of the APN's practice, such as smoking, diet, exercise, correct use of medications, and safety practices. Second, health promotion involves understanding the individual factors that influence risk-enhancing and health-promoting behaviors, as well as the interactions between these behavioral, biological, cultural, and socioeconomic factors. Third, it involves using research-based interventions to support individuals or communities in improving health, and subsequently, evaluating their effectiveness. Clearly, health promotion is an area of APN practice requiring broad application of research competencies.

Cardiovascular disease and cancer are the two leading causes of death in the United States. Smoking is the primary risk factor for both of these conditions, as well as a modifiable risk factor in numerous other common health areas including asthma, pregnancy, and pediatric ear infections. In this exemplar, a cardiovascular CNS developed an interdisciplinary, research-based smoking cessation program with the Heart Center of an academic medical center.

The CNS recognized smoking cessation services are important for patients in the post–myocardial infarction (MI) period. Existing institutional smoking cessation services did not have the capacity to meet the Heart Center's referral needs. Both medical and nursing staff were focused on stabilizing the patient after the acute event and discharging the patient as soon as medically appropriate because of hospital budget constraints, not viewing smoking cessation as part of their counseling role. Effecting change in this arena required application of a wide variety of skills, including evaluation of research findings, interpersonal and group skills, and understanding of political and organizational systems.

The CNS first considered the existing literature, which comprises literally hundreds of research studies addressing behavioral, biological, cultural, and economic factors in smoking cessation. Fortunately, several resources are available to assist APNs in defining a research-based practice in smoking cessation appropriate to their role and patient population. The NGC identifies multiple guidelines that address smoking cessation, with three exclusively focused on this topic. These three guidelines represent the primary sources of clinical practice guidelines used in this exemplar: (1) government (Agency for Health Care Policy and Research, 1996a, 1996b, 1996c); (2) professional organizations (American College of Preventive Medicine [Kattapong, Locher, Secker-Walker, & Bell, 1998]); and (3) private, nonprofit organizations (institute for Clinical Systems Improvement, 1999). The guidelines provide research-based practice standards for both individual and community interventions, incorporating the findings of hundreds of studies.

The CNS identified organizational incentives to expand this service, including improved patient satisfaction, as well as meeting national accreditation requirements. She used a variety of avenues, including personal conversations, staff meetings, and strategic planning forums, to educate and remind staff and administrators about these issues. Recognizing the potential for political turf issues with existing referral resources, she brought them into the discussion early, reassuring them of their continued role as a referral service, and involving them as expert advisors in developing staff's ability to determine appropriate referrals. For example, research indicates that quit rates may be influenced by readiness to change (Prochaska & Velicer, 1997). Recommendations to tailor the intensity of the intervention to readiness to change would ensure the most effective use of limited economic resources.

By sharing with nursing staff the research related to readiness to change theory and the efficacy of minimal intervention counseling, the CNS was able to convince them that they could make a difference with a level of intervention that was feasible within their practice. Through her efforts, smoking cessation services for post-MI patients changed from inconsistent referral to overburdened resources to a consistent practice incorporating (1) assessment of readiness to change, (2) minimal intervention counseling for all patients, (3) referral of patients assessed as being ready to change to the CNS for additional counseling, and (4) CNS referral of such patients who were ready to change and needed more intensive services than she was able to provide.

Evaluation of Practice

The importance of evaluating advanced nursing practice that results from implementation of research-based practice was addressed earlier. This competency is conceptualized as encompassing the process that individual APNs (or groups of APNs) can use to evaluate these aspects of their practice. It is important to distinguish it from outcomes research, outcomes measurement (Deaton, 1998a, 1998b), or the broader based studies of advanced nursing practice outcomes discussed elsewhere in this text (see Chapter 25). It is equally important to emphasize that the individual APN's control over the care delivered is an important aspect of her or his ability to control and assess the outcomes of that care. Obviously, if an APN does not have control over the processes of care under evaluation, the APN will not be able to design and implement strategies capable of attributing outcomes (positive or negative) to her or his practice.

To this end, APNs can use a variety of research methods and approaches to evaluate outcomes of their advanced nursing practice. These activities may involve evaluating specific outcome measures related to general patient management by an APN, specific APN interventions, general nursing practice standards or norms, or programs developed by an APN. Research techniques, although generally used to evaluate outcomes in aggregate, may also be used to assess efficacy of interventions in individual patients. Five components are important in practice evaluation. Each is shown in Table 9–3, along with specific knowledge and skills that are essential for the APN who is evaluating nursing practice.

CRITERIA AND OUTCOME MEASURES

The first component of practice evaluation involves selection of appropriate criteria and outcome measures, which are highly specific to the practice being evaluated. It is important to match these criteria and outcome measures to the interventions being employed. Multiple studies have examined outcomes in groups of patients receiving care from an APN (see Chapter 25). For example, Brooten et al. (1986) described the impact of discharge planning and home follow-up of very-low-birth-weight infants by a perinatal CNS. Naylor and colleagues (1999) demonstrated the value of APNs in discharge planning and home follow-up of hospitalized elders in a study published

TABLE 9-3 COMPETENCY II: EVALUATION OF PRACTICE

PRACTICE EVALUATION COMPONENT	KNOWLEDGE/SKILL
Selection of appropriate criteria and outcome measures	• Familiarity with nursing practice outcome measures • Ability to assess outcome measurement tools • Knowledge of existing databases
Selection of appropriate evaluation research study design	• Knowledge of alternative study designs
Implementation of study or evaluation activity	• Differentiation of research and quality improvement activities and requirements • Data collection and storage techniques
Data collection, storage, analysis, and interpretation	• Selection/application of appropriate statistical techniques • Consideration of bias and generalizability of findings
Dissemination	• Interpersonal and group process skills • Effective written and oral presentation techniques • Audiovisual skills

in a predominantly medical journal, thus endorsing the significant contributions of APNs as members of interdisciplinary teams.

Others have compared outcomes of APN care versus that of other care providers. For example, Lombness (1994) used length of stay as the outcome criterion for a retrospective chart audit comparing patients undergoing elective coronary artery bypass surgery co-managed by a CNS and a cardiac surgeon with historical controls co-managed by a physician assistant and cardiac surgeon. Lydon-Rochelle, Albers, and Teaf (1995) used status of the perineum after birth as an outcome measure in an observational cohort study to describe general outcomes of CNM care, as well as outcomes with specific types of patients and specific interventions. They compared their results to published reports regarding perineal outcomes in births attended by physicians. Similarly, Ramsey, McKenzie, and Fish (1982) examined physiological parameters of weight and blood pressure in adults with hypertension managed by NPs and compared them with those of patients cared for by a physician.

Although such studies have been important to establishing the cost-effectiveness of various APN specialties, they leave many questions unanswered regarding the specific APN interventions that contribute to favorable outcomes, as well as the "dose" of intervention needed (Brooten & Naylor, 1995). Specific APN interventions require evaluation, as do nursing interventions that serve as nursing practice standards or norms. A variety of general outcome criteria can be selected, such as length of stay, number of clinic visits, readmission rates, overall cost of care, patient satisfaction, and many others. Selection of specific parameters relevant to the individual APN's practice may be more appropriate. Brooten and Naylor (1995) suggested using outcome measures more sensitive to nursing interventions, such as functional status, mental status, stress level, and caregiver burden. In describing outcomes that reflected the impact of nursing practice, Lang and Marek (1992) offered several general categories in addition to those previously described, including knowledge, symptom control, quality of life, goal attainment, utilization of services, and safety. Chapter 25 provides further discussion of relevant outcome measures for ANPs, as do several current texts (Bulechek & McCloskey, 1998; Sidani & Braden, 1998).

Issues in the selection of appropriate outcome measures are similar for individual and aggregate decisions. For example, in the Transition of the Preterm Infant to the Open Crib project (Medoff-Cooper, 1994), research outcome criteria were weight gain, maintenance of body temperature, and absence of medical complications such as sepsis, hypoglycemia, and failure to thrive. These same parameters would be useful for effective clinical decision making on an individual basis.

The most appropriate outcomes are those that meet three criteria: sensitivity to nursing interventions, relevance to patients, and feasibility. Two resent studies evaluated the effectiveness of nurse-run clinics for patients with cardiovascular disease (Campbell et al., 1998; Cline, Israelsson, Willenheimer, Broms, & Erhardt, 1998). Outcome measures sensitive to this nursing intervention included aspirin use, blood pressure and lipid management, physical activity, dietary fat intake, number of hospitalizations and time to readmission, shorter length of stay, and lower mean annual health care costs. Additional measures of mortality and quality of life, while not different between the nurse-managed versus routine clinical care groups, were important to measure to determine if the economic benefits were accompanied by a decrease in quality of care.

Stages of readiness to change, as noted earlier, can be used to guide the intensity of health promotion interventions such as smoking cessation. These stages can also be used as an outcome measure. As discussed previously in Exemplar 2, the NGC smoking cessation guidelines suggest that progress from one stage of readiness to quit to the next stage is as valuable an outcome as a quit attempt. Stages of readiness to change are also being explored in other areas of health promotion, such as exercise (Cardinal, 1997).

Traditional disease outcome measures, such as laboratory values or radiologic assessment, often are not the measures most relevant to patients. Increasingly, broad health surveys such as the Short Form-36 Health Status Profile (SF-36) are being used to determine how health plans are improving the overall health of patients (Eisen, Leff, & Schaefer, 1999; Wyrwich, Tierney, & Wolinsky, 1999). The SF-36 comprises eight health scales: physical functioning (10 items), role limitations—physical (4 items), bodily pain (2 items), general health (5 items), vitality (4 items), social functioning (2 items), role limitations—emotional (3 items), and mental health (5 items). Two core dimensions of health, physical and mental, can be derived from these eight scales. There is also a single separate item that is used to assess any change in health from 1 year before (Stewart & Ware, 1992). Overall scores or subscales of the SF-36 may be relevant to an APN's individual, group, or interdisciplinary practice. However, disease specific outcome instruments are more likely to be able to detect changes in the disease as a result of intervention. For example, a symptom index for benign prostate disease was developed after researchers determined that men with identical symptoms related to benign prostate disease had very different opinions about how much their disease bothered them. Furthermore, urine flow rate, the measure most commonly used to evaluate the need for treatment, had almost no relationship to patients' perceptions of their symptoms or need for treatment (Jacobsen et al., 1995).

Similar symptom indices have been developed for a wide variety of clinical problems. For example, the VF-14 index of functional impairment in patients with cataracts considers outcomes such as nighttime driving, seeing steps or stairs, and reading small print (Steinberg et al., 1994). The Functional Assessment of Cancer Therapy–Breast quality of life instrument focuses on outcomes specific to breast cancer patients such as changes in weight, arm swelling, perception of sexual attractiveness, and worry about cancer risk in family members (Brady et al., 1997).

When limited resources are available, fewer outcome measures may be obtainable. Andrews, Tingen, and Harper described 6- and 12-month quit rates as the only outcome measures in the evaluation of a model NP-managed smoking cessation clinic. Fortunately, the model program produced satisfactory 6- and 12-month quit rates of 41% and 36%, respectively. There are few data to guide practitioners, however, in determining which aspects of the program were more or less effective, should they desire to modify the program.

In conclusion, the APN must be able to determine the most appropriate desired outcomes for a given clinical situation as well as how to measure them and, in some cases, assess alternative measures for the same outcome criteria. This process may include selection of (1) equipment (e.g., equipment for monitoring blood pressure); (2) procedures (e.g., techniques for taking central venous pressure measurements, techniques for telephone interviews); and (3) instruments (e.g., those for measuring quality of life or functional status or for scoring subjective physical phenomena). Validity, reliability, sensitivity, and relevance must all be considered in defining appropriate outcome measures. Cost and feasibility of collecting the data must also be considered. To avoid unnecessary effort and duplication, it is essential that the APN know of the data available through existing resources and databases when selecting outcome measures.

RESEARCH STUDY DESIGN

The second component of practice evaluation involves selection of an appropriate evaluation research study design. The purpose of the study design is to minimize the bias inherent in the research process. Nonexperimental designs and methods are often used for evaluation research because they describe "what is." Variables are not deliberately manipulated, and the setting is not controlled (Brockopp & Hastings-Tolsma, 1995). Often, the APN will want to examine relationships among nursing interventions and patient care variables, such as the following:

- What is the relationship between perineal support, hot compresses, alternative positions, and rate of episiotomy and lacerations?
- What is the relationship between telephone support interventions and self-care efficacy in cancer patients receiving treatment at home?
- What is the relationship between implementation of a chest pain management protocol and the timing of the first dose of nitroglycerin?

It is important to remember that nonexperimental designs may suggest relationships but are not strong enough to allow one to attribute causation.

APN practice often includes components of primary prevention and health promotion. Evaluating outcomes of these practice components requires the use of nontraditional research designs because the classic experimental designs for causation may not be feasible. The overall goal of prevention and health promotion studies is to measure things that do not happen (i.e., illness). Because the final outcomes may be the absence of specific events over several decades, the selection of interim outcomes may be based on the rationale that they are predictive of the ultimate prevention outcomes. Interim outcomes measures may include parameters such as changes in knowledge, attitudes, and behavior; functional status or self-care ability; physiological measurements such as blood pressure, cholesterol, or blood sugar; or other outcomes specific to the goal of health promotion. APNs may use interim outcome measures in descriptive studies to describe the outcomes of their prevention and health promotion efforts, such as monitoring client weight changes, smoking cessation rates, and adherence to recommended cancer-screening evaluations in clients participating in a wellness clinic. These approaches may be used to track trends over time, to detect changes following nursing practice innovations, to compare results with published outcomes, or to participate in more formal research studies. In such studies, the study sample consists of a community (such as minority adolescents) in which some participants receive the interventions and are compared with others who do not. For example, a quasi-experimental, nonrandomized two-group study may be used for evaluating outcomes of APN prevention and health promotion efforts.

In addition to evaluating efficacy of nursing interventions within groups of patients, the APN needs to use an organized approach to evaluate individual responses to interventions and subsequent treatment modifications. Although some components of this process are identical to the evaluation of aggregate data, other components differ. In both situations, the parameters for evaluation should be predefined, the interventions and responses carefully documented, and variables that could potentially confound results considered in decision making. However, when evaluating the effectiveness of interventions within groups of patients, the data are generally reviewed retrospectively, with outcomes used to make treatment decisions for future patients. For clinical decision making, data are reviewed in real time, with outcomes affecting the care of a particular patient or group of patients. More data recording is generally required for retrospective analysis, because potentially confounding variables may not be as apparent as in clinical decision making with individual patients.

In some situations, the "n of 1" randomized controlled trial can be used to systematically determine whether an intervention benefits a specific patient. A patient alternately receives an intervention and a placebo. Response is recorded by the patient and health care professional, each one unaware of which cycles consisted of the active intervention versus the placebo. This approach is useful when response to intervention can be defined through measurable outcomes and bias can be controlled through the use of a placebo treatment. Bruera, Schoeller, and MacEachern (1992) described an n of 1 double-blind crossover trial of the benefit of oxygen versus room air in an individual patient. The patient recorded severity of breathlessness during each alternating cycle and both the patient and a blinded investigator chose which of the two gases better relieved dyspnea during each cycle. An unblinded investigator controlled the intervention while monitoring arterial oxygen saturation using a finger oximeter. Although research has demonstrated that oxygen does not benefit most patients with dyspnea, indicators of who will benefit are not clearly defined. This n of 1 methodology allows an APN to use interventions helpful to the individual in the absence of data that clearly guide practice, yet not waste resources on a treatment ineffective for that individual. Similar methodology, used in a large sample of patients, could help define predictors of benefit from oxygen therapy and could certainly be used to study numerous additional clinical problems.

STUDY IMPLEMENTATION

The third component of evaluating practice involves implementation of the study or evaluation activity. In developing the implementation plan, the APN must differentiate between research and evaluative or quality improvement activities. This decision making is linked to the rights and responsibilities of patients and hospitals, respectively. Evaluation data are generally collected to confirm the effectiveness of current standards of care. Patients usually enter the health care arena expecting the quality of their care to be evaluated. Health care administrators expect providers to demonstrate the effectiveness of the care they provide. Although research skills may be used in the process of evaluation, the patient is not exposed to some of the potential risks inherent in traditional research conducted to expand existing knowledge or generate new knowledge. Research studies are often conducted to test new outcomes or examine alternative interventions. Participating patients have a right to expect protection from undue risk and information relevant to decision making. The health care professions have a responsibility to conduct research to improve health care outcomes within the context of patients' rights. Thurston, Watson, and Reimer (1993) provided guidelines for differentiating between these two activities and thus determining the appropriate approval process: departmental review versus institutional review board or another approving body responsible for scientific and ethical review (Table 9–4).

In addition to determining the appropriate approval processes, the APN needs to differentiate between whether the project is research or outcome evaluation. This latter activity will serve as a guide to identifying and acquiring appropriate resources to support the project. Both research and evaluation projects will require a number of resources, including access to existing data, collection of additional data, and management and analysis of the data, in addition to whatever resources are required to deliver the intervention. Outcome evaluation studies are likely to be supported through internal resources and existing organizational mechanisms or structures.

TABLE 9–4 GUIDELINES DIFFERENTIATING RESEARCH FROM QUALITY IMPROVEMENT

Section A
1. Is a risk involved for subjects?
2. Is the intent to ask a new question that will improve or expand knowledge with some generalizability?
3. Is a new therapy, program, or practice to be compared with standard approaches to determine which is better?
4. Are new technologies, interventions, or assessment tools to be compared with those used in providing standard care?
5. Does the patients' involvement change their relationship with the caregiver in terms of patient care?
If the answer is yes to one or more of these questions, the project may require ethical and scientific review as a research proposal.

Section B
1. Is the change in therapy, program, or practice an extension of standard care? (Could include a deviation from normal care where good rationale for the change is readily available.)
2. Is patient/staff satisfaction to be evaluated relative to existing practices?
3. Is a measurement tool for evaluation regularly used in clinical practice?
4. Is data gathering intended to confirm existing standards?
5. Is this development of a new program or refinement of an existing program, with formative or summative evaluation?
6. Is a new technology, intervention, or measurement tool supported by good rationale in the literature, experiences of other professionals, etc.?
Affirmation of these questions suggests a quality improvement project.

Adapted from Thurston, N. E., Watson L. A., & Reimer, M. A. (1993). Research or quality improvement? Making the decision. *Journal of Nursing Administration, 23*(7/8), 46–49; reprinted with permission.

However, unless their institutions have research seed money, APNs initiating research studies will need to consider grant applications as their primary source of funding. Both institutional quality improvement groups and stakeholders in the process (e.g., the department delivering the service, the department or unit affected by poor outcomes in the area, the managed care company) are likely to support APNs' outcome evaluation initiatives.

DATA MANAGEMENT

The fourth component consists of data collection, storage, analysis, and interpretation. Data collection and storage techniques, as well as data analysis strategies, will vary depending on the type of data being collected. Knowledge and skills related to the handling of data are similar regardless of whether the data are collected for evaluation or for the generation of knowledge through research. Such techniques are included among the knowledge and skills necessary for the third research competency, participating in collaborative research (see next section). Because these techniques may be complex, and require computer hardware and software not familiar to many APNs, the authors recommend that APNs seek out appropriate resources or consultants. For example, the institution may have quality improvement or data management personnel who can assist with the design of a data system for the outcome evaluation project (see Chapter 19 for further discussion of data management).

The APN needs a variety of skills in order to use research designs and approaches for evaluating practice. Also needed is an understanding of databases, including the types of data that are stored and retrievable within one's institution, as well as how to plan for the development of additional databases (Wu, Crosby, Ventura, & Finnick, 1994). A wide variety of institutional databases, such as administrative databases for billing and medical records, can provide APNs with clinical data (Bozzo, 1999; Minarik, 1999). Such databases can be invaluable in the evaluation of practice. For example, various databases at the Duke University Medical Center include data related to patient satisfaction following hospitalizations and clinic visits, patients' perceptions of the adequacy of education provided, and assessments of level of pain and functional status. The potential exists for using such data to evaluate the effects of APN practice over time. Aggregate data could be used to track trends related to APN availability or time spent in a specific unit or clinic. A database set up to record APN consults and follow-ups could be linked to existing databases to track parameters and outcomes, relative to APNs' encounters with patients.

The APN also needs an adequate understanding of research methodology to interpret data appropriately and to recognize the potential for confounding variables. For example, in correlating pain and functional status with APN interactions with patients, it would also be important to consider disease status over time. Decreasing functional status in the patient with stable disease has different implications than it would in the context of progressive cancer. The knowledge and skills necessary to interpret data appropriately are also necessary to interpret and use research in practice, as discussed earlier and shown in Table 9-2.

DISSEMINATION

Finally, the fifth component is dissemination, which is related to sharing the results of outcome evaluation projects with relevant individuals, groups, departments, or professional colleagues. Dissemination can be formal (e.g., an oral presentation or a publication) or informal (e.g., a discussion or brief presentation). At a minimum, dissemination of results, including cost and resource implications, to administrators and other key decision makers should be done. Effective dissemination requires that the APN be able to clearly and comprehensively describe the components discussed previously (see Table 9–3). The APN must also be able to explain the outcomes, articulate how or why they were related to advanced nursing practice, and link the findings with current practice or proposals for revised practice.

SUMMARY

A variety of research skills is essential in order to evaluate practice. Some of these skills are developed in learning the previous research competency—interpreting and using research—whereas others must be learned separately in order to select appropriate outcome criteria and measures, develop an appropriate evaluation study design, and implement evaluation within one's practice. The exemplars introduced in the previous section are continued here with discussion of components relevant to the research competency, evaluation of practice.

EXEMPLAR 1: PAIN MANAGEMENT (continued)

In the Bookbinder and colleagues (1995; 1996) CQI pain management project introduced earlier, evaluation was an important component of the project. Baseline assessments of pain management practice and exploration of variability in practice resulted in identification of three areas that were problematic: systems issues such as delays in getting medications to patients, educational issues such as lack of knowledge about assessment or fears of addiction to opioids, and prescribing issues such as inappropriate dosing, routes, or frequency. These three areas provided guidance for selection of specific activities that could be improved. The key process that the interdisciplinary team sought to improve was "administering analgesics in a timely manner" (Bookbinder et al., 1995, p. 334).

Following implementation of the APS quality assurance standards for pain, and extensive in-service education, the interdisciplinary team examined whether it had achieved its goal. Both process and outcome measures were evaluated using the following questions:

1. Was implementation of the APS guidelines feasible?
2. What was the effect of implementing the pain management program on nurses' knowledge and attitudes about pain?
3. What was the effect on patient outcomes such as satisfaction with pain management?
4. What unit-based changes in pain management practice resulted?

Each of these was answered using specific methods. For example, focus groups were used to answer the first question. A 46-item questionnaire measuring attitudes and knowledge related to pain was used to answer question 2. Questionnaires addressing patients' satisfaction and concerns with pain management provided data for question 3. Finally, question 4 was answered by counting the number of pain-related CQI studies initiated by each unit and assessing their effects on practice.

EXEMPLAR 2: HEALTH PROMOTION—
SMOKING CESSATION (*continued*)

This exemplar continues with the example of CNS-driven changes in smoking cessation counseling offered to post-MI patients. Rather than focusing on measuring outcomes of her individual practice by evaluating outcomes in only those patients to whom she provided counseling, the CNS chose to measure outcomes related to the continuum of services provided, in effect measuring outcomes of the programmatic changes she had facilitated. Obviously, quit rates were the logical measurement outcome, and these were evaluated at 6 and 12 months postdischarge, using data readily available through follow-up clinic notes. In addition to the quit rates, the CNS also measured change in readiness to quit, using a standardized questionnaire that had been incorporated into the inpatient clinical assessment forms.

Participation in Collaborative Research

This third research competency involves participation in collaborative nursing or interdisciplinary research studies conducted to generate knowledge that defines optimal nursing or other interventions for particular populations and specific clinical problems (Brooten & Naylor, 1995). In earlier publications, the authors (McGuire & Harwood, 1989, 1996) focused on the actual conduct of research in clinical settings. The emphasis of this competency has evolved in this text to participating in collaborative nursing and interdisciplinary research, which is a more realistic competency. As noted earlier in the chapter, the authors do not define basic and advanced-level activities for this competency. The distinction is impossible to make, because APNs' participation in collaborative research is usually highly context-driven. That is, their particular work setting may be one in which research participation is a major component of the position, or it may be one in which research is not part of the position description at all. Thus this competency is envisioned as one that is important to the APN role, but context-dependent. Generic knowledge and skills important for practicing this competency are shown in Table 9–5.

Why collaborative research? As Martin (1995) wrote, most nurses can find the time for research if they really want to be involved. She emphasized the need to make research a priority, *to collaborate with others,* to break projects into manageable parts, to structure work for multiple outcomes, and to garner the necessary resources. Participating in collaborative research is a reasonably realistic goal for APNs in today's health care environment, although some may elect, with experience and the development of additional skills, to conduct their own individual research (McGuire & Harwood, 1989), which would be considered an advanced level of this competency.

There are several activities conducive to collaborative participation in research, each commensurate with existing APN practice standards (American Association of Critical-Care Nurses and ANA, 1995; ANA 1996; ONS, 1997) that pertain to research. The APN, regardless of type of practice or setting, is the most likely individual to understand the clinical issues and questions in a given patient population. This individual can identify nursing practice problems and work collaboratively as a consultant with academically based researchers to translate these problems into researchable questions. She or he is also a logical individual to work with the research team in identifying nurse-sensitive outcomes. The APN can also be involved in helping to develop methods or study procedures that not only are clinically feasible but help

TABLE 9–5 COMPETENCY III: PARTICIPATION IN COLLABORATIVE RESEARCH

MAJOR PHASES AND STEPS IN THE RESEARCH PROCESS*	KNOWLEDGE	SKILLS
Phase I: Conceptual Phase		
Step 1 Formulating and delimiting the problem	• Understand importance of a good research problem • Understand research problems, purposes, and questions • Understand ethical and practical aspects of research problems	• Identify and document clinical practice problems • Articulate researchable problems, purposes, and questions
Step 2 Reviewing literature	• Have basic understanding of purposes of literature review • Understand generating and building of knowledge	• Identify relevant databases, literature, resources, and consultants • Find and retrieve literature • Use a computer • Critique research • Synthesize research
Step 3 Developing a theoretical framework	• Understand relationship between theory, research, practice, and science (NLN, 1987)	• Assess theories for appropriate "fit" with clinical questions
Step 4 Formulating hypotheses (if appropriate for the research problem)	• Understand relationships between research problems, questions, and hypotheses • Understand quantitative, hypothesis—testing research designs	• Articulate hypotheses in clear, measurable terms
Phase 2: Design and Planning Phase (Developing the Methods)		
Step 5 Selecting a research design	• Have basic understanding of research paradigms, designs, and approaches • Understand distinction between purposes and functions of qualitative and quantitative approaches	• Select an appropriate design or approach that matches research problems and questions • Determine feasibility in a given clinical environment
Step 6 Identifying the population	• Understand basic concepts and principles of population selection in relation to sample selection • Recognize issues related to external validity when selecting sample(s) from population(s)	• Select an appropriate population • Help delineate eligibility and exclusion criteria for sample
Step 7 Selecting measures for the research variables	• Understand principles of measurement • Psychometric properties of measures • Distinction between biophysiologic, self-report, and observational measures	• Determine appropriateness of measures in a given sample • Determine feasibility of measures in a given setting
Step 8 Designing the sampling plan	• Understand probability and nonprobability sampling • Understand issues and methods in determining sample size	• Select an appropriate sample • Help determine procedures for identifying and recruiting sample

Table continued on opposite page

TABLE 9–5	COMPETENCY III: PARTICIPATION IN COLLABORATIVE RESEARCH *Continued*	
MAJOR PHASES AND STEPS IN THE RESEARCH PROCESS*	**KNOWLEDGE**	**SKILLS**
Step 9 Finalizing and reviewing the research plan	• Understand the rationale for developing a full written proposal of the research project: –protection of human subjects –other institutional approvals –submission for funding –methodologic, feasibility, or conceptual critique	• Participate in drafting full proposal • Identify relevant institutional approval mechanisms and assist with applications • Make clinical or administrative arrangements necessary for project implementation (e.g., institutional review; staff education regarding study)
Step 10 Conducting the pilot study and making revisions	• Understand need for and purposes of a pilot study	• Help with implementation in clinical setting • Identify problematic areas (e.g., procedures measures) • Participate in revising research methods if needed
Phase 3: Empirical Phase		
Step 11 Collecting data	• Understand the various time frames required • Understand the need for standardization and quality control	• Help develop a feasible data collection protocol • Monitor data collection and problem-solve when needed
Step 12 Preparing data for analysis	• Understand data preparation and entry procedures • Understand use of computers in data analysis	• Assist with preparing data for entry (e.g., checking, coding, cleaning) • Assist with actual data entry if appropriate
Phase 4: Analytic Phase		
Step 13 Analyzing data	• Understand purposes of analysis • Distinguish between qualitative and quantitative (statistical) analyses	• Assist in determining appropriate analyses
Step 14 Interpreting results	• Understand the process of making sense of results and for examining implications	• Participate in interpreting data and identify implications for practice
Phase 5: Dissemination Phase		
Step 15 Communicating findings	• Understand importance of disseminating research results • Discuss various methods for dissemination	• Participate in decisions regarding when and where to disseminate results • Participate in presentations and publications of results
Step 16 Utilizing findings	• See Competency I, Table 9–2	• See Competency 1, Table 9–2

* The major phases and steps in the research process are from Polit, D. F., & Hungler, B. P. (1997). *Essentials of nursing research: Methods, appraisals, and utilization* (4th ed.). Philadelphia: J. B. Lippincott.

minimize burden to staff and patients. Such collaboration can significantly enhance the clinical relevance and quality of research (McGuire & Harwood, 1989) as well as enhance its scientific rigor (McGuire, Deloney, Yeager, Owen, & Peterson, in press). Another viable collaborative activity is to assist researchers with identification and recruitment of appropriate subjects for a study. In intervention studies, there may be a specific role that the APN could play in implementation of the intervention or measurement of study outcomes.

The main area of knowledge required for this competency is a familiarity with the research process, and an understanding of how it differs from RU and from the nursing process. Polit and Hungler (1997) presented a useful description of the major steps in the research process, grouped into five phases: conceptual, design and planning (methods), empirical, analytic, and dissemination; this framework is used to organize knowledge and skills in Table 9–5. Readers interested in the research process are referred to this text or others often used in master's degree programs (Burns & Grove, 1997; Mateo & Kirchhoff, 1999).

In conclusion, participation in collaborative research is an important competency for APNs, although clearly less critical to the quality and effectiveness of their own practices than are competencies I and II. APN participation in knowledge-generating research can help ground the research firmly in clinical reality, with results that are applicable within and even across settings. The two exemplars continued here provide a brief discussion of participation in collaborative research activities.

EXEMPLAR 1: PAIN MANAGEMENT (continued)

Bookbinder and colleagues (1995; 1996) noted that their CQI project on pain management resulted in a "ripple effect" (p. 342) that led to new collaborative pain management projects in numerous clinical areas. Manifestations of this effect took the form in some instances of systematic research studies testing interventions for pain. For example, some staff began testing the effects of nursing interventions such as patient education and relaxation on anxiety and discomfort. In the postanesthesia care unit, nurses implemented and tested a behavioral pain assessment scale in patients who were sedated. This project highlights the importance of APN leadership in improving practice through the CQI process and fostering new collaborative endeavors, while simultaneously engaging in the research competencies described previously.

EXEMPLAR 3: HEALTH PROMOTION — RISK REDUCTION

The conduct of research extends beyond outcome evaluation of clinical practice to generate new knowledge generalizable to other practitioners. When APNs are involved in the conduct of health promotion research, it is most often as part of an interdisciplinary team. This approach is especially appropriate given that health promotion is most effective when it encompasses a variety of strategies and involves a variety of practitioners. This is exemplified in the work of Hollen, Hobbie, and Finley (1999) describing the evaluation of a risk reduction program for cancer-surviving adolescents. Through collaboration with the NP coordinating a survivor follow-up clinic, a psychologist for the clinic, and a nursing professor, a comprehensive program to decrease risk behaviors in adolescent cancer survivors was designed and tested. Although clearly pertinent to evaluating and guiding the clinical practice of the APN and psychologist seeing these patients, the added rigor of the research design generated knowledge that can be applied in other practice settings.

ACQUIRING AND DEVELOPING RESEARCH COMPETENCIES

This final section discusses the important roles that graduate education and postgraduate research development play in APNs' achievement of meaningful and realistic research competencies that meet the demands placed on them as practitioners. It is unrealistic to expect that any graduate program can, with its temporal and structural constraints, prepare APNs for the full spectrum of possible research competency activities, that is, both basic and advanced levels of activity (Table 9–1). Thus it is important to realize that APNs will develop their research competencies *beginning* in graduate school and *continuing* throughout their careers. Upon graduation, APNs should be able to perform at the basic level of activity shown in Table 9–1 for competencies I and II. With additional experience, continuing education, and mentoring, they may achieve the advanced levels of activity for competencies I and II, and perhaps engage in competency III, depending on their postgraduate positions and their professional goals.

Graduate Education

Graduate programs bear the primary responsibility for teaching necessary knowledge and skills for the basic levels of activity in competencies I and II, and thus preparing their graduates for expansion of competencies when they go out into the workplace. The authors assume, however, that graduate faculty are role models for all three competencies consistent with their respective areas of didactic and clinical expertise. A discussion of this assumption is beyond the scope of this chapter, but such role modeling is critical to the successful teaching of research competencies.

Adoption of this set of research competencies for APNs will require, for many schools, a rethinking of how "research" is conceptualized and taught at the master's degree level. In keeping with the schema for advanced practice nursing presented in Chapter 3, if research is truly a core competency, then it must be internalized by students in APN programs. Internalization of any body of knowledge or set of skills does not occur with brief exposure or admonitions to engage in self-study. Rather, internalization occurs when important material is introduced early, repeated regularly, and integrated into other components of the curriculum at every possible opportunity.

Teaching research competencies effectively may require an overhaul of all APN curricula in a given program, because these competencies need to be integrated throughout the entire curriculum, not just isolated in the "research" course(s). A hypothetical curriculum is shown in Table 9–6 in order to demonstrate how the two major research competencies (I and II) can be integrated throughout an APN curriculum. In some courses, such as research, the specific knowledge and skills listed in Tables 9–2 and 9–3 can be used to develop and organize course content as well as assignments. In other courses, it may be more appropriate to use the specific skills shown in the tables to design and implement student assignments.

A specific example may help to clarify how research competencies can be integrated into the curriculum and taught to APN graduate students. As a member of the graduate faculty at the Emory University Nell Hodgson Woodruff School of Nursing (1993–1999), the first author worked with a number of other faculty to introduce research competencies (McGuire & Harwood, 1996) into the required core research course, and integrate them into subsequent clinical courses in the Adult and Elder

TABLE 9–6	INTEGRATING RESEARCH COMPETENCIES INTO AN ADVANCED PRACTICE NURSING GRADUATE CURRICULUM	
COURSES	COMPETENCY*†	ASSIGNMENTS‡
(Core)§		
Theory/knowledge generation	I. Interpretation and use of research	• Integrative review of literature supporting a given theory
Research/statistics	I. Interpretation and use of research	• Research-based policy, procedure, or protocol
	II. Evaluation of practice	• Short-term individual or group project evaluating a specific intervention and its effects on selected outcomes
	III. Participation in collaborative research	• Design a data collection protocol, develop research questions
Health policy/professional issues	I. Interpretation and use of research	• Write research-based clinical guidelines for a selected problem and make recommendations for implementation at a policy level
	II. Evaluation of practice	• Develop an evaluation plan for a set of clinical guidelines
Ethics	I. Interpretation and use of research	• Write a research-based paper exploring dimensions of a selected ethical issue (e.g., advance directives)
Pharmacology	I. Interpretation and use of research	• Case reports describing selection and use of pharmacologic agents based on existing research
	II. Evaluation of practice	• Written evaluation plan for use of specific pharmacologic agents in treating selected clinical problems (e.g., nonopioid and opioid analgesics for cancer pain)
(Clinical)¶		
Advanced Nursing Practice/ Nurse Practitioner I, II, III, etc. (includes didactic sessions and clinical practice)	I. Interpretation and use of research	• Description of comprehensive assessment and intervention plan for individual cases or groups derived from current research; can include critical pathways, care maps, algorithms, protocols, etc.
	II. Evaluation of practice	• Design and implement an evaluation "study" of a specific intervention; include APN-relevant outcomes; make recommendations for practice based on findings
	III. Participation in collaborative research	• Problem identification, selection of research sample, development of data collection procedures

* Refer to Tables 9–2 and 9–3 for the specific *knowledge* and *skills* required for each competency.
† Note that the specific *knowledge* shown in Tables 9–2, and 9–3 can serve as a foundation for course content in selected courses (e.g., research/statistics).
‡ Note that the specific *skills* shown in Tables 9–2 and 9–3 can be used to design and organize assignments; the examples in this table are more integrative, requiring various combinations of *skills* and building on *knowledge*.
§ It is acknowledged that all ANP programs may not have all of these courses; they are hypothetical only.
¶ These hypothetical courses are assumed to exist in some form in any type of ANP program (e.g., CNA, CNM, CNS, NP).

Health Department. The research course used nursing's circle of knowledge (NLN, 1987) as a conceptual framework for presenting content on the research process and use of research in practice. Three major assignments tapped into the basic level of activities for research competencies I and II. First, students performed individual written quantitative and qualitative research critiques that focused on scientific merit and application of findings to practice. Second, working in small groups, students read about and then selected a research utilization model (e.g., Stetler, 1994) or a research application approach (e.g., EBP) and used it to evaluate a small body of research and make decisions about if and how to apply the findings to practice. Third, again working in small groups (usually aggregated by programmatic specialty, such as family NPs, oncology APNs, or CNMs), students conceptualized and designed an APN outcomes project in which they identified key outcomes attributable to APN practice and then selected methods for measuring the outcomes. In general, students reported that these assignments helped them better understand what research competencies involved and gave them a foundation for subsequent activities in other graduate courses.

Integration of research competencies then occurred in one of the clinical courses required of APN students in the Adult and Elder Health Department. The course focused on chronic care, and included two assignments based on research competencies. In the first one, students wrote a paper describing the formulation and management of a set of data they could use in examining their practice; this assignment was clearly linked with research competency II. In the second assignment, which provided practice with research competency I, students worked with an APN in a clinical setting to conduct a collaborative RU project that resulted in a discrete product, such as a component of a critical pathway or selection of a pain assessment tool for a specific patient population. The assignment required students to identify, retrieve, interpret, and make recommendations for use of the research literature relevant to the problem at hand. Typical feedback from students indicated that this exercise helped cement what research-based practice was all about, and gave them some preparation for repeating the process in other venues. Although this graduate faculty effort to introduce core research competency content early, then reinforce it later in the curriculum, was challenging and required strong collaboration and shared ownership and responsibility, it provides one viable model for how other graduate faculty might attempt to integrate research competencies throughout the curriculum.

Postgraduate Research Development

Much of graduate education is geared toward providing broad knowledge and skills that support future learning and development. Postgraduate research development is highly individualized to the APN's practice setting and specialty and serves to move the APN toward experience with competency III and the advanced levels of activity in research competencies I and II (Table 9-1).

Broad areas of postgraduate research development include (1) expanding knowledge of appropriate clinical research literature, (2) expanding knowledge of appropriate outcome measurement techniques, (3) expanding knowledge of research methodologies, (4) developing and maintaining competency in computer applications related to information access and database management, and (5) honing personal skills as a change agent in complex, fluid environments (see also Chapter 10). There are numerous ways in which an APN can seek further development in these areas, including academic study, mentoring, and self-study.

Formal coursework offers opportunities for development in each of these areas. Relevant courses may be found within graduate programs in nursing, public health, epidemiology, basic sciences (e.g., physiology), social sciences (e.g., psychology), computer sciences, business management, and others. Appropriate courses may also be offered for professional development within one's work environment or by private companies specializing in professional development. APNs can gain needed skills through selection of individual courses to meet their current development needs or pursue an additional academic degree to enhance their research and other competencies.

Pursuing a doctoral degree in nursing or a related field is one means by which an APN can acquire additional research knowledge and skills. Subsequent research roles (not competencies) assumed by APNs who obtain doctoral education must be distinguished. Some APNs will choose to obtain a doctoral degree in order to provide themselves with a more advanced level of research skills that they can apply directly in their clinical practice, providing more research-based care, evaluating their practice, and conducting independent or collaborative research within their specialty areas (J. A. Spross, personal communication, October 1995). Other APNs will choose to obtain a doctoral degree with its attendant advanced research skills so that they can become clinical researchers, not practicing themselves but collaborating with active clinicians such as APNs to address important clinical problems and research questions (Haller, 1990; Kirchhoff, 1993).

The mentor-protégé relationship offers another opportunity for development of advanced research skills. These relationships occur on a continuum ranging from passive role modeling or active precepting of the APN new in a role or new in an institution to the classic mentoring relationship, the professional and personal nurturing of a less experienced person (Kinsey, 1990; Vance & Olson, 1998). APNs can seek out role models both within their organizations and within their practice specialties.

Watching and reading about how others have incorporated research findings into their practice, evaluated their practice, or conducted research can be both instructive and motivating. The APN may thus be able to identify a preceptor to assist in the development of a specific skill or group of skills related to any of the research competencies. For example, an APN may request guidance and feedback from an experienced individual when developing a research proposal for submission to a funding agency or research review board, when selecting or incorporating a new outcome measurement technique, or when designing a database for the collection of outcome data.

Within the mentoring continuum, the classic mentor-protégé relationship offers the maximum opportunity for developing advanced research skills. These relationships are typically initiated by the nurse identifying an individual to be emulated and then approaching the individual with a request for mentorship. If the mentor agrees, she or he then provides teaching, guidance, and feedback in broad areas relative to the protégé's development. The protégé sustains the relationship by providing feedback on how the guidance has been used and by giving status or outcome reports on activities undertaken in this mentoring process. These relationships often provide an opportunity for collaborative research, using the APN's clinical expertise and the mentor's research expertise. APNs may find appropriate mentors among nursing colleagues within their agencies, specialties, professional nursing organizations, or academic faculties. Colleagues from other disciplines may also become research mentors for APNs.

Regardless of the methods chosen to advance one's research skills, self-study is essential to the development of advanced research competencies. This self-study is carefully focused on the individual's specialty area and practice. For instance, in an example provided by the second author's research efforts to determine appropriate treatment of chemotherapy extravasation (K. Harwood, unpublished results, 1995), extensive self-study supplemented graduate education and mentorship support. Graduate work in pharmacology, chemistry, and physiology was supplemented with focused readings in areas such as doxorubicin pharmacology, free radicals and free radical scavenging techniques, and wound healing. This knowledge was used to identify potential antidotes for evaluation in a subsequent research project (Harwood, Stauman, & Gonin, 1994). Determining appropriate animal models for antidote testing required focused self-study in comparative anatomy and physiology (VanSloten, Gee, Bachur, & Wiernik, 1982). In conclusion, the multifaceted and increasingly interdisciplinary nature of clinical practice and research will always require APNs to pursue in-depth knowledge and skills beyond their graduate education to meet research needs and other practice requirements.

SUMMARY AND CONCLUSION

Three research competencies are required for APNs to meet the various research-related demands placed on them in today's health care delivery system: (I) interpretation and utilization of research, (II) evaluation of practice, and (III) participation in collaborative research. The first two of these competencies are operationalized at two levels—basic activities learned through graduate education and advanced activities acquired through postgraduate research development. The third competency does not have basic or advanced levels per se but is context-dependent. As discussed, these competencies are essential to APNs as they define, implement, refine, validate, and evaluate their practices and as they move forward to take visible leadership positions in the health care system of the future.

REFERENCES

Agency for Health Care Policy and Research. (1996b). *Overview: Smoking cessation* (Clinical Practice Guideline No. 18, AHCPR Publication No. 96-0692). Rockville, MD: Author. (Retrieved December 4, 1999 from the World Wide Web: *http://www.ahcpr.gov/clinic/smoview.htm*)

Agency for Health Care Policy and Research. (1996a). *Helping smokers quit: a guide for primary care clinicians* (Clinical Practice Guideline No. 18, AHCPR Publication No. 96-0693). Rockville, MD: Author. (Retrieved December 4, 1999 from the World Wide Web: *http://www.ahcpr.gov/clinic/smokepcc.htm*)

Agency for Health Care Policy and Research. (1996c). *Smoking cessation: a systems approach* (Clinical Practice Guideline No. 18, AHCPR Publication No. 97-0698). Rockville, MD: Author. (Retrieved December 4, 1999 from the World Wide Web: *http://www.ahcpr.gov/clinic/smokesys.htm*)

American Association of Colleges of Nursing. (1996). *The essentials of master's education for advanced practice nursing*. Washington, DC: Author.

American Association of Colleges of Nursing. (1999). Certification and regulation of advanced practice nurses. *Journal of Professional Nursing, 15,* 130–132.

American Association of Critical-Care Nurses and American Nurses Association. (1995). *Standards of clinical practice and scope of practice for the acute care nurse practitioner.* Washington, DC: American Nurses Association.

American Nurses Association. (1981). *Guidelines for the investigative function of nurses.* Kansas City, MO: Author.

American Nurses Association. (1996). *Scope and standards of advanced practice registered nursing.* Washington, DC: Author.

Andrews, J. O., Tingen, M. S., & Harper, R. J. (1999). A model nurse practitioner-managed smoking cessation clinic. *Oncology Nursing Forum, 26,* 1603–1610.

Association of Nurse Executives. (1990). *Current issues and perspectives of differentiated practice.* Chicago: American Hospital Association.

Bookbinder, M., Kiss, M., Coyle, N., Brown, M., Gianella, A., & Thaler, H. (1995). Improving pain management practices. In D. B. McGuire, C. H. Yarbro, & B. R. Ferrell (Eds.), *Cancer pain management* (2nd ed., pp. 321–361). Boston: Jones & Bartlett.

Bookbinder, M., Coyle, N., Kiss, M., Goldstein, M. L., Holritz, K., Thaler, H., Grasella, A., Derby, S., Brown, M., Racolin, A., Ho, M. N., & Portenoy, R. K. (1996). Implementing national standards for cancer pain management: Program model and evaluation. *Journal of Pain and Symptom Management, 12:*334–337.

Bozzo, J. (1999). Databases and nursing outcomes. *American Journal of Nursing, 99*(4), 22.

Brady, M. J., Cella, D. F., Mo, F., Bonomi, A. E., Tulsky, D. S., Lloyd, S. R., Deasy, S., Cobleigh, M., & Shiomoto, G. (1997). Reliability and validity of the Functional Assessment of Cancer Therapy–Breast quality of life instrument. *Journal of Clinical Oncology, 15,* 974–986.

Brockopp, D. Y., & Hastings-Tolsma, M. T. (1995). *Fundamentals of nursing research* (2nd ed.). Boston: Jones & Bartlett.

Brooten, D., & Naylor, M. D. (1995). Nurses' effect on changing patient outcomes. *Image: The Journal of Nursing Scholarship, 27*(2), 95–99.

Brooten, D., Kumar, S., Brown, L. P., Butts, P., Finkler, S. A., Bakewell-Sachs, S., Gibbons, A., & Delivoria-Papadopoulos, M. (1986). A randomized clinical trial of early hospital discharge and home follow-up of very-low-birth-weight infants. *New England Journal of Medicine, 315,* 934–939.

Brown, S. J. (1999). *Knowledge for health care practice: A guide to using research evidence.* Philadelphia: W. B. Saunders.

Bruera, E., Schoeller, T., & MacEachern, T. (1992). Symptomatic benefit of supplemental oxygen in hypoxemic patients with terminal cancer: The use of the *N* of 1 randomized controlled trial. *Journal of Pain and Symptom Management, 7,* 365–368.

Buerhaus, P. I. (1998). Is another RN shortage looming? *Nursing Outlook, 46,* 103–108.

Bulechek, G. M., & McCloskey, J. C. (1998). *Nursing interventions: Effective nursing treatments* (3rd ed.). Philadelphia: W. B. Saunders.

Burns, N., & Grove, S. K. (1997). *The practice of nursing research: Conduct, critique, & utilization* (3rd ed.). Philadelphia: W. B. Saunders.

Campbell, N. C., Richie, L. D., Thain, J., Deans, H. G., Rawles, J. M., & Squair J. L. (1998). Secondary prevention in coronary heart disease: A randomised trial of nurse led clinics in primary care. *Heart, 80,* 447–452.

Cardinal, B. J. (1997). Construct validity of stages of change for exercise behavior. *American Journal of Health Promotion, 12*(1), 68–74.

Carter, J. H., Moorhead, S. A., McCloskey, J. C., & Bulechek, G. M. (1995). Using the Nursing Interventions Classification to implement Agency for Health Care Policy and Research guidelines. *Journal of Nursing Care Quality, 9*(2), 76–86.

Cline, C. M., Israelsson, B. Y., Willenheimer, R. B., Broms, K., & Erhardt, L. R. (1998). Cost effective management programme for heart failure reduces hospitalisation. *Heart, 80,* 442–446.

Cooper, R. A., Laud, P., & Dietrich, C. L. (1998). Current and projected workforce of nonphysician clinicians. *JAMA, 280,* 786–794.

Cronenwett, L. R. (1995). Molding the future of advanced practice nursing. *Nursing Outlook, 43*(3), 112–118.

Deaton, C. (1998a). Outcomes measurement. *Journal of Cardiovascular Nursing, 12*(4), 49–51.

Deaton, C. (1998b). Outcomes measurement: Multidisciplinary approaches and patient outcomes after stroke. *Journal of Cardiovascular Nursing, 13*(1), 93–96.

Doyle, R. L., & Feren, A. T. (1992). *Healthcare management guidelines.* Albany, NY: Milliman & Robertson.

Eisen, S. V., Leff, H. S., & Schaefer, E. (1999). Implementing outcome systems: Lessons from a test of the BASIS-2 and the SF-36. *Journal of Behavioral Health Services & Research, 26*(1), 18–27.

Evidence-Based Working Group. (1992). Evidence based medicine: A new approach to teaching the practice of medicine. *JAMA, 268,* 2420–2425.

Fallowfield, L. J., Hall, A., Maguire, G. P., & Baum, M. (1990). Psychological outcomes of different treatment policies in women with early breast cancer outside clinical trials. *BMJ, 301,* 575–580.

Fawzy, F. I., Fawzy, N. W., Hyun, C. S., Elashoff, R., Guthrie, D., Fahey, J. L., & Morton, D. L. (1993). Malignant melanoma: Effects of an early structured psychiatric intervention, coping, and affective state on recurrence and survival six years later. *Archives of General Psychiatry, 50,* 681.

Firlit, S. L., Walsh, M., & Kemp, M. G. (1987). Nursing research in practice: A survey of research utilization content in master's degree programs. *Western Journal of Nursing Research, 9,* 612–616.

Hadorn, D. C., Baker, D., Hodges, J. S., & Hicks, N. (1996). Rating the quality of evidence for clinical practice guidelines. *Journal of Clinical Epidemiology, 49,* 749–754.

Haller, K. B. (1990). The clinical nurse researcher role in a practice setting. In N. L. Chaska (Ed.), *The nursing profession: Turning points* (pp. 194–201). St. Louis: C. V. Mosby.

Hamric, A. B., Spross, J. A., & Hanson, C. M. (1996). *Advanced nursing practice: An integrative approach.* Philadelphia: W. B. Saunders.

Harwood, K., Strauman, J., & Gonin, R. (1994). Short-term vs. long-term local cooling after doxorubicin (DOX) extravasation: An Eastern Cooperative Oncology Group (ECOG) study [Abstract]. *Proceedings of the American Society of Clinical Oncology, 13,* 447.

Hodgman, E. C. (1983). The CNS as researcher. In A. B. Hamric & J. A. Spross (Eds.), *The clinical nurse specialist in theory and practice* (pp. 73–82). New York: Grune & Stratton.

Hollen, P. J., Hobbie, W. L., & Finley, S. M. (1999). Testing the effects of a decision-making and risk-reduction program for cancer-surviving adolescents. *Oncology Nursing Forum, 26,* 1475–1486.

Institute for Clinical Systems Improvement. (1999, January 21). *Tobacco use prevention and cessation for adults and mature adolescents.* Bloomington, MN: Author. (Retrieved December 4, 1999 from the World Wide Web: *http://www.icsi.org/guide/G29.htm*)

Jacobsen, S. J., Girman, C. J., Guess, H. A., Panser, L. A., Chute, C. G., Oesterling, J. E., & Lieber, M. M. (1995). Do prostate size and urinary flow rates predict health care seeking behavior for urinary symptoms in men? *Urology, 45.*64-69.

Kachoyeanos, M. K. (1995, March/April). Research or else. *MCN, 20,* 111.

Kattapong, V. J., Locher, T. L., Secker-Walker, R. H., & Bell, T. A. (1998). Tobacco-cessation patient counseling: American College of Preventive Medicine practice policy statement. *American Journal of Preventive Medicine, 15,* 160-162. (Retrieved December 6, 1999 from the World Wide Web: *http://www.acpm.org/tobpol.htm*)

Kinsey, D. C. (1990, May). Mentorship and influence in nursing. *Nursing Management,* pp. 45-46.

Kirchhoff, K. T. (1993). The role of nurse researchers employed in clinical settings. *Annual Review of Nursing Research, 11,* 169-181.

Lang, N. M., & Marek, K. D. (1992). Outcomes that reflect clinical practice. In National Center for Nursing Research, *Patient outcomes research: Examining the effectiveness of nursing practice* (NIH Publication No. 93-3411). Bethesda, MD: National Institutes of Health.

Larsen, J. (1980). Knowledge utilization: What is it? *Knowledge Creation, Diffusion, and Utilization, 1,* 421-442.

Lindeke, L. L., & Block, D. E. (1998). Maintaining professional integrity in the midst of interdisciplinary collaboration. *Nursing Outlook, 46,* 213-218.

Lombness, P. M. (1994). Difference in length of stay with care managed by clinical nurse specialists or physician assistants. *Clinical Nurse Specialist, 8*(5), 253-260.

Lydon-Rochelle, M. T., Albers, L., & Teaf, D. (1995). Perineal outcomes and nurse-midwifery management. *Journal of Nurse-Midwifery, 40*(1), 13-18.

Martin, P. A. (1995). Finding time for research. *Applied Nursing Research, 8*(3), 151-153.

Mateo, M. A., & Kirchhoff, K. T. (Eds.). (1999). *Using and conducting nursing research in the clinical setting* (2nd ed.). Philadelphia: W. B. Saunders.

Max, M. (1990). American Pain Society quality assurance standards for relief of acute pain and cancer pain. In M. R. Bond, J. E. Charlton, & C. J. Woolf (Eds.), *Proceedings of the VI World Congress on Pain* (pp. 186-189). Amsterdam: Elsevier.

McCloskey, J. C., Bulechek, G. M., & Donahue, W. (1998). Nursing interventions core to specialty practice. *Nursing Outlook, 46,* 67-76.

McDermott-Blackburn, K. (1998). Role of advanced practice nurses in oncology. *Oncology, 12,* 591-598.

McGuire, D. B. (1992, January). *The process of implementing research into clinical practice.* (Publication No. 92-50M-No. 3320.00-PE. Proceedings of the American Cancer Society Second National Conference on Cancer Nursing Research). Atlanta: American Cancer Society.

McGuire, D. B., & Harwood, K. V. (1989). The CNS as researcher. In A. B. Hamric & J. A. Spross (Eds.), *The clinical nurse specialist in theory and practice* (2nd ed., pp. 169-203). Philadelphia: W. B. Saunders.

McGuire, D. B., & Harwood, K. V. (1996). Research interpretation, utilization, and conduct. In Hamric, A. B., Spross, J. A., & Hanson, C. M. (Eds.), *Advanced nursing practice: An integrative approach* (pp. 184-211). Philadelphia: W. B. Saunders.

McGuire, D. B., DeLoney, V. G., Yeager, K. A., Owen, D. C., Peterson, D. E., Lin L. S., & Webster, J. (in press). Maintaining study validity in a changing clinical environment. *Nursing Research.*

McGuire, D. B., Walczak, J. R., Krumm, S. L., Haisfield, M. E., Beezley, A., Reedy, A. M., Shivnan, J. C., Hanson, J. L., Gregory, R. E., & Ashley, B. (1994). Research utilization in oncology nursing: Application of the Stetler model in a comprehensive cancer center. *Oncology Nursing Forum, 21,* 703-724.

Medoff-Cooper, B. (1994). Transition of the preterm infant to an open crib. *Journal of Obstetric, Gynecologic, and Neonatal Nursing, 23,* 329-335.

Meier, P. P. (1994). Transition of the preterm infant to an open crib: Process of the project group. *Journal of Obstetric, Gynecologic, and Neonatal Nursing, 23,* 321-325.

Minarik, P. (1999). Using hospital databases. *American Journal of Nursing, 99*(2), 54.

Mitchell, P. H., Armstrong, S., Simpson, T. F., & Lentz, M. (1989). American Association of Critical-Care Nurses Demonstration Project: Profile of excellence in critical care nursing. *Heart & Lung: The Journal of Critical Care, 18,* 219-237.

Mundinger, M. O., Kane, R. L., Lenz, E. R., Totten, A. M., Tsai, W-Y., Cleary, P. D., Friedewald, W. T., Siu, A. L., & Shelanski, M. L. (2000). Primary care outcomes in patients treated by nurse practitioners or physicians: A randomized trial. *JAMA, 283,* 59-68.

Murphy, P. A. (1997). Evidence-based care: A new paradigm for clinical practice. *Journal of Nurse-Midwifery, 42*(1), 1–3.

National League for Nursing. (1987). *Nursing theory: A circle of knowledge, Parts I and II* [videotape]. (Available from National League for Nursing, 10 Columbus Circle, New York, NY, 10019.)

Naylor, M., Brooten, D., Campbell, R., Jacobsen, B., Mezey, M., Pauly, M., & Schwartz, J. (1999). Comprehensive discharge planning and home follow-up of hospitalized elders: A randomized controlled trial. *JAMA, 281,* 613–620.

Oncology Nursing Society. (1997). *Statement on the scope and standards of advanced practice in oncology nursing.* Pittsburgh, PA: Oncology Nursing Press, Inc.

Polit, D. F., & Hungler, B. P. (1997). *Essentials of nursing research: Methods, appraisals, and utilization* (4th ed.). Philadelphia: J. B. Lippincott.

Prochaska, J. O., & Velicer, W. F. (1997). The transtheoretical model of health behavior change. *American Journal of Health Promotion, 12*(1), 38–48.

Ramsey, J., McKenzie, J., & Fish, D. (1982). Physicians and nurse practitioners: Do they provide equivalent health care? *American Journal of Public Health, 72,* 55–56.

Sandrick, K. (1993). Out in front: Managed care helps push clinical guidelines forward. *Hospitals, 67*(9), 30–31.

Sidani, S., & Braden, C. J. (1998). *Evaluating nursing interventions: A theory-driven approach.* Thousand Oaks, CA: Sage Publications.

Spiegel, D., Bloom, J. R., Kraemer, H. C., & Gottheil, E. (1989). Effect of psychosocial treatment on survival of patients with metastatic breast cancer. *Lancet, 2,* 888.

Spross, J. A., & Heaney, C. A. (2000). Shaping advanced nursing practice in the new millennium. *Seminars in Oncology Nursing, 16,* 12–24.

Steinberg, E. P., Tielsch, J. M., Schein, O. D., Javitt, J. C., Sharkey, P., Cassard, S. D., Legro M. W., Diener-West, M., Bass, E. B., Damiano, A. M., et al. (1994). The VF-14: An index of functional impairment in patients with cataract. *Archives of Ophthalmology, 112,* 630–638.

Stetler, C. B. (1985). Research utilization: Defining the concept. *IMAGE: The Journal of Nursing Scholarship, 17*(2), 40–44.

Stetler, C. B. (1994). Refinement of the Stetler/Marram model for application of research findings to practice. *Nursing Outlook, 42*(1), 15–25.

Stetler, C. B., & DiMaggio, G. (1991). Research utilization among clinical nurse specialists. *Clinical Nurse Specialist, 5*(3), 151–155.

Stetler, C. B., Bautista, C., Vernale-Hannon, C., & Foster, J. (1995). Enhancing research utilization by clinical nurse specialists. *Nursing Clinics of North America, 30,* 457–473.

Stetler, C., Brunell, M., Giuliano, K., Morsi, D., Prince, L., & Newell-Stokes, G. (1998). Evidenced-based practice and the role of nursing leadership. *Journal of Nursing Administration, 28*(7/8), 45–53.

Stetler, C., Corrigan, B., Sander-Buscemi, K., & Burns, M. (1999). Integration of evidence into practice and the change process: A fall prevention program as a model. *Outcomes Management for Nursing Practice, 3*(3), 102–111.

Stetler, C., Morsi, D., Rucki, S., Broughton, S., Corrigan, B., Fitzgerald, J., Giuliano, K., Havener, P., & Sheridan, E. A. (1998). Utilization-focused integrative reviews in a nursing service. *Applied Nursing Research, 11*(4), 195–206.

Stewart, A. L., & Ware, J. E. (Eds.). (1992). *Measuring functioning and well being: The Medical Outcomes Study approach.* Durham, NC: Duke University Press.

Thurston, N. E., Watson, L. A., & Reimer, M. A. (1993). Research or quality improvement? Making the decision. *Journal of Nursing Administration, 23*(7/8), 46–49.

University of Kent NHS Centre for Reviews and Dissemination. (1999). Getting evidence into practice. *Effective Health Care (Bulletin on the Effectiveness of Health Service Interventions for Decision Makers). 5*(1). (Retrieved [Date] from the World Wide Web: *http://[URL]: www.york.ac.uk/inst/crd/ehc51.htm*)

Vance, C., & Olson, R. K. (Eds.). (1998). *The mentor connection in nursing.* New York: Springer-Verlag.

VanSloten, K., Gee, M., Bachur, N., & Wiernik, P. (1982). Treatment of doxorubicin extravasation in a rat model [Abstract]. In *Proceedings of the Oncology Nursing Society Annual Congress* (p. 70). Pittsburgh: Oncology Nursing Society.

Whedon, M. A. (1996). How is your institution redefining advanced practice roles? *Oncology Nursing Forum, 23,* 711–712.

Wyrwich, K. W., Tierney, W. M., & Wolinsky, F. D. (1999). Further evidence supporting an SEM-based criterion for identifying meaningful intra-individual changes in health-related quality of life. *Journal of Clinical Epidemiology, 52,* 861–873.

Wu, Y. W. B., Crosby, F., Ventura, M., & Finnick, M. (1994). In a changing world: Database to keep the pace. *Clinical Nurse Specialist, 8*(2), 104–108.

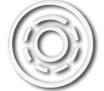

Leadership

EMPOWERMENT, CHANGE AGENCY, AND ACTIVISM

• C H A R L E N E   M.   H A N S O N
• B E V E R L Y   L.   M A L O N E

STRATEGIES FOR IMPLEMENTING PROFESSIONAL AND
CLINICAL LEADERSHIP
Unity Versus Fragmentation
Empowering Others
Networking
Implementing Change Strategies

APNs AS HEALTH CARE LEADERS IN THE
NEW MILLENNIUM

INTRODUCTION

The age of communication and high-tech information systems has markedly changed
the milieu in which advanced practice nurses (APNs) practice and interact with
others. The mantra today is that change is: the only constant in the environment.
This is a time for looking ahead toward new models rather than relying on the
traditions of the past.

In the past, textbooks such as this one carefully set out separate and distinct
chapters that described the knowledge base for leadership, the role of the change
agent, and the development of the political activist. These important components
and competencies were perceived as separate and distinct, with a definitive set of
attributes and skills that were both inherent and learned. However, in today's milieu,
the ability to deal with change and the ability to influence the political process are
inextricably linked with the APN competency of leadership. Change can rarely be
characterized as planned; rather, managing change is continuous and thus embedded
in leadership. In short, effective change agents must be leaders, and effective leadership requires skills as a change agent. These "times" require that all nurses, and most
specifically APNs, play a pivotal role as leaders in the process of change. Thus the
definition of APN leadership has been expanded to include political advocacy and
change agentry in an interdisciplinary environment.

Leadership is a core competency of the APN. As nurses have moved forward
educationally (obtaining master's degrees in nursing), professionally (obtaining certification), and clinically (in patient-focused practice), they have acquired the primary
foundation for advanced nursing practice. Leadership is nurtured and developed
during this advancement process through experiential risk-taking behaviors, reflective
learning, and close association with nurse leaders, mentors, and role models.

To be a leader in the current health care arena requires an understanding of the
personal qualities that are associated with effective leadership, an ability to analyze
health care systems, and the skill to use this understanding to act strategically. In
the chapter, this broader concept of leadership is explored. The essential elements
and skills needed for successful leadership are defined, and how these elements are
transferred into the philosophy and behavior of the APN in both clinical and professional arenas is presented. Obstacles frequently encountered by APNs are examined,
along with strategies to manage these barriers and thus move the leader toward
successful outcomes. In addition, the chapter provides the foundation for effective
leadership within the context of a system fraught with constant change, political
activity, and ideological differences. An "Additional Readings" section is included

that directs the reader to the extensive literature that defines traditional leadership and change concepts and strategies.

FRAMEWORKS THAT DEFINE LEADERSHIP

The nursing literature provides a rich heritage of leadership definitions, concepts, and models that help APNs to develop as effective and dynamic leaders and role models. Concepts such as vision, sharing power, and action-oriented strategies are well defined in nursing's leadership vocabulary. Multiple conceptual models exist that APNs may find useful as a framework for understanding the interactions that occur in the leadership process. Leadership models that empower followers, include others outside of nursing, and allow for change to occur seem to "fit" the best in these unsettled times. Some of these frameworks are briefly explained here; however, it is beyond the scope of this chapter to provide an in-depth discussion of the breadth and depth of nursing leadership. As suggested above, the "Additional Readings" section is provided to broaden understanding of the growth of nursing leadership throughout the 20th century. Concepts are provided as a guide for skill development.

Useful Leadership Definitions and Models

Traditionally, leadership has been defined as an interactive phenomenon of transactions among leaders and followers. For example, Burns (1978) defined *transactional leadership* as occurring when one person takes the initiative to foster the exchange of something of value, either economic, psychological, or political, to another person. The leader and follower may have related purposes but are not necessarily connected by common goals. Leaders incite, stimulate, share with, pacify, and satisfy their followers in an interdependent, interactional exchange. DePree (1989) described leadership as an art form that frees (empowers) people "to do what is required of them in the most effective and humane way possible" (p. 1), and contended that contemporary leadership may be simply viewed as a process of moving the self and others toward a shared vision that becomes a shared reality. By these definitions, the work of both Burns and DePree imply change as a component of leadership. Barker (1994) defined *transformational leadership* as a process whereby change occurs in which "the purposes of the leader and follower become fused, creating unity, wholeness and a collective purpose" (p. 83). Thus transformational leadership occurs when people interact in ways that raise each other to higher levels of motivation and morality. Successful transformational leadership is driven by a common goal or purpose and satisfies the needs of both leader and follower.

The role of follower is important and relevant to any discussions about leadership. Grohar-Murray and DiCroce (1992) included the role of follower in their work exploring the *situational* approach to leadership, which was first defined by Stogdill in 1948 and expanded by Fiedler, Chermers, and Mahar in 1976. Their approach suggests that leadership is situationally dependent, with identified leaders and followers in interchangeable roles based on environmental demands. DePree (1989) enlarged on this idea and used the term *roving leadership* to describe a participatory process that legitimizes the situational leadership of empowered followers through the support and approval of the hierarchical leader. This concept has great relevance for the APN, who continually works in collaborative health care teams that require that the roles of leader and follower be interchangeable to meet the complex needs of the patient. APNs will assume both leader and follower roles, and need to develop skills to know when these different roles are indicated, and when the situation warrants their moving from follower to leader.

However, with full appreciation of the situational approach to leadership, the role of leader extends beyond the immediate situation when the element of vision is addressed. The APN as a leader who has a vision of collaboration among health care team members may facilitate an atmosphere that supports individuals (followers) in assuming the leadership role in various situations. The APN does not cease being the leader by empowering colleagues to appropriately assume a leadership role. In fact, this important approach may be an effective way of both sharing a vision and sharing power.

The concepts in Peter Senge's (1990) *The Fifth Discipline* are very useful as APNs engage in the important work of mastering the competencies surrounding APN leadership. Senge describes a discipline as "a developmental path for acquiring certain skills or competencies" (p. 10). He contends that, although certain people may have innate gifts for playing a musical instrument or running the football, others can develop these proficiencies through practice and commitment to the task. Furthermore, this definition implies that to practice a discipline is to be a lifelong learner. In this case, leadership is a good example because good leaders are constantly striving to become better, to empower others, and to facilitate change.

The five disciplines outlined by Senge provide a framework that effectively integrates the descriptions of leadership provided in the previous paragraphs with the components of learning as they relate to leadership. Because empowerment is key to the previously outlined leadership models, Senge's concepts serve as a useful base upon which leadership and change within complex structures and environments can be understood. The following five disciplines (Senge, 1990) are easily adapted to provide the structure for the leadership competency identified for advanced practice nursing:

Personal mastery is the important work of continually redefining and clarifying one's personal vision, refocusing energies, maintaining objectivity, and committing to personal goals and objectives. The importance of personal growth and development is vital to attaining the competency of APN leadership.

Mental models refers to the images that influence how one views the world and attains new insights; holding one's internal views up for inquiry and scrutiny. This discipline speaks to the need for clear vision about advanced nursing practice and the ability to defend this viewpoint.

Building shared vision refers to the leader's ability to help a team develop and sustain a shared vision of what one seeks to create in the future; the ability to share a vision with others rather than to dictate that vision. The ability to empower others to share the dream and implement change is critical to this discipline.

Team learning is the ability to suspend one's own assumptions, listen to other viewpoints, and genuinely "think together."

Systems thinking is the "fifth discipline"—a conceptual framework for leadership based on the ability to see the whole picture rather than the isolated parts.

This last discipline is an important concept for APNs, who must be able to view advanced practice within the context of health care collectively as one of a team of professionals and patients. As may be noticed, throughout all of these definitions and concepts are the themes of movement, wholeness, and goals. Yet one can also trace from the work of Burns (1978) to more recent definitions the inclusion of integrity, empowerment, and caring, which are more directly related to leadership by APNs. To deliver care in an effective and humane way requires a host of learning organizations with multidisciplinary providers. Nursing is not a solo endeavor, and leadership can be viewed as a way to professionalize nursing within a larger context. Bernhard and Walsh (1995) provided a useful way to understand leadership as a competency within the professional role of APNs. They included eight criteria identified by Pavalko that are essential to the leadership process irrespective of profession: a theoretical base, social values, knowledge, motivation, autonomy, commitment, community, and a code of ethics (Bernhard & Walsh, 1995; Pavalko, 1971). These generic leadership criteria are embedded within APN preparation at the master's level of nursing and subsumed within the essentials of leadership that follow.

Types of Leadership

Certain situations require distinct types of leadership that allow leadership styles to emerge in several unique forms and settings. Leadership begins at the micro, grass-roots level, at "the bedside," if you will. *Clinical leadership* occurs when APNs learn with and from others about how to build appropriate working relationships with health team members, how to instill confidence in patients and colleagues, and how to problem solve as part of a team (Warden, 1997). Clinical leaders are role models and mentors who empower patients and colleagues. They serve as change agents who implement change strategies that improve patient care and enhance APN practice enactment. Some of the direct clinical leadership skills are part of the competencies found in Chapters 7 and 11 in this text. As well, clinical leadership often moves beyond nursing's discipline into the realm of *interdisciplinary leadership,* which occurs across the boundaries of other disciplines. Covey (1989) suggested that inter-disciplinary leadership occurs at a very high level because it requires the ability to interact with issues in another profession's domain. The ability to interact in interdisciplinary leadership positions requires a firm grasp of the issues and differences within the nursing profession while responding to the challenges of the larger society. As clinical leaders gain skill, they develop the attributes needed to interact with other members of the health care team.

Entrepreneurial leadership refers to those APN leaders who go outside of tradi-tional employment systems to create new opportunities to exercise their special abilities (Ballien, 1998). Chapter 1 clearly depicts the role that entrepreneurial nurse leaders have played in creating advanced practice roles in nursing. Creative, entrepre-neurial leadership is necessary for APNs to navigate in the complex managed care system that is the current norm. Ballien (1998) studied entrepreneurial leadership skills as defined by corporate executive officers and senior nurse executives. High-level leadership and communication skills ranked most important in the study, fol-lowed by the ability to build coalitions and to interact with political savvy. Other leadership characteristics of successful entrepreneur nurses ranked as follows: confi-dent, team player, persistent, innovative, risk taker, adjusts to change, decisive, strategic thinker, high integrity, and possesses vision. A conclusion of the study was that nurse leaders must have strong entrepreneurial skills to succeed in today's marketplace. The need to reach out to the community was also perceived as a core requirement. Entrepreneurial leadership is best explained through the use of the following exemplar, which also illustrates the evolving nature of the APN leadership competency and how it expands in breadth over time.

EXEMPLAR 1: ELLIE, APN ENTREPRENEURIAL LEADER

Ellie's dream and goal upon entering a graduate family nurse practitioner (NP) program was to open a practice in the rural community where she and her family lived. She used her health policy course requirements to conduct a needs assessment and to set up interviews with the regional hospital to propose an outreach clinic that would be sponsored by the hospital. She planned to see patients independently and would contract with her physician preceptor to visit once a week for collaboration and to see patients who were beyond her scope of practice. Ellie's entrepreneurial leadership skills allowed her to negotiate with the managed care owner of the hospital and with the medical staff. Her community-based practice was viewed as a model of excellence for other NPs, and she served as a mentor and role model for many. As her clinic gained prominence, Ellie was nominated by the governor to represent APNs and rural interests on the Board of Nursing. She also wrote a column for the local weekly newspaper about prevention and wellness.

After 3 years in practice, Ellie wanted to use extra space in her clinic to broaden the services she offered, so she set up a meeting with the midwifery group in an adjoining town to invite them to use her office as a satellite clinic once a week. She invited two clinical nurse specialists (CNSs) who were seeing mental health and oncology patients in the area to do the same. Her vision and excellent communication skills offered new alliances with other APNs and brought new services for rural patients. The visibility of her successful clinic led to her nomination to membership on the National Rural Health Advisory Committee, which advises the Secretary of Health and Human Services on matters of rural health care. This nationally based committee work allowed Ellie to use well-developed leadership skills to influence the health care system.

Organizational leadership refers to situations in which leaders are formally elected or appointed to positions of power within defined organizations and groups. As with clinical leadership, organizational leadership begins at the grassroots level and proceeds upward to state, national, and international levels. Novice APN leaders need to become involved in the leadership and committee work of local APN coalitions and organizations and move into state and regional leadership roles as they develop their style and strengths as APN leaders. Situations whereby leaders are formally elected or appointed to positions of power within defined organizations and groups are very important to the growth and vitality of advanced practice nursing. The ability to place nurse leaders in key positions is critical to APN visibility and credibility and to establishing the role for APNs within nursing's boundaries and within the larger health care community.

The Process of Change

Subsumed within the competency of leadership for APNs is the competency of being a change agent. Change is a constant within professional and personal life and has continuously escalated within the current health care system. At this point in time, change is a never-ending process that must be woven into the fabric of everyday life and work. Being a successful change agent requires many of the skills and attributes that are needed to be a successful APN leader. However, it is important to understand the complex concepts and forces that drive the health care system, and how APNs take on the important activity of change agentry every time they enact leadership (Klein, Gabelnick, & Herr, 1998).

Steven Covey's work with interdisciplinary groups is very instructive as one studies change and change strategies. Change occurs at both the system and the personal level, and Covey (1989) proposed that one must deal with core values to successfully change or serve as an agent for change:

> *People can't live with change if there is not a changeless core inside them. The key to the ability to change is a changeless sense of who you are, what you are about, and what you value. Real change comes from the inside out.*

(p. 108)

Change for most of us is difficult and painful; at best it can be described as challenging and invigorating (Norton & Grady, 1996). To understand change within today's health care environment, the dynamics of change and the culture within which it occurs must be explored. Peter Senge's seminal work *The Fifth Discipline* (1990), which was described earlier, suggests that systems thinking, which takes into account the notion that change is a given, is the cornerstone that integrates personal mastery, mental modeling, shared vision, and team learning. These are all important constructs when dealing with change and again demonstrate that change is an integral part of the leadership process.

DRIVING AND RESTRAINING FORCES OF CHANGE

Traditional models of the change process are insufficient for addressing change today because these models conceived of change as a linear process that occurred over time. Although they are less useful, certain concepts from these traditional models are still relevant. For example, Lewin's Force Field Analysis model (Figure 10-1) is

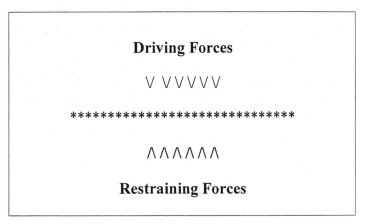

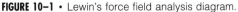

FIGURE 10-1 • Lewin's force field analysis diagram.

helpful in understanding the psychodynamics of change. He described a state of equilibrium between driving and restraining forces that encourage or discourage movement. Driving forces are usually perceived as positive, reasonable, and conscious forces, whereas restraining forces are perceived as negative, illogical, and often subconscious. It is the effect of these opposing forces that make change, especially rapid change, so difficult (Lewin, 1976). These external and internal forces or tensions can also be described as the cognitive dissonance (the conflict between actions and values) that may be evident during change and that cause the uncomfortable feelings that people undergoing change often experience. Driving and restraining forces are useful for APNs in terms of planning for change and evaluating both planned and unplanned changes as they unfold. An example is the movement toward multistate licensure that is gaining momentum as APN practice moves across state lines (see Chapter 22). Forces such as reimbursement and prescriptive authority can serve as both positive and negative influences for APNs as this new form of regulation develops.

PLANNED VERSUS UNPLANNED CHANGE

A major concern for health care stakeholders at all levels is the rapidity with which change has occurred and continues to occur in health care. Change is no longer static and episodic. As the time frame to accomplish change strategies shortens, changes become more and more difficult for individuals and organizations to manage and, therefore, require enhanced strategies to support both leaders and followers. Many of the traditional theory-based models for implementing change do not work because of the speed with which change is occurring. The issues of planned versus unplanned change are based predominately on issues of *time:* time to plan for and think though the desired change, time to orient and allow stakeholders to become comfortable with change, and time to educate and allow the change process to occur.

An illustration of planned change in the clinical setting might be the implementation of evidence-based research innovations in the care of patients by allowing nurses to go through the steps of unfreezing or ending, moving through an educational process to verify new techniques, and then beginning the new procedure. Unfortunately, in unplanned or rapid change, the time frames for the change process to successfully occur are absent or markedly shortened.

The Big Three Model developed by Kantor, Stein, and Jick (1992), and the change processes described by Lewin (1951) and Bridges (1991), all depend on a planned evolution for change that allows for time to work through or bridge the changes over a trajectory that allows for ending of the old order, education to the new order, and then a restructuring of the new version as described previously. Planned change models are helpful in settings where time is not a factor and are useful in helping the APN leader to frame a positive evolution to a new structure for care in certain settings. Further sources for information on planned change are provided in the "Additional Readings" list at the end of the chapter.

Unplanned and constant change is the reality of today's health care environment, and this factor is the basis of the leadership and change discussion that follows. O'Connell (1999) questioned whether health care organizations can sustain fast-paced change unless there is a "culture of change" in place that assists and supports adaptation to new systems and ways of knowing and doing. O'Connell proposed several strategies for developing a culture for change within an organization:

- Maintaining momentum
- Emphasizing managerial support in the process of changing work flow and practice patterns
- Encouraging the question "why" and exercising tolerance for the results
- Emphasizing the importance of concerns on the personal level
- Finding new and different ways to demonstrate administrative support (p. 68)

It is also helpful to consider the techniques used for expert coaching outlined by Norton and Grady (1996) and in Chapter 7 of this text as they relate to providing a positive culture for change. The analogies presented with regard to individuality, sensitivity, and faith when training both athletes and musicians explicate the need for a supportive change environment. It is clear that leaders need to understand the personal implications of change if the culture of change is to be realized. APNs with highly developed psychosocial skills are poised to be pivotal change agent leaders in this process.

Political Activism and Advocacy

Political activism and advocacy is another critical component of APN leadership. Many of the skills needed to successfully navigate in political waters are closely associated with good leadership. The core elements that define contemporary leadership, such as shared vision, systems thinking, and the ability to engage in high-level communication within the context of a changing environment, are all basic to political interaction. Again, change is the common denominator that drives APNs to engage in leadership strategies to advocate for advanced practice and patient issues. In fact, there is little room for discussion about whether APNs need to take on the mantle of policy maker and patient advocate as part of their leadership role (see Chapter 23). For many, it falls within the context of a moral imperative: In order to meet the needs of patients and society, APNs must position themselves strategically at the policy table to advocate for access to care and appropriate interventions for everyone. There is also little question about whether APNs are up to the task. There have been great strides in nurses' skill and acuity as policy makers. Strong mentors have helped along the way, and trial by fire has always been an effective learning tool. The "Acquiring Skills as Leaders, Change Agents, and Activists" section of this chapter offers strategies for developing policy advocacy skills.

KEY ATTRIBUTES OF SUCCESSFUL APN LEADERS

Personal Attributes of Successful Leaders

Several personal attributes are deemed necessary for successful leadership (Table 10–1). These qualities are very broad and support the concept that all leadership today is required to be interdisciplinary. No longer do nurse leaders have the luxury of leading only in nursing circles. A review of Chapter 1 exemplifies the role that nurse leaders have played outside the realm of organized nursing education and practice. The role that certified registered nurse anesthetist (CRNA) leaders played

TABLE 10-1 PERSONAL ATTRIBUTES FOR APN LEADERSHIP

- Vision, coupled with the ability to set priorities
- A good sense of timing
- Self-confidence, assertiveness, and the willingness to take risks
- Expert communication skills and the willingness to connect with others
- Boundary management
- Respect for cultural diversity
- Balance in personal and professional life
- Willingness to collaborate, change and negotiate, fail and begin again

in improving care for anesthetized patients early in the century and the multifaced roles that APNs have played during times of war are good examples of APN leadership potential in interdisciplinary settings.

VISION

Vision is often perceived as the most important component of leadership and the talent that is most coveted. The ability to see into the future and communicate that image to others is a valuable aptitude. Vision encompasses a long-range view of both personal and collective goals that can be shared and that empower others to move forward. Innovation is associated with and closely linked to vision. It is the ability to "think big" or to "think outside the box," the capacity to see alternatives to the current thinking on a given issue. Vision is also grounded in a deep knowledge about the subject and brings with it the responsibility to stay abreast of the field. However, having vision is not enough. A leader must be able to articulate and develop a shared vision, one that others can embrace as their own. In order to do this well, a visionary leader must not get too far out in front of his or her followers because teamwork is critical to shared vision. Tornabeni (1996), a nurse leader, noted that she would not have been able to "hold onto the vision" had she not broadened her scope of influence to include others outside of the discipline of nursing. An important analog to vision is the ability to set priorities so that there is a clear path to the ultimate goal.

A GOOD SENSE OF TIMING

A good sense of timing may be an inherent gift, but for most people it requires painstaking development and practice. Timing is the ability to know when to act and when to hold back. It acknowledges a sense of urgency at times, for example, during an unexpected legislative vote in Congress, or the need during a change in scope of practice to take the time to develop a carefully thought-out plan with careful strategy.

SELF-CONFIDENCE AND RISK TAKING

Taking risks is inherent in the leadership process and is tied inextricably to self-confidence and vision. The willingness to take a chance, to try, to fail occasionally, is the mark of a true leader. The mantra "take a risk, make a decision, pay the price," coined by Helen Mannock in 1959, is worth bearing in mind (Norton & Grady, 1996). Risk-taking behaviors differentiate APNs who will be recognized as leaders and agents for change from other capable APNs. By learning to take risks, the APN enhances her or his leadership repertoire, allowing for more spontaneity and flexibility in response to conflict, resistance, anger, and other reactions to change and high-risk situations (Norton & Grady, 1996). Motivation, which can be described as the desire to move forward, can also be viewed as a component of risk. Staying put is rarely as risky as taking the chance to move ahead.

EXPERT COMMUNICATION

The successful leader must have superb communication skills in order to build the trust and cooperation necessary to negotiate a varied number of difficult intra- and interprofessional issues. The ability to hear another's viewpoint (understand) and respect opposing views is key to being understood and ultimately getting to a win/win outcome. Covey (1989) suggested that one should "seek first to understand and then to be understood" (p. 235). Good leaders listen and really try to hear the other person's viewpoint before they speak. The charisma that is associated with many natural-born leaders is often simply outstanding listening and communication skills. The ability to influence, a key power strategy used to gain the cooperation of others, is an outcome of excellent communication.

A second part of expert communication is relationship building. The art of building strong alliances and coalitions with others and staying connected with colleagues and groups is basic to the sense of community needed within the leadership process. This is true at all levels of leadership, whether at the highest levels of international policy interaction or building coalitions of APNs to solve patient problems at the local level.

BOUNDARY MANAGEMENT

Leadership is cutting-edge behavior and places nurse leaders at the outer boundaries of the profession. The APN leader must not only guard the boundary (as in monitoring appropriate scope of APN practice) but extend it as a bridge in partnering with other groups, and expand the boundary as other client/health care needs are identified. Knowing where the current boundaries of nursing practice are and occasionally going beyond them is another way to define risk taking.

In addition to being a boundary breaker, APN leaders are boundary managers, who teach others how to overlap boundaries with other disciplines and colleagues, build coalitions, and set limits while maintaining their own boundaries—a fine distinction, but strategically important. This process is known as collaboration (see Chapter 11). For example, the certified nurse-midwife (CNM) may delicately negotiate the boundary between the neonatologist, the obstetrician, and the nurse-midwifery staff. Both clinical leadership and professional leadership require the negotiation of boundaries, whether the borders are drawn around patient populations or organizations.

RESPECT FOR CULTURAL DIVERSITY

Cultural competence and valuing diversity are significant attributes for APN leaders. These attributes require sensitivity to one's own biases and the awareness of damaging attitudes and behaviors that surface at all levels of interaction and in all settings. An APN leader needs to be responsive to and serve as role model for the cultural/racial/ethnic milieu of followers and constituencies in any given situation. The following section discusses skill development in this important area.

BALANCE IN PERSONAL AND PROFESSIONAL LIFE

Most people know when they have overextended themselves: their bodies give clues based on fatigue, stress signals, and frustration. One of the negative elements of being a good leader is the provocative realization that one is being asked to play many important cutting-edge roles at the same time. It is very easy to overextend one's abilities well beyond manageable, realistic boundaries. The catchphrase "get a life" may become a sad commentary for many APNs in leadership positions. It is not easy to be both a leader and a competent APN care provider. The skill of being able to delegate tasks, mentor others to take on some of the load, and enlarge the circle of leaders, strategists, and followers is integral to effective leadership. Unfortunately, the inability to set realistic personal boundaries paves the way to stress, frustration, and burnout.

WILLINGNESS TO COLLABORATE, CHANGE, AND NEGOTIATE, TO FAIL AND BEGIN AGAIN

It is not serendipitous that several of the key attributes in Table 10-1 incorporate the word "willingness." The abilities to be open and willing, to take what comes, and to work through differences are key to all levels of leadership. Leadership is about negotiation and interactions with others to reach common goals. To do this may mean failing and trying again and again to reach the desired outcome.

Mentoring and Empowerment

Two major proficiencies, empowerment and mentoring, stand out as important skills in the process of leadership, change, and advocacy. The responsibility to empower and mentor is central to all of the definitions of leadership and change outlined earlier. The ability to help others to grow and to encourage them toward self-actualization requires competent, caring leaders who are interested in the success and well-being of their followers. Coaching and guiding with an awareness and attentiveness to the needs and concerns of followers are basic characteristics of successful leaders. The ideas behind the colloquial statements "taking someone under your wing" or "giving a colleague a leg up" are grounded in the mentoring process. Leading by example, role modeling, enabling followers, and encouraging them to move upward are all leadership aptitudes that must be disseminated.

Mentors have been defined by many as having those qualities that epitomize success in their own careers and the ability and desire to help others achieve success. Mentors are seen as self-confident and competent, with a willingness to share their expertise. Mentees or protégés are viewed as those people who exhibit a desire to learn, are committed to the long course of events, and are open to the process of trial and error. It is important to note that there are two parts to the APN mentorship equation: APNs who are seeking to be mentored by those they aspire to emulate and those APNs who can serve as mentors. "The learning curve [to leadership] is vastly facilitated by exposure to those who display mastery, those who have wisdom" (Koerner, 1997, p. 78). The reward for the mentor is to step back and enjoy the success of the protégé who has succeeded in reaching the next level of competence. Unfortunately, some APNs are reluctant to mentor, perhaps thinking that the protégé will steal expertise or will not work as hard as they did to be successful.

Vance and Olson (1998) suggested the following needed requirements for APNs who want to attract mentors: being dedicated to your cause, marketing yourself, seeking opportunities for networking and meeting other APNs, reaching out to possible mentors who are both leaders and peers, and an attitude of openness. Advanced practice nursing has a wealth of strong nursing leaders and advocates who are willing and able to move new advocates into position to lead the next generation and to make positive change in health care policy. The best way for novice APN leaders to move into the leadership arena is through an experienced nurse advocate.

Closely aligned to, but somewhat different from, the mentoring process is the process of empowerment. As the word implies, empowerment is defined as giving power to another, enabling, giving authority. APNs operationalize this by enabling or giving power to other nurses, colleagues, and patients. Empowerment as a leadership strategy is guided by the shared vision of the leader and follower and a willingness of the leader to delegate power to others. Visionary leaders who empower their followers greatly increase the influence of advanced nursing practice both within nursing and beyond nursing's boundaries.

Attributes of Change Agent Leaders

Leaders are involved with change at many points in the change process, as portrayed in Table 10-2. Visionary change agents intervene early in the change process, before change occurs, and set the stage for the events that follow. They provide the guiding principles and assumptions for the proposed change and begin to introduce themes that position the organization and its members in a positive direction toward the new events. Change implementors, as defined by Kantor, Stein, and Jick (1992) have the difficult task of "making it happen."

TABLE 10–2 KEY CHANGE MAKERS

	ROLE AND MINDSET	ORIENTATION TO CHANGE (KIND OF MOTION)	ACTION FOCUS	TYPICAL ORGANIZATIONAL LEVEL	DOMINANT STAGE OF INVOLVEMENT
Change strategist	Visionary Instigator Corporate view	External environment	Ends Corporate values and business results	Top	Unfreezing
Change implementor	"Project image" Translator Division or department	Internal coordination	Means Overcoming resistance "Project image"	Middle	Changing
Change recipient	User and adapter Institutionalizer Personal view Operational	Distribution of power and proceeds	Means-end congruence Personal benefits	Bottom	Refreezing

From Kantor, R. M., Stein, B. A., & Jick, T. D. (1992). *The challenge of organizational change: How companies experience it and how leaders guide it* (p. 381). New York: The Free Press (an imprint of Simon & Schuster); reprinted by permission. Copyright © 1992 by Rosabeth Moss Kantor, Barry Stein, and Todd D. Jick.

ACQUIRING SKILLS AS APN LEADERS, CHANGE AGENTS, AND ACTIVISTS

Cultural Competence for Nurse Leaders

As noted earlier, a key attribute of APN leadership is the responsibility for cultural competence. The following framework offers helpful strategies for enhancing cultural awareness.

LEVELS OF DIVERSITY

When using a systems framework for understanding a complex concept such as culturally competent leadership, the following levels can be identified: (1) societal, (2) professional, (3) organizational, and (4) individual. For the APN, the responsibility for culturally competent care includes all four levels of the diversity system. Culturally competent care is care delivered with knowledge, sensitivity, and respect for the consumer/family's cultural/racial/ethnic background and reality. This definition is built on the assumption that care providers are fully aware of, sensitized to, and able to integrate their own cultural/racial/ethnic background into their professional delivery of care services. The interactive nature of caregiving requires the engagement and synchrony of the provider's own diversity with the diversity of those receiving the care. To achieve this synchrony, an exploration of the levels of diversity is an appropriate starting point.

Societal. On February 21, 1998, during his radio address, President Clinton announced the U.S. initiative to eliminate racial and ethnic disparities in health by 2010. In order to achieve this goal, six areas were selected in which racial and ethnic disparities in health access and outcomes were significant: cancer screening and management, cardiovascular disease, child and adult immunizations, diabetes, human immunodeficiency virus infection/acquired immunodeficiency syndrome (AIDS), and infant mortality. For the first time in U.S. history, at the highest political level, this initiative acknowledged the reality of the country's racial/ethnic health disparities and articulated a national commitment to eradicate the differences. Concrete examples of the disparity are as follows (Waldrop, 1990):

- An African American baby born today is 2.5 times more likely to die in the first year of life than a white baby, American Indian babies are 1.5 times more likely to die, and Hispanic babies are two times more likely to die.
- The diabetes rate among some American Indians is three to five times higher than that of other groups.
- Asian Americans are struggling with extremely high rates of cancer: Vietnamese American women are five times more likely than other women to be afflicted with cervical cancer, and Asian American men are three to five times more likely than other men to get liver cancer.

These statistics paint a picture that demands the attention of APNs. A color-blind attitude (Malone, 1996, 1997) that acknowledges only the values and norms of the dominant culture as relevant and appropriate disregards the reality of these statistics.

An APN must see in color with all the various hues and shades to provide culturally competent care.

Professional. The nursing profession is highly valued by the public. In a recent poll asking the consumer to identify the most trusted professional care provider, nurses scored higher than any other provider group (Waldrop, 1990). This is a consistent finding. The mission of nursing was perhaps most aptly captured by Virginia Henderson: "to assist the individual sick or well, in the performance of those activities contributing to health or its recovery (or to peaceful death) that he would perform unaided if he had the necessary strength, will or knowledge and to do this in such a way as to help him gain independence as rapidly as possible" (1961, p. 2). With this definition and philosophy of advocacy and respect, the nursing profession is held in high esteem by the American public.

However, APNs must recognize that there is a chasm between the rhetoric and the reality of nursing. Although nursing philosophy espouses statements of idealism and caring, the nursing reality encompasses one's own biases and fears of differences:

> *While the nursing profession speaks strongly to being responsive to differences by individualizing the caring process and tailoring theory-based, scientifically determined patient care principles to the needs of the individual and community, the cloaked vestiges of early parental influence and bias lie unexplored and unidentified within the human heart of the institution of nursing.*

> (Malone, 1997, p. 577).

These dichotomies provide useful lessons as APNs move into positions of leadership and influence.

Organizational. APNs must be able to assess the organizations they work in, manage, and/or own. An organizational assessment is useful in determining the institution's level of commitment to diversity. The areas of assessment need to include the organization's philosophy, goals, or mission statement; strategic plan; budget; and evaluation. The critical assessment factor is usually the consistency between the philosophy/goal/mission statement and the strategic plan. Most institutions clearly profess a philosophy devoted to providing care or access to all regardless of race, creed, or color. Frequently, it is at the strategic level of implementation that the lack of a plan to actualize these noteworthy beliefs becomes visible. Short-term solutions are implemented that will not produce a new organizational culture that values diversity. Likewise, the budget is a sensitive indicator of an organization's priorities. When resources are not allocated to strategies that would increase, retain, or maximize the strength of diversity, the organization's commitment is questionable. Finally, an evaluation plan that does not address diversity is unable to institutionalize the growth and learning from programs and strategic plans.

Individual. For the APN, self-assessment of one's valuing of diversity, such as one's biases and openness to differences of culture, education, opinion, and religion, needs to be a continuous, evolving activity. This self-assessment can be accomplished with self-discipline and an internal awareness of one's strengths and weaknesses. Differences are an issue for every member of the human race. The need to group together along some continuum of sameness is the basis of family structure as well as the basis for stereotyping. Working with colleagues who are different and allowing oneself to be open for feedback and comment from them about race and ethnicity is one method for receiving input about oneself. Once the assessment is completed, initiating desired changes in behavior is the next step. The following strategies are recommended for all APN nurse leaders:

1. Explore and learn about your own racial/ethnic culture and background. For example, there are Italian American nurses, Greek American nurses, Polish American nurses, and many more. Their racial/ethnic family background has contributed to shaping them into the APNs they have become. These roots frequently are unexplored and unceremoniously lumped under the label "white," as if the cultural context and input did not exist.
2. Explore and learn about the different racial/ethnic cultures most frequently encountered in your practice. Read ethnic newspapers, magazines, and books. Listen to the music from this different culture. Learn the language of the culture. Become bilingual with the verbal and the nonverbal behavior of the different culture. Be attentive to the customs and mores of the group. Develop a relationship with a guide, a translator, who can lead you into the mystery and excitement of a different culture.
3. Take advantage of training opportunities for increasing your cultural awareness and sensitivity. Diversity training and development courses are available in most organizations. If not available, the leader's role is to seek out the opportunity and assist the overall organization to value and develop training.
4. Be able to identify personal biases and develop strategies to manage, eliminate, or sublimate those potentially damaging attitudes and behaviors. A leadership strategy may be to use psychiatric APNs as resources to consult in developing a program for valuing diversity.
5. When faced with a difficult patient, determine whether unconscious biases may be operating for you or your colleagues.

Factors Influencing Leadership Development

Allen (1998) explored perceptions of 12 nurse leaders as to the factors and individual characteristics that influenced their leadership development. *Self-confidence,* traced back to childhood and subsequent risk-taking behaviors, was perceived as a critical factor. Feedback from significant others led to enhanced self-confidence over time. The nursing leaders also spoke about having *innate qualities and tendencies of leaders,* such as being extraverted or bossy and wanting to take charge, with roles as team captains and officers in organizations. They were seen as people who "rise to the occasion." A third important factor was a *progression of experiences and successes* that were pivotal in moving them forward. Being at "the right place at the right time" and taking advantage of opportunities that presented in those situations allowed them to progress as leaders. Closely aligned with this factor was the importance of the *influence of significant people* such as mentors, role models, faculty, and parents who had the ability to encourage and provide opportunities for advancement. The final factor in this study dealt with *personal life factors,* defined situationally as ways in which time, family, health, and work schedules influenced their development to a greater or lesser degree. Certainly, study participants who had supportive spouses and relatives who assisted with family and home responsibilities, and employers who were flexible, were assisted in the development process. Allen's findings clearly support the definitions and elements of leadership described in the first part of this chapter.

Educational Strategies for Preparing APN Leaders

Formal educational opportunities such as those experienced during graduate school fit well into the process for leadership development. There are excellent occasions to work with role models and mentors and to set up experiences that offer opportunities to gain personal mastery of skills and to further reinforce self-confidence. Community-based projects such as coordinating health fairs or the Special Olympics offer rich resources for building interpersonal skills and create new opportunities for influence and visibility. Running for graduate student office, local leadership positions in professional organizations, and serving on local boards and coalitions is another good strategy. As well, leadership conferences that foster effective communication and interaction are beneficial. The following exemplar shows how students can practice their leadership development during graduate education.

EXEMPLAR 2: JOAN'S EDUCATIONAL LEADERSHIP EXPERIENCE

Joan was beginning her second year in graduate nursing as an APN student. She had completed her core courses, which gave her a good foundation in the theoretical concepts related to role development, health policy, and research. Now, she was ready to move on to the clinical component of her program and to complete her scholarly project. Joan had thought carefully about this and wanted to focus her project on developing her leadership skills in the policy arena. She knew that one of her faculty, Dr. Wesson, who had taught her health policy course, was a respected state and national leader who was actively engaged in the process of gaining primary care provider (PCP) status for APNs. Joan made an appointment to talk with Dr. Wesson about how she could help with the PCP issue and at the same time complete her scholarly project. Dr. Wesson suggested three things. Joan should use the Internet to become familiar with and articulate about the proposed legislation; she could accompany Dr. Wesson to the next statewide meeting of APNs and offer to carry out the phone survey of APNs that was needed by this group; and she could develop the research proposal, implement the survey methodology, and present the findings as part of testimony at the hearing at the State Capitol in the spring. These activities would allow Joan to interact with leader role models, try out her new leadership skills, and complete her research assignment. Dr. Wesson also suggested that Joan apply for the student scholarship offered by a national APN organization to attend the Washington, DC–based APN Summit.

Throughout the fall and winter, Joan implemented the phone survey with the APN community. She interacted with many practicing APNs and learned a great deal about APN practice. The APN leaders at the state meeting were excellent role models, and Dr. Wesson served as an excellent mentor throughout the year. Joan was extremely proud of her contribution to APNs when she presented her findings at the hearing. Throughout the process, she had used many of the skills that she had read about in her leadership class, such as communication, networking, vision, and timing. Because Joan has a husband and a 4-year-old child, she also learned about balance and boundary management. Her most lasting recollection was how important it was to have a mentor to guide her through the process.

In 1999, the American Academy of Nursing funded a distance learning educational project that brought together four nursing leaders from Georgia to share their ideas about the skills needed to develop successful nurse leaders. These leaders "attended" class over interactive television and offered their experience and expertise to novice APNs. Many of the skills they shared are part of the essentials of leadership as described earlier in this chapter. Table 10–3 is a list of their joint suggestions for students and others who desire to become leaders (Hanson, Boyle, Hatmaker, & Murray, 1999).

Leadership skills are developed and perfected over time and in myriad ways. Communication is one of the strengths often attributed to nurses, and it is a skill that can be augmented through practice. Many of the other skills and attributes shared by Hanson and colleagues (1999) in Table 10–3 are familiar to APNs and just need to be framed within the context of leadership. For example, the notion of staying connected is important for busy APNs and was operationalized by these leaders in a variety of ways, from e-mail list serves and shared projects to planning to attend conferences that allowed for time to interact and problem solve with colleagues about similar professional issues. A sense of timing was described by one leader as negotiating ahead of time with her spouse for time to lobby for prescriptive

---

TABLE 10–3 ATTRIBUTES OF NURSE LEADERS

Expert Communication Skills
- Articulate verbally and in writing
- Ability to get one's point across
- Excellent listening skills
- Desire to hear and understand another's point of view
- Staying connected to other people

Commitment
- Giving of self personally and professionally
- Listening to one's inner voice
- Balancing professional and private life
- Planning ahead, making change happen

Developing One's Own Style
- Getting involved
- Staying involved
- Setting priorities
- Using technology
- Lifelong learning
- Creating a learning environment for self and others
- A good sense of humor

Risk Taking
- Getting involved at any level
- Self-confidence
- Thinking "big"
- Willingness to fail and begin again
- A sense of timing
- Coping with change

Willingness to Collaborate
- Respect for diversity
- Desire to team build
- Sharing power
- Willingness to mentor

Adapted from Hanson, C., Boyle, J., Hatmaker, D., & Murray, J. (1999). *Finding your voice as a leader.* Washington, DC: American Academy of Nursing; reprinted with permission.

authority, with the understanding that she would lessen her load at the end of the legislative session.

The need for faculty and students in graduate programs to become involved in raising the visibility of APN roles in their institutions and communities is extremely important to building APN leaders. Faculty need to serve as resource persons to keep students informed about key legislative issues and introduce them through role modeling to the role of political advocacy. Inviting APNs to accompany faculty who are giving testimony at a legislative hearing is an appropriate way to model the advocacy role.

Gaining local visibility is accomplished through APN students and faculty engagement in local health care activities for special populations such as Special Olympics, AIDS awareness, and support for after-school programs for high-risk youth.

DEVELOPING LEADERSHIP IN THE POLITICAL ARENA

Becoming an Astute Political Activist: The Growth Process

In the political arena, developing power and influence is an imperative that tests APN leadership skill. Leadership strategies used by APNs in the political arena encompass such strategies as developing power, influencing contacts, motivating colleagues to stay abreast of current issues, and providing bridges to other leaders who have access to important resources. Mentoring APNs to understand their power and influence in the health policy arena is a serious role for the APN leader. Taking on the mantle of policy advocate requires a commitment to APN practice and education issues.

The developmental process for becoming a political activist begins during primary school when, as children, one is first introduced to government and the political system. Field trips to Washington, DC, and the state capitol are the first spark toward political activism. Throughout secondary education and by way of the nightly news, young adults continue to be bombarded with policy decisions in many venues. Then, in nursing school, fledgling nurses are further exposed to specific policy related to health care, and they are introduced to professional nursing and specialty nursing organizations. However, serious involvement often begins in graduate school, when health policy is offered as one of the ''core'' courses leading to the role of APN. During master's education, APN students are coached to better understand the power of the policy arena and ways that they can influence the system, both individually and collectively, to better their own practice and to be high-level patient advocates. This is accomplished both though classroom teaching and experientially through interaction with policy makers and nursing leaders and mentors. Exemplar 2, presented earlier in the chapter, exemplifies this educational strategy.

DEPTH OF INVOLVEMENT

Timing is an important consideration for APNs who want and need to be health policy advocates. There is no question that influencing policy is costly in terms of time and energy. Therefore, it is important for APNs to ask themselves several personal and professional questions to determine the degree of involvement and level of sophistication at which advocacy is to be undertaken:

- What are my responsibilities related to wage earning, small children, dependent parents, single parenthood, health issues, school, and gaining initial competence as an APN?
- How can I best serve the APN community at this time?
- What are the learning opportunities for me to be most effective?
- How can I develop a long-term and short-term plan for becoming more politically astute and a better advocate for myself and for my patients?
- What am I able to commit to based on the response to these questions?

Once APNs have made a decision about the depth of involvement they can commit to, they need to find an appropriate mentor. Advanced practice nursing has a wealth of strong nursing leaders and advocates who are willing and able to move new advocates into position to make positive change in health care policy. There is an overwhelming amount of work to be done at every level, whether it be stuffing envelopes in someone's campaign or giving testimony on Capitol Hill. As is true with leadership overall, the best way to move into the policy/political arena is to be socialized or mentored into the process by an experienced nurse advocate.

USING PROFESSIONAL ORGANIZATIONS TO BEST ADVANTAGE

For APNs, close contact with their professional organization is an important link to staying abreast of the national and state policy agendas, for finding a support network of like minds, and for accessing changes in credentialing and practice issues. Unfortunately, in today's complex world, this means being an active member of more than one affiliate organization in order to stay on the cutting edge of pertinent issues. Most APNs are aligned with one or more professional nursing organizations, and those who aspire to an active role in influencing policy often have membership in several. Basic membership brings with it the newsletters, journals, and Internet access needed to stay current, while active membership requires committee assignments and more involvement. As new graduates move from the educational milieu into diverse practice settings, they must align with the APN organizations that best meet their needs and offer the strongest support, choosing to actively engage in some and remain on the periphery in others.

Membership can be at differing levels, from simple financial support through dues to high-level leadership and committee work. Choosing the "right" organizations to belong to is a very personal decision based on particular needs, comfort level, specialty, and experience. Many APNs belong to one organization that meets their particular clinical needs (e.g., the Oncology Nursing Society or the American Association of Nurse Anesthetists) and to another that offers cutting-edge access to pressing professional issues. Examples might be the American College of Nurse Practitioners or the National Association of Neonatal Nurses. Others use their professional organization as a support group that offers nurturing and professional sustenance, a group that "understands" local APN practice concerns. Regional and state affiliations of national organizations often serve this purpose.

The critical factor in interfacing with organizations is getting and staying involved in a very definitive way. Being part of the website list serve or chat room, attending meetings and conferences, reading newsletters and journals, participating on committees, and working up the ladder to leadership positions represent different levels of involvement. Professional organizations offer the source of leadership and collective wisdom necessary to stay the course in today's political and policy arena. The notion of strength in numbers and speaking from one strong voice are not new concepts but are essential to the success of the APN role as an astute policy maker. The number and variety of state and national organizations that are tied to APN education and practice are too numerous to describe here, but it is safe to say that there is something for everyone.

POLITICAL ACTION COMMITTEES

A political action committee (PAC) is the arm of an organization, structured as a separate entity, that finances political campaigns. Federal guidelines dictate how donations and funds are raised and administered (deVries & Vanderbuilt, 1992). The bases of decisions about endorsements are complex and are made at the national professional organization level based on careful research and past support for nursing and health care interests that align with nursing's professional priorities and values. Fund-raising to support candidates is a major function of PACs and requires nursing support at every level. PACs are important to APNs because the decisions about Medicare and Medicaid that undergird APN reimbursement are at stake when supporting political nominees to run for national office. APN leaders are in key positions to influence the endorsement of political candidates who are aligned with APN practice and education issues.

INTERNSHIPS AND FELLOWSHIPS

One excellent way to develop the necessary skills to move into the role of APN policy advocate is to apply for a national or state policy internship or fellowship. These activities, which last from several days to 1 or 2 years, offer a wide range of health care policy and political experiences that are focused to both novice and expert APNs. For example, the Nurse in Washington Internship (NIWI) is a 4-day internship that introduces nurses to policy making in Washington, DC (*www. awhonn.org/intern.htm*). This internship serves as an excellent beginning step toward enacting the APN policy role. Federal fellowships and internships that link nurses to legislators or to the various branches of federal and state government are invaluable in assisting APNs to understand how leaders are developed and how the system for setting health care policy is operationalized.

Raising Awareness Through Communication

The ability to communicate with others accurately, efficiently, and in a timely manner is a driving force in the world of policy and politics. Never before have people had such an opportunity to share information in its original form and to interface with others at great distances. Face-to-face, one-on-one interaction and on-site networking is always the best way to ensure successful communication that satisfies all parties. However, time and distance make this mode of communication a luxury rather than a reality. Few APNs have the time or inclination to serve as full-time policy makers.

The reality is that APNs rely on other modalities such as the Internet to stay connected to the larger professional world.

THE INTERNET

Today's communication networks are wonderful resources for gaining awareness and keeping current on policy initiatives and concerns from a wide variety of perspectives. Probably the most useful tool available to APNs moving into the new millenium is the World Wide Web. The ability to link on line into professional Internet pages, list serves, or chat rooms or to be on extensive mailing lists that target cutting-edge legislation despite great distances has never been better. It is possible to follow committee sessions in Congress via TV or computer as they happen or later the same day via CNN. Government agencies such as the Centers for Disease Control, the Health Care Financing Administration, and the Agency for Healthcare Research and Quality offer rich resources. Internet users can ''bookmark'' favorite search engines and websites that they rely on to keep them abreast of critical happenings. They can also engage in chat rooms and list serves where they can influence change from their home. Table 10-4 is a partial list of Internet sites that offer excellent resources for staying abreast of APN policy and practice issues.

E-MAIL, FAX, AND THE TELEPHONE CONFERENCE

E-mail and fax modalities have revolutionized the ability to communicate rapidly and effectively throughout the world. Board and committee membership can be carried out at any time, day or night. Augmenting skills that are required to intercept attached documents and faxes via computer greatly expands the ability to do business. New telweb conferencing offers yet another mode of communication. Conference calls save countless hours on the road or in the air. Often, grassroots APNs must push for this type of interaction with major policy activists and organizations.

THE MEDIA

The Woodhall Study of Nurses and the Media, a 1997-1998 work commissioned by Sigma Theta Tau entitled ''Healthcare's Invisible Partner,'' makes the point that nurses do not use the media to their best advantage. Mundt (1997) conducted a research study exploring how nurses were represented in 35 books from 13 disciplines about health policy and health care reform. The findings were significant because over half of the books reviewed had no reference to nurses at all and only four books had more than 10 references to nurses in the entire book. The outcomes of this study are clear. APNs must write and publish broadly, integrating nursing's influence into policy decisions (Mundt, 1997). The media in all forms, whether newsprint, television, the Internet, books, or journals, all serve as an important link to information and opinion. Furthermore, the media serve as a springboard for policy initiatives and as a method to communicate with both policy makers, stakeholders, and constituents. The critical issue is, how can APNs use the media as an instrument to enhance policy and professional influence?

Multiple resources are available that provide strategies and pointers for using the media appropriately. Several very basic communication concepts emerge, as shown in Table 10-5. Use the media strategy that works best for you. Most of us know how we present ourselves most effectively and most comfortably. Is it easier to conceive

TABLE 10–4 PARTIAL LIST OF COMMON URLs FOR INTERNET ACCESS	
Agency for Healthcare Research and Quality (formerly Agency for Health Care Policy and Research [AHCPR]):	*www.ahcpr.gov*
American Academy of Nurse Practitioners:	*www.aanp.org*
American Association of Colleges of Nursing:	*www.aacn.nche.edu/*
American Association of Nurse Anesthetists:	*www.aana.com*
American College of Nurse-Midwives:	*www.acnm.org*
American College of Nurse Practitioners:	*www.nurse.org/acnp*
American Medical Association:	*www.ama-assn.org*
American Nurses Association:	*www.ana.org/*
American Nurses Credentialing Center:	*www.nursingworld.org/ancc*
Thomas: Legislative Information on the Internet:	*thomas.loc.govt*
National Association of County and City Health Officials:	*www.naccho.org*
National Association of Neonatal Nurses:	*www.nann.org*
National Certification Board of Pediatric Nurse Practitioners/Nurses:	*www.pnpcert.org*
National Council of State Boards of Nursing:	*www.ncsbn.org/*
National Institute of Nursing Research:	*www.nih.gov/ninr/*
National Institutes of Health:	*www.nih.gov/*
National League for Nursing:	*www.nln.org/*
National Organization/Nurse Practitioner Faculties:	*www.nonpf.com*
National Rural Health Association:	*nrharural.org*
Oncology Nurses Society (ONS):	*www.ons.org/*
Reuters Health Information Services:	*www.reutershealth.com/*
State Government	*www.state.[insert state abbreviation].us/*
U.S. Government Printing Office:	*www.access.gpo.gov*
U.S. Government White House Publications, Executive Orders Search Site:	*www.pub.whitehouse.gov/search/executive-orders.html*
U. S. House of Representatives:	*www.house.gov*
U. S. Senate:	*www.senate.gov*
World Health Organization:	*www.who.int/*

Adapted from Hebda, T., Czar, P., & Mascara, C. (1998). *Handbook of informatics for nurses and health care professionals* (pp. 1–334). New York: Addison-Wesley; reprinted with permission.

of doing a speech or a radio or TV spot, or doing an article for the newspaper? In which mode are you best able to communicate your point using the strategies in Table 10-5? What venue will get the most visibility at the best time? How controversial is the issue? Is it important to pave the way with other stakeholders, in and outside of nursing, before you go public? Is it important to reach many people (the public), or do you need to focus on educating a particular legislator or committee? If you are speaking publicly, are you ready to see your remarks in print the next day? Can you back up what you say? (deVries & Vanderbuilt, 1992; Hassmiller, 1995; Mason & Leavitt, 1998).

TABLE 10–5 BASIC COMMUNICATION STRATEGIES	
Understand how the system works.	Do your homework.
Make your point.	Ask for what you want.
Get the facts straight.	Tell the truth.
Use data to back up your statements.	Personalize the message.
KISS it (keep it simple, stupid).	

EDUCATING POLICY MAKERS AND LEGISLATORS

Educating influential leaders and policy makers requires special consideration. They are usually dealing with a multitude of issues at once and use staffers and aides to stay abreast of the issues. Their work is structured around committees, and so they are much closer to and more informed about some issues than others. They have personal goals as well as responsibilities to their constituents. They are bombarded on every side by multiple special interest groups who want their attention and their vote. The *sine qua non* of educating and influencing busy policy makers can be summed up in four basic strategies:

1. Use their staff to the fullest degree possible. The staffers are following the legislation and have the best insight on the strengths and weaknesses of getting what you want.
2. Be clear, understand the issue fully, and know what you hope to gain and what you are willing to give up.
3. Use multiple strategies.
4. Garner support from others who have a like mission.

The way APNs gain visibility is based on personal style. One APN may write a weekly column in the local newspaper, another may be very visible on local planning and advisory boards, and a third may do a radio talk show. Volunteering for community service or as a member of the local or state speakers bureau also works well. Written materials or videotapes in office waiting rooms provide patients and families with an important introduction to APN health care. As well, personal visits to legislators, policy makers, and health care leaders are critical components to gaining needed visibility. The epitome of gaining visibility is to run for professional or public office.

EDUCATING THE PUBLIC

A common fallacy among APNs is that the public in general is aware of the role and issues surrounding health care and advanced practice nursing. APNs are often amazed to discover that physicians, legislators, and their patients really have very little understanding of what APNs are about, what they can do, and how they fit into the overall scheme of health care. Each and every APN has a primary responsibility for educating people they "touch," and for conducting this education in a clear and articulate manner. Seemingly this is an easy task, but in fact it is fraught with political complexities and varying levels of sophistication. Again, using the strengths of professional associations is key to getting out a message that is clear and appropriate. Most APN organizations have packaged materials and references that grassroots APNs can access from Internet pages or hard copy.

PLAYING BOTH SIDES OF THE STREET

Judy Buckalew, who was the first nurse to be a special assistant to the President of the United States, reminds us that nurses have long been criticized for being very self serving and not "playing both sides of the street" (Pearson, 1987). This phrase refers to the need for the APN to be able to see beyond the issues at hand and to look at the larger scope and differing perspectives about health care legislation of the other stakeholders. It requires careful monitoring of legislation and regulation both in and beyond nursing and knowing the policy makers' philosophy and interests. Buckalew states further, "playing both sides of the street is just smart politics. No matter who is currently in power, you should divide your energy and your power evenly" (Pearson, 1987, p. 54).

Becoming an insider who has a place at the policy and political table happens over time and is predicated on a collegial approach based on mutual respect and valuing of others' points of view. The most highly effective strategy for becoming an insider is networking with colleagues both within the circle of APN peers and with other health care providers who have a stake in the outcomes.

SPECIAL INTEREST GROUPS

One way to offer advocacy and become more visible with the public is to align with and keep abreast of issues that have high priority with special interest groups. For example, using the American Association of Retired Persons (AARP) website is a good way to track the policy and legislative agenda of senior citizens and to share the expertise of APNs. A feature story on the role of the NP in retirement communities or offering information about polypharmacy problems in *Modern Maturity,* the journal for the AARP, gains needed visibility. Likewise, exploring the linkages for the American College of Nurse-Midwives on line can lead you to the issues surrounding home births or birthing center care by APNs. Special interest groups have important connections to legislation and choice of providers, and these groups serve as stepping stones to APN policy influence.

General Political Strategies

In the current political climate, it is critical that the professional posture of every APN be carefully thought out. APNs have come a long way in developing their political acumen at both state and national levels and have considerable power to achieve positive change if they capitalize on their newfound status. An important cohesiveness within nursing has emerged in response to health care system changes. The nursing profession, as a whole, is beginning to recognize its strength at the policy table. As far back as 1984, Nancy Milio cautioned that nurses must be prepared to forge alliances, do their homework, and bring their case before the public, and she predicted that it would be APNs who carry the message forward (Milio, 1984). More than 10 years later, Towers (1995) cautioned the same thing: "It is clear that the contribution that nursing makes in the health-care arena must be brought forward. Nurses need to be heard, their data must be shared, their leadership enhanced. Nurses must take responsibility for education and communicating with legislators" (p. 44). Politics and ethics are inherent in relationships at all systems levels and most obviously in policy development. Therefore, nursing's ethical stance on social mandates that support poor and underserved populations needs to be clearly articulated (Aroskar, 1987). APN leaders have a responsibility to bring their views and perspectives to decision-making and policy forums. They need to turn competitors into partners to make change toward a more interdisciplinary system.

Professional turf issues have plagued APNs since the early days of their clinical practice. A lack of legal empowerment to practice to the fullest extent of knowledge and skills has been a dominant barrier to the optimal practice of NPs (Dempster, 1994). CNMs and CRNAs have the longest track record in dealing with these issues and have many successes to their credit. Health care reform and managed care dialogue have caused physicians and other important health care stakeholders to retrench, which has heightened the perception of APNs as a threat. This has made the current political arena extremely sensitive.

The political agenda that is carried out at the professional level (American Nurses Association/American Medical Association) and between APN specialty organizations is much different from the agenda played out at the grassroots level. There is strong evidence that locally practicing physicians and nurses have strong collaborative relationships and that they are frustrated by the lack of cohesion at the professional level at which policy is made. APNs must closely monitor policy issues through phone trees, newsletters, and regional meetings. There is no question that an important strategy for the removal of barriers is to enlist the grassroots support of physician and nurse teams who are practicing successfully in a collegial manner.

Another strategy to assist in the improvement of practice environments for advanced practice is to create local networks of APNs within state structures that will help to remove barriers and develop workable practice guidelines. Close interaction with local collaborating physicians and leaders of local health care entities is crucial. States that have made the greatest strides in removing practice barriers need to help states that have more serious constraints to advanced nursing practice.

There are a myriad of recent textbooks on the market, as well as a plethora of journal articles, that deal with the issue of grooming APNs with political savvy and know-how to circumvent the land mines of political and legislative action. Most of these resources are well targeted toward helping the nurse gain confidence and expertise as a policy maker. The "Additional Readings" list at the end of this chapter list some of these resources. It is recommended that all APNs, as part of their basic graduate program and through continued seminars and workshops, take advantage of these tools of the trade. Nurses have a formidable voting power base of over 2.2 million. This is an incredible strength for nurses but requires cohesiveness within the ranks in order to make positive change for advanced nursing practice. The notion that someone else will carry the flag is not realistic. Developing political acumen and competence is a required skill for all practicing APNs and most certainly for APN leaders that is nurtured through time and experience. The following list, offered by Lescavage (1995), is a good place for the individual APN to begin developing policy skills:

- *First,* develop political allies in Congress.
- Take part in the numerous fellowships and internships in Washington, DC, and in one's own state.
- Inform lawmakers of APNs' changing goals, ambitions, and needs.
- Become a lobbyist (only 10 of 20,000 staffers are nurses).
- Gain appointments to local, state, and national boards, commissions, task forces, and cabinets.
- Champion causes such as the elderly, teen pregnancy, violence, and AIDS.
- Support nursing organizations and lobby for their interests.
- Write letters and editorials.
- Work on a campaign or, better still, become a candidate.
- Be a strong voice in professional organizations.
- Move at once to address APN issues surrounding regulation, limitations on admitting privileges, limitations to prescriptive authority, and managed care.

OBSTACLES TO SUCCESSFUL LEADERSHIP

There are several obstacles to achieving competence as an APN leader. Most of the obstacles result from conflict and/or competition between individuals or groups. Competition can be both intraprofessional, as between APN groups, and interprofessional, as between physicians and nurses. Grensing-Pophal (1997) identified several pitfalls that present barriers to good leadership and offered some advice. She suggested that being respected rather than being "liked" is one desired criterion for leadership. For most people, this is a difficult reality because being accepted and popular with others is important. Trying to "do it all" rather than delegating to others is a common trap that plagues busy leaders. A good leader is able to encourage a shared work load that recognizes the talents and abilities of followers. Two other pitfalls included avoiding the direct confrontation of difficult issues and a lack of communication with the resulting failure to keep others informed. Communication issues can be partially remedied by e-mails, minutes, and agendas.

One of the most important things that APNs do as leaders is to create community. Creating community in the current health care environment is particularly challenging because of the realignment of clinical decision making, scopes of practice for APNs and physicians, and new roles that blur boundaries between nursing and medicine. Although there are many barriers to leading effectively to create community, three constellations of behavior have been identified that are particularly destructive. Nurses may be particularly vulnerable to these nursing leadership behaviors because of the profession's historic marginalization as a female and relatively powerless group within health care. The first of these constellations is the star complex.

The Star Complex

The star complex is a condition frequently associated with the experienced APN in the clinical setting. As an example, consider the case of Janice, an APN who over the years has become identified with superior patient-focused care. Physician colleagues and other providers consider her to be a partner in the delivery of care. In a recent conversation, a well-respected physician colleague told her how impressed he was with her practice. "In fact," he stated, "you're really not a nurse. You're different from all the other nurses I know." Janice graciously accepted this compliment, knowing that stardom, although overdue, had finally arrived. She had ascended to the heights of provider status and crashed through the nursing ceiling into a zone beyond nursing. Clearly, Janice's understanding of herself as an APN was dormant.

APNs are particularly vulnerable to being seduced into believing they are something other (more) than a nurse. APN specialties that have expanded roles may seek the "status" of medicine. This vulnerability stems from the historical lack of recognition of nursing by physicians, other disciplines, and nurses; the need for approval; and a lack of personal mastery.

A primary strategy for the management of this obstacle is effective mentoring by a powerful APN with an intact nursing identity. An APN with the star complex has usually been mentored exclusively by individuals outside of nursing, such as physicians. Mentors tend to select protégés who remind them of themselves (Bowen, 1985) and then mold their protégés in their own image. The affirmation of the APN's expert clinical skills and even personal mastery are thus validated by a reference group outside of nursing. To acquire a new reference group for validation of worth requires mentoring of the APN by a member of the desired reference group. An additional essential strategy is to use clear and concise communication skills to provide an appropriate response to a colleague who believes that it is a compliment to be identified as other than a nurse. Grohar-Murray and DiCroce's (1992) guidelines for effective communication, discussed earlier in this chapter, are applicable. An appropriate response for Janice to have made would have been, "I'm excellent at what I do; but I'm only one of many excellent nurses."

The existence of the star complex may represent a more fundamental problem for the APN than good communication skills can address. The issue is whether the APN truly desires to be identified as a *nurse,* performing at the boundaries of nursing practice and accepted by other nurses as a valued member of the nursing profession. The resolution of this issue may require counseling and/or group experiential exploration and training. Self-exploration within the context of organizations is provided by various agencies. For example, the Public Health Policy Fellowship at the Health Resources and Services Administration gives individuals opportunities to focus disciplined attention on their role, particularly in terms of authority, power, and leadership, in both small and large interdisciplinary groups. This type of experiential training may prove invaluable to APNs attempting to identify with their professional reference group.

The Queen Bee Syndrome

The Queen Bee Syndrome is best described as a leader who hoards all of the visible leadership tasks for herself. She is threatened by strong individuals and tends to denigrate them instead of sharing power. This type of leader prefers to be surrounded by weak "yes men" who will not challenge her authority. Queen Bee behavior is the antithesis of good leadership, and unfortunately is not uncommon among women and nurses. As APN leaders become more confident in their leadership abilities and as more APNs join the circle of leaders, Queen Bees will have more difficulty remaining as leaders and keeping positions of stature. All effective leadership, as noted previously, requires empowerment of others.

Nurses Not Caring for Their Young

This well-known circumstance is sometimes referred to by the horrific phrase "eating one's young." For example, nurses are often criticized by other nurses for continuing their education and moving into APN roles. This horizontal violence from colleagues hampers others from moving upward in their careers. During orientation to a new position, the process of orienting too often becomes a survival test to see if the new APN can survive without mentoring or a supportive network. Leaders who are aware of this phenomenon can foster mentoring opportunities that can enhance the transition of colleagues in new positions in both practice and leadership roles. APNs need to lead their organizations in a thoughtful evaluation of the nursing environment. Are nurses being supported and mentored to develop their capabilities and professional investment? Are unsupportive comments confronted and addressed? It is not overstatement to claim that the future health of the profession depends on overcoming this barrier and relegating it to history.

STRATEGIES FOR IMPLEMENTING PROFESSIONAL AND CLINICAL LEADERSHIP

Unity Versus Fragmentation

At different times, each subgroup of APNs has emerged as a leader for the nursing profession. Psychiatric CNSs were among the first entrepreneurial APNs to hang out their shingles, despite the litigious climate in which they could be threatened with lawsuits for "practicing medicine." CNMs and CRNAs have led the way in powerfully using data to justify their existence. Both groups began early to record the results of their practices, showing the quality and suitability of their care (Diers, 1992). In the 1990s, NPs, with their flexible, community-based primary care practices, stood at the forefront of the changing health care delivery system. The obstacle to leadership is the tendency for APNs to separate and establish rigid boundaries that distinguish them from one another, thereby blocking opportunities for the increased power that unity would bring.

With this tension and fragmentation, there is a need for leadership by APNs that transcends APN role boundaries. APNs must both manage and bridge boundaries between themselves, among other nursing groups, and within the ranks of the various APN constituencies. Although the uniqueness of each type of APN must be protected, a professional structure that provides a forum for discussing issues pertinent to all types of APNs also needs to be created. This structure may be simply an annual meeting for APNs, or it may be a permanent entity residing within an existing or new professional organization. Progress has been made in this area during the 1990s. Consensus groups at the national level are meeting to discuss policy issues. At the policy level, the power of collective numbers of all APN groups speaking with one voice cannot be overemphasized. APN specialty groups have joined to speak out collaboratively about state regulations regarding reimbursement, prescriptive authority, and managed care regulation. The vision to unify practice and collaborate is calling to every APN.

APN groups are composed of individual APNs. It is critical that each APN, regardless of specialty, take on the burden of moving toward unification. The following guidelines, adapted from Heifetz (1994), may help APNs move from fragmentation to unity:

- Because leadership is a core competency for the APN, the goal of unification must be translated into a shared vision. This is the case whether at high-level policy meetings or in the grassroots clinical setting.
- APNs and their various professional associations need a forum to explore, identify, and regulate the stress related to crossing and perhaps merging boundaries previously viewed as impenetrable. A specific example of this is the blended CNS/NP role discussed in Chapter 16. This redefinition of reality will require taking risks with and without the benefit of a safety net.
- With a legitimate forum established, APNs can direct disciplined attention to the issue of unity. Examples are the national coalitions that have been formed to implement program standards and review and to explore the issues surrounding interstate compacts. A next step is to build unity among all APN groups.
- Each NP, CNS, CNM, and CRNA will return to the referent professional association for continuing dialogue and support of the outcomes from forum discussions. This involves giving the work and dialogue back to grassroots colleagues.

- Each APN will listen with respect and in every humane way possible to leadership voices in the APN and nursing profession communities and in the communities of care recipients, providers, payers, legislators, and citizens.
- Each APN will emerge from this systematic, inclusive exploration of unity with a clear trajectory for building a learning organization to support the continued development of APN leadership in unity.

These strategies lead to the structures upon which unity is built—understanding change, improved communication, coalition building, and collaborative practice. These four building blocks form the foundation of interdisciplinary leadership and practice.

Empowering Others

Earlier in the chapter, empowerment was defined as the ability of the leader to give followers the freedom and authority to act. However, truly empowering others requires more than just giving them permission to act on their own. Empowerment is a developmental process that a good leader fosters over time that leads constituents to feel competent, responsible, independent, and authorized to act. Rajotte (1996) offered a useful six-step method for APN leaders to use to empower other nurses. The first step involves *education,* which in itself provides power through increasing the individual's knowledge base. The process of *leading* is the second step. A leader can "lead" by inspiring, motivating, and encouraging. Providing *structure* is a third method of empowering. Structure provides a framework that offers protection and security as one moves into new territory. The fourth method for enhancing empowerment in followers involves *providing resources* with which one can grow and develop. *Mentoring,* a key skill for leaders, provides the support and direction necessary for change toward empowerment to happen. The last strategy is *actualization,* in which others, whether nurses, patients, or colleagues, are empowered to evoke change. For example, CNMs empower pregnant women by putting them in control of the birthing process though mentoring and providing resources for parenting that nurture self-esteem and enhance family structure.

Networking

Networks are an integral technique used by leaders, change agents, and policy advocates to stay informed and connected regarding APN issues. Networking, both formal and informal, is not a new strategy for APN leaders. Formal networks take the form of committees, coalitions, and consortia of people who come together to share information and plan strategy regarding mutual issues. Formal networks open doors to new opportunities and provide shared resources. Informal networking is a behind-the-scenes format that allows for contact with APNs and others who "speak the same language," have the same viewpoints, and can offer support and critique at critical times. The ability for APNs to stay connected to important practice and education issues through networking is a key component of leadership. The well-known "old boy network" has long been credited as a powerful tool for successful leaders and strategists. The Internet has markedly augmented the busy APN's ability to informally network with professional colleagues and organizations around the world.

Implementing Change Strategies

Jick (1993) suggested an inventory of "10 commandments" that provide a strong base for the APN who is preparing to become an effective change agent (Table 10-6). Many of the skills that were outlined in the earlier "Personal Attributes of Successful Leaders" section, such as shared vision, expert communication, and risk-taking behaviors, are the same skills offered by Jick. However, there are other strategies that assist in the process as follows. First, it is important to analyze the situation and explore the need for change. Second, one must craft an implementation plan that involves everyone. Third, there must be support for capable leadership. Desired change does not happen without strong leadership, both from individuals and from teams (Jick, 1993). In these 10 commandments, one can clearly see the organic link between leadership and change agentry.

One of the current realities in health care is that transition through change is continuous. Change does not have a discrete beginning and ending, but instead appears to be a series of continuous transitions that overlap one another. This phenomenon requires leadership that is continuous and flexible and demands ongoing attention to and redefinition of appropriate strategies. Table 10-7 provides a list of leadership strategies that are useful for moving through these change transitions. These strategies become key leadership skills in times of ongoing

---

TABLE 10-6 10 COMMANDMENTS OF IMPLEMENTING CHANGE

1. *Analyze the organization and its need for change.* Such an analysis involves consideration of the organization's work, its external environment, and its perceived strengths and weaknesses. The history of the organization must also receive consideration.
2. *Create a shared vision and common direction.* This should reflect the organization's philosophy and help articulate what it hopes to become. Implementors have the task of translating the vision to the grassroots so they can appreciate its potential implications for their work or positions.
3. *Separate from the past.* It is important to isolate the structure and the practices that no longer work and determine to move beyond them.
4. *Create a sense of urgency.* People will not go along with change that they see no need for. Currently, the health care system/nonsystem appears to be providing lots of urgency for caregivers as well as other major players. APNs can capitalize on this urgency to focus their practice.
5. *Support a strong leader role.* Desired change does not happen without strong leadership. In these chaotic times, many organizations do not depend on one leader but utilize leadership teams.
6. *Line up political sponsorship.* Once leadership is identified, support must be generated. This is similar to coalition-building, mentioned earlier.
7. *Craft an implementation plan.* A map of the change effort with specific timelines is necessary. It will need to detail clear responsibilities for the various organizational roles.
8. *Develop enabling structures.* Structures that will facilitate and highlight change are necessary. Consider pilot programs, retreats, training workshops, and new reward systems.
9. *Communicate, involve people, and be honest.* A change announcement must be timely, brief, specific, and concise. The necessary follow-up communication must involve listening, repeating, explaining across communication styles, and responding to concerns and resistance.
10. *Reinforce and institutionalize the change.* The commitment to change must be obvious. The new culture must begin to show itself through the reinforcement of new behaviors.

Adapted from Jick, T. D. (1993). *Managing change: Cases and concepts* (p. 195). Burr Ridge, IL: Irwin; reprinted with permission. (Originally published in Jick, T. D. [1991]. *Implementing change* [case no. 491-114]. Boston: Harvard Business School. Copyright © 1991 by the President and Fellows of Harvard College.)

TABLE 10–7 LEADERSHIP STRATEGIES FOR MOVING THROUGH THE TRANSITION OF CHANGE

Developing interim procedures and policies . . . *to create structure*
Fostering group cohesion . . . *so people can draw strength from each other*
Anticipating that old issues/rumors will surface . . . *allow them to be acknowledged*
Reminding folks over and over why change is necessary . . . *to gain support for change*
Creating new communication channels . . . *being honest about uncertainty*
Minimizing unnecessary changes . . . *which can lead to frustration and resistance*
Reminding and showing people what they can count on . . . *to build confidence*

Adapted from Mason, D. J., & Leavitt, J. K. (1998). *Policy and politics in nursing and health care,* (pp. 280–293). Philadelphia: W. B. Saunders; reprinted with permission.

change. Bonalumi and Fisher (1999) suggested that an important component of leadership in an atmosphere of change is the ability to foster and encourage resilience in change recipients. O'Connell (1999) defined the characteristics of resilient people as follows: being positive and self-assured in the face of life's complexities; having a focused, clear vision of what they want to achieve; and having the abilities to be organized but flexible and proactive rather than reactive. Helping colleagues and followers to develop resilience is a major achievement for APN leaders who seek to facilitate the growth of their followers.

APNs AS HEALTH CARE LEADERS IN THE NEW MILLENNIUM

The future is bright for APNs as clinical and professional leaders. The evolution of APNs in the four clinical specialties of advanced practice has had far-reaching influence on this country's health care system as well as on nursing itself. APN leaders have emerged as advanced nursing practice has gained prominence. APNs now hold influential positions of leadership in national organizations and committees as well as state and regional groups. They play important roles as leaders in interdisciplinary clinical practices at the grassroots level. Nursing's model is based on an interactive style that empowers patients. This model holds APN leaders in good stead as they move into the interdisciplinary paradigm of the future. It is very important for new graduates to begin the trajectory for growth and development and for existing APN leaders to mentor their protégés into leadership positions.

As APNs contemplate the demands and opportunities for leadership that the future holds, they must work toward identifying, clarifying, and demystifying reality, for within today's reality lies the basis of tomorrow's change. APNs are change specialists who operate at the boundaries of today's reality. They use collaboration and affirmation as the tools to place nursing and health care in a position to more effectively meet the needs of individuals, families, and communities (Malone, 1996).

APN leaders are poised to move into the next century. As this trajectory occurs, the need to interface with leaders of other disciplines will increase, the need for APN leaders to empower grassroots followers will be ever more important, and the requirement for leadership to be a core competency for all APNs will be paramount.

REFERENCES

Aroskar, M. A. (1987). The interface of ethics and politics in nursing. *Nursing Outlook, 35,* 268–272.

Allen, D. W. (1998). How nurses become leaders: Perceptions and beliefs about leadership development. *Journal of Nursing Administration, 28*(9), 15–20.

Ballein, K. M. (1998). Entrepreneurial leadership characteristics of SNEs emerge as their role develops. *Nursing Administration Quarterly, 22*(2), 60–69.

Barker, A. (1994). An energy leadership paradigm: Transformational leadership. In E. I. Hein & M. J. Nicholson (Eds.), *Contemporary leadership* (4th ed., pp. 81–86). Philadelphia: J. B. Lippincott.

Bernhard, L. A., & Walsh, M. (1995). *Leadership: The key to the professionalization of nursing* (3rd ed.). St. Louis: Mosby.

Bonalumi, N., & Fisher, K. (1999). Health care change: Challenge for nurse administrators. *Nursing Administration Quarterly, 23*(2), 69–73.

Bowen, D. (1985). Were men meant to mentor women? *Training and Development Journal, 39,* 30–34.

Bridges, W. (1991). *Managing transitions: Making the most of change.* Reading, MA: Addison-Wesley.

Burns, J. M. (1978). *Leadership.* New York: Harper & Row.

Covey, S. (1989). *The seven habits of highly effective people: Powerful lessons in personal change.* New York: Simon & Schuster.

Dempster, J. S. (1994). Autonomy: A professional issue of concern for nurse practitioners. *Nurse Practitioner Forum, 5,* 227–232.

DePree, M. (1989). *Leadership is an art.* New York: Doubleday/Currency.

DeVries, C. M., & Vanderbuilt, M. W. (1992). *The grassroots lobbying handbook: Empowering nurses through legislative and political action.* Washington, DC: American Nurses Association.

Diers, D. (1992). Nurse midwives and nurse anesthetists: The cutting edge in specialist practice. In L. Aiken & C. Fagin (Eds.), *Charting nursing's future* (pp. 159–180). Philadelphia: J. B. Lippincott.

Fiedler, F. E., Chermers, M. M., & Mahar, L. C. (1976). *Improving leadership effectiveness: The leader match concept.* New York: John Wiley & Sons.

Grensing-Pophal, L. (1997). Improving your leadership skills: Seven common pitfalls to avoid. *Nursing 97, 27*(4), 41–42.

Grohar-Murray, M. E., & DiCroce, H. R. (1992). *Leadership and management in nursing.* Norwalk, CT: Appleton & Lange.

Hanson, C. M., Boyle, J., Hatmaker, D., & Murray, J. (1999). *Finding your voice as a leader.* Washington, DC: American Academy of Nursing.

Hassmiller, S. (1995). *Legislative logistics for leaders.* Washington, DC: Health Resources and Services Administration.

Hebda, T., Czar, P., & Mascara, C. (1998). *Handbook of informatics for nurses and health care professionals.* New York: Addison-Wesley.

Heifetz, R. (1994). *Leadership without easy answers.* Cambridge, MA: Belknap Press.

Hein, E. I., & Nicholson, M. J. (1994). *Contemporary leadership* (4th ed.). Philadelphia: J. B. Lippincott.

Henderson, V. (1961). *Basic principles of nursing care* (p. 2). Geneva: International Council of Nurses.

Hillesheim, S. J. (1998). The leader meter: A feedback survey. *Nursing Management, 29*(3), 32B–C.

Jick, T. D. (1993). *Managing change: Cases and concepts.* Burr Ridge, IL: Irwin.

Kantor, R. M., Stein, B. A., & Jick, T. D. (1992). *The challenge of organizational change: How companies experience it and leaders guide it.* New York: The Free Press.

Keller, T., & Dansereau, F. (1995). Leadership and empowerment: A social exchange perspective. *Human Relations, 48*(2), 127–146.

Klein, E., Gabelnick, F., & Herr, P. (1998). *The psychodynamics of leadership.* Madison, CT: Psychosocial Press.

Koerner, J. E. (1997). Profiles of leadership: A dialogue with two nursing revolutionaries. *Nursing Administration Quarterly, 22*(1), 1–7.

Lescavage, N. J. (1995). Nurses, make your presence felt: Taking off the rose colored glasses. *Nursing Policy Forum, 1*(1), 18–21.

Lewin, K. (1951). *Field theory in social science.* New York: Harper & Row.

Malone, B. L. (1996). Clinical and professional leadership. In A. B. Hamric, J. A. Spross, & C. M. Hanson (Eds.), *Advanced nursing practice: An integrative approach* (pp. 213–228). Philadelphia: W. B. Saunders.

Malone, B. (1997). Why isn't nursing more diversified. In J. McCloskey & H. Grace (Eds.), *Current issues in nursing* (pp. 574–579). St. Louis: Mosby.

Mason, D. J., & Leavitt, J. K. (1998). *Policy and politics in nursing and health care.* Philadelphia: W. B. Saunders.

Milio, N. (1984). The realities of policymaking: Can nurses have an impact? *The Journal of Nursing Administration, 14*(3), 18–23.

Morrison, R. S., Jones, L., & Fuller, B. (1997). The relation between leadership style and empowerment on job satisfaction of nurses. *Journal of Nursing Administration, 27*(5), 27–34.

Mundt, M. H. (1997). Books on health policy and health reform: How is nursing represented? *Journal of Professional Nursing, 13*(1), 19–27.

Norton, S. F., & Grady, E. M. (1996). Change agent skills. In A. B. Hamric, J. A. Spross, & C. M. Hanson (Eds.), *Advanced nursing practice: An integrative approach* (pp. 249–271). Philadelphia: W. B. Saunders.

O'Connell, C. (1999). A culture of change or a change of culture. *Nursing Administration Quarterly, 23*(2), 65–68.

Pavalko, R. M. (1971). *Sociology of occupations and professions.* Itasca, IL: Peacock.

Pearson, L. (1987). Judi Buckalew: Learning to play political hardball. *The Nurse Practitioner: The American Journal of Primary Health Care, 12*(1), 49–50, 52, 54.

Rajotte, C. A. (1996). Empowerment as a leadership theory. *Kansas Nurse, 71*(1), 1.

Senge, P. (1990). *The fifth discipline: The art and practice of the learning organization.* New York: Doubleday.

Solfarelli, D., & Brown, D. (1998). The need for nursing leadership in uncertain times. *Journal of Nursing Management, 6*(4), 201–207.

Stogdill, R. M. (1948). Personal factors associated with leadership in a survey of the literature. *Journal of Psychology, 25,* 35–71.

Tornabeni, J. (1996). Changes in the advanced practice of administration: A personal perspective of the changes affecting the role. *Advanced Practice Nursing Quarterly, 2*(1), 62–66.

Towers, J. (1995). A call to action: the GNE-GME-NEA debate. *Nursing Policy Forum, 1*(1), 40–45.

Vance, C., & Olson, R. K. (1998). *The mentor connection in nursing.* New York: Springer-Verlag.

Waldrop, J. (1990). You'll know it's the 21st century when . . . *American Demographics, 12*(12), 22–27.

Warden, G. L. (1997). Future organizational leadership. *Journal of Professional Nursing, 13*(6), 334.

Woodhall, N. (1998). Healthcare's invisible partner. *The Woodhall Study on nursing and the media.* Indianapolis, IN: Sigma Theta Tau International.

Additional Readings

Abreu, B. C. (1997). Interdisciplinary leadership: The future is now. *OT Practice, 2*(3), 20–23.

Anderson, R. (1997). The nurse executive: Future organizational leadership. *Journal of Professional Nursing, 13*(6), 334.

Antrobus, S., & Brown, S. (1997). The impact of the commissioning agenda upon nursing practice: a pro-active approach to influencing health policy. *Journal of Advanced Nursing, 25*(2), 309–315.

Barczak, N. L. (1996). How to lead effective teams. *Critical Care Nursing Quarterly, 19*(1), 73–82.

Bessent, H. (Eds.). (1997). *Strategies for recruitment, retention, and graduation of minority nurses in colleges of nursing.* Washington, DC: American Nurses Publishing.

Bowen, W., & Bok, D. (1998). *The shape of the river: Long term consequences of considering race in college and university admissions.* Princeton, NJ: Princeton University Press.

Boykin, A. (1995). *Power, politics and public policy.* New York: National League for Nursing Press.

Buppert, C. (1999). *Nurse practitioner's business practice and legal guide.* Gaithersburg, MD: Aspen Publishers.

Carpenito, L. J. (1998). Redefining the gold standard of health care aka medical care. *Nursing Forum, 33*(3), 3–4.

DePree, M. (1992). *Leadership is an art* (2nd ed). New York: Doubleday/Currency.

Ellis-Stoll, C. C., & Popkess-Vawter, S. (1998). A concept analysis on the process of empowerment. *Advances in Nursing Science, 21*(2), 62–68.

Hamric, A. B., & Spross, J. A., Eds. (1989). *The clinical nurse specialist in theory and practice.* (2nd ed). Philadelphia: W. B. Saunders.

Hamric, A. B., Spross, J. A., & Hanson, C. M., Eds. (1996). *Advanced nursing practice: An integrative approach.* Philadelphia: W. B. Saunders.

Hanson, C. M. (1998). Regulatory issues will lead advanced practice nursing challenges into the new millennium. *Advanced Practice Nursing Quarterly, 4*(3), v–vi.

Jick, T. D. (1993). *Managing change: Cases and concepts.* Burr Ridge, IL: Irwin.

Ketefian, S. (1999). Knowing good and doing good—is there a difference? *Journal of Professional Nursing, 15*(1), 4.

Kleinpell, R. M., & Piano, M. R. (1998). *Practice issues for the acute care nurse practitioner.* New York: Springer-Verlag.

Kissinger, J. A. (1998). Overconfidence: A concept analysis. *Nursing Forum, 33*(2), 18–26.

Lewin, K. (1951). *Field theory in social science.* New York: Harper & Row.

Mahaffey, T. L. (1998). A nursing fellowship: Building leadership skills. *Nursing Management, 29*(3), 30–32.

Malby, B. (1998). Clinical leadership. *Advanced Practice Nursing Quarterly, 3*(4), 40–43.

Manfredi, C. M. (1996). A descriptive study of nurse managers and leadership. *Western Journal of Nursing Research, 18*(3), 314–329.

Mason, D. J., & Leavitt, J. K. (1998). *Policy and politics in nursing and health care* (3rd ed.). Philadelphia: W. B. Saunders.

McGuire, C. A., Stanhope, M., & Weisenbeck, S. M. (1998). Nursing competence—An evolving regulatory issue in Kentucky. *Nursing Administration Quarterly, 23*(1), 24-28.

Mellon, S., & Nelson, P. (1998). Leadership experiences in the community for nursing students: Redesigning education for the 21st century. *Nursing and Health Care Perspectives, 19*(3), 120-123.

Michaels, C. (1997). Leading beyond traditional boundaries: A community nursing perspective. *Nursing Administration Quarterly, 22*(1), 30-37.

Milstead, J. A. (1997). A social mandate: APN leadership for the whole policy process. *Advanced Practice Nursing Quarterly, 3*(3), 1-8.

Milstead, J. A. (1998). *Health policy and politics: A nurse's guide.* Gaithersburg, MD: Aspen Publishers.

Newell, M., & Pinardo, M. (1998). *Reinventing your nursing career: A handbook for success with the age of managed care.* Gaithersburg, MD: Aspen Publishers.

Penney, N. E., Campbell-Heider, N., Miller, B. K., Carter, E., & Bidwell-Cerone, S. (1996). Influencing health care policy: Nursing research and the ANA social policy statement. *Journal of the New York State Nurses Association, 27*(3), 15-19.

Pew Health Professions Commission. (1995). *Critical challenges: Revitalizing the health professions for the twenty-first century, third report.* San Francisco: UCSF Center for the Health Professions.

Safriet, B. (1998). Still spending dollars, still searching for sense: Advanced practice nursing in an era of regulatory and economic turmoil. *Advanced Practice Nursing Quarterly, 4*(3), 24-33.

Simpson, R. L. (1999). Changing world, changing systems: Why managed health care demands information technology. *Nursing Administration Quarterly, 23*(2), 86-88.

Starfield, B. (1997). Primary care and health policy: The future of primary care in a managed care era. *International Journal of Health Services, 27*(4), 687-696.

Sullivan, T. J. (1998). *Collaboration: A health care imperative. Part III, intraorganizational collaboration.* New York: McGraw-Hill.

Triolo, P. K., Pozehl, B. J., & Mahaffey, T. L. (1997). Development of leadership within the university and beyond: Challenges to faculty and their development. *Journal of Professional Nursing, 13*(3), 149-153.

Whitman, M. (1998). Nurses can influence public health policy. *Advanced Practice Nursing Quarterly, 3*(4), 67-71.

Williams, R. P. (1998). Nurse leaders' perceptions of quality nursing: An analysis from academe. *Nursing Outlook, 46*(6), 262-267.

Williamson, S. H., & Hutcherson, C. (1998). Mutual recognition: Response to the regulatory implications of a changing health care environment. *Advanced Practice Nursing Quarterly, 4*(3), 86-93.

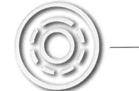

Collaboration

• C H A R L E N E   M.   H A N S O N
• J U D I T H   A.   S P R O S S
• D A N I E L   B.   C A R R

INTRODUCTION

Collaboration works. This simple statement belies the complexity of the phenomenon and the significant interpersonal commitment involved in building collaborative relationships. Research supports the premise that collaboration results in better patient outcomes, including patient satisfaction, and provides personal and professional satisfaction for clinicians. Advanced practice nurses (APNs) must have or acquire interpersonal communication skills and behaviors that make collaboration among a broad range of professionals and clients possible. Today, more than ever before, collaboration between health care providers is an essential component of effective patient care. Historically, discussions about collaboration in the health field have focused on the relationship between physicians and nurses because that is where the most serious tensions have occurred. Although this chapter's discussion is often framed within the context of APN-physician practice, it is important that any discussion of collaborative relationships address both intradisciplinary collaboration among nurses and interdisciplinary collaboration between nurses and members of other disciplines.

The presence or absence of collaborative relationships affects patient care. Clients assume that their health care providers communicate and collaborate effectively. However, client dissatisfaction with care, unsatisfactory clinical outcomes, and clinician frustration can often be traced to a failure to collaborate. The ability to collaborate is a core competency of advanced nursing practice (Brown, 1998; see Chapter 3). Collaboration depends on clinical and interpersonal expertise and an understanding of factors that can promote or impede efforts to establish collegial relationships.

A paradox of the contemporary health care system is that both incentives and disincentives exist for members of different disciplines to collaborate. Incentives and disincentives may be equally powerful, so that motivation to collaborate can be diminished or eliminated by a compelling counterforce. An understanding of this paradox can help APNs and their colleagues approach opportunities for collaboration strategically and build and sustain clinical environments that support collaboration among clinicians. As pressures to change mount in response to ongoing health care reform, and as the proportion of nonphysician health professionals increases, interdisciplinary collaboration at educational, clinical, and institutional levels is essential (Lindeke & Block, 1998).

In this chapter, a conceptualization of collaboration is presented, followed by evidence that collaboration works. Incentives and disincentives for collaborating are identified. A definition and characteristics of collaboration that more fully address values, interpersonal aspects, and goals are offered and strategies for developing and evaluating this competency are suggested. Key collaborative relationships for the APN are those with nurses, physicians, physician assistants, social workers, and other members of interdisciplinary teams. These relationships are used to illustrate important aspects of this core competency.

A CONCEPTUALIZATION OF COLLABORATION

Collaboration can be thought of as one of several modes of interaction that occur between and among clinicians during the delivery of care. To appreciate the complexity of collaboration, it is useful to describe the variety of interactions that can occur. These include parallel communication and functioning, information exchange, coordination, consultation, co-management, referral, and collaboration. Certified nurse-midwives (CNMs) have been credited with creating the clearest definitions of collaboration, consultation, and referral in their practice relationships with obstetricians.

> *Parallel communication:* Providers interact with a patient separately; they do not talk together before seeing a patient, nor do they see the patient together. There is no expectation of joint interactions. For example, the staff registered nurse, the medical student, and the attending physician all ask the patient about the medications the patient is taking.
> *Parallel functioning:* Providers care for patients, addressing the same clinical problem, but do not engage in any joint or collaborative planning. For example, nurses, physical therapists, and physicians document their interventions for pain in separate parts of the patient record.
> *Information exchange:* Informing may be one- or two-sided and may or may not require action or decision making. If action is needed, the decision is unilateral, not a result of joint planning.
> *Coordination:* The establishment of structures to minimize duplication of effort and to maximize efficient use of clients' and providers' resources.
> *Consultation:* The process whereby the clinician who is caring for a client seeks advice regarding a client concern but retains primary responsibility for care delivery (see Chapter 8).
> *Co-management:* This refers to the process in which two or more clinicians provide care and each professional retains accountability and responsibility for defined aspects of care. This process usually arises from consultation in which a problem requires management that is outside the scope of practice of the referring clinician. One clinician usually retains responsibility for the majority of care (as in primary care settings) while the second provider is accountable for managing the problem that is outside the primary provider's expertise. Providers must be explicit with each other about their responsibilities. Co-management may also characterize well-functioning interdisciplinary teams.
> *Referral:* The process by which the APN directs the client to a physician or another practitioner for management of a particular problem or aspect of the client's care when the problem is beyond her or his expertise (see Chapter 8).

With the exceptions of parallel communication and parallel functioning, these processes require some level of interaction and communication among providers. Information exchange, coordination, consultation, co-management, and referral do not require collaboration as it is described here, although collaboration is likely to enhance them.

According to the dictionary, *collaboration* means "to work together, especially in a joint intellectual effort"; it also means to cooperate with the enemy (McKechnie, 1983). The term "collaborative" is often used with other words, such as "teamwork" or "partnership." The description of collaboration in the American Nurses Association's (ANA's) Social Policy Statement (ANA, 1995) informs the definition and discussion of collaboration in this chapter. The ANA recognized that the boundaries of each health professional's practice change and that high-quality care depends on a common focus, a recognition of each other's expertise, an appreciation for the skills and knowledge shared across disciplines, and the collegial exchange of ideas and knowledge. None of these meanings adequately represent this concept as it exists, or should exist, in the provision of health and illness care. On the basis of a review of the literature and their experiences, the authors propose the following definition of collaboration:

> *Collaboration* is a dynamic, interpersonal process in which two or more individuals make a commitment to each other to interact authentically and constructively to solve problems and to learn from each other in order to accomplish identified goals, purposes, or outcomes. The individuals recognize and articulate the shared values that make this commitment possible.

This definition implies shared values, commitment, and goals and yet allows for differences in opinions and approaches. It also acknowledges that collaboration requires individuals to interact holistically (strengths, weaknesses, and emotions), to share power, and to remain open to the possibilities for personal and professional transformation that exist within a collaborative relationship. This definition captures the complexity and challenge of collaboration. Including the notions of shared values and commitment makes clear that collaboration is a process that evolves over time. Tjosvold (1986) and Hughes and Mackenzie (1990) emphasized the importance of goal interdependence to collaboration. By definition, collaboration describes relationships that are positive and work well for professionals and clients. There is room for disagreement in collaborative relationships; partners develop strategies for dealing with disagreement that are mutually satisfactory and enhance collaboration. Because it is an interpersonal process, collaboration cannot be accomplished by mandate.

IMPACT OF COLLABORATION ON PATIENTS AND CLINICIANS

Experience and evidence suggest that collaboration works, yet effective collaboration eludes many clinicians. Why? Some authors link barriers to the history of the health care professions, traditional gender roles, and hierarchical relationships (Christman, 1998; DeAngelis, 1994; Larson, 1999; Wells, Johnson, & Salyer, 1997). Over the years, there have been many reports of successful collaborative relationships involving APNs. Examples include those of Ryan, Edwards, and Rickles (1980), Steele (1986), Littell (1981), Crowley and Wollner (1987), Hilderley (1991), Kavesh (1993), Dressler (1994), Kedziera and Levy (1994), Siegler and Whitney (1994a), Brita-Rossi and colleagues (1996), and Hales, Karshmer, Montes-Sandoval, and Fiszbein (1998).

In a review of the literature on collaboration, Sullivan (1998) noted that collaboration is widely perceived as useful and desirable. Although there are few studies of collaboration that have measured patient outcomes systematically (Sullivan, 1998; Torres & Dominguez, 1998), both patient and provider benefits have been documented. Sullivan (1998) found no reports indicating that collaboration failed when the models or practices had been jointly developed and implemented. Table 11–1 illustrates the types of patient and provider benefits that have been ascribed to clinical collaboration. Of the literature on collaboration, few articles are found in the medical literature. Larson (1999) noted that, of 61 citations on nurse-physician collaboration published between 1990 and 1995, only 29.5% were published in medical journals.

Evidence That Collaboration Works

THE NATIONAL JOINT PRACTICE COMMISSION

In the early 1970s, the ANA and the American Medical Association (AMA) collaborated to form the National Joint Practice Committee (National Joint Practice Commission [NJPC], 1979). The committee was created to respond to tension and conflict between physicians and nurses that was perceived to be due to increased patient loads and cost constraints, which were placing excessive demands on both groups. The NJPC funded several demonstration projects to implement joint practice arrangements within four different hospital settings that were attempting to improve nurse-physician relationships. The NJPC identified five critical elements of collaborative practice in hospital settings: primary nursing, integrated patient records, encouragement of nurse decision making, a joint practice committee, and a joint record review (Devereux, 1981; NJPC, 1979). The NJPC demonstration project was one of the earliest studies to document that collaboration benefited clinicians and patients. Although the data from these NJPC projects indicated improved communication and improved patient care outcomes, the work was never completed. Unfortunately, there has not been widespread implementation of the NJPC's recommendations (Crowley & Wollner, 1987; Fagin, 1992).

TABLE 11–1 BENEFITS OF COLLABORATION	
FOR PATIENTS	FOR PROVIDERS
• Improved quality of care • Increased patient satisfaction • Lower mortality • Improved patient outcomes • Patients feel more secure, cared for, closer to nurses	• Increased sharing of responsibility • Increased sharing of expertise • More mutually satisfying problem solving • Improved communications • Increased personal satisfaction • Increased quality of professional life • Enhanced mutual trust and respect • Bridges care-cure dichotomy • Expands horizons of providers • Avoids redundant care and ensures coverage • Empowers providers to influence health policy

Adapted from Sullivan, T. J. (1998). Collaboration: A health care imperative (pp. 26–27). New York: McGraw-Hill Health Professions Division; reprinted with permission.

OUTCOMES OF INTENSIVE CARE UNIT STAYS

One of the first studies to identify the impact of nurse-physician communication on patient outcomes found that the most significant factor associated with excess mortality in intensive care units (ICUs) was nurse-physician communication patterns. Another factor associated with lower mortality was the presence of a comprehensive nursing education support system in which clinical nurse specialists (CNSs) had responsibility for staff development (Knaus, Draper, Wagner, & Zimmerman, 1986). Hospitals with lower mortality rates had systems that ensured excellent nurse-physician communication.

In an extension of this research, a study of 17,440 patients in 42 ICUs provided additional evidence that interactions among caregivers affect patient care (Shortell et al., 1994). Effective caregiver interactions were associated with lower risk-adjusted length of stay, lower nurse turnover, better quality of care, and greater ability to meet family member needs. In the analytical model the investigators used, caregiver interaction included the culture, leadership, coordination, communication, and conflict management abilities of the unit's staff. "Greater technological availability," a term describing a measure of state-of-the-art treatments, was also associated with lower risk-adjusted mortality. Hospitals that were more profitable, that were involved in teaching activities, and whose unit leaders were more involved in quality improvement activities had greater technological availability.

In another study of ICU outcomes, a threefold increase in in-hospital mortality was associated with not having daily rounds made by an ICU physician (Pronovost et al., 1999). Lack of daily rounds was also associated with an increased risk of complications such as cardiac arrest, acute renal failure, and septicemia. Increased resource utilization was associated with several factors, including lack of daily rounds, having an ICU nurse–patient ratio of less than 1 : 2, not having monthly review of morbidity and mortality, and extubating patients in the operating room. The authors did not cite nurse-physician communication and collaboration in their interpretation of findings. However, absence of daily rounds—an opportunity for nurses and physicians to communicate and plan care—indirectly supports the findings that nurse-physician communication and collaboration affect patient care.

MORTALITY IN MEDICARE PATIENTS

Prior to undertaking an analysis of mortality in magnet and nonmagnet hospitals, Aiken, Smith, and Lake (1994) reviewed the literature on two independent streams of research, magnet hospitals and Medicare mortality. The study examined institutional characteristics in conjunction with characteristics of nurses and physicians working in the same institution (Aiken et al., 1994). A "magnet hospital" is a term used to describe hospitals that have reputations as being good places in which to practice nursing. In the analysis of organizational characteristics of magnet and nonmagnet hospitals, Aiken and colleagues (1994) concluded that the designation of magnet hospital was a proxy for three characteristics of nursing practice in a hospital: nurse autonomy, nurse control over practice, and the relations of nurses with physicians. When mortality data in both types of hospitals were analyzed, these authors found that magnet hospitals had a 5% reduction in excess mortality. The authors concluded that the difference in mortality between the two groups of hospitals was attributable to the organization of nursing care within magnet hospitals. Although this study did not look at advanced nursing practice specifically, the results suggest that organizational characteristics may influence quality of collaboration between nurses and physicians.

OTHER EVIDENCE

In studies of clinical expertise in nurses, Benner, Hooper-Kyriakidis, and Stannard (1999) have identified the myriad ways in which expert nurses, including APNs, contribute to collaboration and teambuilding. Table 11-2 lists the behaviors of expert nurses that represent collaborative activities within specific domains of nursing practice. Wells and colleagues (1997) examined interdisciplinary collaboration on seven inpatient units over time. The authors hypothesized that (1) staff on units using different interdisciplinary strategies would report different levels of collaboration, and (2) staff who perceived high physician involvement in collaborative practice would report greater collaboration than staff who perceived low physician involvement. This study was done at a time when critical pathways were being developed by CNSs. Over time CNSs became APN case managers and the process of critical path development became a collaborative one between APNs and physicians. Degree of use of critical paths was used to categorize collaborative practice strategies. Although there were differences in perceived collaboration based on critical pathway use, the findings suggested that physician involvement was more strongly associated with degree of collaboration than the type of strategy used.

Collaboration has also been associated with decreased costs of care. Lassen, Fosbinder, Minton, and Robins (1997) reported that the complex diagnosis and treatment of septic neonates was enhanced by collaborative nurse-physician relationships and that cost of care was reduced while quality improved. Additional anecdotal benefits of this study included decreased parental anxiety and confusion, enhanced continuity and consistency of care, and a reduction of the need for further consultation. Brita-Rossi and colleagues (1996) showed better patient outcomes and reduced costs when nurses and physicians collaborated to improve orthopedic care.

TABLE 11-2 COLLABORATIVE ACTIVITIES USED BY EXPERT CRITICAL CARE NURSES

Domain: Diagnosing and managing life-sustaining physiologic functions in unstable patients
• Coordinating and managing multiple, instantaneous therapies
The skilled know-how of managing a crisis
• Organizing the team and orchestrating their actions during a crisis
• Exhibiting experiential leadership when a physician is present
• Taking necessary medical action to manage a crisis when a physician is absent
• Recognizing clinical talent and skilled clinicians and marshaling these for the particular situation
• Modulating one's emotional responses and facilitating the social climate
Communicating multiple clinical, ethical, and practical perspectives
• Team building: developing a community of attentiveness, skill, and collaboration
Monitoring quality and managing a breakdown
• Front-line quality improvement, monitoring, and risk management
• Team building in the context of breakdown
• Minimizing health care system failures in destabilized work environments
The skilled know-how of clinical leadership and the coaching and mentoring of others
• Facilitating the clinical development of others
• Building and preserving collaborative relationships
• Transforming care delivery systems

Data from Benner, P., Hooper-Kyriakidis, P., & Stannard, D. (1999). *Clinical wisdom and interventions in critical care* (p. 3). Philadelphia: W. B. Saunders; reprinted with permission.

The importance of collaboration to effective, accessible health care has been recognized by several philanthropies that support health care initiatives. The report of the Pew Health Professions Commission identified the following core competencies for health professionals of the future: community health focus; delivery of contemporary, evidence-based clinical care; expanded accountability; appropriate and cost-effective use of technology; preventive care and promotion of healthy lifestyles; patient and family involvement in decision making; and information management, including lifelong learning (Pew Health Professions Commission, 1995; Gelman, O'Neil et al, 1999). In an earlier initiative, the Pew-Fetzer Task Force on Psychosocial Health Education (1994) advocated a relationship-centered approach to health care. The relationship-centered approach is intended to foster health care that integrates biomedical and psychosocial approaches. The Pew-Fetzer Task Force (1994) described three dimensions of such care: the patient-practitioner relationship; the community-practitioner relationship; and the practitioner-practitioner relationship. The importance of clinician collaboration is illustrated in the description of the practitioner-practitioner relationship:

> *Effective, empathic care requires a community of practitioners who commit themselves to working together to serve the complex matrix of individuals' needs in health and illness. . . . Such relationships serve the needs of practitioners as well as patients: building communities enables health care providers to care for one another and give and receive the support and encouragement that produces personal and professional maturation and more effective patient care.*

> (Pew-Fetzer Task Force, 1994, p. 27)

A guiding principle of this group's work is that the quality of relationships formed with patients, communities, students and fellow practitioners across disciplines "is of primary importance to ensuring effective, comprehensive education and health care"(Pew-Fetzer Task Force, 1994, p. 48). The Robert Wood Johnson Partnerships for Quality Education Project (1998–1999) is another initiative that encourages interdisciplinary collaboration among health care providers and managed care entities.

The Effects of Failure To Collaborate

The failure to communicate and collaborate affects patients and clinician job satisfaction. The absence of collaboration is a source of distress to nurses (Larson, 1999). In addition, failure to collaborate may contribute to inefficiencies in the delivery of patient care (Cooper, Henderson, & Dietrich, 1998; Grumbach & Coffman, 1998). Alpert, Goldman, Kilroy, and Pike (1992) found that job satisfaction and attitude were negatively affected when collaboration failed and that territoriality and competitiveness increased. However, the most important result of failure to collaborate is its negative effect on patient care. The studies of intensive care and the Study to Understand Prognosis and Preferences for Outcomes and Risks of Treatments (SUPPORT), described next, are among the few that document the effects of failure to collaborate on patients.

THE SUPPORT STUDY

The primary purpose of this randomized, controlled trial was to improve end-of-life decision making by improving physician-patient communication and clinical care. This study is relevant because it attempted to manipulate nurse-physician interactions to improve end-of-life care by structuring an intervention using CNSs. The study was conducted at five teaching hospitals across the United States. The intervention consisted of providing physicians with information on the likelihood of specific outcomes for seriously ill patients and the involvement of a specially trained nurse who, although clearly identified as a member of the research team, "had the role and appearance of a typical clinical specialist" (SUPPORT Principal Investigators, 1995, p. 1593). The nurse was free to implement the role in order to achieve the best possible care and outcomes. However, the CNSs' involvement required the approval of physicians, which in all cases was provided. Physicians were free to limit the intervention in any way that they believed would be best for the patient. In general, SUPPORT nurses made relevant information from their interactions with patients and clinicians available to physicians and other caregivers.

This expensive clinical trial had no impact on any of the designated outcomes. Data for 4,742 patients were abstracted from medical records and interviews with patients and families. The authors concluded that providing additional resources, such as the time and expertise of nurses, did not improve collaborative decision making in end-of-life care. Collaboration, or the lack of it, between nurses (APNs) and physicians was not identified as a possible barrier to implementation, nor is it mentioned as an explanation of the findings (Oddi & Cassidy, 1998). The study appears to have been conceptualized from a physician perspective—all of the principal investigators were physicians. The lists of the study team members indicated that nurses delivering the intervention had various education credentials, suggesting that not all SUPPORT nurses were, in fact, CNSs. No data were reported regarding how nursing was organized within the hospital. The failure to analyze and report data on the relationships between organizational characteristics and patient outcomes may contribute to the interpretation that the intervention had no effect and thus, weakens the conclusions drawn by the authors.

Collaboration as an Ethical Issue and Institutional Imperative

Some writers have suggested that the failure to collaborate is an ethical issue. Compassionate, ethical patient care that provides a healing environment requires collaborative working relationships between physicians and nurses (Aroskar, 1998; Larson, 1999; see Chapter 12). Larson (1999) identified key beliefs about collaboration on which nurses and physicians differ: the importance of relationships, what constitutes effective and desirable communication, the degree to which communication and shared decision making occur, the authority nurses have to make decisions, and what strategies would improve communication. The failure to understand each other's perspectives, a prerequisite for collaboration, results in a difficult work environment and contributes to uncoordinated, unsafe care (Larson, 1999).

Gianakos (1997) identified three reasons for nurses and physicians to collaborate, and asserted that the ethical imperative to collaborate is the most important:

- Collaboration is a moral imperative—good patient care requires it.
- Collaboration reinforces commitment to a common goal and reaffirms the message that patient welfare is the goal.
- Collaboration enhances shared knowledge as physicians and nurses educate each other repeatedly about the patient.

The evidence that collaboration works suggests that there are structural as well as interpersonal dimensions to collaboration. That is, although institutional policies or standards do not guarantee collaboration, they can establish expectations for communication and collaboration. As the Knaus and associates (1986) study suggested, such institutional expectations can provide a structure that facilitates interpersonal communication and relationship building. Pellegrino (1996), a physician and medical ethicist, concluded that human organization and relationships are more important than our mutual concerns over resources and technologies. The mutual goal of good patient care and the ethical imperative to collaborate should be at the center of any interdisciplinary effort to plan care or resolve conflicts in approaches to care.

Taken together, the studies and reports on the topic of collaboration suggest that the degree of collaboration is determined in part by one's own personal and professional characteristics and by the culture of the systems in which one practices. Effective collaboration among providers with different perspectives results in a creative and multidimensional intelligence that is emotionally rewarding because patients do better and clinicians derive personal and professional gratification from this work. This conclusion has implications for APNs, administrators, physicians, and others. APNs and their administrative and clinical colleagues need to assess the collaborative climate, determine facilitators and barriers, and work together to strengthen relationships and build an organizational culture that values collaboration. This work is essential and should be a priority for institutions and individuals.

THE CONTEXT OF COLLABORATION IN CONTEMPORARY HEALTH CARE

The pressures on physicians and others to improve quality, work more efficiently, and allow others (e.g., insurers) to be involved in decisions about patient care could be expected to foster collaboration among clinicians. Paradoxically, these same factors may undermine collaboration. In mathematics, there is a phenomenon that occurs in which the closer that organisms, atoms, or attractors move to critical transition, the greater the risk of a catastrophe. In this sense, catastrophe means a sudden transition to a qualitatively different type of organization or state. Catastrophe theory offers a metaphor for understanding the complexity of collaborating effectively in a constantly changing system.

As APNs have acquired more education and are better prepared to practice autonomously and collaboratively, physicians have experienced multiple pressures, including the increasing supply of APN providers (Cooper, Henderson, & Dietrich, 1998; Cooper, Laud, & Dietrich, 1998), that apparently or actually encroach on the physicians' autonomy and willingness to collaborate. The mounting pressures on physicians may lead to fear "undifferentiation"—that no one will be able to tell them from physician assistants, APNs, or other providers—which could be perceived as a sudden transition to a qualitatively different state. These same pressures generate concern about relinquishing authority and power, fears that may cause individuals to withdraw from or sabotage efforts to collaborate. Thus the transition to a (presumably) more effective, accessible, and efficient health care system may actually undermine collaboration, a process many leaders believe is central to achieving the goal of a health care system that is accessible, effective, and affordable.

Confusion about scope of practice can be damaging to collaboration for all involved. Physicians may ask themselves: What's in it for me to collaborate? What areas of my work do I get to expand because other providers can do things I have traditionally done? What do I get to keep that's different from other providers? What do I keep that "looks similar" to what other providers are offering? One physician acknowledged that "certain individuals in our group would have a problem with it . . . saying a nurse can do our job. It bruises egos . . . but I would love [to work with a nurse practitioner]" (Cairo, 1996, p. 415). Physician assistants may be asked to distinguish their role from that of the nurse practitioner (NP) (see Chapter 14). APNs may be uncertain about their scope of practice when a physician or institution asks them to assume responsibility for a new skill, such as performing an invasive procedure. The reality is that managed care and regulatory initiatives are rearranging practice boundaries almost daily. These changes are often at the heart of the tension between players as roles and boundaries of disciplines blur and expand.

Opportunities for Collaboration

There are numerous incentives for nurses, physicians, and other providers to collaborate. APNs, physicians, and other providers share a common purpose—the desire to provide good patient care. This mutual goal should be enough to ensure that collaboration occurs consistently. Each group of clinicians has unique, complementary, and overlapping skills that benefit patients; APNs are eager to make their skills and knowledge available. Although the changes in health care have resulted in numerous pressures that can constrain collaboration, certain opportunities for promoting collaboration exist.

Although it may not be immediately apparent, efforts to reduce costs of health care actually offer APNs and physicians a common goal toward which to work and opportunities for learning from each other. Medicare guidelines that are used to document care for coding and billing encourage physicians and nurses to work together to provide the appropriate level of care necessary to meet the standards for reimbursement. National, interdisciplinary guidelines and standards of care are intended to reduce unwarranted, often expensive, variation in health care. Many guidelines specify interdisciplinary collaboration as a critical component of effective care (Acute Pain Management Guideline Panel, 1992; Management of Cancer Pain Guideline Panel, 1994). Standards and guidelines developed and agreed upon by interdisciplinary groups, whether at the local (office or institution) or national level, offer a sound starting point for jointly determining patient care goals, processes, and outcomes. Reports of interdisciplinary teams charged with developing or adopting clinical practice guidelines indicate that these initiatives have had beneficial effects on interdisciplinary relationships and collaboration (Brita-Rossi, et al., 1996; Weinstein, McCormack, Brown, & Rosenthal, 1998).

Accreditation activities offer another opportunity to build collaborative relationships. The Joint Commission on the Accreditation of Health Care Organizations'

(1992) *Agenda for Change,* requires documentation that demonstrates collaborative, interdisciplinary practice. The premise underlying this initiative is that quality patient care is driven by collegial relationships between members of the health care disciplines (Lumpkins & Veal, 1995). The requirement to document these activities can help providers to develop stronger interdisciplinary approaches to care. Other opportunities for improving interdisciplinary relationships and fostering collaboration include case management (Mahn and Spross, 1996; see Chapter 19), development and implementation of clinical pathways, and interdisciplinary rounds (Felton, Cady, Metzler, & Burton, 1997; Weissman, 1988).

The move toward a more community-based, health promotion/disease prevention model of care is further creating new opportunities for collaborative practice (Simpson, 1998). New alliances both among advanced nursing practice groups and between advanced nursing practice and physician groups need to be developed and nurtured.

Barriers to Collaboration

Although it is easy to discuss professional liaisons and to draw up collaborative arrangements on paper, there are many obstacles to actually implementing serious collaborative professional relationships in the workplace. In addition, research by Sands, Stafford, and McClelland (1990) suggested that team members see themselves primarily as representatives of their own discipline, rather than as members of a collaborative team.

The Robert Wood Johnson initiative entitled Partnerships in Training (1996) is an interdisciplinary project being implemented by stakeholders who are educating health care providers. This 8-year project has identified many of the stresses inherent in building and sustaining interdisciplinary partnerships. Barriers or stresses encountered by participants centered on money, differing agendas, systems that are not integrated, varying philosophies, and long-held beliefs about "how things should be done." This report suggests that building relationships between disciplines will be difficult unless there is a high level of commitment for collaboration to succeed among all participants.

SOCIOCULTURAL ISSUES

Tradition, role, and gender stereotypes are obstacles to collaboration. Safriet (1992) suggested that the field of medicine staked out broad turf early on and considered any movement into this turf by nurses at any level to be unacceptable. Thus turf issues have been a major stumbling block to successful interactions between nurses and physicians. Although nurses are highly valued for the physical care, nurturing, and psychosocial support they provide for patients, it is clear that the physician is perceived and valued as the decision maker about treatment. One writer suggested that physicians are at risk of losing their roles as "quarterbacks" of the health care team (Kuraitis, 1999). Many people think of nurses as second best or as caregivers for the unfortunate or indigent. Such views perpetuate the view that the physician is the supervisor and the nurse is the subordinate. Nursing remains a predominantly female profession and, despite the influx of women into medicine, these role stereotypes still exist. Unfortunately, because of barriers to practice that are difficult to break, APNs may buy into this view, which further hampers collaborative, collegial relationships (Lenz, 1994).

Sexism affects collaboration (Coeling & Wilcox, 1994; Siegler & Whitney, 1994b). Gender stereotypes dominate images of staff nurses in the media, and APNs are rarely portrayed on television. With few exceptions, APNs' contributions are not profiled in health care reports in the lay press. Media bias and the nursing profession's inability to market itself adequately make nursing and advanced nursing practice invisible (Fagin, 1992). The "doctor-nurse game," a phenomenon that is influenced by roles and gender and was first described in the 1970s, continues to operate in many institutions; it is apparent, however, that the rules are changing and nurses do not want to play anymore (Stein, Watts, & Howell, 1990).

Stereotypical images and the invisibility of APNs influence how nursing is viewed by both health professionals and consumers—at best nurses are viewed as kind and nice; at worst, as unintelligent and incompetent. Thus APNs often find that they must actively counter low expectations with interactions and practices that convey their intelligence, competence, confidence, and trustworthiness.

PROFESSIONAL BARRIERS

Each profession is a culture with its own values, knowledge, rules, and norms (Benoliel, 1995; Bray & Rogers, 1997). Often, clinicians differ in their basic philosophy of care based on how they have been socialized into the system. For example, medicine is oriented toward biomedical research, technical solutions, hierarchical relationships, and a strong sense of personal responsibility for patient outcomes (Bray & Rogers, 1997). This sense of responsibility is apparent even among physicians who support APNs but imply or explicitly indicate that physician oversight of APN practice is necessary (Cairo, 1996; DeAngelis, 1994). Fagin (1992) asserted that the stance preferred by physicians is not to collaborate with anyone. This is a strong statement and might seem inflammatory. Yet, the Pew-Fetzer Task Force (1994) (the majority of whose members were physicians) also acknowledged that collaboration was a particular challenge for physicians. In a study of 80 nurse practitioners, physican acceptance and support was the the most frequent factor facilitating NP performance (Hupcey, 1993). The Knaus et al. study (1986), cited prior efforts by organized medicine to discredit APNs. Current efforts to place CRNAs under physician supervision (see Chapter 18), and the review of the literature by Larson (1999) also suggest that collaboration is difficult for physicians.

Supervision of APNs by physicians is often mentioned explicitly or implicitly in some of the literature on advanced practice nursing. The view advanced here is that supervision precludes the development of a collaborative relationship and that physicians cannot truly supervise advanced nursing practice. A study of physicians' supervision of pediatric nurse practitioners (Cruikshank & Chow, 1984) suggested that what is called "supervision" is actually consultation or referral as it is defined in this chapter. Rather than supervision, in this dynamic environment, the authors believe it is preferable to define the scope of autonomous nursing management and identify high-risk populations within a particular population or practice that would require consultation, collaboration/co-management, or referral.

In the past 15 years there had been a slow but steady movement away from language requiring physician supervision and reference to protocols and toward emphasizing consultation, collaboration, peer review, and use of referral. However, the AMA (1995) reaffirmed a policy that *supports* supervision of APNs by physicians and claims that physicians have the responsibility for managing health care needs of patients. Despite rhetoric to the contrary, such a policy does not promote a philosophy of collaboration and reinforces stereotyped views of nurse–physician relationships. Because of such initiatives by organized medicine, the need for nursing to standardize advanced nursing practice educational programs, national certification, and state credentialing is particularly urgent. Chapter 22 explores these issues in greater depth.

ORGANIZATIONAL BARRIERS

Competitive situations arise among APNs and between APNs and other disciplines. In her extensive work in the field of health policy, the first author has observed one group of APNs (e.g., CNMs and CRNAs) align around a common viewpoint early in a debate, while members of other APN groups use precious time debating fine points, delaying or eliminating the possibility of unity on a policy issue that will affect all APN groups. Competitive stances and polarizing statements, whether they occur within or between disciplines, are barriers to collaboration. Managed care has been perceived to have a negative effect on physician-patient as well as physician-APN relationships. The inability of APNs to be part of managed care panels has in many settings made collaboration difficult at best and may contribute to unproductive competition. Patients, as the consumers of health care, are important players in the quest for successful collaboration. Patients are sensitive to the relationships between caregivers and are quick to pick up on the lack of respect or trust between their providers. Some research suggests that collaborative relationships among interdisciplinary health care providers can ameliorate some of these negative effects (Afflitto, 1997; Stichler, 1995; Weinstein et al., 1998). Successful collaborative practices are those in which patients easily move back and forth between providers as their care and situation dictate. Collaboration requires an ability to transform competitive situations into opportunities for working together that are mutually beneficial, where all parties can imagine the possibility of creating a win-win situation.

REGULATORY ISSUES

As noted previously, societies of medical professionals continue to try to limit APN practice (e.g., eligibility for reimbursement, prescriptive authority) through legislative and regulatory reform (Minarik & Price, 1999). Legislation and regulations have been barriers to the implementation of collaborative roles (Fagin, 1992; Inglis & Kjervik, 1993). Although major strides have been made in some states, statutes and regulations often support a hierarchical structure that impedes collaboration between nurses and physicians (see Chapters 8 and 22). Language that mandates the nature of APN-physician relationships can undermine collaborative practice. Using such language to regulate interprofessional relationships presents risks to professional autonomy and effective collaboration for APNs and physicians. Collaboration cannot be mandated; it is a process that develops over time.

Opportunities to create collaborative relationships are lost in the morass of concerns over too-rapid change to new systems of care that affect money, politics, power, and control (Dziabis & Lant, 1998). Furthermore, nurses and other stakeholders who are confronting their own professional concerns may not fully appreciate the stresses physicians experience in today's volatile market. This factor is a serious deterrent to collaborative relationships.

Organized Medicine and Nursing Versus Practice Environment

In an analysis of the evolution of the APN and physician assistant roles, Christman (1998) suggested that responses of organized nursing (e.g., the ANA and the National League for Nursing) to physician efforts to extend advanced practice roles to other specialties in the 1970s were not constructive and contributed to the development of the physician assistant role in medicine. This conclusion is likely to be debated by others who witnessed the same events. However, like the history of the NJPC described earlier, these events suggest that decisions made by leaders of nursing and medical organizations can shape the context and process of interdisciplinary collaboration.

It is fairly well accepted by both medicine and nursing that levels of collaboration at the community "grassroots" level are easier to implement and maintain than those at the professional organizational level. Lack of commitment on the part of organizations' leadership and the continuation of power inequities provide a negative milieu for the interaction between organized medicine and nursing (Stichler, 1995). Although collaboration happens daily among individuals on the home front, at national levels, where it is really needed, the level of collaboration may not be as functional as it needs to be to move toward a coordinated health care system. The positions espoused by "old guard" policy makers from all disciplines may be based on stereotyped beliefs about roles and responsibilities, not reflective consideration of the issues or what is best for consumers. This factor makes it increasingly important for APNs and physicians practicing at local levels, who have learned the art of collaboration, to take an active role in bringing their perspectives and experiences to making policies at institutional, community, state, and national levels that foster collaboration. According to Gianakos (1997), "[f]or physicians and nurses to become more collegial, major medical and nursing organizations must make interdisciplinary collegiality a priority" (p. 58). A broader statutory definition of professional autonomy for APNs than currently exists in many states is necessary if the more complex autonomy of interdependent collaborators is to be exercised effectively (Forbes & Fitzsimmons, 1993; Inglis & Kjervik, 1993).

CHARACTERISTICS OF EFFECTIVE COLLABORATION

Effective collaboration between and among APNs, physicians, and other nurses in an ever-changing health care environment depends on many factors. The definition of collaboration proposed in this chapter demands a radical rethinking of how APNs, physicians, and others are prepared and how clinicians interact to ensure positive patient outcomes. The definition also invites exploration of the characteristics that make up a successful collaborative relationship and the personal and setting-specific attributes that are pivotal to successful professional collaborations.

Some characteristics of collaboration have long been recognized and promulgated, but, as the work of the NJPC indicated, clinicians and organizations have resisted adopting the philosophy and behaviors that promote collaboration. The five components of collaborative practice that the NJPC (1979) identified as critical (see p. 319 in this chapter) acknowledged nurse autonomy and authority for nursing practice, and are still important today. Steele's (1986) analysis of collaboration among NPs and physicians revealed several characteristics: mutual trust and respect, an understanding and acceptance of each other's disciplines, positive self-image, equivalent professional maturity arising from education and experience, recognition that the partners are not substitutes for each other, and a willingness to negotiate. Hughes and Mackenzie (1990) outlined four characteristics of NP-physician collaboration: collegiality, communication, goal sharing, and task interdependence. Spross (1989), based on a review of CNS and interdisciplinary literature, described three essential elements of collaboration: a common purpose, diverse and complementary professional knowledge and skills, and effective communication processes. Although this is not an exhaustive summary of the literature on collaboration, it is clear that shared values, effective interpersonal communication, and organizational structures can promote productive alliances among clinicians and create environments in which collaboration is valued and practiced.

The discussion of characteristics of collaboration that follows elaborates on the definition of collaboration proposed in this chapter. The ability to "make a commitment to interact authentically and constructively" suggests that there are characteristics that are prerequisites—qualities that prospective partners must bring to initial and ongoing encounters. To interact authentically means that partners do not leave some part of themselves behind. For example, partners share the emotional satisfactions and frustrations of clinical work and develop ways of supporting each other. Although not discussed in the literature, the authors have observed that successful collaboration can lead to an intimacy that arises from working closely together over time. In her sixth year in a collaborative practice, one NP compared the relationship to a marriage in terms of the interpersonal ups and downs that occurred and the challenge of dealing with the same person daily over matters of great or negligible, albeit clinical import. Thus mature collaboration can be both rewarding and challenging.

Other essential characteristics are a common purpose, clinical competence, interpersonal skills (or a willingness to learn them), and a sense of humor. Trust, respect, and valuing each other's knowledge and skills reflect the nature of collaboration as an "interpersonal process." They are equally important but only develop fully over time. However, in order for them to develop, prospective partners must enter encounters with a commitment to respect, a willingness to trust, and an assumption that the other's knowledge and skills are valuable. In this sense, these characteristics are also prerequisites, but they are fully realized only after many constructive and productive interactions have occurred. Evans (1994) discussed collaboration as a force for achieving desired outcomes. She confirmed that clinicians who collaborate engage in a communal, intellectual effort on behalf of patients and share problem solving, goal setting, and decision making. Thus collaboration occurs when prospective partners recognize that a problem can be solved *only* when each party's input, expertise, or participation is solicited (Stichler, 1995).

Common Purpose

The notion that a common purpose must be the basis for collaboration is well supported in the literature (Alpert et al., 1992; Arslanian-Engoren, 1995; Spross, 1989). Even if partners have not discussed the purposes and goals of their interactions, the organizations in which they work usually have an explicit mission and goals. These can be the starting point for identifying the goals and purposes of clinical collaboration. Collaboration involves a bond, a union, a degree of patient caring that goes beyond a single approach to care and represents a synergistic alliance that maximizes the contributions of each participant (Evans, 1994). In implementing a model of nurse-physician collaboration at a tertiary care institution, Alpert et al. (1992) affirmed that a special synergy arising from collaborative work improves patient outcomes.

Collaboration, by definition, implies that the participants are interdependent. Recognizing their interdependence, team members can combine their individual perceptions and skills to synthesize more complex and comprehensive care plans (Forbes & Fitzsimmons, 1993). Each member brings a particular set of skills and unique expertise to the table for a combined strength that cannot be matched by individuals working alone. Like other characteristics, the common purpose(s) that initially brought partners together may change over time. For example, the organizational goal or situation that brought two clinicians together becomes subordinate to the deep, personal commitment to work together in ways that improve patient care and are interpersonally satisfying.

Clinical Competence

Clinical competence is perhaps the most important characteristic underlying a successful collaborative experience among clinicians, for without it the trust and desire needed to work together are not possible. Trust and respect are built on the assurance that each member is able to carry out her or his role and function in a competent manner. That clinical competence is a prerequisite for collaboration has been validated in research (Cairo, 1996; Hanson, Hodnicki, & Boyle, 1994; Prescott & Bowen, 1985). Yet stereotyped views of nursing and medical practice may interfere with collaborative efforts. Physicians are perceived as all-knowing and having ultimate responsibility for patient care, whereas nurses may be viewed as nonintellectual, second-best substitutes for excellent health care (Cairo, 1996; Fagin, 1992; Petronis-Jones, 1994; Sands et al., 1990), and having little authority or responsibility for patient care outcomes (Larson, 1999). The status of advanced nursing practice is still such that nurses must prove their competence to the profession and to society (Fagin, 1992; Prescott & Bowen, 1985).

When collaborating clinicians can rely on each other to be clinically competent, mutual trust and respect develops. Partners recognize that leadership is problem based, not team or role based, and are open to sharing power. Instead of one person always being the team leader, in a departure from the traditional "captain of the team" approach, leadership can shift among partners. Thus the person with the most expertise, interest, or talent can respond to the particular demands of the situation or problem. The trust and respect among collaborators are such that they can count on satisfactory resolution of the problem even when they know as individuals that they might have approached the issue differently. In fact, this openness to shared leadership and alternative solutions allows partners to learn from each other. For example, APNs usually have expertise in educating patients about their illnesses and lifestyle choices. Physicians are often expert diagnosticians. Thus collaboration offers APNs and physicians opportunities to model their varied assessment and intervention strategies for each other, fostering mutual learning and appreciation for the contributions of each to the care of patients and families. Because consumers and physicians underestimate nurses' expertise, competence, and authority, APNs need to showcase their competent and exemplary practice in order to build nursing's reputation for competence (Fagin, 1992; Lenz, 1994; see Chapter 25).

Interpersonal Competence

Interpersonal competence is the ability to communicate effectively with colleagues in a variety of situations, including uncomplicated, routine interactions, disagreements, value conflicts, and stressful situations. It requires a level of self-esteem and assertiveness that nurses have begun to acquire only in the past few years (Norton & Grady, 1996). It is imperative that nurses understand and articulate what they bring to clinical practice as members of the health care team. The key to demonstrating interpersonal competence is the APN's ability to communicate clearly and convincingly, both verbally and in writing. This attribute was identified by Hanson and colleagues (1994) in their analysis of the attributes that physicians most valued in their NP colleagues. The ability to communicate well with physicians, other staff members, the patient, and the patient's family was highly regarded by the physicians in this study. After clinical competence, interpersonal competence may be the most important individual characteristic needed for APNs to establish collaborative relationships.

Trust

Implicit in discussions of collaboration is the presence of mutual trust, mutual respect, and personal integrity, qualities evinced in the nature of interactions between partners. In fact, distrust is often cited as a major barrier to successful collaborative relationships (Alpert et al., 1992; Cairo, 1996; Evans, 1994). The development of trust and respect depends on clinical competence; it is very difficult to trust and respect a colleague whose clinical competence is questionable. This does not mean that novice APNs cannot establish collaborative relationships. However, the environments in which APN students and new graduates work must support their "novicehood" so that they can learn and mature clinically. Partners must recognize and appreciate their overlapping and diverse skills and knowledge (Nugent & Lambert, 1996; Spross, 1989; Stichler, 1995) for mutual trust and respect to develop and deepen over time. Partners observe that each other's clinical competence is consistent; that their interactions—even those that involve significant conflict over goals of care and interventions—are respectful, productive, and satisfying; and that patients benefit from their combined talents and efforts. They come to depend on each other to use good clinical judgment and to take appropriate actions.

A central theme of the development of trust is *sharing*. Partners are guided by a shared vision of the possibilities inherent in collaboration; they believe in the value of collaboration, and they are committed to achieving the relationship's potential (Krumm, 1992; Nugent & Lambert, 1996). Collaboration also means sharing in planning, decision making, problem solving, goal setting, and assuming responsibility (Baggs & Schmitt, 1988). Conger and Craig (1998) suggested that shared vision and collaboration between NPs and CNSs could be used to implement a cost-effective model of community-based health care. Thus, even though partners' ideas, opinions, and actions might be different, their belief in each other and their shared vision permit—even value—such differences.

The issue of developing trust presents a particular challenge to APNs because it has been observed that the competence of physicians is assumed and medical incompetence must be proven, whereas nurses must prove themselves and their competence in each new encounter (Fagin, 1992; Prescott & Bowen, 1985). APNs encounter numerous physicians in the course of practice; a lack of positive expectations and the potential assumption of incompetence of APNs until they demonstrate otherwise are major barriers to collaboration (Fagin, 1992). This means APNs require courage and fortitude to challenge such assumptions assertively when they become apparent in disconfirming or aggressive encounters with colleagues (Coeling & Wilcox, 1994).

Valuing and Respecting of Diverse, Complementary Knowledge

Respect for others' practice and knowledge is key to successful collaboration, because it enhances shared decision making. A great deal of successful collaborative work is self-driven. There must be a desire, at a very personal level, to collaborate and to value and respect others' ideas and actions, as well as a personal belief that complementary knowledge will enhance one's own personal plan for patient care. Initially, collaborators have limited knowledge of each other; collaboration is a "conscious, learned behavior" that improves as team members learn to value and respect one another's practice and expertise (Alpert et al., 1992). Medicine and nursing, although overlapping disciplines, are culturally distinct and have diverse goals for patient care. In many cases, they complement each other in their quest to restore patients to health. This complementarity extends beyond the disciplines of medicine and nursing. The Linkages Project, an interdisciplinary educational initiative to promote collaboration between physicians and psychologists, was instrumental in shaping collaborative approaches to clinical care (Bray & Rogers, 1997). Collaboration is built on the respect and valuing of the contributions of each profession to the common goal of optimal health care delivery (Stichler, 1995).

Humor

Another important aspect of the collaborative process is humor. Humor, in which the intent is positive and nonthreatening, is a creative way to set the stage for effective communication and problem solving between disciplines (Balzer, 1993). In collaborative practice, humor serves to decrease defensiveness, invite openness, relieve tension, and deflect anger. It helps individuals keep perspective, acknowledge the lack of perfection, and sets the tone for trust and acceptance among colleagues so that difficult situations can be reframed (Balzer, 1993). Graduate students can be encouraged to observe the ways in which humor is used by preceptors and colleagues and identify those uses that seem effective in improving communication and defusing conflict situations.

Processes Associated with Effective Collaboration

RECURRING INTERACTIONS

In addition to the attributes discussed previously, there are several processes that enable effective collaboration. A theme implicit in the reports of those who have written about their experiences with collaboration is that establishing a trusting and collaborative relationship is a developmental process (Alpert et al., 1992; Bray &

Rogers, 1997; Krumm, 1992; Nugent & Lambert, 1996; Wells et al., 1997). Although this notion of development over time is relevant to all aspects of collaboration, it is particularly important to establishing trust. The fact that effective collaboration is developmental and time dependent explains why collaborative relationships are diffi-cult to develop in organizations where there is a high staff turnover or frequent rotation of clinicians, such as house physicians. A physician wrote that the process seemed to be related to how well the nurse and physician know each other (Alpert et al., 1992).

It seems likely that a series of less complicated interactions, such as information exchange and coordination, that have been satisfactory clinically or personally con-tribute to the development of collaborative relationships. Team members need recur-ring interactions to acquire an understanding of their role requirements and functions and to develop patterns of interaction that are constructive, productive, and support-ive. Several reports illustrate the developmental aspects of interactions that lead to collaborative relationships (Alpert et al., 1992; Bray & Rogers, 1997; Dickinson, Mateo, Jackson, & Swartz, 1995; Hilderley, 1991). Redmond, Riggleman, Sorrell, and Zerull (1999) suggested that projects focused on quality and outcomes of care that involve joint collection and analysis of data build collegiality and foster collaboration. In the authors' experiences, membership on such interdisciplinary committees as pharmacy and therapeutics, performance improvement, institutional review boards, and others with a patient-care focus also fosters communication and collegiality. Recurring inter-actions help clinicians learn the similarities and differences in each discipline's prac-tice. Understanding each other's scope of practice and responsibility enables APNs, physicians, and other colleagues to use their knowledge and skills to benefit patients.

BRIDGING

Krumm (1992) noted that bridging is a component of collaboration. She did not define bridging but implied that it is the ability to develop connections that support positive outcomes for individuals and populations of patients. She described one bridging skill as the "ability to recognize and rearrange boundaries within the practice setting" (Krumm, p. 24).

Two examples illustrate the concept of bridging:

NPs in a gynecological practice noted the length of time it took for patients to get an appointment for colposcopy and the disadvantages to the practice of having only one physician who could do the procedure. They proposed that two of the NPs become trained to do the procedure. They outlined the precedents for such a change in practice and the benefits in terms of clinical outcomes, patient satisfaction, productivity, and cost-effectiveness. The proposal was adopted, two NPs acquired the training, and many of the advantages they anticipated have been realized.

The second author, while a CNS at a tertiary hospital, noted that patients who were admitted directly from the oncology clinic for a short admission were receiving their chemotherapy late at night because members of the house staff were not doing the patients' histories and physicals until last. Lengths of stay were longer, treatments that could have been prepared and given during the better staffed day shift were burdening the evening and night staff, and patients were dissatisfied. House staff left these admis-sions until last because the patients tended to be clinically stable, and to the interns this was an appropriate way of triaging their workload. The CNS and nurse manager met with the physician director of hematology/oncology to propose that short-stay chemotherapy admissions be handled differently from other admissions—an idea for which there was no precedent. All admissions had been done by the interns and residents. Under the new arrangement, patients would come to the unit directly from the clinic with their admission orders written by the attending physician. Intravenous lines could be initiated immediately, prescriptions could be filled by pharmacy as the orders came down, and nurses could initiate teaching and other interventions in a timely fashion.

An important aspect of these examples is that the APNs understood both medical and nursing aspects of care. Brown (1989) called this "shuttle diplomacy." She described the CNS as the person capable of speaking the languages of both medical and nursing subcultures, understanding the problems of each, and assisting in clinical and organizational problem solving. In both cases, boundaries were rearranged in ways that improved patient care and staff job satisfaction, suggesting that bridging creates conditions conducive to collaboration.

CONSULTATION

Consultation is another process that can promote collaboration among clinicians (see Chapter 8). The process of consultation can promote collaboration in several ways. First, it gives the consultant an opportunity to make visible her/his knowledge, competence, and expertise, and the interaction can be used to counter stereotypical views of what APNs and physicians do and how they interact. It is also a situation, when approached with collegiality and an open mind, where one can teach and be taught. CNSs have developed this form of communication to an art form and use it very successfully to interact with nurse colleagues within the hospital setting (Barron, 1989). As APNs mature in their roles, they can observe the ways in which consultation has contributed to a collaborative environment and share these observations with graduate students and staff.

IMPLEMENTING COLLABORATION

Socialization to Collaboration During Graduate Education

Although one might be able to identify a core set of clinical skills that all health professions should possess, it is unusual for graduate health professional students to learn these skills together (Larson, 1995; Stumpf & Clark, 1999). The absence of a common socialization process for health professionals is thought to impede collaboration (Larson, 1995; Pew-Fetzer Task Force, 1994). Predictions about changes in the health care workforce suggest that undertaking initiatives to evaluate and improve interdisciplinary collaboration is critical. Cooper, Henderson, and Dietrich (1998) suggested that medicine and nursing are all in the same "leaky boat" and would do well to pull together. Health care professionals who have been socialized early to value cooperation and collaboration are much better able to understand the strengths and concerns of other groups. The need to focus on collaboration was highlighted in a series of articles on predictions about the interdisciplinary workforce in the new millennium (Cooper, Henderson, & Dietrich, 1998; Grumbach & Coffman, 1998). Reflecting on how patients, policy makers, and educators will deal with the future composition of the interdisciplinary workforce, Cooper, Henderson, and Dietrich

(1998) concluded "it is time for interdisciplinary regulation and clinical integration so that a health care workforce that includes a diversity of disciplines can be assured of providing a uniform level of care in the future" (p. 802).

As part of the socialization process toward building collaboration, it is important that APNs add to the communication skills they learned in their undergraduate nursing programs. Advanced nursing practice curricula need to offer a foundation for collaborative interactions throughout the entire graduate program. Course objectives and specific content should be based on the characteristics of effective intra- and interdisciplinary collaboration and the development of skills to achieve this goal. Professional roles and issues courses need to include content that profiles not only the role sought by the student, but also the roles of the health care providers with whom the student will interact, such as physicians, other nurses, and social workers. It is important that APNs be able to articulate the roles of nurse, NP, CNS, CNM, and CRNA and to explain the nursing profession to consumers and non-nurse health care providers. Content that leads the novice through team interaction, networking, conflict negotiation, and other concepts that build personal self-esteem and confidence are crucial. The theme of collaboration can be woven throughout the major coursework as well as the graduate core curriculum by including objectives that build collaborative skills within other class requirements. For example, an objective for a role development core course that requires the student to build a collage depicting collaborative relationships within nursing would help the student grasp the concept of collaboration.

The curriculum should include content on group dynamics, role theory, organizational theory, change theory, and negotiation strategies to prepare learners for collaborative roles. Students should discuss examples of collaboration and noncollaboration from their own clinical experiences and should be able to identify what factors accounted for success or failure. Furthermore, students need to be aware of the forces, both positive and negative, that influence collaborative efforts. Innovative classroom strategies that allow for interactions, such as role playing and storytelling are extremely worthwhile. Students need opportunities to debrief with peers and faculty their positive and negative experiences of collaboration. This is vital if students are to be able to analyze the personal, social, and organizational variables that affect collaboration.

Most importantly, curricula need interdisciplinary seminars in which students can learn from colleagues in other disciplines. Although it is necessary and valuable for each discipline to structure and clarify role development issues and socialize its members into the profession, it is extremely useful for students in role and policy core courses to be able to discuss and interact with individuals who see policy and practice issues from another perspective. In this way they learn to value each other's contributions and are more able to view differences at a higher level. Furthermore, it is very important for students to observe faculty in collaborative relationships with their interdisciplinary peers. New funding initiatives that allow for interdisciplinary education in both the classroom and the clinical setting offer great promise for improved collaborative relationships between health provider disciplines.

Peer learning approaches that foster socialization to collaboration are enhanced by new technologies such as distance interactive TV and on-line web-based instruction. The capacity for students from various disciplines to interact via problem-based case learning facilitates their ability to learn about and value the style and model by which other health care providers manage patients. The team approach to problem solving and the approach to patient care is enhanced as students learn in interdisciplinary venues. Role behaviors that are negative to collaborative professional relationships are often dispelled before they take root if interdisciplinary learning is started early in the education process.

Peer learning also helps to dispel some of the attitudes physicians and nurses may harbor about the perceived deficits in APN and medical education. Interdisciplinary courses in pharmacotherapeutics, pathophysiology, and the like provide useful tools to alleviate these myths. The way that the health professions are socialized in medical school and nursing school is also important. The underlying principle taught in medical school that physicians must present as confident and "take charge" flies in the face of collaboration. A "captain of the ship" leadership orientation versus the interactive, caring role that nurses are expected to model make for strange bedfellows in practice. Furthermore, the hierarchies present in hospital and academic environments provide a difficult hurdle to overcome.

One of the factors that is critical to socialization is time. Collaborative relationships based on competence, trust, and respect are built as players learn and practice together in various settings and situations both as students and as peers in practice settings. Collaboration cannot be forced and must be allowed to develop over time. Enhancements such as group rounds, team conferences, and joint decision-making activities assist in this process.

Clinical placements for APN students have the potential to set the stage for long-term successful collaboration between APNs and physicians. The key is careful assessment of sites during the preplacement phase in order to match APN students and students from other disciplines with preceptors who support collaboration. Good interdisciplinary clinical educational experiences should be characterized not by parallel processes but by true team approaches to the diagnosis, management, and education of clients and families. Faculty who practice collaboratively with colleagues play a key role in setting up these experiences and can serve as important role models and mentors. Supportive debriefing via journals, patient rounds, and postclinical seminars is an excellent way to instill the concepts of collaboration into long-term student learning, especially when efforts to collaborate are unsuccessful or unsatisfactory.

Final preceptorships and practica offer additional opportunities for APN students to try out collaborative relationships with physicians and to practice newfound collaborative skills. Currently there is broad support for interdisciplinary models of clinician education. There is a need to restructure curricula in order to better understand training and education strategies in non-nursing education models (Bray & Rogers, 1997; Cooper, Henderson, & Dietrich, 1998; Evans, 1994; Fagin, 1992; Larson, 1995; Pew-Fetzer Task Force, 1994). The resurgence of interdisciplinary training for physicians and nurses for primary care practices should have a positive effect on collaboration.

Assessment of Personal Factors

Professionals bring many personal attributes to a professional partnership. Personal characteristics such as clinical and interpersonal competence and well-developed communication skills are vital to the collaborative relationship. Good clinical judgment and a well-developed sense of ethics promote trust. Most important for a good collaborative experience is a shared vision of the desired outcome.

In *The Fifth Discipline: The Art and Practice of the Learning Organization,* Senge (1990) used the metaphors of a superlative basketball team and a fantastic jazz ensemble to illustrate the power of people working in collaboration. It is clear that it takes more than professionals with expert skills, who may have different strengths, working side by side. Senge discussed the energy and power that are produced when teams become aligned to purpose, when they are able to combine energies and harmonize to produce a synergistic effect. Although individuals may come with great skills and expertise, it is the shared vision and the commonality of purpose that lead to success and improved outcome (Senge, 1990). These ideas can inform the work of teams who want to improve collaboration and achieve targeted patient outcomes.

Successful professional collaboration requires work and practice in the same way that personal relationships require time and effort. According to Senge (1990), practice is the hallmark of teamwork. Successful professional relationships, be they basketball teams, a team of primary care physicians and nurses, a birthing center group, or a team of anesthesiologists and CRNAs, need continued work and practice to grow and succeed. Self-assessment is one important component to think about when embarking on a new professional relationship or evaluating the success or failure of current or potential collaborative relationships. The self-directed questions in Table 11–3 may help team members identify their personal strengths and weaknesses vis-à-vis collegiality.

Covey (1989) offered another perspective on moving toward a higher level of interdependence with colleagues. He portrayed interdependence as a higher level of performance than independence. Only individuals who have gained competence and confidence in their own expertise are able to move beyond autonomy and independence toward the higher synergistic level of collaboration. Collaboration appears to have the same meaning as interdependence in Covey's work. This view is provocative when one considers the hierarchical context that often frames clinical collaboration.

Assessment and Monitoring of Environmental Factors

Administrative leadership plays a key role in the development of collaborative relationships between organizational members. Administrators who support team and interdisciplinary administrative models and who are good communicators themselves can do a great deal to increase the momentum of new collaborations. Differing philosophies and standards of care within organizational settings can cause conflict between team members and need to be resolved early (Spross, 1989). The common vision of

TABLE 11–3 PERSONAL STRENGTHS AND WEAKNESSES QUESTIONNAIRE
Am I clear about my role in the partnership?
What values do I bring to the relationship?
What do I expect to gain or lose by collaborating?
What do others expect of me?
Do I feel good about my contribution to the team?
Do I feel self-confident and competent in the collaborative relationship?
Are there anxieties causing repeated friction that have not been addressed?
Has serious thought been given to the boundaries of the collaborative relationship?

quality patient care and staff satisfaction that makes collaboration possible should bring APNs and nursing administrators together to create administrative structures that support collaboration (Krumm, 1992).

Increased acuity of illness in both inpatient and outpatient settings is an obstacle to collaboration. As professionals move from one crisis to another, there is little time to sit down, communicate, analyze data, and make joint decisions (Spross, 1989). The lack of time to communicate remains a significant barrier to collaboration (Coeling & Wilcox, 1994).

Power inequities between medicine and nursing are often apparent. However, power issues also exist among nurses. Elitist stances by APNs set up roadblocks to collaboration with staff nurses. Balancing power differences between groups equalizes the hierarchical differences between members and makes collaboration possible if there is sufficient expertise among players (Stichler, 1995).

STRATEGIES FOR SUCCESSFUL COLLABORATION

Many of the barriers to successful collaboration occur because of values, beliefs, and behaviors that have, until recently, gone unchallenged in society and in the organizations in which nurses practice. There is a need for radical change if the conditions conducive to collaboration are to become the norm. APNs may feel like they are the only ones with an active commitment to collaboration (Spross, 1989). Of all the competencies required for advanced practice, collaboration may be the most difficult to accomplish because it is mediated by social processes (Siegler & Whitney, 1994b) that are ingrained in the larger culture. Efforts to change the environment to one that is more collaborative involve proving oneself over and over and challenging colleagues' behaviors that restrain attempts to work together. These intrapersonal demands, along with the clinical demands of one's job, can be exhausting. Therefore, APNs need to evaluate the potential for collaboration when seeking employment opportunities. Questions about how clinicians work together—the interpersonal climate as well as organizational structures that support collaboration— should be a high priority. A realistic appraisal of the existence of or potential for collaboration is needed to determine whether APNs can provide the standard and quality of care that are characteristic of advanced nursing practice and whether they can expect a reasonable level of job satisfaction.

Individual Strategies

The ability to listen, encourage, and experience someone else's success or failure, and the capability to *know* a colleague well, foster the ability to successfully work as an interactive team (Dziabis & Lant, 1998). The strategies offered by Norton and Grady (1996) for developing and implementing the change agent competency are useful in developing collaborative skills.

One strategy is for APNs to promote their exemplary nursing practices to help other health professionals and consumers better understand their strengths as health care providers (Fagin, 1992; see Chapter 25). In today's health care environment, participating in critical pathway development is one way to do this. Within advanced nursing practice, it is useful for nurses to role-model their practice strategies for other nurses to facilitate intranursing collaboration and consultation. One way to share excellence in practice is to include in grand rounds or team conferences the opportunity for each care team member to describe her or his own decision making about patients and suggest new strategies for care to the team. Furthermore, Garcia, Bruce, Niemeyer, and Robbins (1993) suggested that integrated patient records provide a means to communicate formally about patient care. Joint review and audit of patient care is an important component of collaboration in practice.

Working together on joint projects is another way to facilitate good collaboration. Collaborative research and scholarly writing projects as well as community service projects that tap the strengths of various members open people's eyes to the benefits of collaboration. Federal and private agencies are currently supporting interdisciplinary collaborative studies. Reporting the results in the literature will illustrate the considerable advantages of collaborative interactions. In addition, social opportunities at conferences and receptions allow camaraderie to grow and help reinforce the bond between members of the partnership (Fitzpatrick, Wykle, & Morris, 1990; Hanson, 1993). These strategies move across lines from personal life to organizational settings and from education to practice arenas. New models that foster joint medical and nursing care are needed in primary care as well as within specialty practice in all settings. More importantly, collaboratively developed practice guidelines improve communication and clarify clinicians' roles in patient treatment (Weinstein et al., 1998).

Organizational Strategies

Fagin (1992) and Hanson (1993) identified several strategies that lead toward successful collaboration at all levels. As noted previously, there needs to be a move toward interdisciplinary educational programs that allow for face-to-face interaction between medical and nursing students. Definitive changes in the structure of clinical hours as well as sequencing of content will be required. Given the entrenched bureaucracies involved, this will be a difficult task requiring stronger interactions between schools of medicine and schools of nursing. Health care providers need to be learning about health policy issues from a perspective that offers broad-stroke solutions to health care issues. Faculty in both nursing and medicine need to be evaluating and treating patients and supervising students together. It is important to introduce joint appointments of nursing faculty to medical school clinics to give faculty opportunities to role-model advanced nursing practice care and build rapport (Fitzpatrick et al., 1990).

National and state medical and nursing organizations must endorse the shift toward a more interactive model (Fagin, 1992; Hanson, 1993). Strategies that facilitate this shift, such as retreats, social interactions, communication workshops, joint practice committees, and sensitivity training sessions, are imperative. Again, sharing exemplary nursing innovations is a major factor. Until strategies for this type of change are instituted, barriers to successful interprofessional collaboration will remain.

EXEMPLARS OF SUCCESSFUL COLLABORATIVE PRACTICE

The following are just two exemplars of successful collaboration.

EXEMPLAR 1: THE CNS IN PAIN MANAGEMENT

One of the authors (JS) was hired to start a cancer rehabilitation program. The director of nursing made it clear that she also wanted to improve pain management for all patients in the rehabilitation hospital, not just oncology patients. The CNS began by developing collaborative relationships with the staff on the unit for which she had primary responsibility. As the staff on the unit got to know the CNS's skills, they began to consult her for pain management problems. As the CNS worked with patients, she learned that one of the pharmacists, who was full-time, was very interested in pain management and the two began to work together regularly—jointly evaluating patients and proposing pharmacologic interventions to physicians. This collaboration was particularly beneficial for patients and staff because the CNS only worked half-time. Over time, the head nurse, the unit physician, and the consulting neurologist and physiatrist with whom the CNS and pharmacist had worked on some difficult pain issues began to ask the two clinicians to see patients on other units. The neurologist, in particular, seemed interested in learning more about pain management. The neurologist was also chair of quality improvement. At the CNS' suggestion, the neurologist attended an all-day seminar on pain management that was being offered locally by a nationally known nurse leader in pain management. When she came back from the conference, where she learned about the clinical problems associated with using meperidine, the neurologist immediately sent a memo to clinical staff about its dangers. She then worked with the CNS, the quality improvement committee, and the pharmacy and therapeutics committee to limit the use of the drug for pain management by creating a policy and making the prescription of meperidine a sentinel event, to be evaluated by the CNS, the pharmacist, or the neurologist.

Over time, the CNS, with the support of the director of nursing, the neurologist, and the pharmacist, created an interdisciplinary team for pain management that included, in addition to the initial three disciplines of nursing, medicine, and pharmacy, two nurse educators, a head nurse, a psychologist, a physical therapist, a physical therapy assistant, an occupational therapist, a social worker, and a nurse case manager. Staff from all disciplines learned techniques to assess and treat pain. The team learned more about each other's skills and developed a "transdisciplinary" consultation model so that, regardless of discipline, each member knew the critical elements of patient and chart assessment. An interdisciplinary assessment tool and core interventions that could be initiated by any member of the team was developed. This meant that any member of the team could do an initial evaluation of the patient to determine what steps needed to be taken. For example, although the CNS and psychologist could not make a pain diagnosis, they recognized when one was needed to guide treatment planning. In these situations, they would recommend to the internal medicine (IM) physician or NP that a neurology consult be made if such a diagnosis could not be made by the primary physician or NP. All team members learned how to look at a medication Kardex to evaluate how well prescribed analgesics were being used. If undertreatment was evident from the Kardex review, the psychologist or physical or occupational therapist would involve the CNS or pharmacist. All team members knew some simple nondrug pain management techniques and the criteria for using them.

In analyzing why this collaborative effort worked, there were several organizational and professional factors that were facilitators. Organizationally, the support of the director of nursing and the neurologist, who also had administrative responsibilities, were central. The neurologist's "buy-in" occurred about 6 months after the CNS was hired, resulting from a combination of her personal commitment to improve patient care and the knowledge she acquired at the pain management conference she attended. The fact that she chaired the quality improvement committee was also useful. The interdisciplinary team came together as a team about 18 months after the CNS had begun to work at the hospital. A structural factor that facilitated the development of the pain management program was the existence of weekly team meetings held on each patient. The team meetings provided an opportunity for the CNS to identify pain management issues and report progress on decreasing pain. This structure enabled the team, as a team, to see that managing pain well actually improved patients' participation in therapy, contrary to the widely held belief that patients in rehabilitation should be off their analgesics. This shift in attitude occurred over several months. In addition, the CNS could identify those staff who had a particular interest in pain management and were open to being coached regarding pain management, thus building a community commitment to relieving pain.

Another structural factor was the presence of a NP on each of the patient care units. Units were organized such that an IM physician and a NP were responsible for the medical management of the patients. In fact, some of the IM physicians were among the last to buy in to the institutional efforts to improve pain management. The close collaboration that occurred among NPs and IM physicians facilitated the collaboration of the CNS when she worked with the IM physicians to address patients' pain management issues.

From a process standpoint, the hospital philosophy and staff behavior reflected a commitment to patients. The fact that team meetings were "institutionalized" enabled clinicians to maintain a patient-centered focus even when there were disagreements over how to manage pain. In the beginning of the CNS' tenure, there was great reluctance to use opioids for noncancer pain. Both experiences with patients and discussion of results of pain management efforts in team meetings reinforced the emphasis on patient comfort and progress in therapy as outcomes. Repeated experience with the CNS, observing her competence and the results for patients, served to modify the attitudes of many of the staff. One IM physician's buy-in occurred after the CNS effectively used relaxation, guided imagery, and therapeutic touch to treat the physician's own chronic back pain (he was against use of medication for his own pain, although he had come to prescribe analgesics more frequently for patients because of the advocacy of the staff nurses for their patients).

This was a situation that evolved to an unusually high level of collaboration. Had the team never evolved, the pharmacist and CNS would have still made a contribution to improving pain management. However, the level of interdisciplinary collaboration that ultimately resulted would not have occurred without the administrative, professional, and personal factors that contributed to the success of the initiative.

EXEMPLAR 2: THE NP IN PRIMARY CARE: A PHYSICIAN'S OBSERVATIONS ABOUT COLLABORATION

For several years, Syntex Corporation sponsored a Nurse Practitioner of the Year Award to honor NPs who have achieved high levels of success in their practice. The letters of the physicians and nurses who nominated successful NPs for the award all seem to say the same thing: "The individual exhibits a high level of collaboration." The following is a composite of the nomination letters received by Syntex from physician nominators:

I would like to tell you about MQ, a nurse practitioner who is a member of our group primary care practice. Mary is an extremely competent nurse practitioner and an able diagnostician. I would trust her to care for my own wife and children. She is totally committed to her patients, strives to give them the best possible care, and has many of the same values and ideas about good patient care that my physician partner and I do. Although Mary carries her own panel of patients very successfully, she seems to want and need to consult with me and our other physicians if she is concerned about a complex patient. We all function as a team and we have all learned from Mary's nursing expertise, as she has from ours. All of us work together to give high-quality care. Most importantly, Mary is a team player; all the members of our group practice enjoy her quick wit and willingness to share her expertise. At first, one of the partners did not want a nurse practitioner to join the group, but Mary won him over with her professional and interpersonal competence. I guess that the most important quality that I would share is that Mary is a people person; she works hard to communicate at a high level and it pays off. We trust her as a professional colleague and a friend.

Although this is a composite of typical physician nominations, the content confirms what the literature on collaboration suggests—the burden of proof that collaboration works often depends on APNs' skills and initiatives. APNs and their employers need to recognize that an important component of clinical practice is investing time and energy to build a collaborative climate—immediate results will not be apparent (a disadvantage given the economics shaping health care) but should pay off over time in the form of improved patient outcomes.

CONCLUSION

Collaborative relationships are not only professionally satisfying (e.g., Alpert et al., 1992; Fagin, 1992; Weinstein et al., 1998), they improve access to care (e.g., Siegler & Whitney, 1994a; Waugaman & Foster, 1995) and patient outcomes (e.g., Knauss et al., 1986; Lassen et al., 1997; Rubinstein et al., 1984). Although APNs collaborate with many individuals within and outside nursing and do so successfully, APNs may find that one of their most important collaborative relationships—that with physicians—may also be the most challenging. Despite the fact that there are many successful individual APN-physician collaborative practices, many with data that demonstrate their beneficial effects on health care, tradition and stereotypes are often powerful influences on policy making and in health care and professional organizations, such as hospitals or the AMA.

In the current health care environment, collaboration may flourish regardless of the barriers identified. To meet the demands for cost-effectiveness and quality, clinicians from all disciplines are meeting together to discuss the care they provide and to define ways to deliver it so as to maximize quality and minimize duplication of effort. It is these interactions that foster the trust and respect required for mature collaboration. They enable collaborators to recognize their interdependence and value the input of others, thus creating a synergy that improves the quality of clinical decision making (Lassen et al., 1997; Stichler, 1995; Weinstein et al., 1998). APNs will find that their success as clinicians and leaders often depends on their proficiency as collaborators.

REFERENCES

Acute Pain Management Guideline Panel. (1992). *Acute pain management: Operative or medical procedures and trauma* (Clinical Practice Guideline 92-0032). Rockville, MD: Agency for Health Care Policy and Research.

Afflitto, L. (1997). Managed care and its influence on physician-patient relationship: Implications for collaborative practice. *Plastic Surgical Nursing, 17*(4), 217–218.

Alpert, H., Goldman, L., Kilroy, C., & Pike, A. (1992). 7 Gryzmish: Toward an understanding of collaboration. *Nursing Clinics of North America, 27,* 47–59.

Aiken, L. H., Smith, H. L., & Lake, E. T. (1994). Lower Medicare mortality among a set of hospitals known for good nursing care. *Medical Care, 32*(8), 771–787.

American Medical Association. (1995). *Board of Trustees Report 6-A-95.* Chicago: Author.

American Nurses' Association. (1995). *Nursing's social policy statement.* Washington, DC: Author.

Aroskar, M. (1998). Ethical working relationships in patient care. *Nursing Clinics of North America, 33*(2), 313–324.

Arslanian-Engoren, C. M. (1995). Lived experiences of CNSs who collaborate with physicians: A phenomenological study. *Clinical Nurse Specialist, 9*(2), 68–73.

Baggs, J. G., & Schmitt, M. C. (1988). Collaboration between nurses and physicians. *Image: The Journal of Nursing Scholarship, 20,* 145–149.

Balzer, J. (1993). Humor—a missing ingredient in collaborative practice. *Holistic Nursing Practice, 7*(4), 28–35.

Barron, A. M. (1989). The clinical nurse specialist as consultant. In A. B. Hamric & J. A. Spross (Eds.), *The clinical nurse specialist in theory and practice* (2nd. ed., pp. 125–146). Philadelphia: W. B. Saunders.

Benner, P., Hooper-Kyriakidis, P., & Stannard, D. (1999). *Clinical wisdom and interventions in critical care: A thinking-in-action approach.* Philadelphia: W. B. Saunders.

Benoliel, J. Q. (1995). Multiple meanings of pain and complexities of pain management. *Nursing Clinics of North America, 30*(4), 583–596.

Bray, J. H., & Rogers, J. C. (1997). The Linkages Project: Training health professionals for collaborative practice with primary care physicians. *Families, Systems & Health, 15*(1), 55–62.

Brita-Rossi, P., Adduci, D., Kaufman, J., Lipson, S. J., Totte, C., & Wasserman, K. (1996). Improving the process of care: The cost-quality value of interdisciplinary collaboration. *Journal of Nursing Care Quality, 10*(2), 10–16.

Brown, S. J. (1989). Supportive supervision of the CNS. In A. B. Hamric & J. A. Spross (Eds.), *The clinical nurse specialist in theory and practice* (2nd ed., pp. 285–286). Philadelphia: W. B. Saunders.

Brown, S. J. (1998). A framework for advanced practice nursing. *Journal of Professional Nursing, 14*(3), 157–164.

Cairo, J. M. (1996). Emergency physicians' attitudes toward the emergency nurse practitioner role: Validation versus rejection. *Journal of the American Academy of Nurse Practitioners, 8,* 411–417.

Christman, L. (1998). Advanced practice nursing: Is the physician's assistant an accident of history or a failure to act? *Nursing Outlook, 46,* 56–59.

Coeling, H., & Wilcox, J. (1994). Steps to collaboration. *Nursing Administration Quarterly, 18*(4), 44–55.

Conger, M., & Craig, C. (1998). Advanced nurse practice: A model for collaboration. *Nursing Case Management, 3*(3), 120–127.

Cooper, R. A., Henderson, T., & Dietrich, C. L. (1998). Roles of nonphysician clinicians as autonomous providers in patient care. *JAMA, 280,* 795–800.

Cooper, R. A., Laud, P., & Dietrich, C. L. (1998). Current and projected workforce of nonphysician clinicians. *JAMA, 280,* 788–794.

Covey, S. R. (1989). *The seven habits of highly effective people.* New York: Simon & Schuster.

Crowley, S. A., & Wollner, I. S. (1987). Collaborative practice: A tool for change. *Oncology Nursing Forum, 14*(4), 59–63.

Cruikshank, B., & Chow, T. (1984). Physician supervision/collaboration as reported by PNPs in practice settings. *Pediatric Nursing, 10*(1), 13–18.

DeAngelis, C. (1994). Nurse practitioner redux. *JAMA, 271*(11), 868–871.

Devereux, P. (1981). Nurse/physician collaboration: Nursing practice considerations. *Journal of Nursing Administration, 9*(9), 37–39.

Dickinson, C. P., Mateo, M., Jackson, D., & Swartz, W. (1995). OB-GYN consultants and Sharp, the birthplace: An exemplar of nurse-midwife and obstetrician independence and integration. *Advanced Practice Nursing Quarterly, 1*(2), 40–48.

Dressler, D. (1994). The critical care clinical nurse specialist in joint practice with physicians. In A. Gawlinski & L. Kern (Eds.), *The clinical nurse specialist in critical care* (pp. 51–61). Philadelphia: W. B. Saunders.

Dziabis, S. P., & Lant, T. W. (1998). Building partnerships with physicians: Moving outside the walls of the hospital. *Nursing Administration Quarterly, 22*(3), 1–5.

Evans, J. A. (1994). The role of the nurse manager in creating an environment for collaborative practice. *Holistic Nursing Practice, 8*(3), 23–31.

Fagin, C. (1992). Collaboration between nurses and physicians: No longer a choice. *Nursing and Health Care, 13,* 354-363.

Felton S., Cady, N., Metzler, M. H., & Burton, S. (1997). Implementation of collaborative practice through interdisciplinary rounds on a general surgery service. *Nursing Case Management, 2*(3), 122-126.

Fitzpatrick, J., Wykle, M., & Morris, D. (1990). Collaboration in care and research. *Archives of Psychiatric Nursing, 4*(1), 53-61.

Forbes, E., & Fitzsimmons, V. (1993). Education: The key for holistic interdisciplinary collaboration. *Holistic Nursing Practice, 7*(4), 1-10.

Garcia, M. A., Bruce, D., Niemeyer, J., & Robbins, J. (1993). Collaborative practice: A shared success. *Nursing Management, 24*(5), 72-79.

Gelman, S., O'Neil, E., Kimmey, J., & the Task Force on Accreditation of Health Professions Education. (1999). *Strategies for change and improvement: The report of the Task Force on Accreditation of Health Professions Education.* San Francisco: Center for the Health Professions, University of California at San Francisco.

Gianakos, D. (1997). Physicians, nurses and collegiality. *Nursing Outlook, 45*(2), 57-58.

Grumbach, K., & Coffman, J. (1998). Physicians and nonphysician clinicians. *JAMA, 280,* 825-826.

Hales, A., Karshmer, J., Montes-Sandoval, L., & Fiszbein, A. (1998). Preparing for prescriptive privileges: A CNS-physician collaborative model. Expanding the scope of the psychiatric-mental health clinical nurse specialist. *Clinical Nurse Specialist, 12*(2), 73-80.

Hanson, C. M. (1993). Our role in health care reform: Collegiality counts. *American Journal of Nursing, 93*(12), 16A-16E.

Hanson, C. M., Hodnicki, D. R., & Boyle, J. S. (1994). Nominations for excellence: Collegial advocacy for nurse practitioners. *Journal of the American Academy of Nurse Practitioners, 6,* 471-476.

Hilderley, L. (1991). Nurse-physician collaborative practice: The clinical nurse specialist in a radiation oncology private practice. *Oncology Nursing Forum, 18,* 585-591.

Hughes, A., & Mackenzie, C. (1990). Components necessary in a successful nurse practitioner-physician collaborative practice. *Journal of the American Academy of Nurse Practitioners, 2*(2), 54-57.

Hupcey, J. (1993). Factors and work settings that may influence nurse practitioner practice. *Nursing Outlook, 41,* 181-185.

Inglis, A., & Kjervik, D. (1993). Empowerment of advanced practice nurses: Regulation reform needed to increase access to care. *Journal of Law, Medicine & Ethics, 21*(2), 193-205.

Jones, P. E., & Cawley, J. F. (1994). Physicians assistants and health system reform. *JAMA, 271*(16), 1266-1272.

Kavesh, W. (1993). Physician and nurse practitioner relationships. In M. Mezey & D. McGivern (Eds.), *Nurses, nurse practitioners: Evolution to advanced practice* (pp. 171-184). New York: Springer-Verlag.

Kedziera, P., & Levy, M. (1994). Collaborative practice in oncology. *Seminars in Oncology, 21,* 705-711.

Knaus, W. A., Draper, E. A., Wagner, D. P., & Zimmerman, J. E. (1986). An evaluation of outcome from intensive care in major medical centers. *Annals of Internal Medicine, 104,* 410-418.

Krumm, S. (1992). Collaboration between oncology clinical nurse specialists and nursing administrators. *Oncology Nursing Forum, 19*(1, Suppl.), 21-24.

Kuraitis (1999). *http://www.bhtinfo.com; http://www.scipich.org/pubs/final report.htm*

Larson, E. (1999). The impact of physician-nurse interaction on patient care. *Holistic Nursing Practice, 13*(2), 38-46.

Larson, E. L. (1995). New rules for the game: Interdisciplinary education for health professionals. *Nursing Outlook, 43*(4), 180-185.

Lassen, A. A., Fosbinder, D., Minton, S., & Robins, M. (1997). Nurse/physician collaborative practice: Improving health care quality while decreasing cost. *Nursing Economics, 15*(2), 87-91.

Lenz, C. (1994). Multidisciplinary community-based education and practice. In J. C. McCloskey & H. K. Grace (Eds.), *Current issues in nursing* (pp. 586-602). St. Louis: Mosby.

Lindeke, L. L., & Block, D. E. (1998). Maintaining professional integrity in the midst of interdisciplinary collaboration. *Nursing Outlook, 46,* 213-218.

Littell, S. (1981). The clinical nurse specialist in private medical practice. *Nursing Administration Quarterly, 6*(1), 77-85.

Lumpkins, R., & Veal, J. (1995). Interdisciplinary collaboration: Strengthening documentation. *Nursing Management, 26*(10), 48L-48P.

Mahn, V., & Spross, J. A. (1996). Nurse case management as an advanced practice role. In A. B. Hamric, J. A. Spross, & C. M. Hanson (Eds.), *Advanced nursing practice: An integrative approach* (pp. 445-465). Philadelphia: W. B. Saunders.

Management of Cancer Pain Guideline Panel. (1994). *Management of cancer pain* (Clinical Practice Guideline No. 9, AHCPR Publication No. 95-0592). Rockville, MD: Agency for Health Care Policy and Research.

McKechnie, J. L. (Ed.). (1983). *Webster's new universal unabridged dictionary.* New York: Simon & Schuster.

Minarik, P. A., & Price, L. C. (1999). Collaboration? Supervision? Direction? Independence? What is the relationship between the advanced practice nurse and the physician? States' legislative and regulatory forum III. *Clinical Nurse Specialist, 13*(1), 34–37.

National Joint Practice Commission. (1979). *Brief description of a demonstration project to establish collaborative or joint practice in hospitals* (pp. 2–6) Chicago: Author.

Norton, S. F., & Grady, E. M. (1996). Change agent skills. In A. B. Hamric, J. A. Spross, & C. M. Hanson (Eds.), *Advanced nursing practice: An integrative approach* (pp. 249–271). Philadelphia: W. B. Saunders.

Nugent, K. E., & Lambert, V. A. (1996). The advanced practice nurse in collaborative practice. *Nursing Connections, 9*(1), 5–14.

Oddi, L. F., & Cassidy, V. R. (1998). The message of SUPPORT: Change is long overdue. *Journal of Professional Nursing, 14*(3), 165–174.

Pellegrino, E. D. (1996). What's wrong with the nurse-physician relationship in today's hospitals? A physician's view. *Hospitals, 40,* 70–80.

Petronis-Jones, R. A. (1994). Nurse-physician collaboration: A descriptive study. *Holistic Nursing Practice, 8*(3), 38–53.

Pew-Fetzer Task Force on Advancing Psychosocial Health Education Health Professions Education and Relationship-Centered Care (1994). San Francisco: Pew Health Professions Commission.

Pew Health Professions Commission. (1995). *Critical challenges: Revitalizing the health professions for the twenty-first century, third report.* San Francisco: UCSF Center for the Health Professions.

Prescott, P., & Bowen, S. (1985). Physician-nurse relationships. *Annals of Internal Medicine, 103,* 127–133.

Pronovost, P. J., Jenckes, M. W., Dorman, T., Garrett, E., Breslow, M. J., Rosenfeld, B. A., Lipsett, P. A., & Bass, E. (1999). Organizational characteristics of intensive care units related to outcomes of abdominal aortic surgery. *JAMA, 281,* 1310–1317.

Redmond, G., Riggleman, J., Sorrell, J. M., & Zerull, L. (1999). Creative winds of change: Nurses collaborating for quality outcomes. *Nursing Administration Quarterly, 23*(2), 55–64.

Robert Wood Johnson Foundation (1999). Partnerships for Quality Education. 126 Brookline Avenue, Boston. *www.pqe.org*

Robert Wood Johnson Foundation (1996). Partnerships in Training. Association of Academic Health Centers, Washington, D. C. *pft@acdhlthctrs.org*

Rubenstein, L., Josephson, K., Wieland, G., English, P., Sayre, J., & Kane, R. (1984). Effectiveness of a geriatric evaluation unit. *New England Journal of Medicine, 311,* 1664–1670.

Ryan, L., Edwards, R., & Rickles, F. (1980). A joint practice approach to the care of persons with cancer. *Oncology Nursing Forum, 8*(1), 8–11.

Safriet, B. J. (1992). Health care dollars and regulatory sense: The role of advanced practice nursing. *Yale Journal on Regulation, 9*(2), 417–487.

Sands, R., Stafford, J., & McClelland, M. (1990). "I beg to differ": Conflict in the interdisciplinary team. *Social Work in Health Care, 14*(3), 55–72.

Senge, P. M. (1990). *The fifth discipline: The art and practice of the learning organization.* New York: Doubleday.

Shortell, S. M., Zimmerman, J. E., Rousseau, D. M., Gillies, R. R., Wagner, D. P., Draper, E. A., Knaus, W. A., & Duffy, J. (1994). The performance of intensive care units: Does good management make a difference? *Medical Care, 32*(5), 508–525.

Siegler, E. L., & Whitney, F. W. (Eds.). (1994a). *Nurse physician collaboration: Care of adults and the elderly.* New York: Springer-Verlag.

Siegler, E. L., & Whitney, F. W. (1994b). Social and economic barriers to collaborative practice. In E. L. Siegler & F. W. Whitney (Eds.), *Nurse-physician collaboration: Care of adults and the elderly* (pp. 21–32). New York: Springer-Verlag.

Simpson, R. L. (1998). Bridging the nursing-physician gap: Technology's role in interdisciplinary practice. *Nursing Administration Quarterly, 22*(3), 87–90.

Spross, J. A. (1989). The CNS as collaborator. In A. B. Hamric & J. A. Spross (Eds.), *The clinical nurse specialist in theory and practice* (2nd ed., pp. 205–226). Philadelphia: W. B. Saunders.

Steele J. E. (Ed.). (1986). *Issues in collaborative practice.* Orlando, FL: Grune & Stratton.

Stein, L. I., Watts, D. T., & Howell, T. (1990). The doctor-nurse game revisited. *New England Journal of Medicine, 322,* 546–549.

Stichler, J. F. (1995). Professional interdependence: The art of collaboration. *Advanced Practice Nursing Quarterly, 1*(1), 53–61.

Stumpf, S. H., & Clark, J. Z. (1999). The promise and pragmatism of interdisciplinary education. *Journal of Allied Health, 28*(1), 30–32.

Sullivan, T. J. (1998). *Collaboration: A health care imperative.* New York: McGraw-Hill Health Professions Division.

SUPPORT Principal Investigators. (1995). A controlled trial to improve care for seriously ill hospitalized patients: The Study to Understand Prognosis and Preferences for Outcomes and Risks of Treatment (SUPPORT). *JAMA, 274,* 1591–1598.

Tjosvold, D. (1986). The dynamics of interdependence in organizations. *Human Relations, 39,* 517–540.

Torres, S., & Dominguez, L. M. (1998). Collaborative practice: How we get from coordination to the integration of skills and knowledge. In C. M. Sheehy & M. C. McCarthy (Eds.), *Ad-*

vanced practice nursing: Emphasizing common roles (pp. 217-240). Philadelphia: F. A. Davis.

Waugaman, W. R., & Foster, S. D. (1995). CRNAs: An enviable legacy of patient service. *Advanced Practice Nursing Quarterly, 1*(1), 21-28.

Weinstein, M. E., McCormack, B., Brown, M. E., & Rosenthal, D. S. (1998). Build consensus and develop collaborative practice guidelines. *Nursing Management, 29*(9), 48-52.

Weissman, D. (1988). Cancer pain education: A call for role models. *Journal of Clinical Oncology, 6,* 1793-1794.

Weisman, D., Griffie, J., Gordon, D. B., & Dahl, J. (1997). A role model program to promote institutional changes for management of acute and cancer pain. *Journal of Pain and Symptom Management, 14*(5), 274-279.

Wells, N., Johnson, R., & Salyer, S. (1997). Interdisciplinary collaboration. *Clinical Nurse Specialist, 12*(4), 161-168.

Additional Readings

American Association of Colleges of Nursing. (1999). Certification and regulation of advanced practice nurses. *Journal of Professional Nursing, 15*(2), 130-132.

Bauer, J. C. (1994). *Not what the doctor ordered: Reinventing medical care in America.* Chicago: Probus Publishing Company.

Cooper, R. A., Laud, P., & Dietrich, C. L. (1998). Current and projected workforce of nonphysician clinicians. *JAMA, 280,* 788-794.

Joel, L. A. (1998). Advanced practice nursing in the current sociopolitical environment. In C. Sheehy & M. McCarthy (Eds.), *Advanced practice nursing: Emphasizing common roles* (pp. 47-68). Philadelphia: F. A. Davis.

Joint Commission on Accreditation of Healthcare Organizations. (1992). *Agenda for change.* Oakbrook Terrace, IL: Author.

McCloskey, J. C., & Maas, M. (1998). Interdisciplinary team: The nursing perspective is essential. *Nursing Outlook, 46,* 157-163.

McCoy, S. T., Cope, K. A., Joy, S. J., Baker, R. T., & Brugler, C. I. (1997). Interdisciplinary documentation of patient education: How collaboration can effect change. *Rehabilitation Nursing, 22,* 235-238.

Miller, S., King, T., Lurie, P., & Choitz, P. (1997). Certified nurse-midwife and physician collabora-

tive practice. *Journal of Nurse-Midwifery, 42*(4), 308-315.

Mitchell, P. H., & Shortell, S. M. (1997). Adverse outcomes and variations in organization of care delivery. *Medical Care, 35*(11), NS19-NS32.

Mundinger, M. (1994). Sounding board: Advanced-practice nursing—good medicine for physicians? *New England Journal of Medicine, 330,* 211-214.

Mundinger, M. (1999). Can advanced practice nurses succeed in the primary care market? *Nursing Economics, 17*(1), 7-14.

Mundt, M. H. (1997). Books on health policy and health reform: How is nursing represented? *Journal of Professional Nursing, 13*(1), 19-27.

Reynolds, P. P., Giardino, A., Onady, G. M., & Siegler, E. L. (1994). Collaboration in the preparation of the generalist physician. *Journal of General Internal Medicine, 9*(Suppl. 1), S55-S63.

Safriet, B. J. (1997). Still spending dollars, still searching for sense: Advanced practice nursing in an era of regulatory and economic turmoil. *Advanced Practice Nursing Quarterly, 4*(3), 24-33.

University of York NHS Centre for Reviews and Dissemination. (1999). Getting evidence into practice. *Effective Health Care, 5*(1), 1-16.

Verschuren, P. J. M., & Masselink, H. (1997). Role concepts and expectations of physicians and nurses in hospitals. *Social Science and Medicine, 45,* 1135-1138.

Walker, P. H., Baldwin, D., Fitzpatrick, J. J., Ryan, S., Bulger, R., DeBasio, N., Hanson, C., Harvan, R., Johnson-Pawlson, J., Kelley, M., Lacey, B., Ladden, M. J., McLaughlin, C., Selker, L., Sluyter, D., Vansclow, N. (1998). Commentary: Building community: Developing skills for interprofessional health. *Nursing Outlook, 46*(2), 88-89.

Wocial, L. D. (1996). Collaborative practice: Achieving collaboration in ethical decision making: Strategies for nurses in clinical practice. *DCCN: Dimensions of Critical Care Nursing, 15,* 150-159.

Wood, M., Ferlie, E., & Fitzgerald, L. (1998). Achieving clinical behaviour change: A case of becoming indeterminate. *Social Science and Medicine, 47*(11), 1729-1738.

Woods, L. P. (1998). Implementing advanced practice: Identifying factors that facilitate and inhibit the process. *Journal of Clinical Nursing, 7,* 265-273.

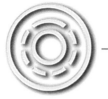

C H A P T E R   1 2

Ethical Decision-Making Skills

- J U A N I T A   R E I G L E
- R O B E R T   J.   B O Y L E

INTRODUCTION

Various factors, including changes in interprofessional roles, advances in medical technology, availability of information on line, revisions in patient care delivery systems, and heightened economic constraints, have increased the complexity of ethical issues in the health care setting. Nurses in all areas of health care routinely encounter disturbing moral issues, yet the success with which these dilemmas are resolved varies significantly. Because nurses have a unique relationship to the patient and family, the moral position of nursing in the health care arena is distinct. As the complexity of issues intensifies, the role of the advanced practice nurse (APN) becomes particularly important in the identification, deliberation, and resolution of complicated and difficult value choices. It is a basic tenet of the central definition of advanced nursing practice (see Chapter 3) that ethical decision-making skills are part of the core competencies of all APNs.

CHARACTERISTICS OF ETHICAL DILEMMAS IN NURSING

In this chapter, the terms "ethics" and "morality" or "morals" are used interchangeably. An ethical or moral dilemma occurs when two (or more) morally acceptable courses of action are present and to choose one prevents selecting another. The agent experiences tension because the moral obligations resulting from the dilemma create differing and opposing demands (Beauchamp & Childress, 1994; Purtilo, 1993). In some moral dilemmas, the agent must choose between equally unacceptable alternatives—that is, both may have elements that are morally unsatisfactory. For example, a certified nurse-midwife (CNM) may oppose mandatory screening of pregnant women for human immunodeficiency virus (HIV) because it violates the central concept of patient autonomy. However, vertical transmission of HIV is often preventable with new therapies, and to exclude screening the mother for HIV may result in transmission of the virus to the fetus. This choice violates the CNM's central tenet to promote good, and thus to choose either alternative results in an unsatisfactory effect on one of the involved parties.

Although the scope and nature of moral dilemmas experienced by nurses reflect the varied clinical settings in which they practice, three general themes emerge when examining ethical issues in nursing practice. First, most ethical dilemmas that occur in the health care setting are interdisciplinary in nature. Issues such as refusal of treatment, end-of-life decision making, cost containment, and confidentiality all have multidisciplinary elements interwoven in the dilemmas, and therefore an interdisciplinary approach is necessary for successful resolution of the issue. Health care professionals bring varied viewpoints and perspectives into discussions of ethical issues, and these differing positions can lead to creative and collaborative decision making. Thus an interdisciplinary theme is prevalent in both the presentation and resolution of ethical problems.

The moral dilemmas that often surround end-of-life decision making provide an excellent example of interdisciplinary issues that call for a collaborative approach. In the Study to Understand Prognosis and Preferences for Outcomes and Risks of Treatments (SUPPORT) investigation, study nurses provided patients and families opportunities to discuss preferences for medical treatments at end-of-life hospitalization (SUPPORT Principal Investigators, 1995). Although the SUPPORT study nurses communicated the patients' and/or families' wishes about resuscitation to the multidisciplinary team, the physicians often neglected to discuss further with the patient or family the patient's treatment preferences. Moreover, when the patient's preferences were known, the multidisciplinary team often did not act in accordance with these wishes. In the 2,534 intervention patients, the prevalence of do-not-resuscitate (DNR) orders and the timing of the orders did not vary significantly from those in the 2,208 control patients. Even terminally ill patients who specifically requested to be designated DNR did not have DNR orders written early in their hospitalization

(SUPPORT Principal Investigators, 1995). In such a situation, nurses experience a moral dilemma with several dimensions. If the patient arrested, the nurses would be obligated to initiate resuscitative interventions and thereby violate the patient's moral and physical boundaries. Additionally, because the physicians failed to acknowledge the nurses' understanding of the patient's wishes, the nurses were excluded from the decision-making process and became marginalized health care providers.

A second theme encountered in many ethical dilemmas is the erosion of open and honest communication. Clear communication is an essential prerequisite for informed and responsible decision making. In fact, some ethical disputes reflect inadequate communication rather than a difference in values (LaMear-Tucker & Friedson, 1997). Clear and definitive communication with patients and families will increase understanding, lead to more knowledgeable decision making, and may improve compliance with current therapies. The skills of communication are applied in several arenas. Within the multidisciplinary health care team, discussions are most effective when members are accountable for presenting information in a precise and succinct manner. The skill of listening is just as crucial in effective communication as having proficient verbal skills. Listening involves recognizing and appreciating various perspectives. To listen well is to allow others the necessary time to form and present their thoughts and ideas. In this way, good communication may be an effective tool in preventing ethical dilemmas. Furthermore, when ethical dilemmas arise, effective communication skills are the key to negotiating and facilitating a resolution.

The third theme that frequently arises when examining ethical issues in nursing practice is the issue of balancing commitments to multiple agents. Nurses have numerous and, at times, competing obligations to various stakeholders within the health care and legal systems (Lynch, 1991; Saulo & Wagener, 1996). Ethical deliberation involves analyzing and dealing with the differing and opposing demands that occur. For example, an acute care nurse practitioner (ACNP) practicing in an acute care setting is writing discharge orders for an elderly woman who is terminally ill with heart failure. The plan of care, agreed upon by the interdisciplinary team, the patient, and her family, is to continue oral medications but discontinue intravenous inotropic support and all other aggressive measures. Just prior to discharge, the social worker informs the ACNP that medical coverage for the patient's care in the long-term care facility will only be covered by the insurer if the patient has an IV in place. Now the ACNP is faced with an ethical dilemma created by multiple commitments and the need to balance obligations. The responsibilities to the patient are to assure that care is provided in a manner that is consistent with the patient's wishes and to minimize the cost burden to the patient. However, the ACNP also has a responsibility to society to practice as a responsible steward of limited resources and to prevent fraud and abuse in the health care system.

The general themes of interdisciplinary involvement, thoughtful communication, and balancing multiple commitments are prevalent in most ethical dilemmas. Although these characteristics emerge as common elements, specific ethical issues may be unique to the specialty area and clinical setting in which the APN practices.

Issues in which personal values contradict professional responsibilities often confront nurse practitioners (NPs) in a primary care setting. Issues such as abortion, teen pregnancy, patient nonadherence to treatment, childhood immunizations, regulations and law, and financial constraints that interfere with care are cited as ethical issues frequently encountered (Turner, Marquis, & Burman, 1996). In one study, primary care NPs interpreted their moral responsibilities as balancing obligations to the patient, family, colleagues, employer, and society (Viens, 1994). Often APNs in a rural setting have fewer resources than their acute care colleagues have to assist with resolution of an ethical dilemma. Thus successful deliberation of complex ethical issues is grounded in the APN's competence to develop an environment that facilitates open communication. Studies of primary care NPs suggest that the patient-practitioner relationship is the central feature in facilitating or hindering ethical decision making (Turner et al., 1996; Viens, 1994).

In the acute care setting, APNs continue to struggle with moral dilemmas involving pain management, end-of-life decision making, advance directives, and assisted suicide (Hall, 1996; O'Connor, 1996; Schlenk, 1997). The prevalence of these issues was described in a 1994 survey of practicing nurses conducted by the American Nurses Association (ANA) Center for Ethics and Human Rights. The practicing nurses identified 10 areas in which moral issues surfaced. Nurses from a variety of practice domains and roles mentioned these contemporary issues. The issues most frequently mentioned by the respondents were issues of cost containment that jeopardized patient welfare; end-of-life decisions; breaches of patient confidentiality; incompetent, illegal, or unethical practices of colleagues; pain management; use of advance directives; informed consent for procedures; access to health care; issues in the care of persons with HIV infection or acquired immunodeficiency syndrome; and providing "futile" care (Scanlon, 1994).

Many of the ethical issues identified in the ANA Center for Ethics and Human Rights study are embodied in the three themes that emerged from discussions with oncology nurses (O'Connor, 1996). The themes of suffering, secrets, and struggle were derived from oncology nurses' descriptions of ethical problems encountered in their practice. The theme of suffering was most frequently cited and involved the issues of pain management and symptom relief. Keeping secrets, the second theme, was a common experience for the study participants. In many situations, the physician communicated to the patient or family information about the patient's condition in a dishonest manner via incomplete disclosure of information or outright dishonesty. Finally, the theme of struggle arose from the oncology nurses' descriptions of situations involving disagreements. Conflict occurred between the nurse and family, nurse and physician, and nurse and other professional colleagues.

The issues of quality of life and symptom management traverse acute and nonacute health care settings (Calkins, 1993; Omery, Henneman, Billet, Luna-Raines, & Brown-Saltzman, 1995; Solomon et al., 1993; Winters, Glass, & Sakurai, 1993). It is not surprising that these issues are central moral concerns for nurses. Typically the nurse monitors the patient, interprets symptoms, and administers medication to provide optimal relief of undesirable and intolerable symptoms. Pain relief and symptom management become problematic for nurses when physicians are reluctant to acknowledge the patient's problem and/or prescribe adequate amounts of medication to alleviate the patient's pain and suffering (Turner et al., 1996; Omery et al., 1995; Solomon et al., 1993). Chronic illness, symptom management, and quality-of-life issues often are central to the ethical dilemmas and conflicts that nurses experience in their relationships with patients and professional colleagues.

The arrival of managed care has significantly changed the traditional practice of delivering health care. Managed care goals of reduced expenditures and services, increased efficiency, enhanced quality of life for patients, and improved treatment and care of patients often compete, creating conflict and tension between parties and among nurses, physicians, and employers with diverse goals (Rowdin, 1995). An example of how managed care goals can create conflict is a situation in which a

CNM practices in a managed care organization where routine obstetrical ultrasound is not approved. This decision by the organization was based on a large randomized study that found no improvement in perinatal outcome when ultrasound was used before 24 weeks' gestation (Ewigman et al., 1993). Although this decision meets the objective of reducing costs and expenditures, by limiting options for the woman, it may conflict with the goal of enhancing care (Chervenak & McCullough, 1995). In some cases, a woman's decision to continue a pregnancy is based on the presence or absence of serious fetal anomalies detected on routine ultrasound. In a managed care environment, the CNM may be faced with several alternatives. The CNM could simply not offer a woman routine ultrasound and thus exclude the option for early detection of fetal anomalies by ultrasound. Another option would be to offer ultrasound to the woman, but state at the outset that this diagnostic test would not be covered by the managed care plan. A third option involves dishonesty on the part of the CNM and would require devising some reason for the woman to be considered at high risk for carrying a fetus with congenital anomalies, thereby sanctioning the use and reimbursement of ultrasound. Each option places the CNM in conflict with some other party, either the patient or the managed care organization.

Technological advances, such as the rapidly expanding field of genetics, will further challenge APNs in the near future. The Human Genome Project is near its goal of mapping the estimated 50,000 to 100,000 genes in the human genome by the year 2005 (Williams & Lea, 1995). This information will be used to identify and further understand inherited disorders. APNs will encounter this information in a variety of settings and may be faced with discussing the need for, and perhaps results of, predictive testing for genetic disorders. Issues such as inadvertent detection of nonpaternity, denial of reimbursement for genetic testing, loss of eligibility for insurance, and the potential for discrimination may surface as the use of genetic technology increases (Williams & Lea, 1995). Because genetic information is crucially linked to the concepts of privacy and confidentiality and the availability of this information is increasing, it is inevitable that APNs will encounter ethical dilemmas related to the use of genetic data.

The complexity of ethical issues in the current health care environment and inability to reach agreement among parties has resulted in participants seeking legal settlement. Ideally, moral rights are upheld or protected by the law, and in some cases it is necessary to have these rights affirmed. For example, the Patient Self-Determination Act (part of the Omnibus Budget Reconciliation Act of 1990) upholds the rights of patients to enact an advance directive to guide future medical treatments. The APN must understand the relevance of current laws and regulations on clinical practice. In some cases, however, political and religious preferences may influence current laws and limit the options available for resolving a moral issue. The tendency to resort to the courts for guidance in ethical decision making is troubling because clinical understanding may be absent from the judicial perspective. It is important that APNs not conflate legal perspectives with ethical decision making.

APNs engage in research as principal investigators, co-investigators, or data collectors for clinical studies and trials. Regardless of the level of involvement, the APN must support the best interests of the patient and uphold the ethical concepts of informed consent and truthfulness. Patients must understand if the research is considered therapeutic or nontherapeutic and that they may withdraw from the study at any time. The use of incentives, such as money or a reduced cost of care, must be balanced with the interests of the subject (Eisenberg, 1999).

ETHICAL DECISION-MAKING COMPETENCIES OF APNs

As described above, the current challenges facing APNs in all practice settings give rise to numerous ethical concerns. Increasingly, APNs are called on to be actively involved with the patient, family, and health care team in understanding and seeking ethical resolutions to complex problems. It is not surprising that a central role in ethical discernment has emerged as an added dimension to nurses' professional roles. At the APN level, ethical involvement follows and evolves from clinical expertise. Ethical involvement requires APNs to extend beyond the technical demands of clinical practice and enter the patient's world (Dreyfus, Dreyfus, & Benner, 1996). As experienced clinicians, APNs are capable of relinquishing this exclusive focus on clinical skills and blending clinical knowledge with humanistic and spiritual knowledge (Dreyfus et al., 1996; Leavitt, 1996).

Another reason that APNs are becoming more involved in clinical ethics is the comfort that they have in working as members of a team. The interdisciplinary approach embraced by bioethics is an increasingly common element in nursing education (Leavitt, 1996). APNs practice in a variety of settings and positions, but in most cases the APN is part of a team of caregivers for the patient. The team may be loosely defined and structured, as in a rural setting, or more definitive, as in the acute care setting. Regardless of the structure, the APN has knowledge and skills to avoid power struggles and facilitate discussion among interdisciplinary team members.

Phases of Core Competency Development

The core competency of ethical decision making for APNs can be organized into three phases. Each phase relies on the acquisition of the knowledge and skills embedded in the previous level. Thus the competency of ethical decision making is reflected in the APN's knowledge and skills in moral reasoning and understood as an evolutionary process in an APN's development. These phases utilize the expert practice domains of monitoring and ensuring the quality of health care practices, teaching/coaching functions, and the consulting role of the nurse (Fenton & Brykczynski, 1993). The essential elements of each phase are described in Table 12–1.

Phase 1: Knowledge Development

The first phase in the ethical decision-making core competency for APNs is developing core knowledge in both ethical theories and principles and the ethical issues common to specific patient populations or clinical settings. This dual knowledge enables the student to integrate philosophical concepts with contemporary clinical issues. A general understanding of ethical theories, principles, and rules is necessary to define and discern the essential elements of an ethical dilemma. A key aspect of this phase is developing the ability to distinguish a true ethical dilemma from a clinically problematic situation. In essence, this first phase incorporates the stages of developing sensitivity to moral issues.

Formal education in ethical theories and concepts should be included in graduate education programs for APNs. Graduate education builds upon the ethical foundation

TABLE 12-1	PHASES OF DEVELOPMENT OF CORE COMPETENCY FOR ETHICAL DECISION MAKING	
	KNOWLEDGE	SKILL
Phase 1: Knowledge Development	Ethical theories Professional code Professional standards	Sensitivity to the ethical dimensions of clinical problems Evaluate practice setting for congruence with literature Identify ethical issues in the practice setting and bring to the attention of other team members Gather relevant literature related to problems identified
Phase 2: Knowledge Application—Moral Action	Ethical decision-making theories Mediation/facilitation strategies	Apply ethical decision-making theory to clinical problems Facilitate decision making using select strategies
Phase 3: Creating an Ethical Environment	Preventive ethics Minimizing barriers to ethical practice	Role-modeling, mentoring others Address barriers to ethical practice through system changes

of professional practice emphasized at the undergraduate level. Moreover, the graduate nursing student brings a knowledge of ethical issues that is blended with clinical experience. The American Association of Colleges of Nursing (1996) proposed that graduate nursing programs provide ethics education and experience for graduate students to understand and analyze the role of personal and professional values in systems of health care. Exposure to ethical theories, principles, and concepts provides the APN an opportunity to develop the language necessary to articulate ethical concerns in an interdisciplinary environment.

The core knowledge of ethical theories should be tempered with an understanding of issues central to the patient populations with whom the APN works. As APNs assume positions in specific clinical areas or with particular patient populations, it is incumbent upon them to gain an understanding of the applicable laws, standards, and regulations, as well as relevant paradigm cases. This information may be garnered from current literature in the field, continuing education programs, or discussions with interdisciplinary colleagues. Ideally this specialized information should be incorporated into the graduate education of APNs. Regardless of how the information is provided, APNs are responsible and accountable for seeking out opportunities to enhance and complement their core knowledge in ethical theories.

Neonatal nurse practitioners (NNPs) practice in a setting that illustrates how ethical knowledge and legal regulations are interwoven in clinical practice. An NNP must understand the current laws and regulations regarding parental rights and resuscitation of preterm newborns. Paradigm cases, such as the cases of "Baby Doe" and "Baby Jane Doe" (United States Child Abuse Protection and Treatment Amendments of 1984) serve as important tools to help the NNP frame ethical dilemmas in neonatal care (Kopelman, Irons, & Kopelman, 1988). Other guidelines regarding the care of this patient population, such as the American Academy of Pediatrics' guidelines for the care of critically ill newborns (American Academy of Pediatrics, Committee on Bioethics, 1996), expand the NNPs understanding and anticipation of ethical issues that arise in these situations.

In this initial stage of developing competence in ethical decision making, ethical conduct or comportment is formed and refined. The emphasis in this stage is on cognitive mastery, in which the APN learns the theories, principles, rules, paradigm cases, and relevant laws that influence ethical decision making. With this knowledge, the APN begins to compare current practices in the clinical setting with the ethical standards described in the literature. In other words, the APN begins to identify and critically examine ethical dilemmas. Phase one is the beginning of the APNs personal journey toward developing a distinct and individualized ethical framework.

Novice APNs are able to recognize a moral problem as an ethical infringement and seek clarification and illumination of the concern. The APN identifies ethical issues and formulates the concerns about which others are uneasy. This step earns credibility and enables the APN to gain self-confidence by bringing the issue to the awareness and attention of others. If the issue remains a moral concern after clarification, the APN may seek additional help to pursue resolution.

Phase 2: Knowledge Application

The second phase of the core competency is applying the knowledge developed in the first level to the practice arena. Phase two begins the APN's journey in assessing real ethical problems and being actively involved in the process of resolving ethical dilemmas. The success and speed with which the APN gains these behavioral skills is related to the presence of mentors in the clinical setting and the willingness of the APN to become immersed in ethical discussions.

Institutional resources such as ethics committees and institutional review boards provide valuable opportunities for APNs to participate in the discussion of ethical issues. Typically, hospital ethics committees serve three functions: policy formation, case review, and education (Spencer, 1997). As a member of the ethics committee, the APN exchanges ideas and gains an understanding of ethical dilemmas from a variety of perspectives. In addition, the APN is informed of current legislation, regulations, and hospital policies that have ethical implications. This is an extremely valuable experience that can accelerate the development of ethical decision-making skills.

Unfortunately, the majority of APNs do not have the opportunity to participate on an interdisciplinary ethics committee, and in some cases may have few professional colleagues available to mentor and develop the skills of ethical decision making. Thus the APN must advance this phase by actively seeking opportunities to engage in ethical dialogue with professional colleagues. Professional organizations offer workshops in which case studies are discussed and analyzed. This format is helpful to the inexperienced APN who needs guidance in applying knowledge to clinical cases.

As the APN acquires core ethical decision-making knowledge the responsibility to take moral action becomes more compelling. Rather than retrospectively analyzing ethical dilemmas, moral action implies that the APN pursues and responds to ethical issues. Moral action requires dedication to work until a resolution is achieved or options are exhausted, and courage to pursue emotionally charged and complex ethical problems. Often the inequities toward or infringements on other persons are enough to motivate moral action, and a timely response can change the course in present as well as future situations. Therefore, the importance of moral action should not be underestimated as a core APN skill, and it should be recognized, fostered, and valued by others.

Often, the more experienced APN has developed professional working relationships with colleagues that are based on trust and mutual respect. Because the preservation of relationships is a significant goal in working toward collaborative ethical decision making, the experienced APN can select strategies that build on this commitment. One way for APNs to maintain the respect of professional colleagues is to acquire ethical knowledge and expertise in their area. Clearly, resolutions that originate from collaborative processes are more satisfactory, generate more creative solutions, and strengthen relationships (Spielman, 1993). This feeling of solidarity empowers others to explore and participate in the ethical decision-making process.

Although the core knowledge of ethical concepts such as respect for persons, truthfulness, and beneficence provide the foundation for moral reasoning, the practical application of these concepts enables the APN to evolve the practical wisdom of moral reasoning. It is the experience in the practice setting and the courage of the APN to openly discuss sensitive issues that enable the APN to assume an active role in dispute resolution.

Phase 3: Creating an Ethical Environment

As the APN becomes more skilled in the application of ethical knowledge, the third phase of competence begins to develop. Teaching and mentoring others regarding ethical decision making and creating an ethical environment are expectations of more experienced APNs. Once the APN transforms ethical knowledge into moral action, the role of mentoring others emerges. Often other nurses and members of the health care team remain silent about ethical issues. In a mentoring capacity, the APN helps others develop the ability to voice ethical concerns. In this way, the APN supports other team members to develop confidence in raising ethical concerns and fosters an environment in which diverse views are expressed.

The experienced APN may initiate informal learning opportunities for nurses and other professional colleagues. Ethics rounds and case review are two ways to engage colleagues in the discussion of moral issues. During this educational process, the APN empowers other professionals by providing knowledge and role modeling to help others understand the broader implications of the issue (Copp, 1986).

APNs with experience in ethical reasoning are considered valuable assets to interdisciplinary bioethics education (Leavitt, 1996). Often the roots of interdisciplinary conflict in the clinical setting are based on preconceived stereotypes of the moral viewpoints of other disciplines (Shannon, 1997). The APN can help professionals from other disciplines understand the perspectives and socialization of nurses in the field of ethics. In addition, the APN models successful negotiation with other disciplines and the resolution of clinical moral dilemmas. Teaching and mentoring functions often are focused on other professional colleagues. This important role of the APN also encompasses aspects of coaching, and teaching patients and families in ethical decision making. It is not sufficient for the APN to simply provide information to patients and families facing difficult moral choices and expect them to arrive at a comfortable decision. The ethical competency is linked closely with the ability to mobilize patients and move those needing help through the necessary steps to reach resolution. The APN helps others appreciate the issues and understand various ways to interpret the problem. Foundational knowledge in ethics and values clarification enables the APN to help others articulate the issue and communicate effectively.

As APNs become more competent and capable in ethical reasoning, they are able to anticipate situations in which moral conflicts occur and recognize the more subtle presentations of moral dilemmas. The ability to look beyond the immediate situation and foresee potential issues directs the APN down a path of preventive ethics.

PREVENTIVE ETHICS

Ethical decision-making skills enable the APN to focus on identifying the values in conflict and developing a course of action suitable to the parties in dispute. This approach, however, concentrates on the resolution of current and ongoing issues rather than preventing the recurrence of moral dilemmas (Forrow, Arnold, & Parker, 1993). An additional important role of the APN is to extend the concept of ethical decision making beyond problem-solving individual cases and move toward a paradigm of preventive ethics.

Preventive ethics is derived from the model of preventive medicine (Forrow et al., 1993). An ethical environment fosters early identification of issues and anticipation of possible dilemmas. The ability to predict areas of conflict and develop plans in a proactive, rather than reactive, manner will avert some potentially difficult dilemmas (Benner, 1991; Forrow et al., 1993). When value conflicts arise, resolution is more difficult because one value must be chosen over another. Preventive ethics emphasizes that all important values should be reviewed and examined prior to the conflict so that situations in which values may differ can be anticipated (Forrow et al., 1993). In other words, the goals of the health care team should be articulated as clearly as possible to avoid potential misinterpretations. For example, a certified registered nurse anesthetist (CRNA) should have an understanding of a terminally ill patient's values regarding aggressive treatment should a cardiopulmonary arrest occur during surgery. However, the CRNA's moral and legal obligations should be openly discussed so that the patient and professional appreciate and recognize each other's values and moral and legal positions.

In addition to the early examination and ongoing dialogue of values, a conscientious inspection of other factors that influence the evolution of moral dilemmas is required. The roles and responsibilities of all parties must be clearly defined to expose any existing power imbalance. During this process, the issues of powerlessness and collaborative practice surface as areas in which the APN can influence change.

By providing knowledge, promoting a positive self-image, and preparing others for participation in decision making, the APN empowers individuals. The skill of the APN is used not to resolve moral dilemmas single-handedly but to mentor others to assume a position of moral accountability and engage in shared decision making. This process of enhancing others' autonomy and providing opportunities for involvement in reaching resolution is a key concept in preventive ethics (Forrow et al., 1993). Although many ethical issues will develop with little warning, the practice of preventive ethics will improve the delivery of morally responsible, innovative, and humanistic patient care.

CREATING AN ETHICALLY SENSITIVE ENVIRONMENT

APNs should strive to develop environments that encourage patients and caregivers to express diverse views and raise questions about the ethical elements of clinical care. Thoughtful ethical decision making arises from an environment that supports and values the critical exchange of ideas and promotes collaboration among members of the health care team, patients, and families. A collaborative practice environment in turn supports shared decision making, shared accountability, and group participation, and it fosters relationships based on equality and mutuality (Pike, 1991). The APN is integral in the development and preservation of a collaborative climate that inspires and empowers individuals to respond to moral dilemmas.

The nature of health care creates a climate in which many workers feel overwhelmed, stressed, and discouraged by the lack of time to care for patients and the increased acuity of patients in both inpatient and outpatient settings. Over time, such climates actually can cause nurses to become accustomed and insensitive to the structures and the dilemmas around them (Chambliss, 1996). An ethically sensitive environment is one in which providers are encouraged to acknowledge when they feel overwhelmed and seek help when they need it (Scott, Aiken, Mechanic, & Moravcsik, 1995). Only when care providers recognize and attend to their personal needs will they be better able to detect and nurture the needs of others.

The APN should advocate for a process of ongoing, rather than episodic, ethical inquiry. This approach to moral reflection sanctions open discussions of values and divergent views and is realized through the reciprocal exchanges of information between members of the health care team and the patient. Throughout this process, the APN incorporates the skills, ethical expertise, and background on issues necessary to facilitate dialogue, mediate disputes, analyze options, and design optimal solutions. Therefore, the ethical decision-making skills of the APN move the resolution of moral dilemmas beyond individual cases toward the cultivation of an environment in which the moral integrity of individuals is respected. Development and preservation of this ethical environment is the key contribution of the APN.

ACQUIRING AND DEVELOPING ETHICAL DECISION-MAKING COMPETENCIES

The skills needed to identify, articulate, and address ethical dilemmas are complex and diverse. Particular strategies, such as those used in values clarification, negotiation, and mediation, provide a foundation for the practice aspects of ethical decision making. The APN must understand the theoretical elements of biomedical ethics and be aware of paradigm cases and relevant law to interpret moral issues in the health care setting. However, successful resolution of moral issues will more likely occur if the application of ethical knowledge is tempered with compassionate and effective communication skills.

Developing an Educational Foundation

Education in ethical theories, principles, rules, and moral concepts provides the foundation for developing skills in ethical reasoning. Through graduate education, the APN studies models of ethical decision making and is introduced to the importance of understanding value systems. Because the APN will apply the theoretical principles in actual encounters with patients, it is imperative that consideration of the contextual factors in specific situations be strengthened. A portion of graduate ethics education should involve discussion of clinical cases involving moral issues. These cases should reflect typical clinical issues encountered by the APN rather than issues that receive extensive media attention yet occur infrequently.

Ethics education is an ongoing process throughout the APN's professional career. Although the foundation for ethical decision-making skills should be provided during graduate education, continuing education programs also are effective and necessary forums to provide current information in a rapidly changing health care environment. Ethical issues are dynamic and re-emerge in altered forms. As technology changes and new dilemmas confront practitioners, the APN must be prepared to anticipate conditions that erode an ethical environment. Knowledge and skills in all phases of developing this competency rely on the application of current ethical knowledge in the clinical setting. Ethical reasoning and clinical judgments share a common process, and each serves to teach and inform the other (Dreyfus et al., 1996; Leavitt, 1996; Solomon et al., 1991). Therefore, the importance of clinical practice cannot be overemphasized.

OVERVIEW OF ETHICAL THEORIES

Although ethical decision making in health care is extensively discussed in the bio-ethics literature, two dominant models are most often applied in the clinical setting. The analytical model of decision making is a principle-based model (see Table 12–2). In this model, ethical decision-making is guided by theories, principles, and rules (Beauchamp & Childress, 1994). In cases of conflict, the principles or rules in contention are balanced and interpreted with the contextual elements of the circumstance. However, the final decision and moral justification for actions are based on an appeal to principles. In this way, the principles are both binding and tolerant of the particularities of specific cases (Beauchamp & Childress, 1994; Childress, 1994).

The principles of respect for persons, autonomy, beneficence, nonmaleficence, and justice are commonly applied in the analysis of ethical issues in nursing. The ANA's current *Code for Nurses* (1985) embraces the principle of respect for persons and underscores the profession's commitment to service (Fowler, 1999). The emphasis on respect for persons throughout the *Code* implies that it is not only a philosophical value of nursing but also a binding principle within the profession.

Although ethical principles and rules are the cornerstone of most ethical decisions, the principle-based approach has been criticized as too formalistic and rigorous for many clinicians (Ahronheim, Moreno, & Zuckerman, 1994). Critics argue that a

TABLE 12–2 PRINCIPLES AND RULES IMPORTANT TO PROFESSIONAL NURSING PRACTICE

Principle of Respect for Autonomy	The duty to respect others' personal liberty and individual values, beliefs, and choices
Principle of Nonmaleficence	The duty not to inflict harm or evil
Principle of Beneficence	The duty to do good and prevent or remove harm
Principle of Formal Justice	The duty to treat equals equally and treat those who are unequal according to their needs
Rule of Veracity	The duty to tell the truth and not to deceive others
Rule of Fidelity	The duty to honor commitments
Rule of Confidentiality	The duty not to disclose information shared in an intimate and trusted manner
Rule of Privacy	The duty to respect limited access to a person

Definitions adapted from Beauchamp, T. L., Childress, J. F. (1994). *Principles of biomedical ethics* (4th ed.). New York: Oxford University Press.

principle-based approach conceals the particular person and relationships and reduces the resolution of a clinical case to simply balancing principles (Gudorf, 1994).
Consequently, when conflicts among principles occur, the description of the principle
is inadequate to provide guidance for resolving the dilemma (Ahronheim et al., 1994;
Childress, 1994).

A second approach to ethical decision making is the casuistic model, in which
current cases are compared with paradigm cases (Ahronheim et al., 1994; Beauchamp & Childress, 1994; Jonsen & Toulmin, 1988; Toulmin, 1994). The strength
of this approach is that dilemmas are examined in a context-specific manner and
then compared with an analogous earlier case. The fundamental philosophical assumption of this model is that ethics emerges from human moral experiences (Ahronheim et al., 1994; Jonsen & Toulmin, 1988). The casuists approach dilemmas from
an inductive position and work from the specific case to generalizations, rather
than from generalizations to specific cases (Ahronheim et al., 1994; Beauchamp &
Childress, 1994; Gaul, 1995).

Some concerns arise when evaluating a casuistic model for ethical decision making.
As a moral dilemma arises, the selection of the paradigm case may differ among the
decision makers, and thus the interpretation of the appropriate course of action
will vary. Furthermore, other than the reliance on previous cases, casuists have no
mechanisms to justify their actions. The possibility that previous cases were reasoned
in a faulty or inaccurate manner is not considered or evaluated (Beauchamp &
Childress, 1994).

Other theories, such as utilitarianism, Kantianism, virtue-based theory, and care-
based theory, provide alternative processes for moral reflection and argument (Beauchamp & Childress, 1994). In particular, the ethics of care has emerged as relevant
to nursing (Cooper, 1989). The care perspective constructs moral problems as issues
surrounding the intrinsic needs and corresponding responsibilities that occur within
relationships (Cooper, 1989; Gilligan, 1982). Moral reasoning involves empathy and
emphasizes responsibility rather than rights. The response of the individual to a moral
dilemma emerges from the affiliate relationship and the norms of friendship, care,
and love (Beauchamp & Childress, 1994; Cooper, 1991).

Although every ethical theory has some limitations and problems, an understanding
of contemporary approaches to ethics and bioethics is a central feature in achieving
a moral resolution. Moral reasoning most often reflects a blend of the various theories
rather than the application of a single theory.

PROFESSIONAL CODES AND GUIDELINES

Frequently the ANA's *Code for Nurses* (1985) is used in undergraduate and graduate
education to introduce the moral beliefs of the nursing profession. The *Code* serves
a worthy function by describing the profession's philosophy and the general ethical
obligations of the professional nurse. However, the *Code* describes broad guidelines
that more reflect the profession's conscience than provide clear directions for specific
clinical situations. In this sense, the *Code* delineates the nurse's overriding moral
obligations to the patient but offers little specific help in balancing competing demands from the institution and other health care professionals. The current ANA
Code is undergoing revision and is expected to address additional professional
obligations.

Professional organizations delineate standards of performance that reflect the responsibilities, obligations, duties, and rights of the members. These standards serve

as guidelines for professional behavior and define desired conduct. Although the general principles are relatively stable, professional organizations often reflect on contemporary issues and assume a proactive posture on pivotal concerns. One example is the ANA's (1994) *Position Statement on Active Euthanasia.* This position statement holds that active euthanasia violates the *Code for Nurses,* and the ANA opposes the participation of the nursing profession in such an act (ANA, 1994). APNs must be familiar with the profession's position on topics relevant to the area of practice. Some degree of involvement with professional and specialty organizations is necessary to strengthen the APN's voice in guiding the profession's moral accountability to the public.

Public policies and legal guidelines may infringe on the process of ethical decision making. It is important to recognize that the law is open to interpretation, and current laws surrounding an issue in conflict may be overemphasized or misunderstood. Unfortunately, there is an increasing tendency to look to the law for the final word. Misinterpretation of legal decisions in precedent-setting cases may diminish the chances of successful negotiation. For example, an APN in Virginia may be involved with a case of withdrawing nutrition and hydration. Parties involved in the case may misunderstand the U.S. Supreme Court ruling in the case of Nancy Cruzan (*Cruzan v. Missouri Department of Health, et al.,* 1990) and incorrectly assume that nutrition and hydration cannot be withdrawn. If the APN is familiar with the Cruzan case, general misconceptions can be explained and clarified. APNs knowledgeable about relevant case law and pertinent state and federal policies are better able to take moral action when dilemmas arise. Information on legal and policy guidelines should be offered during graduate practicum experiences in the area of clinical concentration.

PERSONAL AND PROFESSIONAL VALUES

During graduate education, the APN should be introduced to the concept of value systems and undergo a process of values clarification. Individuals' interpretations and positions on issues are a reflection of their underlying value system. Value systems are enduring beliefs that guide life choices and decisions in conflict resolution (Uustal, 1987). Because values influence behaviors, actions, and choices, an awareness of personal values generates more consistent choices and behaviors.

The APN should be guided through a process of values clarification. Values clarification will enable students to define and analyze their personal and professional beliefs, attitudes, and value systems (Saulo & Wagener, 1996). In addition to personal and professional growth, students can apply the strategies of values clarification to understand care organizations and facilitate the decision making of patients and surrogates in the clinical setting. This approach also is useful during the process of negotiation, in which the APN guides both parties in conflict to identify interests.

Professional and personal communication is based on individual interpretations of the facts, meanings, and significance of the information. Values clarification is an approach to examining the influence that values have on decision making and behavior (Saulo & Wagener, 1996; Uustal, 1987). This process enables APNs to appreciate and articulate the personal and professional values that influence their behavior as well as to recognize and respect the values of other health care team members, patients, and families. Values clarification and values education are practical and effective strategies to expand the health care team's awareness of each other's professional beliefs and to facilitate the decision making of patients and surrogates in the clinical setting.

Values also underlie the decisions of patients and families. Through the process of values clarification, the APN can guide the patient and family toward the recognition and appreciation of previously unconscious value choices. Careful examination of the patient's values enhances treatment decision making and clarifies the motivation underlying the individual's expressed wishes and treatment preferences for the APN and other health care professionals (Doukas & Gorenflo, 1993; Doukas & McCullough, 1991).

Values awareness should include an understanding of how various cultural values affect the decisions made by patients and families and the decisions by care providers to offer particular treatments (Council on Ethical and Judicial Affairs, 1990, 1991; Wright, Cohen, & Caroselli, 1997). When decisions are made that are contradictory to traditional Western medical practice, health care providers may resort to coercive or paternalistic measures to influence choices to be more consistent with the provider's values. The APN and other health care providers must understand the assumptions they make about the decisions of others from different cultures based on their own cultural values and biases. As health care professionals gain an understanding of factors that guide a person's decisions, treatment plans that reflect the patient's value preferences are more easily developed. For example, a patient from a Southeast Asian culture may show respect to authority figures by obeying the APN's treatment suggestions even if the individual disagrees with the plan. In this situation, the APN could assure the patient that questions about the plan of care are welcomed and are not disrespectful (Wright et al., 1997).

Developing Skills in Ethical Decision Making

Acquiring the skills and competence to facilitate the resolution of moral dilemmas is an evolutionary process. Because ethical decision making is not exclusively based on theoretical knowledge, moral reasoning must be tempered with clinical reality. As APNs gain the necessary knowledge and skills in ethical decision making, their involvement should intensify and become more extensive. Once an advanced nursing role is assumed, the APN accepts the function of a full participant in resolution of moral dilemmas rather than simply an interested observer or one of many parties in conflict.

One procedural framework nurses can use in ethical decision making is to adapt the nursing process as a framework to organize and guide the gathering of morally relevant information (Table 12-3). This framework enables the APN to systematically organize the facts and contextual particularities of a dilemma. Although a framework provides structure and suggests a method of examining and studying the ethical issues, the essential component to resolution of ethical dilemmas is moral action. Simply knowing the right course of action does not guarantee that a person has the motivation or courage to act (Rest, 1986). Successful resolution of moral issues requires a blend of knowledge, conviction, emotions, beliefs, and individual character (van Hooft, 1990).

PROBLEM IDENTIFICATION

Ethical dilemmas often are first recognized by the intense emotional reactions they elicit. Emotions are present in all clinical settings, but when personal or professional values are questioned or trespassed, the instinctive response is to react with anger

TABLE 12–3	USE OF THE NURSING PROCESS IN ETHICAL DECISION MAKING
STEP	DESCRIPTION
1: Assessment	Problem identification
	Information gathering
	Medical facts
	Nursing facts
	Values, rights, and obligations of parties
	Other relevant factors
	Culture
	Religion
	Relationships
	Other contextual features
2: Plan	Strategies for resolution
	Collaboration
	Compromise
	Accommodation
	Coercion
	Avoidance
3: Implementation	Initiate a moral action
4: Evaluation	Process
	Outcome

or frustration. Although this is a helpful gauge to awaken an awareness that something may be amiss ethically, too often the individual becomes entangled in the emotions and is unable to move toward an awareness of the consequences for others. It is frequently this point at which the differing parties become polarized and embedded in a particular viewpoint. A difficult but important step in problem identification is to allow and encourage the individuals in conflict to openly express their emotions. This action demonstrates that the perspectives and the emotional responses to the issue are legitimate and meaningful (Fisher & Ury, 1981). As a facilitator, the APN should recognize, understand, and acknowledge the emotions of all parties.

Many conflicts that arise in the clinical setting generate powerful emotional responses yet may not be ethical issues. Ethical issues involve some form of controversy concerning moral values (Ahronheim et al., 1994). It is essential that the APN distinguish and separate moral dilemmas from other issues such as administrative concerns, communication problems, or lack of clinical knowledge. Identifying the cause of the problem and determining why, where, and when it occurred, as well as who or what was affected, will help clarify the nature of the problem (Beare, 1989). For example, less experienced staff may call an APN to resolve a dilemma in pain management. The less experienced nurse's interpretation is that the physician ordered an inadequate dose of an analgesic to manage the patient's symptoms. The nurse requested an increased dosage for the patient, but the physician refused. The APN may determine that the severity of the disease process requires the addition of another analgesic to enhance the effects of the original medication ordered. The issue encountered was not a moral issue but instead reflected problems with nurse-physician communication and the lack of knowledge regarding appropriate pharmacological management.

INFORMATION GATHERING

Once the ethical problem is identified, the APN implements a process to gather and examine the morally relevant facts. Generally, information such as the medical and nursing facts; the values, rights, and obligations of the patient and others; legal factors; and cultural and religious factors should be gathered when initiating the decision-making process. However, these facts are insufficient if not tempered with the contextual features of each case. Only after the unique conditions of the case are considered can an ethically acceptable solution be identified.

Strategies for Resolution

Moral discussions and deliberation can take the form of a debate that degenerates into an assault. One party presents an argument, the other party disputes it, the original party defends, and the second party attacks (Zaner, 1988). Breaking this cycle of destructive interactions is central to arriving at solutions that are resourceful and constructive. Resolutions are most effective when the parties in dispute create the solution.

When the APN is directly involved in a conflict situation, the skills of negotiation are most useful in moving toward a satisfactory settlement. However, in cases where resolution is not easily achieved, it is best to solicit help from a member of the ethics committee or another professional colleague not involved in the case.

The challenge in most cases of ethical disputes is to have all involved listen to each other's perspectives to understand the basis of the disagreement and to work together to create a collaborative solution (Saulo & Wagener, 1996). In many cases, the APN must serve as a facilitator for the parties in dispute and apply the strategies involved in mediation. The key difference between these roles is the level of active involvement in deciding the goals and strategies of resolving the dilemma. As a negotiating party, the APN suggests solutions and identifies acceptable plans (Beare, 1989). In the role of a mediator, the APN guides the process but does not offer opinions or solutions (Ostermeyer, 1991). The process and steps used in negotiation and mediation overlap in many ways, and in both approaches the parties in conflict discover and determine the acceptable solutions (Beare, 1989; Ostermeyer, 1991).

The objective of successful negotiation and mediation is to achieve a mutually satisfactory solution. In reality, however, that is not always possible. The issues of time, cost, available resources, level of moral certainty and the perceived value of the relationship play important roles in the strategy used and likelihood of reaching a desired outcome (Spielman, 1993). These issues are addressed later in the section "Barriers to Ethical Practice and Potential Solutions." The following strategies for negotiation are useful when the APN is facilitating resolution between two parties and when the professional or personal values of the APN collide with the values of others. The key role of the APN in the resolution of moral dilemmas is to guide and stimulate communication between the differing parties.

COLLABORATION

Collaboration is the preferred strategy for achieving a moral resolution. Because it is a fundamental competency of the APN, the steps involved in collaboration will be discussed in some detail. This section focuses on identifying and cultivating the elements necessary for collaboration regarding ethical problems. Additional methods to foster a collaborative environment are discussed in Chapter 11.

The first step in the process of collaboration is to help the disputing parties agree on the issue in conflict and to understand both the cognitive and the emotional perspectives of each party. Because emotions maintain a significant position in moral dilemmas, it is important to provide an environment in which the parties can release unexpressed emotions. An effective method to help others resolve anger or frustration is to listen in a nonjudgmental manner and avoid reacting to the criticisms (Fisher & Ury, 1981). Discussions that occur after the release of emotions are more rational and productive because the emotions have been expressed in an explicit and unambiguous manner (Fisher & Ury, 1981). The APN encourages the parties to discuss their perception of the problem, recognize their emotions, and identify their expectations for resolution (Krouse & Roberts, 1989).

This first step toward moral resolution is particularly difficult, because people in power are often less interested in and less likely to acknowledge the perspectives of those with lesser power (Welton, 1991). This situation is not uncommon in health care environments that traditionally have sanctioned physicians with greater authority and power than nurses. When nurses' ethical reasoning and moral actions are constrained, they react with anger, frustration, and moral outrage (Pike, 1991). The outrage intensifies as nurses sense a violation of their moral integrity. To eliminate this power imbalance, the responsibility and accountability of all parties in the negotiation process must be openly acknowledged and agreed on. One strategy to move other parties toward a collaborative approach is for the APN to be the first to acknowledge her or his understanding of the issue. In this way the APN establishes the ground rule of mutual respect and frames the process in a collaborative and shared model of decision making.

The second step toward successful collaborative moral resolution is to engage all involved parties in active interactions and consensus building (Krouse & Roberts, 1989). Information presented should be questioned, analyzed, and examined. It is important to focus on the interests of each party rather than the positions. Asking the questions "why?" and "why not?" can identify interests of the involved individuals. (Fisher & Ury, 1981). As differing interests emerge, the varying perspectives should be acknowledged with confidence and hopefulness (Ury, 1993). The parties must listen to each other but need not necessarily agree on the others' views or on what is being said. From this stage of active communication and interaction, the process of consensus building begins.

The third step in negotiating or mediating a moral resolution involves formulating a decision and developing a plan of action. The objective of both negotiation and mediation is to generate options and solutions that are consistent with all parties' principles and achieve an outcome that is mutually satisfying (Ostermeyer, 1991; Ury, 1993). During this phase, the parties explore options and together decide on a plan of action. Initially this joint negotiation may seem unlikely, particularly when both parties are attached to their own positions. However, it is possible for the APN to facilitate progression through complex situations by using communication skills such as reframing, identifying shared interests and needs, and examining the differences (Fisher & Ury, 1981; Smeltzer, 1991).

Although implementation of a collaborative process for the resolution of moral dilemmas is most desired, other approaches to manage conflict may be employed. The choice to employ another strategy for resolution may be deliberate or inadvertent. In any case, there are distinct advantages and disadvantages with other methods, and the APN should recognize these factors.

COMPROMISE

When both parties possess a high level of moral certainty in their positions and are committed to preserving the relationship, they may choose to bargain and to have each party relinquish some control over the decision. Compromising and bargaining are time consuming because each party must determine what are acceptable trade-offs. Because time in the clinical setting is limited, both parties must value the relationship and share in the decision making process (Spielman, 1993).

Problems are resolved through compromise when both parties are willing to waive some components of their moral position and embrace a position of cooperation (Spielman, 1993). For example, a chronically ill patient with dilated cardiomyopathy may refuse in-hospital management of the heart failure but agree to a short-term solution, such as a trial of intravenous therapy at home.

The clinical context in which NPs and CNMs practice most often requires collaboration or compromise as approaches to moral resolution. In these situations the patient and clinician maintain high degrees of commitment to the relationship. In addition, most encounters are nonemergent, and thus time is available for engaging in compromise and collaboration.

ACCOMMODATION

In some cases, one party will accommodate and simply agree to support the other's position. This approach may indicate that, to one party, the issue in question was too insignificant for her or him to strive for a mutually acceptable solution (Spielman, 1993). Accommodation frequently occurs when the issue is trivial, time is limited, or one party holds a high level of commitment to preserving the relationship with the other participant (Spielman, 1993). Nurses may resort to this approach if the physician is perceived as too powerful or forceful.

Accommodation is sometimes employed as a tactic in negotiation. The concession is made to dissipate friction and additionally to imply that a reciprocal action is expected in future negotiations with the other party. However, accommodation is an inappropriate strategy when used routinely to gain acceptance or merely to avoid conflict.

COERCION

A coercive and controlling approach may be used when time is short, such as in an emergency, or when the party has little commitment to the relationship. This approach is often aggressive and competitive and reflects a high degree of commitment to a particular moral position (Spielman, 1993). Because control of the decision is assumed by one party and the differing perspectives are discounted, this approach damages the self-esteem of the other party and may result in a sense of powerlessness and moral outrage (Pike, 1991).

An environment in which a coercive and controlling approach is prevalent generates a power imbalance that accentuates vulnerability. Vulnerability damages self-esteem, constrains independence, and restricts choices (Copp, 1986). In this environment, relationships have little importance, and it is unlikely that the group with authority will actively pursue empowering the vulnerable group. Change can occur in this climate, but it often emanates from the constrained party. Redefining one's position (i.e., from victim to involved decision maker) and acknowledging accountability and responsibility for reaching collaborative resolutions are strategies to alter a coercive environment (Pike, 1991).

Although a coercive approach is aggressive and often undesirable, it sometimes is necessary. For example, when a child of Jehovah's Witness parents must emergently receive a blood transfusion and the parents refuse to give consent for the treatment, legal approval is sought. Time, in this case, is limited, and the caregivers are convinced of the moral rightness of their views, just as the parents are convinced of their moral position. Because the child's well-being depends on prompt action, the caregivers are limited to a coercive approach for resolution. In this case, the law usually compels the parents to permit treatment of the minor child.

AVOIDANCE

Participants may avoid, ignore, or deny the dilemma when the moral issue is perceived as trivial or, conversely, is deeply felt by one party and highly charged emotionally. Avoidance is also seen when time is short (Spielman, 1993). If a decision is unnecessary, it may be appropriate for a participant to withdraw from the process of decision making. However, this strategy often is employed when the participant abdicates moral accountability. The APN should consciously monitor avoidance behaviors and pursue the rationale for this technique. It is likely that the individual who practices this technique regularly avoids conflict and would benefit from additional knowledge, support, and role modeling of approaches to conflict management. Individuals who consistently evade moral dilemmas may benefit from values clarification exercises to help them explore deeply held values and to learn ways to deal with them more productively.

EVALUATION OF THE ETHICAL DECISION-MAKING COMPETENCY

The evaluation of ethical decision making should focus on two areas: the process and the outcome. Process evaluation is important because it provides an overview of the moral disagreement, the interpersonal skills employed, the interactions between both parties in conflict, and the problems encountered during the phases of resolution. Whether the APN was the facilitator or a party in conflict, a deliberate and reflective evaluation of the process of resolution should occur (Olczak, Grosch, & Duffy, 1991). It is useful for the APN to assess the type of issue, the inter-relational and situational variables, the conceptual shifts that occurred during the process, and the strategies used by both parties during the negotiation phase (Olczak et al., 1991). As the APN reflects on the process, attention should be given to how similar situations could be anticipated and resolved in the future. Deliberate and consistent review of the process will help the APN assess various approaches to the resolution of ethical dilemmas and identify the onset of moral conflict earlier.

Evaluation of the outcome is also critical because it acknowledges creative solutions and celebrates moral action. Other components of the outcome evaluation include the short-term and long-term consequences of the action taken and the satisfaction of all parties with the chosen solution (Olczak et al., 1991). Unfortunately, a successful process does not always result in a satisfactory outcome. Occasionally the outcome reveals the need for changes within the institution or health care system. The APN may choose to become involved in advancing these identified changes or identifying appropriate resources to pursue the desired objectives. The goal of the outcome evaluation is to minimize the risks of a similar event by identifying predictable patterns and thereby averting recurrent and future dilemmas.

Although evaluation of the ethical problem is an important step in preventing future dilemmas and building ethically sensitive environments, in some situations tension and uneasiness will remain. It is important for the APN to acknowledge that many issues leave a "moral residue" that continues to trouble participants involved in the dilemma. Part of the outcome evaluation must address the reality of these lingering feelings and the related tensions.

BARRIERS TO ETHICAL PRACTICE AND POTENTIAL SOLUTIONS

A number of variables influence how moral issues are addressed and resolved in the clinical setting. Some barriers, once identified, can be corrected and eliminated. Other issues that impede the resolution of ethical issues may require attention at the institutional, state, or national level. Regardless of the nature of the barrier, the APN must identify and respond to the barriers that inhibit the development of a morally responsive environment.

Intraprofessional Barriers

The APN often relies on other nurses and caregivers to recognize ethical issues and initiate dialogue with professional colleagues. In some situations, nurses are uncertain, fearful, insecure, unable to articulate their moral concern, or incapable of taking moral action (Pike, 1991). Nurses who do not feel secure with their ethical knowledge may dismiss an issue as insignificant or discount and minimize their perceptions of the dilemma. Unfortunately, too many ethical issues are "swept under the rug" because a nurse chooses not to raise the concern. It would be far better to raise a concern when it is viewed as insignificant than to wait for the problem to erupt with chaos and conflict.

Conflict between the nurse's personal values and the professional values of nursing may be a source of moral distress. The ANA *Code for Nurses* (1985) elucidates the professional values of nursing, and professional nurses are accountable for practicing in a way that is congruent with the *Code*. In some cases, a nurse's personal values may conflict with the professional values, and the nurse may feel confused and distressed when faced with choosing a response. For example, an emergency room NP may be faced with providing care for a criminal injured in a gunfight that killed innocent bystanders. Although it is disturbing and difficult to provide care for an individual who has caused harm to others, the NP's personal views should not interfere with the quality of the care provided. The process of values clarification is helpful in preparing nurses for this situation. Values clarification uncovers personal values that may have been internalized and not openly acknowledged. Once personal values are realized, the nurse can anticipate more easily situations in which such conflicts will arise and either avoid becoming part of the problem or have a defined strategy to deal with the issue.

Perceptions of powerlessness influence how active nurses become in the resolution of ethical dilemmas (Erlen & Frost, 1991; Gaul, 1995). Power issues between the APN and bedside nurse may evolve as the bedside nurse views the APN as having enhanced decision-making authority and a more direct line of communication to the physician. A sense of powerlessness suggests that the bedside nurse feels incapable or ineffective in changing the situation or correcting the problem. Certainly in some cases the sense of powerlessness is a reality. For example, nurses may not be able to change a managed care organization's perspective on the approved length of stay for a specific DRG. However, all problems can be dissected into smaller parts, and the APN can work on more manageable components of the issue.

The nurse's ethical obligations to maintain a competent and caring relationship with the patient are challenged with the implementation of managed care. As the new health care system alters nurses' roles, several strategies have been proposed to help nurses realize their ethical responsibilities (Erlen & Mellors, 1995). One strategy already discussed is to engage in personal reflection and values clarification. In addition, nurses should assess their competence to provide effective care and address any deficiencies that are exposed. Because patients have shorter hospital stays in a managed care environment, open communication and collaboration with the health care team, patients, and families are essential behaviors for optimal planning. Additionally, nurses should maintain and affirm patient's rights by questioning and challenging changes in the health care system that negatively affect the quality of care delivered. Finally, there is a need to consistently review patient outcomes and quality of nursing care provided (Erlen & Mellors, 1995). These strategies empower the nurse to act on smaller and more manageable parts of the problem.

Feelings of powerlessness can result in individuals feeling vulnerable and defenseless. The APN's role encompasses empowering the professional staff and patients to overcome and avoid the destructive feelings of vulnerability (Copp, 1986). One of the most effective strategies for empowering others is that of role modeling and teaching (Copp, 1986). The APN not only should apply the skills of critical thinking but should demonstrate those skills to other nurses and members of the health care team. Asking and helping nurses and patients to identify, explore, and analyze values and assumptions will cultivate skills in critical reflection and invite the consideration of alternative interpretations of the issue. In this way, the APN helps clarify the interests and obligations of others in ethical decision making.

The APN must address these intraprofessional barriers and educate other caregivers in ways that help them to describe and discuss the ethical concerns. Through role modeling, the APN can illustrate ways to identify and clarify moral problems as well as guide others through the process of moral action. Ethics rounds and retrospective case reviews are two additional strategies the APN can propose to educate and support other nurses in examining ethical issues. Nurses must be able to express diverse views without fearing ridicule or rejection from peers. An environment that supports ethical reasoning and judgment will foster action.

Interprofessional Barriers

Nurses and physicians define, perceive, analyze, and reason through ethical problems from distinct and sometimes opposing perspectives. Although the roles are complementary, these differing approaches may create conflict between the nurse and physician, further separating and isolating the perspectives. The physician either may be unaware of the nurse's differing opinion or does not recognize this difference as a conflict (Gramelspracher, Howell, & Young, 1986). Conflicts are intensified when the physician does not agree with the nurse that certain details and specifics of the situation are important or simply does not feel accountable to resolve the conflict with the nurse (Gramelspracher et al., 1986; Haddad, 1991). The APN must first deal with the interprofessional communication problems between the nurse and physician before seeking resolution of ethical problems.

Although open communication is a necessary component of the collaborative environment, it is not sufficient. Physicians and other members of the health care team must understand the nurse's role and responsibilities. In the traditional hospital setting, physicians viewed and many still view the nurse as subordinate and functioning primarily to carry out the physician's orders (Gramelspracher et al., 1986). In some cases, physicians perceive their authority as threatened when nurses expand their education and assume more autonomous roles as APNs (Haddad, 1991). They may also feel threatened by the level of expertise, beyond that of the physician, that the APN may demonstrate in her or his clinical area, such as pain management or the home management of medical problems. However, respect may increase as the physician realizes the APN's competence and accountability and recognizes that the physician and nurse roles may be very complementary in improving patient care.

Successful collaboration between nurses and physicians is grounded in communication, cooperation, competence, accountability, and trust (Baggs & Schmitt, 1988). These factors may be influenced negatively or positively by the professional relationship that exists between the physician and the APN. For whom does the APN work — the physician, the department, the institution? Who pays the APN's salary? How is the APN paid? Are APNs able to bill for their services, or are they paid from physician or institutional billings? These factors certainly influence the issue of power in the relationship. What role did the physician have in hiring the APN? Was the physician professionally invested in working with APNs initially, or did the institution decide this was a "good idea" and the physicians would now "work with them"? Obviously, the physician who actively seeks to work with an APN is more likely to have a successful and collaborative interaction. However, even in this case the intention may not necessarily be focused toward improvement in patient care by adding another discipline's expertise, but rather bringing an APN on the team to make the physician's job easier. Do the physician and APN work as a team or as two independent agents? What is the level of interaction between APN and physician: constant, side-by-side interaction, or once a day or once a week? When interaction with an APN is a new experience for a physician, more frequent interaction will define the relationship sooner (for better or worse).

Other factors also influence this professional relationship and issues of control. It is more difficult to separate malpractice liabilities when the APN and physician are working together, collaboratively and complementarily, or in an employer-employee relationship, than when the two are entirely independent. The patient's perceptions and expectations of "who's in charge," "whom do I call with problems," and "who has the final say"; the APN's role in the patient's care; and the APN's interaction with the physician will influence the overall interaction between physician and APN. If the patient sees early on that the APN has a role and the physician recognizes and reinforces that role, then in fact the APN will have a more significant and clinically important role. Conversely, if the physician does not refer APN-specific issues to the APN but attempts to handle them herself or himself, or does not define for the patient the importance of the APN's role, the patient is unlikely to see the APN as important to his or her health care. Thus, in a somewhat circular manner, the physician then can influence the patient's perception of the APN's role. The patient's perception of the APN's role and influence in his or her care will in turn influence the professional interaction, balance of power, and level of collaborative behavior between physician and APN.

Again, open communication, cooperation, demonstrated competence, accountability for both role and actions, and trust by both the physician and the APN will facilitate overcoming these barriers to successful collaboration. Finally, time and ongoing interactions in this relatively new (for many physicians) arena will also aid in improving the professional relationship.

Patient/Provider Barriers

Health care providers, employees of the health care institution, and patients and families make up the multicultural clinical setting in which most APNs practice. Nurses are taught to respect the patient's cultural values and beliefs and to avoid imposing traditional Western customs and values in a paternalistic manner. As noted earlier, APNs may encounter a cultural conflict when they are confronted with a cultural practice that they regard as harmful (Kikuchi, 1996). For example, parents may inform a NP in a pediatric outpatient setting that, because of cultural and religious reasons, they do not want their child immunized. In this case, the NP is faced with a cultural belief that places both the child and community at risk (Kikuchi, 1996). The NP wants to preserve the parent's rights and preferences but is concerned about the child's best interests and the potential harm to other children should they be exposed to an illness from a nonimmunized child. Issues that result from cultural diversity are difficult to resolve without help from others more familiar with the specific cultural practices and beliefs. Occasionally contact with the language department of a local university can direct the APN to helpful resources. In troubling cases, when the risk of harm is great, the APN should consult with clergy and other resources to help distill some reasonable options that preserve the rights and dignity of the patient and family.

The absence of an advance directive may be a barrier to upholding the patient's wishes regarding end-of-life care. Advance directives are legal documents that support the rights of patients to determine in advance their wishes for future end-of-life treatment. There are two types of advance directives, the living will and the durable power of attorney for health care or health care proxy. For patients who have executed an advance directive, the APN should discuss with the patient and family how the advance directive will guide end-of-life decision making. APNs should encourage patients without an advance directive to consider completing the health care proxy portion. This section allows the patient to appoint an individual who will make health care treatment choices for the patient in the event the patient becomes incapacitated. If no advance directive is executed, the decision maker for the incapacitated patient is based on the state statute and an estranged relative may be assigned this responsibility.

Another barrier to ethical practice that challenges many APNs is the issue of patient noncompliance. Patients may choose not to be actively involved in their care or in improving their well-being. A patient's actions may be entirely contradictory to the APN's instructions, which raises numerous ethical questions. Once the underlying reason for noncompliance is explored, the APN has several choices. Certainly the first response is to determine if the reason for the noncompliance can be rectified, such as obtaining financial support to assist in purchasing medications. However, if the patient simply chooses to ignore the agreed upon plan of care, the APN may be faced with terminating the patient-provider relationship, maintaining the relationship with less optimal objectives for care, or continuing to try to persuade the patient to comply with the best treatment plan. Often the APN spends a disproportionate amount of time with noncompliant patients, attending to preventable exacerbations of their illness or in follow-up conversations attempting to convince the patient to follow the recommended treatment. These patients are unsettling to the APN because other patients, who are more amenable to the plan of care, receive less time than the noncompliant patient receives. There are no easy solutions to managing the noncompliant patient. In many cases, patients do not intentionally choose to ignore the provider's recommendations. Other factors, such as impaired thinking and concentration, financial issues, emotional disorders, and other priorities, conflict with the patient's ability to follow the prescribed treatment plan. Members of the health care team often view patient compliance as a direct responsibility of the APN, and APNs may feel pressure from the team when efforts to enhance patient compliance are unsuccessful. In these cases, the APN should solicit help from other resources, such as social workers or home health nurses, to help uncover the causes of noncompliance.

In some cases, the health care team, including the APN, has one perspective based on common values and beliefs. When the team presents a unified perspective that challenges the patient's and family's values, feelings of intimidation surface and the patient and family may become silent. Rather than first trying to elicit the patient and family perspectives, the health care team often states the plan of care and goal of treatment without a clear understanding of the patient's wishes. The process of intimidation is subtle and unintentional. The health care team does not strive to repress the patient's autonomy. However, the act of presenting information in a clear, direct, and straightforward manner is interpreted by some as the right way and only way to manage the patient's condition. This practice is often seen in fast-paced environments with significant time constraints on providers.

It is often easier for patients and families to express diverse views when someone solicits their position and genuinely listens to their perspectives. The APN can help patients and families overcome feelings of intimidation by asking what they think should be done, clarifying any misconceptions, and accepting their understanding and interpretation of the situation. Unconditional acceptance can break down barriers and lead to communication that is open and honest and facilitates shared decision making.

Organizational/Environmental Barriers

Although other strategies can yield successful resolutions, the approaches of collaboration and compromise are usually more satisfactory to all parties. These methods require more time from the patient and health care team, and, unfortunately, time often is so limited that the benefits of collaboration or compromise are seldom realized. To overcome this barrier, the APN may need to resolve the dilemma in stages, with the most central issue addressed first. For example, if a patient is not receiving adequate pain management because the bedside nurse is concerned about hastening death, the clinical nurse specialist (CNS) should first focus on relieving the patient's pain. Once the immediate need is addressed, the CNS can help the nurse identify nonpharmacological interventions to promote comfort and educate the nurse about the dosage and timing of medications to avoid wide fluctuations in pain management. An additional strategy such as arranging for the nurse to rotate to a hospice unit represents a preventive approach to avert similar dilemmas in the future.

The issues of continuity of care and knowing the patient and family are significant problems in acute care settings. Many institutions continue to push for shorter lengths of stay and more streamlined and "efficient" management of patients. Typically, this environment does not embrace the concept of "knowing the patient." Rather, care in this climate is based on knowing the expected response to illness and treatment of a select population of patients. In other words, individualized care is not standard practice. Although this philosophy has numerous financial advantages, often the patient and family loses the necessary individualized attention that can greatly enhance their recovery. The APN struggles in this environment to better meet the needs of patients and families. Certainly the APN must advocate for providing individualized care to patients and families; however, this position is difficult and risky when it contradicts the objectives of the institution or third-party payers. Despite the institutional or third-party payer goals, the APN is morally obligated to work toward improving the work environment if current conditions are not in the patient's best interests. Fortunately, many institutions are willing to make some concessions in the delivery of patient care if there are clear outcome data that support a change in practice.

It would also be wise for the APN to identify resources both within and outside the institution to assist with the process of resolution. The recognition of a moral dilemma does not commit the APN to conducting and managing the process of resolution. APNs should engage appropriate resources to address the identified needs and work toward agreement. In many situations, such as in rural clinics, resources within the organization are not available. Without another professional colleague to help decipher the problem, the APN is sometimes left with little more than intuition. Guidelines from professional organizations regarding the APN's moral obligations (see "Additional Resources") are helpful in providing some direction for action. APNs practicing in isolation should network with colleagues and establish resources for providing direction in ethical reasoning.

Moral resolution and open reflection cannot occur in an environment that devalues the perspectives of some professionals. When one group of individuals is empowered to act and other parties are constrained, a distrustful and hostile environment results. Moral issues should be addressed with an interdisciplinary approach, and the APN provides a valuable voice for nursing during dispute resolution.

CONCLUSIONS

The changing health care environment has placed extraordinary demands on nurses in independent practice settings as well as in acute care settings. The limitations of time, reimbursement, and resources conflict with nursing's moral imperatives of involvement, connection, and commitment. Ethical decision-making skills are a core competency for the APN and reflect both the art and science of nursing. The APN is in a key position to assume a more decisive role in managing the resolution of moral issues. The skills of problem identification, values clarification, negotiation, collaboration, and evaluation empower the APN to critically analyze and direct the decision-making process. The identification of patterns in the presentation of moral issues will enable the APN to engage in preventive strategies to improve the ethical qualities of patient care.

REFERENCES

Ahronheim, J. C., Moreno, J., & Zuckerman, C. (1994). *Ethics in clinical practice*. Boston: Little, Brown.

American Academy of Pediatrics, Committee on Bioethics. (1996). Ethics and the care of critically ill infants and children (RE9624). *Pediatrics, 98*(1), 149.

American Association of Colleges of Nursing. (1996). *The essentials of master's education for advanced practice nursing*. Washington, DC: Author.

American Nurses Association. (1985). *Code for nurses with interpretive statements*. Kansas City, MO: Author.

American Nurses Association. (1994). *Position statement on active euthanasia*. Washington, DC: Author.

Baggs, J. G., & Schmitt, M. H. (1988). Collaboration between nurses and physicians. *Image: The Journal of Nursing Scholarship, 20*(3), 145-149.

Beare, P. G. (1989). The essentials of win-win negotiation for the clinical nurse specialist. *Clinical Nurse Specialist, 13*(3), 138.

Beauchamp, T. L., & Childress, J. F. (1994). *Principles of biomedical ethics* (4th ed.). New York: Oxford University Press.

Benner, P. (1991). The role of experience, narrative and community in skilled ethical comportment. *Advances in Nursing Science, 14*(2), 1.

Calkins, M. E. (1993). Ethical issues in the elderly ESRD patient. *ANNA Journal, 20*(5), 569.

Chambliss, D. F. (1996). *Beyond caring: Hospitals, nurses, and the social organization of ethics*. Chicago, IL: University of Chicago Press.

Chervenak, F. A., & McCullough, L. B. (1995). The threat of the new managed practice of medicine to patients' autonomy. *Journal of Clinical Ethics, 6*(4), 320-323.

Childress, J. F. (1994). Principles-oriented bioethics: An analysis and assessment from within. In E. R. DuBose, R. Hamel, & L. J. O'Connell (Eds.), *A matter of principles?* (pp. 72-98). Valley Forge, PA: Trinity Press International.

Cooper, M. C. (1989). Gilligan's different voice: A perspective for nursing. *Journal of Professional Nursing, 5*(1), 10-16.

Cooper, M. C. (1991). Principle-oriented ethics and the ethic of care: A creative tension. *Advances in Nursing Science, 14*(2), 22.

Copp, L. A. (1986). The nurse as advocate for vulnerable persons. *Journal of Advanced Nursing, 11*(3), 255-263.

Council on Ethical and Judicial Affairs. (1990). Black-white disparities in health care. *JAMA, 263*(17), 2346.

Council on Ethical and Judicial Affairs. (1991). Gender disparities in clinical decision making. *JAMA, 266*(4), 559.

Cruzan v. Missouri Department of Health, et al., 110 S. Ct. 2841 (1990).

Doukas D. J., & Gorenflo, D. W. (1993). Analyzing the values history: An evaluation of patient medical values and advance directives. *Journal of Clinical Ethics, 4*(1), 41-45.

Doukas, D. J., & McCullough, L. B. (1991). The values history: The evaluation of the patient's values and advance directives. *Journal of Family Practice, 32*(2), 145-153.

Dreyfus, H. L., Dreyfus, S. E., & Benner, P. (1996). Implications of the phenomenology of expertise for teaching and learning everyday skillful ethical comportment. In P. Benner, C. A. Tanner, & C. A. Chesla (Eds.), *Expertise in nursing practice: Caring, clinical judgment and ethics* (pp. 258-279). New York: Springer-Verlag.

Eisenberg, L. (1999). The social imperatives of medical research. In T. L. Beauchamp & L. Walters (Eds.), *Contemporary issues in bioethics* (5th ed., pp. 449-456). London: Wadsworth.

Erlen, J. A., & Frost, B. (1991). Nurses' perceptions of powerlessness in influencing ethical decisions. *Western Journal of Nursing Research, 13*(2), 397-407.

Erlen, J. A., & Mellors, M. P. (1995). Managed care and the nurse's ethical obligations to patients. *Orthopaedic Nursing, 14*(6), 42-45.

Ewigman, B. G., Crane, J. D., Frigoletto, F. D., LeFevre, M. L., Bain, R. P., & McNellis, D. (1993). Effect of perinatal ultrasound screening on perinatal outcome; Radius Study Group. *New England Journal of Medicine 329*(12), 821-827.

Fenton, M. V., & Brykczynski, K. A. (1993). Qualitative distinctions and similarities in the practice of clinical nurse specialists and nurse practitioners. *Journal of Professional Nursing, 9,* 313-326.

Fisher, R., & Ury, W. (1981). *Getting to yes*. New York: Viking Penguin.

Forrow, L., Arnold, R. M., & Parker, L. S. (1993). Preventive ethics: Expanding the horizons of clinical ethics. *Journal of Clinical Ethics, 4*(4), 287-294.

Fowler, M. D. (1999). Relic or resource? The Code for Nurses. *American Journal of Nursing, 99*(3), 56-58.

Gaul, A. L. (1995). Casuistry, care, compassion and ethics data analysis. *Advances in Nursing Science, 17*(3), 47.

Gilligan, C. (1982). *In a different voice.* Cambridge, MA: Harvard University Press.

Gramelspracher, G. P., Howell, J. D., & Young, M. J. (1986). Perceptions of ethical problems by nurses and physicians. *Archives of Internal Medicine, 146,* 577–578.

Gudorf, C. E. (1994). A feminist critique of biomedical principlism. In E. R. DuBose, R. Hamel, & L. J. O'Connell (Eds.), *A matter of principles?* (pp. 164–181). Valley Forge, PA: Trinity Press International.

Haddad, A. M. (1991). The nurse/physician relationship and ethical decision making. *AORN Journal, 53*(1), 151–154, 156.

Hall, J. K. (1996). Assisted suicide: Nurse practitioners as providers? *Nurse Practitioner 21*(10), 63–66, 71.

Jonsen, A. R., & Toulmin, S. (1988). *The abuse of casuistry: A history of moral reasoning.* Berkeley: University of California Press.

Kikuchi, J. F. (1996). Multicultural ethics in nursing education: A potential threat to responsible practice. *Journal of Professional Nursing, 12*(3), 159–165.

Kopelman, L. M., Irons, T. G., & Kopelman, A. E. (1988). Neonatologists judge the "Baby Doe" regulations. *New England Journal of Medicine, 318*(11), 677–683.

Krouse, H. J., & Roberts, S. J. (1989). Nurse-patient interactive styles: Power, control, and satisfaction. *Western Journal of Nursing Research, 11*(6), 717–725.

LaMear-Tucker, D., & Friedson, J. (1997). Resolving moral conflict: The critical care nurse's role. *Critical Care Nurse, 17*(2), 55.

Leavitt, F. J. (1996). Educating nurses for their future role in bioethics. *Nursing Ethics, 3*(1), 39.

Lynch, V. A. (1991). Forensic nursing in the emergency department: A new role for the 1990's. *Critical Care Nursing Quarterly, 14*(3), 69–86.

O'Connor, K. F. (1996). Ethical/moral experiences of oncology nurses. *Oncology Nursing Forum, 23*(5), 787–794.

Olczak, P. V., Grosch, J. W., & Duffy, K. G. (1991). Toward a synthesis: The art with the science of community mediation. In K. G. Duffy, J. W. Grosch, & P. V. Olczak (Eds.), *Community mediation* (pp. 329–343). New York: The Guilford Press.

Omery, A., Henneman, E., Billet, B., Luna-Raines, M., & Brown-Saltzman, K. (1995). Ethical issues in hospital-based nursing practice. *Journal of Cardiovascular Nursing, 9*(3), 43–53.

Omnibus Budget Reconciliation Act of 1990, PL, 101-508, 42 U.S.C. § 4206.

Ostermeyer, M. (1991). Conducting the mediation. In K. G. Duffy, J. W. Grosch, & P. V. Olczak

(Eds.), *Community mediation* (pp. 91–104). New York: The Guilford Press.

Pike, A. W. (1991). Moral outrage and moral discourse in nurse-physician collaboration. *Journal of Professional Nursing, 7*(6), 351–362.

Purtilo, R. (1993). *Ethical dimensions in the health professions* (2nd ed.). Philadelphia: W. B. Saunders.

Rest, J. R. (1986). *Moral development: Advances in research and theory.* New York: Praeger.

Rowdin, M. A. (1995). Conflicts in managed care. *New England Journal of Medicine, 332*(9), 604.

Saulo, M., & Wagener, R. J. (1996). How good case managers make tough choices: Ethics and mediation. *Journal of Care Management, 2*(1), 8.

Scanlon, C. (1994). Survey yields significant results. *American Nurses Association Center for Ethics and Human Rights Communiqué, 3*(4).

Schlenk, J. S. (1997). Advance directives: Role of nurse practitioners. *Journal of the American Academy of Nurse Practitioners, 9*(7), 317.

Scott, R. A., Aiken, L. H., Mechanic, D., & Moravcsik, J. (1995). Organizational aspects of caring. *The Milbank Quarterly, 73*(1), 77–95.

Shannon, S. E. (1997). The roots of interdisciplinary conflict around ethical issues. *Critical Care Nursing Clinics of North America, 9*(1), 13.

Smeltzer, C. H. (1991). The art of negotiation: An everyday experience. *Journal of Nursing Administration, 21*(7/8), 26–30.

Solomon, M. Z., Jennings, B., Guilfoy, V., Jackson, R., O'Donnell, L., Wolf, S. M., Nolan, K., Koch-Weser, D., & Donnelly, S. (1991). Toward an expanded vision of clinical ethics education: From individual to the institution. *Kennedy Institute of Ethics Journal, 1*(3), 225.

Solomon, M. Z., O'Donnell, L., Jennings, B., Guilfoy, V., Wolf, S. M., Nolan, K., Jackson, R., Koch-Weser, D., & Donnelley, S. (1993). Decisions near the end of life: Professional views on life-sustaining treatments. *American Journal of Public Health, 83*(1), 14–23.

Spencer, E. M. (1997). A new role for institutional ethics committees: Organizational ethics. *Journal of Clinical Ethics, 8*(4), 372–376.

Spielman, B. J. (1993). Conflict in medical ethics cases: Seeking patterns of resolution. *Journal of Clinical Ethics, 4*(3), 212–218.

SUPPORT Principal Investigators. (1995). A controlled trial to improve care for seriously ill hospitalized patients: The Study to Understand Prognosis and Preferences for Outcomes and Risks of Treatments (SUPPORT). *JAMA, 274,* 1591–1598.

Toulmin, S. (1994). Casuistry and clinical ethics. In E. R. DuBose, R. Hamel, & L. J. O'Connell (Eds.), *A matter of principles?* (pp. 310–318). Valley Forge, PA: Trinity Press International.

Turner, L. N., Marquis, K., & Burman, M. E. (1996). Rural nurse practitioners: Perceptions of ethical dilemmas. *Journal of the American Academy of Nurse Practitioners, 8*(6), 269.

United States Child Abuse Prevention and Treatment Amendments of 1984, 42 USCS § 5101.

Ury, W. (1993). *Getting past no.* New York: Bantam Books.

Uustal, D. (1987). Values: The cornerstone of nursing's moral art. In M. D. Fowler & J. Levine-Ariff (Eds.), *Ethics at the bedside* (pp. 136–153). Philadelphia: J. B. Lippincott.

van Hooft, S. (1990). Moral education for nursing decisions. *Journal of Advanced Nursing, 15,* 210.

Viens, D. C. (1994). Moral dilemmas experienced by nurse practitioners. *Nurse Practitioner Forum, 5*(4), 209–214.

Welton, G. L. (1991). Parties in conflict: Their characteristics and perceptions. In K. G. Duffy, J. W. Grosch, & P. V. Olczak (Eds.), *Community mediation* (pp. 105–118). New York: The Guilford Press.

Williams, J. K., & Lea, D. H. (1995). Applying new genetic technologies: Assessment and ethical considerations. *Nurse Practitioner, 20*(7), 16, 21–26.

Winters, G., Glass, E., & Sakurai, C. (1993). Ethical issues in oncology nursing practice: An overview of topics and strategies. *Oncology Nursing Forum, 20*(Suppl. 10), 21–34.

Wright, F., Cohen, S., & Caroselli, C. (1997). Diverse decisions: How culture affects ethical decision making. *Critical Care Nursing Clinics of North America, 9*(1), 63.

Zaner, R. M. (1988). *Ethics and the clinical encounter.* Englewood Cliffs, NJ: Prentice-Hall.

Joint Commission for Accreditation of Healthcare Organizations. (1900). *Accreditation manual for hospitals: Standards on patient rights and organization ethics.* Oakbrook, IL: Author.

Kennedy Institute of Ethics. (1999). *New titles in bioethics.* Washington, DC: Georgetown University Press.

National Institutes of Health Office of Extramural Research, Office for Protection from Research Risks. (1993). *Protecting human research subjects: Institutional review board guidebook.* Washington, DC: National Institutes of Health.

President's Commission for the Study of Ethical Problems in Medicine and Biomedical and Behavioral Research. (1983). *Deciding to forego life-sustaining treatment.* Washington, DC: Author.

President's Commission for the Study of Ethical Problems in Medicine and Biomedical and Behavioral Research. (1983). *Making health care decisions.* Washington, DC: Author.

President's Commission for the Study of Ethical Problems in Medicine and Biomedical and Behavioral Research. (1983). *Screening and counseling for genetic conditions.* Washington, DC: Author.

Ross, J. W., Bayley, C. M., & Pugh, D. (Eds.). (1986). *Handbook for hospital ethics committees.* Chicago: American Hospital Association.

Task-Force to Improve the Care of Terminally-Ill Oregonians. (1998). *The Oregon Death with Dignity Act: A Guidebook for Health Care Providers.* Portland OR: OHSU Center for Ethics in Health Care.

Additional Resources

American Hospital Association. (1994). *Values in conflict: Resolving ethical issues in health care.* Chicago: Author.

American Medical Association, Council on Ethical and Judicial Affairs, (1996). *Code of medical ethics: Current opinions with annotations.* Chicago: American Medical Association.

American Nurses Association. (1985). *Code for nurses with interpretive statements.* Kansas City, MO: Author.

American Society for Bioethics and Humanities. (1998). *Core competencies for health care ethics consultation.* Glenview, IL: Author.

Campbell, M. L. (1998). *Foregoing life-sustaining therapy.* Aliso Viejo, CA: American Association of Critical-Care Nurses.

Encyclopedia of bioethics. (1995). New York: Simon & Schuster Macmillan.

Hoffman, D. E., Boyle, P., & Levenson, S. A. (1995). *Handbook for nursing home ethics committees.* Washington DC: American Association of Homes and Services for the Aging.

Websites with Ethics Policy Statements or Guidelines

American Academy of Neurology, Practice Statements: *www.aan.com/resources.html*

American Academy of Pediatrics, Policy Statements: *www.aap.org/policy*

American Association of Nurse-Anesthetists (AANA): *www.aana.com*

American College of Nurse-Midwives: *www.acnm.org/*

American College of Medical Genetics, Policy Statements: *www.faseb.org/genetics/acmg*

American College of Physicians, Center for Ethics and Professionalism: *www.acponline.org/ethics*

American College of Surgeons, Statements: *www.facs.org*

American Medical Association, Council on Ethical and Judicial Affairs: *www.ama-assn.org*

American Nurse's Association: *www.ana.org*

American Society for Law, Medicine and Ethics: *www.aslme.org*

American Society for Reproductive Medicine: *www.asrm.org*

American Society of Anesthesiologists, Policy Statements: *www.asahq.org/standards*
American Society for Transplantation, Policy Statements: *www.a-s-t.org/index.html*
Americans for Better Care of the Dying: *www.abcd-caring.org*
Center to Improve the Care of the Dying: *www.gwu.edu/~cicd*
Institute of Medicine, National Academy of Sciences: *www4.nas.edu/IOM/IOMHome.nsf*
National Bioethics Advisory Commission: *www.bioethics.gov*
National Hospice Organization: *www.nho.org*
National Institutes of Health, Office for Protection from Research Risks: *grants.nih.gov/grants/oprr/oprr.htm*
National League for Nursing: *www.nln.org*
Project on Death in America: *www.soros.org/death.html*

Society for Critical Care Medicine: *www.sccm.org*
United Network for Organ Sharing, Policy Statements: *www.unos.org*
University of Pennyslvania Center for Bioethics: *www.bioethics.net*

Ethics and Legal Search Sites

Bioethicsline database on Internet Grateful Med (literature search): *igm.nlm.nih.gov*
Legal Information Institute: *www.law.cornell.edu*
Medical College of Wisconsin Center for the Study of Bioethics, Bioethics Online Service (literature search): *www.mcw.edu/bioethics*
National Reference Center for Bioethics Literature: *www.georgetown.edu/research/nrcbl*
State laws on the Internet: *www.legalonline.com*

PART III

Advanced Practice Roles:
The Operational Definitions of
Advanced Nursing Practice

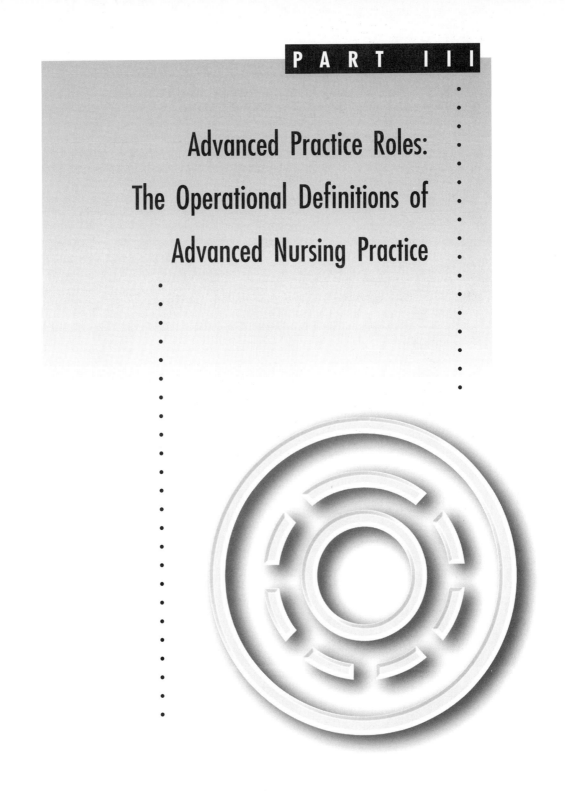

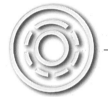

The Clinical Nurse Specialist

• P A T R I C I A   S.   A.   S P A R A C I N O

INTRODUCTION

The clinical nurse specialist (CNS) role was created to keep expert nurses in clinical practice and to improve patient care. Because the role was developed to keep the clinical expert at the bedside, without traditional staff nurse responsibilities, the context of its development and implementation has been primarily in hospital settings. The CNS is a registered nurse "who, through study and supervised practice at the graduate level (master's or doctorate), has become expert in a defined area of knowledge and practice in a selected clinical area of nursing" (American Nurses Association [ANA], 1980, p. 23). The dimensions of the CNS role are expert clinician, consultant, educator, and researcher. Integrating these dimensions is difficult but essential to sustain the role's integrity, yet differentiating between the components is necessary to keep responsibilities clear and contributions distinct. Within these four dimensions there are competencies, including, but not limited to, direct clinical practice, consultation, expert teaching and coaching, scholarly or scientific inquiry, clinical and professional leadership, collaboration, and ethical decision making (ANA, 1986; Hamric, 1989a). The impact and influence of the CNS is most clearly felt within these three spheres: patients or clients, nursing personnel, and organizations or networks (National Association of Clinical Nurse Specialists [NACNS], 1998). Competencies and spheres of influence are discussed later in this chapter.

The role's historical development in the United States has been described previously (Bigbee, 1996; Hamric, 1983b, 1989a; Hoeffer & Murphy, 1984; Sparacino, 1990) and in this text (Chapter 1). The nurse specialist or CNS role also exists in other countries, such as Canada, the United Kingdom, Australia, Japan, and China. However, both the definition and implementation in each country are influenced by culture, education, standards, and practice differences that are not discussed in this chapter.

The role's professional development has confronted many challenges. Its evolution has not been logical or linear. The role was implemented before the existence of a coherent curriculum for educational preparation, criteria for certification, consistent use of capabilities, agreement about regulatory control, or implementation of third-party reimbursement. Much has been expected of role incumbents, and too often evaluation of the CNS's impact has not been tied to improving patient outcomes, efficient use of resources, cost efficiency, or revenue generation. Yet the CNS is best prepared to respond to rapid systems changes. Not surprisingly, over the past 20 years the popularity of the CNS role has waxed and waned; positions have been cut when the role was deemed expendable, and reinstituted when its contributions were considered invaluable. However, the role has survived. Its effectiveness is derived from its flexibility, but the role's versatility has made it vulnerable to restructuring and retitling. Role flexibility has been taken too far when CNS and case manager titles are alternately applied several times to the same nurse within a year. The CNS role is not interchangeable with other roles; no other advanced practice role is subject to the expectation of interchangeability (Boyle, 1996). The value of the CNS role is questioned when CNSs and administrators do not understand the role, and disparate and arbitrary implementation and utilization dissipate its impact.

The intent of the CNS role is to improve patient care and influence others. CNSs are successful when they deliver high-quality care that can be measured in terms of cost-effectiveness, patient outcomes, and improvements in nursing practice. The CNS's clinical reasoning is not limited to the consideration of physiological and psychological variables, but extends beyond the boundaries of clinical practice to incorporate education, research, social policy, organizational factors, and political change. Historically, CNSs focused primarily on direct care and patient responsibilities, and considered the systems context in which care was given. The emphasis has shifted to system obligations with little responsibility for patient care. Currently the emphasis on health care reform and the restructuring of health care reimbursement is on cost containment and care-efficient strategies. Health care reform has influenced the shift in emphasis from extraordinary to ordinary, from costly to more cost-efficient, from curative to preventive. CNSs have been integral to this effort, designing and implementing practice guidelines and innovative practice models, evaluating the cost efficiency and fiscal impact of technology and its impact on patient care, the quality of care given, and the protection of continuity of care and patient satisfaction.

PROFILE OF THE ROLE

Role Definition

The nursing profession, specialty organizations, and nurse authors have developed and refined the definition of the CNS role. In 1976, the ANA provided an operational definition of the CNS (ANA, Congress of Nursing Practice, 1976). In 1980, the ANA published *Nursing: A Social Policy Statement.* This document was the first to differentiate between the specialist prepared at the graduate level and the nurse with a baccalaureate degree who is a specialist in nursing practice but "a generalist in providing the full range of nursing practice"; it promulgated the classic CNS definition presented above. In 1983, Hamric further developed the definition by making the distinction between the direct care functions (e.g., expert practitioner, role model, and patient advocate) and indirect care functions (e.g., change agent, consultant/ resource person, clinical teacher, supervisor, researcher, liaison, and innovator) (Hamric, 1983b). In 1986, the ANA's Council of Clinical Nurse Specialists expanded the established definition to delineate the multifaceted dimensions of the role, including expert clinical practice, education, consultation, research, and administration components, and to define the flexible boundaries as determined by the needs of complex patient populations, evolving nursing specialties, and the needs of the health care market. In 1989, Hamric proposed the CNS role definition, using a three-dimensional model to delineate the role's defining characteristics and the relationships between primary criteria for the role (e.g., graduate study in the specialty, certification, and focus of practice on the patient/client/family), the four subroles (clinical expert, consultant, educator, and researcher), and skills or competencies (e.g., change agent, collaborator, clinical leader, role model, patient advocate) (Hamric, 1989a).

For more than a decade, there has been discussion about the feasibility of singular titling (Cronenwett, 1996; Sparacino & Durand, 1986; Spross & Hamric, 1983), analyzing the commonalities and differences between the CNS and nurse practitioner (NP) roles (Fenton & Brykczynski, 1993; Keane & Richmond, 1993). The singular titling proposal attempted to address educational, regulatory, and other related issues with some uniformity and efficiency. Although the proposal for singular titling generated significant debate and opposition, the generic advanced practice nurse (APN) designation became widely accepted as nomenclature for the CNS, NP, certified nurse-midwife, and certified registered nurse anesthetist. By 1995, the umbrella APN title was reflected in the ANA's *Nursing's Social Policy Statement,* and the APN definition was remarkably similar to the CNS definition in the 1980 edition of the ANA's social policy statement: "The nurse in advanced practice acquires specialized knowledge and skills through study and supervised practice at the master's or doctoral level in nursing. The content of study in the specialty area includes theories and research findings relevant to the core of specialization" (ANA, 1995, p. 14).

Distribution

Determining how many CNSs are currently practicing in the United States has been an elusive goal. The ANA's database from 1980 listed 19,070 nurses who identified themselves as CNSs, but only 5,245 of the 19,070 were prepared at the graduate level (ANA, 1985). By 1993, it was estimated that CNSs numbered between 40,000

(American Association of Colleges of Nursing, 1993) and 58,000 (ANA, 1993). The difficulty in reporting more recent estimates for numbers of CNSs is twofold: most CNSs are members of specialty nursing organizations rather than general professional organizations, and specialty nursing organizations now use the generic APN category for reporting numbers of APN members, which include CNSs, nurse practitioners, and other APN roles.

CNS COMPETENCIES AND SPHERES OF INFLUENCE

The classic dimensions or subroles of the CNS role are expert clinician, consultant, change agent (leader), educator, and researcher. Integrating these dimensions is difficult but necessary, yet maintaining distinction between the elements is important to keep role responsibilities clear (Sparacino & Cooper, 1990). There are competencies, or skills, that a CNS must master to accomplish and integrate the subroles. Some competencies are common threads that weave throughout core competencies, such as clinical and professional leadership, collaboration, and ethical decision making. The core competencies include direct and indirect clinical practice, consulting, expert teaching and coaching, and scholarly or scientific inquiry. What the CNS does (e.g., the four subroles) and how the CNS performs the role (e.g., competencies) can have a substantial impact on the practice setting (e.g., spheres of influence). Practice in each sphere of influence (patients/clients, nurses, and organizations/networks) (NACNS, 1998), in combination with mastery of CNS competencies, is essential to be a successful CNS.

CNSs have been challenged by maintaining patient care as the focus while successfully integrating the essential role dimensions, competencies, and multiple clinical and organizational responsibilities. Various texts (Gawlinski & Kern, 1994; Hamric & Spross, 1989; Hamric, Spross, & Hanson, 1996; Sparacino, Cooper, & Minarik, 1990) and the professional journal *Clinical Nurse Specialist* offer many practical suggestions for successfully implementing the CNS role. Rather than repeating those recommendations, this section emphasizes key elements and pragmatic implementation of the competencies, with examples of CNS impact within the spheres of influence.

CNS Competencies

CLINICAL PRACTICE

Clinical practice is the heart of advanced nursing practice. The genesis of the CNS role was specialized and expert clinical practice with responsibility for direct care of patients. Many authors have described strategies for successfully implementing the expert clinician subrole, building on the foundations laid by earlier authors (Felder, 1983; Koetters, 1989; Sparacino & Cooper, 1990). Each strategy is dependent on the individual CNS, particular practice setting, and prevailing health care environment. Patient care can be direct or indirect. For many years, the CNS's direct clinical practice was imbedded in the multidisciplinary care of the hospital setting and was not linked to patient outcomes or resource utilization (Hamric, 1995). Thus there were few tangible or useful data to justify the role when health care systems that were restructuring looked at the bottom line. However, most of the patients currently cared for in settings where CNSs practice (hospital, home care, or community) are sicker and frailer and in need of specialized, expert care. Students or colleagues have questions that include, What patient is a CNS most likely to care for directly? What sort of care does a CNS give? How does a CNS decide to allocate time for direct care, or guide other nurses delivering that care? How does the CNS's direct care responsibilities differ from those of staff nurses and of other APNs?

A CNS is most likely to directly care for a patient whose diagnosis or care is complex, unique, or problematic. A CNS's clinical expertise and specialty influence the patient population to whom care is given. Examples of complex or problematic patients include a very-low-birth-weight infant, a frail older person with multiple hospital readmissions, a child with complex congenital heart disease, a young pregnant woman with a transplanted organ, or a child with multiple trauma and no payer source who is in need of extensive rehabilitation. Examples of unique situations are the care of a patient with the rarely used Eloesser flap for treatment of a tuberculous empyema; an evaluation and implementation of a new intervention, such as continuous renal replacement therapy; or an introduction of an experimental chemotherapy.

Direct clinical practice is also a means by which the CNS can assess the quality of care for a specific patient population; it provides a qualitative assessment that enhances the interpretation of quantitative data and directs the change in care provided. For example, when a field nurse notes that older home care patients are not consistently taking medications, a CNS's clinical expertise and involvement with the direct care of the same patients can provide a more detailed and complex assessment. The result of a CNS's assessment may be that the older patients are cognitively impaired and therefore unable to remember to take their medications, the medication regimen is too complex and so doses are missed, or the medicines prescribed are too expensive and not covered by supplemental insurance or Medicaid and so doses are halved or skipped or prescriptions not filled. Outcomes of the CNS's evaluation might include integrating advanced assessment skills such as cognitive screening into the admission assessment of all older patients, identifying therapeutic alternatives such as a simpler or more economical medication regimen to improve treatment adherence, or other creative interventions to promote health and quality of life.

The type of care a CNS gives is either regular or episodic (Koetters, 1989). Examples of regular care are providing nursing care for all patients with newly diagnosed diabetes in a community clinic, delivering total patient care for the first patients in a fetal surgery program, or visiting all patients with congestive heart failure in a home care agency who have had more than one hospital readmission within 60 days of the initial hospitalization. A CNS in private practice certainly provides regular patient care. Episodic care helps a CNS assess and intervene in a particular problem. Examples of episodic care include planning and coordinating a patient's complex hospital discharge, facilitating a support group for patients with primary pulmonary hypertension, or providing total patient care (having the same responsibilities as a staff nurse) to determine the feasibility of proposed changes in the patient care or other system changes. Involvement in regular or episodic care enables CNSs to identify problems that interfere with care and require CNS intervention. Examples include lack of staff knowledge, need for clinical policies or procedures, or the need for conflict mediation among team members. For each clinical situation, a CNS takes a comprehensive approach and uses a high level of discriminative judgment, advanced knowledge, and expert skill, including expertise in the technical and humanistic aspects of care. Although clinical expertise is the cornerstone of CNS practice, a CNS will not be successful because of knowledge or technical expertise alone.

There are advantages and disadvantages to providing direct patient care. The advantages of regular and consistent direct patient care are that it provides a CNS the opportunity to demonstrate clinical competency, maintain clinical expertise, identify staff learning needs, role model important clinical behaviors, evaluate resource utilization, and ensure CNS visibility and accessibility. Certain clinical skills, particularly psychomotor ones such as administering chemotherapy or troubleshooting ventricular assist devices, become less proficient over time if not periodically used. Regular clinical practice helps a CNS to maintain the expertise and clinical competence needed to practice and to develop the skills of other nurses. In addition to maintaining and refining clinical skills, direct clinical practice is imperative at two particular points: during a CNS's orientation to establish credibility, and prior to and occasionally throughout the implementation of organizational change to assess the impact of changes on patient care. CNSs must weigh the benefits and costs of different ways to implement the direct care competency. Advantages such as developing credibility with staff or maintaining one's skills are evaluated against potential disadvantages such as financial costs, competing demands, time pressures, and other factors. For example, with economic constraints, unless the CNS can make a compelling justification, administrators are unlikely to see direct care as an organizational priority, forcing the CNS to limit the amount of time spent in direct care.

A CNS's clinical practice interventions may be continuous or time limited, but should result in improvements in clinical outcomes, patient/family satisfaction, resource allocation, staff knowledge and skills, health care team collaboration, and organizational efficiency. A CNS intervention may be as simple as assisting a patient and family to navigate a hospital's bureaucratic maze; a successful outcome usually occurs because the CNS knows how and when to break the rules, bypass organizational or philosophical roadblocks, and focus on the patient and family.

A CNS also regularly provides indirect care, for example, when a CNS delegates care to but guides the direct care given by a staff nurse. Another type of indirect patient care is when a CNS selects a patient population in which there are recurrent problems or themes, poor outcomes, or recidivism, and then collaborates with other members of the health care team to develop and implement standards of care, critical pathways, clinical procedures, or quality or performance improvement plans. Implementation and adherence should be evaluated in order to compare outcomes; refine critical pathways, algorithms, or guidelines; improve clinical management; and further promote consistent adherence. A pathway or guideline is rarely self-sustaining, and requires a key person who continuously champions its dependable implementation if it is to be successful and achieve its intended outcome. A CNS is often the primary coordinator of such an effort.

Another type of indirect patient care provided by the CNS is related to system responsibilities for evaluating technology and its impact on patients and resources. Technology's advances have made significant changes in health care delivery. However, technological advances, the shift in health care delivery to managed care, increased competition, changing and greater consumer expectations, and capped budgets create conflicting demands and priorities. Technology has provided objective criteria with which to make clinical judgments (e.g., medication titration based on hemodynamic indices), devices with which to remotely assess a patient (e.g., telemonitoring of vital signs and weights), and interventional alternatives with which to treat (e.g., fiberoptic, robotic, and virtual reality surgery). Yet technology warrants close scrutiny, for with technology comes a responsibility to evaluate the fiscal impact, quality, environmental impact, risk versus benefit, and patient response.

CONSULTING

The literature cites many examples of the essential components of consultation (Barron & White, 1996; Hamric, 1983b) and strategies for ensuring the success of a CNS as a consultant (Noll, 1987; Sparacino & Cooper, 1990). The CNS is a content expert and so assists in suggesting a wide range of alternative approaches or solutions to clinical or systems problems, whether internal or external to the practice setting. The CNS is a resource consultant and provides pertinent information that enables nurses and others to make decisions based on a range of relevant and appropriate alternatives. The CNS is a process consultant and facilitates change so that decisions can be made for particular and future situations (Sparacino & Cooper, 1990).

A CNS can be an internal and external consultant. Internal consultation is part of a CNS's job description and includes assisting with organizational development in one's own practice setting, especially the creative use of resources and alternative strategies to bypass perceived system obstacles. A CNS may recognize that an internal consultation needs the collaboration of multiple consultants, with more than one CNS and other disciplines participating; a CNS often initiates the plan, mobilizes the resources, defuses the politics, and facilitates the resolution. Unless consultation is a CNS's primary responsibility (e.g., a psychiatric consultation liaison CNS), there may be a problem if a CNS's time is used more for consultations than direct care; the impact on patient care is less visible, unless the strategies are well documented and the outcomes measured. External consultation assists the nursing profession, a specialty organization, other health providers, and health systems external to the practice setting with approaches or solutions for specific problems.

The consultant aspect of the CNS role is not necessarily a given; it is an expectation, but each CNS's consultative skill varies. Consultation requires interpersonal skills of flexibility and trust, and a nonjudgmental and nonthreatening demeanor. Likewise, consultation requests more often are informal and occur when a CNS is already present on a patient care unit. Informal consultations are just as likely to be initiated in the hall or stairwell. Of course, actual consultation occurs in a more private location, because respect for patient confidentiality cannot be overemphasized. The goal of a consultation is to help the consultee become more knowledgeable, and so the most successful approach is to recognize the vulnerability of a nurse who initiates the consultation and to focus on the problem as perceived by the consultee. However, nursing consultation does not need to be done in isolation. Collaborative consultation with CNSs in different specialties or other health care providers, together with the staff nurses involved, results in a staff nurse learning from expert clinicians' shared and collective knowledge, consultation colleagues learning from questioning one another, and a patient benefiting from the collective wisdom and expertise. Collaborative consultation results in both the development of a plan for the effective and efficient care of a patient with complex problems, and the support and education of staff caring for a patient. See Chapter 8 for further discussion of consultation.

EXPERT TEACHING AND COACHING

There are many descriptions in the literature of the essential components of the educator role (Priest, 1989; Sparacino & Cooper, 1990) and of expert teaching and coaching skills (Clarke & Spross, 1996; see Chapter 7 in this text). Expert teaching and coaching is a part of direct clinical practice and is influenced by scholarly inquiry and research utilization. A CNS's teaching and coaching function is both formal and informal. A CNS teaches staff nurses, patients and families, graduate nursing students, clinical nurse specialists, health professionals, and consumer groups. Expert coaching implies "the existence of a relationship that is fundamental to effective teaching" (Clarke & Spross, 1996, p. 140).

A CNS is a role model for nurses, demonstrating the practical integration of theory and evidence-based practice. By maintaining a focus on continuously improving clinical practice and integrating new knowledge into practice, a CNS influences the further development of the proficient and expert nurse, and increases the staff nurse's accountability and autonomy. A CNS is not effective when she or he is or is perceived to be territorial, omnipotent, or omniscient. A CNS's time is better used by teaching others the why, what, and how of a patient care intervention than being constrained by repeatedly providing the same patient interventions. Developing standards for patient education and providing resources to ensure that patient education is consistent across populations are also important educational activities of the CNS. As a staff nurse applies the new knowledge and skills taught by a CNS, the CNS can move on to new or more complex responsibilities. A staff nurse can become the role model for the skill mastered or the knowledge gained, and so the influence of the CNS continues to improve patient care. This growth cycle is never complete. Whenever there is a major staff turnover or a CNS enters a new practice setting, the cycle must begin anew.

A CNS's expert teaching and coaching skills are pivotal in providing or influencing patient and family education. Teaching or coaching complements the care given to a patient and family by other nurses and health professionals. CNSs continually look for better ways to teach patients and families, using diverse combinations of cognitive, educational, and behavioral strategies to improve patient education and compliance. However, a CNS may not be able to teach every patient and family and so must assess whom to teach. A CNS could delegate routine preoperative teaching for a cardiac surgical patient to the practice case manager or presurgical program educator. A CNS could therefore allocate more time to teach high-risk or complex patients—for example, an octogenarian who is undecided about an aortic valve replacement, or a young adult with prosthetic valve endocarditis and a relapse of intravenous drug use.

The restructuring of health care systems has placed a greater burden of accountability for their health care on patients. This is one of many factors that has contributed to greater health care activism on the part of consumers; patients are aware of the need to be better informed and educated about health risk factors, preventive self-care, treatment options, and risks vs. benefits of treatments. Nonetheless, behaviors are influenced by a variety of sociocultural characteristics. A CNS must determine which patients (or populations of patients) are more appropriate for the CNS to teach such as a prenatal patient with poor social support living in an economically depressed community, an urban African-American male with hypertension, or a teen who is newly diagnosed with Type I diabetes.

A CNS has a professional responsibility to serve as an educator for graduate nursing students and, when the opportunity arises, as a mentor. By working with graduate nursing students in the classroom or in the clinical setting, a CNS shares knowledge, demonstrates the level of advanced nursing practice to which a student can aspire, and role models the integration of practical and scientific knowledge into expert clinical practice. A CNS can provide opportunities for a graduate nursing student to do a clinical practicum or residency; the reward of working with an excellent student is being able to do more, to extend one's influence more broadly, and to be in more places at one time. A graduate student's presence benefits the practice setting as well; in addition to providing patient care the student completes projects (e.g., writing patient education materials or clinical procedures) or tasks (e.g., a research literature review to support a proposed change in clinical practice) that benefit the practice setting.

A CNS also has many opportunities to educate other health care providers and consumer groups. The focus should be within a CNS's specialty area only, or the demands will extend beyond a focused area, and a CNS will become overextended and recognition of specialty expertise will be dissipated. A CNS must carefully balance obligations for teaching within her or his practice setting with teaching outside of the practice setting or the immediate community. The more a CNS is pulled away from the needs of the practice setting, the greater is her or his risk of becoming an invisible and, therefore, unnecessary health care provider.

SCHOLARLY OR SCIENTIFIC INQUIRY

The essential components of the researcher role (McGuire & Harwood, 1989; Sparacino & Cooper, 1990) and advanced practice research competencies (McGuire & Harwood, 1996) are described in the literature. The competency of scholarly or scientific inquiry encompasses the continuum from scholarly inquiry to research utilization and research conduct. A CNS fosters the spirit of inquiry by documenting problems to determine research needs or by generating or refining research problems. Inherent to the CNS role is the responsibility to interpret and apply research findings. A CNS analyzes and evaluates the appropriateness of the research, and applies research findings to clinical practice. Evidence-based practice is realized in clinical procedures, administrative policies, educational materials for patients and staff, and clinical pathways. Evaluating outcomes of practice is another important example of research application (McGuire & Harwood, 1996; see also Chapter 9).

In order to be effective, CNSs must be able to apply research to practice. Many CNSs will want to participate in conducting nursing research, a goal usually accomplished when a CNS is more experienced in the role. Research is essential to build and extend the knowledge base for nursing practice, and to better understand the impact of nursing interventions on patient outcomes. Before becoming involved in research, a CNS must assess the practice setting's readiness and receptiveness, the administration's support, and whether research is a realistic performance goal at the given time. Most often the practical level of involvement is collaborative nursing and interdisciplinary research (McGuire & Harwood, 1996). By being a member of a research team, a CNS is in the unique position to contribute to the generation of clinically based knowledge, to create a link between practical application and theoretical design, and to bridge the gap between how nursing ought to be and what is practiced. A CNS is the clinical expert, understands the clinical issues, and has access to patients; a nurse researcher is the research expert, knows research methodology, and has access to the resources that support the research. CNSs and nurse researchers should be actively involved in research that documents the impact of advanced nursing practice, managed care, and other health care changes on the quality of patient care. There are consequences when CNSs are not involved in the design and conduct of a study or the discussion of its results; its outcomes may be disappointing, recommendations misguided, and money misspent (Oddi & Cassidy, 1998). A professional concern is whether the priorities of nurse researchers are different than those of the nurses providing patient care who are struggling with health care delivery reorganization and the changing burdens of care (Fagin, 1998).

In addition to applying research findings to clinical practice, CNSs must use research to influence public policy. It would be ideal to anticipate public policy needs in sufficient time to conduct research to influence the regulatory process. However, such foresight and the necessary time to conduct prospective research that might have policy implications are rare, but that does not mean that research results cannot be used to provide the substantive and objective facts that are more powerful and meaningful than impassioned pleas. The research literature is extensive, and professional, state, and national agencies have extensive data banks. This research must be used wisely, translating the findings to commonly understood and generally applicable language (Hamric, 1998).

CLINICAL AND PROFESSIONAL LEADERSHIP

The leadership competency is one of the three common threads that weave throughout the core competencies. It is integral to the role because a CNS has responsibility for clinical innovation and change within the patient care system. A CNS has significant formal and informal impact and influence; a CNS must be visionary yet practical. A CNS is a change agent. Through the CNS's influence and authority, nursing practice improves (Hamric, 1983b). As change agent, a CNS is the link between a variety of resources and nursing staff (Girouard, 1983), and asserts clinical and professional leadership in the practice setting or health care system, in health care policy and delivery decisions, or in the administration of direct care programs. A CNS authors and actuates clinical procedures, practice guidelines, and clinical pathways; designs and directs quality and performance improvement initiatives; chairs interdisciplinary committees or manages clinical projects; and influences or guides institutional health care policy decisions.

Clinical and leadership competencies are integrated with the other CNS competencies to support the overall purpose and goals of an organization. Most health care organizations are a bureaucratic maze; a CNS works with staff, patients, and families to help them comprehend the complexities and wend their way through the system. A CNS can serve as an advocate or "shuttle diplomat" between administrators and clinical staff, helping both groups understand the vagaries and particulars of organizational change, listening and supporting when appropriate and explaining decisions when needed (Brown, 1989).

COLLABORATION

Collaboration is the second common thread, and it is an essential competency, particularly because there are so many people with whom a CNS regularly works and interacts. A CNS collaborates with nurses, physicians, other health care providers, and patients and their families. A CNS is a nurse attending, a teacher and role model for nursing staff. The outcome of CNS-coordinated collaboration is empowerment of nurses and a recognition of the nurse as a critical member of the health care team (Boyle, 1994). This results in team building, synergism, and integrative solutions. CNSs and physicians also collaborate, although some practice settings and working relationships are more enlightened or conducive to partnership than others. When boundary issues and the pragmatic considerations of jobs and income are put aside, the differences in physician and CNS practice are complementary, afford integrative solutions, and further strengthen collaboration (Minarik & Sparacino, 1990). The outcome is high-quality and cost-efficient patient care. Integrated care management, especially in controlling capitated risk in current health care delivery systems, is best achieved by a collaborative team approach (Moss, Steiner, Mahnke, & Cohen, 1998). A CNS builds collaborative relationships with patients and families and provides an interface between patient, family, and physician. Many patients have health care needs that are so complex that no one health care professional can manage them all. A CNS is in the unique position to assist a patient and family to determine their needs, learning how to ask questions, assess treatment options, and ensure a positive outcome. CNS advocacy often prevents adversarial situations and their negative sequelae.

Collaboration between a CNS and other health care professionals contributes the necessary expertise to provide effective and efficient health care. CNSs can integrate the insights of many individuals with different perspectives, each providing theoretical and applied knowledge. Collaboration is an essential competency, but it is the well-earned result of clinical competence, effective communication, mutual trust, valuing complementary knowledge and skills, collegiality, and a favorable organizational structure (Hanson & Spross, 1996; Hughes & Mackenzie, 1990; Steele, 1986; see Chapter 11).

ETHICAL DECISION MAKING

Ethical decision-making is a specific APN competency; it is also a common thread running through all core competencies. A CNS has significant influence on the negotiation of moral dilemmas, direction of patient care, access to care, and allocation of resources. CNSs consider numerous factors when making ethical decisions, including professional and religious codes, cultural values, bioethical principles, the casuistic model, and ethical theories (Reigle, 1996; see Chapter 12). CNSs play critical roles in preventive and applied ethics. In promoting preventive ethics, a CNS is responsible for anticipating ethical conflicts when possible, teaching ethical theories, helping staff and patients clarify values, serving as a role model in discussions with patients about treatment preferences and options, demonstrating critical thinking in the analysis of moral dilemmas, and enhancing others' autonomy (Forrow, Arnold, & Parker, 1993, cited in Reigle, 1996).

CNSs have similar responsibilities when applying ethical decision-making skills to patient and organizational issues. They can articulate moral dilemmas. They can interpret and mediate patient, family, and team members' perspectives to ensure as complete a discussion as possible. They recognize the need for consultation with an ethics committee and often initiate the consult. When necessary, CNSs validate staff nurses' concerns and help nurses present their concerns to other team members, ensuring that the nursing perspective is considered when ethical issues are discussed. When CNSs are excluded from interdisciplinary processes involving ethical decisions, opportunities for effective nursing care are minimized and outcomes such as timely and appropriate end-of-life care are compromised (Oddi & Cassidy, 1998).

Spheres of Influence

Having described CNS competencies, it is apparent that there are three spheres of CNS influence: patient/clients, nursing personnel, and organizations or networks (NACNS, 1998). CNSs influence the patient/client sphere through activities such as assessment; diagnosis, planning, and outcome identification; interventions; and evaluation. CNSs influence nursing personnel by helping to identify and define problems and opportunities in delivering care, nurse-specific outcomes, and collaborative practice; developing innovative solutions; and evaluating the effect of solutions. The organization/network sphere of influence includes identifying problems and opportunities, identifying resource management needs and developing innovative solutions, and evaluating the quality and cost-effectiveness of patient care technologies and care processes (NACNS, 1998).

The delineation of spheres of influence is theoretically intended to avoid the overlap of subrole competencies and the perception of role ambiguity by distinguishing CNSs from other APNs (NACNS, 1998). Each sphere of influence requires various CNS competencies, so what a CNS does (e.g., the four subroles) and how a CNS performs the role (e.g., competencies) affects the practice setting through the effective use of influence (e.g., spheres of influence). Understanding each sphere of influence and mastering CNS competencies are essential for a CNS to be successful.

EXEMPLAR OF CNS PRACTICE

This exemplar illustrates how a CNS (the author) used the CNS competencies and spheres of influence to care for a complex and critically ill patient, her distraught but divided family, a concerned but overwhelmed physician, and a large group of caring but inexperienced nursing staff.

EXEMPLAR

Mrs. H. was an 82-year-old woman who was brought by paramedics to the emergency department with acute abdominal pain and severe pulmonary congestion. She was the matriarch of a large, supportive family who had differing opinions about the degree of her prehospital independence and state of health. For several weeks before admission, she had been experiencing dyspnea on exertion and was unable to walk more than a few steps. These symptoms progressively worsened. She was having severe respiratory distress at rest, was unable to walk more than a few steps without stopping to rest, and slept elevated on three pillows. Mrs. H. had worked her entire life until she retired about 20 years previously. Her husband had died at a young age. She had three children and a large extended family.

Her past medical history included insulin-dependent diabetes mellitus, hypertension, atrial fibrillation, coronary artery disease, critical aortic stenosis, congestive heart failure (American Heart Association class IV), mild chronic obstructive pulmonary disease, chronic renal insufficiency, chronic urinary tract infections, and obesity. Pertinent findings on admission included:

1. *Physical examination:* alert and oriented but somnolent, coarse rales to midlung bilaterally, respiratory rate 26–34 and labored, accessory muscle use, 3+ bilateral pitting edema to the knees, jugular venous distention
2. *Chest x-ray:* mild cardiac enlargement, bilateral interstitial pulmonary edema, calcification of the aortic valve, and a left pleural effusion
3. *Cardiac echo and catheterization:* severe aortic calcification not amenable to balloon valvuloplasty, peak aortic gradient 66 mm Hg, CO 7.67 L/min, aortic valvular area 0.7 cm^2; no ejection fraction was recorded
4. *Laboratory:* white cell count 11.9/μL, hemoglobin 8.2 gm/dL, hematocrit 25.1%, sodium 126 mEq/L, fasting blood sugar 237 mg/dL, blood urea nitrogen 51 mg/dL, creatinine 1.9 mg/dL; urinalysis: yeast $\oplus$

Mrs. H. stated that she could not go on as she was presently living and requested surgery. There was extensive discussion with the family, surgeon, and myself about surgery, emphasizing that the risks outweighed the benefits. The patient participated little in the discussion, only interjecting periodically that she wanted an operation to fix her aortic valve. Several days after hospital admission, Mrs. H. had surgery for an aortic valve replacement, using a tissue valve. Her postoperative course was complicated by reoperation for bleeding and she needed pharmacological and pacer support for hypotension, complete heart block, and low urine output. The remainder of her 6-month hospital stay included reintubation and prolonged failure to wean from the ventilator, with a subsequent tracheostomy; ventricular ectopy and atrial fibrillation; drainage from her sternal wound and sepsis; and renal failure requiring dialysis. She was in the critical care unit for most of the 6 months because of ventilator dependency until, after one of many family conferences, she was extubated and transferred to an acute care unit, where she died about a week later.

Mrs. H.'s care was also confounded by various extended family dynamics. One son and one daughter shared unofficial power of attorney for health care. The son was very vocal about his preferences for his mother's future care, while the daughter, who had many personal crises, deferred to her two sons (Mrs. H's grandsons). Another daughter had financial power of attorney, but she felt culturally powerless to influence decisions because she was the youngest sibling. A nephew was an active participant in family conferences, and he opined that everything should be done.

Commentary

This was a difficult and challenging case, and it required using each of the CNS competencies and affecting each sphere of influence. There were numerous factors to consider in this case, and there were both successes and failures. Because of the nature of the CNS role as well as the complexity of the case, it is nearly impossible to discuss each competency or influence separately. Rather, this section discusses key issues, interventions, successes, and failures, and the reader is referred to Table 13–1 to observe the overlapping nature of competencies and influence. The principal issues and interventions were the following:

1. Mrs. H. specifically stated that she did not want to continue to live as a cardiac cripple and demanded the surgery, despite the risks being clearly outlined. Her family did not want her to have the surgery but supported her decision. Her physician and I spent several hours with Mrs. H. and her family discussing the risks versus benefits of the surgery. In addition, her physician and I, together and independently, spent significant time with other physicians and nurses discussing the conflict between the patient's right to request treatment and the questionable chance for her survival or recovery. Specifically, could this elderly patient with multiple co-morbidities demand cardiac surgery, and at what level of risk could her surgeon conscionably refuse to perform the surgery? The key ethical principle we considered was the patient's autonomy, her preferences, and her freedom to act on her choice. We tried to clarify the sources of conflict and reviewed the primary ethical principles and theories involved in the decision-making and consent process.
2. Mrs. H. had multiple nursing care needs postoperatively. Because of her multisystem failure, she
   - Had numerous episodes of hemodynamic instability as a result of the stress of hemodialysis on a depressed myocardium

TABLE 13–1 OVERLAPPING COMPETENCIES AND INFLUENCE

KEY ISSUES	CORE COMPETENCIES				COMMON COMPETENCIES			SPHERES OF INFLUENCE		
	Clinical Practice	Consultation	Expert Teaching and Coaching	Scholarly or Scientific Inquiry	Clinical and Professional Leadership	Collaboration	Ethical Decision Making	Patients/ Clients	Nurses	Organization
1. Preoperative surgical consent	✓	✓	✓	✓		✓	✓	✓	✓	✓
2. Postoperative nursing care	✓	✓✓	✓		✓	✓✓	✓✓	✓	✓✓	✓
3. Family discord		✓✓		✓✓					✓✓	
4. Overwhelmed nurses										
5. Ethical dilemmas										
6. Appropriateness of cardiac surgery in the octogenarian	✓	✓	✓		✓	✓			✓	
7. Patient's limited ability to communicate								✓		

- Required a tracheostomy because of respiratory failure
- Had complex dressing changes to her open sternal wound
- Had difficulty communicating about the adequacy of pain control and comfort because of a variable level of consciousness, English as a second language, and her tracheostomy
- Developed breakdown of the skin over her sacrum and was placed on a special bed to reduce pressure and prevent further breakdown

The amount of direct care I provided depended on whether Mrs. H. was in the critical care unit (experienced nurses) or the surgical floor (transitional care from critical care to acute care, where there were less experienced nurses), whether the adequacy or appropriateness of a procedure (sternal wound care, tracheostomy care) needed to be reassessed, or whether a new product needed application (protection of the sacral wound). More often I provided indirect care, working with the nurses to re-evaluate her care, revise her nursing care plan, and influencing the direction of care.

3. The patient's family was large and divided in their opinions, and so I facilitated many family conferences, sometimes just with family members and other times with the physician or other nursing staff, depending on the issue and the family's requests. The discussion in each of the many family conferences easily strayed from the meeting's intended purpose, and instead became distracted by concerns about smaller but more tangible issues, such as Mrs. H.'s sacral wound instead of her ventilator dependency; the need to look for long-term placement, despite the grandson's lack of follow-through; unrealistic expectations for Mrs. H.'s recovery, arguing that she was a candidate for dialysis in an ambulatory care center, despite her bedbound status; and, as the poor chance for recovery became clearer, the family's clearly stated message of "you did the surgery—you cure her," forgetting the extensive preoperative discussion about the high risks and potential for a poor outcome.

4. The nursing staff felt overwhelmed with the extensive physical care combined with the various ethical issues involved. I, too, felt overwhelmed and wondered whether I was remaining objective but supportive. I therefore asked for a consultation with my psychiatric liaison CNS colleague; she provided support to me and to the nursing staff in private consultations as well as to the various health care providers in the many interdisciplinary care planning conferences.

5. Because of the various ethical issues involved, the physician and I asked for a consultation with representatives of the hospital's Ethics Committee. Ethical principles and theories discussed included
   - Autonomy, related to Mrs. H.'s preferences and her freedom to act on a choice
   - Beneficence, in relation to the right of the surgeon to refuse to perform a high-risk operation when the alternative of medical support has even higher risks
   - The theory of utilitarianism, in relation to the issues of rationing health care by age and allocation of resources. The relationship of the influence of resource allocation decisions on clinical judgment was also explored.

6. The nursing staff had numerous questions about the conflict between the reasons for and the reasons against surgery in someone who was 82 years old. Specifically, they asked whether cardiac surgery in an elderly and ill patient was appropriate. I conducted an extensive literature search, discussed the findings with the surgeon to corroborate my conclusions and his opinion, and then provided in-services for the nursing staff to discuss the results and practical application to Mrs. H.'s care.

7. Ironically, Mrs. H's earlier request that she did not want to become ventilator dependent was "lost" and confounded subsequent medical and nursing decisions

because of her inability to communicate for much of the postoperative period. Mrs. H. was awake and appeared alert when, many months later, the family made the decision to take her off the ventilator, transfer her to the surgical floor, and institute a "do not resuscitate" order. After discussion with the CNS and physician, the family agreed to a fenestrated tracheostomy tube so that Mrs. H. would have some chance for limited communication during her remaining life.

There were various successes and failures in this case. The noteworthy successes included the excellent care that Mrs. H. and her family received from each provider; the knowledge (e.g., ethical priniciples, appropriateness of cardiac surgery in the elderly) and skills (e.g., tracheostomy care, complex sternal wound care, appropriate use of specialty beds) that many nurses acquired in the 6 months of caring for Mrs. H.; the collaboration between the CNSs (cardiovascular surgery CNS and psychiatric liaison CNS), nurses, physicians, and Ethics Committee consultants; and the fact that the dilemmas of caring for such a complex patient were supported by the medical center's mission and vision. There were failures from which valuable lessons for the future were learned, such as the physician's—and CNS's—dilemma of considering surgical risk versus benefit in this elderly patient with multiple co-morbidities; intervening sooner to assist the family in reaching consensus about long-term treatment options; and understanding the emotional and financial impact of prolonging Mrs. H.'s inevitable death.

IMPACT AND INFLUENCE

Health care delivery models have shifted the emphasis from specialized to primary care, from curative to preventive interventions, from uncontrolled costs to expense accountability, and from individually controlled practice to consensus-derived, evidence-based practice guidelines. Yet affordability of health care has the greatest influence on access to health care and the care a patient receives. Affordability of health care influences treatment options, health outcomes, access to health care providers, and the burden of cost for noncovered types of care (Moore, 1997). A CNS plays a significant role in any health care delivery system by keeping a comprehensive focus on quality care and extensive documentation to facilitate quality patient outcomes. Managed care has provided CNSs with an opportunity that has long eluded them: linking their services to patient outcomes and resource utilization. A CNS's particular impact has been on patient and family outcomes, outcomes management, care efficiency, and cost-effectiveness. However, prevention of patient care variance is difficult to quantify.

Evidence-Based Practice

Knowledge is the basis for practice. When research is evaluated for its applicable scientific evidence, informed decisions are made in providing patient care and achieving good patient outcomes, and credible nursing practice is documented (McPheeters & Lohr, 1999). A CNS is the ideal clinician to assess the contextual factors that are barriers and facilitators to change, and to develop and implement evidence-based practice. In addition, a CNS's involvement in the development of clinical pathways and procedures means that the CNS can ensure research evidence informs clinical processes and standards. Examples of evidence-based practice range from using an outcome-driven clinical pathway developed by a multidisciplinary effort to improve patient outcomes and reduce cost of care (Patton & Schaerf, 1995), to initiation of an evidence-based falls prevention program in an acute care setting (Stetler, Corrigan, Sander-Buscemi, & Burns, 1999).

Outcomes Management

Management of outcomes is driven by the rapid movement to managed care, and the need for national standards for measuring performance in health care. Traditionally, key outcome indicators have been linked more to organizational structures than to organizational or clinical processes. However, although key outcome indicators are influenced by patient variables more than organizational variables, less attention has been given to the relationship between organizational attributes and patient outcomes (Mitchell & Shortell, 1997). The traditional model linking structure, processes, and outcome is a linear one, but Mitchell, Ferketich, and Jennings (1998) proposed a dynamic model that posits reciprocal relationships between the care delivery system, interventions, client, and outcomes. Assuming responsibility for using outcome data to improve patient care delivery is a prime opportunity for the CNS to assess patient care strategies and community systems, analyze interdisciplinary communication and collaboration, coordinate care, monitor patient and system progress, and evaluate patient and system outcomes. The challenge is to facilitate cost-effective patient care interventions that are effective with all populations.

CNS Impact on Outcomes

Measuring and reporting the impact of a CNS on patient and family outcomes has been slow, but the evidence is mounting and the impact irrefutable. Classic studies include evaluation of the impact of CNS interventions on low-birth-weight infants and hospitalized elderly (Brooten et al., 1986; Neidlinger, Kennedy, & Scroggins, 1987; see also Chapters 9 and 25). More recent studies have also demonstrated the impact of CNS interventions on patients who received transitional care services from a CNS and were discharged from the hospital earlier than the norm. The various patient populations analyzed included women delivered by unplanned cesarean delivery (Brooten et al., 1994), high-risk childbearing women (York. et al., 1997), and the hospitalized elderly (Naylor et al., 1994, 1999). In each of the studies, the transitional care, discharge planning, and home follow-up given by a CNS resulted in safe, feasible, and cost-effective care; the outcomes included decreased cost of care, fewer rehospitalizations, fewer multiple rehospitalizations, fewer hospital days per patient, and no group differences in functional status. In the study by Brooten and colleagues (1994), there were improved clinical outcomes, including improved infant birth weight and more immunizations. The study by York and associates (1997) also analyzed the mean total hospital charges, and found that charges for the intervention group were 44% less than for the control group.

Other more recently published studies of the impact of CNS practice specifically related to case management or outcomes management demonstrate cost savings, patient satisfaction, and increased staff knowledge. Geropsychiatric patient outcomes were improved, length of hospital stay and cost of care were reduced, and nursing staff knowledge and attitudes were improved when a geropsychiatry CNS facilitated various interventions (Mathew, Gutsch, Hackney, & Munsat, 1994). Patients with congestive heart failure whose care was managed by CNSs had significantly shorter lengths of hospital stay and lower hospital expenses than those patients receiving usual care (Topp, Tucker, & Weber, 1998). CNSs have developed and implemented structured interventions for pain management, using an outcomes approach to improve pain management. The results were improved patient satisfaction with pain management during hospitalization, consistency in patients' ability to identify a perceived level of acceptable pain, significant increase in staff nurses' knowledge of pain management, and more consistent pain management practice patterns by staff nurses (Barnason, Merboth, Pozehl, & Tietjen, 1998). The evaluation of a CNS-directed outcomes management program for patients undergoing total hip and total knee arthroplasty demonstrated reduced length of hospital stay and hospital costs, and a significant reduction in complications (Wammack & Mabrey, 1998).

ISSUES AND CHALLENGES

Patient care has always been and will continue to be the very essence of the CNS role. A CNS's flexibility is well suited to adapt to systems changes while keeping the patient as the central focus. However, a CNS's ability to maintain a focus on patient care has been threatened by the changing demands of the health care environment. A number of issues currently challenge the CNS role. These issues include but are not limited to educational preparation; factors influencing role evolution, such as health care organizational changes and forced changes in role focus and titling; second licensure; and legal barriers.

Educational Preparation

The dilemma in defining appropriate CNS education has been the identification of and agreement about a core body of knowledge for practice. All agree that basic CNS preparation requires a master's degree in nursing. Despite the efforts of the ANA's Council of Clinical Nurse Specialists and subsequently its Council for Advanced Practice Nursing, uniformly accepted standards for educational preparation have not been established. Uniformity in educational preparation would permit uniformity in licensure (Safriet, 1998). The NACNS (1998) has made recommendations for education for core CNS competencies, which should help to standardize curricula.

Graduate preparation of the CNS varies substantially, and the operative variable seems to be individual institutional educational philosophy that influences faculty philosophy and program emphasis. Without a common basis or standards for the educational preparation of a CNS, it is difficult to define consistent standards of practice and to provide uniform certification at the advanced level. Much of the recent debate about curricular design has centered on the similarities and differences in the core curriculum of graduate nursing programs preparing CNSs and NPs. The greatest difference is found in the practice setting (Forbes, Rafson, Spross, & Kozlowski, 1990). The intent of developing a core curriculum is not homogenization but standardization (see Chapter 4).

The knowledge and skills acquired in a graduate program should prepare a CNS to practice at an advanced level, regardless of setting or patient population.

There is general agreement that such a program should address the different advanced nursing practice role components and competencies. There has been less agreement about teaching the skills of the role competencies versus professional cultivation that prepares a student to continue to learn the core competencies (Sparacino, 1994).

Factors Influencing CNS Role Evolution

ORGANIZATIONAL CONSIDERATIONS

The constant threat of organizational redesign and other critical elements, including organizational structure and climate, administrative justification, and forced changes in role focus and role titling, can significantly affect a CNS's practice. A classic but recurring debate is whether a CNS should be in a staff or a line position (Prouty, 1983; Baird & Prouty, 1989). In a staff position, a CNS is freed from more administrative responsibilities and allowed to focus on patient care delivery and related issues, and the less threatening consultative capacity. The disadvantage of such a position is a lack of formal authority, such that power is referent or exercised by virtue of clinical expertise and knowledge. The advantage for a CNS in a line position is formal authority, but the distinct disadvantage is that administrative responsibilities may dominate one's activities and erode the time available for clinical issues and patient care.

Recently there has been serious discussion about the need for a CNS to acquire NP skills for job security. The basis for this challenge may be that CNSs have been increasingly pulled from the bedside to address competing demands and other organizational needs. Those who disagree with this proposal argue that an acute care NP's (ACNP) primary emphasis is on patient care, limited to the particular practice setting and to the exclusion of a CNS's flexibility to care for patients across the continuum of care. In addition, the ACNP has less opportunity to participate in the other areas of usual CNS influence, such as staff education and development, nurse mentorship, change agent leadership, consultation, research, and outcomes management. A CNS's decision to learn NP skills may be based on clinical and practical concerns. For example, NP skills may enable the CNS to provide better patient care in a CNS job or the CNS may make a deliberate decision to prepare for another APN role (NP or blended role). The CNS may believe that such preparation is needed to ensure job security in a changing environment. It may be that a state requires such preparation in order to be licensed as an APN. When a CNS makes this decision, it should be based on an assessment of personal, clinical, institutional, and statutory factors. Despite many ups and downs, the CNS role has not disappeared. The need for APNs who can care for patients, develop staff nurses, build interdisciplinary teams, and implement evidence-based practices and other systems changes is not going away.

THE CNS AS CASE MANAGER

The minimum educational requirement endorsed by the Case Management Society of America for a nurse case manager is a baccalaureate degree. However, a master's prepared case manager who also has experience as a CNS is very effective because case management includes many CNS responsibilities, such as patient care, collaboration with a multidisciplinary team, clinical system orchestration, administration of the interface between a patient and the health care system, and involvement with, if not direction of, resource management and clinical system development. Mahn and Spross (1996) proposed nurse case management as an advanced practice role; most of the APN case manager descriptors are based on CNS competencies. However, managed care's impact affects resource management and CNS impact and influence, especially if a CNS is used exclusively as a case manager. In such situations, the APN case manager is forced to neglect CNS responsibilities such as coaching of nurses.

THE CNS AS OUTCOMES MANAGER

There is a theoretical but subtle distinction between a case manager and an outcomes manager. A case manager's responsibilities are unit or setting based and involve coordinating patient-focused care and resource management. An outcomes manager's responsibilities are broader, including additional obligations that focus on the continuum of care that is beyond a specific case load. An outcomes manager is responsible for clinical and financial analysis and outcomes for a particular patient population, including development and revision of organizational systems. The literature suggests that a CNS, with her or his expert clinical and consultant competencies, is best qualified to be an outcomes manager and to undertake the responsibilities of patient and quality measurement and research, financial analysis, provider education, and development and implementation of interdisciplinary practice improvements (Houston & Luquire, 1997; Weiss, 1998). Advanced educational preparation and clinical expertise lend credibility to an outcomes manager's ability to develop, implement, and evaluate an outcomes management program. Houston and Luquire (1998) are most specific when they state that "most outcomes managers must function in five roles: clinical practice, consultation, administration, research, and education" (p. 2), the classical description of the CNS. However, the outcomes manager, as described by Houston and Luquire (1997) is most like the APN case manager (see Chapter 19), a role that is different from the CNS. One must ask, is the "outcomes manager" title yet another permutation of "clinical nurse specialist"? There is no reason for yet another title. Clinical nurse specialist is an honorable title, and to continually introduce alternatives to legitimize this APN role and use titles that are descriptors of responsibility is confusing and a disservice to CNSs who perform the same work. As described by Mahn and Zazworsky (Chapter 19), the APN case manager is a different APN role than the CNS.

Second Licensure

An alternative to second licensure is a multistate licensure system proposed by the National Council of State Boards of Nursing (NCSBN) in 1997 (NCSBN, 1998). An interstate compact addresses the more general licensure issues that hinder interstate practice, making mobility between two or more states possible while keeping a state-based licensure and discipline arrangement. The interstate compact has not yet addressed advanced practice, in part because there is little licensure uniformity for advanced practice (Williamson & Hutcherson, 1998) (see Chapter 22).

Legal Barriers

Legal barriers for a CNS are similar to those encountered by other advanced practice nurses: restrictions on scope of practice, authority to prescribe drugs, and reimbursement. Sole authority for defining the scope of advanced practice nursing should rest with a state's Board of Nursing. Nurse Practice Acts should be amended at the state level to define and acknowledge advanced practice nursing, and there should be fewer references to specific titles. Statutory requirements for physician supervision or formalized APN-physician collaboration should be eliminated; APNs' prescriptive authority should be defined and controlled by Boards of Nursing regulations; and there should be a change in state and federal reimbursement and valuation of services provided (Safriet, 1992). Although Safriet's classic monograph addressed NP and certified nurse-midwife issues, her recommendations are also applicable to a CNS's expanding domain and scope of practice. However, CNSs must consider how general or specific desired regulatory changes should be. For example, some CNSs may not need or desire to prescribe drugs, or may not have sufficient opportunity to prescribe often enough to do so safely. Nonetheless, CNS advocates should support legal efforts to obtain CNS prescriptive authority for those who can or must prescribe.

The significant health care system changes that have occurred in the past several years have had various effects on CNSs and other APNs, in some states more than others. Previous barriers to advanced practice were related to scope of practice and reimbursement, and the sources were state and federal laws. The Legislative/Regulatory Committee of the NACNS is drafting model statutory and regulatory language to regulate CNS practice (A. Hamric, personal communication, October 1999). Once developed, this document can further assist in standardizing state regulation of CNS practice, and in decreasing interstate regulatory barriers. Although progress has been made in overcoming the barriers imposed by state statutes and administrative dicta, the financial changes in the current health care market have created new challenges for APNs in general, and CNSs in particular (Safriet, 1998).

EVALUATING THE ROLE

There are various ways to evaluate CNS performance, such as appraisal of competencies or activities including self-evaluation, administrative and peer review, certification, and program and outcomes evaluation (Cooper & Sparacino, 1990; Girouard, 1996; Hamric, 1983a, 1989b; Sample, 1983). Although each method has merit, evaluating CNS effectiveness in a way that links structural and process variables is useful only if the procedure also addresses CNS impact on cost, quality, and patient outcomes (Girouard, 1996). Common elements include CNS impact on patient care quality and cost of patient outcomes, with similar results regardless of specialty area or practice setting (Barnason et al., 1998; Broussard, 1996; Mathew et al., 1994; McAlpine, 1997; Smith & Waltman, 1994; Topp et al., 1998; Wammack & Mabrey, 1998).

CONCLUSION

CNSs have learned hard lessons from the many travails they have endured. Although the future of the health care market is uncertain, there is no better time to advance the CNS position and its influence. CNSs have weathered many challenges, including forced changes in role responsibilities and title, decreased involvement in direct patient care, increased responsibility for directing other health care providers, constant organizational redesign oblivious to the CNS's diverse contributions, and undeserved attacks caused, until recently, by the qualitative nature of a CNS's work. However, these threats to the CNS role and developmental changes in the health care system have also created exciting opportunities.

A CNS embodies unique talents and skills: clinical expert, pragmatic visionary, and change agent. The preceding discussion chronicles in detail a CNS's competencies and spheres of influence. The central focus of every CNS remains the patient. Now that a CNS's influence and impact can be measured, what APN role is better than a CNS to improve patient outcomes, cost efficiency, and performance improvement? Who is better prepared than a CNS to integrate new knowledge into practice, and influence and implement practice guidelines and innovative practice models? Carpe diem!

REFERENCES

American Association of Colleges of Nursing. (1993). In search of the advanced practice nurse. *AACN Issue Bulletin,* March.

American Nurses Association. (1980). *Nursing: A social policy statement.* Kansas City, MO: Author.

American Nurses Association. (1985). *Facts about nursing 84–85* (p. 27). Kansas City, MO: Author.

American Nurses Association. (1986). *The role of the clinical nurse specialist.* Kansas City, MO: Author.

American Nurses Association. (1993). *Nursing facts: Registered nurses: A distinctive health care profession.* Washington, DC: Author.

American Nurses Association. (1995). *Nursing's social policy statement.* Washington, DC: Author.

American Nurses Association, Congress of Nursing Practice. (1976). Description of practice: clinical nurse specialist. In *The scope of nursing practice.* Kansas City, MO: Author.

Baird, S. B., & Prouty, M. P. (1989). In A. B. Hamric & J. A. Spross (Eds.), *The clinical nurse specialist in theory and practice* (2nd ed., pp. 261–284). Philadelphia: W. B. Saunders.

Barnason, S., Merboth, M., Pozehl, B., & Tietjen, M. J. (1998). Utilizing an outcome approach to improve pain management by nurses: A pilot study. *Clinical Nurse Specialist, 12*(1), 28–36.

Barron, A-M., & White, P. (1996) Consultation. In A. B. Hamric, J. A. Spross, & C. M. Hanson (Eds.): *Advanced nursing practice: An integrative approach* (pp. 165–183). Philadelphia: W. B. Saunders.

Bigbee, J. L. (1996). History and evolution of advanced nursing practice. In A. B. Hamric, J. A. Spross, & C. M. Hanson (Eds.), *Advanced nursing practice: An integrative approach* (pp. 3–23). Philadelphia: W. B. Saunders.

Boyle, D. McC. (1996). The clinical nurse specialist. In A. B. Hamric, J. A. Spross, & C. M. Hanson (Eds.), *Advanced nursing practice: An integrative approach* (pp. 299–336). Philadelphia: W. B. Saunders.

Brooten, D., Kumer, S., Brown, L. P., Butts, P., Finkler, S. A., Bakewell-Sachs, S., Gibbons, A., & Delivoria-Papadopoulos, M. (1986). A randomized clinical trial of early hospital discharge and home follow-up of very-low-birth-weight infants. *New England Journal of Medicine, 315*(15), 934–939.

Brooten, D., Roncoli, M., Finkler, S., Arnold, L., Cohen, A., & Menuti, M. (1994). A randomized trial of early hospital discharge and home follow-up of women having cesarean birth. *Obstetrics and Gynecology, 84*(5), 832–838.

Broussard, B. S. (1996). The role of the perinatal home care clinical nurse specialist. *Home Healthcare Nurse, 14*(11), 855–860.

Brown, S. J. (1989). Supportive supervision of the CNS. In A. B. Hamric & J. A. Spross (Eds.), *The clinical nurse specialist in theory and practice* (2nd ed., pp. 285–298). Philadelphia: W. B. Saunders.

Clarke, E. B., & Spross, J. A. (1996). Expert coaching and guidance. In A. B. Hamric, J. A. Spross, & C. M. Hanson (Eds.), *Advanced nursing practice: An integrative approach* (pp. 139–164). Philadelphia: W. B. Saunders.

Cooper, D. M., & Sparacino, P. S. A. (1990). Acquiring, implementing, and evaluating the clinical nurse specialist role. In P. S. A. Sparacino, D. M. Cooper, & P. A. Minarik (Eds.), *The clinical nurse specialist: Implementation and impact* (pp. 41–75). Norwalk, CT: Appleton & Lange.

Cronenwett, L. R. (1995). Molding the future of advanced practice nursing. *Nursing Outlook, 43*(3), 112–118.

Fagin, C. M. (1998). Nursing research and the erosion of care. *Nursing Outlook, 46*(6), 259–260.

Felder, L. (1983). Direct patient care and independent practice. In A. B. Hamric & J. Spross (Eds.), *The clinical nurse specialist in theory and practice* (pp. 59–72) New York: Grune & Stratton.

Fenton, M. V., & Brykcyznski, K. A. (1993). Qualitative distinctions and similarities in the practice of clinical nurse specialists and nurse practitioners. *Journal of Professional Nursing, 9*(6), 313–326.

Forbes, K. E., Rafson, J., Spross, J. A., & Kozlowski, D. (1990). The clinical nurse specialist and nurse practitioner: Core curriculum survey results. *Clinical Nurse Specialist, 4*(2), 63–66.

Gawlinksi, A,. & Kern, L. S. (Eds.). (1994). *The clinical nurse specialist role in critical care.* Philadelphia: W. B. Saunders.

Girouard, S. (1983). Theory-based practice: Functions, obstacles, and solutions. In A. B. Hamric & J. A. Spross (Eds.), *The clinical nurse specialist in theory and practice* (pp. 21–37). New York: Grune & Stratton.

Girouard, S. A. (1996). Evaluating advanced nursing practice. In A. B. Hamric, J. A. Spross, & C. M. Hanson (Eds.), *Advanced nursing practice: An integrative approach* (pp. 569–600). Philadelphia: W. B. Saunders.

Hamric, A. B. (1983a). A model for developing evaluation strategies. In A. B. Hamric & J. A. Spross (Eds.), *The clinical nurse specialist in theory and practice* (pp. 187–206). New York: Grune & Stratton.

Hamric, A. B. (1983b). Role development and functions. In A. B. Hamric & J. Spross (Eds.), *The clinical nurse specialist in theory and practice* (pp. 39–56). New York: Grune & Stratton.

Hamric, A. B. (1989a). History and overview of the CNS role. In A. B. Hamric & J. A. Spross, (Eds.), *The clinical nurse specialist in theory and practice* (2nd ed., pp. 3–18). Philadelphia: W. B. Saunders.

Hamric, A. B. (1989b). A model for CNS evaluation. In A. B. Hamric & J. A. Spross (Eds.), *The clinical nurse specialist in theory and practice,* (2nd ed., pp. 83–104). Philadelphia: W. B. Saunders.

Hamric, A. B. (1995). Creating our future: Challenges and opportunities for the clinical nurse specialist. *Oncology Nursing Forum, 22*(3), 547–553.

Hamric, A. B. (1998). Using research to influence the regulatory process. *Advanced Practice Nursing Quarterly, 4*(3), 44–50.

Hamric, A. B. & Spross, J. A. (Eds.). (1989). *The clinical nurse specialist in theory and practice* (2nd ed.). Philadelphia: W. B. Saunders.

Hamric, A. B., Spross, J. A., & Hanson, C. M. (Eds.). (1996). *Advanced nursing practice: An integrative approach.* Philadelphia: W. B. Saunders.

Hanson, C. M., & Spross J. A. (1996). Collaboration. In A. B. Hamric, J. A. Spross, & C. M. Hanson (Eds.), *Advanced nursing practice: An integrative approach* (pp. 229–248). Philadelphia: W. B. Saunders.

Hoeffer, B., & Murphy, S. A. (1984). Specialization in nursing practice. In *Issues in professional nursing practice* (pp. 1–10). Kansas City, MO: American Nurses Association.

Houston, S., & Luquire, R. (1997). Advanced practice nurse as outcomes manager. *Advanced Practice Nursing Quarterly, 3*(2), 1–9.

Hughes, A., & Mackenzie, C. (1990). Components necessary in a successful nurse practitioner-physician collaborative practice. *Journal of the American Academy of Nurse Practitioners, 2*(2), 54–57.

Keane, A., & Richmond, T. S. (1993). Tertiary nurse practitioners. *Image: The Journal of Nursing Scholarship, 25*(4), 281–284.

Koetters, T. L. (1989). Clinical practice and direct patient care In A. B. Hamric & J. A. Spross (Eds.), *The clinical nurse specialist in theory and practice* (2nd ed., pp. 107–124). Philadelphia: W. B. Saunders.

Mahn, V. A., & Spross, J. A. (1996). Nurse case management as an advanced practice role. In A. B. Hamric, J. A. Spross, & C. M. Hanson (Eds.), *Advanced nursing practice: An integrative approach* (pp. 445–465). Philadelphia: W. B. Saunders.

Mathew, L. J., Gutsch, H. M., Hackney, N. W., & Munsat, E. M. (1994). Promoting quality and cost-effective care to geropsychiatric patients. *Issues in Mental Health Nursing, 15*(2), 169–185.

McAlpine, L. A. (1997). Process and outcome measures for the multidisciplinary collaborative projects of a critical care CNS. *Clinical Nurse Specialist, 11*(3), 134–138.

McGuire, D. B., & Harwood, K. V. (1989). The CNS as researcher. In A. B. Hamric & J. A. Spross (Eds.), *The clinical nurse specialist in theory and practice* (2nd ed., pp. 169–204). Philadelphia: W. B. Saunders.

McGuire, D. B., & Harwood, K. V. (1996). Research implementation, utilization, and conduct. In A. B. Hamric, J. A. Spross, & C. M. Hanson, (Eds.), *Advanced nursing practice: An integrative approach* (pp. 184–212). Philadelphia: W. B. Saunders.

McPheeters, M., & Lohr, K. N. (1999). Evidence-based practice and nursing: Commentary. *Outcomes Management for Nursing Practice, 3*(3), 99–101.

Minarik, P. A. (1992) Second licensure for advanced nursing practice? *Clinical Nurse Specialist, 6*(4), 221.

Minarik, P. A., & Sparacino, P. S. A. (1990). Clinical nurse specialist collaboration in a university medical center. In P. S. A. Sparacino, D. M. Cooper, & P. A Minarik (Eds.), *The clinical* nurse specialist: Implementation and impact (pp. 231–260). East Norwalk, CT: Appleton & Lange.

Mitchell, P. H., Ferketich, S., & Jennings, B. M. (1998). Quality health outcomes model. Image: The Journal of Nursing Scholarship, 30(1), 43–46.

Mitchell, P. H., & Shortell, S. M. (1997). Adverse outcomes and variation in organization of care delivery. Medical Care, 35, 19–32.

Moore, K. (1997). Socioeconomic status as quarantine: Unfortunate consequences of the inability to afford health care. Outcomes Management for Nursing Practice, 1,(1) 41–48.

Moss, J. K., Steiner, K., Mahnke, K., & Cohen, R. (1998). A model to manage capitated risk. Nursing Economics, 16, 65–68.

National Association of Clinical Nurse Specialists. (1998). Statement on clinical nurse specialist practice and education. Glenview, IL: Author.

National Council of State Boards of Nursing. (1998). Interstate compact for a mutual recognition model of nursing. Chicago: Author.

Naylor, M., Brooten, D., Jones, R., Lavizzo-Mourey, R., Mezey, M., & Pauly, M. (1994). Comprehensive discharge planning for the hospitalized elderly. A randomized trial. Annals of Internal Medicine, 120, 999–1006.

Naylor, M., Brooten, D., Campbell, R., Jacobsen, B. S., Mezey, M. D., Pauly, M. V., & Schwartz, J. S. (1999). Comprehensive discharge planning and home follow-up of hospitalized elders. JAMA, 281, 613–657.

Neidlinger, S., Kennedy, L., & Scroggins, K. (1987). Effective and cost efficient discharge planning for hospitalized elders. Nursing Economics, 5(5), 225–230.

Noll, M. (1987). Internal consultation as a framework for clinical nurse specialist practice. Clinical Nurse Specialist, 1, 46–50.

Oddi, L. F., & Cassidy, V. R. (1998). The message of SUPPORT: Change is long overdue. Journal of Professional Nursing, 14(3), 165–174.

Patton, M. D., & Schaerf, R. (1995). Thoracotomy, critical pathway, and clinical outcomes. Cancer Practice, 3(5), 286–294.

Priest, A-R. (1989). The CNS as educator. In A. B. Hamric & J. A. Spross (Eds.), The clinical nurse specialist in theory and practice (2nd ed., pp. 147–168). Philadelphia: W. B. Saunders.

Prouty, M. P. (1983). In A. B. Hamric & J. Spross (Eds.), The clinical nurse specialist in theory and practice. New York: Grune & Stratton.

Reigle, J. (1996). Ethical decision-making skills. In A. B. Hamric, J. A. Spross, & C. M. Hanson (Eds.), Advanced nursing practice: An integrative approach (pp. 273–295). Philadelphia: W. B. Saunders.

Safriet, B. J. (1992). Health care dollars and regulatory sense: The role of advanced practice nursing. Yale Journal on Regulation, 9(2), 149–220.

Safriet, B. J. (1998). Still spending dollars, still searching for sense: Advanced practice nursing in an era of regulatory and economic turmoil. Advanced Practice Nursing Quarterly, 4(3), 24–33.

Sample, S. A. (1983). Justifying and structuring the CNS role in the nursing department. In A. B. Hamric & J. Spross (Eds.), The clinical nurse specialist in theory and practice (pp. 117–128). New York: Grune & Stratton.

Smith, J. E., & Waltman, N. L. (1994). Oncology clinical nurse specialists' perceptions of their influence on patient outcomes. Oncology Nursing Forum, 21(5), 887–893.

Sparacino, P. S. A. (1990). A historical perspective on the development of the clinical nurse specialist role. In P. S. A. Sparacino, D. M. Cooper, & P. A. Minarik (Eds.), The clinical nurse specialist: implementation and impact (pp. 3–10). East Norwalk, CT: Appleton & Lange.

Sparacino, P. S. A. (1994). Issues and future trends for the critical care clinical nurse specialist. In A. Gawlinski & L. S. Kern (Eds.), The clinical nurse specialist role in critical care (pp. 293–307). Philadelphia: W. B. Saunders.

Sparacino, P. S. A., & Cooper, D. M. (1990). The role components. In P. S. A. Sparacino, D. M. Cooper, & P. A. Minarik (Eds.), The clinical nurse specialist: Implementation and impact (pp. 11–40). Norwalk, CT: Appleton & Lange.

Sparacino, P. S. A., Cooper, D. M., & Minarik, P. A. (Eds.). (1990). The clinical nurse specialist: Implementation and impact. Norwalk, CT: Appleton & Lange.

Sparacino, P. S. A., & Durand, B. A. (1986). Editorial on specialization in advanced nursing practice. Momentum, 4(2), 2–3.

Spross, J., & Hamric, A. B. (1983). A model for future clinical nurse specialist practice. In A. B. Hamric & J. Spross, (Eds.): The clinical nurse specialist in theory and practice (pp. 291–306). New York: Grune & Stratton.

Steele, J. E. (Ed.). (1986). Issues in collaborative practice. Orlando: Grune & Stratton.

Stetler, C. B., Corrigan, B., Sander-Buscemi, K., & Burns, M. (1999). Integration of evidence into practice and the change process: Fall prevention program as a model. Outcomes Management for Nursing Practice, 3(3), 102–111.

Topp, R., Tucker, D., & Weber, C. (1998) Effect of a clinical case manager/clinical nurse specialist on patients hospitalized with congestive heart failure. Nursing Case Management, 3(4), 140–147.

Wammack, L., & Mabrey, J. D. (1998). Outcomes assessment of total hip and total knee arthroplasty: Critical pathways, variance analysis, and continuous quality improvement. *Clinical Nurse Specialist, 12*(3), 122–129.

Weiss, M. E. (1998). Case management as a tool for clinical integration. *Advanced Practice Nursing Quarterly, 4*(1), 9–15.

Williamson, S. H., & Hutcherson, C. (1998). Mutual recognition: Response to the regulatory implications of a changing health care environ-

ment. *Advanced Practice Nursing Quarterly, 4*(3), 86–93.

York, R., Brown, L. P., Samuels, P., Finkler, S. A., Jacobsen, B., Perseley, C. A., Swank, A., & Robbins, D. (1997). A randomized trial of early discharge and nurse specialist transitional follow-up care of high-risk childbearing women. *Nursing Research, 46*(5), 254–261.

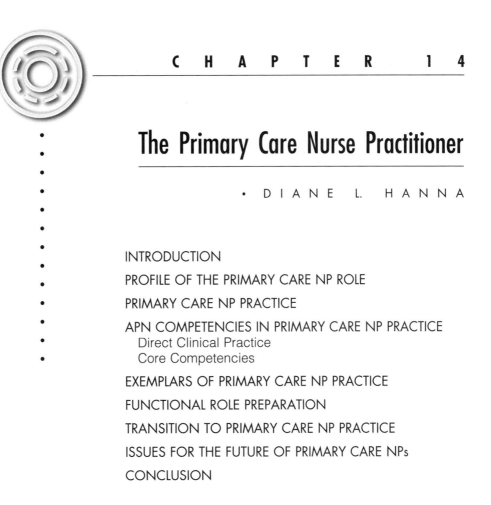

The Primary Care Nurse Practitioner

• D I A N E   L.   H A N N A

INTRODUCTION

This chapter provides an overview of the primary care nurse practitioner (NP) role. With today's emphasis on primary health care within managed care systems, this advanced practice nurse (APN) role has gained widespread attention in today's health care system. This chapter explores the evolution of primary care NP roles and settings. Primary care NP practice as it relates to the Institute of Medicine (IOM) definition of primary care is discussed. APN competencies as operationalized in primary care NP practice are described. Exemplars of a pediatric and family NP practicing in an urban and a rural setting are provided to demonstrate the integration of NP competencies in diverse primary care settings. An overview of an adult NP practicing in a large health maintenance organization (HMO) provides a third and contrasting example. Finally, comments about functional role preparation, transition to professional practice, and key issues for primary care NPs are presented.

PROFILE OF THE PRIMARY CARE NP ROLE

The first primary care NP role, that of pediatric NP, focused on the care of children and was conceived to increase access to pediatric primary care (Ford & Silver,

1967) (see Chapter 1). Since then, a variety of primary care NP roles have evolved, emphasizing care to specific populations such as families, adults, the elderly, and women.

In general, these roles have evolved over time as the ability of nurses in advanced practice to address the needs of varied populations has been recognized. Frequently, the primary care NP role has been acknowledged for increasing access to care for underserved populations (Clawson & Osterweis, 1993). With growing concerns over rising health costs, NPs have come to be recognized as cost-effective providers of quality primary care (Brown & Grimes, 1993; Cook & Nolan, 1996; Kane et al., 1991; Kornblit, Senderoff, Davis-Ericksen, & Zenk, 1990; Mabrook & Dale, 1998; Mundinger et al., 2000).

Overlapping of specialty areas, blended and dual NP practice roles, and varied titling by states make it difficult to determine the number of primary care NPs in the nation. Policy makers at both the state and federal levels have cited the difficulty in obtaining accurate information on NPs in the workforce (Virginia General Assembly, 1999; National Advisory Council on Nurse Education and Practice [NACNEP], 1997). A survey of NP programs nationwide by the National Organization of Nurse Practitioner Faculties (NONPF) and the American Association of Colleges of Nursing (AACN) showed a total of 8,144 students completing NP programs from August 1997 to July 1998. The majority (80%) graduated from master's-level programs, and 18% completed post-master's NP programs. Only 2% of the graduates had completed postbasic registered nurse (certificate) NP programs. The large majority of NP graduates had completed programs in primary care specialties. Breakdowns, by primary care specialty area, of combined graduates of master's, post-master's and certificate graduates are as follows: family NP, 51.5%; adult NP, 17.4%; and pediatric NP, 10%. Significantly smaller percentages of graduates were noted in the following categories: gerontological/geriatric (4.3%), women's health (4.2%), school (0.2%), and occupational health (0.2%) (AACN and NONPF, 1999).

Earlier data from the National Sample Survey of Registered Nurses in March 1996 revealed an estimated 71,000 registered nurses had formal preparation to practice as NPs (Division of Nursing, Bureau of Health Professions, 1997). Almost 90% of the 71,000 estimated NPs nationwide were employed in nursing. Of the 63,000 employed as NPs, about 36,800 (58%) had the position title "nurse practitioner." Slightly more than 10% were employed in nursing education positions and the remaining were distributed among a variety of nursing positions. Most of the 36,800 with NP titles worked in ambulatory care settings, including physician practice sites (36%), school health sites (16%), community health centers (14%), hospital outpatient departments (10%), and HMOs (almost 4%) (Division of Nursing, 1997). As managed care plans continue to penetrate the health care market and HMO care expands, it is anticipated that growing numbers of NPs will be employed in this setting (Cooper, 1997). The 1996 national survey also noted that approximately 24% of the 36,800 registered nurses working with NP titles worked in rural areas (Division of Nursing, 1997).

Between 1992 and 1997, there was a striking increase in the number of institutions offering master's-level NP programs from less than 100 nationwide to more than 250. This trend was sparked by discussions of major federal health reforms and a renewed interest in primary care. The result was a fourfold increase in the number of NPs graduating annually, with further increases anticipated in the future (Cooper, Laud, & Dietrich, 1998; see Chapter 4). Future workforce requirements for NPs are difficult to predict in a rapidly changing health care system where the nature of the NP role itself is evolving. As the NACNEP Nurse Practitioner Workforce Report stated, "The rapid proliferation of NP educational programs and graduates and the extensive changes in the health care delivery system do not provide a solid base from which to predict demand for NPs. Careful monitoring is needed to develop a body of knowledge sufficient to determine supply and requirement trends and to identify factors influencing these trends" (NACNEP, 1997, p. 2). The major NP member organizations, national certifying bodies, and the Department of Health and Human Services, Division of Nursing continue to work together to determine the supply and demand for NP primary care providers across all settings and populations.

PRIMARY CARE NP PRACTICE

What do family, adult, pediatric, obstetric/gynecological, gerontological, and other primary care NPs have in common? The answer to this question lies in a more in-depth analysis of the terms "primary care" and "nurse practitioner." Definitions of primary care have evolved over time. As part of a 2-year study on the future of primary care, the IOM developed an updated definition of primary care. The definition is intended to help health professionals, policy makers, educators, and the public confront the rapid changes underway in health care as primary care is re-emphasized in the United States. The IOM Committee on the Future of Primary Care (1996) offered this updated definition:

> *Primary care is the provision of* **integrated, accessible health care services** *by clinicians who are* **accountable** *for addressing a large* **majority of personal health care needs,** *developing a* **sustained partnership** *with* **patients,** *and practicing in the* **context of family and community.**

> (p. 31)

Within this definition, the emphasized words clarify the nature of services, those involved in the delivery of care, and the nature of the relationship between clinician and patient. Each of the terms in the IOM definition is summarized and explained in the IOM report (1996).

Of note is the broad base of input into this definition of primary care. The IOM Committee on the Future of Primary Care was composed of 19 members representing medicine, nursing, dentistry, health professions educators, health insurers, public health professionals, health care administrators, health economists, and health care consumers. Both NPs and physician assistants were represented on the committee. The definition reflects a broad perspective of health care. It is based on a 1978 IOM definition, but the newer version emphasizes the importance of the patient-clinician relationship in the context of family and community. It also recognizes the facilitation of primary care delivery by teams and integrated delivery systems. The integration of primary care is crucial as the health care paradigm in the United States shifts from a fee-for-service to a managed care reimbursement mechanism and providers change relationships with employers and payers. The role of the primary care NP in collaboration with medical subspecialists offers a provocative approach to health care in this milieu.

An overview of the selected terms in the IOM definition of primary care (1996, pp. 32–50) assists in describing the role of NPs in primary care:

Integrated care refers to "the provision of comprehensive, coordinated, and continuous services" that address any health problem at any stage in the life cycle, combines health services and information to meet a patient's needs, and provides care over time by an individual or team of professionals ("clinician continuity") with effective and timely communication of health information ("record continuity").

Accessibility describes the ease with which the care can be attained. Here, there is a specific emphasis on the elimination of barriers to care. Patient barriers include geographic location, administrative hurdles, reimbursement, culture, and language.

Clinician is defined as "an individual who uses a recognized scientific knowledge base and has the authority to direct the delivery of personal health services to patients."

Accountable applies to both individual clinicians and the systems in which they operate. They are accountable for the care provided, including quality of care, patient satisfaction, efficient use of resources, and ethical behavior.

Majority of personal health care needs is interpreted as a competency to manage the large majority of patient health problems without restriction by problem or organ system. Consultation or referral to other health professionals is made if further evaluation or management is needed.

Sustained partnership refers to a relationship between patient and clinician continued over time. It is based on mutual trust, respect, and responsibility.

Context of family and community references an understanding of the circumstances and facts surrounding a patient. Living conditions, resources, family dynamics, work situation, and cultural background are considered when patients are evaluated. In a broader sense, community refers to the population potentially served, whether or not its members are patients. A group residing within a defined geopolitical boundary, enrollees in a health plan, and a neighborhood with a common heritage are all examples of community. Here the emphasis is on an awareness of public health trends within a community (e.g., leading causes of morbidity and mortality, immunization rates) and their implications for health promotion and disease prevention strategies.

This updated IOM definition of primary care encompasses much of the essence of advanced nursing practice with its emphasis on accountability, a holistic approach to patient care, inclusion of health promotion and disease prevention activities, and description of a patient-clinician relationship "predicated on the development of mutual trust, respect, and responsibility" (IOM, 1996, p. 37). A primary care NP certainly brings these attributes and activities to the primary care setting. The APN's use of *professional caring* with patients as *partners* in health care sets nursing's contributions to primary care apart from other providers' practice (Green-Hernandez, 1997). In Chapter 6, the use of a holistic framework and the forming of partnerships with patients are identified as two of the major characteristics of the APN style of care.

By engaging in the *nursing* process in the primary care setting (i.e., data collection, assessment, planning, implementation, and evaluation) with defined advanced practice skills and competencies, an NP can effectively provide primary care. The population of patients for which the NP is prepared to provide care (e.g., families, adults, children, women, the elderly) serves to differentiate the types of primary care NPs practice (e.g., family NPs; adult NPs; pediatric NPs, including school NPs; obstetric-gynecological NPs; women's health care NPs; and gerontological NPs). The American

Nurses Association (ANA) document concerning the scope and standards of primary care NP practice also reflects the integration of primary care delivery and the nursing process in this APN role (ANA, 1996).

The concept of *integrated, accessible health care services* described by the IOM also underscores the importance of a team approach in primary care delivery, with collaboration between the professionals providing health services. Traditional medical models of care delivery have emphasized the diagnosis and treatment of disease (i.e., curing). Nursing models of care have emphasized developmental and systems theories in considering human responses to illness (i.e., caring over time). Using a holistic approach to assessment and treatment, the primary care NP addresses illness, promotes health, and prevents disease. Interpersonal skills, patient and family education, and coaching and guidance are critical elements of practice. APNs integrate elements of care from nursing and medical models in a collaborative approach to clinical practice that enhances the comprehensiveness and quality of care rendered. Many of the skills and competencies in primary care NP practice are based on the knowledge and skills needed to manage common acute and chronic health problems encountered in primary care settings. By employing expert clinical reasoning and utilizing diverse management approaches (see Chapter 6), the NP renders appropriate cost-effective primary care.

At times, the complexity of health care problems may exceed the NP's scope of practice. In these instances, consultation with physicians or other appropriate team members is indicated. However, it is important to note that the diagnosis and treatment of disease is still integrated with nursing expertise related to the patient's experience of illness. Again, the importance of a team approach to care is emphasized. By the same token, medical practitioners and other professionals on the primary care team may and should consult NPs when issues concerning adherence to therapy, patient and family responses to illness, and health promotion strategies arise. Thus the collaborative efforts of both medical and nursing professionals on primary care teams can assure the provision of high-quality, comprehensive, and holistic patient care (Arcangelo, Fitzgerald, Carroll, & Plumb, 1996; Cook & Nolan, 1996; Hollinger-Smith, 1998; Leveille et al., 1998).

APN COMPETENCIES IN PRIMARY CARE NP PRACTICE

The overview of primary care NP practice provided so far reflects an inclusion of the primary criteria for advanced nursing practice as described in Chapter 3: graduate education, certification, and practice focused on patient/family. Given this overview of the scope of primary care NP practice, its differentiation from medicine and general nursing practice, and the differentiation of various NP roles in primary care, a closer examination of practice competencies enhances understanding of the role. APNs in primary care NP roles bring a variety of skills and competencies to their practice that build on a foundation of basic nursing education. These competencies, initially introduced in basic and graduate education programs, are *continually* developed through clinical experience and ongoing professional education. In Chapter 3, the synergistic impact of graduate education and clinical practice experience on APN development is described, and a set of core competencies in each APN role are identified. An overview of each of the APN competencies in primary care NP practice follows.

Direct Clinical Practice

Primary care services encompass the entire life span of patients. Primary care NPs may be broadly prepared to care for patients at any stage of life (e.g., family NPs) or may have a particular population focus in their practice (e.g., pediatric NPs). No matter what the focus, primary care NPs are involved in the management of health and illness status using the nursing process.

Advanced patient history-taking and physical assessment skills are critical tools for primary care NPs during the data collection stage of the nursing process. Effective communications skills and the ability to establish partnerships enhance the NP's ability to obtain a comprehensive history. A working knowledge of cultural diversity provides an important foundation for this process. Particular attention is paid to personal health habits, stressors, genetics, and an assessment of health risk factors to identify appropriate health promotion and disease prevention strategies.

Evaluating the subjective and objective data collected requires critical thinking and diagnostic reasoning skills on the part of the primary care NP. These aspects of clinical decision making are required not only in the identification of problems but in the further evaluation and management of health needs of primary care clients. Specific health promotion needs based on stages of physical and psychosocial development may be assessed. Much of primary care NP practice involves the diagnosis and management of acute, self-limiting, minor illnesses and stable chronic diseases. However, primary care practice requires an ability to recognize signs and symptoms of complex and unstable health problems requiring medical or other consultation. It also calls for the recognition of emergency situations and initiation of effective emergency care.

Following the initial assessment phase of the nursing process, primary care NPs may plan for care in the form of additional diagnostic studies, specific therapeutic measures, and coaching and guidance strategies. Clinical practice guidelines such as those cited on the Agency for Healthcare Research and Quality (2000) website *http://www.AHRQ.gov/clinic* can help to guide the clinician in planning for appropriate intervention. The efficacy and safety of therapy over time as well as the client's health goals, risk factors, and illness experience are also considered as plans are developed.

Further diagnostic tests (e.g., laboratory, radiography, or other diagnostic studies) may be required to more accurately assess the patient's health status. Age-specific screening examinations may be recommended as a part of clinical preventive service guidelines. Specific therapeutic measures may encompass both pharmacological and nonpharmacological therapies. If pharmacological therapy is initiated, the NP determines the appropriate treatment and counsels the patient about drug regimens and side effects (NONPF, 1995).

Many of the primary care NP's therapeutic recommendations may be nonpharmacological (e.g., specific dietary or activity recommendations, stress management strategies). In fact, primary care NPs are more likely to use nonpharmacological therapies than are traditional medical practitioners (Moody, Smith, & Glenn 1999). Patient education and counseling strategies in the management of health and illness status include anticipatory guidance related to normal growth and development for patients and families as well as potential changes they may experience in terms of specific health problems. Additional coaching and guidance competencies utilized in NP practice are discussed in the following section.

Once plans of care are developed and implemented, the primary care NP uses expected outcome criteria to evaluate the effectiveness of interventions. Scheduling phone or office follow-up visits to appropriately monitor clients is an important aspect of ongoing evaluation. When outcome criteria are not achieved, the plan of care is revised accordingly, and further consultation may be indicated (NONPF, 1995). Careful documentation of all services provided forms the basis for professional reimbursement. Outcome data for groups of patients are a critical measure of practice safety and efficacy. These data are closely monitored by the payers of health care and help to validate professional practice. The Health Plan Employer Data and Information Set (HEDIS) is one example of performance measures used to evaluate primary care practice (Buppert, 1999; see Chapter 25).

Core Competencies

COACHING AND GUIDANCE

As mentioned in the discussion of direct clinical practice, coaching and guidance competencies are critical elements of NP practice. An emphasis on these activities helps to differentiate NP practice from that of other primary care providers. Coaching and guidance in NP practice is based on a variety of psychosocial theories such as learning theory, communication theory, and family dynamics. Competency in this aspect of practice may be reflected in a variety of ways. For example, the NP demonstrates competency in patient education by assessing a patient's readiness to learn and level of motivation and then providing an environment that promotes learning. Interactions with patients in ways that are nonjudgmental and culturally sensitive facilitates a sense of partnership in the primary care setting.

The explanation of a client's condition, treatment choices, and rationale for procedures is another important competency in this aspect of practice. The NP helps patients to understand their own body and symptoms and responds to their questions. Relevant lifestyle adjustments and other measures for health promotion are also discussed. When combined, these strategies can help to maximize patients' participation in their own care. As a patient counselor, the primary care NP may assess and support patients experiencing crisis, loss, or grief situations and determines whether referral to mental health professionals may be indicated (NONPF, 1995).

Coaching and guidance activities become the backbone of health promotion and disease prevention activities. Once lifestyle patterns are assessed and risk factors for illness and injury are determined, the NP is positioned to work with the patient to identify and individualize appropriate health promotion strategies. Exercise, nutrition, stress management, injury prevention, safe sexual practices, and elimination of smoking and other substance abuse habits are areas frequently addressed. Again, creating a partnership with the client lays the groundwork for prioritizing risk reduction strategies and planning realistic interventions that contribute to success. Expert coaching and guidance in APN practice is fully discussed in Chapter 7.

CONSULTATION

Three types of advanced nursing practice consultation are most common: APN–staff nurse consultation, APN-APN consultation, and APN-physician consultation (see Chapter 8). All three of these consultative relationships can foster more effective patient care and are important tools in primary care NP practice. For example, NPs in primary care may have the opportunity to work with home health nurses to coordinate and deliver health care services to homebound patients. Community-based nursing professionals offer valuable insights into family and home environment issues impacting patient health. Furthermore, community health nurses have a wealth of knowledge regarding available community resources and insurance coverage for home care services. It is also the wise primary care NP who will seek another NP as consultant when additional advanced nursing practice expertise is needed. This might entail validation of a clinical finding or advice related to a particular area of clinical practice such as pediatrics, geriatrics, or women's health. Finally, as previously discussed, physician consultation can become a critical tool for practice when complex medical conditions or those requiring medical specialist referrals are encountered.

RESEARCH SKILLS

Clinical practice in this "age of information" offers both exciting opportunities and challenges for the primary care NP. Health care knowledge resources are increasingly available in electronic form, especially on the Internet. However, current information systems are not always easily integrated into clinical practice and contain content of varying quality (Hersh, 1999; Stange, 1996). Health care informatics have facilitated the development of clinical practice guidelines based on current research and the consensus of clinical experts (Fonteyn, 1998; Pearson, 1998). Today's primary care NP must have research savvy to retrieve available information and to critically appraise important practice innovations (Tsafrir & Grinberg, 1998; Worrall, 1999).

Clinical practice guidelines developed from evidence-based, clinically effective practices can be used to improve primary care. With the advent of managed care systems, practice guidelines have also been used to reduce costs, standardize practice, and decrease medical liability. Clinical practice guidelines in primary care should be used as a tool to assure best practices in care delivery. When combined with outcome and performance measures that provide feedback to clinicians, guidelines can be modified to meet the needs of the local patient population (Bergman, 1999).

As experts in preventive and patient-centered care, primary care NPs should take an active role in clinical practice research, the development of clinical practice guidelines, and review of outcome and performance measures. Stange (1996) cited opportunities for interdisciplinary collaboration in primary care research and the creation of primary care research centers. These activities require a mastery of basic research skills, as discussed in Chapter 9.

CLINICAL AND PROFESSIONAL LEADERSHIP

A more general set of skills related to the NP role and the individual, groups, and organizations to which they relate comprise this core competency. Here, an understanding of the NP role, health policy, change and conflict theory, business and marketing, and professional leadership is a critical foundation (NONPF, 1995). Of all the related competencies described, clinical and professional leadership may require the most experience and professional maturity to develop (see Chapter 10). Professional leadership requires an ability to see the big picture and to interact with multiple participants in the health care system. In an era of rapid change through marketplace reform and dynamic health policy debates, the ability to market the NP role to managed care systems and policy makers is an example of professional leadership critical to the profession's future (see Chapters 21 through 23).

At the patient care level, an NP demonstrates clinical leadership through the coordination of care to meet multiple client health needs and requests. The importance of the interdisciplinary team and collaboration in primary care has been cited. The primary care NP assists in the development of such a team to provide optimal therapy. Establishing priorities for care and ensuring continuity of care is yet another example of leadership in patient care. Finally, serving as a role model, mentor, and preceptor for novice practitioners is an important way to ensure a viable future for the NP role (NONPF, 1995).

From a broader health policy perspective, participation in professional organizations as well as health legislation and policy-making activities can result in important strategies to improve the health of populations. NPs have an important perspective to share through analysis of contemporary health policy and its impact on consumers, providers, and the nation. Historically, NPs have advocated for the needs of underserved populations in the health policy arena. In an era of rapidly evolving health care systems, advocating for accessible, affordable primary care for the underserved continues to be of major importance.

COLLABORATION

Each of the competencies in primary care NP practice discussed so far requires the development of collaborative relationships with patients and other health care professionals. Direct clinical practice in primary care with expert coaching and guidance has a collaborative relationship between patient and NP at its core. The IOM definition of primary care (1996) implies the use of professional collaboration to deliver "integrated" and "accessible" care. Effective collaboration results in more comprehensive, patient-focused care (Hughes and Turner, 1996) that promotes quality, cost-effective outcomes (Brita-Rossi et al., 1996; Stichler, 1995). Expert coaching and guidance also requires the establishment of a collaborative relationship between patient and provider. Professional consultation and research entails collaborative relationships between a variety of health care providers with common goals and purposes (Conger & Craig, 1998; Weinstein, McCormack, Brown, & Rosenthal, 1998). On a broader level, primary care NPs engaged in clinical and professional leadership must also utilize effective collaborative skills to assist groups and organizations to envision preferred futures, achieve consensus, and implement change. (See Chapter 11 for an in-depth discussion of collaboration.)

ETHICAL DECISION-MAKING SKILLS

Ethical decision-making skills are frequently considered in the context of acute care settings or end-of-life issues, but these skills are also an integral part of primary care NP practice. The IOM definition of primary care refers to the primary care clinician as being "accountable" for addressing health care needs. Accountability refers to both clinicians and the systems in which they operate and includes a responsibility for ethical behavior. Care that respects and protects patient dignity as well as ensures that an individual's presenting complaint is addressed is a hallmark of accountability in primary care (IOM, 1996).

The primary care NP may encounter patient care issues with significant ethical overtones. Examples include reproductive issues, informed consent, and conflicting health care goals among family members. The primary care setting also provides an opportunity to discuss other ethical issues such as advance directives and organ donation with patients in a relaxed and thoughtful manner. Primary care NPs are accountable first and foremost to their patients, with patient confidentiality honored at all times. In an era of managed care, the primary care clinician's accountability to the health care system in which she or he practices may create tension, especially where the use of resources for patient care is concerned. Primary care NPs must always be ethically accountable for their actions, especially where financial incentives related to resource utilization are involved (Abel, 1994; Aroskar, 1998; Coolican & Swanson, 1998; IOM, 1996; see Chapter 12).

EXEMPLARS OF PRIMARY CARE NP PRACTICE

Having considered the scope of primary care NP practice along with its competencies, specific examples are provided here to demonstrate how an NP can assist in meeting the primary care needs of a particular community. The first two exemplars illustrate NPs engaged in the delivery of primary care to underserved populations in two very different settings, a low-income urban community and a rural health center. In community-based practices such as these, the importance of community assessment has been recognized as a way for primary care practitioners to more effectively meet the needs of the population they serve (Abraham & Fallon, 1997; Courtney, 1995; Reece, 1998). A community needs assessment can identify existing and potential health problems as well as health promotion needs (Reece, 1998). Once these needs are identified, collaboration with other health care professionals, educators, and community leaders can provide a critical link in empowering individuals, families, and communities to improve their health status.

The third exemplar describes an adult NP's practice in a large HMO. As NPs increasingly become involved with managed care systems, an understanding of the business and legal aspects of practice is critical to survival as a primary care provider in a competitive marketplace. The value-added aspects of NP care in a collaborative practice system continue to make the NP a preferred primary care provider. Chapter 26 provides several examples of innovative practice opportunities. These examples describe the wide variety of practice settings available to the primary care NP.

EXEMPLAR 1: URBAN PEDIATRIC NP PRACTICE

Jane is a pediatric NP caring for children in a low-income urban community. This community once thrived as part of a major industrial center but was devastated by factory closings and a declining local economy. Recent health status indicators for this urban area reveal increasing rates of teen pregnancy. There is growing concern in the community about substance abuse, school dropouts, and community violence.

This setting is a challenging one, but Jane feels that, by working with children and families through the community Child Health Clinic, she might be able to help them deal with the risks that poverty introduces to their health. The clinic is a public-private venture jointly funded by the local health department, the community hospital, and various charitable organizations in the greater metropolitan area. It serves as a source of primary care to many of the community's children whose health care is subsidized by Medicaid and who are now enrolled in a statewide managed care program. The clinic also provides services to non-Medicaid recipients using a sliding-scale fee.

Jane sees a variety of infants, children, and adolescents who come to the clinic for both well-child visits and acute/episodic health problems. Her care entails thorough health assessments by history taking, physical assessment, and appropriate diagnostic studies or screening examinations. She then recommends appropriate interventions (both pharmacological and nonpharmacological) for the child. These are in keeping with established clinical guidelines used in the clinic. Much of Jane's time is spent discussing normal childhood growth and development with parents as well as effective parenting skills, nutritional needs, immunizations, and age-specific injury prevention guidelines. If the child is ill, she describes ways to monitor the child's health status. Jane's days take on a busy pace as she sees children for regularly scheduled well-child visits and manages a variety of episodic health problems during the clinic's walk-in hours.

At times, Jane may consult with the clinic pediatrician about acute health problems or abnormal health screening findings. For children and families with complex health problems, she may also consult with other members of the clinic team for further evaluation and management. Public health nurses are available for home assessment and case management services, and the clinic social worker provides additional outreach services. A nutritionist and eligibility worker from the Women, Infants, and Children's nutrition program are on site to address nutritional needs in depth.

Jane also engages with this community outside the walls of the clinic. Involvement with community activities enhances her credibility and acceptance among this low-income population. On occasion she is asked to assist with health screening examinations for the local Head Start program. Recently there has been growing concern about unmet needs for child health services in the greater urban area. Inappropriate use of local emergency rooms for episodic health care and a rising incidence of asthma and lead poisoning have contributed to a renewed commitment to pediatric primary care. As a respected primary care provider for an underserved community, Jane has been asked to serve on a local Child Health Task Force. She will work with other health care providers and community leaders to identify ways to more effectively use public and private resources in addressing children's health needs. Together, they hope to promote a healthier future for the community at large.

EXEMPLAR 2: RURAL FAMILY NP PRACTICE

With 3 years of experience as a family NP at the Mountain Breeze Rural Health Center, Mary realized how much she had developed as a primary care provider. She had worked as a public health nurse for 10 years in this coal mining and industrial community of Appalachia and was familiar with its poverty and limited access to health care. In fact, the mountains themselves, with narrow winding roads, posed one of the major barriers to care in this area—transportation.

Before the local family physician of 40 years retired, Mary had been able to pursue her NP education through a master's degree program offered by the state university satellite program on the community college campus 40 miles away. The hour commute to school grew long, but that trip was short when compared with the additional 300 miles traversed by teleconferencing to provide for interaction with faculty on the main campus. Mary was fortunate to have been the recipient of a state scholarship for her graduate education. For this educational funding she had agreed to practice in a medically underserved area of the state. This was easy for Mary because Appalachia had been home to her for all of her life.

Anticipating the loss of their longstanding physician, the community had worked hard to support the establishment of a rural health center in the area. Mary was well known to the local citizens as a public health nurse, and they readily accepted her in her new role as an NP. The nearest hospital, 30 miles away, had recently been engaged in the development of rural health networks and provided physician coverage in the center 3 days per week. The retiring family physician had been a real asset for Mary to work with in her first year following graduation as she made the transition to her new role. Now, on the 3 days per week that physicians were on site, she could be sure that patients requiring more complex medical management were scheduled. These days also provided an opportunity to review and discuss other patient management issues and to develop skills and knowledge related to the medical issues in her practice.

Mary's days at the center were always full but never predictable. As an FNP she provided care for a wide range of episodic health concerns for patients across the lifespan. She cared for many adults with chronic health problems such as diabetes and hypertension. She devoted much of her effort to working with patients and their families on improved nutritional status and other health promotion strategies. One of her diabetic patients had recently started insulin therapy. After teaching him how to monitor his glucose at home, she was able to adjust his initial insulin therapy over the phone. The phone proved to be a valuable tool for her practice because many families had no regular source of transportation to the clinic. As the only female primary care provider in the area, Mary found much of her time devoted to women's health care. Women found it easy to share their concerns with her, and Mary frequently discussed family health problems with them during these visits. She also followed many children from infancy through childhood for well-child and episodic visits.

One afternoon a week, Mary left the clinic and made rounds on patients in the local nursing home. She worked closely with the staff there to identify ways to assist this elderly population in maintaining as much independence as possible. She also enjoyed occasional trips to the local high school to assist with sports physicals. From time to time she was invited to be a speaker at the employee health seminars held at the nearby packaging plant.

Her work was rewarding and there were many challenges ahead. She had recently discussed the area's low childhood immunization rates with local leaders. They were now developing a proposal for a mobile health unit to increase access to immunizations and other primary preventive services to remote sections of the tri-county area. Mary was asked to portray some of this Appalachian community's health needs to a contingency of state and federal legislators visiting the area. She hoped to make a compelling case for a mobile health unit so that funding for the project could be secured.

EXEMPLAR 3: ADULT NP IN AN HMO

Terry, an experienced adult NP, had worked in a private family health practice on the East Coast with three physicians and another NP for 10 years. When her family was relocated to the West by her husband's employer, she found a very different kind of job market for NPs. Now, instead of working with a small group practice, she had taken a job as an adult NP with a large HMO.

Although the types of health care problems she encountered in her new practice were similar to those she dealt with previously, the new work environment was quite different. Centralized scheduling created shorter patient visit times than those in her previous practice. Terry had to find new ways to streamline visits and still maintain her personalized approach as a health care provider. Well-developed clinical guidelines were available for reference when needed. Prescriptive practice in this HMO necessitated familiarity with medications on formulary. Referrals to specialists required completion of a special form and approval by the medical director on site.

Health records were maintained electronically, thus facilitating easy retrieval and transmission of patient data. These electronic databases were also used to track utilization and outcome data for the panel of patients assigned to her. Terry received monthly reports on the number and type of patient visits, utilization of services, costs of care, and her overall clinical productivity.

There are several NPs employed at this large primary care site. Terry enjoys a collegial relationship with them and the other team members. The physicians in this practice are familiar with the primary care NP role and the value NPs have added to the health care team. Terry also participates in new opportunities to evaluate her primary care team's practice. Reviewing utilization and outcome data assists the team in developing special strategies to address the needs of their patient population. Using HEDIS measures to track results, they engage in a process of continuous quality improvement.

FUNCTIONAL ROLE PREPARATION

Based on the exemplars, it is clear that the scope of primary care NP practice is broad and requires a high level of clinical competency and professional accountability. Students in graduate NP education programs must develop a solid foundation of knowledge in primary care and management skills in order to facilitate more autonomous clinical practice than was required in their previous generalist nursing roles. They must understand the professional accountability that is assumed when undertaking this APN role and demonstrate a commitment to continuous professional growth and development. Skills as a team member are also essential to the primary care NP because the role calls for collaboration with a variety of health professionals (see Chapter 11).

To prepare students for collaborative practice, interdisciplinary approaches to education should be undertaken (Felten, Cady, Metzler, & Burton, 1997). In the classroom, clinical content can be effectively presented by NPs, physicians, and other members of the primary care team as one way to facilitate understanding of the perspective and expertise that each brings to patient care. Clinical experiences for students are also enhanced by an interdisciplinary approach. By seeing first-hand how collaborative approaches to patient care can facilitate cost-effective, comprehensive care, students will be better prepared for interdependent primary care practice.

A strong curriculum that provides an in-depth clinical knowledge base and skill level is required based on the NP specialty and scope of practice. In addition to basic role and clinical competencies developed in primary care NP programs, an understanding of other professional practice issues related to advanced nursing practice is critical. NPs must be familiar with statutes and regulations governing practice in their state as well as appropriate licensing, professional credentialing, and clinical privileging procedures. A clear understanding of one's professional scope of practice is directly related to professional regulation and reimbursement issues. Résumé development and interview and contract negotiating skills are important tools for securing a rewarding clinical practice position. Familiarity with risk management procedures and appropriate professional liability coverage will help to provide protection from costly malpractice litigation. Finally, changes in the health care environment for NP practice require higher levels of understanding about the practice setting's billing and reimbursement policies and procedures. This awareness is essential for the development of economically sound primary care practice (see Chapters 20, 22, and 23).

The emphasis on cost-effectiveness of care will continue to grow as managed care markets expand. Reimbursement will be more closely tied to clinical productivity. NPs must have an understanding of cost-efficient practices and clinical decision-making skills to be able to establish appropriate priorities in clinical care. In busy practice settings, the use of telephone triage and management skills is another tool in addressing both acute and chronic health problems. The NP may require additional guidance and experience to develop telephone interview and follow-up skills. An ongoing emphasis on clinical preventive services for health promotion and disease prevention promotes cost-effective care (Ryan, 1993). The NP must learn ways to incorporate these services into routine patient visits and seize teachable moments with clients for effective health education. An "ethic of caring" must continue to undergird NP practice in order to bridge the gap between cost-containment strategies reducing quantity of services and those concerns related to quality of services (Abel, 1994).

Marketplace forces and health policy debates continue to create rapid change in primary care delivery systems. The primary care NP must understand the forces that are driving change and the ways they may shape practice in the future. Furthermore, student APNs should begin to develop an understanding of how they can influence health policy to assure that quality health care services are made accessible, affordable, and available to all.

TRANSITION TO PRIMARY CARE NP PRACTICE

With so many professional practice issues to consider, as well as the need for well-developed APN competencies, it is no surprise that newly prepared primary care NPs may feel overwhelmed as they face the realities of advanced practice. The initial year of NP practice is an important transitional year that provides the critical foundation for developing professional expertise and delivering high-quality health care. Brown and Olshansky (1997) have studied the experiences of new NP graduates during their first year of primary care practice. From their data collection and analysis they constructed a theoretical model representing the transition to the primary care NP role (see Chapter 4). Their research has important implications for the first year of clinical practice as a primary care NP. First, the new graduate may experience a considerable amount of anxiety and general sense of disequilibrium. The first 6 months of practice is a time for redefinition of one's professional self and a time of being "in limbo." Realistic expectations for practice knowledge, skills, and performance must be maintained by the new practitioner, professional mentors, and others in the practice setting. As Brown and Olshansky noted, "the vital contribution of the first year of clinical practice experience and skill repetition to expanding knowledge and strengthening practice skills cannot be overemphasized" (1997, p. 51).

ISSUES FOR THE FUTURE OF PRIMARY CARE NPs

Negotiating the evolving health care marketplace and moving from an "invisible" provider status in many managed care systems to recognized members of provider panels are the major challenges facing primary care NPs today. NPs have long been recognized as providers of cost-effective, high-quality care. These attributes are in keeping with managed care's emphasis on prevention and cost savings. However, access to primary care NPs has been increasingly controlled by managed care organizations. Many managed care organizations do not extend contracts to NPs directly. Instead, physicians who hire them are responsible for NP performance and compensation. This invisible provider status makes it difficult for health care consumers to access NP care directly and, equally challenging, to evaluate the impact of NP services on costs and outcomes in capitated systems of care (Cohen, Mason, Arsenie, Sargese, & Needham, 1998; Yurkowski, 1997).

Managed care organization executives have reported a high degree of satisfaction with NPs serving as primary care providers and recognize their value in providing expert coaching and guidance (Mason, Cohen, O'Donnell, Baxter, & Chase, 1997). However, there is still confusion about the scope of NP practice among health care professionals, managed care executives, and the public. NPs must continue to educate these groups about their role in primary care delivery. The development of sound marketing strategies that clearly define NP care and its benefits are essential in negotiating with managed care plans (Pakis, 1997). Identifying a "professional niche" that contributes to decreased costs and improved outcomes may be of particular benefit in marketing efforts (see Chapter 21). To be successful in today's health care marketplace, NPs must also have a proficient understanding of accounting, finance, economics, and reimbursement practices (Wing, 1998). Whether reimbursed by Medicare, Medicaid, indemnity insurers, or managed care organizations, the primary care NP must be familiar with the reimbursement policies of third-party payers, including documentation and billing guidelines (Buppert, 1998).

The development of more formal contracting, credentialing, and privileging processes for NPs in managed care systems is likely as the health care system evolves. The primary care NP must be familiar with organizational credentialing measures and complete them. It is likely that NPs will need to provide data on the outcomes of care they have provided. The HEDIS, with specific performance measures for primary care, has been developed by the National Committee for Quality Assurance, a nonprofit organization that accredits health plans. An understanding of HEDIS measures and how HEDIS scores will affect clinicians and is critical to the future of all primary care providers (Buppert, 1999; Rustia and Bartek, 1997; Yurkowski, 1997; see Chapters 20, 22, 24, and 25).

Practice opportunities and perceived differences in NP scope of practice are largely related to state regulations and the practice environments they create (Cooper, Henderson, & Deitrich, 1998; Mason et al., 1997; Sekscenski, Sansom, Bazell, Salmon, & Mullan, 1994). NPs must continue to address restrictions on their scope of practice, prescriptive authority, and eligibility for reimbursement that create barriers to professional practice. The committed efforts of NP leaders at state and national levels, combined with support from nursing organizations to educate policy makers and effect change in these areas have been commendable. However, much remains to be done to remove remaining legal and regulatory restrictions to practice (see Chapter 22). Furthermore, ongoing professional vigilance to protect the gains of the past is required. Professional unity with APNs, coalition building, and strong leadership at state and national levels are critical to achieve these goals. NPs in primary care practice must be willing to invest in these organizations and activities to protect and promote their professional futures.

The advent of telehealth technologies offers exciting possibilities for health care delivery and education. Along with these developments come new professional challenges related to interstate licensure and professional reimbursement for telehealth services (Sharp, 1996, 1997; Williamson & Hutcherson, 1998). NPs will have many continuing education opportunities available to them via the Internet, cable television, and other evolving modalities. By the same token, they will need to become familiar with the new sources of electronic health care information available to their patients and counsel them about reliable resources to use.

CONCLUSION

As stated earlier, primary care NPs have been recognized as pioneers in NP practice. This APN role was conceived to enhance access to cost-effective health care practice for underserved populations. The cost, quality, and competence benefits of primary care NPs have been well validated since the role's inception in the mid 1960s. As the nation moves toward prepaid, managed systems of care with an emphasis on primary care and health promotion, the NP becomes an ideal provider of primary care for all patient populations. The IOM's updated definition of primary care (1996) encompasses much of the essence of advanced practice nursing and highlights the major role of NPs in primary care delivery.

The APN competencies of primary care NP practice have been described to provide a comprehensive overview of this advanced practice role. As with other APN roles, the continued professional development of NPs will lead to greater proficiency in each of the competencies over time. The traditional period from student to professional primary care NP provides an important time to expand knowledge and strengthen clinical practice.

The health care system, no doubt, will continue to evolve with marketplace and policy reforms as well as emerging communications technologies shaping its future. NPs will assume a critical role in the primary care workforce of the future if they take an active role in developing health policy and care delivery systems today. Both professional unity and interdisciplinary collegiality must undergird these efforts.

R E F E R E N C E S

Abel, E. (1994). Productivity versus quality of care: Ethical implications for clinical practice during health care reform. *Nurse Practitioner Forum, 5*(4), 238–242.

Abraham, T., & Fallon, P. J. (1997). Clinical exemplar. Caring for the community: Development of the advanced practice nurse role. *Clinical Nurse Specialist, 11*(5), 224–230.

Agency for Healthcare Research and Quality. (2000). *Clinical information. http://www.ahrq.gov/clinic*

American Association of Colleges of Nursing and the National Organization of Nurse Practitioner Faculties. (1999). *1998-1999 Enrollment and Graduations in Baccalaureate and Graduate Programs in Nursing.* Washington, DC: American Association of Colleges of Nursing.

American Nurses Association. (1996). *The scope and standards of practice of advanced practice registered nursing.* Washington, DC: Author.

Arcangelo, V., Fitzgerald, M., Carroll, D., & Plumb, J. D. (1996). Collaborative care between nurse practitioners and primary care physicians. *Primary Care, 23*(1), 103–113.

Aroskar, M. A. (1998). Ethical working relationships in patient care: Challenges and possibilities. *Nursing Clinics of North America, 33*(2), 313–324.

Bergman, D. A. (1999). Evidence-based guidelines and critical pathways for quality improvement. *Pediatrics, 103*(1, Suppl. E), 225–232.

Brita-Rossi, P., Adduci, P., Kaufman, J., Lipson, S. J., Totte, C., & Wasserman, K. (1996). Improving the process of care: The cost-quality value of interdisciplinary collaboration. *Journal of Nursing Care Quarterly, 10*(2), 10–16.

Brown, M. A., & Olshansky, E. F. (1997). From limbo to legitimacy: A theoretical model of the transition to the primary care nurse practitioner role. *Nursing Research, 46*(1), 46–51.

Brown, S. A., & Grimes, D. E. (1993). *Nurse practitioners and certified nurse midwives: A metaanalysis of process of care, clinical outcomes, and cost-effectiveness of nurses in primary care roles* (#NP-85). Washington, DC: American Nurses Association.

Buppert, C. (1998). Reimbursement for nurse practitioner services. *Nurse Practitioner, 23*(1), 67, 70–74, 76 passim.

Buppert, C. (1999). HEDIS for the primary care provider: Getting an "A" on the managed care report card. *Nurse Practitioner, 24*(1), 84, 86, 88–89, 92–94, 97–99.

Clawson, D. K., & Osterweis, M. (Eds.). (1993). *The roles of physician assistants and nurse practitioners in primary care.* Washington, DC: Association of Academic Health Centers.

Cohen, S. S., Mason, D. J., Arsenie, L. S., Sargese, S. M., & Needham, D. (1998). Focus groups reveal perils and promise of managed care for nurse practitioners. *Nurse Practitioner, 23*(6), 48, 54, 57-60 passim.

Conger, M., & Craig, C. (1998). Advanced nurse practice: A model for collaboration. *Nursing Case Management, 3*(3), 120-127.

Cook, T., & Nolan, W. (1996). A nurse practitioner-led, collaborative, out-patient practice: A case study in outcomes management. *Seminars for Nurse Managers, 4,* 154-162.

Coolican, M. B., & Swanson, A. (1998). Primary health-care physicians: Vital roles in organ and tissue donation. *Connecticut Medicine, 62,* 149-153.

Cooper, R. A. (1997). The growing independence of nonphysician clinicians in clinical practice. *JAMA, 277,* 1092-1093.

Cooper, R. A., Henderson, T., & Dietrich, C. L. (1998). Roles of nonphysician clinicians as autonomous providers of patient care. *JAMA, 280,* 795-802.

Cooper, R. A., Laud, P., & Dietrich, C. L. (1998). Current and projected workforce of nonphysician clinicians. *JAMA, 280,* 788-794.

Courtney, R. (1995). Community partnership primary care: A new paradigm for primary care. *Public Health Nursing, 12*(6), 366-373.

Division of Nursing, Bureau of Health Professions. (1997). *Nurse practitioners* (based on data from the National Sample Survey of Registered Nurses, March 1996). Prepared by Evelyn B. Moses, Chief, Nursing Data Analysis Staff. Washington, DC: Health Resources and Services Administration.

Felten, S., Cady, N., Metzler, M. H., & Burton, S. (1997). Implementation of collaborative practice through interdisciplinary rounds on a general surgery service. *Nursing Case Management, 2*(3), 122-126.

Fonteyn, M. (1998). The Agency for Health Care Policy and Research guidelines: Implications for home health care providers. *American Association of Colleges of Nursing Clinical Issues, 9*(3), 338-354.

Ford, L. C., & Silver, H. K. (1967). The expanded role of the nurse in child care. *Nursing Outlook, 15,* 43-45.

Green-Hernandez, C. (1997). Application of caring theory in primary care: A challenge for advanced practice. *Nursing Administration Quarterly, 21*(4), 77-82.

Hersh, W. (1999). "A world of knowledge at your fingertips" The promise, reality, and future directions of on-line information retrieval. *Academic Medicine, 74*(3), 240-243.

Hollinger-Smith, L. (1998). Partners in collaboration. *Journal of Professional Nursing, 14*(6), 344-349.

Hughes, A. M., & Turner, L. C. (1996). Nurse-physician collaboration: Historical review and impact today. *CACCN, 7*(3), 24-28.

Institute of Medicine Committee on the Future of Primary Care. (1996). *Primary care: America's health in a new era.* Washington, DC: National Academy Press.

Kane, R. L., Garrard, J., Buchanan, J. L., Rosenfeld, A., Skay, C., & McDermott, S. (1991). Improving primary care in nursing homes. *Journal of the American Geriatrics Society, 39,* 359-367.

Kornblit, P., Senderoff, J., Davis-Ericksen, M., & Zenk, J. (1990). Anticoagulant therapy: Patient management and evaluation of an outpatient clinic. *Nurse Practitioner, 15*(8), 21-26, 29, 32.

Leveille, S. G., Wagner, E. H., Davis, C., Grothaus, L., Wallace, J., LoGerfo, M., & Kent, D. (1998). Preventing disability and managing chronic illness in frail older adults: A randomized trial of a community-based partnership with primary care. *Journal of the American Geriatrics Society, 46*(10), 1191-1198.

Mabrook, A. F., & Dale, B. (1998). Can nurse practitioners offer a quality service? *Journal of Accident and Emergency Medicine, 15*(4), 266-268.

Mason, D. J., Cohen, S. S., O'Donnell, J. P., Baxter, K., & Chase, A. B. (1997). Managed care organizations' arrangements with nurse practitioners. *Nursing Economics, 15*(6), 306-314.

Moody, N. B., Smith, P. L., & Glenn, L. L. (1999). Client characteristics and practice patterns of nurse practitioners and physicians. *Nurse Practitioner, 24*(3), 94-96, 99-100, 102-103.

Mundinger, M. O., Kane, R. L., Lenz, E. R., Totlen, A. M., Tsai, W., Cleary, P. D., Friedewald, W. T., Siu, A., L., & Shelanski, M. L. (2000). Primary care outcomes in patients treated by nurse practitioners or physicians: A randomized trial. *Journal of the American Medical Association, 283*(1), 59-68.

National Advisory Council on Nurse Education and Practice. (1997). *Nurse practitioner workforce report executive summary.* Washington, DC: Author.

National Organization of Nurse Practitioner Faculties. (1995). *Advanced practice nursing: Nurse practitioner curriculum guidelines and program standards.* Washington, DC: Author.

Pakis, S. (1997). Managing the marketing function for advanced nurse practitioners in a managed care environment. *Seminars for Nurse Managers, 5,* 149-153.

Pearson, K. C. (1998). The role of evidence-based medicine and clinical practice guidelines in treatment decisions. *Clinical Therapeutics, 20*(Suppl. C), C80-C85.

Reece, S. M. (1998). Community analysis for health planning: Strategies for primary care practitioners. *Nurse Practitioner, 23*(10), 46-59.

Rustia, J. G., & Bartek, J. K. (1997). Managed care credentialing of advanced practice nurses. *Nurse Practitioner, 22*(9), 90-92, 99-100, 102-103.

Ryan, S. A. (1993). Nurse practitioners: Educational issues, practice styles, and service barriers. In M. Osterweis & S. Garfinkel (Eds.), *The roles of physician assistants and nurse practitioners in primary care* (pp. 41–49). Washington, DC: Association of Academic Health Centers.

Sekscenski, E. S., Sansom, S., Bazell, C., Salmon, M. E., & Mullan, F. (1994). State practice environments and the supply of physician assistants, nurse practitioners, and certified nurse-midwives. *New England Journal of Medicine, 331,* 1266–1271.

Sharp, N. (1996). Nurse practitioners, telemedicine, and the Federal Communications Commission. *Nurse Practitioner, 21*(7), 99–100.

Sharp, N. (1997). Medicare reimbursement: For NPs, CNSs, MDs, and telehealth. *Nurse Practitioner, 22*(8), 143–146.

Stange, K. C. (1996). Primary care research: Barriers and opportunities. *Journal of Family Practice, 42*(2), 192–198.

Stichler, J. F. (1995). Professional interdependence: The art of collaboration. *Advanced Practice Nursing Quarterly, 1*(1), 53–61.

Tsafrir, J., & Grinberg, M. (1998). Who needs evidence-based health care? *Bulletin of the Medical Library Association, 86*(1), 40–45.

Virginia General Assembly, House Joint Resolution No. 682, *Directing the Joint Commission on Health Care to study the need to collect workforce data on nurse practitioners, clinical nurse specialists, registered nurses, licensed practical nurses, and certified nurse aides.* (1999).

Weinstein, M. E., McCormack, B., Brown, M. E., & Rosenthal, D. S. (1998). Build consensus and develop collaborative practice guidelines. *Nursing Management, 29*(9), 48–52.

Williamson, S. H., & Hutcherson, C. (1998). Mutual recognition: Response to the regulatory implications of a changing health care environment. *Advanced Practice Nursing Quarterly, 4*(3), 86–93.

Wing, D. M. (1998). The business management preceptorship within the nurse practitioner program. *Journal of Professional Nursing, 14,* 150–156.

Worrall, G. (1999). Clinical practice guidelines: Questions family physicians should ask themselves. *Comprehensive Therapy, 25*(1), 46–49.

Yurkowski, W. (1997). The use of nonphysician providers in managed care settings. *JAMA, 277,* 1095.

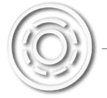

The Acute Care Nurse Practitioner

- D E B O R A H   M.   R U S T
- K A T H Y   S.   M A G D I C

INTRODUCTION

As changes in the health care environment have occurred, the acute care nurse practitioner (ACNP) has emerged to provide care for acutely and chronically ill patients in a variety of settings. ACNPs entered advanced practice nursing and have rapidly expanded their roles in practice settings. The ACNP provides comprehensive care in a collaborative model with physicians, patients, families, staff nurses, and other health care providers. The ACNP role can differ depending on geographic location, as well as private practice settings. This chapter presents an overview of the role, role competencies, definition of the scope of practice, and aspects of role implementation and development. Exploration of these topics will assist individuals who are considering the role to better understand an ACNP's scope of practice and allow for successful role implementation within the acute care health system or private practice. Environmental issues that are unique to ACNP practice are discussed.

OVERVIEW OF THE ACNP ROLE

The role of nurse practitioners (NPs) in ambulatory care has been well documented since the 1960s (see Chapter 14). The role of the ACNP has not been as extensively documented in the literature because it is a relatively new role. The neonatal NP (NNP) role, which originated in the 1970s, is the oldest ACNP role. The NNP arose as a result of cutbacks in the numbers of pediatric residents based on a perceived overabundance or maldistribution of pediatricians in the United States, coupled with increasing acuity and complexity of neonatal patients. These factors resulted in shortages of bedside care in neonatal intensive care units (NICUs) (Lott, Polak, Kenyon, & Kenner, 1996).

At about the same time, the need for NPs evolved to include care of adult patients in acute and critical care settings, and primary care NPs were recruited and prepared for hospital-based practice. Later, ACNPs were adult NPs who adopted a clinical practice in the inpatient setting. In the late 1980s, the popularity of the ACNP role developed within tertiary care centers (Barber & Burke, 1999). In order to meet this market need, graduate ACNP programs began to emerge in the late 1980s. Currently, there are over 73 ACNP programs in existence (American Association of Colleges of Nursing, 1998). The role of the ACNP was originally developed to fulfill a need for inpatient care of acutely and chronically ill patients, mostly in specialty areas. Factors that were influential in the development of this novel advanced practice nurse (APN) role included hospital restructuring secondary to managed care, a decrease in residency coverage for both infant and adult patients, and the paradigm shift in health systems of care toward primary care (Daly & Gent, 1997; Ingersol, 1995; Keane, Richmond, & Kaiser 1994; Parrinello, 1995). Research studies have demonstrated that the care that ACNPs provide is effective, is of high quality, is cost-effective, and results in patient satisfaction (Piano & Zerwic-Johnson, 1998; Prescott & Driscoll, 1980; Kubala & Clever, 1974; Spitzer et al., 1974).

The ACNP role emerged in response to societal changes such as anticipated changes in health care delivery and cost containment. Silver and McAtee (1988) proposed to address the shortage of physicians, residents, and fellows in specialty practices by using NPs in the hospital setting. The goal of this proposal was to provide high-quality acute care in the face of physician reductions, particularly in teaching hospitals.

To meet this need, ACNPs were educated to identify health risks and health promotion needs and to manage acute and chronic illness in collaboration with and under the supervision of a physician (i.e., intensivist, internist, or cardiologist). Silver and McAtee (1988) envisioned that these NPs would develop clinical decision-making skills and technical skills in order to admit patients to the hospital, complete the history and physical examination, assess patients' clinical status, and manage subsequent changes in a patient's clinical condition. ACNPs would also write medical orders, perform a variety of diagnostic and therapeutic tests, order and interpret laboratory studies, and counsel patients and their families in collaboration with physicians.

As has been true in the past, nurses were asked to fill the gaps during times of health care change. To evaluate the potential of using APNs to compensate for reduced availability of residents, Knickman, Lipkin, Finkler, Thompson, and Kiel (1992) conducted a time and motion study of internal medicine residents at two large urban New York City hospitals. They demonstrated that 46% of the resident's time was spent in activities only a physician could perform. When an APN was added to the team, this time requirement for physician-based tasks decreased to 20%. Moreover, nonacademic institutions have also expanded services, and they have needed to find an approach to provide sufficient medical care. Hospital administrators were looking for the best way to provide that medical care. One solution was to prepare NPs to practice in acute care settings. All of these factors within the recent economic and political health care environment have been instrumental in the movement of the NP into the acute care setting to fill perceived gaps in the health care system (Keane & Richmond, 1993).

SCOPE OF PRACTICE FOR THE ACNP

The education, titles, certification, and scope of practice of the early NNPs varied widely depending on local custom, hospital policy, or the state nurse practice act. Education of these nurses was institutionally based, with primary responsibility assumed by neonatologists and previously "trained" NNPs. As the demand for NNPs increased in the early 1980s, there was a need for more educational programs to prepare them. Unfortunately, this need was not met within existing graduate programs. The majority of NNP education programs were hospital based or operated under the auspices of medical departments that awarded a certificate of continuing education units upon completion. Requirements for entry and type and amount of preparation received varied widely. Some of these programs have subsequently made the transition to graduate nursing education (Lott et al., 1996). The National Association of Neonatal Nurse Practitioners (NANN) issued a position paper supporting graduate education for NNPs and has provided guidelines outlining specific scope of practice and competency statements (NANN, 1994).

Today, the scope of practice of the ACNP encompasses the professional function privileges and responsibilities associated with acute care advanced nursing practice. These activities are performed in collaboration with qualified and legally authorized professional health care providers. In addition, ACNPs are prepared to recognize situations in which care requirements are beyond their individual scope and to seek consultation when such situation arises. The *Standards of Clinical Practice and Scope of Practice for the Acute Care Nurse Practitioner* is a publication resulting from a collaborative effort by the American Nurses Association (ANA) and the American Association of Critical-Care Nurses (AACN). This publication describes the practice of the ACNP, focusing on the adult patient and delineating the scope, functions, and role of the ACNP in clinical practice (ANA and AACN, 1995). It also establishes clinical practice standards that are organized along the lines of the nursing process that will be explored later in the chapter. (see Table 15–6). Scope of practice for the ANCP includes six general categories: (1) the ACNP's role in acute care, (2) the practice environment, (3) patient population, (4) educational preparation, (5) regulation of practice, and (6) ethical issues in acute care.

Within the *Standards of Clinical Practice,* the term "advanced practice nurse" refers to "nurses who have acquired the knowledge base and practice experience to prepare them for specialization, expansion, and advancement in selected practice roles" such as the ACNP. The curriculum of an ACNP program is taught within the nursing paradigm and should contain advanced health assessment, physiology, advanced pathophysiology, pharmacology, diagnostic reasoning, clinical decision making, advanced therapeutics, and specialty preparation, as well as instruction in research methods and utilization (ANA and AACN, 1995, p. 9). Advanced assessment includes health history and risk appraisal; physical and mental status examination; interpretation of diagnostic studies; psychosocial assessment, including family and social support systems; assessment of the patient's home and community resources; and consideration of disease prevention applicable to the patient. Physiology is emphasized as a foundation for ACNP diagnostic reasoning skills. It is the basis for pathophysiology, pharmacology, and advanced therapeutics, with pathophysiology providing a detailed study of mechanisms of disease. When coupled within the conceptual framework of nursing, physiology provides the basis for ACNP therapeutic management of patient problems. Pharmacology includes pharmacokinetics, pharmacodynamics, and drug therapies along with content needed to prescribe medications and assess a patient's response. Furthermore, integrated into the ACNP program is a precepted clinical practicum that provides opportunities to integrate and synthesize health and disease theory, clinical research findings, bioethical decision making, and cultural diversity, along with knowledge of advanced therapeutics (nonpharmacologic therapies) (ANA and AACN, 1995).

The scope of ACNP practice is influenced on five levels: national, government (state), institution, service related, and individual (see Figure 15–1).

National

At the national level, the scope of ACNP professional practice was developed collaboratively by the ANA and the AACN (1995). In this publication, "scope of practice" defines the ACNP as a provider of advanced nursing care across the continuum of acute care services to patients who are acutely and critically ill using a collaborative model. The focus of care is restorative, with the short-term goal being patient stabilization, provision of physical and psychological care, and minimization of complications. The long-term goal is restoration of the patient's maximal health potential (with concurrent evaluation of risk factors in achieving this outcome) (ANA and AACN, 1995). The practice environment for the ACNP is "any setting in which patient care requirements include complex monitoring and therapies, high-intensity nursing interventions, or continuous nursing vigilance within the full range of high-acuity care" (ANA and AACN, 1995). The "standards of clinical practice" include not only standards of care, but also standards of professional performance for ACNPs. These

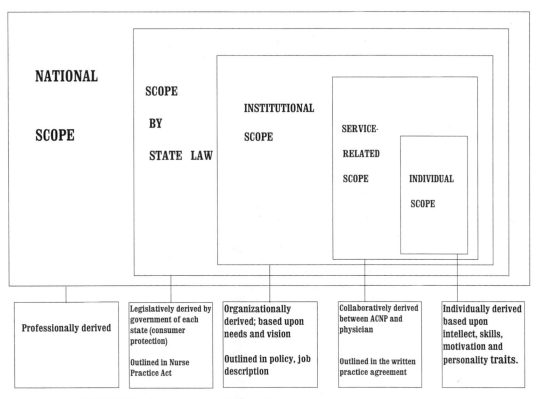

NATIONAL

SCOPE

SCOPE BY STATE LAW

INSTITUTIONAL SCOPE

SERVICE-RELATED SCOPE

INDIVIDUAL SCOPE

| Professionally derived | Legislatively derived by government of each state (consumer protection)

Outlined in Nurse Practice Act | Organizationally derived; based upon needs and vision

Outlined in policy, job description | Collaboratively derived between ACNP and physician

Outlined in the written practice agreement | Individually derived based upon intellect, skills, motivation and personality traits. |

FIGURE 15–1 • The scope of ACNP practice.

standards describe a level of care and performance common to the ACNP by which the quality of ACNP practice can be judged (ANA and AACN, 1995).

In addition to the *Scope of Practice and Standards of Clinical Practice for the Acute Care Nurse Practitioner,* the ANA and AACN jointly developed a national certification examination for ACNPs. Certification in Adult Acute Care is conducted through the American Nurses Credentialing Center (ANCC) with a purpose to provide documentation to the public that a licensed professional has demonstrated mastery of knowledge and skills to practice the profession (Kristeller, 1995). Certification is usually voluntary and suggests a quality of service higher than what is necessarily required for licensure (Hravnak & Baldessari, 1997). However, new regulations regarding Medicare reimbursement for NP services stipulate that national certification is required for all new NP graduates to obtain reimbursement. The first Adult Acute Care certification examination was administered in December 1995 (ANA and AACN, 1995). Eligibility criteria and the test blueprint provide guidance to ACNP graduates preparing to sit for the examination, and serve as a resource for faculty developing an ACNP program. Examination topics include system-specific health problems, common problems in acute care, ethics and scope of practice, and health promotion and disease prevention (ANCC, 1999). Successfully passing the ACNP certification exam entitles the ACNP to use the credentials ''CS,'' or certified specialist. Recertification is a mechanism that provides evidence that the individual reaffirms this mastery over time.

As of August 1999, there were more than 1,376 ACNPs who had taken the national ACNP certification (ANCC, 1999). Eligibility criteria include holding a master's degree or higher in nursing and having been prepared as an adult ACNP in an ACNP master's degree in nursing program or a formal postgraduate ACNP program within a school of nursing granting graduate-level academic credit. National certification for NNPs through the National Certification Corporation has been in effect since the early 1980s.

Government (State)

The government or individual state level is the second mechanism that has a voice in the professional scope of practice for the ACNP. The nurse practice statute in each state governs ACNP practice. APN practice regulations are intended to be global and are meant to define practice within a specific state, and these regulations vary from state to state (Cummings, 1997; Hall, 1993). At times, confusion exists regarding the meaning of licensure versus certification. *Licensure* statutes exist to limit practice to people with specific qualifications. *Certification* statutes only provide a definition and limits as to who can use the ACNP title; these statutes do not limit practice. Licensure differs from certification in that licensure is granted by the state, is required to practice the profession, guarantees a safe level of practice, and is generally not specialty specific (Hravnak & Baldisseri, 1997). In granting authority for ACNPs to practice as APNs, the state boards rely upon mechanisms such as graduation from an approved educational program and successful passing of a specialty certification exam. States have different requirements regarding physician supervision of the NP and varying degrees of prescriptive authority. The majority of states do not differentiate between NP practice specialties (family, adult, pediatric), nor do they provide a list of skills, tasks or procedures permissible within the scope. When trying to examine a particular practice act to determine what an ACNP can and cannot do within her or his scope, it is best to interpret the act as broadly as possible (assume can unless cannot is described) and give plain and ordinary meanings to the words used in the statutes. When in doubt regarding interpretation of the nurse practice act, it is always prudent to consult with the employing hospital's legal counsel (Hravnak, Rosenzweig, Rust, & Magdic, 1998b).

Institutional

The institution in which the ACNP practices will identify the scope of practice within that institution by delineating the patient population the ACNP is hired to serve and the process for collaboration with other health care providers in the institution (Parinello, 1995). An employer is responsible for the acts of its employee while the employee performs on behalf of the employer. However, an employer cannot be held responsible for an employee should the employee step beyond the bounds that it has set forth (Cummings, 1997; Prosser, 1971). This "scope of employment" may take the form of a job description, hospital policy, or both (Cummings, 1997; Hravnak et al., 1998b). In addition to the job description, the ACNP will also need to go through the process of hospital credentialing. The credentialing process verifies the qualifications and skills of the prospective ACNP employee. The privileging process grants the ACNP the right to enact the performance standards and skills and results from a written agreement that has been collaboratively developed by the ACNP and the physician(s) with whom the ACNP will work.

In settings where the ACNP role is being newly introduced, a job description may not exist. Depending on the practice setting, the responsibility for developing the job description may be undertaken by the ACNP or performed jointly with the employer. In general, the job description should include ACNP responsibilities as they relate to patient care, collaborative relationships, professional conduct, and professional development. A sample job description used at the University of Pittsburgh Medical Center is found in Table 15–1. Performance standards included in the job description delineate the responsibilities for which the ACNP is accountable and provide a template against which both the ACNP and the employer can evaluate performance (Hravnak et al., 1998b). Once the job description is in place, a plan for conducting an ongoing performance evaluation should be outlined, reflecting individual ACNP performance within the context of ACNP scope of practice and competencies.

Institutional credentialing is a process whereby the professional and technical competence of licensed providers may be formally recognized by the institution (Kristeller, 1995). This process is essential because the accrediting bodies of an institution, such as the National Practitioner Data Bank and the Joint Commission on the Accreditation of Healthcare Organizations, also play a role in defining NP scope of practice. (Refer to Chapter 22 for general information pertaining to credentialing and privileging.) The medical model for credentialing and privileging is used in most instances to provide institutional credentialing and/or privileging for the ACNP because of the traditional medical nature of many of the role responsibilities. The ACNP is required to provide proof of licensure, certification, educational preparation, malpractice insurance, and skill performance (Hravnak & Baldessari, 1997). This information is then reviewed and verified by the credentialing board and is periodically reviewed according to an established policy within the institution. Credentialing is necessary in order for the ACNP to perform certain medical skills within the institution, although the ACNP may or may not hold a medical staff appointment.

Once an individual is credentialed, a determination is made as to the privileges that may be granted. Privileging is a process whereby the institution, through its credentialing board, determines which medical procedures may be performed and which conditions may be treated by the ACNP (Kristeller, 1995). These privileges are partly based on the individual ACNPs professional license and inherent scope of practice, documented training, experience, competence, and health status. For example, an ACNP who has received educational preparation for performing invasive diagnostic procedures such as insertion of central line catheters, lumbar puncture, chest tube placement, and intubation can request that these privileges be a part of her or his "institutional" scope of practice. An ACNP may periodically request new privileges based upon evolving mastery of skills, further training, and changes in services needed by the patient population and institution (Hravnak & Baldessari, 1997). It is important to understand that, although an ACNP may be qualified to perform certain procedures, privileges to perform these acts may not necessarily be granted.

Service Related

Scope of ACNP practice is also regulated by the needs of a specific population or care delivery team (i.e., service) within the organization. The written practice agreement or

TABLE 15-1 SAMPLE ACNP JOB DESCRIPTION

University of Pittsburgh Medical Center

Job Title: Certified Registered Nurse Practitioner
Department: Clinical Administration
Reports to: Clinical Administrator

Function

The certified registered nurse practitioner (CRNP) functions as a member of the medical care management team. The CRNP diagnoses medical conditions, plans and implements interventions, and evaluates patient responses under the direction of and in collaboration with a physician supervisor or designated attending physician.

Qualifications

1. Licensure as a professional nurse in the Commonwealth of Pennsylvania.
2. Certification as a nurse practitioner by the Commonwealth of Pennsylvania (CRNP) or completion of submission of all required materials.
3. Certification by the American Nurses Credentialing Center as a nurse practitioner (preferred).
4. Minimum of 2 years' nursing experience.
5. Master's degree in nursing.
6. Advanced cardiac life support certification preferred.

Qualifications are reviewed annually and clinical privileges authorized through the Medical Staff credentialing process.

Scope

Clinical privileges for individual CRNPs are recommended by the supervising physician to the Allied Health Credentialing Committee through the Medical Staff approval process. CRNPs may engage in activities that normally constitute the practice of nursing without credentialing, provided they have the preparation, knowledge, and experience necessary to properly execute the practice. Medical diagnostic, therapeutic, and management functions will be instituted under medical supervision using protocols or guidelines developed by the individual services/programs.

Responsibilities

The CRNP is responsible for

1. *Assembling* a complete medical database, including health history, history of chief complaint, and physical examination upon patient admission of selected patients, and *documenting* the findings in the patient record.
2. *Assessing* selected patients using physically and technologically derived data, including the evaluation of diagnostic test results, and *documenting* this assessment in the patient record.
3. Under the direction and in consultation/collaboration with the physician preceptor, or designee, *diagnosing* medical conditions and *planning* medical therapeutics and interventions based on the medical database. *Documenting and communicating* the diagnosis and plan to other members of the health care team.
4. Under the direction of, and in consultation/collaboration with the physician preceptor, or designee, *ordering* medical consultations, therapies, and interventions including, but not limited to, medications, diagnostic tests, respiratory care including ventilator management, nutrition, fluid and electrolyte support, and blood and blood products. *Documenting* these orders and directives in the patient record and *communicating* them to other members of the health care team.

432

5. *Performing* invasive diagnostic and therapeutic procedures based on the needs of the specific patient population as determined collaboratively by the CRNP, physician preceptor, and service or unit medical director and approved by the Allied Health Credentialing Committee of the medical staff. *Documenting* the procedures and the patient responses and results in the patient record.

6. *Evaluating and analyzing* patients' responses to disease processes and therapeutic interventions, and *determining* the effectiveness of care and the need to alter the plan of care.

7. *Presenting* selected patient's assessments, diagnoses, and plans of care during medical team rounds.

8. *Providing* information and support to patients and family members. *Facilitating* communication between patients and family members and members of the health care team.

9. *Collaborating* with nurses and nurse managers to implement and evaluate holistic patient care delivery.

10. *Serving* as a resource to members of the health care team to facilitate patient delivery by using an in-depth pathophysiologic and psychosocial knowledge base.

11. *Participating* in activities that contribute to the education of other health care professionals, including *presenting and publishing*.

12. *Acting* as a role model, and, in selected cases, *precepting* nurses and other advanced practice nurses, including other nurse practitioners.

13. *Participating* in medical and nursing research projects, including *presenting and publishing* the findings.

14. *Promoting and practicing* economical and effective health care.

15. *Demonstrating* behavior that models the UPMC's service vision/philosophy.

16. *Teaching and promoting* practices to improve or maintain health to patients and family members, and others within and outside the UPMC.

17. *Participating in or initiating* activities necessary for annual reappointment and privileging. *Documenting* evidence of continuing competency in the areas of medical diagnoses, therapeutics, invasive procedures, and management, as well as required certification(s).

18. *Participating* in activities that enhance professional development with role as an advanced practice nurse, such as
    a. *serving* on UPMC committees related to CRNP utilization, including regularly updating medical management protocols;
    b. *reading* professional journals and texts to maintain currency on the latest clinical, professional, and legislative trends, *sharing the* knowledge gained with other members of the health care team;
    c. *attending* continuing education programs; and
    d. *participating* in professional organizations.

19. *Serving* on departmental and interdisciplinary committees.

20. *Performing* other duties as determined collaboratively by the physician preceptor, the CRNP, and the clinical administrator that are within the scope of practice of CRNPs and the policies of the UPMC.

From Burkholder, J., & Dudjak, L. (1994). The midlevel practitioner role: One medical center's experience. *AACN Clinical Issues in Critical Care Nursing, 5*(3), 372–374; reprinted with permission.

service-related scope outlines the clinical functions and tasks of the individual ACNP and the medical regimens that may be administered by the individual ACNP (Burkholder & Dudjak, 1994; Hravnak et al., 1998b). The written agreement serves as a contract between the physician and the ACNP and is derived through a collaborative effort of the ACNP and physician(s). The written agreement serves as the basis for application of clinical privileges. It contains a more detailed and specific description of the types of activities the ACNP will perform as a member of the practice. Because the written agreement is created through a collaborative effort, it ensures that the ACNP and the physician(s) have agreed to the skills and tasks included. Once developed, the written agreement is submitted to the institution's credentialing board. In turn, the written agreement is used to communicate this information to other members of the health care team. Examples of items contained in a written agreement include the following: a NP working with a cardiology service may interpret electrocardiograms and initiate treatment for patients experiencing dysrhythmias, the NP working with an oncology service may perform bone marrow aspirations, the NP on the renal medicine service may write orders for hemodialysis, and the NP with the cardiovascular surgery service may harvest the vein grafts for coronary artery bypass surgery (Hravnak et al., 1998b).

The written agreement may also include parameters as to the level of communication between the ACNP and the physician that is required before the performance of a specific function. This may be referred to as "degree of supervision required." Degree of supervision may range from a level of no supervision being required to a level that requires direct supervision by the physician. For example, an ACNP may require no supervision in conducting an admission history and physical exam, but may require direct supervision by the physician when performing central line insertion. The written agreement also provides a means by which the responsibilities of the ACNP may be titrated in the event that new skills are acquired or improved. Continuing with the previous example, an NP with novice skills in central line insertion may require direct supervision for a specified period of time or number of successful attempts. However, as the ACNP approaches expert status, the level of supervision may be changed to that of none required. In this case, the written agreement will need to be modified.

Written agreements, often formatted as a checklist, are necessary because the detail included in a written agreement usually cannot be spelled out in a job description. Job descriptions, by their very nature, tend to be global in order to cover NPs working in a variety of settings within the institution. When negotiating the written agreement, both the ACNP and the physician need to ensure that no function is in conflict with the individual state's nurse practice act and the policies of the particular institution.

Individual

The final determinant of scope of practice relates to the individual characteristics of the ACNP. These include such things as prior experience, specialization, motivation, self-esteem, personal ethics, personality traits, and communication style (Hravnak et al., 1998b). In order to provide safe, quality, efficient care, the ACNP must continually pursue ongoing education to be knowledgeable of recent advances in health care and judicious in the application of research findings. ACNPs should not only read the literature, but also publish in the literature. Sharing their clinical expertise and experiences can benefit their peers as those peers seek to develop and enhance their roles. It is important that ACNPs be involved in their specialty and professional organizations. ACNPs need to become involved so that the unique issues related to ACNP practice gain recognition by the leaders of the national organizations and also so ACNPs can have a voice in the decisions to be made. Becoming an ACNP does not stop at graduation.

COMPETENCIES OF THE ACNP ROLE

Core Competencies

The core APN competencies that have been explained in Chapter 3 are clearly evident in the ACNP role. ACNPs practicing in intensive care units (ICUs) and NICUs sit on interdisciplinary ethics teams that are required to determine the course of action in highly difficult patient situations. A strong foundation in the concepts surrounding ethical decision making is a requirement for ACNP role implementation. As well, the core competency of coaching and teaching is played out at the highest levels when ACNPs prepare patients who have had serious illnesses for discharge, and as they assist family members in caring for loved ones who have undergone catastrophic or debilitating health problems.

"Collaboration" is a term that is frequently used when discussing the ACNP's practice. Broadly speaking, collaboration is defined as working together (King & Baggs, 1998). Collaborative practice in the clinical setting means "cooperatively working together, sharing responsibility for solving problems and making decisions to formulate and carry out plans for patient care" (Baggs & Schmitt, 1988). In the acute care setting, collaboration needs to occur between all members of the health care team. Collaboration is the future for health care providers and is one of the critical elements of the ACNP role. The key elements that define collaborative practice include (1) cooperation, (2) assertiveness, (3) shared decision making, (4) communication, (5) planning together, and (6) coordination. In order for collaboration to be operationalized, trust is the essential element that must be garnered. When trust is the foundation for a collaborative relationship, cooperation can exist, assertiveness does not become threatening, shared decision making is not avoided, communication is not hampered, and coordination of care is not haphazard (King & Baggs, 1998; Norsen, Opladen, & Quinn, 1995).

In a collaborative practice model, the emphasis is on patient outcomes. Each professional should be responsible for providing the care for which she or he was best prepared. A collaborative practice model in acute care focuses on the idea that each patient needs the services of different types of providers simultaneously (King et al., 1998). It has been suggested that the dyad of APN and physician forms the core of collaborative practice in acute care (King & Baggs, 1998; Norsen et al., 1995). The advantage to this model is the ongoing continuity and coordination of care (Norsen et al., 1995). To formulate a collaborative dyad between the ACNP and physician, it is essential that each partner achieve full professional status. This means that each partner has completed basic and postgraduate education, which, in turn, allows them to take advantage of and use the full scope of practice of each of the partners. In turn, this assumption refutes the resident replacement model that has been put forth by some as a role for APNs (King & Baggs, 1998).

Although there has been much support for collaborative practice between nurses and physicians, barriers still exist. Unfortunately, these barriers are created between those for whom collaborative practice should be the focus—nurses and physicians. There is still the tenet that health care is heirarchical and that the physician is "captain of the ship," delegating to others responsibilities that the physician does not have the time or interest to do. Incomplete understanding of the ACNP role may fuel the concern of both physicians and nurses that, perhaps, ACNPs are selling out to the medical model and trying to practice like "mini-doctors" (King & Baggs, 1998). This belief can and does lead to protection of one's turf. However, there is growing recognition that physicians cannot do it all and that there are other providers who can effectively deliver a wider and more comprehensive range of care. Additional barriers focus on nurses being threatened by the increased responsibility and account-ability involved in collaborative practice and the perceived differences in educational preparation and skills between nurses and physicians (King & Baggs, 1998).

Specialty Competencies

The ACNP is prepared to provide direct care in the acute care setting for patients who are acutely and critically ill and whose conditions are complex. The short-term goal of the ACNP is to stabilize patients with episodes of acute illnesses, minimize complications, and provide physical and psychological care. The long-term goal is to restore maximal health potential by evaluating risk factors to achieve a positive outcome (ANA and AACN, 1995). Similar to other APNs, ACNPs are required to assess patients, think critically, perform diagnostic reasoning, manage cases, and prescribe therapeutic interventions (Clochesy, Daly, Idemoto, Steel, and Fitzpatrick, 1994; Keane & Richmond, 1993, see Chapter 6). Although no model has been developed defining ACNP competencies, there appears to be an evolving set of competencies that encompass both the ACNP specialty and the APN core competencies discussed previously. Key competencies of the ACNP include six elements (Table 15–2): demon-strate knowledge of advanced pathophysiology, complete a health history, conduct physical exams, demonstrate the ability to order and interpret diagnostic tests, demon-strate technical competence with procedures, and collaborate with other care provid-ers to facilitate positive outcomes (Shah & Sullivan, 1998). Individual elements of the ACNP role vary depending on the practice setting and patient population served, but the basic elements remain.

The ACNP needs to develop and apply skills unique to the needs of a specific patient population based upon clinical specialty or practice setting. ACNPs emphasize their specialty knowledge balanced with generalist nursing preparation and holistic care. In addition, the ACNP is uniquely qualified to identify problems for which the acute care population is at risk to implement strategies to minimize or prevent that risk. Some of the risk factors imposed by an inpatient stay are physiologic in nature; these include immobility, decreased nutritional intake, fluid and electrolyte imbalance, altered immunocompetence, existing or developing co-morbid disease states, and risk associated with invasive diagnostic and therapeutic interventions. Other risks have a psychological foundation; these include physical limitations, environmental sleep deprivation, changes in body image, role reversal, financial challenges, and knowledge deficits. Additionally, some risk factors are related to discontinuation of care, polypharmacy, and conflict of communication among the family and/or care team. Although the ACNP may need to utilize specialty skills and knowledge of advanced pathophysiology, physical exam skills, and diagnostic test interpretation to assist a patient with particular needs or disease, what they have in common with

TABLE 15-2 COMPETENCIES FOR ACNPs

Demonstrates knowledge of advanced pathophysiology in the following areas:
  Neurology
  Cardiology
  Pulmonary concerns
  Renal concerns
  Endocrinology
  Gastrointestinal concerns
  Fluid balance
  Acid/base balance
Completes a health history
Conducts a partial or complete physical exam
Demonstrates ability to appropriately order and interpret the following:
  Arterial blood gases
  Venous blood analyses
  Cardiac enzymes
  Coagulation measures
  Liver function tests
  Urinalysis/culture
  X-rays—abdominal/chest/routine
  12-lead EKG
Demonstrates technical skill with the following procedures:
  Cardiovascular: Arterial puncture/cannulation/line removal
                  IAPB management
                  Pulmonary artery catheter: management/removal/insertion
                  Resuscitation management
                  Vasoactive drugs: initiation/management
  Pulmonary: Airway management
                  Endotracheal tubes: insertion/management/removal
                  Oxygen devices
                  Chest tube-insertion/management/removal
                  Thoracentesis
                  Ventilator management: initiation/maintenance/weaning parameters
  Gastrointestinal: Nasogastric/intestinal tube: insertion/removal
                  G-tube: re-insertion/management/removal
                  Paracentesis
                  Nutritional therapies: initiation/maintenance
  Neurological: Lumbar puncture
  Renal: Peritoneal dialysis: management/removal of catheter
                  Bladder suprapubic aspiration
  Miscellaneous: Institutes blood component therapies
                  Administration of intradermal tests
                  Cutaneous suturing
                  Venous catheter insertion/management central/peripheral
  Wounds: Management/debridement/packing
                  Apply local anesthesia
                  Perform cultures
Collaborates with other care providers to facilitate positive patient outcomes.
  Consultations: initiation
  Discharge planning initiation

From Shah, H., & Sullivan, D. T. (1998). Evaluation of the acute care nurse practitioner's role. In R. Kleinpell & M. Piano (Eds.), *Practice issues for the acute care nurse practitioner* (pp. 111–143). New York: Springer-Verlag; reprinted with permission.

other APNs is (1) a generalist nursing foundation, (2) a health promotion basis to their practice, and (3) the development and appreciation of diagnostic reasoning skills. These skills make the ACNP a bona fide member of the health care team and a desirable commodity in the health care industry (Hravnak & Madgic, 1997).

PROFILE OF THE ACNP ROLE

The managed care environment has allowed ACNPs to move into a variety of practice settings to fulfill the need of inpatient care to the acutely ill. With increased managed care market movement, hospitals have investigated methods to decrease fixed costs. Additionally, with decreases in medical resident numbers and with medical education shifting to primary care, the evolution of the ACNP role occurred. The majority of ACNP practice is in ICUs and acute care settings, with speciality area practice sites continuing to expand (Kleinpell, 1998). ACNPs have transitioned into a variety of roles with diverse responsibilities. Two types of ACNP roles exist, one focusing on episodic management of patients in a particular clinical setting and the second involving case management of patients throughout their hospitalization. Rural clinics and hospitals employ only 5% of ACNPs (Kleinpell 1999).

As positions for ACNPs emerged predominantly in ICUs and acute care areas within health care systems, ACNPs came to focus on episodic care of patients on a particular clinical unit with acute care problems. Initially, both NNPs and ACNPs functioned in physician extender roles, performing the work of residents or house staff (Kleinpell, 1998; Lott et al., 1996). In collaboration with a physician, an ACNP would manage the care of a patient admitted to an ICU with an acute medical condition. Once the patient was stabilized, patient care would be transferred to another care provider. ACNP roles such as these have been described in specialty ICU settings: cardiothoracic, surgical, coronary, medical, neurologic and trauma, and neonatal. Providing episodic care allows ACNPs the opportunity to develop their skill and knowledge about specific conditions in a delineated setting. However, the limitation of this model is that it does not allow for continuity of care.

In the second model, the case management approach, the ACNP directly manages patient care throughout the patient's hospitalization, providing individualized ongoing care with continuity to the patient and family. This model requires a broader knowledge base beyond that related to the patient's initial condition. The goal of this model is to facilitate and coordinate a patient's hospital stay in order to provide quality and cost-effective care (Clochesy et al., 1994). ACNPs can be based on a cardiology heart failure service or a medical or surgical unit with a homogeneous population of patients. Care is provided in a systematic, collaborative approach. The ACNP will admit the patient to the hospital in collaboration with a physician, complete the history and physical examination, assess the patient's initial clinical status, order and interpret diagnostic and therapeutic tests, perform procedures, and prepare the patient for discharge.

As medical centers continue to reorganize in an attempt to contain costs and streamline patient care services, the ACNP employment market will continue to be dynamic. In medical teaching centers where residents rotate monthly, it is imperative that the ACNP be able to establish relationships and maintain flexibility to work with a team that changes, because re-establishing relationships is necessary. The ACNP provides a vital role of continuity that is balanced by the availability of attending and consulting physicians along with other medical team members, such as social workers and dietitians and where strong permanent relationships provide a supportive network.

Recent studies involving ACNPs have explored the evaluation of the ACNP role and the function of the ACNP within a practice setting (Kleinpell, 1998; Shah & Sullivan, 1998). They found that ACNP clinical practice varies with the individual and the institution in which clinical practice occurs but that all ACNPs collect a database and manage client care (Shah, Sullivan, Lattanzio, & Bruttomesso, 1993).

Although skill differences exist among ACNPs nationally, regionally, and locally, there are strong commonalties that exist. As with other APN roles, the ACNP is proficient in advanced physical assessment, clinical decision making (diagnostic reasoning), ordering and interpreting laboratory studies and procedures, and collaborating in the development and implementation of a treatment plan that includes prescribing medication. Diagnostic reasoning and advanced therapeutic interventions, consultation, and referral to other physicians, nurses, and providers are intrinsic components of this role as described by the ANA and AACN (1995). The ACNP role, as is true of other APN roles, is one of evidenced-based practice as it relates to the basic sciences. Specifically, ACNPs should be able to demonstrate knowledge of pathophysiology for their decision making when ordering and interpreting diagnostic tests and in making treatment decisions.

Typically an ACNP carries a case load of patients, admitting patients directly to her or his respective service, obtaining the history, performing the physical exam, and managing her or his particular case during the patients' hospitalization (Shah & Sullivan, 1998). The ACNP diagnoses the origin of a complex medical problem that develops in an acutely or critically ill patient. In order to arrive at a diagnosis, diagnostic reasoning must be utilized (see Chapter 6). The skills inherent in effective diagnostic reasoning include the fundamental skills of the ACNP role: history taking, physical examination skills, pattern recognition, the ability to analyze and synthesize data, and the ability to generate a working diagnosis. This requires the ACNP to have an in-depth understanding of pathophysiology as it relates to the patient's disease process, as well as strong verbal presentation and defense skills. Failure to diagnose because of a lack of understanding of the disease process can lead to progression of the primary disease condition and/or the development of complications. Incorrect diagnosis may lead to inappropriate or suboptimal therapy or unnecessary toxicity secondary to the side effects of treatment. In the event of a delay in diagnosis, disease progression may result (Kassirer, 1989; Szaflarski, 1997). There are a number of factors that can affect the quality of diagnostic reasoning (see Table 15–3). All of

TABLE 15–3 FACTORS AFFECTING QUALITY OF DIAGNOSTIC REASONING	
PATIENT FACTORS	CLINICIAN FACTORS
• Increasing level of patient acuity • Multisystem disease • Poor historians • Altered mental status • Unavailability of significant other	• Clinical experience • Knowledge of the disease • Knowledge of complex diagnostic technologies • Incomplete history database as a result of unavailable medical records or diagnostic test results • Increasing workload • Demands for cost-effective diagnostic evaluation

Adapted from Szaflarski, N. L. (1997). Diagnostic reasoning in acute and critical care. *AACN Clinical Issues, 8*(2), 291–302; reprinted with permission.

these factors challenge the ACNP's ability to accurately and expeditiously diagnose a patient's ever-changing physical condition.

Kleinpell (1997) surveyed 126 ACNPs and described role components that reflected the elements of advanced therapeutic management. In order to have an impact upon quality patient care outcomes, professionals assume responsibility for the provision of care for which they are prepared. In acute care, patients require services from different types of providers simultaneously. These different types of providers include physicians, APNs, and nurses. Each provider has a function and skill set that can make a unique contribution affecting the outcome of a patient's condition. For example, a physician would have primary responsibility for the patient during a cardiac arrest; however, the ACNP has primary responsibility related to family teaching and initiation of a consultation. Specific role aspects and procedures performed by the ACNP are identified in Table 15–4.

Differences and Commonalities with Other APN Roles and Physician Assistant Role

The ACNP role differs from other ANP roles by the type and acuity of the patient as well as the setting in which the care occurs (Lott et al., 1996). For example, the clinical nurse specialist (CNS) enacts the APN role through three spheres of influence: at the patient level in direct care, at the nurse level, as with staff development; and at the institutional level, providing oversight for care. In comparison, the ACNP utilizes clinical assessment skills to assess complex and acutely ill patients through health history taking, physical and mental status examination, performing procedures,

TABLE 15–4 PROCEDURES PERFORMED BY THE ACNP

MOST FREQUENTLY		LESS FREQUENTLY	
Direct care		**Direct care**	
Discuss care with family	95%	Manage patient receiving ventilation	49%
Order/interpret laboratory tests	90%	Suture superficial lacerations	48%
Initiate discharge planning	88%	Initiate and adjust intravenous lines	43%
Perform cultures	85%	Perform cardioversion	42%
Place nasogastric feeding tubes	84%	Perform incision/drainage	40%
Institute and adjust intravenous lines	82%	Adjust temporary pacemaker	37%
Interpret 12-lead electrocardiogram	81%	Manipulate pulmonary artery catheter	33%
Initiate specialty consultation	79%	Initiate arterial lines	32%
Examine and clean wounds	77%	Initiate peripherally inserted catheters	29%
Adjust nutritional feedings	65%	Remove intracardiac catheter	29%
Perform defibrillation	64%	Initiate central venous pressure lines	18%
Institute blood therapies	60%	Adjust cardiac assist devices	17%
Perform wound packing	60%	Perform lumbar puncture	16%
Apply local anesthesia	58%	Insert pulmonary artery catheter	16%
Perform wound debridement	57%	Perform endotracheal intubation	15%
Initiate vasoactive drips	54%	Perform needle thoracentesis	11%
Manage resuscitation	52%		
Indirect care		**Indirect care**	
Give nursing inservices	78%	Case manage inpatients	24%
Initiate QA/QI study	53%		

From Kleinpell, R. M. (1997). Acute care nurse practitioner: Roles and practice profiles. *AACN Clinical Issues, 8*(1), 156–162; reprinted with permission.

and risk appraisal for complications. Both APN roles are targeted to a patient-centered approach to care, but the continuous on-unit presence of the ACNP at the bedside of intensive care patients often differentiates the role of the ACNP from other NP roles. However, the role differentiations between ACNPs and CNSs are not always clear cut because of institutional variations, blurring of roles, and the skills of the particular APN (Lott et al., 1996).

Table 15-5 can assist one in conceptualizing where the main focus of ACNP practice falls within the health care continuum as compared to the primary care NP. In addition, it can help one understand where overlap between the roles occurs. Within the table are examples of management strategies of common health care problems traditionally encountered in primary, secondary, and tertiary health care settings (Hravnak et al., 1995). To use diabetes as an example, ACNP practice predominantly involves strategies directed toward management of the patient during an acute exacerbation of his or her diabetes (i.e., diabetic ketoacidosis). Because of the severity of symptoms, the patient needs to be admitted to the hospital, where he or she can be continuously monitored and where management strategies may change from hour to hour (tertiary care). However, during this same hospitalization, the patient may need to have an infected foot ulcer treated with intravenous antibiotics (secondary care). Once the crisis is over, the ACNP may provide teaching on routine foot care (primary care). However, at this point the patient is referred back to his or her

TABLE 15–5 PATIENT CARE PROBLEMS AND MANAGEMENT INTERVENTIONS TRADITIONALLY ASSOCIATED WITH HEALTH CARE DELIVERY SETTINGS

	CARE PROBLEM AND INTERVENTIONS		
DELIVERY SETTING	Diabetes	Hypertension	Pneumonia
Tertiary care management (ICU setting)	Diabetic ketoacidosis management Fluid replacement Electrolyte titration IV insulin	Continuous vasoactive drugs Arterial pressure monitoring Evaluation/management of possible intracerebral bleed	Mechanical ventilation Pulmonary toilet Culture assessment Sepsis management Continuous monitoring
Secondary care management (inpatient setting)	Insulin administration and monitoring Hydration Etiology workup Empiric infection treatment	Additional antihypertensives Adjunct therapy as needed	IV antibiotics Oxygen therapy Advanced assessment Chest roentgenogram, arterial blood gases, S_{PO_2}
Primary care management (outpatient setting)	Oral antihyperglycemics or subcutaneous insulin Diet Prevention/monitoring of associated complications Foot care Risk factor management	Diet Oral agents Lifestyle changes Prevention/assessment of associated complications Risk factor management	Oral or intramuscular antibiotics

Adapted from Hravnak, M., Kobert, S. N., Risco, K. G., Baldisseri, M., Hoffman, L. A., Clochesy, J. M., Rudy, E. B., & Snyder, J. V. (1995). Acute care nurse practitioner curriculum: Content and development process. *American Journal of Critical Care, 4*(3), 179–188; reprinted with permission.

primary care provider for further follow-up and management. In comparison, the primary care NP's practice predominantly involves strategies directed toward management of the patient's diabetes when it is stable (primary care). This would include ongoing surveillance of the patient's self-management of his or her diabetes along with education on diabetic risk factors, and assessing for signs of disease progression and complications. The primary care NP may also assess when the diabetic patient is not in good control and requires adjustment of insulin or oral hypoglycemic agents (secondary care). At the point where the patient is not responding or becomes acutely ill, the primary care NP will need to refer the patient to a setting where continuous monitoring and management is provided (tertiary care). Using this example helps educators and clinicians to understand that there is a natural overlap of knowledge and practice between acute care and primary care NPs. However, each also has her or his own distinct focus.

APNs, including the ACNP, are different from physician assistants (PAs). The PA role is under the jurisdiction of physician licensure, which is supervisory rather than collaborative and does not allow for independent functions. Although some of the care provided by PAs is similar to that provided by ACNPs, there are differences in philosophy, education, scope of practice, and patient approach between the APN and the PA (Lott et al., 1996).

ACNP Collaboration with Physician Hospitalists

The hospitalist is a physician specialist in inpatient medicine, who is responsible for managing the care of hospitalized patients in the same manner that a primary care physician is responsible for managing her or his outpatients. This newly emerging role was first described by physicians in 1996 as a consequence of the explosive growth of the primary care and internist role secondary to managed care. Hospitalist specialists have a central role in hospitals in Great Britain and Canada, but until recently such a specialist has been a scarce commodity in the United States (Wachter & Goldman, 1996). However, this physician role is now being incorporated in academic teaching centers and community settings. The physician hospitalist role has been based in internal medicine and, recently, the ACNP has been added as a member of this health care team. An admitting physician refers the patient to the hospitalist team for management during the acute care admission. This team provides care for the patient during hospitalization and refers the patient back to the primary care provider at the time of discharge. The goal of this service is to provide seamless, cost-effective care. This can be an advantage for a physician in private practice with busy office hours who may have limited time to make hospital visits and may not be sufficiently familiar with acute care management. The specific role of the ACNP, as a member of the hospitalist team, is similar to the roles previously described, including obtaining an admission history and physical exam, performing daily physical exams, rounds with the physician, developing a treatment plan, reviewing laboratory studies and x-rays, and performing procedures. Furthermore, coordinating patient care management when many consultants are involved in decision making is a significant part of the role, as is consultation with the case managers to effectively facilitate discharge planning (Wachter & Goldman, 1996). This new role for ACNPs can be viewed as direct competition to physicians and, as with other APN roles, will emerge based on need for providers to care for patients and positive interactions with physicians. As has been seen with NNPs, the ACNP can function as a valuable colleague in the emerging role as hospitalist.

Outcome Studies Related to ACNP Practice

In today's health care market, the driving force is the provision of health care at the lowest cost. Lawmakers and insurers want to know why any health care provider should be incorporated into patient care systems (Buppert, 1995). Although NPs may have known for a long time that they care for patients safely, offer excellent prevention services, and score high on studies of patient satisfaction, hard facts and figures are needed to justify the role (Buppert, 1995). Because the ACNP role is in its early stages of development, there have been few studies reporting health care outcomes as a consequence of ACNP practice. Outcome studies have grouped NPs with other nonphysician providers. Consequently, it has been difficult to understand the differences an ACNP makes in care. If ACNPs are to maintain and justify their existence, sound, outcome-based evidence is needed.

Over the past 20 to 30 years, the majority of research on NPs has been focused in the area of primary care. More recently, there have been several studies that have focused on ACNPs. There has been evidence suggesting that, in areas of subacute transitional care (von Sternberg et al., 1997), neonatal intensive care (Mitchell-Di Censo et al., 1996), perioperative care (Hylka & Beschle, 1995), and trauma services (Spisso, O'Callaghan, McKennan, & Holcroft, 1990), NPs provide care better than or equivalant to that of a physician (Rudy et al., 1998). Piano and Zerwic-Johnson (1998) identified eight studies (Carzoli, Martinez-Cruz, Cuevas, & Murphy, 1994; Cintron, Bigas, Linates, Aranda, & Hernandez, 1983; Hooker & McCraig, 1996; Lombness, 1994; Mitchell-Di Censo et al., 1996; Spisso et al., 1990; Weinberg, Liljestrand, & Moore, 1983; Ziemer et al., 1996) that explored ACNP effectiveness in several types of tertiary care settings. In their analysis, these authors reported that NP-directed outcomes were similar to those of their respective comparison group and that NP-directed care was cost effective. It was noted, however, that methodological flaws, including lack of randomization and appropriate control of comparison groups and insufficient sample size, limit the interpretations of these studies (Piano & Zerwic-Johnson, 1998). Rudy and colleagues (1998) published a study comparing NPs and PAs to residents in two academic medical centers. They concluded that tasks and activities performed by ACNPs and PAs are similar to those performed by resident physicians. It was noted that residents treated patients who were sicker and older than those treated by ACNPs and PAs; however, patient outcomes were similar for both groups (Rudy et al., 1998). However, the issue of cost of care provided by ACNPs/PAs compared to resident physicians was not addressed.

As stated previously, if ACNPs are to justify their existence, it is imperative that their worth be supported by careful research. Many nurse researchers are advocating the development of more rigorous guidelines for conducting outcome studies related to ACNP practice. Studies of ACNP effectiveness can be organized into the categories of processes of health care, outcomes of health care, patients' satisfaction with care, and agreement between NP and physician decisions. In addition, methodological concerns need to consider provider sample and setting, patient sample, and the design itself (Piano & Zerwic-Johnson, 1998; Sox, 1979).

ACNP ROLE IMPLEMENTATION

An Exemplar of ACNP Practice

Caring for patients in an intensive care setting is used as an exemplar for ACNP practice.

◎ EXEMPLAR

In the cardiothoracic intensive care unit (CTICU), Marie, an ACNP, functions collaboratively with the critical care team. The day typically begins with a report from the previous shift's ACNP on the patient's condition. Following this, Marie performs a focused assessment and physical examination on each of her patients and reviews the medication regimen and any ordered laboratory or diagnostic reports. She will then document a daily progress note along with appropriate orders. In addition, Marie will participate in patient-focused rounds with the health care team. During these rounds, all members of the team review each patient's progress and diagnostic results, and provide input to the management plan. A major component of the role is reassessment. This allows Marie to evaluate and modify therapeutic modalities, assess patient status, and make or update plans according to significant clinical findings. Marie's on-unit ACNP availability provides continuity and subsequently will impact outcomes. Like the primary care NP or CNS, Marie must be adept at time management. However, unlike the primary care NP, she must deal with ongoing hour-by-hour patient care management of her particular patient population with complex acute care problems.

Marie's other daily responsibilities may include performing procedures such as central line placement, arterial line insertions, or chest tube removal. The procedures performed will be determined by the ACNP skill set for which she has received hospital/unit privileges. Admission and transfer of patients into and out of the unit is also a part of her day. A very important part of Marie's role in the CTICU is communication with families. She may communicate with the family either directly or by telephone. Meeting daily with families to communicate the plan of care affords the opportunity to provide the information and teaching needed by the family. Throughout the day, Marie may attend a variety of teaching conferences such as grand rounds.

The role of the CTICU ACNP is unique in that Marie manages the patient from admission to discharge from the unit and manages the acute phase of their illness. However, Marie's patients also require holistic management of both medical and nursing problems (skin care, bowel management, etc.) and health promotion (i.e., the prevention of complications related to immobility). As a consequence, Marie provides both acute and primary care to her patients, an issue that has confused many ACNPs. Because Marie, as an ACNP, has cared for the patient since admission to the unit and is aware of her patient's history and baseline health status, she is better able to detect subtle changes in the patient's clinical condition.

Clinical Practice Settings

The ACNP can function in diverse settings in which patients require the use of complex technologies, including hospitals, health care systems, intensive care units, trauma centers, and emergency departments (ANA and AACN, 1995; Keane & Richmond, 1993). The needs of patients influence the clinical practice setting and subsequently influence the role responsibilities of the ACNP. As one might surmise, key elements of advanced assessment, diagnostic reasoning, collaboration, and health promotion are integral to ACNP practice regardless of the setting. In order to effectively illustrate ACNP practice, examples of successful role implementation are presented in the following section.

Specialty Settings

BONE MARROW TRANSPLANTATION SERVICES

The ACNP working as a member of the bone marrow transplantation service has an autonomous role while functioning as a part of a collaborative practice model; the team is composed of a resident, a fellow, an attending physician, and the ACNP. The ACNP provides the continuity of care for the service by being the only constant member of an academic health care team where physicians rotate clinical responsibilities. The ACNP carries a caseload of patients and follows them through their hospital stay until discharge. Role responsibilities include prerounding daily on each patient, performing physical examinations, interpreting laboratory tests (electrolytes and x-rays), and consulting specialists (gastroenterology, infectious disease, pulmonary medicine) to assist in patient management. Based on the information gathered, the ACNP collaborates with the team to develop the daily treatment plan. In addition, the ACNP provides teaching to the house staff and nursing staff and incorporates health teaching and health promotion (risk associated with immunosuppression) into her or his practice.

CARDIOLOGY

The role of the ACNP working on the heart failure service is similar to those previously described. Responsibilities include obtaining a patient history, performing a physical examination, performing preprocedure evaluation, ordering and interpreting laboratory and diagnostic tests, reviewing these with the physician team, and collaborating with consultative services (pulmonary, renal, or critical care services) to develop the management plan. Additional role responsibilities include teaching patients and families relative to heart failure and treatment procedures (i.e., coronary artery bypass graft surgery) and facilitating discharge planning.

ORTHOPEDICS

The role of the ACNP working with patients with orthopedic problems has been reported to include role responsibilities shared among several team members. This team provides coverage for the emergency room and orthopedic clinic and the orthopedic service. The orthopedic ACNP works closely with the attending physicians, staff nurses, and residents to coordinate care from preadmission testing to discharge. Each of the ACNPs carries a case load of hospitalized patients and outpatients undergoing short procedures. This role may include perioperative management as first assistant in the operating room (Gates, 1993).

DIAGNOSTIC AND INTERVENTIONAL SERVICES

In preadmission surgical services, the major clinical functions of an ACNP include history taking and physical examinations; performing preprocedure evaluations; providing patient and family education; obtaining and interpreting laboratory, electrocardiographic, and radiological data; identifying at-risk individuals in need of preadmission discharge planning; initiating contacts with social services; and discharge planning and making management recommendations for patients in the holding area. Because it is possible to foresee the growth of this type of ACNP role, research evaluating the cost- and time-effectiveness of an ACNP and ACNP collaboration is needed.

EDUCATIONAL PREPARATION OF THE ACNP

Educational preparation for the ACNP has been evolving over the past 20 years. As previously described, adult NPs were educated in the primary care model, then received "on the job training" in acute care settings. This role was followed by the NNP, which emerged in the late 1970s. It was the neonatal group that recognized the need for a specialized educational background in acute care. Educational preparation of the NNP was initially institutionally based, with neonatologists and previously "trained" NNPs assuming the teaching responsibility (Lott et al., 1996). As the demand for the NNP increased and nursing graduate programs did not respond, NNP programs became more hospital based or operated under the auspices of medical departments. Graduates were awarded a nondegree certificate. Then, in 1994, under the leadership of the NANN, concerns regarding inadequate numbers of NNPs, lack of NNP programs, inconsistency in educational preparation, and variable competency of program graduates were addressed in a position statement that supported graduate education as the entry level for the NNP. NANN also developed and published the *Program Guidelines for Neonatal Nurse Practitioner Educational Preparation* (NANN, 1994). NANN's primary goal was to facilitate the development and evaluation of graduate NNP programs through recommendations on general curriculum content and entry-level competency statements. In addition, it provided a guide for developing academic programs that could also be used by regulatory, accrediting, and certifying bodies in the evaluation of NNP programs (Lott et al., 1996). During this time, the National Organization for Nurse Practitioner Faculties (NONPF) published a document entitled *Advanced Nursing Practice: Nurse Practitioner Curriculum Guidelines* (NONPF, 1990). This document delineates content and competencies for primary care NP preparation and practice and also supports the preparation of the NP at the graduate level.

As the need for health care providers for adults in acute and critical care grew, increasing numbers of primary care NPs were recruited into the acute care setting and, once again, received on-the-job training to manage these patients. Although primary care NP programs provide an admirable background for advanced clinical assessment skills, development of the clinical decision-making process, and patient care management in primary care settings, curricula do not provide experience in making clinical decisions and the advanced assessment skills and management strategies unique to patients who are acutely and critically ill (Hravnak et al., 1995). In the late 1980s, formal dialogue began between graduate-level nursing faculty and national nursing organizations for the purpose of developing educational guidelines for the ACNP. Faculty seeking to develop ACNP programs focused upon identifying and incorporating role components common to all APNs in addition to those components specific to NPs, while distinguishing content, skills, and clinical requirements necessary for the ACNP to meet the unique needs of acutely ill patients and their families. A wide variety of clinical practice settings has made it difficult to reach consistency among ACNP educational programs. Early on, faculty drew from curricula models that prepared primary care NPs while drawing from curricula that educated CNSs, who have historically functioned in acute care. In an attempt to define the content, skills, and clinical requirements for ACNP preparation, it has been necessary to differentiate components of ACNP practice from those of the CNS. There is still a diversity of opinion regarding distinction between these two roles and how this should be reflected in curricula. Many believe that the CNS lacks some of the needed advanced preparation skills such as physical assessment, diagnostic reasoning, and pharmacologic management necessary to function as an NP. Some schools have blended the curricula to preserve the CNS focus but are adding courses, such as physical diagnosis and pharmacology, that will enhance the ACNP role. Other schools clearly separated CNS and ACNP programs.

As the process of developing guidelines for ACNP education progressed, a significant debate surfaced. This debate focused on the question "What constitutes acute care?" If NPs are going to be educated to function in the acute care setting, how should that be defined? Early on, the debate centered on the differences between "acute" and "primary" care, and then extended to the difference between "acute" and "critical" care. Is the issue geography or patient acuity? What part of the ACNP's practice is unique from that of NPs practicing in primary versus critical care settings? Are there areas of overlap? It is important to reach some general agreement on these questions because the answers help to narrow the areas of content skills and clinical requirements needed by ACNPs. Traditionally, primary care NPs have practiced in outpatient settings performing well-care visits and health promotion and education, in addition to managing patients with stable chronic illnesses (e.g., diabetes) and common acute, episodic complaints (e.g., flu symptoms or sinusitis). It would follow, then, that an ACNP would practice in a setting, such as a hospital, where the patients are in need of more intense care because they are more acutely ill than what can be managed in an outpatient area. Yet, are there not sicker patients outside of the hospital setting that require closer monitoring? In today's managed care environment, acutely ill patients are often managed on an outpatient basis, with hospital admission being reserved for those who do not respond to outpatient care. It is not uncommon for NPs in outpatient care settings to manage patients who present with an acute exacerbation of a chronic illness and who also have multiple co-morbid conditions that must be monitored (e.g., a patient with chronic obstructive pulmonary disease who develops a community-acquired pneumonia and is also diabetic and hypertensive). Which NP is best suited to provide care for these patients?

The second part of this debate relates to whether or not "acute care" really means "critical care" (i.e., intensive care). No one would question that patients in the ICU who are on mechanical ventilation and vasopressor drugs would clearly fit under the purvue of an ACNP, but does this mean that ACNPs should only function in ICUs? Certainly, there are patients who require long-term mechanical ventilation, and even receive intravenous positive inotropic medications (e.g., dobutamine), who are being managed outside the ICU in places such as subacute care facilities and clinics. There are also the issues surrounding care in rural communities where the intensivist is not needed, although care for complex patients exists. Many believe that, while these issues remain controversial, faculty will experience much difficulty in developing a curriculum if they focus on trying to determine the "divisions" among primary, acute, and critical care content (Hravnak et al., 1995). These concerns will remain educational priorities for ACNP faculty into the new millennium.

Development of the ACNP Curriculum Guidelines and National Standards for Education

In 1993, Keane and Richmond made recommendations for ACNP educational preparation. It was their opinion that curricula must reflect the strengths of both the NP and the CNS. They stated that critical aspects to the delivery of care by an NP in a highly specialized setting include "an indepth knowledge of the specialty's health problems and the technology used, coupled with the generalist approach reflecting nursing's holistic view of the individual with health care problems" (Keane & Richmond, 1993, p. 283).

Development of national standards for ACNP education was initiated as a result of the "Preparing Nurses for Advanced Practice in Acute Care Consensus Conference" held in 1993. The attendees, consisting of individuals representing 11 academic institutions, nine clinical agencies, and five professional organizations, met to draft standards for educational programs preparing ACNPs. The outcome included statements about philosophy, title, and core curriculum with the purpose of providing guidance to schools developing similar programs and to provide a starting point for preparation of a mechanism for certification (Clochesy, 1994). The recommendation from this group was that the curriculum for ACNPs should include advanced assessment, physiology, advanced pathophysiology, pharmacology, diagnostic reasoning, clinical decision making, and advanced therapeutics. These standards were later refined by the Acute Care Nurse Practitioner Task Force of the ANA in collaboration with the American Association of Critical-Care Nurses (AACN). The outcome of this task force was a document, published in 1995, entitled *Standards of Clinical Practice and Scope of Practice for the Acute Care Nurse Practitioner*. In addition, the Acute Care Nurse Practitioner Certification Examination was developed and offered for the first time in 1995. Both of these actions helped to gain official recognition of the ACNP role (ANA and AACN, 1995).

Further guidance for development of the ACNP curriculum came from the NONPF's revised guidelines, *Advanced Nursing Practice: Curriculum Guidelines and Program Standards for Nurse Practitioner Education* (NONPF Curriculum Guidelines Task Force, 1995), and the *AACN Taskforce on the Essentials of Master's Education for Advanced Practice Nursing* (AACN, 1996). The revised NONPF guidelines set forth a recommendation of 500 hours as the minimum number of clinical hours for all NP programs, inclung ACNP programs. The AACN's *Essentials of Master's Education* defined the content that forms the foundation of all graduate nursing education irrespective of specialty. It is important to note that specialty content for inclusion in ACNP programs has not yet been developed or published by any national organization. At this point, most educators utilize the content encompassed by the ACNP certification examination as a guide for specialty content.

Invasive Procedures

The issue of ACNPs performing invasive procedures has been the subject of many debates among ACNPs and faculty. Some believe that the more skills a student can master before entering the workforce, the more marketable that graduate ACNP will be. Others believe that skill acquisition can occur once the student is employed. To date, there has been no consensus reached as to which skills should be considered core skills necessary for any ACNP student to have upon graduation. The needed skills tend to vary within the specialty focus of any given program.

Teaching various skills requires not only time but also many resources, not the least of which is competent faculty. Building in time for teaching skills adds to the length of a program. Clinical time needs to be focused on learning the process of diagnosing and managing patients. In addition, there is no guarantee that procedures will be available for instruction and, even when the opportunity does present itself, an ACNP student frequently has to compete with medical students and interns for access to the procedure.

Nursing Standards of ACNP Clinical Practice

Standards of practice for the ACNP build upon the generalist standards of care discussed in *Standards of Clinical Nursing Practice* (ANA, 1991). The nursing process, which includes assessment, diagnosis, outcome identification, planning, implementation, and evaluation, is used as the foundation (see Table 15-6). ACNP practice standards are written very broadly to allow for a wide diversity of ACNP practice. At first blush, the reader may question how ACNP standards of care differ from other NP standards. Certainly, use of the nursing process is not unique to acute care. What is important to remember is that for ACNPs these standards must be interpreted within the framework of restorative care. It is this focus that differentiates an ACNP from other NPs. Although these standards are very broad, there are statements that more precisely differentiate ACNP practice as outlined in Table 15-6. For example, standard I deals with assessment. Measurement criterion number V states "The data collection process is continuous, in acknowledgement of the dynamic nature of acute illness" (ANA and AACN, 1995). What is unique to ACNP practice in this statement is

---

TABLE 15-6 STANDARDS FOR ACUTE CARE NURSE PRACTITIONER

Standard I: Assessment
The acute care nurse practitioner collects the patient data.
Measurement criteria example: The data collection process is continuous, in acknowledgment of the dynamic nature of acute care illness.
Standard II: Diagnosis
The acute care nurse practitioner analyzes data in determining diagnoses.
Measurement criteria example: Diagnoses are re-evaluated as new or additional assessment data become available.
Standard III: Outcome Identification
The acute care nurse practitioner identifies expected outcomes individualized to the patient.
Measurement criteria example: Expected outcomes are modified based on changes in the patient's condition.
Standard IV: Planning
The acute care nurse practitioner develops a plan of care that prescribes interventions to attain expected outcomes.
Measurement criteria example: The plan of care is individualized, recognizes the dynamic nature of the patient's illness, and reflects the patient's needs across a full continuum of acute care.
Standard V: Implementation
The acute care nurse practitioner implements the interventions identified in the multidisciplinary plan of care.
Measurement criteria example: Interventions are prescribed consistent with the multidisciplinary plan of care.
Standard VI: Evaluation
The acute care nurse practitioner evaluates the patient's progress toward attainment of expected outcomes.
Measurement criteria example: Evaluation is systematic and ongoing.

Adapted from ANA and AACN (1995). *Standards of clinical practice and scope of practice for the acute care nurse practitioner* (pp. 19–23). Washington, DC: American Nurses Publishing; reprinted with permission.

the word "continuous." What is also evident, in standard V, is the repeated use of the term "multidisciplinary." The very nature of acute illness mandates the need for continuous patient assessment and mobilization of a variety of health care professionals and resources to provide restorative care to the acutely ill patient. Often, a primary care NP is the sole provider of patient care and only refers the patient to a physician or other health care provider when the patient's condition warrants it. With acutely ill patients, use of multidisciplinary health care teams is the norm. There is never the expectation that one person can provide all the care an acutely ill patient requires.

ROLE DEVELOPMENT ISSUES

Although ACNPs have championed many successes in their quest for role development and growth, there are still real and potential barriers to overcome. Kleinpell (1997) conducted a study that explored the aspects of the ACNP role. Identified advantages of the ACNP role included role autonomy, broad scope of practice, and contributions to collaborative care. Barriers included obstacles to obtaining clinical privileges and role expansion, lack of time to perform job responsibilities, and gaining physicians' acceptance of the role. These issues will continue to escalate as workforce issues, as described in the Pew 4th Report about oversupply of the physicians and APN workforce (Finocchio et al., 1998) and with the evolution of the physician hospitalist role.

Opportunities for expanding the ACNP role include identifying potential practice arenas and meeting the market demand for the role. There have been basic similarities among ACNP roles; however, there can be significant differences in the role's development based on the practice setting. Being aware of the similarities in roles and having flexibility and vision will minimize barriers to role implementation and expansion. Limiting the ACNP scope to a specific hospital setting does not permit care to be provided across the continuum of services, outpatient to inpatient. An ACNP initially hired to work in a cardiology private practice covering cardiac catheterization, including managing patients using protocol orders and performing precatheterization and postcatheterization teaching and planning, could expand her or his role to include coverage of overflow patients in the coronary care unit. This would expose the ACNP to a variety of patients with different diagnoses. This example portrays the developing nature of ACNP practice. Once an ACNP is integrated into a practice, role changes or expansion can provide developmental opportunities for ACNP practice.

Success related to performing job responsibilities in an efficient manner is largely dependent upon the individual ACNP's time management and comfort with the skills required. Performing procedures can be initially time intensive because of undeveloped psychomotor skills. Repetition will enhance the ACNP's efficiency in performing procedural skills and also diagnostic reasoning when formulating a plan of care and interpreting diagnostic test results. An intrinsic component of the role is optimizing patient outcomes. Initial focus on the key elements of the ACNP role, especially through presenting patient cases and exposure to diagnostic reasoning and critical thinking, allows the ACNP to build a strong platform that demonstrates her or his contributions to the practice group or system.

Reimbursement

Reimbursement for NP services has been a challenging process and is not an issue unique to ACNPs. Almost every encounter between an NP and a patient is associated with a private or public payer. Despite the setting, reimbursement mechanisms will decide whether an ANCP will continue to provide care on a long-term basis.

The four major types of payers that ACNP services can be billed under are Medicare, Medicaid, indemnity-type insurance, and managed care organizations. Each type of payer has its own reimbursement policies and fee for service operating under a separate body of regulations. Some payers have a history of reimbursing for ACNP services in the same manner as they reimburse for physician services; for other payers this is a new practice. In the past, most reimbursers have paid the hospital for total operating costs, combining the costs of ACNP services together with other operating costs. In this situation, the hospitals then pay the ACNP as a salaried employee. Currently, the federal government programs, Medicare and Medicaid, provide reimbursement for all health care providers utilizing this program. However, individual states control which reimbursement providers are eligible for payment. Health care reform brought about industry-related health care changes, specifically capitation, which provides a specific dollar amount for health care services regardless of the actual cost. The focus of care is placed upon the actual cost of care; therefore, the fewer the diagnostic tests, the healthier the system is financially. ACNPs need to be attentive to billing and coding schemes and be judicious about pharmacologic and diagnostic treatment decisions. In addition, when providing care to the complex patient, the ACNP must be aware of the need to collaborate with physician colleagues versus utilizing physician consultation services. In a capitated system, physician consultation services lead to excessive expense that may not be fully reimbursed.

Medicare reimbursement provisions for APNs in the Balanced Budget Act of 1997 made it necessary for the ACNP to have an understanding of reimbursement guidelines and to be able to articulate these guidelines to their employers. The framework for current ACNP reimbursement has been developed from the guidelines, understanding that individual states have wide latitude in the division of federal money (Hravnak, Rosenzweig, Rust, & Magdic, 1998a).

In accordance with the Balanced Budget Act of 1997, the restrictions on the type of areas and settings in which NPs can receive direct Medicare payments were removed, allowing ACNPs to bill Medicare Part B directly, regardless of the setting or geographic location. The new payment structure allows for direct payment for ACNP services in areas or settings authorized under state licensure laws. Therefore, an ACNP can bill for Medicare services in independent practice states providing the requirements for physician collaboration or "incident to" are fulfilled. (See Chapters 20 and 23 for a detailed understanding of Medicare and Medicaid issues.)

A second area of concern relates to nonduplicate billing for ACNP and physician services. The Health Care Financing Administration (HFCA) has indicated that payments will not be provided if a "facility is paid any amount with respect to furnishing such services" (Department of Health and Human Services, 1998). An ACNP must communicate with physician provider(s) to clearly understand who will be submitting the bill for reimbursement. Claims submitted twice for the same services could imply fraud. In the instance where ACNPs are hospital employees, they are not eligible for individual reimbursement. In this case, Medicare supplements their salary to the hospital under Medicare Part A (American College of Nurse Practitioners, 1998; Hravnak et al., 1998a).

ACNPs, like other APNs, should contact the provider relations department of their local Medicare carrier in their state in order to request an application for a provider number. Practice managers who bill Medicare will be aware of the local Medicare carrier. Once the ACNP obtains a provider number, entering the provider number on the HFCA-1500 form, if she or he is the person providing services for a particular patient, enables the ACNP to receive reimbursement for services at 85% of the payment structure (American College of Nurse Practitioners, 1998).

Private payers such as Blue Cross/Blue Shield have varied reimbursement structures. Familiarity with the rules of the company in order to obtain reimbursement for the ACNP or to the practice is to the ACNP's benefit. Vigilant monitoring of payment mechanisms is necessary to assure appropriate reimbursement.

Managed care organizations require ACNPs to establish a provider contract in order to be paid for services rendered. To receive reimbursement from a health maintenance organization (HMO), an ACNP is required to be a part of a managed care panel. The ACNP can expect that reimbursement rates will generally be less because access to patients is based on cost effectiveness. This decrease will impact acute care reimbursement in all practice settings. If the ACNP is an employee of the HMO, the provider payment structure will be salaried. If the ACNP practices in an acute care setting that utilizes a particular HMO, the ACNP must apply to become a member of a provider panel. Processing of the application may be lengthy because of unfamiliarity with the role. Contacting the provider relations department every 2 to 4 weeks will assist in clarifying information and enhance the timely processing of the application. If the application is rejected because of "the provider panel being closed," this means that there are no more providers needed to serve a given population of patients. In this case, making an inquiry about what types of providers are needed will assist in the application process. For example, the HMO may need more specialty care providers like ACNPs instead of primary care providers, but the documentation may not reflect this need. Another approach is to involve a patient as an advocate, because the patient's employer is the purchaser of the provider services. As members of provider panels, ACNPs are assigned a provider relations representative. This person's role is to familiarize ACNPs with procedures for claim authorization, filing, and processing and to share information about system changes (Workman, 1998).

ACNPs need to be fluent with reimbursement regulations and have an understanding of the International Classification of Diseases, 9th Revision diagnostic coding system (ICD-9) and procedures codes because they may be responsible for admitting patients and required to provide an admitting diagnosis (O'Donahue, 1996; see Chapter 20). All visits must be coded for a specific disease or sign/symptom; there is no capacity to code for a "rule out" diagnosis. Diagnostic codes need to accurately reflect the level of services provided. The Physician's Current Procedural Terminology (CPT) code book provides standard descriptions of diagnoses and procedures. These procedures codes are referred to as evaluation and management (E & M) codes, which define seven components of inpatient and outpatient visits: history, examination, medical decision making, counseling, coordination of care, nature of the presenting problem, and time (Bryan 1996; Hravnak et al., 1998a). ACNPs have been trained to understand how to formulate a diagnosis and fully understand the seven components of the E & M codes; therefore, with assistance from the organization, the ACNP should be able to accurately reflect the care delivered in order to secure the most appropriate reimbursement.

Reimbursement rules and regulations for all APNs are being built into licensure and credentialing mechanisms. By January 1, 2003, all NPs, including ACNPs, applying for Medicare numbers for the first time will need both to have a master's degree in nursing and to meet the state requirements for licensing and certification (Peters, 1999).

Challenges for the ACNP Role

Gaining acceptance of the role will depend largely upon combating barriers to practice. The role of the ACNP is currently evolving and gaining recognition. Practicing ACNPs report that many physician and hospital administrators are unfamiliar with the role and the differences between a primary care NP and an ACNP. Additionally, some physicians feel threatened by the role. Misperceptions about the role and labeling the role as a physician extender have stemmed from the perception that ACNPs are replacements for house staff. Indeed, one of the earliest publications on the ACNP fueled this perception (Silver & McAtee, 1988). It is extremely important for ACNPs to frame acute care practice within the nursing paradigm, one that uses the admitting history and physical examination to put forth a plan a care that includes the patient's holistic problems as well as the medical diagnosis; to address these nursing and medical problems throughout the hospital stay; and to frame the discharge summary so that patients have a continuum of nursing as well as medical care as they return to the community.

ACNPs need to develop strong collaborative relationships with physicians to provide optimal patient care. Understanding the position physicians face as they move from specialty to primary care practices is important for ANCPs. Some physicians are frustrated as health care moves to a corporate structure that dictates physician salaries and practices, thus placing stress on the physician-ACNP relationship. It is essential that both communicate and work through differences in order to support each other so that the ultimate outcome is to improve patient care.

Exposure to the comprehensive care that ACNPs provide and marketing of the role to all members of the health care team will lead to role recognition and role acceptance. Relying on personal experience or exposure to the role is an inactive means of marketing the role. Furthermore, ACNPs should recognize that, because the role is relatively new, active marketing must include describing role capabilities and role effectiveness in terms of outcome data relative to a population served by the ACNP. Resistance to the role has been reported from physicians and other health care professionals (Kleinpell, 1997). Such resistance primarily stems from uncertainty of the functions of the role and perceived blurring of professional boundaries. Certainly, as the role of physician hospitalist emerges, tensions with ACNPs will become more evident. As well, the perceived threat that the CNS role will be replaced by the ACNP has added to role resistance among some nurses. It appears likely that hospital employment will be less common as hospitals decrease fixed costs, such as payroll. ACNPs will be either self-employed contractors or, more likely, employees or partners in a private physician practice. This will depend on dynamics of local markets. Educating administrators and nurses can facilitate acceptance of the role, which will in turn provide an opportunity for independent contracting for ACNP professional services. It will be imperative that ACNPs be aware of their worth in terms of billable revenue and the care they are able to provide for contract negotiations and marketing purposes.

In the future, ACNPs may practice in multiple settings with individually negotiated contracts. Managing episodes of acute illness or exacerbation of chronic illness in home health care, subacute care, and outpatient settings might be directed by the ACNP, as is already the case in some areas. These areas are natural extensions of acute care services and encompass the scope of ACNP practice, the stabilization of acute and chronic disease. A myriad of opportunities relative to acute and chronic therapeutic management exist—for example, the management of renal dialysis or ventilator-dependent patients.

Cost reduction of acute care services will continue. The traditional team of physician, resident(s), and ACNP collaborating may change to a staffing ratio of one physician with several ACNPs. Looking at patient acuity relative to the population served will determine the composition of the team. Currently there has been one physician for every ACNP in most practice settings, with the relationship being a collaborative one. In the future, certain patient populations may be managed by several ACNPs with one physician, as is already the case in some settings such as the heart failure service described earlier.

As this NP role continues to evolve, it will be the responsibility of ACNP nurse leaders to encourage standardization of education for the ACNP based on the acute care setting in which the ACNP will be practicing. Standard clinical competencies that provide consistency in education and training must be developed. ACNPs also need to belong to a strong nursing organization that could oversee the political and educational needs of ACNPs. Having several organizations that offer membership for all NPs does a disservice to the unique issues facing ACNPs.

The future for the ACNP role is promising. Many ACNPs report that their current positions were created by their employers. Being able to develop a role has a distinct advantage for ACNP practice and provides a strong position for negotiating a contract and a position in a practice setting. With more ACNPs holding graduate degrees, there is potential to apply basic science knowledge to clinical practice to effectively demonstrate diagnostic reasoning skills and therapeutic management, clinical skills central to the ACNP role. Participation with researchers in clinical and bench research settings is another future direction for ACNPs. Collaboration with public policy makers to influence legislation issues related to the ACNP role or, on a larger scope, health policy issues (i.e., ACNP prescriptive authority and reimbursement for ACNPs) is an imperative for all ACNPs (AACN, 1995; see Chapters 22 and 23).

SUMMARY

The ACNP's focus of care is primarily restorative, with the short-term goal being patient stabilization, provision of physical and psychological care, and minimization of complications. The role of the ACNP, although primarily enacted in acute and critical care settings, continues to broaden to a variety of clinical sites and specialty practice settings. The workforce of ACNPs is steadily increasing. Some ACNPs report that their role includes system-focused responsibilities: teaching, research, or projects; however, the majority of ACNPs find direct patient care management the focus of the role. The growth of ACNP educational programs speaks to the current market demand for APNs in the acute care setting. With increasing numbers of ACNPs being educated and employed to work in acute care settings, the trend toward using ACNPs in such settings appears to be spreading.

The ANCP role has developed over the past 30 years. The movement of NPs into acute care settings was developed as a response to a need for acute care services in critical care areas. Educational preparation for the ACNP has progressed over the years from hospital-based training programs to master's education. ACNPs have been involved in the development of acute care delivery along with physicians, practicing in a collaborative comprehensive care model. They are capable of providing a full spectrum of acute care services. ACNPs have been among nurse leaders in obtaining third-party reimbursement for professional services and coping with the challenges of managed care.

The ACNP role provides an opportunity for APNs to have a significant impact on health care outcomes at a dynamic time in health care. As the role continues to evolve along with the market, and as health care systems respond to economic change, opportunities to develop the ACNP role as a new position or with a focus different than an existing role will arise. Further development of the ACNP role should be based on the evaluation of the need for the role, understanding the scope of the role, and assessment of the practice or organization and the service needs of the patient population. Because the adult ACNP role is still evolving, participation in national organizations to develop consensus regarding role components, course curricula, marketing, and evaluation of the role to grant full recognition is necessary to assure that the elements of the ACNP role are fully represented. ACNPs must be strong activists in efforts to gain full recognition of the role within their proper scope of practice across acute care settings.

REFERENCES

American Association of Colleges of Nursing. (1996). *AACN taskforce on the essentials of Master's education for advanced practice nursing.* Washington, DC: Author.

American Association of Colleges of Nursing. (1998). *Peterson's guide to nursing programs: Baccalaureate and graduate nursing education in the U.S. and Canada.* Princeton, NJ: Peterson's Guide, Inc.

American Association of Critical-Care Nurses. (1995). *Advanced nursing practice: Facts and strategies for regulation, reimbursement and prescriptive authority.* Washington, DC: Author.

American College of Nurse Practitioners. (1998). How to bill for Medicare. *Nurse Practitioner World News, 3*(2), 1, 20.

American Nurses Association. (1991). *Standards of clinical nursing practice* (ANA Publication no. NP 79). Kansas City, MO: Author.

American Nurses Association and American Association of Critical-Care Nurses. (1995). *Standards of clinical practice and scope of practice for acute care nurse practitioner.* Washington, DC: American Nurses Publishing.

American Nurses Credentialing Center. (1999). *Nurse practitioner board certification examination catalog.* Washington, DC: Author.

Baggs, J. G., & Schmitt, M. H. (1988). Collaboration between nurses and physicians. *Image: The Journal of Nursing Scholarship, 20,* 145–149.

Barber, P. M., & Burke, M. (1999). Advanced practice nursing in managed care. In M. D. Mezy & D. O. McGivern (Eds.), *Nurses, nurse practitioners* (pp. 203–218). New York: Springer-Verlag.

Bryan, V. (1996). *Breaking the code of health care reimbursement with ICD-9-CM.* Leesburg, VA: The Regis Group, Inc.

Buppert, C. K. (1995). Justifying nurse practitioner existence: Hard facts to hard figures. *Nurse Practitioner, 20*(8), 43–48.

Burkholder, J. S., & Dudjak, L. J. (1994). The mid-level practitioner role: One medical center's experience. *AACN Clinical Issues in Critical Care Nursing, 5*(3), 369–403.

Carzoli, R. P., Martinez-Cruz, M., Cuevas, L. L., & Murphy, S. (1994). Comparison of neonatal practitioners, physician assistants, and residents in the neonatal intensive care unit. *Archives of Pediatric and Adolescent Medicine, 148,* 1271–1276.

Cintron, G., Bigas, C., Linates, E., Aranda, J. M., & Hernandez, E. (1983). Nurse practitioner role in a congestive heart failure clinic: In-hospital time, costs, and patient satisfaction. *Heart and Lung, 12,* 237–240.

Clochesy, J. M., Daly, B. J., Idemoto, B. K., Steel, J., & Fitzpatrick, J. J. (1994). Preparing APNs for acute care. *American Journal of Critical Care, 3*(4), 255–259.

Cummings, C. M. (1997, July). Scope of employment vs. scope of practice. *Advance for Nurse Practitioners,* pp 17–18.

Daly, B., & Gent, C. (1997). Influence of the health care environment. In B. Daly (Ed.), *The acute care nurse practitioner* (pp. 29–56). Washington, DC: American Nurses Publishing.

Department of Health and Human Services. (1998). Medicare program: Revisions to payment policies and adjustments to the relative value units under the physician fee schedule for 1999. 63 *Federal Register* 58813, p 58:73.

Finocchio, L. J., Dower, C. M., Blick, N. T., et al., and the Taskforce on Health Care Workforce Regulation. (1998). *Strengthening consumer protection: Priorities for health care workforce regulations* (pp. 27–30). San Francisco: Pew Health Professions Commission, October 1998.

Gates, S. J. (1993). Continuity of care: The orthopaedic nurse practitioner in tertiary care. *Orthopaedic Nursing, 12*(5), 48–50, 66.

Hall, J. K. (1993). How to analyze nurse practitioner licensure laws. *Nurse Practitioner, 18*(8), 31–34.

Hooker, R. S., & McCraig, L. (1996). Emergency department uses of physician assistants and nurse practitioners: A national survey. *American Journal of Emergency Medicine, 14,* 245–249.

Hravnak, M., & Baldiserri, M. (1997). Credentialing and privileging: Insight into the process for acute care nurse practitioners. *AACN Clinical Issues, 8*(1), 108–115.

Hravnak, M., Kobert, S. N., Risco, K. G., Baldisseri, M., Hoffman, L. A., Clochesy, J. M., Rudy, E. B., & Snyder, J. V. (1995). Acute care nurse practitioner curriculum: Content and development process. *American Journal of Critical Care 4*(3), 179–188.

Hravnak, M., & Magdic, K. (1997). Marketing the acute care nurse practitioner. *Clinical Excellence for the Nurse Practitioner, 1,* 9–13.

Hravnak, M., Rosenzweig, P., Rust, D., & Magdic, K. (1998a). Reimbursement, liability and insurance. In R. Kleinpell & M. Piano (Eds.), *Practice issues for the acute care nurse practitioner* (pp. 27–40). New York: Springer-Verlag.

Hravnak, M., Rosenzweig, P., Rust, D., & Magdic, K. (1998b). Scope of practice, credentialing, and privileging. In R. Kleinpell & M. Piano (Eds.), *Practice issues for the acute care nurse practitioner* (pp. 41–46). New York: Springer-Verlag.

Hylka, S. C., & Beschle, J. C. (1995). Nurse practitioners, cost savings, and improved patient care in the department of surgery. *Nursing Economics, 13*(6), 349–351.

Ingersol, G. (1995). Evaluation of the advanced practice nurse role in acute care and specialty care. *Critical Care Nursing Clinics of North America, 7,* 25–34.

Kassirer, J. P. (1989). Diagnostic reasoning. *Annals of Internal Medicine, 110,* 893–900.

Keane, A., & Richmond, T. (1993). Tertiary NPs. *Image: The Journal of Nursing Scholarship, 25*(4), 281–284.

Keane, A., Richmond, T., & Kaiser, L. (1994). Critical care nurse practitioners: Evolution of the advanced practice nursing role. *American Journal of Critical Care, 3,* 232–237.

King, K. B., & Baggs, J. G. (1998). Collaboration: The essence of acute care nurse practitioner practice. In R. Kleinpell & M. Piano (Eds.), *Prac-*

tice issues for the acute care nurse practitioner (pp. 67–78). New York: Springer-Verlag.

Kleinpell, R. M. (1997). Acute care nurse practitioner: Roles and practice profiles. *AACN Clinical Issues 8*(1), 156–162.

Kleinpell, R. M. (1998). Acute care nurse practitioner: Reports from the practice settings profiles. In R. Kleinpell & M. Piano (Eds.), *Practice issues for the acute care nurse practitioner* (pp. 1–9). New York: Springer-Verlag.

Kleinpell, R. M. (1999). Evolving role descriptions of the acute care nurse practitioner. *Critical Care Nurse Quarterly, 21*(4), 9–15.

Knickman, J. R., Lipkin, M., Finkler, S. A., Thompson, W. G., & Kiel, J. (1992). The potential for using non-physicians to compensate for the reduced availability of residents. *Academic Medicine, 67,* 429–428.

Kristeller, A. R. (1995). Medical staff: Privileging and credentialing. *New Jersey Medicine, 92,* 26–28.

Kubala, S., & Clever, L. H. (1974). Acceptance of the nurse practitioner. *American Journal of Nursing, 74,* 452–453.

Lombness, P. M. (1994). Difference in length of stay with care management by clinical nurse specialists or physician assistants. *Clinical Nurse Specialist, 8,* 253–260.

Lott, J. W., Polak, J. D., Kenyon, T. B., & Kenner, C. A. (1996). Acute care nurse practitioner. In A. B. Hamric, J. A. Spross, & C. M. Hanson (Eds.), *Advanced practice nursing: An integrative approach* (pp. 351–373). Philadelphia: W. B. Saunders.

Mitchell-Di Censo, A., Guyatt, G., Marrin, M., Goeree, R., Willan, A., Southwell, D., Hewson, S., Paes, B., Rosenbaum, P., Hunsberger, M., & Baumann, A. (1996). A controlled trial of nurse practitioners in neonatal intensive care. *Pediatrics, 98,* 1143–1148.

National Association of Neonatal Nurses. (1994). *Program guidelines for neonatal nurse practitioner educational preparation.* Petaluma, CA: Author.

National Organization of Nurse Practitioner Faculties Curriculum Guidelines Task Force. (1995). *Advanced nursing practice: Curriculum guidelines and program standards for nurse practitioner education.* Washington, DC: National Organization of Nurse Practitioner Faculties.

National Organization of Nurse Practitioner Faculties Education Committee. (1990). *Advanced nursing practice: Nurse practitioner curriculum guidelines.* Washington, DC: National Organization of Nurse Practitioner Faculties.

Norsen, L., Opladen, J., & Quinn, J. (1995). Practice model: Collaborative practice. *Critical Care Nursing Clinics of North America, 7,* 43–52.

O'Donahue, W. (1996). *Accurately coding for critical care services and pulmonary medicine.*

Northbrook, IL: American College of Chest Physicians.

Parrinello, K. (1995). Advanced practice nursing. *Critical Care Nursing Clinics of North America, 1*, 9–16.

Peters, S. (1999). Degrees of success: Federal Master's requirement speeds graduate movement. *Advance for Nurse Practitioners, 24*(1), 63–64.

Piano, M. R., & Zerwic-Johnson, J. (1998). Demonstrating the effectiveness of the acute care nurse practitioner: Current and future research. In R. Kleinpell & M. Piano (Eds.), *Practice issues for the acute care nurse practitioner* (pp. 10–26). New York: Springer-Verlag.

Prescott, P. A., & Driscoll, L. (1979). Evaluating nurse practitioner performance. *Evaluation and the Health Professions, 2*(4), 387–418.

Prescott, P. A., & Driscoll, L. (1980). Evaluating nurse practitioner performance. *Nurse Practitioner, 5*(4), 28–29, 31–32.

Prosser, W. L. (1971). *Law of torts* (4th ed., p. 460). West Publishing, Inc.

Rudy, E. B., Davidson, L. J., Daly, B., Clochesy, J. M., Sereika, S., Baldesseri, M., Hravnak, M., Ross, T., & Ryan, C. (1998). Care activities and outcomes of patients cared for by acute care nurse practitioners, physicians assistants and resident physicians: A comparison. *American Journal of Critical Care, 7*(4), 267–281.

Shah, H., & Sullivan, D. T. (1998). Evaluation of the acute care nurse practitioner's role. In R. Kleinpell & M. Piano (Eds.), *Practice issues for the acute care nurse practitioner* (pp. 111–143). New York: Springer-Verlag.

Shah, H. S., Sullivan, D. T., Lattanzio, J., & Bruttomesso, K. (1993). Preparing acute care nurse practitioners at the University of Connecticut. *AACN Clinical Issues, 4*(4), 625–629.

Silver, H. K., & McAtee, P. (1988). Speaking out: Should nurses substitute for house staff? *American Journal of Nursing, 88*, 1671–1673.

Sox, H. C., Jr. (1979). Quality of patient care by nurse practitioners and physicians assistants: A ten-year perspective. *Annals of Internal Medicine, 91*, 459–468.

Spisso, J., O'Callaghan, C., McKennan, M., & Holcroft, J. W. (1990). Improved quality of care and reduction of housestaff workload using trauma nurse practitioners. *Journal of Trauma, 30*, 660–663.

Spitzer, W. O., Sackett, D. L., Sibley, J. C., Roberts, R. S., Gent, M., Kergin, D. J., Hackett, B. C., & Olynich, A. (1974). The Burlington randomized trial of the nurse practitioner. *New England Journal of Medicine, 290*, 251–256.

Szaflarski, N. L. (1997). Diagnostic reasoning in acute and critical care. *AACN Clinical Issues, 8*(2), 291–302.

von Sternberg, T., Hepburn, K., Cibuzar, P., Convery, L., Dokken, B., Haefemeyer, J., Rettke, S., Ripley, J., Vosenau, V., Rothe, P., Schurle, D., & Won-Savage, R. (1997). Post-hospital sub-acute care: An example of a managed care model. *Journal of the American Geriatric Society, 45*, 87–91.

Wachter, R. M., & Goldman, L. (1996). The emerging role of "hospitalists" in the American health care system. *New England Journal of Medicine, 335*, 514–517.

Weinberg, R. M., Liljestrand, J. S., & Moore, S. (1983). Inpatient management by a nurse practitioner: Effectiveness in a rehabilitation setting. *Archives of Physical Medicine and Rehabilitation, 64*, 588–590.

Workman, L. (1998). Third party reimbursement. *Nurse Practitioner 6*(5), 11, 111.

Ziemer, D. C., Goldschmid, M. G., Musey, V. C., Domin, W. S., Thule, P. M., Gallina, D. L., & Phillips, L. S. (1996). Diabetes in urban African Americans. III. Management of type II diabetes in a municipal hospital setting. *American Journal of Medicine, 101*, 25–33.

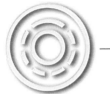

The Blended Role of the Clinical Nurse Specialist and the Nurse Practitioner

· K A R E N S K A L L A
· A N N B. H A M R I C

INTRODUCTION

This chapter describes the evolution and implementation of blended role advanced nursing practice. The blended role advanced practice nurse (APN) is defined as a graduate of a master's degree program in nursing that fully includes both clinical nurse specialist (CNS) and nurse practitioner (NP) preparation. Therefore the blended role APN is eligible for certification in a specialty area as well as certification as a NP. The blended role APN demonstrates the core advanced nursing practice competencies through the provision of comprehensive primary and specialty care to a specific population and crosses settings from primary through tertiary care. In practice, blended role preparation combines the strengths of two traditional roles: the primary health care skills of NPs and the in-depth, specialty and systems knowledge of CNSs. The blended role APN thus maximizes expertise to meet expanded responsibilities for the more complex health problems experienced by patients today (Hockenberry-Eaton & Powell, 1991). Issues related to role preparation and implementation are discussed and illustrated by clinical case presentations and role exemplars.[1]

EVOLUTION OF THE BLENDED ROLE

Historical Forces Driving Development of the Blended Role

The development of an APN role that blends the practice of the CNS and NP cannot be traced to any particular event. Davitt and Jensen (1981) provided one of the earliest job descriptions in the literature that parallels the blended role APN practice described in this chapter. Some authors believed that the skills and strengths of NP and CNS roles should or would be combined to meet projected health care needs (Kitzman, 1989; Spross & Hamric, 1983). Spross and Hamric (1983) proposed a model describing future CNS practice. According to their projections, a time would come when there would be a need for a nurse with a master's degree who had the clinical and scholarly skills of both the NP and the CNS. These authors proposed the title of advanced registered nurse practitioner (ARNP) for this future role. This title, in use in some state statutes, would reflect the role that emerged from combining NP and CNS preparation and practice. The practice of this future APN combined the domains of service and scopes of practice of NPs and CNSs. The ARNP was seen as a practitioner who would be client based rather than setting based, providing care in primary, secondary, and tertiary settings to ensure continuity of services to a specialty-based patient population. Through independent and interdependent practice with physicians, the ARNP would deliver direct care, such as advanced clinical assessment, manage acute and chronic problems associated with a specific patient population, and provide ongoing guidance about potential diagnosis-specific problems as well as generic primary prevention education. The ARNP would also provide vital indirect patient care through expert clinical consultation, coordination and facilitation of client services, and support for improved nursing practice (Spross & Hamric, 1983).

Gleeson and coworkers (1990) reported a model of collaborative practice that suggests how and why a blended role APN, who is different from either a CNS or a NP, may be the most appropriate APN for a defined population. Kitzman (1989) pointed out that CNSs and NPs have contributed significantly to the growth of each other's practice. CNSs have been credited with cultivating a climate within nursing

[1] Portions of this chapter appeared in the previous edition of this book. The authors and editors gratefully acknowledge the work of Allison Weber Shuren, MSN, RN, CCRN, CPNP, for her important contribution to the first edition of this text (Shuren, 1996).

open to expanded nursing practice (Kitzman, 1989), for developing theory-based practice, and for establishing the behavioral expectations of a nurse in advanced practice. NPs can take credit for expanding practice beyond traditional nursing boundaries; fostering lay recognition of APNs, which has promoted consumer acceptance of advanced nursing practice (Hanson & Martin, 1990); and developing collegial relationships with physicians (Kitzman, 1989). Currently, the blended role is a natural evolution of two APN roles that have expanded and matured, yet it is an APN role distinct from either the CNS or the NP role.

Historically, the CNS has been viewed as a specialist in nursing care who provides specialized nursing care for a specific patient population, staff development, and systems change in secondary and tertiary inpatient care settings. In contrast, NPs have been viewed as generalists who provide primary and preventative care and treat illnesses for a broad patient population in outpatient care settings. However, as Kitzman (1983) presciently observed, CNSs are found in outpatient settings providing extensive primary and preventative services and assessment and management of illness (Brooten et al., 1991; Damato et al., 1993; Sawyers, 1993). Also, NPs are practicing in tertiary care centers managing acute and chronic illnesses for specific patient populations and improving nursing care through education, consultation, and research (Dale, 1991; Davitt & Jensen, 1981; Gleeson et al., 1990; Hunsberger et al., 1992; Keane & Richmond, 1993; Nemes, Barnaby, & Shamberger, 1992; Weinberg, Likestrand, & Moore, 1983). As the CNS and NP roles have crossed, so have their practice settings (Deane, 1997). This has contributed to the current development of the blended role APN.

Despite this crossover of CNS and NP roles, merged roles and reconceptualized advanced practice educational models have been and continue to be much-debated topics among nursing leaders, educators, and APNs. Numerous articles and editorials both in support of and in opposition to merging APN roles (Deane, 1997; Page & Mackowiak, 1997; Redekopp, 1997; K. B. Wright, 1997) appear in the literature. Some authors believe that the debate is more theoretical and based on minimal research (Fenton & Brykczynski, 1993). Others suggest that the merger is inevitable and believe that blending the roles would be advantageous for health care organizations, patient care, and graduate nursing education (Cooper, 1990; Elder & Bullough, 1990; McGivern, 1993; J. E. Wright, 1990). Still others assert that the roles are distinctly different in scope of practice and setting and should be maintained as such (Beecroft, 1994; King & Ackerman, 1995; Lyon, 1996; Page & Arena, 1994; Zimmer et al., 1990). What is notable in these articles is the either-or tone asserting that either the roles must blend or they must stay distinct.

The position advanced here is that the blended role is a distinct role that can coexist with traditional CNS and NP roles, and that it has developed in response to the growing needs of specific patient populations. Most nursing leaders and APNs agree that a common core of knowledge, skills and competencies, and professional attributes exists that should be required of all APNs (see Chapter 3; Hamric, 1996). Differences between the CNS and NP are largely based on focus of service (Forbes, Rafson, Spross, & Kozlowski, 1990; Jackson, 1995; Pearson, 1990; Sawyers, 1993).

Health Care Trends Driving Evolution of the Blended Role

Current development of the blended role has been driven by a variety of forces. Patient needs and health care system needs have contributed to the way in which this role is being implemented. Patient needs have changed within the context of the current health care system. The system's complexity increasingly requires the skills of both the CNS and the NP to manage the growing populations of specialty and chronically ill patients—for example, the oncology patient, the congestive heart failure patient, or the patient requiring palliative care. These skills are required to provide quality care at a lower cost as treatment shifts from inpatient to outpatient settings. With this shift comes an increasing need to improve access to more complex chronic care in a way that primary care patient issues can also be monitored. Implementation of the blended role provides access to complex care while decreasing costs in a variety of ways. Complex care provided by blended role APNs improves access not only for people in urban or suburban areas but for rural populations that are currently underserved because of distance and costs. Health care economics cannot support both specialists and primary care medical providers to these areas, but blended role APNs can enhance physician practice or provide a reasonable alternative to help bridge this gap and improve access to quality care.

POPULATION TRENDS AND THEIR EFFECT ON CARE SETTINGS

Current population dynamics are driving the effort for cost containment in the health care system. The population base of the United States is changing and aging. This aging population has grown, creating the need and demand for affordable primary care and chronic disease management. Prosperity and subsequent medical advances have produced better health care, resulting in a population that is living longer with chronic disease (Lynn & Harrold, 1999). The need to keep health care costs down necessitates that these chronically ill patients be managed in outpatient rather than inpatient settings, at the same time that specialty inpatient services are being downsized or abandoned. This has resulted in the movement of specialty care to the outpatient setting.

These forces have caused a shift in the focus of care from younger people with more acute care health needs to older people with more chronic disease issues (Porter-O'Grady, 1997). Therefore, the nature of outpatient care has changed dramatically. There are more patients to be seen, they are more acutely ill, and increasing numbers are being treated for chronic disease. Additionally, patients are treated in a wide variety of settings, including hospitals, freestanding clinics, private offices, public clinics, and rural outreach clinics.

Clinically, this evolution has created new demands on the traditional APN roles of NP and CNS. The need for a provider who has both specialty nursing skills and basic primary care skills for certain populations of patients has emerged. Functionally, this APN requires skills of staff education, consultation, and leadership to assist chronically ill patients to navigate a complex care system. Increasing numbers of patients are living with multiple chronic illnesses as they age, requiring a type of provider who can bring basic primary care to a specialty setting. The blended role APN can meet this need.

MANAGED CARE AND COST CONTAINMENT

The rapid pace of change in today's health care system from an illness-driven health care industry to one emphasizing primary health care and prevention means that organizations and individuals must accommodate multiple, simultaneous changes. Cost-effective health care that prevents disease and provides quality care to those who are acutely and chronically ill is the bottom line. Reengineering, redesign, and restructuring (i.e., redefinition of roles and of work and the use of less expensive care providers) are the focus of many institutional initiatives designed to respond to these pressures. Efforts to control costs and to forge a new balance between primary care and illness services are changing the availability and types of positions in health care.

Managed care continues to be a driving force in health care. In managed care, the patient is viewed as part of the system from birth to death, moving along a continuum of health care (Mayer, 1997). Each point on the continuum represents different levels of care and cost; therefore, it is critical that the patient is matched with the right continuum point from both a quality and cost point of view. One role of each health care practitioner is to identify where her or his particular patient's problem fits most appropriately on the health care continuum, with respect to both care and cost, at any particular time in the patient's life. This system of care clearly supports the practice of the blended role APN. Blended role APNs are well suited to "match" patients to the right point on the continuum to maximize appropriate care that is cost-effective. Familiarity with both inpatient and outpatient systems allows blended role APNs to cross care settings to provide the continuity that serves as the foundation of managed care. Specialty expertise enables them to recognize critical turning points in a patient's illness course and prevent unnecessary use of health care resources through early intervention and prevention. For example, a palliative care blended role APN may recognize an ambulatory cancer patient as having abdominal pain from narcotic-related constipation and prescribe aggressive bowel management, whereas a primary care provider might assume a bowel obstruction and admit the patient as a surgical emergency.

The blended role can address many of the clinical management challenges raised by managed care systems while demonstrating cost-effectiveness. Patients get accessible, timely, and appropriate specialty medical care when necessary. Routine follow-up and symptom management is done by the blended role APN in collaborative practice with physicians. Interestingly, many of the cases that appear in the literature are not explicitly stated as being "blended practice," but in fact, on examination of education and function, these APNs may be practicing a blended role. One excellent example is the efforts by one health care system to address the costs incurred by readmission of cardiac patients to the hospital (Paladichuk, Brass-Mynderse, & Kaliangara, 1997). A clinic staffed by blended role APNs saved 160 readmissions per year across two hospitals at a cost savings of $1.2 million. They reported patients to be very satisfied and more adherent to treatment because of their ability to access blended role APNs. Another example of the potential impact of APNs (which included blended role APNs) is a study that implemented a comprehensive discharge planning and home follow-up program for hospitalized elders (Naylor et al., 1999). The gerontological specialty background of these practitioners enabled them to devise a program that reduced readmissions, lengthened the time between discharge and readmission, and decreased the costs of providing health care. At 24 weeks, the total and per-patient reimbursements for acute health services in the control group were approximately twice as much as those of the group receiving the APNs' intervention ($1,238,928 versus $642,595).

There are many specific functions (Mayer, 1997) that must occur in a cost-effective manner in managed care. The best example is care of the chronically ill. Chronic illness care is expensive. These patients require intense follow-up, and in some cases multiple hospital admissions (for an example, see George et al, 1999). In general, their experiences in the healthcare system have made these patients more sophisticated consumers. They have higher expectations of providers and health care systems with respect to continuity of care, access to health care providers, and decision-making power. The blended role APN meets the needs of these consumers by providing continuity of care for patients in need of specialized long-term follow-up and by coordinating complex services cost-effectively. Blended role practitioners can play a pivotal role in assisting the patient to navigate the health care system by providing direct care and care coordination.

Various other APN competencies are needed and valuable in managed care settings. Health maintenance organizations (HMOs) have received a great deal of attention in the press, not all of it positive (Mayer, 1997). Blended role APNs can use their consultative and educational skills in improving system problems and marketing effective programs to counter negative press and promote quality health care. The effectiveness of managed care depends, in large part, on educated consumers. Because blended role APNs have in-depth specialty knowledge and are deeply involved with individual patients across settings, they are well positioned to be highly credible to consumers. They are able to blend medical and nursing therapeutics to "bring every-thing together" in their educational activities and programs. Within managed care, blended role skills are also suited to the tasks of demand management and case management, as illustrated earlier in the acute care clinic (Paladichuk et al., 1997).

There are many roles within managed care that can be played by different kinds of providers, but the skills of blended role APNs make them well suited to provide a wide variety of functions. The blending of CNS and NP clinical, leadership, and system competencies makes this APN's marketability quite high, as predicted by Cronenwett (1995). If current health care trends continue, one would expect that the number of blended role APNs will significantly increase in the future.

THE PHYSICIAN WORKFORCE AND THE NEED FOR PRIMARY CARE PROVIDERS

Managed care is driving the medical community to re-examine physician training and workforce needs. There are greater demands for general practitioners to manage overall patient care and act as "gatekeepers" to costly specialty care. To meet this need, the Council on Graduate Medical Education has advocated a decrease in spe-cialty residency programs and a restructuring of medical training to attract more physicians to primary care. The goal for the future is to have a more even distribution of physician expertise, with 50% of physicians being generalists and 50% being specialists (Kindig, Cultice, & Mullen, 1993). This change dramatically reduces avail-able hospital resident coverage and has already left some institutions in a quandary as to how they will meet patient care needs.

Three needs can be clearly identified from this trend, each of which opens an opportunity for implementation of various APN roles. The first is for an increase in general primary care providers. These providers are the "gatekeepers" and provide primary care to a broad population. This role is well suited for the traditional primary care NP. The second need is for the provision of care on specialty inpatient units, formerly met by residents. Ideally, this need is met by the acute care NP (ACNP) if direct care is needed, or by the CNS if staff and systems issues are present. The CNS, in contrast to the ACNP, has a major focus on nursing staff support and changing staff practice while taking an active role in system changes needed as a result of the changes driven by cost containment. The last need is for coordinated and comprehensive care across primary and specialty settings. This role is uniquely suited for the blended role APN. The same emphasis on wellness and prevention found in traditional primary care settings needs to be maintained in light of populations who are living longer with complex chronic illnesses. The duality of the blended role enables the patient to be managed by a practitioner with an ability to maintain a holistic perspective while assisting in negotiating multiple life stages and chronic disease processes. The ability of blended role APNs to manage complex patients necessitates that they also be able to manage and influence the systems within which they function. The following exemplar demonstrates how the blended role APN might collaborate with other APN providers.

E X E M P L A R   1

A patient presents to her family NP (FNP) with a breast lump that she has found on her monthly breast self-exam taught to her by her FNP. On exam, the FNP finds a 3-cm hard lump. She refers the patient to a surgeon who, upon exam and biopsy, diagnoses the patient with breast cancer. The surgeon performs a lumpectomy and node dissection, whereupon he finds that 10/12 nodes are positive. The patient is referred by the surgeon to a medical oncologist and a radiation oncologist, who both initiate treatment. The patient is enrolled in a clinical trial using aggressive high-dose chemotherapy and stem cell rescue. The patient is monitored by the blended role APN, who educates her about her treatment, coordinates her initial chemotherapy in the outpatient infusion room, and communicates the plan back to the FNP. During the course of her therapy, the patient develops a fever and cough and is evaluated by the blended role APN, who realizes that the patient's illness, given her normal white count, is an acute, self-limited problem unrelated to her treatment. By exam, she diagnoses the patient with a community-acquired pneumonia and, after confirming the diagnosis with a chest x-ray, prescribes the appropriate antibiotic. The patient proceeds through her treatment regimen and contacts the blended role APN about refilling a prescription for an inhaler. The blended role APN refers the patient back to her FNP for follow-up because the treatment of her asthma is a chronic problem managed by her primary care provider and is unrelated to her cancer treatment.

   The patient then reaches the point where she begins the high-dose chemotherapy portion of her treatment. She is admitted to the oncology inpatient unit for this phase. The blended role APN contacts the ACNP on the unit to update her on the patient's progress to date. The ACNP then follows the treatment regimen planned by the medical oncologist and makes rounds on the patient daily with the attending physician covering the unit. The patient is discharged after 3 days, and the ACNP alerts the blended role APN that the patient has been discharged and will require follow-up to assess her neutropenic status and development of problematic symptoms related to her high-dose therapy. Five days later the patient calls with mouth pain and is seen by the blended role APN, who initiates first-line symptom management for mucositis. At the patient's 2-week follow-up visit, the blended role APN, in collaboration with the medical oncologist, admits the patient for worsening pain related to mucositis from her treatment. The unit's CNS is consulted to assist with pain management. The patient is managed and discharged again by the ACNP. The patient completes her treatment course with no further issues and is referred back to the FNP for primary care. She continues to see both the medical oncologist and blended role APN in follow-up on alternating visits to assess for evidence of disease progression.

   This example illustrates the need for coordinated care for patients facing complex illness. The blended role APN fills this need because these practitioners are educationally and functionally prepared to understand the intricacies of the system and the roles of other providers in both inpatient and outpatient settings. As a result, they can anticipate the need for and can provide continuity of care as the patient passes from one setting to another.

This role can also enhance job satisfaction by enabling the use of an expanded repertoire of skills. The blended role APN is able to make more of an impact on patient outcomes because long-term continuous relationships with patients across settings can be established.

PROFILE OF THE BLENDED ROLE APN

The profession's understanding of and consensus about the blended role is in active evolution. Currently, many nurses who practice this blended role may not identify it as such, and may identify themselves as either CNSs or NPs, although by education and role they function as both. Within the Oncology Nursing Society, for example, there is no specific designation for a blended role APN to be identified in their demographic database. The most accurate estimate of blended role practitioners within the specialty that could be obtained was 2,128. This number was generated by accessing those providers who identified themselves as both CNSs and NPs on the demographic portion of their membership application. Similar information was sought from the specialties of gastroenterology, pulmonary care, and critical care; however, this information was not available because it had not been collected in a way to give an estimate of blended role providers. It is very important that this role be articulated and tracked within professional organizations so that accurate numbers of blended role APNs can be followed over time.

Several key characteristics define the blended role, such as setting, education, and competencies. The competencies include both those that are core to APN practice and those that make the blended role distinct from either the NP or the CNS role.

Settings

The current health care environment has encouraged the development of both CNS and NP roles to the point where patient populations are being identified whose complex needs require an APN with dual preparation and the ability to cross settings. Blended role APNs are able to both deliver limited primary care in the specialty setting and bring specialist skills to the primary care setting. At this time, blended role APNs function primarily in outpatient specialty settings but may incorporate a component of inpatient care depending on patient care needs and institutional demands. Practice settings for blended role APNs range from hospitals to private practice, from intensive care units to the home setting, and from rural outreach clinics to tertiary care centers. Patient care needs dictate both the settings and the focus of practice. Regardless, crossing settings to provide continuity of care is a key distinguishing characteristic of the blended role APN.

The rich diversity of settings illustrates the practice demands placed on the blended role APN. Despite the challenges, many settings in which the skills of the blended role APN have positively affected patient care have been identified. Most involve complex patient populations within a specialty. For example, blended role APNs can be found staffing congestive heart failure clinics in the acute care setting (Paul, 1997), delivering comprehensive care in an outpatient oncology clinic (Jacobs & Kreamer,

1997), managing symptoms in a palliative care research program, managing complex elderly patients in a life-care community, or functioning in rural oncology outreach settings. These practice settings require both specialty knowledge gained in CNS programs and primary care skills gained in NP programs. However, when blended role APNs bring primary care skills to the specialty setting, their function as primary care providers is limited when practicing as specialists. Conversely, they may bring specialty skills to a primary care setting, but their specialty practice is limited when functioning in this setting. Functions of the blended role APN in these various settings include highly technical tasks, delivery of basic primary care and specialty care, staff education and research, and system improvements.

A wide variety of professionals collaborate with the blended role APN in these various practice settings. Allied health care professionals, physicians, patients and families, and peers all participate in the practice of the blended role APN. For example, the practitioner may consult a dietitian regarding the nutritional status of a cancer patient who is losing weight, then collaborate with a physician regarding chemotherapy for that patient's disease, participate in a family meeting with a social worker to plan the transfer home, and finally return to the clinic to examine the patient in follow-up of a pain problem. This scenario illustrates the strength of the role: an APN who has the skills to manage complex patients by providing specialty care across practice settings, thereby facilitating the patient through the health care system.

Education

A primary feature of the blended role APN is educational preparation. Theoretically, there are many ways to prepare for a blended role. Commonly, preparation generally begins with specialist training in a master's degree CNS program. Master's preparation is followed by a post-master's certificate program enhancing core CNS skills with the clinical skills of a NP. Conversely, NPs can return to graduate programs to gain CNS skills. Students can also be prepared concurrently in graduate programs as CNSs and NPs in order to practice in a blended role. The end result is a blended role APN who is able to apply these skills across care environments with a specialty patient population in collaboration with specialists in other disciplines.

Educational preparation is a cornerstone to blended role practice and identity. Several criteria should be considered when choosing programs for blended role education. The quality of faculty is critical. Instructors should be active leaders in their field and well known through presentations and publications. The availability of appropriate clinical sites is also critical. Many programs now exist that compete for clinical sites and preceptors. In addition, CNSs seeking to obtain NP certification should investigate both the quantity and nature of clinical time necessary to complete the program. The ideal program will look at students individually, identify their weaknesses, and strengthen them to fulfill a blended role. Requirements for repeating previous work and courses are not useful and are expensive, and should be approached carefully. The CNS, as an expert in a specialty, may find the transition from expert to novice in a NP program stressful (see Chapter 5 for more discussion of this phenomenon), but it enables the blended role APN to bring primary care skills to the specialty setting. Additionally, programs should be evaluated for proximity as well as cost. Lost wages for practicing nurses should be considered in factoring educational costs. Negotiation with employers to share the cost and provide time for training can be undertaken using the value-added aspects of blended practice as a rationale for funding. As new research providing outcomes data becomes available, this negotiation should become easier. Comprehensive education in research theory and implementation is critical for this role because it enhances thinking, reasoning, conceptualization, and the ability to solve problems (O'Flynn, 1996). It also enables practitioners to improve, expand, and apply research in practice as well as process data to make decisions (O'Flynn, 1996; see Chapter 9).

Continuing education for the blended role is currently a challenge. Most educational opportunities for didactic learning through conferences are targeted to either the NP or the CNS. Interestingly, however, current offerings are beginning to target blended role APNs by providing topics relevant to this APN role. For example, one general APN conference offered such topics as "Coding for Reimbursement: Are We Doing It Right?" along with "Bugs & Drugs: Antimicrobial Therapy in Primary Care." Conferences given by specialty organizations are beginning to recognize the trend as well and are providing sessions addressing blended role practice.

Core Competencies: Framework for Practice

A framework for practice of the blended role remains the biggest challenge facing these practitioners. Practice has not yet been standardized across practice settings but is currently evolving with the role. It is critical to articulate blended role practice for several reasons. First, blended role APNs have a broad range of skills. Those skills must be identified in collaborative practice to clearly define the scope of practice for the blended role APN. Second, in order to properly market themselves, both to potential employers and to the public, a framework for practice must be developed and communicated so that others can understand this role. Third, blended role APNs themselves must be educated to have an understanding of their unique role so that they identify themselves as blended role APNs and track outcomes resulting from their practice. This understanding is necessary both for present providers in outcome measurement and for future providers in education and role socialization.

Blended role APN practice exemplifies the core competencies common to APN practice, with features unique to the blended role as well. This discussion of APN competencies illustrates the common APN core competencies (see Chapter 3) as they are implemented in a blended role. The ways in which blended role practice includes elements of CNS and NP practices yet is distinct from the practice of these other APNs are also described (see Figure 16-1). As noted earlier expert specialty practice to a narrowly defined and complex patient population, crossing settings to deliver care, and dual CNS/NP educational preparation are three distinguishing characteristics of the blended role. Although the next sections describe core competencies characteristic of all APN roles, the reader can clearly see that they are operationalized in distinct ways in blended role APN practice.

EXPERT CLINICAL PRACTICE

Direct care of a narrowly defined population of complex patients is the primary component of blended role practice. Patient care is holistic and delivered by the blended role APN as an individual and/or as a member of a formal team. Tasks associated with clinical responsibility vary depending on the practice setting and specialty. Core characteristics include expert clinical reasoning and ethical decision making to provide basic wellness and preventive care, diagnosis and management

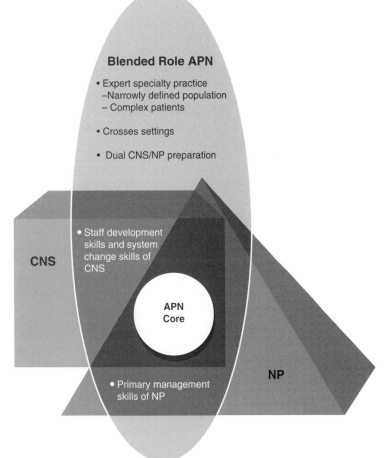

Blended Role APN

• Expert specialty practice
  – Narrowly defined population
  – Complex patients

• Crosses settings

• Dual CNS/NP preparation

CNS

• Staff development skills and system change skills of CNS

APN Core

• Primary management skills of NP

NP

FIGURE 16–1 • Conceptual model of the blended role: framework and competencies.

of illness at the level of a primary care practitioner, and management of the sequelae of chronic illnesses within specialty settings.

The blended role APN most often functions within a team to deliver care. Team members range from dyad models of physician–blended role APN in collaborative practice to group practices or hospital services. Team responsibilities may include patient rounds, case presentations at weekly team meetings, cross-coverage, and on-call duties. As integral members of health care teams, blended role APNs must delineate the expanded scope of their practice and negotiate patient coverage during off time in collaboration with peers and physician colleagues. Criteria should be agreed on to identify the inpatients and outpatients whose care will be the APN's responsibility. To avoid overextension of the APN and to enable the APN to provide the range of services that she or he can offer, a maximum caseload of patients must be determined. In addition, time and activities relating to ambulatory patient care should be stipulated. Specifically, the APN should have standard clinic schedule limitations on numbers of patients seen per clinic, guidelines for decision making, and criteria for patient phone call triage. Human and other resources, such as clinical assistants and computers to address clerical functions, need to be negotiated during the hiring process. Ignoring this aspect of providing care may mean that the APN performs these functions by default, compromising productivity and cost-effectiveness. Other personal and political consequences may ensue, such as job dissatisfaction and devaluation of APN contributions.

Emphasis on the direct care component of the blended role necessitates that a shift be made with respect to other role components to compensate for the time required to address direct patient care issues. For example, system responsibilities, including staff consultation, form a smaller component of blended role APN practice than that of the CNS role. Alternatively, there is less emphasis on the direct care component for a blended role APN than for an ACNP, because of the blended role APNs' emphasis on other role components. Within the direct care component, there is more emphasis on primary care for a primary care NP than for a blended role APN whose main focus is specialty care and secondary focus is primary care.

Ethical decision-making skills are part of the holistic approach of care provided by blended role APNs to assist patients through their illness process. One example of this is the first author's experience in a palliative care setting, helping family members make choices consistent with the patient's preferences for end-of-life care when the patient is terminally ill and not able to state those preferences. These skills may also be used on an organizational level by the blended role APN who is a member of an ethics committee to address institutional issues such as allocation of a drug in short supply.

This holistic approach to direct care is particularly well suited to the skills of blended role APNs as they assist patients in decision making; however, it can be a challenge, particularly when the patient is faced with a complex chronic illness. This challenge is compounded as patients age and face a variety of chronic illnesses to manage, as shown in the following exemplar.

EXEMPLAR 2

AB is a 79-year-old female who has Alzheimer's disease that was initially diagnosed 9 or 10 years ago when she moved into an apartment in a continuing care retirement community. She has been a resident in the health center's Alzheimer's unit for the last 3 years. Her level of dementia is considered to be moderate to severe, with language disturbance, severely impaired memory/recall, and dependence in all activities of daily living. Her days are filled with walking in the halls, singing, and occasional interchange with staff during therapeutic activities.

AB has had numerous falls without injury but, after an unwitnessed fall in the evening, was unwilling to stand and was holding onto her right hip/thigh. The registered nurse present was unable to examine the leg because of AB's agitation. The blended role APN who was on call that evening was contacted and the situation described. It seemed very likely from the description of the fall and the limited examination that AB had sustained a fracture. She had been lifted into bed and seemed comfortable if she was not moved. Knowing the risk of delirium inherent in sending a patient with dementia to the emergency department for evaluation, the blended role APN concluded that it was preferable to keep AB in familiar surroundings. Consequently, she prescribed oral medications to treat the pain and ordered an x-ray of the hip using a mobile x-ray unit in the morning. The next day, together with AB's brother, the physician, and an orthopedic consult, the blended role APN determined a course of action/plan of care. The x-ray confirmed a nondisplaced intertrochanteric fracture, and plans were made to admit AB to the acute care facility at 6 A.M. on the second day postfracture for a multiple pinning procedure, with recovery in the evening and immediate transport back to the extended care facility. The orthopedic surgeon also understood that AB would begin physical therapy immediately after surgery so that she would not experience muscular atrophy resulting from immobility and would maintain baseline cognition.

Prior to admission, the blended role APN communicated with the hospital, providing great detail about AB, her dementia, and those interventions that could be used to calm her, such as singing if she became agitated while hospitalized. It was clearly communicated that AB should not receive psychotropics and should not be restrained. AB was readmitted to the long-term care unit at 9 A.M. the morning after surgery and began touch down weight-bearing on day 2 postoperatively. The staff was supported with education regarding the orthopedic procedure done and why she would resume activity so quickly. Her baseline cognition remained unchanged, and within 3 weeks she was walking with assistance and was singing in the halls.[2]

The specialized knowledge of the geriatric CNS combined with the skills and responsibility of the NP made a difference in the specialized care needed for this woman. Continuity of care was maintained across care settings, an emergency room visit was prevented, and both patient and staff benefited from the experience.

EXPERT GUIDANCE AND COACHING OF PATIENTS, FAMILIES, AND OTHER CARE PROVIDERS

Blended role APNs, as all APNs, must be skilled educators as they fulfill a variety of educational functions. Patients and families, communities, and professionals all benefit from their guidance and coaching. Graduate training as educators gives them the skills to translate their clinical expertise into effective coaching. Specialty training enhances these skills. Because their scope of practice crosses both medicine and nursing, blended role APNs are in a strong position as educators to influence the delivery of health care by educating providers across disciplines.

The modern patient is expected to take an active role in health maintenance, and so patients must be effectively educated in order to be partners in their care. Many have subsequently become information seekers. At a time when patients now need more information, providers have less time to educate because of the reimbursement constraints imposed by the health care system. Adding to the burden, medical advances have produced a wealth of knowledge about which patients, as well as providers, need to be informed. Blended role APNs, because of their specialty knowledge and training in education, are in an excellent position to offer both individual and programmatic patient education. Training in both primary and specialty care enables them to identify the patient education needs for a defined patient population and subsequently assist in development of programs and materials. They may also function in the review of existing material for applicability and appropriateness particular to a given setting. Funding these educational programs is frequently a challenge. Familiarity with the research process enables blended role APNs to identify and act on potential sources of grant funding for such projects, while contacts made

[2] The authors gratefully acknowledge Brenda Jordan, MS, ARNP, CS, Kendall at Hanover, NH, for her assistance with this exemplar.

in the role of educator and consultant help them pursue private or corporate sources of funding.

Information seeking on the Internet is becoming an integral part of patient education today. The Internet is used by both providers and patients to identify resources, referrals, and educational material. Much of this information can be overwhelming and misleading to patients. Blended role APNs, in utilizing their research and coaching competencies, can act as resources to filter and validate much of this information while providing the expertise to explain complex information in a way that patients can understand. As APNs, they have received formal training as educators that few medical programs provide. Patient education addresses both primary care for wellness concerns and specialty issues for patients with complex illnesses. The blended role APN has the opportunity to effectively educate patients with chronic illness about both illness and wellness, at a level that the patient can understand. In addition, blended role APNs integrate teaching and coaching activities into the time they spend with patients. As pressures mount to see more patients in less time, this critical activity must be safeguarded.

Education of health care professionals is provided by blended role APNs both formally and informally. Formal education practices such as the mentoring of both graduate students and staff nurses are within the blended role scope of practice. Informal teaching and role modeling of behavior for staff nurses, home care nurses, and ambulatory care nurses makes this blended role unique. In caring for their complex specialty populations across settings, it is critical that blended role APNs communicate how to provide the best possible nursing care for individual patients to the nurses that care for those patients on a daily basis. Conducting similar activities with medical students and residents may fall informally within the scope of practice, but the practitioner must evaluate whether or not to make it a formal part of her or his practice. Blended role APNs may teach in formal educational institutions as guest lecturers or clinical instructors. They are frequently asked to assist in staff development via presentations at in-services and conferences, particularly for issues within their clinical specialty. Informally, education of peers and other providers occurs during consultation for specific patient issues as specialty knowledge is shared.

Community education is also an important point of practice for blended role APNs. Their credibility and accessibility as nurses make them ideal for educating groups and organizing specialty screening clinics and events. Their expert practice within the specialty gives them the added ability to provide direct care diagnostic services and make referrals to specialists based on the findings of the screening.

CONSULTATION

Blended role APNs may find themselves in the role of consultant, although in blended practice this activity will likely play a smaller part than for a CNS. In a review of consultation in nursing (Berragan, 1998), two trends are described, internal and external consultation. Internal consultation occurs within the context of the practitioner's role. External consultation occurs when the practitioner is an independently practicing consultant. Although prepared to do both, the blended role APN primarily functions as an internal consultant. As practitioners across health care settings, these APNs are consulted on a variety of patient and family issues. Consultation usually focuses on specific patient problems such as symptom management, but may address broader problems such as initiating and delivering palliative care. Consultation frequently occurs between blended role APNs and physicians or other nonspecialty providers over specific patient care issues with respect to diagnosis and treatment. This is in contrast to the CNS, who most frequently consults with nursing staff for nursing care or organizational issues. Opportunities for external consultation are uncommon but may occur depending on the practitioner. One example is an oncology blended role APN hired as an outside consultant to assist in the development of a chemotherapy program at a local community hospital. As with other competencies, consultation skills are integrated into practice and allow the blended role APN to take advantage of opportunities to provide support through practice-based interventions on a patient level, and future planning and development on an organizational level (Berragan, 1998). Additionally, consultation provides a rich source of professional satisfaction and credibility when the outcomes are successful.

RESEARCH SKILLS

A variety of opportunities exist for integrating research into blended role practice. Practitioners are prepared by graduate education to utilize research in clinical practice and to collaborate with researchers. One way to conceptualize this practice is to understand research competencies as involving three levels of reader, evaluator, and doer of research, as presented in Chapter 9.

Blended role APNs, along with their other APN colleagues, have an important opportunity to identify research questions directly from their clinical practice. Additionally, they collaborate both in research ventures within institutions and in large multicenter cooperative studies. As an expert clinician and trained problem solver, the blended role APN is well suited to identify research topics that investigate complex patient problems, then follow through in research utilization and dissemination. For example, many nationally developed clinical guidelines provide answers to clinical questions such as how best to manage pain or incontinence, which may take on added complexity when applied to a particular patient group. Blended role APNs are in good positions to utilize and disseminate these guidelines as they clinically manage patients whose chronic problems cross care settings. Blended role APNs can provide continuity in following through with national guidelines as the patient passes from one setting to another. For example, a blended role APN in oncology would help the staff identify a pain management plan based on the Agency for Healthcare Research and Quality guidelines for a terminal patient admitted to the hospital, then follow-up with that patient in the ambulatory setting to modify the plan as the patient's condition changes. In collaboration with staff, the blended role APN can identify areas of practice that are problematic and subsequently model evidence-based practice. As a researcher faced with a clinical question, the practitioner can locate current research to solve it or alternatively assist in development of a study to answer the question (Redekopp, 1997). Involvement in professional activities develops contacts to use as potential sources of research funding. Furthermore, the blended role APN is educationally prepared to professionally present or publish the findings in order for others to benefit from the experience.

In addition to research utilization and dissemination, the blended role APN may have the opportunity to collaborate in large organizational research efforts. As front-line providers, blended role APNs are in an excellent position to recruit patients to studies. The following exemplar illustrates the integration of research and clinical blended role practice.

EXEMPLAR 3

The Neuropathic Pain Project was initiated in the first author's institution to improve the assessment and treatment of neuropathic pain caused by chemotherapy-related nerve injury in adult lung cancer patients, beginning with the first chemotherapy cycle pain assessment and ending with pain relief or control. As a member of the project, the blended role APN helped develop and pilot an assessment and treatment algorithm for patients at high risk for developing neuropathic pain. After final implementation of the algorithm, outcome measurements are planned in the areas of cost, patient satisfaction, functional level, and clinical benefit.

Mrs. R is a 50-year-old white female with stage IIIB non–small cell lung cancer, receiving third-line chemotherapy for her disease. She presented to the oncology blended role APN with worsening tingling and pins and needles in her hands and feet. She has a 12-year history of diabetes mellitus for which she now takes insulin, although her last hemoglobin A_{1c} level was high. In performing a physical exam, the blended role APN noted that Mrs. R's cranial nerve examination was essentially normal. Motor examination revealed a weakness of the intrinsic muscles of her hands, digit extensors, and wrist extensors. In addition, there was weakness of the fifth dorsiflexors. Strength was otherwise normal. Reflexes were absent throughout. Sensory examination demonstrated loss of two-point discrimination on her fingertips, and decreased vibration in the ankles. The blended role APN, in collaboration with a physician member of the pain service, concluded that Mrs. R had sensorimotor polyneuropathy affecting the upper and lower extremities.

Utilizing her background in primary care, the blended role APN explained to Mrs. R and her husband that, although there could be a component of neuropathy related to the cisplatin that may slowly improve, the motor component was likely related to her uncontrolled diabetes mellitus. They discussed possible strategies to try to improve her neuropathy. Good control of her diabetes could help reverse some of the symptoms. The blended role APN planned to have Mrs. R document her blood glucose level on a daily basis so that they could work to control her diabetes. In addition, physical therapy and occupational therapy consults were arranged. The blended role APN planned to have Mrs. R's hemoglobin A_{1c} checked the next time she came for chemotherapy. Neurontin was prescribed at a dose of 300 mg p.o. t.i.d. for her paresthesias and dysesthesias, but when Mrs. R returned for follow-up she told the practitioner that the side effects of the drug decreased her quality of life so she stopped taking it. She was re-evaluated and started on Elavil, which was effective and well tolerated. Mrs. R was able to function at a higher level as a result of her pain control.[3]

This exemplar demonstrates two important points: the importance of active participation in research in order to utilize the findings in clinical practice, and the value of a blended role APN in a specialty setting to deliver primary care within the context of a patient's chronic illness.

The future of research by blended role APNs rests in part on these APNs contributing to the current body of nursing literature. A large amount of research by NPs in the primary care setting already exists. The profession needs literature that describes blended role APN functions in varied settings. Additionally, descriptive studies identifying various practice functions need to be published to assist other blended role APNs to develop their practice models. Subsequently, those studies need to be

[3] The authors gratefully acknowledge Louise Meyer, RN, MS, ARNP, OCN, Dartmouth Hitchcock Medical Center, for her assistance with this exemplar.

expanded to link these roles to outcomes and cost analysis. This work is critically important to successfully establish and market blended role practice.

LEADERSHIP: CLINICAL, PROFESSIONAL, AND SYSTEMS

The variety of activities fulfilled by blended role APNs gives them the broad skills necessary to be credible leaders. Leadership activities can be conducted locally, such as in organizational committees or professional groups, and leadership can also occur nationally. As noted in Chapter 10, on the national level, the blended role demands participation in shaping public policy, and this should be reflected in educational preparation (O'Flynn, 1996). Education and practice (see also Chapter 23) must impart knowledge and skill regarding the process of policy development (Milstead, 1997) in order for APNs to be effective in policy endeavors.

Diverse experiences help mold blended role APNs into expert practitioners, change agents, and negotiators who communicate effectively. They have organizational as well as patient responsibilities, depending on how they are utilized within their organization. They may be asked to provide staff development programs in their area of specialty or participate in a committee that forms practice guidelines for a particular patient population. In working with a particular population, they can identify system-atic changes that affect the care of their patients. For example, a palliative care blended role APN may identify an urgent need for designated beds within her or his institution as the population she or he works with increasingly needs inpatient placement. This need has arisen because financial concerns have forced family mem-bers to work rather than provide care at home. This blended role APN would then work at the administrative levels necessary to effect the required changes identified.

Management and negotiation of the health care delivery system is critical to success-ful implementation of the blended role. This component develops over time with practice and experience. It includes management of patient care through the health care continuum and so requires the practitioner to manage diverse systems of care in order to manage the patient. Skill at working the system is gained by utilizing familiar activities of the blended role APN: problem solving, negotiation, collaboration, and education. The complexity of the health care delivery system demands creative management approaches to patient problems, while the complexity of the modern patient demands expert clinicians. Therefore, the current challenge is management of patients with complex illnesses through health care systems in such a way as to deliver high-quality care at a lower cost while maintaining patient satisfaction (Paladichuk et al., 1997).

Utilization of leadership in the political arena enables APNs to be particularly effective in legislative advocacy and lobbying for health care reform. One way to do this is to catch the attention of legislators (Milstead, 1997) by developing connections with them, providing fact sheets, statistics, and personal vignettes. One concrete example of this was the effort by a large group of blended role APNs in the author's oncology department to write letters to their congress members to address ambulatory payment classifications (Mortenson, Edwards, & Bowers, 1998), an issue that greatly affected APN reimbursement. They were able to speak as providers of direct care who understood the complexities of the financial interests of the government, insurers, and their institution and the effect the legislation would have on their patients.

As nurses, blended role APNs are innately trusted by the public as patient advocates. As clinicians, they have the specialty expertise to identify problems, particularly related to their respective specialty, and the experience across care settings to identify creative solutions. Considerable impact on health care systems is possible if APNs utilize their skills in policy development and implementation.

COLLABORATION

Interdisciplinary care has received increased attention as a model of health care delivery in managed care systems (Simpson, 1998). Interdisciplinary care is integrated into blended role practice as demonstrated by the variety of peers and providers with whom blended role APNs interact; collaboration occurs on many levels with various providers. Collaborative efforts facilitate patients across care settings, aid in problem solving, and provide many professional opportunities. Interdisciplinary care environments open opportunities to develop true collaborative practice with physicians, because patients such as those with chronic illness are in need of integrated care from both medicine and nursing. Chapter 11 discusses the collaboration competency in detail.

The following exemplar demonstrates the integration of the collaboration and research competencies and provides a particularly successful outcome.

E X E M P L A R   4

Acute confusion in hospitalized patients was identified by the blended role APN as a problem in the first author's institution. In collaboration with CNSs who also encountered these patients, a group of APNs designed a research project to assess and address this problem. Utilization of this research plus review of other research in this area led to numerous consultations on the acute care units to identify the etiology and appropriate treatment of specific cases of acute confusion. After assessing the prevalence of the problem, the blended role APN used the information for multiple lectures to nursing staff on the care of the delirious patient both inside and outside the institution. Cases like this prompted an effort by the APN group to address the issue on an organizational level. The blended role APN contributed to the development and implementation of a nursing treatment algorithm: "Assessment and care of the confused/ agitated patient: etiologies and interventions for consideration." Implementation of the algorithm plus a collaborative research utilization project on an organizational level had a tremendous financial impact, reducing the usage and subsequent costs of "patient sitters" from $232,056 to $113,640 during a 10-month period without untoward effects on patient care.[4]

Collaboration with physicians is important in blended role practice because physicians provide medical support for the APN's clinical practice. Each provider must be supportive of the other's clinical skill while recognizing that differences in style exist. Many issues may arise in development of this collaborative practice (for an excellent example, see Hilderly, 1991). Good negotiation and communication skills are critical to work through areas that may become difficult. The issue of time is among the most problematic. Time must be negotiated between providers to maximize the potential of each professional. Negotiated time is vital for two reasons: first, when seeing a patient, both physician and blended role APN must negotiate tasks so that reimbursement is maximized for the time spent with the patient; and second, each

[4] The authors gratefully acknowledge Peggy Plunkett, MSN, ARNP, CS, Dartmouth Hitchcock Medical Center, for her assistance with this exemplar.

professional must have protected time for professional activities and development. Collaboration between providers in clinical practice is important so that tasks are not duplicated or missed. Skills in conflict resolution and communication are useful in developing and articulating clear roles. Collaborative practice is a partnership in every sense of the word, and to be successful each provider must function as two complementary parts of a whole.

Differentiating Blended Role Practice from Other APN Roles

What differentiates blended role practice from other APN roles? Three characteristics distinguish the blended role APN, as noted in Figure 16-1. First, blended role APNs are educationally prepared differently than other practitioners, because they learn both CNS and NP roles and expectations. Second, because of this preparation, blended role clinical practice differs from that of both CNS and NP in that the blended role APN crosses settings while clinically managing specialty populations. These two characteristics have created the third, in that the blended role APN cares for a more narrowly defined complex patient population than other APNs. This narrow focus is necessary to enable staff education and support and system change activities characteristic of the blended role. Incorporating all of the competencies described previously with these characterisitcs means that blended role APNs are continually challenged by issues of balance and emphasis of role components in their practice. Individual blended role APNs must be clear on their role and scope of practice in order to continue to meet patient needs and to avoid becoming subject to the restructuring of positions as institutions struggle with a dynamic health care system.

EDUCATIONAL PREPARATION

Educational preparation of blended role APNs is fundamentally different from that of other practitioners, as described earlier. The educational goal for the blended role APN is to prepare a practitioner who can deliver basic primary care within a specialty setting, have the expertise to manage clinically complex populations across settings and effectively influence systems of care in order to facilitate the management of these populations, and encourage staff development within her or his area of expertise. Currently, practitioners most frequently enter the process already prepared as CNSs. Subsequently, they complete a post-master's NP certificate program in family, adult, or pediatric medicine to enhance clinical skills of assessment, diagnosis, and treatment of primary care illness and reinforce basic prevention and wellness concepts.

ROLE IMPLEMENTATION IN PRACTICE

It is challenging to clarify the role differences between NP, CNS, and blended role APN. One particular primary care setting was described by a critical care CNS who became a FNP:

> *Without my knowledge of secondary care, hospital practice . . . it would be very difficult and uncomfortable [practicing in my new primary care role]. Additionally, it was quite helpful when two [patients with] acute myocardial infarctions, two hemorrhages, and one case of acute, severe respiratory distress presented in the office during my first seven months of practice. . . .*

the most frequent questions asked me [by patients] had to do with my experiences in critical care, cardiology, and trauma. Few questions were asked about my family practice experience. This seemed a little odd at first. However, the reason for the interest in secondary care experience soon became clear. Many patients in our practice have chronic disease like chronic obstructive pulmonary disease, coronary artery disease, and congestive heart failure that require hospitalization at times. They wanted to make sure I knew what to do when [it was my turn to make] rounds.

(Crotty, 1998, pp. 19–20)

This FNP, although utilizing CNS specialty knowledge in this setting, is not practicing in a blended role because he is functioning as a primary care clinician. The distinction is that the blended role APN utilizes the NP role and all dimensions of the CNS role in a specialty setting. Various examples of blended role practice are beginning to appear in the literature, such as an outpatient congestive heart failure clinic implemented by a blended role APN (Paul, 1997). This APN described clinical responsibility for this specialty population across settings, the educational role with patients and families, and the research role of evaluating clinical outcomes.

BALANCE AND ROLE DIFFERENTIATION

The true blended role APN has responsibility for executing traditional CNS subroles in addition to the focus on primary care in a specialty setting. There are CNSs and NPs currently in practice who identify their role as blended but who may not practice in a true blended role because their role has not fully developed balance. For example, the blended role APN's scope of clinical practice differs from the ACNP's scope in the amount of outpatient follow-up that is incorporated into clinical responsibilities as well as the CNS activities of staff support and systems change. Unlike the ACNP, who is responsible for a variety of acutely or critically ill patients and for limited ambulatory care activities (if any), the blended role APN is responsible for ongoing follow-up of a particular patient population across settings. The blended role APN has a greater focus on primary care than does the ACNP. The blended role is defined by this clinical focus. This difference in focus is illustrated by a descriptive report of the ACNP role (Kleinpell, 1998) in which mean time spent in the clinical practice component was reported to be 89%. Other activities played a much smaller part in ACNP practice: teaching, 13%; research, 11%; and staff education, 1%. In contrast, the CNS is prepared for a different role as educator, consultant, and researcher with a limited direct care clinical role. These roles are different yet complementary. The blended role APN is distinguished from the CNS who completes a certificate NP program but returns to her or his current position functioning strictly as a CNS without an expanded focus on direct and primary care. One example is presented in the literature of a NP and a CNS who worked collaboratively in building a pediatric diabetes program (Page & Mackowiak, 1997). They each needed a part of the other's role to meet the needs of their population.

The blended role APN differs the most from the APN case manager. Both are educationally prepared for the role of primary coordinator of care by virtue of their master's degrees and share some role overlap (Papenhausen, 1990). The APN case manager is accountable for clinical and fiscal outcomes; the blended role APN cannot afford to be oblivious to fiscal outcomes, but primary responsibility will fall to someone else. With APN case managers, there is greater emphasis on organization, coordination, and monitoring of patient care (Smith, 1994) and on system-level interventions to enhance quality of care and contain costs. The most notable difference in practice is evident in the level of direct tertiary clinical management of patients. Most APN case management models (Schroer, 1991) include elements of direct patient assessment and clinical decision making in ambulatory care settings but end there. Although APN case managers closely follow established patients when they are admitted to the hospital, they typically relinquish direct patient management to the hospital-based team.

ISSUES IN IMPLEMENTATION OF THE BLENDED ROLE

Many issues are raised in blending the CNS and NP roles that, if unaddressed, will create confusion both inside and outside the profession. To make sense of this confusion regarding APN roles, it is critical to focus on the "role" and not on the job title (Ackerman, 1997) because focus on the title leads to confusion. The blended "role" is relatively new, so the degree of clarity that facilitates a consensus as to titling does not yet exist. This lack of clarity in the blended role is the first hurdle to overcome to strengthen its implementation in practice. Examining the advantages and disadvantages to blending from the perspective of a variety of stakeholders can help address issues of role development and identity. Blending the CNS and NP roles affects not only individual practitioners but the disciplines of both medicine and nursing. In addition, examination of the issue from a broader perspective reveals that health care consumers have a stake in how this role evolves, and indeed may affect future role implementation.

Titling

Difficulties with APN titling (Fitzpatrick, 1998) and a summary of efforts to build consensus around the meaning of advanced nursing practice (see Chapter 3) have been described. However, it must be acknowledged that, if and when the term "advanced practice nurse" is accepted by the profession and policy makers embracing a variety of APN positions, the issue of titling the blended role APN will remain difficult. Spross and Hamric (1983) proposed the ARNP title for the role described in this chapter. Since that time, the ARNP title has been increasingly used in state regulations to refer to the NP. Consequently, it has significant problems as a title that would readily convey that the APN possesses blended role skills. The blended role is an APN role that is in need of a clear title in order to articulate the uniqueness of the role to both professionals and the public.

One review of the advanced practice literature suggests designating blended role APNs as advanced NPs (Dunn, 1997). This idea has merit because it could distinguish the blended role from both the CNS and NP roles through the designation "advanced," or through naming the specialty, such as oncology NP. An example of how this might work is provided by the psychiatric nursing specialty. In 1994, the American Nurses Association (ANA) and other organizations wrote a practice statement that made the psychiatric CNS eligible for NP certification and titling as a psychiatric NP (Caverly, 1996). This is not necessarily a blended role, but it does highlight the specialty skills of the APN. The difficulty with this title is the absence of any explicit CNS designation.

Some leaders have advocated using the generic title of APN for the blended role (Snyder & Mirr, 1995). This stance supports the merging of CNS and NP roles into one APN role. Combining the skills and competencies of the CNS and NP has been the focus of this chapter and is an important trend in the continuing evolution of advanced nursing practice. However, the title APN is more appropriately used as an umbrella term to describe all APN roles, including CNS, certified nurse-midwife, certified registered nurse anesthetist, NP, ACNP, APN case manager, and the blended CNS/NP role (see Chapter 3). Titles should reflect the actual practice and should be unique if the practice is unique. Because the blended role APN is a distinct APN role, it needs a distinct title.

This leaves the possibilities of "blended role APN" or "CNS/NP". In practice, the first author uses NP when introducing herself to clients because the public is more likely to be familiar with this term. When interacting with other health care professionals, this author endeavors to explain and clarify the blended role by explaining the similarities and differences between her practice and the practices of CNSs and NPs. In professional identification, this author and most of her departmental colleagues use the credentials "MSN, ARNP" (New Hampshire's regulatory designation for the adult NP) to designate a blended role. The alternative title of CNS/NP has not been widely explored, nor has it been used often in the literature. This possibility deserves to be considered, because it explicitly denotes both CNS and NP roles merged into one practice. However, this option may be viewed as cumbersome and confusing to consumers. As the blended role is becoming more clearly definable as a distinct APN role, this lack of a consensus title represents an increasing problem in marketing. As noted, examples of blended role practice were found with authors referring to themselves as NPs, or just APNs. Nursing leaders, including those in practice and in education, need to come to consensus on the title and preparation for the blended role APN if it is to become a fully legitimate APN role.

Impact of Blending the NP and CNS Roles

The impact of blending, both positive and negative, is felt not only by CNSs and NPs but by the nursing profession as a whole. Many advantages to blending CNS and NP roles exist for nursing. Identifying a blended role can create a stronger professional affiliation by decreasing role confusion among APNs within diverse settings. Clarification of a blended role opens up a number of different role opportunities to explore and expand to fulfill a variety of health care needs. In addition, blended role practice can create a forum for these APNs to participate in nursing research and education addressing complex patient problems and systems. Blended role APNs can focus on topics that explore how attention to basic primary care in the context of chronic illness improves the quality of life for chronically ill patients. Intensive and ongoing education of this population is critical to successful clinical management. Blended role APNs bring their unique perspective to develop programs that meet the educational needs of these patients. Furthermore, this perspective can be applied to increase political power from which to successfully lobby for such things as prescription of specialty restricted drugs. Political power can also be utilized to increase reimbursement potential and strengthen nursing's financial foundation. The Balanced Budget Act (BBA) of 1997 put the CNS on equal footing with the NP with respect to billing for the Medicare program. CNSs can now participate in Medicare as do NPs and bill the program directly for their services. Unfortunately, the BBA did not address any other payer, such as Medicaid. Each Medicaid program and each commercial insurer can set its own rules, and many do not "recognize" the CNS as independent for billing purposes. Blended role APNs can use their ability to bill various payers to lobby for needed resources for their patient populations.

There are few disadvantages to the nursing profession for a blended role, but they are important to consider. Both CNSs and NPs come with special skills and role identity developed through education, experience, and socialization. Therefore, both will need to recreate a new identity as blended role APNs (K. B. Wright, 1997). This may present a challenge as the role itself evolves. Role identification and clarification require both a degree of tolerance for ambiguity and the determination to define a new role. In the quest to define this role, CNS/NPs must be careful to maintain their nursing focus. Blended role APNs frequently work within a medical model in collaborative practice with physicians. It would be easy to adopt a medical model, but the greatest strength of the role is the nursing focus that it brings to health care. One example of this concept is an effort by one specialty department to encourage blended role APNs to cover an inpatient unit using a model similar to the monthly physician rotation. This model had been identified as a frequent source of complaints by patients, who sought more continuity in inpatient care. The group, recognizing the discontinuity, is currently designing an alternative plan to provide an ACNP position to address this situation. The power of a nursing focus in bringing CNS and NP skills to address a problem enables the blended role APN to augment and complement the care delivered by a physician rather than be a physician extender.

There are many issues to consider specific to CNSs. Historically, their clinical expertise has been limited to the inpatient setting, where the critical roles of educator, consultant, and researcher have been relatively "invisible" both publicly and politically. The public sees the benefits of these efforts, but rarely sees the individual responsible for them. Their interaction with a CNS is generally limited to management of a clinical issue in the inpatient setting. In response to a need for specialty nursing care in the outpatient setting, some CNSs have developed a practice in the outpatient setting. The public may have more contact with the few CNSs who work in collaborative practices, but the limitations of lack of prescriptive privileges and inability to provide overall clinical management frequently are difficult to overcome. One clear advantage for CNSs to developing a blended CNS/NP practice is increased public acceptance and visibility for the CNS (Knutson, 1991) component. Blending the roles helps CNSs address many of these issues while expanding their scope of APN practice across settings. In contrast to the outpatient setting, one result of blending in the inpatient setting is a trend toward requiring additional CNSs dedicated to staff support, as blended role providers primarily move across settings. Blended role providers spend significant time with outpatients and so are limited in the amount of time they have to support staff because they are more involved in direct care. It is critical for institutions to recognize this; otherwise the gains made in improving the care of chronically ill patients by blended role APNs will be offset by patient readmissions caused by a lack of staff education, increased staff turnover, and/or poor nursing care resulting from lack of support by a CNS (Page & Arena, 1994). Therefore, the development of the blended role must progress with concurrent support of CNS positions. Alternatively, Shuren (1996) suggested that her outpatient activities enabled her to identify and resolve a problem with inpatient staff's patient education practices.

Several issues of particular concern to NPs have been identified in the past (K. B. Wright, 1997), but few are currently relevant. NPs stand to strengthen their credibility with the specialty focus brought by the CNS role. In addition, having been accused of losing their nursing roots by training within a medical model, blending strengthens their alliance with the nursing profession. One real concern should focus on the inevitable time when NPs and blended role APNs both become increasingly subject to the demands of the system to see more patients in less time, as is currently experienced by physicians. This needs to be addressed by NPs and blended role APNs on both an institutional and a national level to advocate that critical nursing functions remain a part of patient care. Research documenting outcomes of successful educational programs will assist in this effort (see George et al, 1999).

The blended CNS/NP role clearly affects physicians. Within primary care, the blended role APN can strengthen what the primary care physician presently has to offer. For example, the first author, as an oncology CNS, completed a clinical rotation with a primary care physician for her NP program. She was able to help educate that physician, also a new hospice director, about current pain management strategies. The blended role APN prepared in a specialty can extend the ability of a primary care practitioner to manage a wide range of chronic illnesses and the symptoms resulting from those illnesses. Alternatively, blended role APNs can ensure that primary care issues are addressed and appropriately managed in the specialty setting. Even though a medical specialist does not have primary care training, patients seen on a frequent basis use their physician specialist as a primary care practitioner (Rosenblatt, Hart, Baldwin, Chan, & Schneeweiss, 1998). In the study by Rosenblatt and colleagues (1998), pulmonologists, oncologists, and gynecologists each had a substantial proportion of patients—27%, 21%, and 20%, respectively—for whom they provided care outside their specialty domain. In general, specialists provided out-of-domain care to patients with whom they had a majority-of-care relationship. This intuitively makes sense and points to a system of care that has not been explicitly addressed. Patients whose care is usually delivered by a specialist do not want to make another trip to a generalist if the specialist is willing to take care of their primary care problem. An example of the blended role APN improving care in the first author's institution is an oncology APN who performs routine Pap smears on patients seen by the oncologist with whom she collaborates. This phenomenon is seldom acknowledged but is a reality of the current system. Blended role APNs are able to address this reality in a competent and efficient way by providing primary care in specialty settings. Over time, the blended role provider could potentially become the provider of record for selected chronically ill populations. This system would maintain continuity of care focused on both specialty and primary care needs of the chronically ill patient. It is a value-added role for systems with potential improvements in patient satisfaction, adherence to therapy, and improved health maintenance. These outcomes should be studied in settings where blended role APNs practice.

The blended role can be perceived to have both negative and positive effects on the medical profession. Physicians have expressed a perceived loss of identity; if blended role APNs can do the tasks of a physician, then what is left for that physician to do? This can lead to the perception of being threatened and can result in conflict over issues related to competition. In response to this concern, it is important to note that clear role limitations have been established by state nurse practice acts as to what is and is not within nursing's scope of practice. In addition, the blended role APN's ability to function is different when doing primary care versus specialty care. For example, blended role APNs licensed to function as primary care NPs can diagnose and treat primary care problems in the specialty setting. However, they are not licensed to diagnose and treat a disease within the specialty. This limits their practice within specialty settings and therefore should reduce any perception of competition with physicians. Finally, there are role limitations dictated by the credentialing and privileging system within many institutions. Within specialty practice, these role limitations must be maintained because nurses are not physicians and there are certain tasks that may not be within the scope of blended role nursing practice. These tasks may need to be formally defined for each specialty (e.g., the ACNP may perform more medical procedures), but at the present time they are negotiated by each practitioner within the existing institution's privileging policy. The blended role APN, by definition more limited in specialty practice, can participate in that portion of patient care that is within her or his scope of practice, providing advanced nursing care (e.g., managing pain medication in terminal stages of cancer) and freeing the physician specialist to be a specialist. This can provide both practitioners with time to keep current and pursue professional interests.

The Blended Role—Mixing versus Matching of the CNS and NP

The debate continues: Why blend the CNS and NP roles? The answer to this question lies both in the present needs of patients with complex problems and the demands of the evolving health care system, and in how the profession chooses to shape the future of advanced nursing practice.

Cronenwett (1995) pointed out the lack of clarity among current roles. The ANA's *Nursing's Social Policy Statement* suggested describing advanced practice in terms of specialization, expansion, and advancement, rather than roles (ANA, 1996; Cronenwett, 1995; see Chapter 3). Alternatively, clearly defined roles continue to be needed for the pure NP and CNS (see Chapters 13 through 15). However, in the current health care system, the difficulty at times lies in attempting to match either CNS or NP to positions that may require the skill of both roles. Many of these skills can be acquired on the job, but this assumes competent preceptorship with collaborating practitioners who may or may not have the time to adequately impart those skills. A CNS functioning in a pulmonary clinic is an expert in pulmonary care, but may lack the primary care skills to ensure comprehensive care. Similarly, a NP in the same setting may have the skills to provide good primary care but would require years of on-the-job training to function on the level of a CNS specialized in pulmonary care. The health care system can no longer pay for the time required for those practitioners to acquire skills they lack. It is becoming increasingly evident that both expert clinical skills of the NP and interpersonal, collaborative, research, and leadership skills of the CNS are needed to manage certain complex patients in today's dynamic health care system (K. B. Wright, 1997). This system has produced advanced technology that requires more specialized training and education to provide complete care. Both primary treatment and symptom management have increased in complexity. It is important to note that not all complex patients need a blended role APN. They may be better served by an APN case manager or CNS. The issue of which provider is appropriate depends on the source of the patient's complexity. However, certain complex patients may need a blended role APN to deliver specialty primary care across settings.

This point is illustrated in the literature by the account of a CNS who had used CNS-specific skills to initiate and maintain a chronic disease clinic (Paladichuk et al., 1997) but found she could not practice independently in diagnosis and treatment and so returned to a NP program to gain those skills. The niche for the blended role may in fact lie with chronic disease management, where the combined skills of the blended role APN are critical to ensure holistic care and state-of-the-art symptom management for patients facing longer lives with chronic disease.

Duality and Accountability

Implementation of the blended APN role is a challenge. The practitioner faces a variety of issues that need to be addressed to be successful. Confrontation of the role's duality is the first issue to address because it illustrates many challenges. Duality creates the biggest challenge in meeting the demands of diverse role activities in a blended role position. Although diversity is a central component of role success, excellent time management skills are required to balance the demands that this diversity creates.

By definition the blended role APN is both CNS and NP. Therefore, to whom is the blended role APN accountable? Various possibilities should be thoroughly considered when implementing this role. Historically, the CNS has been accountable to nursing, and this is a strong reason to implement the blended role position under the direction of nursing. Those functions of educator, consultant, and researcher are likely to be most utilized by nursing. However, the clinical component of the position may be more logically aligned with medicine. Collaborative practice models and many NP positions are often structured with accountability to medicine. In addition, it can be argued that medicine has the most to learn about advanced practice nursing from the blended role APN, and so greater impact on the system can be made by accountability to medicine. There is no one correct answer for this question. Each practitioner must use her or his negotiation skills to establish an appropriate route of accountability for a given position and setting. It is critical, however, that the accountability structure supports a balanced practice so that both CNS and NP components are visible. Developing interdisciplinary and intradisciplinary relationships and lines of support are also critical to role success.

Evaluation of Blended Role Practice

Accountability raises the issue of practice evaluation. When implementing the blended APN role, evaluation is necessary for financial justification of the position and future role development. Cost analysis should focus not only on dollars saved by virtue of having a blended role APN but on clinical outcomes, so that value can be demonstrated. Nurses must support their practice by aggressive use of computer technology to track data in local and national databases to demonstrate accountability for their outcomes (see Chapter 25). A lack of specific historical measures upon which to base blended role practice evaluation has slowed research for the blended role; such measures are important to provide validity and illustrate the value of the role to health care institutions.

The first step is development of a valid and reliable tool that can be used in a variety of settings. Many tools exist to standardize health care data collection, such as the Uniform Needs Assessment Instrument (UNAI) for posthospital discharge, the IMSystem, the Minimum Data Set (MDS) for nursing facility resident assessment and care screening, and the Nursing Minimum Data Set (NMDS) (Carroll & Fay, 1997). None of these tools currently captures the blended role, but each may contain useful outcome markers that can help develop patient outcomes to demonstrate the impact of blended role practice. Byers and Brunell (1998) proposed using Donabedian's model (see Chapter 25) together with the common understanding that value is equal to quality divided by cost. In evaluation of quality, the structure and process of care delivery are evaluated along with the impact of care on objective and perceived outcomes. This model would help support the role of the CNS/NP because it captures many different aspects of care, both direct and indirect. Consultation with outcome managers (Fleschler & Luquire, 1998) in hospital quality improvement departments and outcome management programs can help the blended role APN address such issues as when to measure an outcome, to what level of analysis the research should be taken, and how to achieve appropriate scientific rigor (Carroll & Fay, 1997) for what is being studied. In order to conduct complete outcome studies, the issue of admission privileges for blended role APNs must be addressed. For example, tracking admission and readmission rates could be very useful for evaluating a practitioner's ability to clinically manage a patient population across settings over time. However, because admission privileges are restricted, most likely by state or institutional policy that restricts scope of practice (Kinney, Hawkins, & Hudman, 1997), admission rates cannot be accurately determined. Measured outcomes would likely be improved by improving continuity of care through blended role practice, but it is exceedingly difficult to conduct outcome studies when one cannot measure the admission rates for blended role APNs because they cannot directly admit patients.

It is clear that comprehensive practice evaluation must be a priority among APNs (Byers & Brunell, 1998) in order to describe their role and measure their practice. Performance measures specific for blended role APNs must be developed. Efforts have begun for other nursing roles (Herman, 1998; Irvine, Sidani, & McGillis-Hall, 1998), including NP and CNS roles, that can be adapted to create models for blended role performance measures. Measures such as the Health Plan Employer Data and Information Set (HEDIS), which measure performance, are useful as tools both to address liability issues and to demonstrate a blended role APN's impact on quality care (these issues are discussed more extensively in Chapter 25).

Potential Problems in Role Development

Specific challenges can be identified in development of the blended role. The challenge of role strain is of most concern. An important question to ask is, is the blended role APN trying to be everything to everyone? The NP and CNS roles are each valuable roles in themselves. The blended role APN must give up a piece of each of these roles in the blending process in order to be successful. The risk for role strain leading to burnout is a serious one. APNs who try to be everything to everyone will soon find themselves with more responsibility than can be handled. They run the risk of doing an inferior job with too broad a scope of practice rather than doing a good job with a limited scope of practice. These risks are analogous to those experienced by CNSs in the 1980s (Hamric, 1989).

One example of how this issue arises is in the performance of medical procedures such as a lumbar puncture, paracentesis, or special surgical technique. When evaluating whether or not to include either a medical task or any other responsibility into blended role practice, the provider must decide whether doing the task will meet the ultimate goal of quality patient care. Several strategies may be utilized in this evaluation process. How much time will be spent doing the task versus how much will it benefit the specific patient population? What aspect of practice will the provider have to give up to make room for the added responsibility? What is the risk-benefit ratio of the task for the provider and/or the patient? What are the political ramifications of agreeing or declining the responsibility? Is the task within the state's nurse practice act, and is it legal? Is the task nursing or medical, and is this issue important? Will adequate training be provided to take on this new task or responsibility? Investigation of these questions can be used to clarify limits on practice that are consistent with meeting the needs of both patients and institution.

Another challenge to blended role providers is educational preparation and continuing education (Conger & Craig, 1998). Graduate programs that plan to offer a combined CNS/NP blended role curriculum will likely have to incorporate a year of extra education and increased clinical hours unless a very well-integrated and well-defined program is developed. Generic programs that do not prepare students for specific CNS and NP competencies needed for blended role practice are doing their students a disservice. This difficulty also raises the issue of continuing education. The practitioner must take responsibility to maintain continuing education in both traditional specialty and primary care practices. This can be a challenge but should become easier as more blended role APNs are educated and begin practicing. Continuing education is also an issue facing physician specialists. The amount of new information to process in order to keep current in their profession is getting beyond the ability of the specialists to manage, particularly within the current health care system. The value of a blended role APN in this context is in augmenting the practice of the physician specialist, leaving time for both to pursue appropriate continuing education. One strategy to successfully define a realistic practice is to negotiate regular protected time for professional activities, particularly those of education and research. This may be difficult to do, and is most successful when negotiated at the time of hire.

Keys to Successful Role Development

Keys to success in development of the advanced practice nursing role, outlined by Brown (1998), can be applied specifically to the blended role. First, a clear scope of practice mutually agreed upon in a collaborative practice is critical to function efficiently and avoid turf issues. Second, there must be consensus regarding scheduling and workload. This consensus must be negotiated at the time the provider is hired and should be formally reviewed on a regular basis. Third, organizational support for the role must exist. The organization must value the blended role APN and provide support for a balanced role. Finally, interdisciplinary networks for collaboration, consultation, and referral should be available for the practitioner to be most effective. These networks may not exist in some settings but can be made available through Internet access and formal organizational affiliations for the blended role APN to create a network.

One priceless asset in development of the successful blended role is peer support. Peer support is critical to assist in problem solving, provide support, and collaborate in outcomes research. The blended role is among the newest APN roles to be developed. Therefore, it is critically important that opportunities for sharing issues regarding development and implementation of the role are provided in order to facilitate problem solving. A setting without multiple peers is common, but developing a regional peer network through on-line discussions, formal meetings, and informal consultation should be integral to the practice of any blended role APN.

Successful development depends on two concepts. First, the diversity of skills defined by each role (Jacobs & Kreamer, 1997) is critical to successful implementation of the role. Second, successful time management is critical to both professional success and personal satisfaction. As noted, success in the blended role requires balance and time management. Core preparation involves graduate education to provide competency as a NP and clinical expertise as a CNS. Balance in this role may be difficult to achieve, but the balanced practice as described earlier must be maintained. This necessitates considerable skill at negotiation and time management for these APNs. Negotiation with administrators and colleagues to balance activities such as patient care, research, patient and staff education, and improving system practices is critical. The goal is to avoid excessive emphasis on any one activity, and this presents a challenge, particularly because the clinical component generates revenue. However, a balance must be created in order to successfully maintain the diversity that the blended role offers. Bringing such a diverse set of skills to the health care setting challenges the blended role APN to manage many competing priorities.

The value of the blended role is in the ability of these practitioners to fulfill a variety of functions. They are ''value added'' because they bring primary care skills to the specialty setting. The specialty practice of the CNS is necessary to understand the chronic illness, as well as its impact on the patient and on society, and to act in proactive ways to improve care within systems and across settings. The primary care training of the NP facilitates the delivery of primary care within the specialty and enables the practitioner to maintain continuity in delivering comprehensive care. Blended role practice is beyond the limitations of either of the original roles. The impact of blended role APN care on the health care system can be measured by examining the outcomes of blended role practice. Initial research supports the validity of this role (Naylor et al., 1999), as described earlier, but future studies need to focus on outcomes related to a variety of practice settings.

CONCLUSION

The journey to the blended APN role can be long and painful. Discarding a former role socialization in favor of a new one can be uncomfortable, and transitioning from expert to novice to expert can be frustrating. New models of education will be needed for this role to develop to its full potential. Ultimately, the quality of the APN depends on the quality of mentoring, preceptorship, and role modeling that occurs in education and in practice (O'Flynn, 1996). Therefore, it is critical that practitioners of the blended role identify themselves as such, so that they can be available to APNs and students interested in blended role practice. ''For APNs who embrace change, there are unlimited opportunities to actively participate in the redefinition of health care, the transformation of practice settings, and the creation of provider roles'' (O'Malley & Cummings, 1995, p. 6).

Despite demands by the health care system, nursing as a profession must maintain control over the development of the blended role. The risk of losing control over development is to lose the diverse components of the role that are not billable but that make the role valuable to many settings. The role cannot be driven by medicine or by the need for providers (Deane, 1997), and it must not be driven by adjustment to a medical gap or surplus (K. B. Wright, 1997). Development must also not be driven by outside forces that may seek to diminish the ability of APNs to coalesce into a political force, which is necessary to change restrictive state statutes (Caverly,

1996). Instead, the role must be driven by the need for quality patient-centered care delivered by nurses who bring a wide variety of special skills to patients across settings. As leaders and change agents, blended role APNs may face criticism, but they must maintain these characteristics in order to improve patient care and move the profession of nursing forward.

On a societal level, patient satisfaction and quality improvement are becoming increasingly important goals in a competitive health care market. As consumers, patients are demanding high-quality care while, as taxpayers, those patients are demanding lower costs. In order to thrive, nursing must adjust to these trends. The blended role APN is one such promising adjustment.

It can no longer be adequate to react or to respond too late in the cycle of change. No longer can the APN (the nurse practitioner and clinical specialist) of the past be configured or prepared in the same way for the future. Clearly, for the APN, integrating many of the characteristics of both nurse practitioner and clinical specialist will be required to create an effective, meaningful role for the nurse in advanced practice.

(Porter-O'Grady, 1997, p. 10).

The "effective meaningful role" of the blended role APN has evolved to augment the ranks of NP and CNS to meet the needs of specialty populations who require complex coordinated care in a dynamic health care system.

REFERENCES

Ackerman, M. H. (1997). The acute care nurse practitioner: Evolution of the clinical nurse specialist? *Heart & Lung, 26*(2), 85–86.

American Nurses Association. (1996). *Nursing's social policy statement.* Washington, DC: Author.

Beecroft, P. C. (1994). CNS: Thriving or heading for extinction? *Clinical Nurse Specialist, 8*(2), 63.

Berragan, L. (1998). Consultancy in nursing: Roles and opportunities. *Journal of Clinical Nursing, 7*(2), 139–143.

Brooten, D., Genaro, S., Knapp, H., Jovene, N., Brown, L., & York, R. (1991). Functions of the CNS in early discharge and home follow-up of very low birthweight infants. *Clinical Nurse Specialist, 5*(4), 196–201.

Brown, S. J. (1998). A framework for advanced practice nursing. *Journal of Professional Nursing, 12*(3), 117–120.

Byers, J. F., & Brunell, M. L. (1998). Demonstrating the value of the advanced practice nurse: An evaluation model. *AACN Clinical Issues, 9*(2), 296–305.

Carroll, T. L., & Fay, V. P. (1997). Measuring the impact of advanced practice nursing on achieving cost-quality outcomes: Issues and challenges. *Nursing Administration Quarterly, 21*(4), 32–40.

Caverly, S. (1996). The role of the psychiatric nurse practitioner. *Nursing Clinics of North America, 31*(3), 449–463.

Conger, M., & Craig, C. (1998). Advanced nurse practice: A model for collaboration. *Nursing Case Management, 3*(3), 120–127.

Cooper, D. (1990). Today—assessments and intuitions: Tomorrow—projections. In P. S. Sparacino, D. M. Cooper, & P. A. Minarik (Eds.), *The clinical nurse specialist: Implementation and impact* (pp. 285–311). Norwalk, CT: Appleton & Lange.

Cronenwett, L. R. (1995). Modeling the future of advanced practice nursing. *Nursing Outlook, 43,* 112–118.

Crotty, G. (1998, April). Clinical nurse specialist to nurse practitioner: Personal observations. *Tennessee Nurse,* pp. 19–20.

Dale, J. C. (1991). New role for pediatric nurse practitioners in an in-patient setting. *Journal of Pediatric Health Care, 5*(6), 336–337.

Damato, E. G., Dill, P. Z., Gennaro, S., Brown, L. P., York, R., & Brooten, D. (1993). The association between CNS direct care time and total time and very low birth weight infant outcomes. *Clinical Nurse Specialist, 7*(2), 75–79.

Davitt, P., & Jensen, L. (1981). The role of the acute care nurse practitioner in cardiac surgery. *Nursing Administration Quarterly, 3,* 16–19.

Deane, K. A. (1997). CNS and NP: Should the roles be merged? *Canadian Nurse, 93*(6), 24-30.

Dunn, L. (1997). A literature review of advanced clinical nursing practice in the United States of America. *Journal of Advanced Nursing, 25*(4), 814-819.

Elder, R. G., & Bullough, B. (1990). Nurse practitioners and clinical nurse specialists: Are the roles merging? *Clinical Nurse Specialist, 4*(2), 78-84.

Fenton, M. V., & Brykczynski, K. A. (1993). Qualitative distinctions and similarities in the practice of clinical nurse specialists and nurse practitioners. *Journal of Professional Nursing, 9*(6), 313-326.

Fitzpatrick, E. R. (1998). Analysis and synthesis of the role of the advanced practice nurse. *Clinical Nurse Specialist, 12*(3), 106-107.

Fleschler, R., & Luquire, R. (1998). Advanced practice role of the outcomes manager. *Outcomes Management for Nursing Practice, 2*(2), 54-56.

Forbes, K. E., Rafson, J., Spross, J. A., & Kozlowski, D. (1990). The clinical nurse specialist and nurse practitioner: Core curriculum survey results. *Clinical Nurse Specialist, 4*(2), 63-66.

George, M. R., O'Dowd, L. C., Martin, I., Lindell, K. O., Whitney, F., Jones, M., Ramondo, T., Walsh, L., Grissinger, J., Hansen-Flashen, J., & Pennettieri, R. A. (1999). A comprehensive educational program improves clinical outcome measures in inner-city patients with asthma. *Archives of Internal Medicine, 159,* 1710-1716.

Gleeson, R. M., McIlvain-Simpson, G., Boos, M. L., Sweet, E., Trzcinski, K. M., Solberg, C. A., & Doughty, R. A. (1990). Advanced practice nursing: A model of collaborative care. *MCN, 15*(1), 9-12.

Hamric, A. B. (1989). History and overview of the CNS role. In A. B. Hamric & J. A. Spross (Eds.), *The clinical nurse specialist in theory and practice* (2nd ed., pp. 3-18). Philadelphia: W. B. Saunders.

Hamric, A. B. (1996). A definition of advanced nursing practice. In A. B. Hamric, J. A. Spross, & C. M. Hanson (Eds.), *Advanced nursing practice: An integrative approach* (pp. 42-56). Philadelphia: W. B. Saunders.

Hanson, C., & Martin, L. L. (1990). The nurse practitioner and clinical nurse specialist: Should the roles be merged? *Journal of the American Academy of Nurse Practitioners, 2*(1), 2-9.

Herman, J. (1998). Documenting acute care nurse practitioner practice characteristics. *AACN Clinical Issues, 9*(2), 277-282.

Hilderly, L. (1991). Nurse-physician collaborative practice: The clinical nurse specialist in a radiation oncology private practice. *Oncology Nursing Forum, 18*(3), 585-591.

Hockenberry-Eaton, M., & Powell, M. L. (1991). Merging advanced practice roles: The CNS and NP. *Journal of Pediatric Health Care, 5,* 158-159.

Hunsberger, M., Mitchell, A., Blatz, P., Paes, B., Pinelli, J., Southwell, D., French, S., & Soluk, R. (1992). Definition of an advanced nursing role in the NICU: The clinical nurse specialist/nurse practitioner. *Clinical Nurse Specialist, 6*(2), 91-96.

Irvine, D., Sidani, S., & McGillis-Hall, L. (1998). Linking outcomes to nurses' roles in health care. *Nursing Economics, 16*(2), 58-64, 87.

Jackson, P. L. (1995). Opportunities and challenges for PNPs. *Pediatric Nursing, 21*(1), 43-46.

Jacobs, L. A., & Kreamer, K. M. (1997). The oncology clinical nurse specialist in a post-master's nurse practitioner program: A personal and professional journey. *Oncology Nursing Forum, 24,* 1387-1392.

Keane, A., & Richmond, T. (1993). Tertiary nurse practitioners. *Image: The Journal of Nursing Scholarship, 25*(4), 281-293.

Kindig, D., Cultice, J., & Mullen, F. (1993). The elusive generalist physician: Can we reach a 50% goal? *JAMA, 270,* 1069-1073.

King, K. B., & Ackerman, M. H. (1995). An educational model for the acute care nurse practitioner. *Critical Care Nursing Clinics of North America, 7,* 1-8.

Kinney, A., Hawkins, R., & Hudman, K. S. (1997). A descriptive study of the role of the oncology nurse practitioner. *Oncology Nursing Forum, 24,* 811-820.

Kitzman, H. J. (1983). The CNS and the nurse practitioner. In A. B. Hamric & J. Spross (Eds.), *The clinical nurse specialist in theory and practice* (pp. 275-290). New York: Grune & Stratton.

Kitzman, H. J. (1989). The CNS and the nurse practitioner. In A. B. Hamric & J. A. Spross (Eds.), *The clinical nurse specialist in theory and practice* (2nd ed., pp. 379-394). Philadelphia: W. B. Saunders.

Kleinpell, R. M. (1998). Reports of role descriptions of acute care nurse practitioners. *AACN Clinical Issues, 9*(2), 290-295.

Knutson, K. (1991). Merger of ANA advanced practice councils clarified. *Nurse Practitioner, 16*(8), 10.

Lynn, J., & Harrold, J. (1999). *Handbook for mortals.* New York: Oxford University Press.

Lyon, B. L. (1996, June 15). Meeting societal needs for CNS competencies: Why the CNS and NP roles should not be blended in master's degree programs. *Online Journal of Issues in Nursing (Adult Practice Nursing),* pp. 1-6.

Mayer, G. (1997). The impact of managed care on hospital nursing. *Best Practices and Benchmarking in Healthcare, 2*(4), 162-167.

McGivern, D. O. (1993). The evolution to advanced nursing practice. In M. D. Mezey & D. O. McGivern (Eds.), *Nurses, nurse practitioners:*

Evolution to advanced practice (pp. 3–30). New York: Springer-Verlag.

Milstead, J. A. (1997). Using advanced practice to shape public policy: Agenda setting. *Nursing Administration Quarterly, 21*(4), 12–18.

Mortenson, L. E., Edwards, J. J., & Bowers, M. L. (1998, November/December). APCs threaten hospital outpatient cancer programs, use of new agents, and supportive care drugs. *Oncology Issues,* pp. 25–29.

Naylor, M. D., Brooten, D., Campbell, R., Jacobsen, B. S., Mezey, M. D., Pauly, M. V., & Schwartz, J. S. (1999). Comprehensive discharge planning and home follow-up of hospitalized elders. *JAMA, 281,* 613–620.

Nemes, J., Barnaby, K., & Shamberger, R. (1992). Experience with a nurse practitioner program in the surgical department of a children's hospital. *Journal of Pediatric Surgery, 27,* 1038–1042.

O'Flynn, A. I. (1996). The preparation of advanced practice nurses: Current issues. *Nursing Clinics of North America, 31,* 429–438.

O'Malley, J., & Cummings, S. H. (1995). Change . . . more change . . . and change again. *Advanced Practice Nursing Quarterly, 1*(1), 1–6.

Page, N. E., & Arena, D. M. (1994). Rethinking the merger of the clinical nurse specialist and the nurse practitioner roles. *Image: The Journal of Nursing Scholarship, 26*(4), 315–318.

Page, N. E., & Mackowiak, L. (1997). Role play: The clinical nurse specialist and nurse practitioner: complementary roles. *Journal of the Society of Pediatric Nurses, 2*(4), 188–190.

Paladichuk, A., Brass-Mynderse, N., & Kaliangara, O. (1997). Chronic disease management: An outpatient approach. *Critical Care Nurse, 17*(6), 90–95.

Papenhausen, J. L. (1990). Case management: A model of advanced practice? *Clinical Nurse Specialist, 4*(4), 169–170.

Paul, S. (1997). Implementing an outpatient congestive heart failure clinic: The nurse practitioner role. *Heart & Lung, 26,* 486–491.

Pearson, L. J. (1990). 25 years later 25 exceptional NPs look at the movement's evolution and consider future challenges for the role. *Nurse Practitioner: The American Journal of Primary Health Care, 15*(9), 9–31.

Porter-O'Grady, T. (1997). Over the horizon: The future and the advanced practice nurse. *Nursing Administration Quarterly, 21*(4), 1–11.

Redekopp, M. A. (1997). Clinical nurse specialist role confusion: The need for identity. *Clinical Nurse Specialist, 11*(2), 87–91.

Rosenblatt, R. A., Hart, L. G., Baldwin, L. M., Chan, L., & Schneeweiss, R. (1998). The generalist role of specialty physicians: Is there a hidden system of primary care? *JAMA, 279,* 1364–1370.

Sawyers, J. E. (1993). Defining your role in ambulatory care: Clinical nurse specialist or nurse practitioner? *Clinical Nurse Specialist, 7*(1), 4–7.

Schroer, K. (1991). Case management: Clinical nurse specialist and nurse practitioner, converging roles. *Clinical Nurse Specialist, 5*(4), 189–194.

Shuren, A. (1996). The blended role of the clinical nurse specialist and nurse practitioner. In A. B. Hamric, J. A. Spross, & C. M. Hanson (Eds.), *Advanced nursing practice: An integrative approach* (pp. 375–394). Philadelphia: W.B. Saunders.

Simpson, R. L. (1998). Bridging the nursing-physician gap: Technology's role in interdisciplinary practice. *Nursing Administration Quarterly, 22*(3), 87–90.

Smith, L. D. (1994). Continuity of care through nursing case management of the chronically ill child. *Clinical Nurse Specialist, 8*(2), 65–68.

Snyder, M., & Mirr, M. P. (Eds.). (1995). *Advanced practice nursing: Guide to professional development.* New York: Springer-Verlag.

Spross, J. A., & Hamric, A. B. (1983). A model for future clinical specialist practice. In A. B. Hamric & J. A. Spross (Eds.), *The clinical nurse specialist in theory and practice* (pp. 291–306). New York: Grune & Stratton.

Weinberg, R. M., Likestrand, J. S., & Moore, S. (1983). In-patient management by a nurse practitioner: Effectiveness in a rehabilitation setting. *Archives of Physical Medicine and Rehabilitation, 64,* 588–590.

Wright, J. E. (1990). Joining forces for the good of our clients. *Clinical Nurse Specialist, 4*(2), 76–77.

Wright, K. B. (1997). Advanced practice nursing: Merging the clinical nurse specialist and nurse practitioner roles. *Gastroenterology Nursing, 20*(2), 57–60.

Zimmer, P., Brykczynski, K., Martin, A. C., Newberry, Y. G., Price, M. J., & Warren, B. (1990). *Advanced nursing practice: Nurse practitioner curriculum guidelines (Final Report: NONPF Education Committee).* Paper presented at the National Organization of Nurse Practitioner Faculties, Washingon, DC.

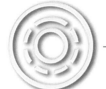

The Certified Nurse-Midwife

· M A R G A R E T   W.   D O R R O H
· M A U R E E N   A.   K E L L E Y

BARRIERS TO PRACTICE
Legislative, Regulatory, and Financial Barriers
Workload

CONCLUSION

INTRODUCTION

Nurse-midwifery has made many contributions that have paved the way for advanced nursing practice to flourish. These efforts have included the development of standards, core clinical competencies, and successful legislative and regulatory initiatives. Nurse-midwifery activities that have been instrumental in securing prescriptive authority and direct reimbursement by insurers for certified nurse-midwives (CNMs) have also had an indirect and favorable impact on all advanced practice nurses (APNs). Nurse-midwifery has its roots in nursing and has been supportive of nursing. The American College of Nurse-Midwives (ACNM) recently put a proposal before its membership to change its name to the American College of Midwives. In a demonstration of allegiance to nursing, the membership voted overwhelmingly to retain "Nurse" in the name of the organization (Kraus, 1997b).

Despite these contributions, there are tensions between the ACNM and advanced practice nursing. Organized nurse-midwifery has not been viewed as joining forces with the nursing profession's efforts to organize and align all advanced practice roles. Several factors may account for this. The profession has set a high priority on increasing availability of and access to midwifery services. Much effort has gone into meeting the increasing demand for nurse-midwives. Because the ACNM defines the CNM as an individual educated in the two disciplines of nursing and midwifery (ACNM, 1997i), new graduates are viewed as *beginning-level practitioners of midwifery,* not as APNs. Herein may lie one of the fundamental philosophical differences with the larger nursing profession. Paradoxically, availability and access are central arguments for health care reform initiatives that promote APN roles.

In this chapter, the authors are discussing midwives who are practicing in an advanced nursing role. When the issue of non-nurse midwives is addressed, an attempt will be made to make that clear. While remaining mindful and respectful of the rich history and groundwork laid by nurse-midwifery, the authors support all of the criteria for practice put forth in this text. The pioneering efforts of CNMs have helped to cultivate a clinical and political climate of acceptance not only for them, but also for clinical nurse specialists (CNSs), certified registered nurse anesthetists (CRNAs), and nurse practitioners (NPs) as legitimate and visible providers of care across all settings. The task is to describe nurse-midwifery practice so that the reader can appreciate why it can be seen as an APN role. As authors, we offer our own perspectives on the issues that prevent full integration of nurse-midwifery into advanced nursing practice.

Nurses and nurse-midwives alike have a stake in issues related to this level of professional practice. The reflections offered in this chapter are meant to foster dialogue, understanding, and wisdom as nurses and nurse-midwives work to accomplish their goals related to practice. It is our hope that all in nursing will continue to work productively and collaboratively on activities that promote advanced nursing practice.

HISTORICAL PERSPECTIVE

The word "midwife" has had the same meaning in all times and in all cultures. In Biblical times, the midwife assisted a woman in labor, helped with the delivery, and provided aftercare for the mother and child. Novice midwives acquired knowledge and skill from practical training with experienced midwives and through their own observation and experience. Skilled midwives provided emergency medical or surgical assistance as needed and, in recognition of their importance, were exempted from injunctions against work on the Sabbath when performing their duties. Present-day midwives are granted the same privilege!

In colonial times, midwives were an integral part of community life and were highly respected. By the early 1900s, a number of developments had considerably diminished that respect and led to an ebb in the practice of midwifery. A key factor was the medicalization of childbirth. By the early 1900s, the medical field had become highly competitive; attending labor and delivery was a way physicians could establish a practice. Families pleased with the medical care provided at childbirth would return to the same physician for other care. This phenomenon combined with women's low social status made it difficult for midwives to compete against physicians. Although the arrival of physicians on the childbearing scene was late, this accident of history continues to influence the regulation and practice of nurse-midwifery.

The renaissance of midwifery in the United States was not to occur for more than two decades, although it remained part of mainstream health care in many European, Asian, and African countries. Like the emergence of other forms of advanced nursing practice, the resurgence of midwifery and the evolution of nurse-midwifery occurred in response to the need for care by the underserved. By the late 1960s, the contributions of nurse-midwifery were accepted and recognized. The profession was inundated with requests for nurse-midwives and was criticized for not having enough CNMs trained to meet the needs of women in this country. This led to a proliferation of nurse-midwifery educational programs and the development of more nurse-midwifery practices. Table 17-1 presents a timeline of key events that influenced the development of modern nurse-midwifery as described by Varney (1996).

THE NURSE-MIDWIFERY PROFESSION IN THE UNITED STATES TODAY

There are currently more than 6,700 active and student members of the ACNM. Of that number, approximately 5,700 are in clinical practice. Overall, 68% of CNMs hold a master's degree; 4% have a doctoral degree (J. Bougass, ACNM, personal communication, 1999). Approximately 2% of nurse-midwives are men (ACNM Public Relations Department, personal communication, October 3, 1995). In 1997, the most current year for which data are available, nurse-midwives attended 258,227 births, which constitutes 8.47% of the nation's vaginal births (Dower et al., 1999). It has been estimated that by 2000, 10% of all births in the United States will be attended by CNMs (Nitzsche, 1995).

Education/Accreditation

The ACNM established a national mechanism for the accreditation of education programs in 1962. Because the organization wanted to have its process subject to

TABLE 17-1 THE EVOLUTION OF NURSE-MIDWIFERY: A TIMELINE OF CRITICAL EVENTS

YEAR	EVENT	SIGNIFICANCE
Colonial times to early 1900s	Midwives traveled to the colonies. They were respected in communities and trained in apprenticeships. Practices were often handed down from mother to daughter.	Midwifery had a strong basis in service to others. Went beyond an occupation—often seen as a "calling." The women who practiced midwifery tended to be rich in life experience if not in formal education.
Early 1990s	Midwifery was co-opted by organized medicine.	Decreased number and experience of practitioners effectively put midwives "in the closet."
1925	Frontier Nursing Service was founded in Hyden, Kentucky.	Imported British-trained midwives utilized the nursing model. Designed to meet the specific needs in an underserved area. Births took place in homes. Neonatal mortality rate 9.1/1,000 births from 1925 to 1951 (not matched by United States at large until 1990s).
1931	The Maternity Center Association, in New York, opened the Lobenstine Clinic.	Provided care for immigrant families in upper Manhattan tenements.
1932	The first nurse-midwifery education program was developed at the Lobenstine Clinic.	Offered advanced preparation in midwifery to public health nurses. Acknowledged relationship of nursing and midwifery.
1941	The Tuskegee School of Nurse-Midwifery opened in Alabama.	Access to nurse-midwifery education for minorities.
1943	The Catholic Maternity Institute was founded in Santa Fe, New Mexico.	
Mid-1940s	The National Organization of Public Health Nurses (later absorbed into the American Nurses Association) was established for nurse-midwives.	Recognition of midwifery as having a foundation in nursing.
1955	The American College of Nurse-Midwives was founded.	Began formalizing standards for education, certification, and practice. The basic certificate program was the norm. Also provided a formal voice for nurse-midwives.
Early 1960s	A certified nurse-midwife pilot project was conducted in Madera County, California.	
Late 1960s and 1970s	Nurse-midwifery services and educational programs (mostly certificates) proliferated; autonomous birth centers were developed.	Increased utilization of and demand for CNMs in a variety of settings.
1980s	Malpractice crisis arose.	Closed some practices and threatened closure at some programs until issue resolved.
1980s and 1990s	Certified nurse-midwives moved to graduate-level education.	Majority of programs now prepare students at master's level
1990s	The milieu for health care practice is changing; certified nurse-midwives are moving toward primary care of women.	CNMs adapting to environment in which quality, access, and cost must all be addressed.

peer review and recognition, it applied to the Department of Education for recognition as an accrediting agency. This recognition was granted in 1982, and has been maintained since that time. ACNM-accredited programs must receive preaccreditation status prior to enrolling students and, once initial accreditation is granted, programs are revisited at least every 8 years.

There are currently 44 programs accredited by or with preaccreditation status from the Division of Accreditation (DOA) of the ACNM. Five of these programs are certificate-level programs and 39 are master's programs. The profession supports preparation of midwives at both the certificate and the degree level. This position is based on two rationales. The first is that differences in preparation have not resulted in differences in certification test results (Fullerton & Severino, 1995). Second, it is based on the concern that "mandatory degree requirements would limit access to maternity and gynecological services for women who have been shown to benefit from midwifery care by denying [them] practice opportunities" (Carrington & Decker, 1997). Although the DOA supports different educational pathways, it requires that all ACNM-accredited education programs must either require a baccalaureate upon entrance or grant no less than a baccalaureate upon graduation (ACNM, 1993).

The accreditation process rests on two cornerstones. The first are the Criteria for the Evaluation of Education Programs (ACNM, 1997h). These criteria specify the elements necessary to develop and maintain a nurse-midwifery program. Because they evaluate the specialty content of midwifery (i.e., content that addresses the *hallmarks and components of midwifery,* including but not limited to intrapartum care), these criteria apply regardless of the academic "house" in which the program resides (i.e., nursing, public health, allied health, medicine). In addition, they apply regardless of the level at which the student is being prepared (baccalaureate, master's, doctoral, certificate) (Bellack, Graber, O'Neil, & Musham, 1998; Carr, 1999). This approach to education is not without difficulties, such as when state laws require a certain level of education to practice or to perform certain aspects of practice such as prescribing medication. The ACNM criteria are revised every 5 years in order to maintain currency. The criteria do require that a midwifery program be directed by a midwife, that midwifery faculty have at least 1 year of clinical nurse-midwifery experience prior to teaching, and that the faculty maintain currency in clinical practice.

The second cornerstone of the accreditation process is the *Core Competencies for Basic Midwifery Practice,* most recently revised in 1997 (ACNM, 1997g). This document represents the delineation of the fundamental knowledge, skills, and behaviors expected of a new practitioner. It is divided into four major sections: (1) hallmarks, which speak to the underlying philosophy of the profession; (2) professional responsibilities, which delineate the nonclinical requirements of the professional midwife; (3) the midwifery management process, which is the clinical decision-making framework for practice; and (4) the components of clinical care. This document ensures equivalent preparation for all graduates of midwifery education programs accredited by the ACNM's DOA. It likewise contributes to the blueprint for the certification examination for CNMs (ACNM, 1997j).

Certification/Certification Maintenance

A national certification examination for entry into practice was instituted in 1971. The ACNM Certification Council Inc. (ACC) develops and administers this examination. The examination has a multiple-choice format, and is based on both the core competencies and a periodically conducted task analysis of currently practicing midwives. Each year, approximately 400 students graduate from an ACNM-accredited program and take the certifying examination.

As of January 1, 1996, the certificate became a time-limited one, valid for 8 years from date of issue. Mechanisms for certification maintenance, administered by the ACC, include such options as certification maintenance modules, continuing education units (CEUs), and retaking the certification examination. At this juncture, the time-limited certificate does not apply to midwives certified prior to 1996, and therefore the certification maintenance program is optional for this group. Instead, the continuing competency assessment mechanism, which was developed in 1987, may be used.

Continuing Competency Assessment

In 1987, the ACNM developed a continuing competency assessment mechanism for its members in clinical practice. Its purpose was to demonstrate that clinicians continued to maintain contemporary knowledge, and met a national standard for practice. This 5-year cycle requires that practicing midwives either acquire 50 contact hours of continuing education appropriate for midwifery practice or retake the certification examination. There is no ongoing clinical practice requirement for maintaining certification. The ACNM Continuing Education Committee grants CEUs for programs that meet the guidelines of the International Association for Continuing Education and Training. The ACNM initially "mandated" competency assessment but modified this position in 1995, placing the decision to mandate participation in the hands of state regulators or employers. The ACNM still sets the standard that all CNMs must demonstrate continuing competency, and a number of states and employers have adopted evidence of ACNM continuing competency as a requirement for licensure or employment (ACNM, 1997f). There is no requirement for ongoing clinical practice for either certification maintenance or continuing competency assessment.

Regulation, Credentialing, and Reimbursement

As with all health professions in the United States, midwives are regulated on a state-by-state basis. CNMs must comply with the legal requirements for the practice of nurse-midwifery in the jurisdiction in which they practice. (The term "jurisdiction" reflects the inclusion of the District of Columbia, the Virgin Islands, and Puerto Rico as well as the 50 states.) The practice of nurse-midwifery differs in the various jurisdictions because of legal, regulatory, and other influences. Such influences include statutes, rules and regulations, opinions of the state attorney general, court decisions, licensure, registration, and certification. This results in differences in such parameters as what state agency regulates midwifery practice, whether midwives have prescriptive authority, what educational degrees are required for practice, and what types of employer and practice arrangements are permitted. States may also have regulations about private insurance reimbursement, and are required to set the Medicaid reimbursement schedule for nurse-midwives. The effect that this variation in state law and regulation has on midwifery practice was examined by Declercq, Paine, Dejoseph, and Simmes (1998). They found that, when compared to states with low regulatory support for nurse-midwifery practice, states with high regulatory support had a nurse-midwifery workforce three times larger, three times the number of midwife-attended births, and two times as many midwife-patient contacts.

The political climate affects nurse-midwifery practice and can promote or restrain the practice of CNMs. For example, the relative power of constituencies such as medical and nursing organizations and consumer groups and the relationships among them can shape legislation and patterns of referral to CNMs. Laws and other ordinances that regulate CNM practice should ensure that all practitioners are qualified to practice nurse-midwifery. The ACNM recently reaffirmed the autonomy with which the CNM practices. The ACNM's official clinical practice statement on independent nurse-midwifery practice is presented in Box 17-1.

In addition to state regulation, hospitals and health plans have established credentialing requirements for health care professionals. The impact of these credentialing standards is to determine who may have hospital admitting privileges, who may be employed by health systems, and who may be listed on managed care provider panels. An optimum system would create a mechanism that was consistent with the profession's standards, recognize midwifery as distinct from other health care professions, and recognize processes that permit midwives to build upon entry-level competencies within their statutory scope of practice (Dower et al., 1999).

The Pew Health Professions Commission on the Future of Midwifery made a number of recommendations about the practice environment (Dower et al., 1999). These recommendations reflect the understanding that the professional and regulatory environments combine to significantly impact the ability of nurse-midwives to be part of the health care team. Table 17-2 contains a summary of these recommendations.

The American College of Nurse-Midwives

The growth and development of American nurse-midwifery owes much to the ACNM, founded in 1955. The mission of the ACNM is to promote the health and well-being

---

BOX 17-1 • CLINICAL PRACTICE STATEMENT ON INDEPENDENT MIDWIFERY PRACTICE
(American College of Nurse-Midwives, 1997)

It is the position of the ACNM that midwifery practice is the independent management of women's health care, focusing particularly on pregnancy, childbirth, the postpartum period, care of the newborn, and the family planning and gynecologic needs of women. The practice occurs within a health care system that provides for consultation, collaborative management or referral as indicated by the health status of the client.

Independent midwifery enables certified nurse-midwives (CNMs) and certified midwives (CMs) to utilize knowledge, skills, judgment and authority in the provision of primary women's health services while maintaining accountability for the management of patient care in accordance with the ACNM *Standards for the Practice of Nurse-Midwifery.*

The ACNM believes that independent practice is not defined by the place of employment, the employee-employer relationship, requirements for physician co-signature, or the method of reimbursement for services. Nor should *independent* be interpreted to mean *alone,* as there are clinical situations when any prudent practitioner would seek the assistance of another qualified practitioner.

The ACNM also believes that collaboration is the process whereby health care professionals jointly manage care. The goal of collaboration is to share authority while providing quality care within each individual's professional scope of practice. Successful collaboration is a way of thinking and relating that requires knowledge, open communication, mutual respect, a commitment to providing quality care, trust, and the ability to share responsibility.

TABLE 17–2 PRACTICE ENVIRONMENT RECOMMENDATION

PRACTICE	REGULATION & CREDENTIALING	EDUCATION	RESEARCH	POLICY
Four recommendations are offered to health care system administrators and practitioners—including midwives and other professionals—to help ensure that practice structures are designed to provide the best health care possible by making the midwifery model of care readily available to women. 1. Midwives should be recognized as independent and collaborative practitioners with the rights and responsibilities regarding scope of practice authority and accountability that all independent professionals share. 2. Every health care system should integrate midwifery services into the continuum of care for women by contracting with or employing midwives and informing women of their options.	RECOMMENDATIONS: 5. State legislatures should enact laws that base entry-to-practice standards on successful completion of accredited education programs, or the equivalent, and national certification; do not require midwives to be directed or supervised by other health care professionals; and allow midwives to own or co-own health care practices. 6. Hospitals, health systems, and public programs, including Medicare and Medicaid, should ensure that enrollees have access to midwives and the midwifery model of care by eliminating barriers to access and inequitable reimbursement rates that discriminate against midwives. 7. Health care systems should develop hospital	The following recommendations will challenge educators to continue to develop faculty, programs, curricula and recruitment policies to meet consumer demands in a changing health care arena. 8. Education programs should provide opportunities for interprofessional education and training experiences and allow for multiple points at which midwifery education can be entered. This requires proactive intra- and interprofessional collaboration between colleges, universities and education programs to develop affiliations and complementary curriculum pathways. 9. Midwifery education programs should include training in practice management and the impact of	12. Midwifery research should be strengthened and funded in the following areas: • Demand for maternity care, demand for midwifery care, and numbers and distribution of midwives; • Analyses of how midwives complement and broaden the woman's choice of provider, setting, and model of care; • Cost benefit, cost effectiveness, and cost utility analyses, including the relationship between knowledge of economic/cost analyses and provider practices; • Midwifery practice and benchmarking data (among midwives) with a goal of developing appropriate productivity standards;	14. A research and policy body, such as the Institute of Medicine, should be requested to study and offer guidance on significant aspects of the midwifery profession including • Workforce supply and demand; • Coordination of regulation by the states; • Funding of research, education, and training; and • Coordination among the federal agencies whose policies affect the practice of midwifery.

498

3. When integrating midwifery services, health care organizations should use productivity standards based on the midwifery model of care and measure the overall financial benefits of such care.
4. Midwives and physicians should ensure that their systems of consultation, collaboration and referral provide integrated and uninterrupted care to women. This requires active engagement and participation by members of both professions.

privileging and credentialing mechanisms for midwives that are consistent with the profession's standards, recognize midwifery as distinct from other health care professions, and recognize established processes that permit midwives to build upon their entry-level competencies within their statutory scope of practice.

health care policy and financing on midwifery practice, with special attention to managed care.
10. The profession should recognize and acknowledge the benefits of teaching midwifery model of care in a variety of education programs and affirm the value of competency-based education in all midwifery programs.
11. The midwifery profession should identify, develop and implement mechanisms to recruit student populations that more closely reflect the U.S. population and include cultural competence concepts in basic and continuing education programs.

- Descriptions and outcomes analyses of midwifery methods and processes;
- Analysis of midwifery practice outcomes, from preconception through infancy, using an evidence-based perspective;
- Normal pregnancy, normal labor and birth, healthy parent-infant relationships, and breastfeeding; and
- Satisfaction with maternity and midwifery care.

13. Federal and state agencies should broaden systematic data collection, which has traditionally focused on medicine and physicians, to include midwifery and midwives.

From Dower, C. M., Miller, J. E., O'Neil, E. H., and the Taskforce on Midwifery. (1999). *Charting a course for the 21st century: The future of midwifery.* (pp. i–v). San Francisco: Pew Health Professions Commission and the UCSF Center for the Health Professions; reprinted with permission.

of women and infants within their families and communities through the development and support of professional midwifery. The organization establishes clinical standards, creates liaisons with state and federal agencies and members of Congress, administers and promotes continuing education programs, supports midwifery-relevant research and practice, and supports the accreditation mechanism.

The ACNM Philosophy (Box 17-2) and Code of Ethics embody the spirit of the profession. The Code of Ethics (Ad Hoc Committee on Code of Ethics, 1990) aligns with the American Nurses Association's Code of Ethics. A CNM has professional moral obligations. The code identifies the obligations that guide the CNM in the practice of nurse-midwifery and clarifies what consumers, the public, other professionals, and potential practitioners can expect of the profession. Nurse-midwifery exists for the good of women and their families; this good is safeguarded by practice that is consistent with the ACNM Philosophy (ACNM, 1989) and ACNM Standards for the Practice of Nurse-Midwifery (ACNM, 1993). The belief that pregnancy and childbirth are normal life processes is at the heart of nurse-midwifery practice. The nurse-midwife learns to be "with woman" (the original meaning of midwife) without having to "manage" pregnancy, labor, or delivery. The patience to allow normal processes to proceed at an unhurried pace is one of the nurse-midwife's skills. This is one of the key differences between nurse-midwifery and medical approaches to the care of women. Adherents of the medical model tend to intervene even when things are proceeding normally. In nurse-midwifery, when intervention is indicated, CNMs ensure that it is integrated into care in a way that preserves the dignity of the woman and her family. The Code of Ethics further describes expectations regarding

BOX 17-2 • ACNM PHILOSOPHY
(American College of Nurse-Midwives, 1989)

Certified nurse-midwives believe that every individual has a right to safe, satisfying health care with respect for human dignity and cultural variations. ACNM further supports each person's right to self-determination, to complete information and to active participation in all aspects of care. ACNM members believe the normal process of pregnancy and birth can be enhanced through education, health care and supportive intervention.

Nurse-midwifery is focused on the needs of the individual and family for physical care, emotional and social support and active involvement of significant others according to cultural values and personal preferences. The practice of nurse-midwifery encourages continuity of care; emphasizes safe, competent clinical management; advocates non-intervention in normal processes; and promotes health education for women throughout the childbearing cycle. This practice may extend to include gynecological care of women throughout the life cycle. Such comprehensive health care is most effectively and efficiently provided by nurse-midwives in collaboration with other members of an interdependent health care team.

ACNM assumes a leadership role in the development and promotion of high quality health care for women and infants both nationally and internationally. The profession of nurse-midwifery is committed to ensuring that certified nurse-midwives are provided with sound educational preparation, to expanding knowledge through research and to evaluating and revising care through quality assurance. The profession further ensures that its members adhere to the *Standards of Practice for Nurse-Midwifery* in accordance with the *ACNM Philosophy*.

practice competence, nurse-midwife–client relationships, ethical responsibilities, collegial practice, and nondiscrimination. Responsibilities for conducting research in nurse-midwifery and for supporting community and political activities that promote access to health care are also delineated.

IMPLEMENTING APN COMPETENCIES

Advocacy and Client Education: Cornerstones of Nurse-Midwifery Practice

Nurse-midwifery is multifaceted, constantly evolving, and broader in scope than its pioneers first envisioned it. It is a dynamic discipline (Bergstrom, 1997). Nurse-midwives have, in common with all APNs, the characteristics of using a holistic perspective, establishing a partnership with the client, involving significant others and family members in care, using clinical reasoning, managing health and illnesses, and using processes to perform self-evaluation. To further understand nurse-midwifery practice, it is helpful to take a close look at the core competencies related to advocacy and client education.

Advocacy

Advocacy is central to nurse-midwifery practice. Client education and support of clients' rights and self-determination inform every aspect of nurse-midwifery care. These values have been challenged by the burgeoning growth of medical technology in the last two decades and the incursion of managed care in the 1990s. The availability of highly technical interventions for many aspects of childbearing, such as infertility, monitoring pregnancies, and delivery, conflicts with the traditionally low-technology, low-interventionist approach of CNMs. Vulnerable populations (e.g., women who have not had access to early prenatal care or low-income women receiving care at a teaching hospital clinic) are more likely to be exposed to high-technology interventions. This presents CNMs with several challenges: to evaluate technologies to determine whether and how they can be incorporated into nurse-midwifery care, to incorporate such therapies into practice in ways that are consistent with nurse-midwifery's values, to explain technology in a way that empowers women to make informed decisions, and to provide equal access to the technology. Creativity is required to enact the midwifery model of care across many settings (ACNM, 1997b; Corry & Rooks, 1999).

The advent of managed care has often restricted the choices that women can make for their personal health care. The ACNM is strongly supportive of legislation ensuring that consumers have access to the full spectrum of qualified health care professionals and providers. To that end, women should be able to designate a CNM as their primary care provider (ACNM, 1998a).

Client Education

Client education is another cornerstone of nurse-midwifery practice and is integral to the CNM's advocacy role. CNMs best fulfill the role of advocate when they invest time, effort, and caring in establishing a partnership with the client and provide her with the teaching and counseling that is characteristic of nurse-midwifery practice. A study of 1,181 women suggests that this emphasis on education explains some differences between nurse-midwives' and obstetricians' care processes (Oakley et al., 1995). Although many processes were similar, the nurse-midwives emphasized educational/psychosocial care and restrained use of technology tailored to the individual, whereas the obstetricians' practice reflected routine use of state-of-the-art technology. CNMs' emphasis on education enables women to participate knowledgeably and fully in their care. The value of a partnership that has been built over the course of the pregnancy becomes eminently clear during labor, when decisions have to be made. CNMs understand that a woman in the midst of labor may not be in the best position to make good, coherent decisions. The CNM and informed significant others can act in the client's best interests at this time, because the woman's goals and her contingency plans for events that might interfere with them have been jointly determined by the time labor begins.

Client education, never an easy task, is made even more daunting by the rapidity with which new technologies are developed, tested, and offered to women. Many women make decisions about their care without adequate information and are then left to suffer any consequences (Franklin, 1994). The CNM is often a pregnant woman's best hope of receiving adequate information and of ensuring that she is not left bewildered and alone. Nurse-midwives bring the gifts of skill, knowledge, and love to a health care setting that can be devoid of human warmth, all the more so as the technological aspect of care becomes more and more complex. There can be few more noble tasks than providing every woman a safer passage to motherhood and a better future for her children and family (Hsia, 1991).

THE CURRENT PRACTICE OF NURSE-MIDWIFERY

Scope of Practice

Originally, midwifery practice was limited to prenatal, intrapartum, postpartum, and newborn care. Today, although some CNMs limit their practice or are limited by their practice settings to pregnancy care alone, nurse-midwifery care has expanded to include the primary care of women, preconception, gynecologic, contraceptive, and infertility care. Nurse-midwives care for teenage women, women in their childbearing years, women in midlife or those who are elderly. This expansion is due largely to consumer demand and the need for greater access to these services. Interestingly, in many other countries midwifery practice continues to be somewhat restricted to care related to childbirth only.

"Scope of practice" refers to what CNMs are actually doing in practice once the core competencies have been met. The ACNM (1992) provides a guide for the evaluation and addition of other skills and procedures to nurse-midwifery practice. Thus procedures such as circumcision, vacuum extraction delivery, endometrial biopsy, colposcopy, and elective termination of pregnancy can be included in some CNMs' practice. The term "scope of practice" is also used to differentiate nurse-midwifery practice that is office based, providing no labor and delivery care, from full-scope practice, which includes labor and delivery care. Both types of practice may or may not include the additional procedures previously mentioned.

The ACNM Core Competencies (1997g) codify knowledge and practice expectations of the graduate CNM, serve as a guide for education programs, and represent basic CNM practice to other organizations, health care professionals, and practice settings (Roberts, 1997). Table 17–3 offers an overview of nurse-midwifery practice, including the knowledge needed and the processes used to provide care. Care of women at other developmental stages or with other health care needs follows similar guidelines. Nurse-midwifery practice incorporates knowledge of the following: normal human physical and psychological development, anatomy and physiology, physiological and psychological deviations from normal, embryology and genetics, reproduction, sexuality, and pharmacology. CNMs recognize indicators of developmental changes throughout women's life cycles and can counsel women regarding health promotion measures specific to these changes. They recognize indicators of problems with sexuality and can provide counseling or initiate consultation or referral for problems outside the scope of nurse-midwifery practice. Like all APNs, CNMs are familiar with deviations from normal, risk factors, appropriate preventive measures, and interventions for selected pathology. Whatever a woman's developmental stage or health care concern, CNMs are expected to teach and counsel clients regarding self-care practices, health promotion, nutritional issues, emotional concerns, and sexuality. Nurse-midwifery practice includes well-defined processes for interacting with physicians and other colleagues to ensure high-quality care. The core competencies, practice guidelines, and agency- or practice-specific policies establish the standards of care within the scope of practice for a particular agency or practice setting. Readers will also recognize many similarities in the values and philosophy guiding CNM practice to that guiding care in other advanced practice roles, especially obstetrical-gynecological (OB-GYN) NPs.

Although nurse-midwifery practice overlaps with aspects of care provided by other health professionals, elements of care provided by CNMs are unique to this group of health care providers. CNMs adhere to the belief that the life processes they deal with are *normal;* therefore, the midwifery approach, at least initially, is noninterventive. When interventions are indicated, CNMs may not limit themselves to modern allopathic (medical) approaches and may advise clients to use measures from older traditions that women have found comforting and effective. Such treatments may include acupressure, herbals, homeopathics, healing touch, bodywork, and nutritional interventions. These complementary interventions are most likely to be used for the common discomforts of pregnancy, during labor, for premenstrual problems, or for menopausal symptoms. Nurse-midwifery alone among other professions gives credence to the *presence of the midwife* as being therapeutic in and of itself.

Nurse-Midwifery Management Processes

Regardless of practice setting, the process of nurse-midwifery management has four aspects: independent management, consultation, co-management (collaborative management), and referral (ACNM, 1997e). Implicit in the process are timely action and documentation of the three aspects other than independent management (Avery, 1992; Keleher, 1998). The key differences among these aspects of management relate to accountability.

TABLE 17–3 OVERVIEW OF NURSE-MIDWIFERY PRACTICE

	GENERAL WOMEN'S HEALTH	PREGNANCY	INTRAPARTUM	POSTPARTUM	CARE OF THE NEWBORN
Knowledge needed	Bioethics Interpersonal communication Culture and community resources Counseling Normal reproductive biology Scientific bases of prescriptions to prevent or facilitate pregnancy	Genetics Physiology of normal pregnancy Embryology Pathophysiology Risks Clinical indicators for complications Pharmacokinetics of medications commonly used in pregnancy	Anatomy of normal and abnormal labor in all stages Anatomy of fetal skull and its landmarks Prescription of medications and solutions	Anatomy and physiology (A & P) of the puerperium involutional process Lactation and methods for facilitation or suppression Recognition of deviations from normal	A & P and indications of normal adaptation to extrauterine life Stabilization of the neonate
Assessment and diagnosis	History, physical, lab data, and health risks	Parameters and methods for assessing progress of pregnancy and fetal well-being	Progress of labor Maternal and fetal status	Emotional, psychosocial, and sexual factors	Neonatal physical assessment Neonatal gestational age assessment
Teaching	Health promotion Preventative self-care	Childbirth education Parenting Nutritional education	Reinforcing labor comfort measures taught in childbirth classes Hygiene	Anticipatory guidance re: self-care, infant care, family planning, family relationships	Infant care Nutritional needs of the infant

Comforting	Drug and nondrug measures for discomforts related to menstruation and menopause Information on coping with stress	Drug and nondrug measures for the discomforts of pregnancy	Sensitivity to emotional changes Hands-on care Drug and nondrug measures for pain Local and pudendal anesthesia administration	Managing discomforts of puerperium	Enhancing bonding
Supporting	Active listening	Assisting and supporting the woman in decision making	Physical and emotional support	Supporting woman in breastfeeding and self- and infant care	Support for the changes in family structure with a new member
Treatment and management	Promotion of family-centered care	Monitoring progress of pregnancy	Monitoring progress of labor Managing abnormal birth events Placental expulsion Repair of lacerations or episiotomy	Appropriate interventions for any deviation from normal	Facilitating adaptation of newborn to extrauterine life
Coordination and complex management	Collaboration, referral Practice/business management Promotion of the continuity of care Consultation and co-management	Advocacy Care jointly planned with woman Developing a birth plan Managing deviations from normal	Back-up plans for emergencies in place Promotion of continuity of care	Providing for continuity of care for the woman and neonate	Resuscitation and emergency care when needed Referrals as necessary

INDEPENDENT MANAGEMENT

CNMs are responsible and accountable for the management decisions they make in caring for clients. CNMs provide independent management when they systematically obtain or update a complete and relevant database for assessment of the client's health status. This includes the history, the results of the physical examination, and laboratory data. On the basis and interpretation of these findings, CNMs accurately identify problems and diagnoses and implement a plan of action. They delineate health care goals and formulate and communicate a complete needs/problem list in collaboration with the woman. CNMs know when consultation, co-management, or referral is needed and initiate these interactions in a timely manner.

CONSULTATION

When CNMs identify problems or complications, they seek advice from another member of the health care team, often a physician but not always an obstetrician. When they retain independent management responsibility for the client while seeking advice, this is called consultation (ACNM, 1997d, 1997e). A consultation may center on an ongoing health problem (e.g., hypothyroidism); a nonobstetrical, time-limited problem that arises during pregnancy (e.g., bronchitis or food poisoning), or an obstetrical complication (e.g., size-date discrepancy). After consultation, the CNM and the woman discuss the recommendations, if any, and modify the plan of care accordingly. In the process of consultation, CNMs do not abdicate responsibility for decisions. If they seek consultation from another professional and the suggestions the other professional makes do not seem to be in the client's best interests, they will not be used. Thus the process of consultation used by CNMs is consistent with the consultation process described in Chapter 8. It is fair to say that novice CNMs are likely to consult often and to use most of the recommendations they receive until they acquire more experience. Consulting is one way of continuing to learn. The experienced CNM is likely to have a tentative plan in mind when consulting and uses consultation to verify the approach or to seek alternatives. It is important to emphasize that CNMs assume direct responsibility for implementing the plan of care in light of their independent management role.

CO-MANAGEMENT OR COLLABORATIVE CARE

One outcome of consultation may be the decision to shift to co-management or collaborative care. This usually occurs if part of the woman's care is an ongoing medical, gynecological, or obstetrical complication beyond the scope of the CNM's practice. In this situation, the CNM and physician *collaboratively manage* the patient, with the CNM defining and retaining accountability for nurse-midwifery aspects of care (ACNM, 1997e) (see Chapters 8 and 11 for further discussions of consultation and collaboration, respectively).

REFERRAL

When CNMs identify the need for comprehensive management and care outside the scope of nurse-midwifery practice, they direct the client to a physician or another professional for management of the particular problem (ACNM, 1997d, 1997e). Referral involves the transfer of some or all of the care and some or all accountability to another provider. This management aspect is usually temporary, and, once the client's condition returns to that which is within the CNM's scope of practice, the CNM resumes independent management or co-management. For example, the CNM would refer a woman to an internist for hospitalization for pneumonia, to a surgeon for appendicitis, or to an obstetrician for a cesarean birth. Once the woman regains her health or recovers from surgery, she could return to the care of the CNM.

The details of these aspects of management are developed by individual CNMs in concert with obstetrical consultants/backups and the practice settings in which nurse-midwifery practice takes place. In addition to these patterns of care, CNMs also serve as consultants to or co-managers with other providers, including physicians, APN colleagues, registered nurses, physical therapists, and mental health colleagues (Hunter & Lops, 1994).

Practice Settings

One soon learns that there are many different practice styles and roles in nurse-midwifery, from full-scope CNMs to office-based CNMs who are not on a call schedule and do not do deliveries. CNMs practice in urban, suburban, and rural areas in a variety of settings. They practice in tertiary and secondary hospitals, often as part of a group practice of CNMs or CNMs and OB-GYN or family practice physicians. CNMs are employed by health maintenance organizations and neighborhood health centers. Many CNMs are in private practice, either self-employed or employed by physicians or other CNMs. In some settings, the CNM is the primary care provider; in others, the CNM may have a much more circumscribed practice (Kraus, 1997a; Miller, King, Luric, & Choitz, 1997). The CNM's actual practice depends on the needs of the population being served, the CNM's willingness to undertake a variety of functions, the availability of educational resources for the many different functions a CNM performs in a specific setting, the particular needs and requests of clients, the availability of physician and CNM colleagues for backup and coverage, and other organizational variables (Ament, 1998).

Some of the settings in which nurse-midwives provide labor and delivery care are clients' homes; autonomous birth centers; birth centers within hospitals; and traditional labor and delivery units of community, regional, and tertiary care hospitals. For clients, the choice of setting may be a matter of philosophy, comfort, convenience, degree of medical risk, or a combination of these factors. Each setting has its unique advantages and disadvantages, and the ACNM has published a position statement on practice settings (ACNM, 1997a).

Using the client's home as the setting for birth seems in many ways ideal. What could be more family centered? The CNM is in a position to evaluate the client's resources and help her prepare for childbirth and motherhood within her own setting. Any problems the client might have will be much more apparent if she is seen in her own home. Risks of iatrogenic complications or nosocomial infections are minimized. After the birth of the baby, the client can rest or sleep in her own bed, comfort and nurse her baby at will, and enjoy the attention and support of her loved ones. Birth at home certainly makes inclusion of family members in the birth (if the mother desires it) a simpler matter than in some other settings.

There are disadvantages to home birth as well. The client's home may be too far from emergency services. It might be difficult to have the degree of privacy needed for the birth if the house is crowded. Depending on the mother's other responsibilities and support system, her ability to rest may be promoted or compromised. The nurse-midwife's resources may be spread too thin, for instance, when two clients are in labor at the same time on opposite sides of town. It can be difficult to get medical backup (either house calls or admitting privileges) for home births in some areas (Scupholme & Walsh, 1994).

The *autonomous birth center* offers solutions to some of the problems with home births. It usually has homelike, attractive birth rooms. Selected emergency equipment is available, which can save crucial seconds that in a less controlled environment might be spent searching for such items. The CNMs and clients are at one location, and more than one client can be cared for at a time. The disadvantages of the autonomous birth center are similar to those of home birth. When an emergency exceeds the birth center's resources, the client must be transported to a hospital for care. Another important factor is that the client has to get up and take her baby home in a relatively short time, because birth centers do not generally have the ability to keep clients more than 24 hours.

The *birth center within the hospital* would seem to offer safety in emergencies as an advantage, but many believe that the simple proximity of epidural anesthesia, operating rooms, and other highly interventive technologies leads to their increased use. It is easy to lose sight of the "high-touch/low-tech" approach when one is located in the midst of multitudinous technical devices (Fullerton, 1994). However, being within the hospital setting does eliminate some of the problems nurse-midwives have encountered in obtaining medical backup when needed.

Differences in Practice Between Nurse-Midwives and Other Providers

The most significant difference between CNMs and OB-GYN NPs and family NPs (FNP) is the management of labor and delivery and the care of the newborn infant. OB-GYN NPs and FNPs do not provide independent care or co-management of care during labor and delivery. Some OB-GYN NPs and CNMs may have practices that are evenly divided between pregnancy-related and gynecologic services. Others limit their practices to pregnancy-related care. FNP practices are usually even more varied and include the care of men and children as well as women's health care.

The practices of maternal-child health CNSs and nurse-midwives also overlap in many ways. Like FNPs or OB-GYN NPs, maternal-child health CNSs do not provide independent management of labor and delivery. However, they are likely to be involved with specific patients and programs related to mother-infant services. Brooten and colleagues' (1986) study of CNS interventions with premature infants is an example of such intervention. The maternal-child health CNS often has more preparation in the care of older infants and children than does the CNM. Unlike the CNM or the OB-GYN NP or FNP, the maternal-child health CNS is also likely to be responsible for some staff development related to mother-infant care. She or he is more likely to practice in a hospital or community health or public health agency.

There are midwives who are not nurses (Johnson et al., 1998). In the United States, they are known as professional midwives (preferred term), independent midwives, apprentice midwives, community midwives, or lay midwives. They are most likely to practice within their communities, providing care to pregnant women and attending home births. Their practices are determined partly by the degree to which a particular jurisdiction regulates midwifery and partly by what the prevailing consumer demand and level of medical support are for this type of care. CNMs and midwives relate to each other differently depending on the perceived quality of care provided by both groups, the ability to recognize mutual interest in providing high-quality women's health care, and the consumer demand and medical support for each group within a particular community. The debate over non-nurse midwifery is discussed further in the "Professional Issues" section.

Research suggests that CNMs and OB-GYN physicians differ most in the processes they use in providing care (Oakley et al., 1995). Many differences between CNMs and obstetricians can be explained by the differing values between medicine and nursing/midwifery. CNMs approach the care of women, particularly during pregnancy, with the expectation that all will occur normally until proven otherwise. OB-GYN physicians are trained to diagnose and treat abnormalities and approach the care of women with the expectation that problems commonly will occur. Each professional group has expertise of value to the other. Successfully meeting the challenges of working together with OB-GYN physicians is as essential to providing nurse-midwifery care as are the core competencies for practice.

Summary

It should be evident from this discussion of nurse-midwifery care, scope of practice, management processes, and practice settings that CNMs have many opportunities to influence women's health care. Nurse-midwifery allows its practitioners to provide client-focused care that is both autonomous and collaborative within or across a variety of settings (Crofts, 1994). It offers a woman the opportunity to obtain, throughout her life as well as during her childbearing years, accessible, understandable, high-quality care that will be safe, satisfying, and individualized to her and her family's needs and desires.

AN EXEMPLAR OF NURSE-MIDWIFERY PRACTICE

The day-to-day practice of midwifery is similar in all settings. In this section, the first author (MWD) describes her own practice in an autonomous nurse-midwife–owned birth center to illustrate how the components of nurse-midwifery care are enacted in this setting.

EXEMPLAR

The client education process begins before a client is accepted into the practice. Orientation sessions are held to provide prospective clients with information to assist them in determining whether they want to have their baby in a birth center. These sessions conducted by the CNM are designed to provide both information and a tour of the physical facility. Prospective clients can see firsthand the comfort measures (such as the whirlpool tub) and the equipment on hand to handle normal deliveries and emergencies. Finances are discussed. The cost of care in the birth center is approximately half of that for obstetrical care in a hospital setting with a physician. Many insurers, Medicaid, and Medicare provide reimbursement; managed care entities have been slower to embrace this form of safe, satisfying and cost-effective care.

Clinical documentation must be meticulous, and an individualized health record assures that accurate, consistent, and complete information is obtained. Thorough health and family histories are taken. The questions asked elicit information about the woman's physical health and her psychological well-being. How does she feel about being pregnant? What kind of support system does she have in place? What resources might she have that are not currently being called upon? Was the pregnancy planned or a surprise? What are her family circumstances? Is there a stable relationship? Are there other children? It is important to document both positive and negative influences that can have an impact on the client's health and the health of her baby. Once the assessment is complete, risk factors that would prevent us from being able to accept a client are reviewed; if we cannot accept a client, we make a referral. If no risk factors are identified, we schedule the client's first visit.

When clients are accepted into the practice, they are told that they are equal partners in their care. It is the role of client education to bring this to reality. To be active participants in their care, clients are taught to weigh themselves and do their own urine dipstick test. They participate in charting the information, thus noting the progress of their pregnancy firsthand. The program of care for pregnant clients at our birth center includes 10 to 15 prenatal visits, childbirth classes, labor and delivery in the birth center, a home visit within 72 hours, and two office follow-up visits for mother and baby—one at 1 week and the other at 6 weeks postpartum.

Clinical hours are held daily. The CNMs in the practice share in doing client visits, teaching classes, and on-call time. Other responsibilities include administration and facility maintenance. We see pregnant clients, postpartum clients with their babies, and gynecological clients. The amount of time scheduled for a visit is based on need. A first visit for a pregnant patient is an hour long. An established gynecological client who is coming for her contraceptive injection requires only a few minutes, long enough to establish that she's having no problems.

A pregnant client is given the CNM pager number and instructions on how and when to use it. When a client is in active labor or her membranes have ruptured, she calls the CNM on duty. She is met at the birth center and examined. Most often when the woman arrives she is in active labor. We attribute this largely to the educational process that has taken place. On the rare occasion of false labor or very early labor, we are able to individualize care. If a client lives far away, we may elect to observe progress for a number of hours. If the woman is sleep deprived, she and her labor may benefit from some sedation. We remain with our clients in the birth center while they labor. There is a registered nurse (RN) on call for every delivery. If the CNM attending the client is tiring from having been up for a long labor, or several labors, the RN can be called to come in early to care for the client while the CNM rests. Sometimes, the RN is not needed until close to time for the birth.

The mother-to-be helps us to accommodate her wishes by preparing a birth plan. As her due date nears, one of her tasks (along with packing a bag to bring to the birth center and readying her home for a baby) is to write a birth plan, which will become a part of her record. This form allows her to tell us who she wants with her in labor, what she imagines labor will be like, what she *hopes* labor will be like, and what comfort measures would assist her in labor. We use this tool in several ways. We evaluate the effectiveness of our teaching by reading what the woman thinks labor will be like. Fears not previously revealed give us an opportunity to resolve any emotional factors that could hinder a successful labor. Knowing the person(s) the client wants with her during labor informs us about her support system. The people present at labor are an important factor in enhancing the woman's experience of labor.

The list of comfort measures is mainly a reminder to us, although a key contribution from the client. In the midst of labor, a woman may forget that she was looking forward to the whirlpool tub for relaxation and pain relief. A glance at the birth plan helps us try the things the client has already identified as potentially helpful to her. The birth-plan helps to emphasize to the client that this is *her* labor, with its inherent responsibilities and rights. Her dignity and worth as a human being are underscored. We try to nourish the woman's self-esteem and strengths that help in labor, life, and motherhood. The stronger the woman is in every way, the better her outcome is going to be.

Clients are given plenty of written material to help with their recall of information covered in classes. (If a client is unable to read, extra time is spent individually giving information verbally and making sure of understanding.) To help the client assume responsibility for herself and her labor, she is expected to bring with her to the birth center food and beverages that she would like while laboring and certain supplies, such as perineal pads, bed pads, and diapers. Clients take their babies home dressed in their own clothes and wrapped in their own blankets. They take with them an instructional booklet that they were given in the postpartum class. The booklet describes mother and baby care in detail for the first few days. Because mothers and babies are discharged early, often in 4 to 6 hours, it is imperative that the mother is prepared to check the baby's temperature and respirations, to check her own uterus, and to be able to recognize signs of complications that require attention. These are all enumerated in the instructions, and there is room for notes and questions. Having a reference helps new moms feel more secure—if something needs attention, they can always call the nurse-midwife, but they usually find what they need to know in the booklet. It often confirms what they sensed—either that everything was okay or that they need to get in touch with the nurse-midwife. Thus new mothers start out having faith in their own perceptions reinforced regarding their infants.

Empowering our clients, enhancing their decision-making abilities, reinforcing the mind-body connection, and enhancing family life by helping women find their personal power are goals of CNM care at the birth center. When I think of the enormous effects of empowerment, two new moms come particularly to mind.

M. L.'s case is proof positive of the benefits of teaching new mothers to trust their feelings and make decisions based on them. On the third or fourth day, M. L.'s baby ceased nursing well. He had been nursing vigorously and now was not. Nursing poorly is one of the signs listed in our booklet as requiring professional help. M. L. insisted to her husband that they had to go to the emergency room immediately. (They lived a long distance from the birth center, and it had been decided earlier that, if there should be a problem that seemed serious, she should go to a nearby emergency room, rather than try to get to the CNM.) Initially, doctors could find nothing wrong, but M. L. insisted they keep looking. As it turned out, the baby had a congenital heart defect that does not show up on clinical examination until 3 or 4 days after birth. M. L. said she was glad she had been given the information at the birth center; it gave her the confidence to trust her feelings that something very serious was wrong. The baby had heart surgery and is doing well.

A woman with confidence and trust in herself can do almost anything, as the case of S. J. shows. S. J. was 26 years old and came to the birth center soon after it opened to have her fourth child. She had a high school education and was home with her children, all of whom were under the age of 5. Her self-esteem was negligible. Her husband came to a few of the prenatal classes but was sullen and unsupportive. S. J. seemed to droop, but she was an excellent mother and was an attentive and fast learner at everything to do with childbirth, childrearing, and health in general. Her interest and enthusiasm grew as we reinforced her abilities and strengths. By the time she gave birth to her son, she seemed a different person from the withdrawn, self-effacing young woman we'd met 7 months earlier. Two years after this baby's birth, S. J. paid a visit to the birth center. "I just wanted to thank you," she said. "Before I came here, I never felt I was any good at anything. You told me I was a good mother, you noticed how well cared for my children were, and you encouraged me to learn all about birth and even let me borrow books and tapes. Well, I learned I was good—at a lot of things! You all showed me that. And I wanted you to know I'm in nursing school now because I want to be able to do what you do—not just take care of people physically, but help people grow."

The ability to have such a positive impact on others is very satisfying. However, it is clear that being a nurse-midwife does not entail "doing it all" for our clients. It is far more important, and healthier for all concerned, to teach our clients so that they are empowered to provide themselves and their families with the best possible care for every situation. We cannot be there for every health difficulty our clients may have, but we can give them the confidence to *know* when something is wrong and the knowledge of what to do in various situations. Nurse-midwives *give* from the core of their being. They listen, which is one of the crucial skills nurse-midwives bring to their practice. The listening is more than an auditory experience. Nurse-midwives listen observantly to hear clearly. They communicate confidence in the care of their clients in everyday matters. They hear clearly, and their clients respond.

The rewards of our practice are many, but we have faced some challenges, too. On the rare occasions that things go wrong, we are scrutinized intensely. Vacation coverage is difficult to find. Other challenges include complying with regulations and legislation, finding appropriate resources for medical consultation and referral, and dealing with misperceptions of our practice within the larger health care system. These issues are not unique to our practice, as the next section shows.

PROFESSIONAL ISSUES

Image

Although there is universal recognition of the term "midwife," the word also conjures up a variety of images, some positive and others negative. After their first encounter with a nurse-midwife, many people comment that they are surprised at how "normal" and/or how "professional" she or he was, but most are unable to say just what they expected. Stereotypes that have been voiced about nurse-midwives include "old, stooped, with stringy gray hair," "someone shuffling around in jeans and Birkenstocks," "someone practicing illegally," and "backward." These images are damaging and misleading. In contrast, actual experiences with nurse-midwives are judged overwhelmingly positive. A commonly heard refrain from clients of nurse-midwives is that every woman should have the privilege of being cared for by a nurse-midwife.

Part of the confusion about the image of the midwife stems from the different types of midwives that can be found in the United States. In addition to certified nurse-midwives, people may have heard about direct-entry midwives, lay midwives, and granny midwives. A direct-entry midwife is someone who has completed formal academic midwifery preparation without a nursing background. These individuals tend to have baccalaureate degrees in areas other than nursing, and are more likely to practice in the home or birth center. Lay midwives are typically associated with home birth practice and informal training or apprenticeship experience. A new type of this practitioner evolved in response to a counterculture movement in the 1960s. Over time, some of this group developed training courses, ranging from weekend workshops to intense academic programs. An unfortunate result of this lack of standardization has been marked variation between practitioners, and thus difficulty in characterizing this practice as professional. Granny midwives are women who attended births of women in communities throughout the Southeastern United States from the founding of the country until the middle 20th century. The granny midwife was likewise apprentice trained, and was responding to a need in her community (Rooks, 1997).

From this discussion, it is no wonder that the public image of the nurse-midwife is unclear. In addition to consumer confusion, there has been a fair amount of professional resistance to nurse-midwives from the medical community. This is not unlike the response to other APNs. Despite both confusion and resistance, the ACNM is committed to ensuring that a positive image of the professional midwife emerge, and seeks media opportunities to educate consumers about the role of the nurse-midwife. Even with these efforts, each nurse-midwife in clinical practice also spends a portion of the day explaining who she or he is and striving to both educate and improve the image of the midwife—one patient at a time.

Credentialing

In 1994, the ACNM made the difficult decision to develop a mechanism to accredit midwifery education programs that do not require a nursing credential. The reader is advised to carefully weigh this decision in the context of advanced practice nursing as described throughout this book. In addition, the certification body, the ACC, similarly decided to give graduates of these programs the same examination administered to graduates of nurse-midwifery education programs (Burst, 1995; Shah & Hsia, 1996). These decisions were based on political realities. First, an increasing number of states or hospitals were granting recognition to attend births to individuals whose credentials to practice were less than those established by the ACNM. Second, New York passed a midwifery practice act with the intent of having all midwives take the same examination. The assumption was made that, with equivalent educational criteria, a sound program could be developed for those who desired midwifery without a nursing degree (Williams & Kelley, 1998). The ultimate reason for the ACNM's decision was to advance a single standard for professional midwifery in this country.

Once that decision was made, the ACNM's DOA developed accreditation standards that included skills, knowledge, and competencies in health science that would be prerequisite to midwifery practice. In addition, each graduate must successfully complete college-level courses in biology, chemistry, microbiology, anatomy and physiology, human development, psychology, epidemiology/statistics, pathophysiology, and nutrition (Burst, 1995). The profession also supported research to examine the quality of education and practice of these early graduates. A pilot study at the State University of New York Health Science Center "confirmed that direct-entry students could acquire and demonstrate the basic health skills at a level equivalent to their RN classmates" (Fullerton, Shaw, Holmes, Roe, & Campau, 1998).

This decision by the ACNM has been met with mixed reactions. There are those who believe that these initiatives further obscure advanced nursing practice and make it even more difficult for APNs to attain some of the regulatory and legislative supports they seek. However, the ACNM may be at the cutting edge of developing a transdisciplinary workforce, a legion of people with different backgrounds but the same core set of midwifery competencies. It is difficult to predict where this type of cross-training will go. Part of its ability to succeed will rest on the state regulatory agencies. In 16 states, midwifery, without an RN credential, is regulated by a state agency. In 11 more states, the practice of midwifery by non-nurses is legal but unregulated. There are 15 states in which one must have an RN credential to practice legally as a midwife (ACNM, 1999). If the demand for this type of practitioner grows, and states use the ACNM national standards, which demonstrate equivalent preparation, the public will be assured of a well-qualified provider. Such a group does seem consistent with projections regarding the type of workforce needed in the future (Senge, 1990).

Congruence/Incongruence with APNs

In our opinion, the ACNM's commitments to expand the pool of available midwives and to include non-nurse midwives in a diverse midwifery workforce make it difficult for the organization to advocate master's-level preparation for all CNMs. In this sense, midwifery is diverging from the vision of advanced nursing practice advocated in this text. Several observations can be made, however, that suggest that the mainstreaming of nurse-midwifery within advanced nursing practice may be inevitable. Despite the fact that there are inconsistencies regarding the CNM role within advanced nursing practice, CNMs are developing in ways congruent with the vision that is bringing together CNSs, CRNAs, NPs, and other APNs. The core competencies defined by the ACNM and their operationalization are consistent with the core competencies of advanced practice described in Chapter 3. Most nurse-midwifery education is delivered in master's-level programs. Clinical and regulatory issues such as access to and availability of services as well as second licensure for APNs are likely to engage CNMs in collaborative efforts to promote the values and vision driving advanced practice. Some states already require a master's degree for licensing as an APN (including CNMs) and/or for prescriptive authority; others have established a date by which a master's degree will be required. These precedents could well affect federal funding for nurse-midwifery education. It is unlikely that nurse-midwives will risk the legal privileges for which they fought so hard by resisting efforts to ensure a common definition of advanced nursing practice across state and federal laws and regulations. Appeals to the ACNM have been made by CNMs in states that have passed the requirement for a master's degree. The ACNM Board of Directors has responded by reaffirming support for certificate programs and referring members to other resources and offering specific strategic suggestions. Safriet (1992), an attorney, has argued that consistency in the definition of advanced nursing practice and in the criteria for being licensed as an APN is needed if APNs are to be able to practice with the autonomy that other professionals enjoy. In the current climate, however, it is difficult to anticipate how nurse-midwifery will address the regulatory complexity that is likely to result from the entry of non-nurses into midwifery. Whether the regulatory climate will be more or less open to innovative programs such as those contemplated by the ACNM is not clear.

These are the driving forces that are likely to carry CNMs and nurse-midwifery along in their currents or wake as APN roles are defined and regulated at federal and state levels. Failure to be involved or opposition to the changes will undermine nurse-midwifery's efforts to secure accessible health care for individuals and may well undo its historical legislative achievements, which have enabled CNMs to practice autonomously.

Collegial Relationships and Autonomy

It will come as no surprise to the reader that the factors that have been associated with job satisfaction are often the areas in which barriers to nurse-midwifery practice exist. These factors include working with competent personnel, having high-quality client interactions, having the time to provide a preferred style of care, being involved with clients' care plans and decision making, having good interpersonal relationships with other CNMs and with backup physicians, having professional autonomy, experiencing feelings of personal worth, and participating in teamwork (Collins, 1990). Although nurse-midwives can enjoy many of these rewards, as the earlier description of practice at the birth center shows, they often encounter difficulties in securing them, especially with regard to relationships with physicians, professional autonomy, and workload. For both the nurse-midwifery profession and individual CNMs, the goal is to pursue productive, collaborative relationships with all involved.

PHYSICIANS

Individual CNMs and individual physicians often get along and develop the kind of mature collaborative relationships described in Chapter 11. However, the current health care environment, in which organizations and providers are scrambling to cut costs and services, is not conducive to building the kind of CNM-physician rapport that has made so many CNM-run practices successful. Barriers to effective working relationships between CNMs and physicians often arise within organizations. Although there may be individual members of organized medical groups with whom CNMs work well, the organizations themselves often spend time and money on efforts to restrict APNs' ability to practice autonomously. These efforts include lobbying against federal and state laws and regulations that are favorable to CNMs and other APNs. Chapter 21 describes the American Medical Association's recent public relations campaign to convince the public that APNs and other nonphysician providers are quacks. In a recent document, the American Medical Association described "integrated" practice with APNs, declaring that the physician is still "captain of the ship." Some state medical and nursing associations have found common ground on which to base organizational collaboration. However, CNMs who enjoy excellent collaborative relationships with individual physicians should be alert to the activities of organized medical groups both nationally and within their jurisdictions, so that they can protect their rights to practice nurse-midwifery and encourage their physician colleagues to speak out against limitations on CNM practice.

In hospitals and communities in which physicians continue to have (or are seen as having) power over who can and cannot practice, entrepreneurial CNMs may have more difficulty gaining clinical privileges or medical backup. Often, CNMs need to apply to a hospital's medical board if they wish to be able to attend laboring women in that hospital. A CNM who is the first APN to apply for these privileges in that hospital must be prepared to blaze a trail in everything, from attempting to change hospital bylaws and educating labor and delivery nursing staff regarding CNM practice, to obtaining a chart box in medical records, to negotiating for a locker in a changing room! (Scoggin, 1997).

Whether they need clinical privileges or not, CNMs must have medical consultation and backup available. This requirement may be incorporated into a state practice act, but, even if it is not, clinical practice and ACNM standards demand it. For the CNM working in an agency, formal and informal structures to ensure physician availability are likely to be established. If the CNM is the first one to practice in the organization, these structures will have to be developed. Regardless of practice setting, CNMs need to have a physician with whom they can consult or to whom they can make a referral when needed. Entrepreneurial CNMs will find physicians who are quite willing to be available and welcome the opportunity to collaborate. However, one may find oneself in the position of negotiating for such backup with physicians who are reluctant at best and actively hostile at worst. Many times, it is a matter of education, public relations (see Chapter 21), and consumer demand. Just seeing the care provided at a CNM-run birth center can diminish resistance and elicit support. A combination of interpersonal skills, business savvy, and marketing strategies can help CNMs overcome barriers that arise from lack of knowledge, lack of trust, and power imbalances.

BARRIERS TO PRACTICE

Legislative, Regulatory, and Financial Barriers

Last but not least, there continue to exist barriers to full-scope nurse-midwifery practice. Restrictions to practice can be found at the local, state, and federal levels. If interpersonal, marketing, and public relations efforts fail to secure admitting and clinical privileges for CNMs, legislation that ensures CNMs and other APNs access to these privileges will be needed (ACNM, 1997c). Inequitable reimbursement for their services remains a problem for CNMs in many states. Legislation and regulations that mandate reimbursement equitable to the value of CNMs' work, practice costs, and malpractice expenses must be enacted. Nurse-midwifery care should be an option in managed care systems, but it may not be if APNs and consumers do not make their voices heard. Nurse-midwives must have prescriptive authority, and greater uniformity and consistency of regulations at the federal and state levels for prescribing and dispensing medications are needed. Nurse-midwives must be assured of a continuing source of professional liability insurance. Allocations for nurse-midwifery education from federal and state funding agencies are at risk in the current political climate, in which many politicians are seeking to minimize government initiatives that promote health and education. Medicare and Medicaid must ensure facility fee payment for birth centers.

Workload

When there is a full complement of CNMs to share the work of night call (e.g., being on call one or two nights a week), clinics, and other responsibilities, the unpredictable timing of labor and delivery and the erratic sleep patterns that result are manageable (Flanagan, 1993). For many CNMs, especially those in solo or independent practices, however, a full complement of staff is a luxury. To give their best to their clients and to stay healthy, CNMs with a heavy on-call schedule need to develop self-care strategies that enable them to balance work with personal responsibilities and relationships. The sabbatical has been proposed as one way to promote professional development while decreasing the demands of full-scope practice (Keleher, 1993). This is likely to work only in large, well-funded practices. In addition, finding other CNMs who can cover for vacation and sick time can become a minor crisis. The physical and emotional demands of "catching" babies, in addition to the long hours and periods of sleep deprivation, mean that nurse-midwifery is not for everyone. For those who love it, the satisfaction of watching pregnancy progress, the physical and mental demands of labor and delivery, the element of unpredictability in the timing of birth, and the joy of birth make nurse-midwifery fascinating, exciting, and personally rewarding (Lubic, 1997).

CONCLUSION

In spite of the resistance from the established medical community, there is a growing demand and need for nurse-midwives' unique services. Nurse-midwives are woman centered and family centered (VandeVusse, 1997). They have been thinking globally and acting locally long before it became trendy to do so. They are called to do what they do. As long as there are pregnant women who wish to give birth in an informed and caring fashion, there will be a need for nurse-midwives. Indeed, there are those in the profession who feel that midwifery holds the key to contemporary obstetrical problems (Baldwin, 1999; Rooks, 1998).

Nurse-midwifery, advanced nursing practice, and the profession of nursing in general are at a critical juncture. Although nurse-midwifery is standing somewhat apart from advanced practice efforts, it seems clear that there is a need to recognize the interdependence of advanced nursing practice and nurse-midwifery. By examining the separate yet related courses being charted by the nursing profession (related to advanced nursing practice) and by nurse-midwives (to meet demands for midwifery services), one sees that there is great potential for divisiveness at a time in our history when we need to be unified. The directions nurse-midwives are pursuing may seem unfathomable to those outside nurse-midwifery. The authors have each been involved in political battles for the right to practice and have watched nurse-midwifery evolve from different regions of the United States. We believe there is vision and wisdom in the ACNM's initiatives that will benefit advanced nursing practice and APNs in the long run. However, there appear to be many forces driving the nursing profession toward requiring a master's degree for second licensing, and opposition to this requirement is unlikely to be successful. Mounting such an opposition will drain energy away from CNMs and all APNs whose main goals are to improve access to health care and to provide that care. More important, it could undermine every hard-won political and legislative victory. All CNMs need to give serious consideration to the insights of Safriet (1992), who maintains that APNs will only be able to practice autonomously when there is a uniform definition of advanced nursing practice on which laws and regulations are based.

CNMs have often led the nursing profession into the future, and many of the initiatives mentioned in this chapter indicate that the profession continues to move forward. It may now be time for CNMs to join forces with the nursing profession, which is investing its energy and resources in preserving and expanding the climate for autonomous nursing practice that CNMs helped to create.

ACKNOWLEDGMENT

The authors wish to acknowledge Dorroh and Norton for their important contribution to the first edition of this text (Dorroh & Norton, 1996).

REFERENCES

Ad Hoc Committee on Code of Ethics. (1990). *Code of ethics for certified nurse-midwives.* Washington, DC: American College of Nurse-Midwives.

Ament, L. (1998). Reimbursement, employment, and hospital privilege data of certified nurse-midwifery services. *Journal of Nurse-Midwifery, 43,* 305–309.

American College of Nurse-Midwives. (1989). *Philosophy of the American College of Nurse-Midwives.* Washington, DC: Author.

American College of Nurse-Midwives. (1992). *Expansion of nurse-midwifery practice and skills beyond basic care competencies.* Washington, DC: Author.

American College of Nurse-Midwives. (1993). *Standards for the practice of nurse-midwifery.* Washington, DC: Author.

American College of Nurse-Midwives. (1997a). *ACNM statement on practice settings.* Washington, DC: Author.

American College of Nurse-Midwives. (1997b). *The appropriate use of technology in childbirth.* Washington, DC: Author.

American College of Nurse-Midwives. (1997c). *Barriers to midwifery practice.* Washington, DC: Author.

American College of Nurse-Midwives. (1997d). *Certified nurse-midwives and certified midwives as primary care providers/case managers.* Washington, DC: Author.

American College of Nurse-Midwives. (1997e). *Collaborative management in nurse-midwifery practice for medical, gynecological, and obstetrical conditions.* Washington, DC: Author.

American College of Nurse-Midwives. (1997f). *Continuing competency assessment.* Washington, DC: Author.

American College of Nurse-Midwives. (1997g). *Core competencies for basic nurse-midwifery practice.* Washington, DC: Author.

American College of Nurse-Midwives. (1997h). *Criteria for preaccreditation and accreditation of education programs in nurse-midwifery and midwifery.* Washington, DC: Author.

American College of Nurse-Midwives. (1997i). *Definition of a certified nurse-midwife/definition of midwifery practice.* Washington, DC: Author.

American College of Nurse-Midwives. (1997j). *Midwifery education.* Washington, DC: Author.

American College of Nurse-Midwives. (1998a). *Healthcare/managed care reform.* Washington, DC: Author.

American College of Nurse-Midwives. (1998b). *Mandatory degree requirements for midwives.* Washington, DC: Author.

American College of Nurse-Midwives. (1999). *Nurse-midwifery today: A handbook of state laws & regulations.* Washington, DC: Author.

Avery, M. D. (1992). Advanced nurse-midwifery practice. *Journal of Nurse-Midwifery, 37,* 150–154.

Baldwin, K. A. (1999). The midwifery solution to contemporary problems in American obstetrics. *Journal of Nurse-Midwifery, 44,* 75–79.

Bellack, J., Graber, D., O'Neil, E. H., & Musham, C. (1998). Curriculum trends in nurse-midwifery education: Views of program directors. *Journal of Nurse-Midwifery, 43,* 341–350.

Bergstrom, L. (1997). Midwifery as a discipline. *Journal of Nurse-Midwifery, 42,* 417–420.

Brooten, D., Kumar, S., Brown, L. P., Butts, P., Finkler, S. A., Bakewell-Sachs, S., Gibbons, A., & Delivoria-Papadopoulos, M. (1986). A randomized clinical trial of early hospital discharge and home follow-up of very-low-birth-weight infants. *New England Journal of Medicine, 315,* 934–939.

Burst, H. V. (1995). An update on the credentialing of midwives by the American College of Nurse-Midwives. *Journal of Nurse-Midwifery, 40,* 290–296.

Carr, K. C. (1999). Creating off-campus/distance learning courses for midwifery education: A brief introduction. *Journal of Nurse-Midwifery, 44,* 57–64.

Carrington, B. W., & Decker, B. (1997). A master's degree for entry-level ACNM certified-midwives: An option or necessity? *Journal of Nurse-Midwifery, 42,* 364–366.

Collins, C. (1990). *CNM job satisfaction: Luxury or necessity?* Presented at the ACNM Convention, Atlanta, GA.

Corry, M. P., & Rooks, J. (1999). Public education: Promoting the midwifery model of care in partnership with the Maternity Center Association. *Journal of Nurse-Midwifery, 44,* 47–56.

Crofts, A. J. (1994). Entrepreneurship—the realities of today. *Journal of Nurse-Midwifery, 39,* 39–42.

Declercq, E. R., Paine, L. L., Dejoseph, J. F., & Simmes, D. (1998). State regulation, payment policies, and nurse-midwife services. *Health Affairs, 17,* 190–200.

Dorroh, M. W., & Norton, S. F. (1996). The certified nurse-midwife. In A. B. Hamrick, J. A. Spross, & C. M. Hanson (Eds.), *Advanced practice nursing: An integrative approach* (pp. 395–420). Philadelphia: W. B. Saunders.

Dower, C. M., Miller, J. E., O'Neil, E. H., and the Taskforce on Midwifery. (1999). *Charting a course for the 21st century: The future of midwifery.* San Francisco: Pew Health Professions Commission and the UCSF Center for the Health Professions.

Flanagan, J. (1993). Speaking up and talking out—barriers to nurse-midwifery practice. *Journal of Nurse-Midwifery, 38,* 246–251.

Franklin, M. (1994). The nurse-midwifery challenge. *Journal of Nurse-Midwifery, 39,* 110–111.

Fullerton, J. T. (1994). Reflections on nurse-midwifery role and functions. *Journal of Nurse-Midwifery, 39,* 107–109.

Fullerton, J. T., & Severino, R. (1995). Factors that predict performance on the national certificaton examiniation for nurse-midwives. *Journal of Nurse-Midwifery, 40,* 19–25.

Fullerton, J. T., Shah, M. A., Holmes, G., Roe, V., & Campau, N. (1998). Direct entry midwifery education: Evaluation of program innovations. *Journal of Nurse-Midwifery, 43,* 102–105.

Hsia, L. (1991). Midwives and the empowerment of women. *Journal of Nurse-Midwifery, 36,* 85–87.

Hunter, L. P., & Lops, V. R. (1994). Critical thinking and the nurse-midwifery management process. *Journal of Nurse-Midwifery, 39,* 43–46.

Johnson, P. G., & The Midwifery Research Project Group. (1998). Midwife and nurse-midwife: The effect of title on perception and confidence in services provided by professional midwives. *Journal of Nurse-Midwifery, 43,* 296–304.

Keleher, K. C. (1993). Sabbatical leaves for nurse-midwives in clinical practice. *Journal of Nurse-Midwifery, 38,* 165–167.

Keleher, K. C. (1998). Collaborative practice, characteristics, barriers, benefits, and implications for midwifery. *Journal of Nurse-Midwifery, 43,* 8–11.

Kraus, N. (1997a). Practice profile of members of the American College of Nurse-Midwives: Findings of a direct mail survey. *Journal of Nurse-Midwifery, 42,* 355–363.

Kraus, N. (1997b). What's in a name: Defining the professions of midwifery. *Journal of Nurse-Midwifery, 42,* 69–70.

Lubic, R. W. (1997). Principles for a successful professional life. *Journal of Nurse-Midwifery, 42,* 53–58.

Miller, S., King, T., Lurie, P., & Choitz, P. (1997). Certified nurse-midwife and physician collaborative practice: Piloting a survey on the Internet. *Journal of Nurse-Midwifery, 42,* 308–315.

Nitzsche, R. E. (1995). 40 years old and still growing. *Quickening, 26*(2), 2.

Oakley, D., Murtland, T., Mayes, F., Hayashi, R., Petersen, B. A., Rorie, C., & Andersen, F. (1995). Processes of care: Comparisons of certified nurse-midwives and obstetricians. *Journal of Nurse-Midwifery, 40,* 399–403.

Roberts, J. (1997). The core competencies for basic midwifery practice: Critical ACNM document revised. *Journal of Nurse-Midwifery, 42,* 371–372.

Rooks, J. P. (1997). *Midwifery and childbirth in America.* Philadelphia: Temple University Press.

Rooks, J. P. (1998). Unity in midwifery: Realities and alternative. *Journal of Nurse-Midwifery, 43,* 315–319.

Safriet, B. (1992). Health care dollars and regulatory sense: The role of advanced practice nursing. *Yale Journal of Regulation, 9,* 417–488.

Scoggin, J. (1997). The historical relationship of nurse-midwifery with medicine. *Journal of Nurse-Midwifery, 42,* 49–52.

Scupholme, A., & Walsh, L. (1994). Home-based services by nurse-midwives. *Journal of Nurse-Midwifery, 39,* 358–362.

Senge, P. M. (1990). *The fifth discipline: The art and practice of the learning organization.* New York: Doubleday/Currency.

Shah, M. S., & Hsia, L. (1996). Direct entry midwifery education: History in the making. *Journal of Nurse-Midwifery, 41,* 351–353.

VandeVusse, L. (1997). Sculpting a nurse-midwifery philosophy: Ernestine Wiedenbach's influence. *Journal of Nurse-Midwifery, 42,* 43–48.

Varney, H. (1996). *Nurse-midwifery* (3rd ed.). Boston: Blackwell Scientific Publications.

Williams, D. R., & Kelley, M. A. (1998). Core competency-based education, certification and practice: The nurse-midwifery model. *Advanced Practice Nursing Quarterly, 4,* 63–71.

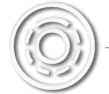

The Certified Registered Nurse Anesthetist

- M A R G A R E T   F A U T - C A L L A H A N
- M I C H A E L   J.   K R E M E R

INTRODUCTION

As noted in Chapter 1, nurse anesthesia is the oldest organized specialty in nursing. Standardized postgraduate education, credentialing, and continuing education were all areas pioneered by certified registered nurse anesthetists (CRNAs). CRNAs were among the first nurse specialists to receive direct reimbursement for their services, and have a history of activism in legislative and regulatory matters, such as prescriptive authority. This chapter discusses professional definitions of nurse anesthesia practice and issues important to the specialty. The American Association of Nurse Anesthetists (AANA) is described, and its model of professional competence for CRNAs is presented. Nurse anesthesia education, credentialing, certification, and recertification processes are all explored. A profile of current CRNA practice is presented, reimbursement mechanisms are delineated, and projections for future trends are proposed.

PROFESSIONAL DEFINITIONS

A CRNA is a registered nurse who is educationally prepared for, and competent to engage in, the practice of nurse anesthesia. CRNAs are both responsible and accountable to others for their individual professional practices. As well, nurse anesthetists are capable of exercising independent professional judgment within their scopes of competence and licensure (Jordan, 1994).

Nurse anesthesia is not a medically delegated act (Jordan, 1994). The practice of anesthesia is not exclusively the practice of medicine or the practice of nursing. It has been said that, if anesthesia is administered by a nurse, it is the practice of nursing, whereas physician-administered anesthesia is the practice of medicine (Gunn, 1991).

Licensure for CRNAs and other advanced practice nurses (APNs) varies by state, as discussed elsewhere in this text (see Chapter 22). No state requires that nurse anesthetists be supervised by anesthesiologists. CRNAs work in collaboration with providers from a variety of backgrounds: surgeons, dentists, podiatrists, and anesthesiologists. The degree to which CRNA practice is addressed in state nurse practice acts is not consistent; for example, in New Jersey, nurse anesthesia practice is regulated to a higher degree than in other states. Legislated prescriptive authority variability affects CRNA practice. Debate continues as to whether CRNAs need prescriptive authority to work in most settings. Conventional wisdom holds that CRNAs do not require prescriptive authority protection because CRNAs are most commonly institutionally based and administer, but do not independently prescribe, medications. Federal law indicates that nurse anesthesia practice and related drug administration is not prescriptive but is rather a request for anesthesia services. Choosing anesthesia techniques and selecting and ordering drugs by nurse anesthetists are not construed as prescriptive behavior by the federal courts (M. Tobin, personal communication, 1995).

Nurse anesthesia practice is, by historical and legal precedents, part of nursing practice. Two precedent-setting cases were *Frank v. Smith,* 175 Ky. 416, 194 S.W. 375 (1917) and *Chalmers-Francis v. Nelson,* 6 Cal. 2d 402, 57 P.2d (1936) (cited in Thatcher, 1953). The latter case involved Dagmar Nelson, a California nurse anesthetist. Legal challenges to Nelson's right to provide anesthesia came from local anesthesiologists, with resulting litigation eventually going to the U.S. Supreme Court. The professional organization representing CRNAs at that time, the National Association of Nurse Anesthetists, filed an amicus curiae brief with the Supreme Court. The case was a watershed in deciding the legality of nurse-administered anesthesia (Bankert, 1989). Case law is replete with other examples of successful challenges by nurse anesthetists for their right to practice.

The question of which professional group CRNAs should be aligned with has been a topic explored legally, ethically, and educationally since the inception of the practice of nurse anesthesia. Some courts of law have held that nurse anesthesia is not the practice of medicine; rather, it is by virtue of nursing licensure that CRNAs are able to practice anesthesia legally. Other courts have found that anesthesiology cannot be easily classified within either the discipline of nursing or the discipline of medicine (Waugaman, 1991).

The roles of physicians and nurses in anesthesia overlap. The components of this overlap include a similar educational heritage, comparable socialization into the specialty, constant time and space in the operating room environment, and like relationships and therapeutic interventions with patients. The noncurative nature of surgical anesthesia is more similar to the practice of nursing than it is to medicine (Faut, 1984).

Callahan (1995) reported that there was an 88% role overlap in the practice of nurse anesthetists and anesthesiologists as evaluated by experts in both fields. The findings of Callahan mirror those of Cromwell and Rosenbach (1988), health care economists who extensively studied economics in anesthesiology and cost-effective anesthesia provider mixes. These investigators found that CRNAs were underutilized, close substitutes for anesthesiologists and that full utilization of CRNAs would result in significant savings in health care expenditures. Nurse anesthetists frequently work with anesthesiologists. There is ongoing debate about the merits of the "anesthesia care team" (e.g., CRNAs practicing with anesthesiologists). Publications on this topic in the anesthesiology literature have at times advocated team anesthesia from both economic and safety perspectives (Abenstein & Warner, 1996), implying that anesthesiologist involvement in anesthesia care improves outcomes, although existing outcomes research does not uniformly support this contention.

Acknowledging that the practices of nurse anesthetists and anesthesiologists are similar, the courts had to decide if nurse anesthetists and anesthesiologists indeed compete in practice settings (*Oltz v. St. Peter's Community Hospital*, 861 F.2d 1440, 1443 [9th Cir. 1988]; cited in Bankert, 1989]). There is no other area of health care in which a provider can substitute for a physician as does the CRNA in the provision of anesthesia services. Institutional credentialing may limit the ability of CRNAs to perform functions such as discharging patients from the facility or in components of prescription writing. However, strategies have been developed to overcome these barriers in various settings.

CRNA PRACTICE PROFILES

In 1998, 95% of the 27,807 practicing American nurse anesthetists were AANA members. The AANA surveys its members annually, with a response rate of 62% for fiscal year 1998. For the same year, AANA survey data showed that 39.3% of CRNAs were hospital employed, 36.4% worked in groups composed of CRNAs and anesthesiologists, 14.3% were self-employed or CRNA group employed, and 10.1% were in other types of practices. These data reflect a 5% decrease in hospital employment over 4 years (Garde, 1998).

With increased managed care market penetration, hospitals endeavor to decrease their fixed costs, such as payroll. Surgical case volumes have remained constant while reimbursement rates have fallen. An initial reaction to this trend was decreasing the number of available beds and licensed staff in acute care settings. However, to deal with current surgical patient volumes, some hospitals have found it necessary to aggressively recruit professional nursing staff and re-open previously closed units. Economic considerations such as decreased reimbursement have caused hospital employment for CRNAs and other APNs to be less common as cost shifting of these providers out of hospitals occurs. This cost-shifting may lead to managing caseloads with fewer practitioners who may be group employed or independent contractors.

Regarding practice locations, 62% of AANA members are employed in urban settings. In smaller localities, 12% of CRNAs work in towns with fewer than 50,000 residents and 22% of CRNAs practice in rural areas (Garde, 1998). These rural CRNAs significantly increase access to health care for rural citizens. For example, in downstate Illinois, 58 hospitals serving 300,000 citizens have anesthesia services solely provided by CRNAs. Over 70% of anesthesia in rural areas is provided by nurse anesthetists. Orkin (1998) repored on a survey of rural hospital administrators regarding their satisfaction with anesthesia outcomes in settings where most anesthesia was provided by CRNAs. There was strong satisfaction with anesthesia services provided by CRNAs reported by the administrators in this dataset. Another study compared morbidity and mortality for gallbladder surgery in one rural hospital for over 25 years, with anesthesia provided by the same CRNA, against gallbladder surgery morbidity and mortality in urban hospitals. Controlling for significant variables such as patient acuity, there was no statistically significant difference in morbidity and mortality between the two groups (Callaghan, 1995).

Employment Factors

The CRNA Manpower Study from the National Center for Nursing Research (1991) projected a need for over 35,000 CRNAs by the year 2010. The current average CRNA age of 45 reflects this major potential for increased demand for CRNAs in the near future (Garde, 1998; Jaffee & Revak, 1998).

The anesthesia provider employment marketplace will be dynamic for the near future because of the impact of managed care. Trends in physician practice include unionization and hospital employment. Multiple variables affect anesthesia provider mixes in various settings. The term "provider mix" refers to the following variations in anesthesia practice: physicians may practice anesthesia without nurse anesthetists; in team anesthesia, physicians may collaborate with one or more CRNAs; or CRNAs may practice anesthesia collaborating with the operating surgeon, dentist, or podiatrist.

Team anesthesia is the predominant model within which CRNAs practice. Although some anesthesiologists may be ambivalent about nurse anesthesia, Dr. Robert Dripps, a pioneering academic anesthesiologist, had very positive beliefs about CRNAs.

It is apparent that the physician anesthesiologist offers greater depth of training than the nurse anesthetist, but this does not necessarily qualify the physician as a better anesthetist. By achieving the technical skills and the appropriate experience and knowledge, a conscientious nurse can easily surmount the gap in training. An anesthesiologist, acting as a technician, who fails to keep abreast of advances in medicine soon loses the advantage. In most large hospital departments, nurse and physician anesthetists and technicians work in harmony. . . . Considering the extensive national demands for anesthesia care, it is unlikely that all anesthestics will ever be given solely by physicians. As paralleled by the trend toward midwifery in obstetrics, there is and always will be a need for nurse anesthetists.

(Dripps, 1977, p. 3)

Nurse anesthesia education and anesthesia practice have advanced tremendously in the time since these thoughts were recorded. Although medical anesthesiology residency programs take longer, educational requirements for the two provider groups are similar (Jordan, 1994; Kaye, Scibetta, & Grogono, 1999).

Another factor impacting employment is the anesthesia assistant. Programs at Emory and Case Western universities prepare anesthesia assistants, who go directly from their undergraduate education in nonclinical disciplines to training as anesthesia assistants. Therefore, the preparation for this role is different from that of physicians, nurses, or physician assistants. Practice privileges of anesthesia assistants, who are legally recognized in only four states at this writing, are linked to a sponsoring physician.

Access to Care

As stated earlier, nurse anesthetists are involved in the administration of 65% of the 26 million anesthetics given in this country each year. Furthermore, nurse anesthetists provide approximately 70% of anesthesia given in rural settings. CRNAs collaborate closely with other providers, such as surgeons and primary care practitioners, in all settings. Without the services of CRNAs in these communities, many small hospitals would close, leaving few alternatives for health care. Some rural CRNAs have completed additional training in the management of acute and chronic pain and offer services such as pain clinics so that patients do not have to travel to distant centers for pain treatment.

CRNAs have traditionally been represented in other underserved population setting areas. Urban and county hospitals frequently use CRNAs. Nurse anesthetists are actively involved in anesthesia care in settings such as the Maryland Institute for Emergency Medical Services, Chicago's Cook County Hospital, and San Francisco General Hospital. Many CRNAs practice in the Veterans Administration hospital system, dealing with complex surgical patients. The military heavily relies on and actively recruits nurse anesthetists. A CRNA may be the only anesthesia provider on a Navy vessel. In such a situation, knowledge of regional anesthesia and the ability to practice independently enable the CRNA to capably respond to mass casualty situations, in which many trauma victims simultaneously require anesthesia.

Settings in Which CRNAs Practice

With most surgery currently conducted on a same-day admission or outpatient basis, patients may not meet their anesthetist until shortly before surgery. Multiple mechanisms, such as telephone interviews or preanesthesia clinics, can be used to conduct preanesthesia assessment and allow anesthesia providers to discuss care options, procedures, and risks with patients. Patients and health care providers continue to readjust to this reimbursement-driven shift in services. Clinical information obtained through telephone interviews is confirmed when patients arrive; detailed physical assessment and establishing rapport also occur on the day of surgery.

Anesthesia services can facilitate diagnosis, as in the case of the "curare test" for myasthenia gravis. Anesthesia as a therapeutic modality is seen in the treatment of acute and chronic pain; it is also used in psychiatry for conducting interviews under the influence of ultra-short-acting intravenous barbiturates, and for accelerated detoxification of opioid-dependent patients. However, the most common use of anesthesia resources is for the administration of surgical anesthesia.

Anesthesia is frequently used in obstetrics, for providing analgesia and anesthesia to parturients. Regional anesthesia and applied pharmacology have greatly advanced obstetrical anesthesia, which in the past relied on systemic drugs that could cause neonatal depression. Epidural analgesia has become increasingly common for vaginal and cesarean section delivery, often obviating the need for general anesthesia and its attendant risks (Bader & Datta, 1994). In addition to utilizing regional anesthesia in obstetrical and postpartum settings, CRNAs work collaboratively with other clinicians in these areas to manage intra- and postpartum pain with a variety of pharmacological and nonpharmacological modalities (Faut-Callahan & Paice, 1990).

International Practice

Internationally, nurse anesthesia practice exists in western Europe, portions of eastern Europe, Scandinavia, and parts of Africa and Asia. The International Federation of Nurse Anesthetists (IFNA) was chartered in 1989 with 11 founding member countries, and has grown to 20 member countries representing over 30,000 nurse anesthetists worldwide. The AANA, under the leadership of past president and IFNA executive director Ronald Caulk, CRNA, FAAN, has spearheaded this fledgling organization. The IFNA meets every 3 years to discuss issues related to practice and education. Although the practice of nurse anesthesia reaches around the globe, the scope of practice and educational processes for nurse anesthetists vary from one country to another (Kelly, 1994). CRNA volunteers participate in charitable surgical services throughout the third world through services such as Operation Smile and the Orbis Project. These volunteer surgeons, nurses, and CRNAs provide services such as cleft lip and palate repair for children in underserved areas. Health Volunteers Overseas also provides voluntary anesthesia and surgical services in addition to teaching clinical anesthesia in third-world countries (M. Catchpole, personal communication, 1995).

A study by McAuliffe and Henry (1998) demonstrated that nurses were providing anesthesia services in more than 100 countries that comprise 60% of the member states of the World Health Organization. Data were collected from 96 countries, in all world regions, at four levels of development, and were analyzed for commonalities and differences. The authors found that the use of nurses to provide anesthesia was not related to a country's level of development. Nurses provided anesthesia in two thirds of developed, developing, and least developing countries, working with and without anesthesiologists. Nurses in this sample performed all the critical tasks required in the administration of anesthesia. Nurse anesthetists worldwide are making a significant contribution to health.

SCOPE OF PRACTICE

Anesthesiology is the art and science of rendering a patient insensible to pain by administration of anesthetic agents and related drugs and procedures. Anesthesia and anesthesia-related care are those services that anesthesia professionals provide on request, assignment, or referral by the patient's physician (or other health care professional authorized by law), most often to facilitate diagnostic, therapeutic, or surgical procedures. In other instances, the referral or request for consultation or assistance may be for management of pain associated with labor and delivery, management of acute and chronic ventilatory problems, or management of acute or chronic pain through the performance of selected diagnostic or therapeutic blocks or other forms of pain management (AANA, 1992a).

The scope of practice of the CRNA encompasses the professional functions, privileges, and responsibilities associated with nurse anesthesia practice. These activities are performed in collabortion with qualified and legally authorized professional health care providers. CRNAs are prepared to recognize situations in which health care requirements are beyond their individual competencies and to seek consultation or referral when such situations arise (AANA, 1992a).

Anesthesia care is provided by CRNAs in four general categories: (1) preanesthetic evaluation and preparation; (2) anesthesia induction, maintenance, and emergence; (3) postanesthesia care; and (4) perianesthetic and clinical support functions. Parallels between nursing and nurse anesthesia can be seen. CRNAs perform preanesthetic assessments, plan appropriate anesthetic interventions, implement planned anesthetic care, and evaluate patients postoperatively to determine the efficacy of their interventions. CRNAs working alone routinely perform all of these aspects of clinical practice. When CRNAs and anesthesiologists work together in "team" anesthesia, a variety of factors, such as local anesthesia practice patterns, determine to what extent each practitioner is involved in specific anesthesia care areas.

Preoperative evaluation has become more complex with the increasing acuity of surgical patients. Thorough preanesthetic assessments, combined with specialty consultation as needed, are essential activities at which nurse anesthetists must be proficient. Other aspects of preanesthetic patient preparation are requesting indicated diagnostic studies; selecting, obtaining, ordering, or administering preanesthetic medications and fluids; and obtaining informed consent for anesthesia (AANA, 1992a).

Developing and implementing an anesthetic care plan is another aspect of CRNA practice. This care plan is formulated with input from the patient, the surgeon, and, in team anesthesia settings, the collaborating anesthesiologist. Similarly, the choice of administering regional or general anesthesia is not solely the province of any one of the aforementioned participants. Input from the patient, the surgeon, and the anesthetist is relevant in the important decision about which type of anesthetic to administer in a given situation. Compromise and flexibility may be necessary to achieve the goals of surgery and anesthesia without incident.

CRNAs select, obtain, or administer the anesthetics, adjuvant drugs, accessory drugs, and fluids necessary to manage the anesthesia, to maintain physiological homeostasis, and to correct abnormal responses to anesthesia or surgery (AANA, 1992a). When CRNAs perform these activities, they are recognized legally to be providing anesthesia services on request, not to be prescribing as defined by federal law. With the advent of legislated prescriptive authority for CRNAs and other APNs, these providers can prescribe legend and in some cases Schedules II through V controlled substances.

Monitoring is another vital area in which CRNAs participate. Nurse anesthetists select, apply, and insert appropriate noninvasive and invasive monitoring modalities for collecting and interpreting physiological data. These activities are all recognized components of anesthesia services performed on request by CRNAs and are not prescriptive. Criteria for the use of invasive monitors and who places them vary by institution and geographical region. Professional fees associated with the placement of devices such as pulmonary artery catheters at times leads to conflict over which practitioner (e.g., anesthetist or surgeon) will place invasive monitors and receive the associated reimbursement.

Nurse anesthesia practice also includes airway management using endotracheal intubation, mechanical ventilation, and pharmacological support both within and outside the operating room. In some settings, CRNAs are the sole providers of this service. A combination of technical skills required for airway management utilizing a variety of instruments and knowledge of respiratory anatomy and physiology and pharmacology is important. For example, indiscriminate use of muscle relaxants in critically ill ventilator-dependent patients can occur (Loper, Butler, Nessly, & Wild, 1989), leading to undesirable outcomes such as post-traumatic stress syndrome. CRNAs need to remind clinicians caring for ventilator-dependent patients that sedative/amnestic drugs and analgesics need to be included when critically ill patients are mechanically ventilated. As well, the role of the CRNA in helping patients and families to understand these procedures is important.

Nurse anesthetists manage emergence and recovery from anesthesia by selecting, obtaining, ordering, or administering medications, fluids, or ventilatory support in order to maintain homeostasis, to provide relief from pain and anesthesia side effects, and/or to prevent or manage complications (AANA, 1992a). These activities also fall within the scope of providing anesthesia services and are not prescriptive in the traditional sense (e.g., where a practitioner would write a prescription that a pharmacist would fill). Releasing or discharging patients from a postanesthesia care area can be performed by the CRNA. Providing postanesthesia follow-up evaluation and care related to anesthetic side effects or complications are other CRNA functions.

Regional anesthesia is used by many CRNAs in the management of surgical anesthesia, labor pain, and postoperative pain. CRNAs are increasingly involved with pain management services. The use of epidural analgesic infusions and patient-controlled analgesia has greatly contributed to the effective treatment of preventable pain. Nurse anesthetists should have a role in the formulation of protocols and staff education when acute pain protocols are introduced.

Nurse anesthetists respond to emergency situations by providing airway management skills and by implementing basic and advanced life support techniques. CRNAs can provide leadership in these settings, away from the operating room, reinforcing the need for nationally promulgated standards of anesthesia care. One of these standards of care, for example is the measurement of end-tidal carbon dioxide to rule out esophageal intubation (AANA, 1992a).

Nurse anesthetists are bound by the standards of practice adopted by the profession as shown in Table 18–1.

TABLE 18–1 STANDARDS FOR NURSE ANESTHESIA PRACTICE

Introduction

These standards are intended to:

1. Assist the profession in evaluating the quality of care provided by its practitioners.
2. Provide a common base for practitioners to use in their development of a quality practice.
3. Assist the public in understanding what to expect from the practitioner.
4. Support and preserve the basic rights of the patient.

These standards apply to all anesthetizing locations. While the standards are intended to encourage high quality patient care, they cannot assure specific outcomes.

Standard I.

Perform a thorough and complete preanesthesia assessment.

Interpretation:
The responsibility for the care of the patient begins with the preanesthetic assessment. Except in emergency situations, the CRNA has an obligation to complete a thorough evaluation and determine that relevant tests have been obtained and reviewed.

Standard II.

Obtain informed consent for the planned anesthetic intervention from the patient or legal guardian.

Interpretation:
The CRNA shall obtain or verify that an informed consent has been obtained by a qualified provider. Discuss anesthetic options and risks with the patient and/or legal guardian in language the patient and/or legal guardian can understand. Document in the patient's medical record that informed consent was obtained.

Standard III.

Formulate a patient-specific plan for anesthesia care.

Interpretation:
The plan of care developed by the CRNA is based upon comprehensive patient assessment, problem analysis, anticipated surgical or therapeutic procedure, patient and surgeon preferences, and current anesthesia principles.

Standard IV.

Implement and adjust the anesthesia care plan based on the patient's physiological response.

Interpretation:
The CRNA shall induce and maintain anesthesia at required levels. The CRNA shall continuously assess the patient's response to the anesthetic and/or surgical intervention and intervene as required to maintain the patient in a satisfactory physiologic condition.

Standard V.

Monitor the patient's physiologic condition as appropriate for the type of anesthesia and specific patient needs.

A. **Monitor ventilation continuously.** Verify intubation of the trachea by auscultation, chest excursion, and confirmation of carbon dioxide in the expired gas. Continuously monitor end-tidal carbon dioxide during controlled or assisted ventilation. Use spirometry and ventilatory pressure monitors.
B. **Monitor oxygenation continuously** by clinical observation, pulse oximetry, and if indicated, arterial blood gas analysis.
C. **Monitor cardiovascular status continuously** via electrocardiogram and heart sounds. Record blood pressure and heart rate at least every five minutes.
D. **Monitor body temperature continuously** on all pediatric patients receiving general anesthesia and when indicated, on all other patients.
E. **Monitor neuromuscular function and status** when neuromuscular blocking agents are administered.
F. **Monitor and assess the patient's positioning** and protective measures.

Interpretation:
Continuous clinical observation and vigilance are the basis of safe anesthesia care. The standard applies to all patients receiving anesthesia care and may be exceeded at any time at the discretion of the CRNA. Unless otherwise stipulated in the standards a means to monitor and evaluate the patient's status shall be immediately available for all patients. As new patient safety technologies evolve, integration into the current anesthesia practice shall be considered. The omission of any monitoring standards shall be documented and the reason stated on the patient's anesthesia record. The CRNA shall be in constant attendance of the patient until the responsibility for care has been accepted by another qualified health care provider.

Standard VI.

There shall be complete, accurate, and timely documentation of pertinent information on the patient's medical record.

Interpretation:
Document all anesthetic interventions and patient responses. Accurate documentation facilitates comprehensive patient care, provides information for retrospective review and research data, and establishes a medical-legal record.

Table continued on following page

TABLE 18-1 STANDARDS FOR NURSE ANESTHESIA PRACTICE *Continued*

Standard VII.

Transfer the responsibility for care of the patient to other qualified providers in a manner which assures continuity of care and patient safety.

Interpretation:
   The CRNA shall assess the patient's status and determine when it is safe to transfer the responsibility of care to other qualified providers. The CRNA shall accurately report the patient's condition and all essential information to the provider assuming responsibility for the patient.

Standard VIII.

Adhere to appropriate safety precautions, as established within the institution, to minimize the risks of fire, explosion, electrical shock, and equipment malfunction. Document on the patient's medical record that the anesthesia machine and equipment were checked.

Interpretation:
   Prior to use, the CRNA shall inspect the anesthesia machine and monitors according to established guidelines. The CRNA shall check the readiness, availability, cleanliness, and working condition of all equipment to be utilized in the administration of the anesthesia care. When the patient is ventilated by an automatic mechanical ventilator, monitor the integrity of the breathing system with a device capable of detecting a disconnection by emitting an audible alarm. Monitor oxygen concentration continuously with an oxygen supply failure alarm system.

Standard IX.

Precautions shall be taken to minimize the risk of infection to the patient, the CRNA, and other health care providers.

Interpretation:
   Written policies and procedures in infection control shall be developed for personnel and equipment.

Standard X.

Anesthesia care shall be assessed to assure its quality and contribution to positive patient outcomes.

Interpretation:
   The CRNA shall participate in the ongoing review and evaluation of the quality and appropriateness of anesthesia care. Evaluation shall be performed based upon appropriate outcome criteria and reviewed on an ongoing basis. The CRNA shall participate in a continual process of self evaluation and strive to incorporate new techniques and knowledge into practice.

Standard XI.

The CRNA shall respect and maintain the basic rights of patients.

Interpretation:
   The CRNA shall support and preserve the rights of patients to personal dignity and ethical norms of practice.

From the American Association of Nurse Anesthetists. (1996). *Scope and Standards for nurse anesthesia practice.* Park Ridge, IL: Author; reproduced with permission.

Accountability

CRNAs are legally liable for the quality of the services they render. They make independent judgments and decisions as to the appropriateness of their professional services and the probable effects of those services on the patient. A CRNA who believes that the health care plan as it relates to anesthesia for a particular patient is inappropriate should seek consultation for more appropriate direction. CRNAs should be patient advocates and always seek resolution to these issues. If reasonable doubt continues, it is the responsibility of the CRNA to consider withdrawal from rendering the service, provided that the well-being of the patient is not jeopardized (AANA, 1992a).

Credentialing of CRNAs

CRNAs practice according to their expertise, state statutes or regulations, and local institutional policy. Institutional credentialing procedures may require additional evidence of clinical and didactic education in areas such as cardiothoracic or regional anesthesia. State nurse practice acts and practice patterns in the anesthesia community contribute to variability in the scope of nurse anesthesia practice in different settings.

To be a nurse anesthetist, one must meet four requirements:

1. Graduation from an approved nursing school with current state registered nurse licensure
2. Graduation from a nurse anesthesia educational program accredited by the Council on Accreditation of Nurse Anesthesia Educational Programs or its predecessor
3. Successful completion of the certification examination administered by the Council on Certification of Nurse Anesthetists or its predecessor
4. Compliance with criteria for biennial recertification

These criteria are defined by the Council on Recertification of Nurse Anesthetists (AANA, 1992b).

Competence can be partially assured through institutional credentialing processes. A hospital may delineate procedures that the CRNA is authorized to perform by the authority of the governing board. Guidelines for granting CRNAs clinical privileges are found in the *Guidelines and Standards for Nurse Anesthesia Practice* (AANA, 1992a). Recommended clinical privileges for CRNAs are in the areas of preanesthetic preparation and evaluation; anesthesia induction, maintenance and emergence; post-anesthetic care; and perianesthetic and clinical support functions.

ROLE DEVELOPMENT AND MEASURES OF CLINICAL COMPETENCE

The role of the nurse anesthetist encompasses many facets. Callahan (1994) described a competency-based model for nurse anesthesia practice that demonstrated areas in which nurse anesthetists must strive to achieve competence (Fig. 18–1). The unifying themes of caring, collaboration, communication, and technology are defined in Table 18–2. Many of the characteristics of advanced nursing practice described in Chapter 3 are found in this model. Although the model is in its infancy and further research with its use is in progress, it depicts the many facets of the CRNA role. Munguia-Biddle, Maree, Klein, Callahan, and Gilles (1990) defined components of the model and suggested that the nurse anesthesia process is a problem-solving model that utilizes assessment, analysis, planning, implementation, and evaluation in the complex decision making and actions that exemplify CRNA practice within the health care environment. They further define lifelong learning as a part of the nurse anesthesia process. This essential process function is in concert with the changing characteristics of nurse anesthesia practice.

Additional clarification of the components of the model is found in Table 18–3. The nurse anesthesia process parallels the nursing process and emphasizes the importance of this approach to comprehensive anesthesia care following the model and its components; 2 exemplars are provided which describe CRNA practice.

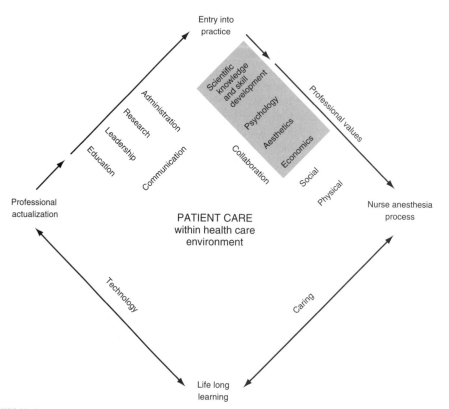

FIGURE 18–1 • Nurse anesthesia practice model. (From Munguia-Biddle, F., Maree, S., Klein, E., Callahan, L., & Gilles, B. [1990]. *Nurse anesthesiology competence evaluation: Mechanism for accountability.* Unpublished document, American Association of Nurse Anesthetists, Park Ridge, IL; reproduced with permission.)

TABLE 18–2 NURSE ANESTHESIA PRACTICE MODEL

The advanced practice of nursing in the specialty of nurse anesthesia has special attributes that speak to the strength and uniqueness of the CRNA role in the provision of anesthesia care in the health environment.

Caring for the patient as a holistic being is an important tenet of CRNA professional behavior. CRNAs strive to be altruistic human beings, believing that caring is essential to one's personal development.

Collaboration between the nurse anesthetist and other members of the health care team takes place in separate and joined activities and responsibilities that are directed at attaining mutual goals of excellence in patient care.

Communication is sharing information to achieve mutual understanding. Communication skills are a cornerstone of patient interviews, imparting information to other health professionals, documentation of practice, and participation as a contributory member in meeting society's health needs.

Technology denotes an area rich in technological advances and scientific content that requires strengthening and updating through the professional life. Practitioners have the ability to apply the nursing process to complex problems at a high level of competence.

From Munguia-Biddle, F., Maree, S., Klein, E., Callahan, L., & Gilles, B. (1990). *Nurse anesthesiology competence evaluation: Mechanism for accountability.* Unpublished document, American Association of Nurse Anesthetists, Park Ridge, IL; reproduced with permission.

TABLE 18–3 DEFINITION OF NURSE ANESTHESIA PRACTICE MODEL COMPONENTS

Professional Actualization

Professional actualization is a dynamic, ongoing endeavor to realize maximum development of professional potential.

Education provides an environment that allows for exploration and application of strategies to facilitate the preparation of future practitioners, thereby assuring continuance.

Leadership demonstrates the ability to define reality, set goals, communicate a vision, and influence the willing participation of others in purposeful action that is directed to goal achievement.

Research encourages active involvement in scientific inquiry as a consumer, participant, or contributor. It is the driving force of actualization that validates our role in the provision of anesthesia services, enhances growth for the nurse anesthetist and the profession, and leads to new knowledge and improved safety in patient care.

Administration provides the interface between people, groups, departments, organizations, professions, and society that enhances individual and collective professional growth.

Professional Values

A **profession** may be defined in terms of the domains of human endeavor valued by the members of the profession. Such are the following domains within the profession of nurse anesthesia practice.

Intellectual. Integral concepts within this domain are based on advanced knowledge in the fields of anatomy, physiology, pathophysiology, technology, and pharmacology as applied to anesthetic practice. The continued development of technical expertise and competence in practice are inherent in this area of concern.

Psychological. The professional nurse anesthetist is concerned with enhancement of the patient's coping skills in a time of possible physical and emotional disruption produced by the perioperative experience. Recognition of the needs of the practitioner are expressed as concern with issues such as communication, autonomy, counseling, and impairment or incompetent practice within the workplace and the profession as a whole.

Aesthetics. Spiritual growth and religious preferences are recognized and respected as inherent to full development of human potential within the patient and the nurse anesthetist. Ethical development and involvement within the political realm encompassing the nurse anesthetist as a member of society is held to be a continual and necessary growth process.

Economics. CRNAs place great value on the historical role of the nurse anesthesia profession in providing continuity of anesthesia care that supports an economically viable health care industry. The exploration of strategies leading to resolution of liability issues as well as mechanisms to increase feelings of potential job security are recognized as valuable to continued professional and personal growth and well-being.

Social. Valued concepts within this domain include enhancement and preservation of the professional role of nurse anesthetists in the societal health-care delivery system, legal and legislative responsibility for competent patient care, constant development of improved standards of care, patient education, and continued liaison with other health care providers.

Physical. Patient safety and the interface between technology and humankind or machines and the patient are of paramount concern. The appropriateness of physical work that considers the impact of schedules, stress, fatigue, and vigilance must be demonstrated in the clinical setting as important factors in securing the patient care environment.

From Munguia-Biddle, F., Maree, S., Klein, E., Callahan, L., & Gilles, B. (1990). *Nurse anesthesiology competence evaluation: Mechanism for accountability.* Unpublished document, American Association of Nurse Anesthetists, Park Ridge, IL; reproduced with permission.

CRNA PRACTICE EXEMPLARS

EXEMPLAR 1: RURAL COMMUNITY HOSPITAL

David and Patty are hospital-employed CRNAs at a community hospital in central Illinois. David has practiced as a CRNA for 20 years, and Patty for 22 years. Their practice includes a physician anesthesiologist, who is also hospital employed. The hospital has four operating rooms and an active obstetrics department, where labor epidurals are provided by the CRNAs and the anesthesiologist. All three anesthesia providers rotate taking call. They act as backups for each other if additional help is needed, such as caring for a multiple trauma patient.

The nurse anesthetists have deep ties with the community in which they practice. Because it is a town of 30,000, many people know each other. David and Patty are active in church and community groups. They are very cognizant of the perceptions of their professional and personal lives. They work with the same surgeons and obstetricians routinely. Competence, caring, and dependability are qualities that David and Patty convey; these attributes help solidify their roles as trusted APNs in the community.

Because the majority of their surgical cases are performed on an outpatient basis, preanesthetic assessment takes place on the outpatient unit, one floor below surgery. The CRNAs or the anesthesiologist conduct a preoperative interview in a private room with the patient. This time is crucial for establishment of the rapport necessary between the patient and their anesthesia providers. The health history is obtained and patients are prompted for additional information as necessary. Anesthetic options are explained using easily understood language. The risks and benefits associated with each anesthetic option are described. Sometimes, surgeons indicate preferences for particular anesthetic techniques; however, the anesthesia provider ensures that patients are comfortable with the proposed anesthetic, its benefits, and potential risks.

On a typical day, several elective surgical cases are scheduled. Emergency cases may be scheduled at any time later in the day. Other clinical activities for David and Patty include the placement and management of labor epidurals, helping with venous access, emergency airway management, and acting as team leaders during cardiac arrests. The CRNAs are consulted on pain and ventilator management. They serve on the pharmacy and therapeutics committee because perioperatively administered medications constitute a large part of the hospital formulary. They are also members of the operating room committee. This committee has representation from operating room nursing, surgery, and anesthesia. Time and resource allocation are two of the priority areas for this committee. These clinical and leadership roles emphasize the core APN competencies:

1. *Expert clinical practice:* The CRNAs have to be highly competent because the other anesthesia providers are frequently busy when they are performing their duties. When taking call, the CRNAs, collaborating with the staff physicians and nurses, are responsible for expert anesthetic assessment, crisis management, decision making, implementation, and evaluation skills.

2. *Expert guidance and coaching of patients, families, and other care providers:* This core competency is evident in both the perioperative and obstetrical arenas. In the obstetrical area, the CRNAs provide expert guidance and coaching of patients and their families regarding labor analgesia that they provide with labor epidurals. The guidelines used for implementation and management of labor epidurals were collectively developed by the anesthesia department, the staff obstetricians, and the labor and delivery unit nurses.

3. *Consultation:* The CRNAs are consulted for pain management; treatment of postoperative/postprocedure nausea and vomiting; ventilator management; acquisition of new equipment for the operating room and intensive care units; oral intake guidelines for surgery and other diagnostic and therapeutic procedures; and their expertise with sedation techniques.

4. *Research skills:* The CRNAs read anesthesia journals and visit anesthesia websites regularly. The rapid development of new technology and pharmacology in anesthesia mandates an ability to critique and utilize these developments to assure evidence-based practice. CRNAs also collaborate in clinical research about anesthesia and pain management.

5. *Clinical and professional leadership:* This core competency is evident on multiple levels. The CRNAs are regarded as clinical leaders in the operating room. Their counsel on positioning, monitoring, and fluid management is important to surgeons and operating room nurses. Professional leadership opportunities exist both in the hospi-

tal and through local forums, as well as in state and national organizations. David and Patty have served on committees for their state professional organization, and stay actively involved in developments affecting their national organization (e.g., writing letters to legislators).

6. *Collaboration:* Collaboration is key to nurse anesthesia practice. The CRNAs collaborate with surgeons, dentists, podiatrists, and the anesthesiologist in their department. There is significant mutual respect between the CRNAs and these clinicians. The long record of clinical competence, dependability, and affability that David and Patty exhibit helps maintain their position as valued collaborators in their practice setting.

7. *Change agent skills:* The CRNAs bring their knowledge, skills, and abilities in perioperative monitoring, pain management, and airway management to their colleagues. One example of how David and Patty brought about change was to advise the hospital to purchase two anesthesia machines with computerized record-keeping capabilities. Rather than having to keep an anesthetic record by hand, this technology only requires the anesthetist to enter patient demographics, drugs and fluids administered, and other information deemed necessary for the case. A laser-printed anesthetic record is printed at the end of each case. The information entered into the computer can also be used for billing and continuous quality improvement.

On a typical day, Patty or David may deal with cases as diverse as an elective cesarean section, a hip pinning in an elderly patient, a closed reduction of a Colles' fracture in a 10-year-old, and placement of labor epidurals. The labor epidurals require monitoring for adequate analgesia as well as potential side effects. Each patient has unique requirements for anesthesia management; often, family members will have questions for the anesthesia providers.

Many of the observations of Dorroh and Norton (1996) and Dorroh and Kelley (Chapter 17) about the role of the certified nurse-midwife (CNM) pertain to the CRNAs depicted in this exemplar. There are many rewards associated with their practice, but there are also challenges. Surgical or anesthetic morbidity and mortality understandably result in close internal and some external scrutiny. CRNAs must be able to defend their actions in terms of congruence with standards of care and existing hospital policies. Vacation coverage can be difficult to find and expensive, given the current undersupply of CRNAs. As with CNMs, CRNAs find that complying with regulations (e.g., Medicare/Medicaid) and legislation can be challenging. Fortunately, state and national professional associations are available for consultation on these issues. Like CNMs, CRNAs deal with "misperceptions of our practice from within the larger health-care system" (Dorroh & Norton, 1996, p. 214). The ongoing challenges for CRNAs and other APNs is to have effective public relations and government relations strategies in place to minimize these misperceptions.

EXEMPLAR 2: ACADEMIC MEDICAL CENTER

Paul is a 38-year-old CRNA employed in a tertiary-level academic medical center. He has practiced in this setting for 10 years. He is a teaching associate in the department of anesthesiology in the school of medicine. His salary is derived from two sources: the medical center pays two thirds, and the physician practice group affiliated with the university pays one third. Paul could earn more working at the local health maintenance organization (HMO) or providing locum tenens anesthesia coverage. He stays at the university because his position there offers a wide scope of practice, challenging patients, complex procedures, a collegial atmosphere, and the opportunity to share his expertise with students.

Paul provides expert guidance and coaching to patients and families when he rotates through the preanesthesia evaluation clinic. When surgery is scheduled, patients and their families have scheduled appointments in this clinic, where an anesthesia provider obtains their health history, performs physical assessment, and develops an anesthesia care plan with the patient. Additional guidance and coaching occurs during the postoperative period, when questions related to pain management and control of postoperative nausea and vomiting arise.

Expert guidance and coaching of other care providers occurs on several levels: with newly hired peers, with surgical and anesthesia house staff, and with perioperative nursing colleagues. Paul may be assigned to help orient a new CRNA, especially to areas where the CRNA may not have recently worked, such as in cardiovascular anesthesia. Surgical house staff may work with Paul during their anesthesia rotation. Surgeons frequently ask for advice regarding postoperative pain management. In some tertiary centers, Paul and his CRNA colleagues will be asked by the staff anesthesiologists to work as clinical perceptors with beginning anesthesiology residents, and with medical students completing their anesthesia clerkships. Paul works closely with perioperative nurses on issues such as patient positioning, coordinating, sending laboratory specimens, obtaining medications, and issues related to operating room turnover times.

Consultation occurs with peers, attending physicians, and other colleagues such as operating room nurses and educators. Another CRNA may want to compare experiences with Paul regarding certain types of procedures. Paul is respected because of his experience in this health care system, and attending physicians will ask him what his experience has been with particular treatment regimens. Paul is also a member of the quality assurance committee in his department, and is consulted on his knowledge of standard of care issues. Because Paul is known as a clinical expert in nurse anesthesia, nursing colleagues frequently consult with him on areas as diverse as conscious sedation and reimbursement for APNs.

Because Paul works in an academic environment, he is constantly challenged to be aware of current anesthesiology literature. Case reports and clinical and basic research papers are discussed formally and informally with attending and resident physicians and nurses in the department. His department is involved in clinical and basic research. Although Paul has not been a primary investigator, he has helped collect data on numerous clinical studies and has been asked for his input on clinical research protocols. Part of the mission of Paul's department is to conduct research, and he feels strongly that he should be an informed user of applicable research findings in his practice.

Clinical and professional leadership come naturally to Paul and some of his colleagues at the medical center. The CRNAs are considered clinical leaders because they are a clinical constant in their department: residents, fellows, and some attending physicians are transient. New attending physicians are usually told when working with an experienced CRNA that the CRNA is knowledgeable about the surgical procedures and anesthetic requirements, so that the attending physician can concentrate on resident education. Attending physicians typically are assigned to work with a resident or fellow in one operating room, and will also provide coverage for a second room staffed by a CRNA.

In terms of professional leadership, Paul and his colleagues are often asked to plan continuing education meetings for their state nurse anesthesia association. The clinical and academic resources at their tertiary medical center allow these CRNAs access to high-quality speakers who draw from extensive clinical experiences. Some of Paul's colleagues hold elected or appointed offices with their state and national professional organizations. Another CRNA Paul works with is active in a state-level APN coalition.

Because CRNAs always collaborate with physicians when they practice, the academic medical center is similar to other practice settings with respect to professional relationships. Paul and his colleagues interface with surgeons, perioperative nurses, anesthesiologists, and technicians routinely. At this tertiary center, patients always have input regarding their anesthesia management, so Paul and his colleagues collaborate with patients to formulate an anesthetic care plan.

As a highly motivated professional, Paul has well-developed change agent skills. He is well aware of the departmental hierarchy in which he works and has found niches within the department where he has been especially interested in practicing, such as cardiovascular anesthesia. Within this specialty area, Paul has been a change agent with regard to the standardization of the management of vasoactive drips. He had colleagues who did not routinely use infusion pumps for all their vasoactive drips, which occasionally resulted in drug overdoses. Another area where he has been influential is in developing expertise with the management of patients with difficult airways and sharing techniques he has learned with other clinicians in the department.

NURSE ANESTHESIA EDUCATION

Nurse anesthesia education occurs in diverse settings. This is demonstrated by the many academic units that house nurse anesthesia educational programs. Educators in nurse anesthesia are proud of the educational diversity of their graduates. However, the relative value of this diversity has never been quantified in terms of an academic power base or educational credibility. This diversity exists because the nurse anesthesia educational community values various undergraduate degrees for entrance into nurse anesthesia programs and because of the initial difficulty nurse anesthesia educators met when trying to move certificate nurse anesthesia programs into schools of nursing. The AANA promotes graduate education for entrance into practice. Since 1998, all nurse anesthesia programs have been at the graduate level. This requirement does not dictate the movement of programs into one academic discipline. This may stem from those programs that in the 1970s established relationships with whichever academic unit was open to affiliating with a nurse anesthesia program. The first four graduate programs in nurse anesthesia all had different academic affiliations: medicine, nursing, allied health, and education. Programs that pioneered nurse anesthesia education at the graduate level established relationships with those departments in colleges and universities that were willing to take risks with the small numbers of students in nurse anesthesia programs. This diversified model of nurse anesthesia education has proliferated in the last 15 years, and many of these long-established programs would find it difficult to change their academic affiliations.

As described in Chapter 1, the Catholic Franciscan sisters offered one of the first organized nurse anesthesia courses at St. John's Hospital in Springfield, Illinois, in 1912. Although other nurse anesthesia programs opened in the early 20th century, curricula and clinical experiences were not standardized. At the first meeting of the National Association of Nurse Anesthetists, educational standards for the specialty were discussed by founding members. Nurse anesthesia educators agreed that the minimum length of academic programs in the specialty would be 6 months. Formal accreditation of nurse anesthesia programs began in 1952 (Bankert, 1989; Thatcher, 1953).

In the mid-1970s, over 170 nurse anesthesia educational programs existed. Currently, 90 CRNA educational programs operate in the United States and Puerto Rico. A rapid decline in the numbers of nurse anesthesia programs occurred in the 1980s. This change was of great concern to the specialty. The closures were attributed variously to physician pressure, declining support, the inability of hospitals to continue support of small programs, and lack of a geographically accessible university with which a nurse anesthesia program could affiliate (Faut-Callahan, 1991). Those who argued that nurse anesthesia programs closed solely because of the graduate degree mandate offered little evidence to support that claim. One can surmise that, if the requirement for graduate education were the only reason for program closures, those programs would have remained open until 1998, when the master's degree was required.

Despite the decline in the overall numbers of nurse anesthesia programs, many of which were certificate programs that had enrollments of less than five students, the level of educational programs changed dramatically (Figure 18-2). Through the 1990s, the overall number of CRNA graduates has leveled at approximately 950 annually (Figure 18-3). After an initial decline in graduates, the newer graduate programs increased their admissions. To accomplish this, programs had to increase the numbers of clinical training sites (Figure 18-4). The result has been a strengthened educational system, deeply entrenched in an academic model.

Colleges of nursing are more frequently becoming the sites for nurse anesthesia programs as nurse anesthesia and other APN groups increasingly collaborate on legislative, policy, and educational matters. Agatha Hodgins' expressed desire for a separate professional organization and education process for nurse anesthesia has been partially supplanted by the rapprochement between nursing and nurse anesthesia (Mungia-Biddle et al., 1990). Coalitions of APNs have been effectively working together on the state and federal levels with health care reform issues.

Nurse anesthesia educational curricula include time requirements for both didactic and clinical activities that reflect minimum standards for entry into practice. Academic content areas are crucial to the preparation of practitioners for beginning-level competence in a highly demanding, rapidly changing specialty. Various colleges and schools that administratively house nurse anesthesia programs may have additional academic requirements. Nurse anesthesia programs in colleges of nursing include core graduate-level courses taken by all graduate-level nursing students. These courses include graduate-level nursing theory, nursing research, advanced physical assessment, and

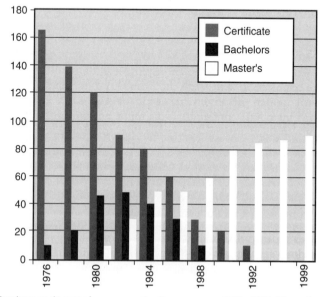

FIGURE 18-2 • Numbers and types of nurse anesthesia programs, 1976–1999. (From Council on Accreditation of Nurse Anesthesia Educational Programs, Park Ridge, IL, [1999]; reprinted with permission.)

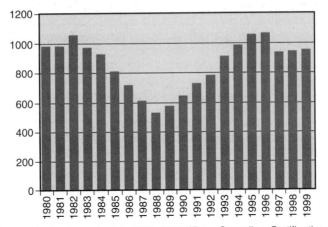

FIGURE 18–3 • Nurse anesthesia graduates, 1974–1999. (From Council on Certification of Nurse Anesthetists, Park Ridge, IL, [1999]; reprinted with permission.)

pharmacology. The content areas and mandated time allocations for the nurse anesthesia core courses are listed in Table 18-4. These course requirements constitute 330 didactic hours.

The clinical component requires that the student administer a minimum of 450 anesthetics, or 800 hours of actual anesthesia administration time. An external agency, the Council on Certification of Nurse Anesthetists, requires that students complete given numbers of surgical procedures and anesthetic techniques. For example, all students must administer at least 45 general anesthetics using a mask airway (versus endotracheal intubation). Similarly, a required number of endotracheal intubations or thoracic surgical cases must be met for nurse anesthesia graduates to be eligible to take the national certification examination.

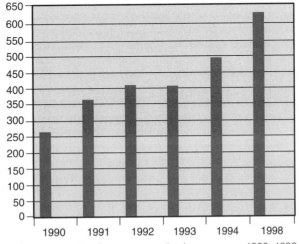

FIGURE 18–4 • Number of clinical sites for nurse anesthesia programs, 1990–1998. (From Council on Accreditation of Nurse Anesthesia Educational Programs, Park Ridge, IL, [1999]; reprinted with permission.)

TABLE 18-4 ACADEMIC COURSE REQUIREMENTS

TOPIC	REQUIRED CONTACT HOURS
Professional aspects of nurse anesthesia practice	45
Advanced anatomy, physiology, and pathophysiology	135
Chemistry and physics of anesthesia	45
Advanced pharmacology	90
Principles of anesthesia practice	90
Clinical and literature review conferences	45

Most programs exceed these minimum requirements. In addition, many require study in methods of scientific inquiry and statistics, as well as active participation in student-generated and faculty-sponsored research (AANA, 1992b).

The Council on Accreditation of Nurse Anesthesia Educational Programs accredits nurse anesthesia educational programs. Council members include CRNAs, physicians, and other members of the professional community. The Council on Accreditation conducts mandatory, on-site program reviews every 10 years. Nurse anesthesia educators and the Council on Accreditation have found that retaining a prescriptive curriculum in terms of hours and types of clinical experiences has helped the survival of educational programs. That is, when documented deviations from established standards for nurse anesthesia educational programs occur (e.g., physicians restricting clinical access), program directors can cite COA standards mandating these experiences.

Nurse anesthesia was the first nursing specialty to have mandatory certification. This process began in 1945, when the first certification examination in nurse anesthesia was given. The Council on Certification, like other AANA councils, is administratively independent of the AANA. The mission of the certification council is to certify nurse anesthesia graduates by examination, thus protecting and assuring the public regarding CRNA competency. The Council on Certification utilizes psychometricians, an academy of test item writers, and computer adaptive testing to assess beginning-level competence in nurse anesthesia graduates.

Another AANA council, the Council on Recertification, was developed in the late 1960s. The impetus for its development was the need to document for the public continued professional excellence for practicing CRNAs. The certification period for CRNAs is every 2 years and is renewable. Documentation of anesthesia practice and continuing education activities is required for recertification. Continuing education programs must be approved by the council to meet requirements for recertification (AANA, 1992b).

These three councils, plus the Council for Public Interest in Anesthesia, endeavor to assure the public that the education and practice of CRNAs is more than adequate for the demands of the specialty. Nurse anesthesia education continues to evolve along with education in other APN areas.

AMERICAN ASSOCIATION OF NURSE ANESTHETISTS

Since its organization as the National Association of Nurse Anesthetists in 1931, the AANA has placed its responsibilities to the public above or at the same level as its responsibilities to its membership. The association has produced education and practice standards, implemented a recertification process for nurse anesthetists (1945), and developed an accreditation program for nurse anesthetists (1952). It was a leader in forming multidisciplinary councils with public representation to fulfill the profession's autonomous credentialing functions (AANA, 1992b).

When founder Agatha Hodgins became ill, Gertrude Fife, who provided anesthesia for pioneeing heart surgeon Claude Beck, assumed the burden of developing the young National Association of Nurse Anesthetists (Thatcher, 1953). The Association's name was changed to the American Association of Nurse Anesthetists in 1939. Helen Lamb, who served two terms as AANA president (1940–1942), worked exclusively with Dr. Evarts Graham, one of the first modern thoracic surgeons (Bankert, 1989). The first anesthesia administered for correction of tetralogy of Fallot was given by a nurse anesthetist. Early CRNA leaders were involved in complex practice settings with surgeons who were also influential in their fields.

In addition to developing a professional identity for nurse anesthesia, early CRNA leaders developed curricular standards for nurse anesthesia educational programs. These standards included a minimum program length of 6 months and, later, institution of mandatory certification and recertification policies.

The AANA was among the first nursing specialty organizations. At a 1931 regional nurse anesthesia meeting, Agatha Hodgins put forth the essentials for a national organization of nurse anesthetists as she saw them:

> *Improvement of the present situation is in the hands of the nurse anesthetists themselves. If the work is to be properly safeguarded and hoped-for progress attained, it is necessary that remedies be applied to certain detrimental conditions now acknowledgedly existing. It would seem that the first step should be the awakening of deeper interest and the development of constructive leadership. Following in logical order would be: self-organization as a special division of hospital service . . . educational standards, post-graduate schools of anesthesia . . . required to conform to an accepted criteria of education; state registration, putting right the nurse anesthetist to practice her vocation beyond criticism; constant effort toward improving the quality of work by means of study and research, thus affording still greater protection to the patient; [and] dissemination of information gained through proper channels.*

(Thatcher, 1953, p. 183).

The division between nurse anesthesia and nursing service has occurred in many practice settings in which CRNAs are responsible to the hospital rather than to the nursing administration.

Early affiliation with the American Nurses Association did not occur, as noted earlier, because each organization had different ideas of what such an affiliation would entail (Gunn, 1991; Thatcher, 1953). With time, the breach between nursing and nurse anesthesia has narrowed considerably. Legislative and regulatory advances for APNs, such as direct reimbursement, prescriptive authority, and expanded scope of practice, have involved coalitions of APNs. As more nurse anesthesia programs have moved into schools of nursing, shared values have readily been identified by nurse anesthesia educators. These values include concepts such as ensuring access to primary and specialty care for all citizens that can be provided by APNs.

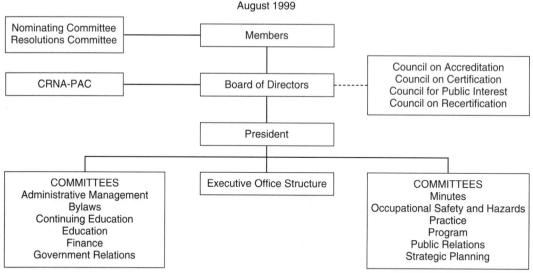

AMERICAN ASSOCIATION OF NURSE ANESTHETISTS
Organizational Chart
August 1999

FIGURE 18–5 • AANA organizational chart—committees of interest. (From American Association of Nurse Anesthetists; reprinted with permission.)

The AANA represents 95% of the practicing CRNAs in this country (Garde, 1998). This is an unusually high percentage of members for any professional organization. It is believed that this is because the AANA endeavors to be responsive to member concerns. The AANA allows multiple venues for direct member input rather than relying on a delegate system for member feedback to leadership (Foster & Garde, 1994).

The AANA has steadily grown, responding to member needs and legislative, regulatory, practice, and educational concerns. The organization has 10 major departments at its Park Ridge, Illinois, headquarters and in a Washington, DC, office (Figure 18–5). AANA affairs are handled by an elected board of directors in conjunction with AANA staff members. More than 20 committees and subcommittees conduct activities directed by the board. The AANA conducts business at six national meetings each year held at various sites. Additionally, four autonomous councils function independently of the executive office. These councils have been developed autonomously of the AANA to avoid potential conflicts of interest in the areas of accreditation, certification, recertification, and public interest.

PROFESSIONAL ISSUES FOR CRNAs

Reimbursement for Nurse Anesthesia Clinical Services

In the early years of the 20th century and through the 1950s, CRNAs were usually paid employees of either the surgeon or the hospital for whom they worked. In rural areas, CRNAs often contracted with hospitals to provide services based on fee-for-service structures—that is, a set amount of compensation per case as opposed to a straight salary for hours worked (Simonson & Garde, 1994). With the advent of private payers such as Blue Cross/Blue Shield, only physician providers and hospitals were paid by the plan. Other health care providers, such as CRNAs, psychologists, and physical therapists, would submit charges to the hospital or treating physician. The hospital or physician would then obtain reimbursement for services as "incident to" their own and pass the money on to the nonreimbursed provider (Simonson & Garde, 1994).

Because of escalating health care costs in the 1970s and 1980s, Medicare instituted a prospective payment system (PPS) in 1983. Although initially this legislation affected only Medicare Part A (hospital costs), it ultimately affected Medicare Part B (physician and nonphysician costs). PPS legislation mandated a fixed payment rate for all hospital care, covering Part A services paid to hospitals based on a patient's diagnosis-related classification group (DRG). This fixed rate was to cover all costs associated with hospital admission, including services provided by nonphysician health providers. CRNAs were in great jeopardy under this system because, in their effort to cut costs, hospitals had no incentive to hire CRNAs, because their cost would come directly from the hospital DRG payment. Congress inadvertently created reimbursement disincentives for the use of CRNAs while bolstering incentives for the use of anesthesiologists. AANA lobbying efforts caused the Health Care Financing Administration (HCFA) to rewrite portions of this legislation, enabling all CRNAs to obtain direct Medicare reimbursement or to sign over their billing rights to their employer (Simonson & Garde, 1994).

Historically, anesthesia charges have been based on direct time involvement, either as a charge for simple time or as a charge based on a combination of time and the complexity of the anesthetic. The resource-based relative value scale, developed in the 1960s, is used to determine anesthesia charges based on the complexity of the surgical procedure. The result is charges for "base units," or surgical procedures described by anatomical or functional units. Additional "modifier units" can be added to base units for factors such as emergency procedures, extremes of age, or anesthetic risk. After adding base and modifier units, time units are calculated at one unit per 15 minutes. The value of time units is determined by the payer (e.g., Medicare or Blue Cross/Blue Shield) and the market. One unit of anesthesia time may be billed at from $15 to over $70. The total of base, modifier, and time units determines the professional fee for the administration of anesthesia. Many third-party payers, such as Medicare and some Blue Cross insurers, completely ignore the practitioner's charges and base payments on their own fee schedules. These payments are often determined by what providers charge "on average" for their services (Simonson & Garde, 1994).

Attempts to control spiraling health care costs and improve access to care have resulted in the previously mentioned proliferation of managed care contracts and a resurgence of interest in HMOs. CRNAs can expect their reimbursement rates to decrease in the near future. This decrease will affect anesthetists in any practice setting—self-, group or hospital employed. Fee-for-service reimbursement structures, as described earlier, may become things of the past as managed care increasingly dominates health care markets. All providers, including physicians, may eventually be salaried. Despite the trend of increased managed care, organized medicine continues to advocate the fee-for-service system as the only means to maintain the integrity of the physician-client relationship and fights vigorously to maintain the status quo

(Simonson & Garde, 1994). The economics of managed care do not ensure APNs access to clients based on their cost-effectiveness. Because of the desire to maintain fee-for-service payment in some settings, the most cost-effective provider may not be the one chosen to participate in managed care. Transitional mechanisms in vertical integration strategy (e.g., combining payers, provider, and a wide spectrum of services in the same network, such as physician-hospital organizations) still focus on physicians and hospitals as principal health care resources. Some sources consider this a stopgap measure, not addressing all players, such as insurance providers, in the system. Cost-effectiveness and provider practice profiles are increasingly considered in managed care contracting, but there may be a reticence to disrupt traditional local practice patterns as managed care increasingly influences some markets (Kongstvedt, 1994).

Impact of Managed Care on CRNA Education and Practice

Historically, APNs and physician assistants have practiced collaboratively with physicians in HMOs, providing both primary and specialty care. HMO physicians acknowledge the continued role for APNs in HMOs (Bowser, 1994).

A paradigm shift in acute care has occurred, wherein hospitals are no longer financial profit centers but are now recognized as cost centers. Critical pathways and other utilization review mechanisms are used to minimize the average length of hospital stay. The need for inpatient beds is less because early discharge, home health, and outpatient care services are increasingly the norm.

Increasingly, capitated payments are made to health care providers. Under capitation, a per member per month allotment of money is paid to cover the health care needs of a predefined population. Providers are expected to treat patients within this cost or incur a loss of income. Thus financial risk for health care has shifted from insurance companies to health care providers. For example, a surgical inpatient who spends 2 hours of a 5-day hospitalization in the operating room finds that operating room costs comprise 35% to 40% of the entire hospitalization cost. Today's anesthesia providers have to keep pace with the huge growth in knowledge, medicolegal pressures, greater financial complexity, and new ethical dilemmas associated with managed care organizations (Kaye et al., 1999).

Some of the effects of managed care on anesthesia practice include the need to demonstrate value by improving quality of care at a reduced cost, or by maintaining quality while reducing cost. Suggested strategies (Kaye et al., 1999) include

1. Fostering more appropriate use of anesthesia drugs
2. Using anesthesia information management for pharmaceutical cost containment
3. Fast-tracking patients who need coronary artery bypass grafting and ambulatory surgical patients

Nurse anesthesia education programs have been affected by the restructuring of health care organizations. Traditional certificate programs were based in hospitals that paid for significant portions of overhead expenses. As hospitals have downsized or joined corporate entities, some remaining hospital-based, university-affiliated programs have had to develop alternative fiscal management strategies. CRNA educators must be able to demonstrate the value added to the organization by the nurse anesthesia program, its faculty, and its students.

CRNAs and APNs can play significant roles in the shift from inpatient acute care to outpatient and home health services. It seems likely for CRNAs that hospital employment will be less common as hospitals decrease their fixed costs, such as payroll, and wish to outsource services such as anesthesia to private groups. However, there is also a recent trend toward hospital employment of some specialty health care providers. It is imperative that CRNAs and other APNs track these trends closely and negotiate for a place at the decision-making table.

Whether CRNAs will be self-employed, employed by CRNA groups, or employed by physician-CRNA groups will depend on local market dynamics. Independent contracting by CRNAs for their professional services will continue to increase. It will be imperative for CRNAs and other APNs to know their worth in terms of billable revenue and quality of care provided for contract negotiation and public relations purposes.

In the future, each CRNA may practice in multiple settings with individually negotiated contracts. Home health services such as parenteral infusion therapy and management of chronic pain might be directed by CRNAs, as is already the case in some areas. These settings are natural extensions of anesthesia, pharmacology and clinical skills. Myriad opportunities will exist for CRNAs and other APNs to collaborate in the management of acute and chronic pain and the treatment of respiratory and nutritional disorders.

Continued Challenges for CRNAs

A current major challenge to the profession is that of physician supervision of CRNAs under Medicare and Medicaid. Supervision rules were developed to quantify reimbursement, but at times have been incorrectly construed as standards of care. Deferral to state law is compatible with the position of the Joint Commission on Accreditation of Healthcare Organizations (JCAHO). The JCAHO does not require physician supervision of nurse anesthetists. When CRNAs were given direct Medicare reimbursement in 1989, there was no statutory requirement for CRNAs to be supervised by physicians in order to receive reimbursement. Twenty-nine states do not require supervision of CRNAs in nurse practice acts or board of nursing rules (Foster, 1998).

The American Society of Anesthesiologists (ASA) has used the HCFA proposal to foster debate on whether anesthesiologists should supervise CRNAs. Physician supervision is not the pertinent issue, because the current HCFA conditions do not require anesthesiologist involvement. Many ASA members believe that each CRNA should practice under anesthesiologist supervision. The reality of practice in rural and underserved areas, however, is that in those settings CRNAs collaborate safely and effectively with the operating physician, dentist, or podiatrist (Foster, 1998; Callaghan, 1995). Some anesthesiologists have incorrectly informed hospitals and/or surgeons that surgeons are automatically liable for the acts of the CRNA because of the supervision requirement. This creates a disincentive for hospitals to use CRNAs, who may be the lower cost providers giving the same quality of care (Cromwell, 1998; Foster, 1998).

To date, the AANA has found that a number of physicians, patient groups such as the Center for Patient Advocacy, and the National Rural Health Association have decided to support the proposed rule change. Approximately 100 members of Congress have written letters of support or are otherwise sympathetic to the proposed rule change (Foster, 1998). This issue involves AANA utilization of its legal, policy, education, and research resources to deal with a major public policy and public relations challenge. Resolution of the supervision issue is pending at this writing. The tradition of strong leadership meeting challenges directly continues. AANA Executive Director John Garde, CRNA, MS, FAAN, said

> *[T]he profession has an optimistic future. I point out with pride the commitment that AANA members have toward [the future of their profession]—a commitment that encompasses being outstanding anesthesia practitioners who belong to their Association. I am reminded, too, what each of you brings every day to your patients. Dick Davidson, president of the American Hospital Association, said when asked about what will remain in health care 100 years from now, "There will always be personal contact and caring. We will always have hands touching patients. Everything we do is about human need. That's the constant over time." And, that is the legacy of the nurse anesthesia profession.*

(Garde 1998, p. 15)

Another current issue impacting nurse anesthesia education is reimbursement inequity under Medicare and some private insurance plans. Compensation for cases performed by student nurse anesthetists is less than the reimbursement for resident anesthesiologists, producing an economic disincentive for the education of nurse anesthetists. This issue is being addressed by AANA.

In the educational arena, there is continued debate about the preparation of CRNAs. Currently, the minimum length of nurse anesthesia programs is 24 months. However, because of the combination of didactic and clinical time requirements, many programs are 27 to 36 months long. Nurse anesthesia curricular requirements can overload the typical master's curriculum. Because of the time commitment and academic rigor necessary for this specialty area, there is increasing interest in a clinical doctoral degree as the exit degree in nurse anesthesia. The vision of nursing leader Dr. Luther Christman for nurses to be prepared with advanced degrees both in their discipline and in a basic science reflects the trend to propose preparation beyond the master's degree for entry into this and other advanced practice specialty areas (Christman, 1977). Doctoral programs in nurse anesthesia are being developed. Approximately 1% of practicing nurse anesthetists possess doctoral degrees in disciplines including education, nursing, physiology, and pharmacology.

The future of nurse anesthesia education and research is promising. With more CRNAs holding graduate degrees, there is more potential for basic and applied research to be conducted by CRNAs. More graduate education in nursing, the basic sciences, and business will better enable CRNAs to collaborate with other investigators in the arenas of clinical and bench research; practice, legislation, and policy formulation will also be enhanced by this additional educational preparation. A greater nurse anesthesia voice in policy formulation has already been felt, with CRNA members securing places on state boards of nursing and other governmental positions.

SUMMARY

Nurse anesthesia, the earliest nursing specialty, was also the first nursing specialty to have standardized educational programs, a certification process, mandatory continuing education, and recertification. Nurse anesthetists have been involved in the development of anesthetic techniques along with physicians and engineers. Nurse anesthetists have been nursing leaders in obtaining third-party reimbursement for professional services and in coping with challenges such as the prospective payment system, managed care, and physician supervision.

Nurse anesthetists provide surgical and nonsurgical anesthesia services in a variety of settings both in the United States and in other parts of the world. CRNAs work in collaboration with physicians as do other APNs, and are capable of providing the full spectrum of anesthesia services.

Activism in the state and federal legislative and regulatory arenas is a recognized CRNA activity. Increasing coalition building between nurse anesthetists, other APNs, and nursing educators is congruent with a shared nursing vision. This vision values health care for all Americans provided in a safe and cost-effective manner by APNs collaborating with other health care professionals.

REFERENCES

Abenstein, J., & Warner, M. (1996). Anesthesia providers, patient outcomes, and costs. *Anesthesia & Analgesia, 82,* 1273–1283.

American Association of Nurse Anesthetists. (1992a). *Guidelines and standards for nurse anesthesia practice.* Park Ridge, IL: Author.

American Association of Nurse Anesthetists. (1992b). *Qualifications and capabilities of the CRNA.* Park Ridge, IL: Author.

Bader, A., & Datta, S. (1994). Obstetric anesthesia. In M. C. Rogers, J. Tinker, & B. Covino (Eds.), *Principles and practice of anesthesiology* (pp. 2065–2104). St. Louis: C. V. Mosby.

Bankert, M. (1989). *Watchful care: A history of America's nurse anesthetists.* New York: Continuum.

Bowser, R. (1994). Lecture from HMO physician administrator in Managed Care Course in Health Systems Management [unpublished]. Chicago: Rush University.

Callaghan, J. (1995). Twenty-five years of gallbladder surgery in a small rural hospital. *American Journal of Surgery, 169*(3), 313–315.

Callahan, L. (1994). Establishing measures of competence. In S. Foster & L. Jordan (Eds.), *Professional aspects of nurse anesthesia practice* (pp. 275–290). Philadelphia: F. A. Davis.

Callahan, L. (1995). *Development of a single blended anesthesia provider: An exploratory study.* Unpublished doctoral dissertation, Florida State University, Tallahassee.

Christman, L. (1977). Doctoral education: A shot in the arm for the nursing profession. *Health Services Manager, 10*(5), 6, 7.

Cromwell, J. (1998, November 15). *Barriers to achieving the optimal workforce mix.* Paper presented at the AANA Fall Assembly of States, Colorado Springs, CO.

Cromwell, J., & Rosenbach, M. (1988). The economics of anesthesia delivery. *Health Affairs, 7*(4), 118–131.

Dorroh, M., & Norton, S. (1996). The certified nurse-midwife. In Hamric, A. B., Spross, J. A., & Hanson, C. M. (Eds.), *Advanced nursing practice: An integrative approach* (pp. 395–420). Philadelphia: W. B. Saunders.

Dripps, R. (1977). Preface. In R. D. Dripps, J. E. Eckenhoff, & L. D. Vandam Dripps, (Eds.), *Introduction to anesthesia* (5th ed., pp. 1–11). Philadelphia: W.B. Saunders.

Faut, M. (1984). *Doctoral education for nurse anesthesia practice.* Unpublished clinical defense paper, Rush University, Chicago.

Faut-Callahan, M. (1991). Graduate education for nurse anesthetists: Master's versus a clinical doctorate. In *National Commission on Nurse Anesthesia Education Report* (pp. 110–115). Park Ridge, IL: American Association of Nurse Anesthetists.

Faut-Callahan, M., & Paice, J. (1990). Postoperative pain control for the parturient. *Journal of Perinatal and Neonatal Nursing, 4*(1), 27–41.

Foster, S. (1998). *Comments of the American Association of Nurse Anesthetists on the proposed rule regarding the Medicare and Medicaid programs; hospital conditions of participation; provider and supplier approval.* Unpublished document, American Association of Nurse Anesthetists, Park Ridge, IL.

Foster, S., & Garde, J. (1994). The American Association of Nurse Anesthetists: The role of the professional organization. In S. Foster & L. Jordan (Eds.), *Professional aspects of nurse anesthesia practice* (pp. 35–48). Philadelphia: F. A. Davis.

Garde, J. (1988). Preface. In W. Waugaman, S. Foster, & B. Rigor (Eds.), *Principles and practice of nurse anesthesia* (p. i–xiv). Norwalk, CT: Appleton & Lange.

Garde, J. (1998, November). Annual report of the executive director. *AANA News Bulletin,* pp. 14–16.

Gunn, I. (1991). The history of nurse anesthesia education: Highlights and influences. In *National Commission on Nurse Anesthesia Education Report* (pp. 33–41). Park Ridge, IL: American Association of Nurse Anesthetists.

Jaffe, J., & Revak, G. (1998, November 13). *CRNA manpower recruitment to retirement.* Paper presented at the AANA Fall Assembly of States, Colorado Springs, CO.

Jordan, L. (1994). Qualifications and capabilities of the certified registered nurse anesthetist. In S. Foster & L. Jordan, (Eds.), *Professional aspects of nurse anesthesia practice* (pp. 3–10). Philadelphia: F. A. Davis.

Kaye, D., Scibetta, W., & Grogono, A. (1999). Anesthesia manpower and recruitment 1998: An update. *Advances in Anesthesia, 16,* 1–27.

Kelly, J. (1994). An international study of educational programs for nurses providing anesthesia care. *AANA Journal, 62*(6), 484–495.

Kongstvedt, P. (1994). *The managed care handbook* (2nd ed.). Gaithersburg, MD: Aspen Publishers.

Loper, K., Butler, S., Nessly, M., & Wild, L. (1989). Paralyzed with pain: The need for education. *Pain, 37,* 315–316.

McAuliffe, M., & Henry, B. (1998). Survey of nurse anesthesia practice, education, and regulation in 96 countries. *AANA Journal, 66*(3), 273–286.

Munguia-Biddle, F, Maree, S., Klein, E., Callahan, L., & Gilles, B. (1990). *Nurse anesthesiology competence evaluation: Mechanism for accountability.* Unpublished document, American Association of Nurse Anesthetists, Park Ridge, IL.

National Center for Nursing Research. (1991). *CRNA manpower study.* Washington, DC: U.S. Department of Health and Human Services.

Orkin, F. (1998). Rural realities. *Anesthesiology, 88*(3), 1597–1598.

Simonson, D., & Garde, J. (1994). Reimbursement for clinical services. In S. Foster & L. Jordan (Eds.), *Professional aspects of nurse anesthesia practice* (pp. 129–142). Philadelphia: F. A. Davis.

Thatcher, V. (1953). *History of anesthesia with emphasis on the nurse specialist.* Philadelphia: J. B. Lippincott.

Waugaman, W. (1991). Nurse anesthesia: The practice of nursing, medicine, or something else? *Nurse Anesthesia, 2*(4), 157–159.

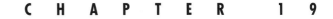

C H A P T E R   1 9

The Advanced Practice
Nurse Case Manager

• V I C K Y   A.   M A H N
• D O N N A   Z A Z W O R S K Y

INTRODUCTION

OVERVIEW OF CASE MANAGEMENT, NURSE CASE
MANAGEMENT, AND APN CASE MANAGEMENT
    Case Management
    Nurse Case Management
    APN Case Management

MANAGED CARE TRENDS
    Care Reimbursement Trends
    Regulatory Requirements
    Risk-Assessing a Population for Targeted Case
      Management Interventions

DISEASE MANAGEMENT AND THE APN CM
    Disease Management Interventions
    Tools of Disease Management
    Disease Management Outcomes

PROFILE OF NURSE CASE MANAGEMENT PRACTICE
    Types of Nurse Case Management
    Functions That Distinguish Nurse Case Management
      from APN Case Management

APN CM COMPETENCIES
    Direct Care, Expert Coaching, and Guidance
    Consultation, Collaboration, and Leadership
    Change Agency
    Ethical Decision Making and Conflict Resolution
    Research Utilization and CQI
    Exemplar of APN CM Practice

EDUCATION, EXPERIENCE, AND CERTIFICATION:
PREPARING FOR THE APN CM ROLE

549

INTRODUCTION

Over the last decade, managed care has infiltrated almost every aspect of the health care system. Driven largely by economics, the goal to deliver cost-effective care through prudent use of resources and the elimination of redundant and unnecessary services was the predominant theme of the 1990s. A variety of medical management techniques to improve care and contain costs in the competitive health care market have been implemented. These include utilization management, critical pathways, patient care guidelines, and case management. Despite these resource management strategies, global fiscal performance in the health care market place was not significantly affected. Why? Because, to put it into simplest terms, *the horse is already out of the barn.* The patient or health plan member has already become sick or needs costly intervention. The health care system can try to save a few dollars through prudent use of pharmaceuticals or diagnostics or by restricting access to care; however, the largest gain will be in preventing costly health problems from occurring in the first place.

In the new millennium, case managers (CMs), including nurse case managers (NCMs), will experience a more proactive and systematic approach to managing care. Not only will they perform the traditional case management activities of assessing, planning, implementing, and coordinating activities for individuals with immediate health care needs, they also will find themselves engaged in population-based programs for high-risk client groups who have no active symptoms or complications. NCMs will be educating, supporting, coaching, and advocating for clients at risk for chronic disease and other high-risk health problems so that those clients adopt behaviors known to reduce disease, limit chronicity or progression, and prevent complications. Such an approach should reduce health care resource consumption over time. Finally, NCMs will share accountability with other stakeholders in the health care industry to demonstrate the overall value of case management. Not only will advanced practice nurse (APN) CMs be challenged to demonstrate cost savings, they also will be called upon to use empirical techniques to show that the case management process does indeed influence client behaviors, clinical outcomes, and physical and emotional functioning.

In this chapter, a conceptual overview of managed care organizational incentives and a description of the population enrolled in health plans are discussed in order to identify leverage points for APN CM intervention. Disease management, a strategy used to influence care processes and outcomes within the traditional hospital setting and across the continuum of care, is discussed. Disease management is particularly relevant to the contributions APNs can make in the broader realm of APN CM strategies. The APN CM role and related core skills, competencies, and accountabilities are described within the context of population-based care and systems evaluation. In addition to describing advanced education, clinical functions and exemplars are used to distinguish the APN CM role from the non-APN CM role. Current certification programs relevant to APN CMs are also described. The authors hope this chapter will contribute to the evolution of the APN CM role and stimulate further critical thinking and research on the contributions of APN CMs. Finally, this chapter identifies opportunities for the APN CM to influence health care and set the stage for innovations that will ultimately improve the health of our communities and reduce the economic burden on our health care system.

OVERVIEW OF CASE MANAGEMENT, NURSE CASE MANAGEMENT, AND APN CASE MANAGEMENT

Case Management

Case management is a practice framework that has been implemented in a variety of settings by nurses, social workers, and other health care providers (see Chapter 1). To foster a common understanding of the work done by professional case managers, the interdisciplinary Case Management Society of America (CMSA) has defined case management as "A collaborative process which assesses, plans, implements, coordinates, monitors and evaluates options and services to meet an individual's health needs through communications and available resources to promote quality cost-effective outcomes" (CMSA, 1994, p. 8). This definition incorporates the system, clinical, and fiscal aspects that are central to case management approaches to providing care.

The CMSA's definition is apropriate for all disciplines that practice case management; it is not specific to nurses. An interdisciplinary definition is useful because it applies to a range of health care systems and service settings. Some patient populations, such as indigent patients, may be best served by social work CMs. Other populations, such as patients with mild head injuries, may be best served by rehabilitation counselors. Although the definition of case management is consistent with the nursing process framework, it does not fully address the specialized clinical nursing expertise that seems essential to achieve optimal cost and quality outcomes in certain patients who require health promotion or illness management.

Nurse Case Management

Nurse case management is a health care delivery process that aims to provide quality health care, enhance quality of life, diminish fragmentation, and contain costs (American Nurses Association [ANA], 1988). Furthermore, nurse case management has been characterized as a set of "goal-oriented activities that organize, coordinate, and monitor health care delivery based on measurable objectives designed to meet the needs" of chronically ill or complex patients (Doell Smith, 1994, p. 65). The primary reasons for using nurse case management to deliver care are to control costs, enhance quality of care, decrease fragmentation and duplication of services, and ensure accountability for achieving cost and quality outcomes through nursing interventions that are based on holism, scientific and experiential knowledge, and partnership with the patient. Other benefits of nurse case management have also been identified. It can increase provider control over the practice, enhance provider satisfaction, improve standards of care, promote interdisciplinary communication and collaboration, and increase the volume of cases and market share (Zander, 1993).

Acute, primary, and community care settings are implementing innovative nurse case management programs as a way to promote quality outcomes in a cost-effective manner. While traditionally nurse case managers (NCMs) practiced in environments linked to the hospital setting, new avenues of influencing health care have surfaced. For example, NCMs may practice telephone case management by following the client's progress over time and ensuring timely and appropriate utilization of health care benefits (Bushnell, 1992; Friedman, Gleeson, Kent, Foris & Rodriguez, 1998). Sponsored by the payer, provider, or the employer, NCMs establish relationships with clients over the telephone. A NCM monitors a client's health status based on telephone interviews. Depending on the client's responses, the NCM determines whether interventions are needed. Referrals to local resources are initiated when necessary, and in general, the telephone NCM serves as an advocate to the client, with the incentive of lowering health care costs over time. NCMs also practice in physician offices, educating patients and facilitating appropriate utilization of physician-prescribed health care resources based on local or national evidence-based guidelines.

APN Case Management

Contemporary nurse case management reflects a natural evolution from nursing's history of client advocacy, social service, and public health (see Chapter 1). Nurse practitioners (NPs), certified nurse-midwives (CNMs), and clinical nurse specialists (CNSs) also provide care that is congruent with case management concepts; their care can improve health care access, coordination, and continuity across settings (Brooten et al., 1991; Newman, 1990; Office of Technology Assessment, 1986). Such studies suggest that APN case management is a means of improving access to care in a timely manner. APN case management has also been viewed as a way of enhancing the visibility of advanced nursing practice (Cooper, 1990; Hamric, 1992; Mahn & Spross, 1996). Many arguments have been made for having nurse case management done by APNs (Connors, 1993; Fralic, 1992; Hamric, 1992). Currently, the APN CM is an evolving advanced practice role, and has yet to be formally recognized by the ANA as advanced nursing practice. The APN CM is master's prepared and must have expert knowledge in a clinical specialty, the skills to establish mutually agreeable goals between the client and other members of the health care team, and the ability to establish an intervention schema that will help the client reach his or her goals. However, the scope of influence of the APN CM differs from other APN roles, in that the APN CM is expected to influence care at a systems level through establishing disease management strategies, health promotion, disease prevention, and complication management programs across the continuum of health care services. Finally, the APN CM is accountable for evaluating the effectiveness of the case management intervention, both at the level of an individual patient/client and at a system-wide level.

Based on the previous discussion, the following definitions of a NCM and an APN CM[1] guide the discussion of APN case management.

> *Nurse Case Manager:* A NCM is an experienced bachelor's-prepared registered nurse (RN) who is accountable for managing a defined group of patients/clients in order to optimize clinical and cost outcomes. Outcomes are achieved through clinical practice and partnership and collaboration with patients and other members of the interdisciplinary team. The NCM is responsible for matching the patient's/client's care needs to the most appropriate level of service based upon predefined guidelines, clinical protocols, and payer-based criteria in order to achieve optimal clinical outcomes in the most resource-efficient manner.
>
> *APN Case Manager:* An APN CM has graduate preparation in nursing with established expertise in a clinical specialty. The APN CM is accountable for managing high-risk, clinically complex, or resource-intensive clients/patients within her or his specialty in order to optimize clinical, functional, and cost outcomes. The APN CM also establishes programs and system improvements within a continuum of health care services in order to improve care rendered to her or his "at-risk" populations. In addition, the APN CM is accountable for evaluating the cost and quality outcomes associated with the case management intervention.

The differences between the APN CM and the NCM are discussed later in the section "Functions That Distinguish Nurse Case Management from APN Case Management."

MANAGED CARE TRENDS

The impact of managed care on case management practice, care reimbursement issues, and regulatory requirements related to managed care is described in this section. In addition, economic and clinical risk assessments as part of case and disease management strategies are presented.

Care Reimbursement Trends

Managed care is an integrated network that combines the financing and delivery of health care services to covered individuals. Conceptually, there is a triad of players associated with any managed care organization—the payer, the hospital providers, and the physician providers. Generally, the managed care organization serves as the payer, and contracts with health care organizations and physicians to furnish health care services to members of the plan. In managed care, financial incentives exist that encourage members to use providers associated with the plan and to follow procedures that help the plan to control costs. Financial incentives also encourage providers to control expenditures. For example, shared risk pools may be established whereby unused portions of designated moneys for specialty services would be distributed among primary care providers. Thus, managed care is a system of controlled resource

---

[1] The reader will note that these definitions have been revised from their previous forms in Mahn and Spross (1996).

use and coordination of care that may be applied to *all* clients within a delivery system in order to optimize quality and cost-effective care.

Oftentimes, the NCM must make decisions based upon the reimbursement structure that exists between the client's payer and providers. *Indemnity plans,* often understood as "fee-for-service" plans, mean that the member pays a premium for health care coverage and has a wide selection of providers and health care settings. Typically, the provider or health care facility will bill the expenses to the insurance company, and a varying percentage of the charges will be reimbursed within reasonable limits for the geographic region. This payer structure encourages the provider and health care facility to increase admissions and length of stay (LOS); resource consumption generally goes up because the majority of charges will be reimbursed. Indemnity plans are costly to the member and are decreasing in availability. Regions in the United States that are heavily saturated with managed care may have as little as 3% to 5% of their health care market covered by indemnity insurance. A modification of indemnity insurance that preserves the client's ability to choose a provider within a cost containment framework is the preferred provider organization. This system contracts with providers at a discounted fee-for-service rate.

Since the mid 1980s, Medicare reimbursements have been structured by *diagnosis-related group* (DRG) pricing (see Chapter 23). Thus, reimbursement is fixed for each retrospectively assigned DRG based upon the final analysis of diagnoses and procedures found in the patient's medical record following discharge. Frequently, DRG reimbursement fails to cover the health care organization's expenses, particularly for complicated or extended stays. Under this reimbursement structure, the health care facility has incentives to increase admissions; however, they are at risk for absorbing the costs when LOS or resource utilization exceeds reimbursable amounts. Thus, NCMs working within a DRG-based reimbursement structure have a greater need to reduce LOS and resource consumption for their sponsoring organizations. As a result, the NCM must be in a position to assist the patient to adjust to shorter hospital stays and to find alternative methods to facilitate recuperation, such as skilled nursing facilities (SNFs) and home health care (HHC).

As managed care has begun to dominate the health care market in both the commercial and the Medicare sectors, two other methods of reimbursement have emerged. *Per diem reimbursement* means the health care organization receives a fixed dollar amount for services provided, such as hospital bed days, home care visits, or SNF days. This reimbursement structure encourages the facility to increase admissions and utilize resources sparingly. However, for each day the patient stays, the institution receives more dollars. Thus, under this structure, the NCM may be far less concerned with decreasing LOS than she or he might be under other structures. In fact, the NCM must recognize that, in many case types, such as total joint replacement procedures, the majority of costs are incurred the first day of admission. Subsequent days of care are less expensive for hospitals because fewer costly resources are used. In order for the hospital to cover its costs for such a procedure under a fixed per diem structure, a longer length of stay is desirable. To complicate this payment structure, the health care organization may have risk pools built into the contract, which provide economic incentives when costs or hospital bed days fall under certain targets. Each contract between payer and provider may be different, and NCMs must stay informed about managed care contractual agreements made by their sponsoring organizations.

Capitated reimbursement structures place the greatest amount of fiscal risk upon the health care facility. Unlike the former three structures, there are incentives to avoid hospital admissions and service utilization altogether. In capitated structures, the health care organization receives a fixed amount per member per month regardless of which members are utilizing service. Thus, the fewer members who require services, the more profit the health care organization can realize. When members require hospitalization, the NCM has incentives to move the patient out as quickly as possible, with limited resource consumption. Health care organizations may have numerous capitated agreements with payers within their communities. In addition, the degree of financial risk may vary among contracts. Some capitated contracts may be for "global risk," which means that the health care organization has agreed to accept full economic responsibility for all contracted services for a population of covered lives. This may include accountability for resource management (e.g., service authorization, utilization management, and case management services). In contrast, "partial risk" means that the managed care organization (payer) may retain account-ability for resource management. Under the terms of some contracts, selected services such as community case management may be "carved out" as a separate contract with separate reimbursement structures. For example, The Carondelet Health Care Network had a partial risk contract with a Medicaid based managed care plan for hospital, physician, and ancillary services. A carved out contract for community case management services was arranged in a fee-for-service reimbursement structure. The managed care organization would refer and authorize visits for high-risk clients to the case management program. Case management visits (meaning visits to the client's home or the care setting, or accompanying the client to the doctor's office) were reimbursed at $50 per visit. When the contract with the health care system was renegotiated, and evolved into a global risk structure, case management services were no longer reimbursed as fee-for-service. Instead, case management was included in the monthly capitation reimbursement.

The NCM must be able to recognize the discrepancies among multiple reimbursement structures that affect decision making for the clients for whom she or he is responsible. To complicate the matter even further, the NCM must also be aware that financial incentives among hospitals, providers, and payers are often far from aligned. For example, an agreement may exist between a hospital and a payer to provide services under a capitated agreement. However, if the patient's physician is reimbursed under a traditional fee-for-service structure, it may be difficult to motivate the physician to reduce admissions or LOS. In addition, there may be few economic incentives for the physician to limit use of medically prescribed resources, which account for most health care expenses. NCMs may then find themselves in a situation of conflict between the medical providers and the health care organization. Likewise, NCMs may find themselves in a situation of conflict between the needs of the patient and the payer. In these situations, NCMs need to be able to influence decisions made by other stakeholders through their expertise in clinical assessment and articulation of the patient's needs in order to secure the most appropriate health care settings and services. Table 19–1 summarizes the diverging incentives of four common payer arrangements that exist between hospitals and payers.

Regulatory Requirements

The constraints of a cost-managed system are becoming increasingly problematic. Consumers of health care are voicing dissatisfaction with the myriad restrictions placed on them as members of a health plan. The health plan can regulate which

TABLE 19-1 DIVERGENT INCENTIVES OF VARIOUS PAYMENT STRUCTURES			
REIMBURSEMENT TYPES	ADMISSION TARGETS	LOS TARGETS*	RESOURCE TARGETS
Indemnity	Increased	Increased	Increased
DRG	Increased	Decreased	Decreased
Per Diem	Increased	Increased	Decreased
Capitation	Decreased	Decreased	Decreased

* LOS = length of stay.

doctors members may see and which medications will be allowed, and can exclude alternative treatment options as a covered benefit. Although such restrictions originally were designed to better manage care while saving money, the public is quickly starting to ask for scrutiny of the overall value of the care being provided. A new focus is being placed on the quality of the care being purchased (see Chapter 25).

Managed care systems are expected to have explicit standards for selection of their care providers and formal programs for quality improvement and utilization review. Increasingly, regulatory requirements are being applied to managed care organizations, who not only have to prove a profit margin to their stockholders, but must be able to demonstrate quality of care to employers and other purchasers of health care. The National Committee for Quality Assurance (NCQA) accredits managed care organizations. NCQA accreditation is an evaluation of how the health plan ensures that its members are getting high-quality care, and is based on precise data reporting of measures known as the Health Plan Employer Data and Information Set (HEDIS). With over 70 predefined measure sets, HEDIS examines specific indicators on the effectiveness of care, access and availability of care, satisfaction with the experience of care, health plan stability, utilization of services, the plan's ability to provide its members with informed health care choices, and the cost of care. For example, managed care organizations have to report rates for childhood immunization, mental health utilization, and annual eye examinations to assess for retinopathy in diabetics. Although the collection of HEDIS measures is not typically the direct responsibility of a NCM, a managed care organization's performance data give some clues as to where there may be opportunities for APN CMs to educate clients, manage diseases, facilitate access and referral, or influence alternative care choices. (See Chapter 25 for additional information on HEDIS and other measures of performance.)

Risk-Assessing a Population for Targeted Case Management Interventions

A small percentage of individuals often account for a disproportionate share of health care expenditures. In a typical population, 5% of the members (most of whom are severely, chronically ill) consume 60% of the health care costs, 45% of the members consume 37% of the costs, and the remaining 50% of the population account for only 3% of the costs (unpublished data from Value Health Sciences, Inc., Santa Monica, CA, June, 1995, cited in Eichert, Wong, and Smith, 1997, p. 41). A closer review of these resource-intense populations reveals three subgroups of patient/member types. First, there are those patients who have had a single high-expense episode, such as organ transplant, total joint replacement, or heart valve surgery. A second group are those patients with terminal disease who are resource intensive for a finite period of time. The third group are those patients with chronic disease, such as diabetes, renal failure, hypertension, or asthma, who ultimately utilize a large portion of health care goods and services (C. J. Heller, personal communication, 1999).

Within the chronic disease group, there are three further subcategories of individuals. The first subcategory are those patients/members who are medically unstable and who are already using numerous resources for the management of disease symptoms and sequelae. An example is the long-term diabetic patient who requires costly revascularization procedures or experiences renal complications. With this group, episodic case management may have a small impact on cost and quality outcomes; even significant gains that can result from proactive interventions may be of minimal impact on long-term outcomes.

The second subcategory includes those patients/members who have no active symptoms or complications that require immediate attention. The members of this group are typically active participants in their treatment regimens and have adequate self-management skills. Although this group would certainly be receptive to case management, education, or disease management strategies, case management may not yield the greatest return on investment, because these individuals are already actively engaged in preventive or effective health care behaviors.

Finally, a third subcategory of the chronic disease population include those who are medically stable but have not adopted health care behaviors that limit disease progression and prevent serious complications. Such "passive participants," commonly referred to in the health care literature as being "noncompliant" or "nonadherent," may not engage in effective health care behaviors because of inability to access services, lack of education regarding the disease, or a clinician's failure to diagnose, prescribe, or coordinate. Additional reasons for "passive participation" may be related to depression, limited literacy skills, social isolation, economic constraints, cognitive disorders, lack of motivation, or conflicting health care beliefs. It is this population of "passive participants" who may yield the greatest return from appropriate case management intervention.

To achieve the greatest impact on costs in the most efficient manner, it is critical to target the high-utilization/expenditure groups within a larger population for early interventions to prevent complications or treat them promptly (Eichert, Wong, & Smith, 1997). A variety of methodologies may be used by a health care network or managed care organization to begin to sift through the larger population of enrollees in order to identify those individuals most amenable to case management. These include the use of the payer's claims data to identify those clients with various comorbidities, diagnoses, or procedures. Software applications exist that can search historical claims data on patients/members with selected diagnoses and Current Procedural Terminology (CPT) codes and identify those clients who are actually underutilizing health care services that are associated with health promotion and effective disease management (Mahn, 1999; Rieve, 1999). For example, if a patient/member with a diagnosis of diabetes type II is being managed according to the American Association of Diabetes guidelines, he or she would be expected to have CPT codes in their claims data for fasting blood sugars and hemoglobin A_1C blood tests within the last 6 months. If the codes were missing, it would trigger the software to identify the patient/member for case management follow-up.

Other risk assessment tools are available to identify high-risk populations. The Short Form (SF)-36 or SF-12 health status profiles may be useful to identify patients/members who are most at risk for a decline in health status (Ware, Snow, Kosinski, & Gandek, 1994). Originally developed by the Rand Corporation, this tool may be administered in any setting within the health care continuum and can be used to assess changes in physical and emotional functioning over time. Normative values for a wide range of disease types have been established through Quality Metrics (formally known as the Medical Outcomes Trust), and can be useful as a comparison benchmark (Ware et al., 1994). The Probability for Repeated Admissions (PRA+) is another tool that is frequently used to identify patients/members who are most likely to become heavy users of health care services (Boult, Pacala, & Boult, 1995). This questionnaire can be used to risk-stratify new health plan enrollees. For example, low- to moderate-risk members may then be referred to a telephone case management program, and high-risk members may be referred to a home case management program for long-term follow-up. The PRA+ may be used in conjunction with disease-specific surveys, such as the Medical Research Council Dyspnea Scale to assess severity of breathlessness in chronic obstructive pulmonary disease populations (Wedzicha et al., 1998).

The APN CM must be knowledgeable about the advantages and disadvantages of surveying techniques. For example, the SF-36 or PRA+ may be more cost-effective to administer via a mailed survey; however, the reliability of these instruments decreases when administered in this fashion. Administering these tools via telephone survey increases the reliability, while a face-to-face interview with the client yields maximum reliability. Although the methodologies associated with obtaining claims data or administering risk assessment surveys are beyond the scope of this chapter, these approaches are quickly becoming industry standards and are currently mandated by the Health Care Financing Administration (HCFA) for senior risk members. They can be effective tools to identify case management leverage points within the total risk population.

DISEASE MANAGEMENT AND THE APN CM

Whether in a hospital or health plan environment, disease management strategies drive the care management team to control costs across the continuum and reduce long-term disease complications. Disease management has been described as a "proactive case management program" in which "the CM is accountable for cost-benefit and acuity management across the entire continuum" (Ward & Rieve, 1997, p. 256). However, an argument can be made that case management is a distinct strategy within the larger strategy of disease management. In this view, disease management may be seen as an organized process in which a community of health providers from many disciplines work together to ensure the appropriate management of a particular disease or population of patients. Although APN CMs may be instrumental in coordinating the efforts of a team developing such programs, they may simultaneously focus their case management practice within a specific point of care in the continuum. Thus, APN CMs collaborate with other providers to improve health care processes.

For example, one APN CM may work in the area of health promotion and disease prevention, assessing the population and developing longitudinal interventions to prevent costly debilitation associated with chronic disease in patients at risk. Another APN CM may practice in acute care and focus on complication management to achieve desired outcomes associated with hospital care. Finally, there are opportunities for the APN CM to practice within the community, following high-risk clients with pre-existing conditions, chronic disease, or terminal disease. At any point on the continuum, the APN CM may collaborate with physicians, NPs, and other providers to promote optimal treatment decisions and reduce costly variations among practitioners and health care delivery processes. The APN CM must have a working knowledge of all disease management system components including the people, the tools, and the evaluation methods.

Eichert and Patterson (1997) described the key elements of disease management as:

- Clinical management through the use of risk assessments and evidence-based guidelines
- Behavior modification through the application of theories and practices that apply to the particular population being managed for the specified disease
- Outcomes research for ongoing measurement that reflects behavior change, cost savings, and quality of clinical practice
- Financial management that can demonstrate cost of care across the continuum

In essence, the APN CM facilitates the development and implementation of a systematic approach to disease management that incorporates these elements for one or more points on the continuum of care. For a more comprehensive review of disease management, the reader is referred to *Disease Management: A Systems Approach to Improving Patient Outcomes* (Todd & Nash, 1997).

Disease Management Interventions

Disease management interventions focus on behavior modification and outpatient activities. The APN CM addresses these components through staff education and team coordination. Whether the disease management program is for chronic low back pain, diabetes, multiple sclerosis (MS), or congestive heart failure (CHF), the APN CM assumes a leadership role in establishing evidence-based practice guidelines and identifying appropriate patient interventions, such as telephone case management, selection of educational media for small group education/activities, or home visits. The intent of these interventions is to augment physician/NP visits and redirect care to an outpatient, less costly environment (Plocher, 1996).

Tools of Disease Management

It is essential to determine the appropriate vehicle to communicate the disease management strategy. APN CMs must be able to select the most effective tool to encourage an evidence-based approach to care. Is a critical pathway more practical than a care guideline? When is a protocol necessary? Would standardized medical orders guide the team to select recommended diagnostic and treatment practices? The APN CM needs to evaluate the process being altered and select the tool that will best guide decision making and influence clinical practice. The authors of this chapter offer the following definitions of three common disease management tools:

Care Guidelines: Care guidelines are established based on formal research or substantial clinical evidence. The information within the guideline is what should be *done most of the time* in the management of a particular disease or population of patients, such as patients with diabetes, pneumonia, or CHF. Variances in practice are to be expected and should be documented because they may teach health care providers something new.

Critical Pathways: Critical pathways are elements of practice or key decision points that are *time ordered* and *presumed* to influence clinical or economic outcomes. They have an interdisciplinary focus, and are designed to promote standardization; however, variations are expected. The authors of this chapter suggest that it is probably not necessary to collect variance data on a routine basis unless a particular process or outcome is under focus review.

Protocols: Protocols are standards of practice, such as advanced cardiac life support protocols or weight-based heparin or aminoglycoside protocols. They are things that should be done *nearly all the time.* Minimal variation should occur, and collection of variances need not occur once the process is stabilized within the organization.

Disease Management Outcomes

The success of a disease management program is reflected in the following evaluation areas:

- *Return on investment:* How much did it cost to implement the program versus how much the organization saved during the period of time that the program was being evaluated?
- *Changes in utilization patterns:* Have admissions, readmission rates, or bed-days/1,000 covered lives decreased significantly?
- *Clinical outcomes:* Is the diabetic patient staying within a desired range of glucose control as evidenced by the hemoglobin A_1C blood test?
- *Satisfaction of the patients, providers, and plans:* Are patients more satisfied with their health, providers, and plans? Are the providers satisfied with their patients' health status and support services? Is the plan satisfied with the program? Did the disease management program demonstrate value for future marketing?

PROFILE OF NURSE CASE MANAGEMENT PRACTICE

NCMs are employed in a wide range of health care entities, including hospitals, home care, behavioral health settings, managed care organizations, health insurance companies, clinics, physician offices, long-term care agencies, public health organizations, schools, rehabilitation agencies, occupational health settings, and independent case management companies. Profiles of existing NCM practice remain difficult to obtain because of wide variation in job titles, work settings, and backgrounds of NCMs. In addition, a variety of credentialing bodies for case management have sprung up within the past 4 to 5 years, each with its own standards and descriptive profiles, making a global assessment of nurse case management difficult.

A survey conducted by Pace University in order to understand the current and future employment patterns of NCMs in New Jersey, New York, and Connecticut (Falter, Cesta, Concert, & Mason, 1999) provided some insight into contemporary nurse case management. A total of 69 facilities was randomly selected to be interviewed, including hospitals, home health care (HHC) agencies, managed care companies, and long-term care facilities. It was found that 52 (75%) of the 69 facilities employed NCMs. Six of the facilities (9%) employed nurses with different titles who performed case management functions. Titles included intake nurse, resident care coordinator, discharge planner, home care coordinator, patient care manager, and primary care nurse. When asked what the single most important qualification for the nurse case management role was, clinical experience was the most frequently identified criterion, followed by experience in home care and utilization management. Seventy-seven percent of the facilities hired NCMs with a Bachelor of Science degree. Only three facilities (5%) said that an advanced degree was an important qualification to perform successfully in the current case management role; however, 31 (53%) agreed there is a need to educate case managers at the master's level. Of greatest interest, however, was the finding that 39 facilities (67%) reported that their case managers are involved with the management of outcome data. Another 19 facilities (32%) reported that their case managers are not involved in data management, simply because they do not possess the technology to store and report outcome data.

Although this study was confined to three northeastern states, it may well be representative of national trends. It would appear that health care organizations are beginning to see the link between the case management role and outcomes data management. As regulatory bodies such as HCFA and the Joint Commission for the Accreditation of Healthcare Organizations (JCAHO) begin to enforce the collection of outcomes data, such as the Minimum Data Set for Long Term Care, the OASIS Data Set for Home Care, and the collection of core measure sets for hospitals, more and more health care agencies will be forced to obtain the necessary technology to support such data collection and reporting initiatives. With this rise in technology, there will be a greater demand for case managers to manage and interpret data, and to serve as change agents for their organizations in order to improve quality and cost performance.

Types of Nurse Case Management

Nurse case management models may be health or illness focused. Although community and acute care models differ in terms of practice setting, target populations, and span of accountability, the success of nurse case management interventions relies on the nurse's clinical knowledge and expertise. Some populations for which nurse case management has been used include acute care populations such as cardiovascular surgical patients (Mahn, 1993), the chronically mentally ill (Bryson, Naqvi, Callahan, & Fontenot, 1990); human immunodeficiency virus–positive women (Riley, 1992); perinatal clients (Ladden, 1991); clients in rural settings (Parker et al., 1990); trauma patients (Daleiden, 1993); and community health centers for health assessment, counseling, education, and screening (Ethridge, 1991). Which nurse case management model a health care agency chooses depends on the agency's goals and the creativity of the NCMs. Furthermore, a health care agency may elect to implement multiple models of nurse case management simultaneously. Common organizational goals that justify the use of nurse case management include reducing lengths of acute care stay, readmissions, resource use, and costs; increasing access to services and market share; and becoming a recognized center of excellence for a particular product line. Table 19–2 illustrates the span of accountability and common functions for five types of NCM. The reader should note that functions appearing in bold type represent APN CM functions.

TABLE 19–2 SPAN OF ACCOUNTABILITY AND COMMON FUNCTIONS ASSOCIATED WITH FIVE COMMON NCM MODELS

NCM TYPE	TYPICAL SETTING	SPAN OF ACCOUNTABILITY	COMMON FUNCTIONS
Utilization resource manager	Hospital Clinic	Patients assigned within a geographically defined unit or department *Typically carries a case load of 20–30 patients.*	• Daily chart review for LOS and medical appropriateness • Ensure payer-based criteria are met (e.g., Interqual or Milliman & Roberts) • DC planning • Referral and authorization procurement • Claims monitoring • Collaboration with nursing, medicine, social work, payer • Minimal patient contact
Staff nurse case manager	Hospital Clinic Primary care Physician office	Patients assigned within a geographically defined unit or department *Typically carries a case load of 8–12 patients.*	• Direct patient care during a shift • 24-hour care planning • Patient/family education • DC planning in collaboration with other care members • Daily review of pathway/guidelines • May participate in pathway, guideline, or protocol development • May participate in quality improvement initiatives (e.g., quality committees, CQI teams)
Telephone nurse case manager	Payer office (e.g., HMO, insurance company) Hospital Clinic	Caseload may be organized by physician groups, clinical specialty, or payer *Typically carries an active case load of 150–200 clients.*	• Intake/triage • Identify and prioritize client problems • Referral, coordination, and authorization for services • Periodic follow-up phone contact with patient or family depending upon need • Evaluation of patient's adherence to prescribed or recommended health care behaviors following disease management guidelines or protocols • Patient/family education • May participate in the development of disease management guidelines and protocols • May have additional utilization management responsibilities depending on employer

Role	Setting	Case load	Responsibilities
Clinical nurse case manager	Hospital Ambulatory care setting Home care	Patients assigned by case type, product line, or physician service. Crosses geographical boundaries to follow patient throughout an episode of care. *Typically carries a case load of 8–20 patients.*	• Limited day-to-day bedside care • Comprehensive assessment (e.g., admission, preoperative, periodic, postdischarge) • Patient/family teaching • 24-hour accountability • Daily assessment of patient status and response to treatments • Facilitation of care plan through multidisciplinary collaboration • Coordination of DC plan • **Staff education and expert consultation** • **Oversight of pathway, guideline, and protocol development, implementation, and aggregate evaluation** • **Evaluation of clinical and financial outcomes for aggregate population** • **Facilitate, coordinate, and lead process improvement initiatives within the care delivery system** • **Influence nursing practice and health care policy through publications, lecturing, and consultation in academic and practice environments**
Community nurse case manager	Hospital Home Physician office SNF Community centers Industry	Predefined geographic region within community or by client case type if specialized. Follows clients across multiple settings and over time. *Typically carries an active case load of 30–40 clients.*	• Comprehensive assessment upon referral • Evaluate client's level of risk and appropriateness of referral • Identify and prioritize client problems • Establish mutually agreed upon goals with client and care team • Coordinate needed resources • Collaborate with client to determine frequency of follow-up contacts to evaluate client's status (e.g., face-to-face visits and telephone follow-up) • Patient/family education • Ongoing evaluation to establish interventions most appropriate to client's disease trajectory • **Oversight of disease management guideline development, implementation, and evaluation** • **Evaluation of clinical and financial outcomes related to aggregate population** • **Facilitate, coordinate, and lead process improvement initiatives within local care delivery systems** • **Influence nursing practice and health care policy through publications, lecturing, and consultation in academic and practice environments**

CQI = continuous quality improvement; DC = discharge; HMO = health maintenance organization; LOS = length of stay; SNF = skilled nursing facility.

Regardless of the type of NCM or the organizational model of nurse case management used, nurses who provide case management bring an understanding of disease processes, therapies, and responses to illness and treatment that other disciplines may not offer. The goal of both nurse case management and case management is to accomplish the quality and fiscal outcomes sought by managed care systems. Increasingly, one finds that NCMs are sharing direct and indirect fiscal risk with their sponsoring organizations. In some organizations, continued employment of the NCM is contingent upon the person's ability to demonstrate a cost savings of at least her or his annual salary, in addition to the demonstration of measurable outcomes that improve patient function, patient, provider, and payer satisfaction and other clinical and fiscal outcomes. However, in nurse case management the methods for accomplishing quality and cost outcomes rely on a nursing perspective: advocacy for access, holistic assessment, partnership with patients and families over time, interventions related to health promotion and self-care skills, and coordination of care across settings (Smith, 1993). Table 19-3 illustrates activities common to most nurse case management models.

Health care organizations that provide nurse case management resources to their clients, patients, or plan members must be cognizant of the potential for role confusion, redundancy, and duplication when multiple models of nurse case management are used within the health care network. All nurse case management services must be clearly defined and well integrated into the health care environment. Patients, families, and other members of the health care team may become confused when faced with multiple staff with the title "case manager."

Functions That Distinguish Nurse Case Management from APN Case Management

In Table 19-2, the functions of five different types of NCM reveal that not all types of nurse case management are consistent with advanced nursing practice. Nurses who perform case management functions, whether at the basic or the advanced practice level, must have sufficient clinical expertise to understand the needs and clinical management of specific patient populations. Clinical interventions are often

---

TABLE 19-3 ACTIVITIES COMMON TO NURSE CASE MANAGERS

- Collaboration with administrative, management, and clinical staff who are responsible for specified patient groups
- Assessment, planning, implementation, coordination, referral, and evaluation of patients and families in assigned target populations
- Provision of internal consultation to other disciplines and departments with the goal of managing care of patients and families expeditiously
- Participation in the development of documentation systems and tools (i.e., critical pathways or practice guidelines) to monitor clinical and fiscal outcomes
- Collecting, analyzing, and sharing of data and information in order to influence process improvements and support integration of core systems and processes within the care environment
- Development of partnerships with physicians in order to achieve clinical and fiscal outcomes
- Teaching and coaching other caregivers on the health care team regarding clinical, fiscal, and system processes related to patient care management
- Role modeling of professional nursing practice

directed toward enhancing patients' and their families' self-care skills by helping them access appropriate health care services and community resources. Prior clinical experience is critical for (1) anticipating the likely trajectory of certain illnesses; (2) understanding and making choices among alternative interventions; (3) analyzing variances from standards of care, guidelines, and critical pathways; (4) understanding and respecting the clinical judgments of other providers; and (5) negotiating among patients, providers, and payers. The NCM must also be able to influence the delivery system in which the care is provided; this is essential. The interpersonal skills nurses bring to the care of patients are just as important in their relationships with other members of the health care team. Those that are particularly important to the NCM role at the system level of intervention are collaboration, communication, and conflict resolution (Connors, 1993). The reader must realize that, in contemporary NCM practice, these activities are carried out by NCMs with varying levels and types of preparation and experience; current practice does not routinely require the NCM to have advanced nursing education. Research (Ethridge & Lamb, 1989; Lamb & Stempel, 1994) and anecdotal reports (Connors, 1993) suggest that there are some patients whose care can be effectively managed and coordinated by nurses who are not APNs. However, research also indicates that there are patients who require APN CMs. Although the NCM role may be considered to be advanced practice when the NCM possesses advanced education and a clinical specialty, and when NCMs demonstrate APN competencies and functions, the distinguishing features between the NCM and the APN CM have yet to be sufficiently supported by research or endorsed by professional nursing organizations.

Using work by Calkin (1984) and Connors (1993), Mahn and Spross (1996) recommended some approaches for differentiating basic nurse case management from APN case management. Calkin (1984) differentiated advanced nursing practice from basic nursing practice on three dimensions: education, experience, and patient complexity. She used a bell curve as a way of understanding the different problem-solving skills of novices, experts-by-experience, and APNs, specifically CNSs. She postulated that nurses deal with a range of human responses that exist in a normal distribution. Calkin described the knowledge and skills of the novice nurse as best suited to managing a narrow range of typical and predictable human responses to health and illness. Experts-by-experience demonstrate skills superior to novices when dealing with the same situations that the novice is able to handle (e.g., earlier recognition of problems and faster problem solving). In addition, they are capable of assessing and intervening in a broader range of human responses than the novice. When compared with APNs, experts-by-experience are more likely to describe their expert interventions in terms of intuition. Calkin characterized the APN (CNS) as academically and clinically prepared to intervene effectively for a full range of human responses to actual or potential problems. Thus, in addition to education and experience, basic nurse case management could be differentiated from APN case management along the dimensions of patient complexity (physical, emotional, or social) and predictability of clinical course.

Connors (1993) suggested that care management could be conceptualized as a continuum anchored by care coordination on one end and case management on the other. She asserted that every patient needs care coordination but not all patients need case management. "Case management, in its most limited application, is usually reserved for patients or clients with more complex health care needs, that is, high-risk, high-volume, high-costs patients and those with catastrophic illnesses" (Connors, 1993, p. 192). In the continuum description, care coordination is linked with health and case management with illness. In Mahn and Spross' (1996) opinion, this was a limitation of the continuum Connors described. As an example, a mother and baby who are healthy but live in a crime-ridden area may be considered high-risk clients because of limited social supports and a risk of exposure to drugs or violence. Furthermore, the APN CM practice is not limited to the illness side of the continuum. APN CMs may be actively engaged in program development and clinical practice associated with health promotion and prevention strategies.

The authors have observed that case management by APNs is characterized by greater complexity of clinical decision making and greater skill in managing constraints of care related to organizational bureaucracy than is the practice of nurse case management at the basic level. Unlike NCMs, APN CMs have greater autonomy — they can perform more extensive assessments and initiate a variety of treatments which may include prescribing. In addition, APN CMs are recognized as experts based on experience and advanced education, an understanding of the relevant research literature, research utilization skills, and an extensive network of community and care management resources related to their specialty.

On the basis of the contributions of Calkin (1984) and Connors (1993), Mahn and Spross (1996) concluded that basic and advanced nurse case management can be differentiated along several dimensions. They suggested that care coordination (or nurse case management practiced by experts-by-experience) may best describe the processes used to achieve clinical and fiscal outcomes when clinical situations are simple, common, time limited, or predictable, or require few and inexpensive resources. Clinically, patients with novel or uncommon diagnoses and patients whose care is complex, resource intensive, or unpredictable are likely to need an APN. High-volume or high-risk populations may need an APN CM initially so that disease management processes can be established, such as guidelines, pathways, and standards of care that ensure achievement of clinical and fiscal outcomes appropriate for the population. As experience with the population accumulates and the disease management program is successfully diffused across the health services continuum, the care for such high-risk patients, although complex, may become more routine and no longer require an APN CM.

Mahn and Spross (1996) also suggested that the type of NCM needed might depend on organizational variables: the numbers and types of clinicians involved in the network (the more clinicians there are, the less predictable behaviors and interactions will be); the status of guideline use and development (the greater the number of people who need to be brought together to learn to use existing guidelines or to develop new guidelines, the more complex the scenario); and the degree to which existing practices must be changed to ensure that clinical and fiscal outcomes are reached or the need for concurrent program development as nurse case management is implemented (the more change needed, the more organizationally and interpersonally complex the scenario). Thus, as Mahn and Spross (1996) suggested, the more complex and uncertain the organizational variables, the more an organization needs APNs practicing within their case management systems. Their conclusion remains true: some nurse case management can be done by experts-by-experience, whereas other nurse case management must be done by APNs.

Research is needed to validate these ideas on differentiating basic and advanced nurse case management presented in the first edition of this book (Mahn & Spross, 1996) and in the current discussion. At this stage in the evolution of nurse case management, health care agencies do employ experts-by-experience as NCMs to oversee care for patients who fit the preceding descriptions of populations needing APN case management. This is particularly so when staff turnover is high or when primary staff nurses need ongoing education and support to manage these more complex case types. Moving experienced nurses into nurse case management roles is seen as a way to recognize and retain experienced nurses while promoting a successful, professional practice model (Zander, 1990). As experience with nurse case management accumulates, the profession will be in a better position to determine what mix of APNs and experts-by-experience is needed to provide care coordination and case management services that ensure that clinical, fiscal, and system goals are met.

APN CM COMPETENCIES

APNs have been valued for their specialized knowledge and their training in complex decision making (Madden & Reid Ponte, 1994). Parallels between traditional APN roles and the NCM role have been observed (Connors, 1993; Fralic, 1992; Hamric, 1992; Newman, cited in Smith, 1993). Hamric (1992) analyzed the nurse case management literature and suggested that the NCM role be viewed as an APN role. She exhorted APNs to "confront the challenge of case management forcefully and articulate their role to this practice modality" (Hamric, 1992, p. 13). Interestingly, NCM functions (see Table 19–3) closely align with the traditional subroles of the CNS (clinical practice, consultation, education, and research) (Hamric, 1989) and incorporate the CNS's change agent, management, and leadership skills (Gournic, 1989). The parallels between the APN CM role and the traditional CNS role are also reflected in the number of nurse case management articles published by CNSs (e.g., Cronin & Maklebust, 1989; Flynn & Kilgallen, 1993; Lynn-McHale, Fitzpatrick, & Shaller, 1993; Nugent, 1992; Sherman & Johnson, 1994; Strong, 1992; Trinidad, 1993; Wagner & Menke, 1992). Patient populations who have been cared for by CNSs include multisystem failure patients in critical care (Strong, 1991), long-term care patients (Schroer, 1991), trauma patients (Daleiden, 1993; Rotz, Yates, & Schare, 1994), pediatric patients with cardiac defects or chronic illness (Doell Smith, 1994; Gaedeke-Norris & Hill, 1991), and patients who have undergone coronary artery bypass graft (Tidwell, 1994). Jenkins and Sullivan-Marx (1994) proposed a primary care delivery model in which NPs would practice as NCMs.

Because the APN CM continues to evolve, this section focuses on how the APN competencies are currently operationalized in APN case management and additional competencies that APN CMs need to perform well in the role. Table 19–4 outlines eight APN CM competencies to help the reader see that APN CM functions are congruent with the APN competencies described throughout Part II of this text. Additional competencies are included to demonstrate how the APN CM is likely to be different from more established APN roles. Figure 19–1 illustrates the flow of competencies and skills required for the APN CM to perform within a complex health care system and is consistent with the conceptual model described in Chapter 3. Although the health care system is understood as a continuum of care, the system as it relates to case management practice is depicted as a triad of case management strategies. The APN CM may practice at any point in the continuum, with an emphasis on developing disease management strategies for her or his population, establishing health promotion or prevention programs, or serving in the acute care environment

TABLE 19-4	APN COMPETENCIES AND RELATED SKILLS AND FUNCTIONS	
APN COMPETENCY	APN CM KNOWLEDGE/SKILL	APN CM FUNCTIONS
Direct care	• In-depth, holistic assessment skills • Expert, clinically relevant knowledge and skills • Formation of client-nurse partnership • Expert clinical reasoning • Application of diverse management approaches	• Find and screen cases • Conduct health assessments • Establish client goals • Coordinate interventions among other providers • Link patient with appropriate resources • Monitor patient's progress toward goals • Evaluate effects of interventions
Expert guidance and coaching	• Behavioral change theory • Teaching-learning theory • Ability to communicate in a nonjudgmental style	• Assess level of client readiness to modify health care choices • Coach patients and families through developmental, health, and illness transitions • Educate other providers about clinical, fiscal, and system processes
Change agency	• Assessment of processes, systems, and organizations • Social marketing theory	• Assess community or population needs • Plan new services/programs • Establish program objectives and interventions • Develop marketing materials • Program implementation and evaluation
Consultation	• Provision of case consultation • Securing of consultation to enhance care and nurse case management	• Participate in work redesign • Initiate system-wide process improvements (e.g., CQI teams, documentation tools, electronic medical record)
Collaboration	• Communication, coordination, and negotiation	• Monitor service plan regarding quality, timeliness, quantity, costs of services, and effectiveness • Develop protocols of care, guidelines, critical pathways, and other disease management tools
Ethical decision making	• Recognition and raising of ethical dilemmas • Conflict resolution stratgies • Negotiation • Affirmation of others	• Identify all options available to client • Evaluate risks and benefits of decision options • Balance system/fiscal and client goals • Maintain satisfaction of both internal and external customers
Research utilization and CQI	• Research interpretation and utilization • Research design, data collection, analysis and synthesis	• Review and interpretation of the literature • Design and implementation of evaluation plan • Facilitation of CQI teams • Interpretation of process and outcome data
Data analysis and information management	• Health care finance • Billing codes and procedures • Health care information systems • Database query • Statistical process control	• Prioritize data collection activities • Facilitate strategies to capture data and information • Analyze cost, quality, and satisfaction outcomes • Analyze trends in care delivery processes • Prepare and present data findings to stakeholders • Collaborate with information systems experts in the implementation of automated, electronic case management systems

Revised and expanded upon based on the original work of Hamric (1992), Connors (1993), and Mahn and Spross (1996).

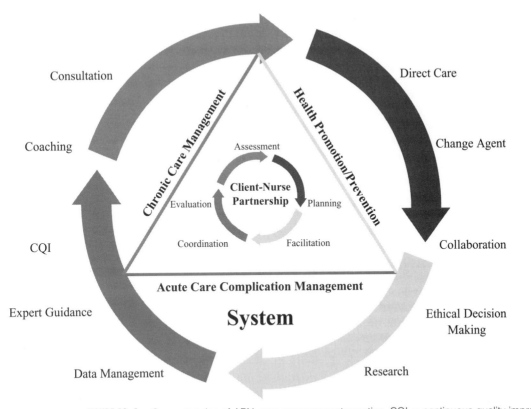

FIGURE 19–1 • Competencies of APN case management practice. CQI = continuous quality improvement. (Copyright 1999 by MIDS, Inc., Tucson, AZ; reprinted with permission.)

to manage high-risk, complex patients. Regardless of the APN CM's practice focus, the case management processes of assessment, planning, facilitation, coordination, and evaluation are applied to the management of all clients. All case management interventions occur within the context of the client-nurse partnership, which is the centerpoint of the model. APN CMs need to be assertive, confident clinicians who are recognized by others as having exemplary clinical skills.

Direct Care, Expert Coaching, and Guidance

The central competency of an APN CM is direct clinical practice. The APN CM's direct care is consistent with the characteristics outlined in Chapter 6. In addition to assessment of physical issues, functional status, and symptom distress, the APN CM might be more likely than other APNs to perform more detailed assessment of environmental, organizational, psychosocial, sociocultural, spiritual, economic, ethical, and other contextual factors that affect individual patients and their health care choices. Based on assessment data, APN CMs use diverse management approaches. A comprehensive, holistic, and integrated synthesis of assessment information is necessary for the APN CM to develop a successful care management plan and achieve a greater degree of well-being for her or his client. APN CMs are responsible for monitoring a client's progress toward his or her goals, evaluating the effects of their interventions, and linking the client with appropriate resources for ongoing management as warranted by the intensity and severity of the client's illness. APN CMs may retain the client as a primary client if the case remains complex, or delegate the care of the client to other care providers who are capable of managing the routine aspects of care and who will keep the client "anchored" to the health care system as needed.

The nurse case management literature consistently advocates a relationship focus (Fralic, 1992; Lamb & Stempel, 1994; Newman, Lamb, & Michaels, 1989). This is consistent with the discussion of formation of partnerships with patients (in Chapter 6; see also Brown, 1996). Analysis of interviews with patients experiencing nurse case management suggested that the process used in nurse case management practice is one in which the NCM becomes a "trusted insider" to the client. As the process unfolds, patients integrate the nurse's teaching and coaching so that they become their own "insider experts," able to make judgments about their needs for care (Lamb & Stempel, 1994). Until the NCM becomes a "trusted insider," interventions to optimize wellness or foster self-care skills may have limited impact. Within the partnership context, patient and family values and health perceptions must be honored. Lamb and Stempel (1994) suggested that successful outcomes such as fewer days in the hospital and critical care unit, fewer readmissions, and reduced use of emergency room services are related to "monitoring and teaching activities of the nurse case managers, which occur in the context of a caring nurse-client relationship" (p. 9).

This understanding of how the nurse-client relationship contributes to the success of the nurse case management intervention has theoretical support (Newman, 1994), and is also directly linked to the APN CM competency of expert coaching and guidance (see Chapter 7). Being able to translate clinical knowledge into patient action is one of the greatest challenges for the APN CM, and extends far beyond the scope of delivering educational materials to the patient or his or her family. Likewise, the APN CM must be careful not to assume responsibility for clients' health care decisions, but rather assist them to more actively participate in self-care behaviors. Newman and colleagues (1992) described this role as a facilitator and collaborator. In this process, the APN CM helps the patient understand his or her behavior patterns, acknowledge the options and choices in relation to his or her problem, and be aware of the consequences of selecting one of those options.

Although the ability to facilitate health care behaviors and decisions may be based upon the art of "connecting" with the patient, it is also a skill based upon demonstrated research in the areas of patient education and behavioral change theory. Chapter 6 points out that among APNs' knowledge utilization skills is the ability to use middle-range theories to influence practice. Responsibility for analyses of processes and outcomes of care, core job responsibilities in APN CM practice, gives these APNs a unique opportunity to apply middle-range theories to clinical practice. The following exemplars illustrate the use of middle-range theories and the integration of the direct care and expert coaching competencies of APNs.

The APN CM must be able to make a distinction among a client's current health care behaviors, current health care status, and knowledge of his or her disease process. This distinction is essential to determining the most appropriate intervention to meet the client's needs.

EXEMPLAR 1

The APN CM is caring for Ms. Mallory, who has smoked two packs of cigarettes a day for the past 25 years and happens to be a retired military nurse. The APN CM recognizes that it will do little good to instruct her on the dangers of smoking. In fact, the presentation of educational materials may be viewed by the client as insulting and could undermine the development of a therapeutic relationship. The APN CM recognizes that the client's behaviors are incongruent with her level of understanding of the disease and will begin to explore other avenues of intervention. The APN CM has taught smoking cessation classes using the Stages of Change behavior theory (Prochaska, DiClemente, & Norcross, 1992), and decides to use this to guide her assessment. Stages include precontemplation (becoming aware that a change in behavior is needed), contemplation (thinking about making a change), action (making the change), and maintenance (maintaining the new behavior) or relapse (going back to the old behavior). During the APN CM's initial contact with the client, they reviewed Ms. Mallory's signs and symptoms together—shortness of breath, wheezing, sputum production, and seeking—in order to understand the client's experience with the disease thus far and determine her level of readiness to change. The APN CM worked on establishing a therapeutic client-CM relationship and fostering greater self-care management skills for the client. Without communicating judgement or criticism, the APN CM asked the client about her experience with smoking (i.e., when she began, how smoking makes her feel, triggers for smoking, past attempts at smoking cessation, the cost of cigarettes, and social inconveniences). In this manner, the APN CM set the stage for Ms. Mallory to become more aware of her behavior. Care providers in a situation such as this often try to assume control of the patient, asserting their credibility as the "health care professional," which may actually create disincentives for the patient to change. The APN CM operated from a different philosophy, understanding that the ultimate goal is to move the client toward greater control of his or her own disease process.

In another situation, an APN CM used the Health Belief Model (HBM) (Becker, 1974) to coach a client. Key elements of the HBM include individual perception, cues to action, and likeliness for action. Individual perception refers to whether a patient perceives the illness or health problem to be of a serious nature and his or her own perceived degree of susceptibility to the illness. Cues to action refer to factors that affect clients' choices—who influences their health care behaviors and decisions and how. Likeliness for action refers to the benefits and barriers of adopting a new behavior identified by the client. It is important for the APN CM to distinguish between the benefits that she or he perceives for the client and the benefit that the client perceives. An assessment of barriers such as cost, time, distance, accessibility, language, culture, and physical ability must also be taken into consideration. Assessing barriers can assist the APN CM when establishing a plan of care with the client.

EXEMPLAR 2

The APN CM was caring for a client (Mr. Hernandez) with CHF, whom she encouraged to attend a free class about CHF at a local clinic. Mr. Hernandez declined, stating that he did not have transportation. The APN CM then offered to coordinate transportation for this client; however, the client gave another reason for why he could not attend the class, stating that he did not feel comfortable leaving his wife alone while he went to the class. The APN CM suggested that they arrange for a volunteer "friendly visitor" from a local church to sit with his wife while he attended classes; the client again declined, stating that he did not feel comfortable with a stranger. The APN CM realized that she was unlikely to convince Mr. Hernandez to attend class because of a variety of personal beliefs and perceived barriers. She recognized that this client was at risk for complications, hospitalization, and a diminished ability to care for his wife; he required more monitoring and disease surveillance than was possible through routine doctor's office visits. She also recognized that more frequent, direct home monitoring by clinicians was impractical and expensive, and so offered an alternative to attending CHF class. The client agreed to start working with a telephone NCM to monitor his diet, medications, weight changes, and symptoms.

These exemplars illustrate the ways in which APN CMs integrate interpersonal skills with knowledge of disease, illness trajectories, treatment responses, and experience with an individual to encourage clients to adopt effective self-care behaviors. APN CMs must also decide when they should intervene directly and when to delegate to other members of the health care team. Knowledge and application of middle-range theories (see Chapter 6) may be helpful to the APN CM for analyzing clinical situations and determining opportunities for intervening effectively with individual clients.

Consultation, Collaboration, and Leadership

The APN CM also influences care on a broader level than individual patients. Their collaborative, consultative, and leadership skills enable APN CMs to influence direct care and health care delivery systems. This may be one of the reasons so many CNSs have moved into APN CM roles; case management positions directly link APNs to outcomes. The APN CM's accountability for accomplishing clinical, fiscal, and organizational outcomes on a system-wide level significantly influences the expression of these particular competencies. This accountability is one key difference between the APN CM and other APNs.

As a recognized clinical expert in a specialty, the APN CM functions as a clinical consultant in the development of population-specific process improvements within her or his health care system. Serving as a consultant across the delivery system is probably one of the key differences between the APN CM and other APN roles, although this role function is most similar to the blended CNS/NP role. One of the advantages of being an APN CM is that one's practice influence can be exercised at multiple points along the continuum and is not limited to one department or point of service. The APN CM may also lead or participate in CQI teams. These activities indicate the importance of leadership, consultation, negotiation, research, data analysis, communication, and change agent skills. APN CMs must have enough autonomy and control over their daily work and schedule to be able to shift back and forth between involvement with direct care and involvement with system issues in order to achieve desired outcomes for individual patients and the aggregate population. The APN CM provides continuity for both individual patients and providers across the settings in which care is delivered.

Work redesign and process improvements within clinical services or care settings are strategies for achieving quality and cost outcomes in health delivery systems (Baird, 1995). APN CMs often lead such system changes by exercising leadership on clinical, financial, and political issues that affect patient care and evaluating the care delivery system. The APN CM must identify stakeholders and cultivate their interest in and commitment to designing, implementing, and evaluating changes aimed at improving care delivery. Prior to implementing a change, the APN CM collaborates with stakeholders to establish mutually agreed upon goals, accountabilities, and a process for evaluation, including responsibilities for data collection and analysis. APN CMs have leadership skills that enable them to build the interdisciplinary consensus that is required to develop and implement care guidelines, protocols, standard order sets, critical pathways, decision algorithms, or comprehensive disease management programs.

Because APN CMs are members of a team that is accountable for treating, comforting, and administering care within specified time frames to meet both quality and economic targets, they can become champions for CQI within their areas of clinical accountability. Their involvement in providing direct care, analyzing the care delivery system for costly inefficiencies and inconveniences, and initiating process improvements makes APN CMs ideal consultants to other health care associates who are charged with system re-engineering or process improvement. Although some could argue that leadership for establishing system-wide case management programs lies with the APN CM, it may be a specialty in and of itself. The Center for Case Management now offers certification in Administrative Case Management, which focuses on the business and operational aspects of a case management program. This certification is discussed further in this chapter in the section "Education, Experience, and Certification: Preparing for the APN CM Role."

Change Agency

Although change agency is part of leadership for all APNs, because of the APN CM's responsibility for process improvement, the change agent role is discussed separately here. In order to influence cost and quality outcomes for a population of patients, it may become necessary for the APN CM to act as a change agent and develop a formal program or other systematic approaches to organize the new care processes that will be applied to the population. Social marketing theory has been used as a framework for developing programs to influence care for a population. Social marketing is the design, implementation, and control of programs seeking to increase the acceptability of a social idea, cause, or practice among members of a target group (Kotler & Zaltman, 1971). (For further discussion of marketing, a key element of the APN CM's change agent role, see Chapter 21.) Because program development and evaluation is an important component of the APN CM's approach to change, social marketing is outlined here.

Social marketing reflects the nursing process with a marketing focus; the target group may include patients, providers, and purchasers of health care goods and services. The first step is planning. The objectives must be clearly defined and supported by a literature review and evidence-based practice. It is important for APN CMs to compare and contrast the demographics of their community to that of other communities that have been successful with a similar innovation, and determine the level of community support required to initiate such a program. Next, they would define their interventions. A detailed analysis of the services that are to be provided should be conducted. The third step is a thorough assessment of the population targeted to receive the services, including demographics, frequency of the disease, and prior health care utilization patterns when known. The results of this assessment will serve as crucial baseline data for program evaluation. An implementation plan and the required resources must be defined. The implementation plan includes a description of projected improvements, explicit time frames, and actual performance measures that will determine whether the program objectives were met. Pretest or evaluation instruments and marketing materials need to be developed (or selected from existing ones). Prior to full implementation, the instruments, marketing materials, and intervention/program are piloted. Based on the pilot results, the program, instruments, and marketing materials would be modified as necessary. Collaboration with interdisciplinary care providers, administrative leaders, insurance partners, and financial and informatics specialists throughout the process of program development and implementation is essential to ensure the program's success. Hospodar and Zazworsky (1997, 1999) described their use of social marketing theory to create a case management program as part of a national Medicare Demonstration Project called The Community Nursing Organization.

Ethical Decision Making and Conflict Resolution

Embedded in the concept of partnership with patients and families is the APN CM's role as client advocate. If the organization is truly committed to quality and customer satisfaction, the barriers to effective advocacy are fewer. The APN CM's dual account-ability for patient and organizational outcomes may give rise to ethical dilemmas with somewhat different features than those encountered by other APNs. For exam-ple, patient and organizational outcomes can come into conflict, and these conflicts are likely to be more visible because the costs of clinical decisions are monitored. The APN CM must be able to articulate the risks and benefits of choices and decisions for both the patient and organization. Within the NCM process, APNs have opportuni-ties to apply "preventive ethics" (see Chapter 12). For example, a well-designed critical pathway may indicate that a particular patient population can be discharged to home within a week of admission. However, if successful discharge depends on adequate social supports and a patient does not have these, the pathway and the data used to develop it can provide the justification for deviating from the pathway. Knowledge of fiscal variables and costs of services also enables the APN CM to articulate the costs of *not* pursuing a decision that is in the patient's best interests, in order to persuade others to do what is best for the patient. Finally, the APN CM must be able to anticipate situations in which her or his clinical decisions or those of other health care professionals may conflict with the goals and concerns of other stakeholders, such as third-party payers. In these situations, the APN CM can reaffirm the value of other care providers without diminishing their contributions and interven-tions, while negotiating for options that are truly in the best interest of the patient. The APN CM's ability to influence others is more likely to result from her or his clinical expertise and ethical decision-making skills, rather than from an explicit position of authority.

Research Utilization and CQI

Much of nurse case management is data driven. The advanced education, research skills, and specialized knowledge of APN CMs allow for the application of research methodologies and CQI principles to practice. Nurse case management and CQI are linked in philosophy and process (Cesta, 1993). It is essential that APN CMs be able to lead an interdisciplinary team toward data-based conclusions and process improvements. They must be able to influence practice patterns and develop meaningful standards, practice protocols, clinical pathways, or health care programs that promote teamwork, improve customer satisfaction and clinical outcomes, and reduce costs. APN CMs must be able to review current literature and research findings, and assist other health care team members to draw meaningful conclusions and see potential applications to their own practices.

In addition, the APN CM will be instrumental in designing evaluation plans that identify the overall value of specific case management interventions (i.e., a link between the intervention and the outcome). An understanding of how extraneous or confounding variables influence an outcome must be clearly expressed in the evaluation plan. Increasingly, APN CMs are engaged in national demonstration projects with rigorous evaluation components. Such programs typically involve federal funding or national endowments, and generally require the presence of a doctorate-level researcher to guide the project; however, APN CMs may be actively involved with all phases of such a demonstration.

DATA ANALYSIS AND INFORMATION MANAGEMENT

One of the positive outcomes of managed care is the recognition of the value of data and the need to invest in technology to collect and analyze data. Increasingly, case managers are assuming responsibility for the oversight of clinical, economic, and quality outcomes data associated with the provision of care within their sponsoring organizations. The APN CM must be able to analyze data and manage information—a competency not currently part of the traditional APN core skills and competencies. One of the unique skills of expert nurses and APNs is the ability to recognize patterns of client responses to health and illness. APN CMs bring this pattern recognition skill to the analysis of aggregated hospital or claims data in order to identify patterns in resource utilization. Patterns in resource utilization become leverage points for future case management interventions or system improvements. The APN CM must be able to quantify, track, and control cost and quality indicators in both the inpatient and outpatient environment. This is a core competency for the APN CM.

One of the first considerations of the APN CM in using data to design an evaluation plan for a case management program is to develop an understanding of the stakeholders in the processes of care, and the audience who will ultimately be reviewing the outcome findings. In other words, what questions might a group of physicians ask regarding the impact of the case management system on their patients? Likewise, what performance data will be necessary to demonstrate the value of the case management program to representatives from the payer who is contracting for services? The APN CM must first have an understanding of the information needs of the sponsoring organization and other stakeholders in order to design the evaluation plan for the case management program. This will help prioritize the data collection and analysis efforts that will be necessary in order to demonstrate program effectiveness. Data collection efforts should be evaluated in terms of the "value in knowing" the answer, and the "ease in obtaining the data." Data that are collected through automated, electronic means, such as the patient's social security number or marital status, may be easy to collect, but should be weighed against the overall "value of knowing." Likewise, there may be data elements that are difficult to collect, such as PAR+ or

SR-36 scores; however, there is great benefit in knowing this information. Data collection efforts must be prioritized so that finite information system (IS) resources can be put to the best use. Once incremental measures are established, the source of the data needs to be identified. Continuum-based case management programs may require multiple sources of data, and the cooperation of many different care providers to collect the information. If information needs are prioritized and limited to only the most relevant process steps in caring for the population of interest, a concise data plan can be developed to communicate the evaluation plan. Figure 19–2 illustrates a conceptual data plan for the evaluation of congestive heart failure (CHF) management across the care continuum. The central circle indicates that CHF is the focus of the performance evaluation plan. The wedges within the second circle identify points of service delivery (e.g., primary care) to CHF patients, specific care processes (e.g., risk assessment), and care focus (e.g., patient and family) that are being monitored. Key performance measures for each of these aspects of service delivery are specified in the third circle. The sources of data for each measure that will be used to evaluate the care of CHF patients are indicated on the perimeter of the wheel. The CHF conceptual data plan addresses several processes and outcomes of interest to the multiple stakeholders across the care continuum. This particular ''scorecard'' format not only permits one to examine the impact of selected interventions on patient outcomes, resource utilization, and costs, but effectively illustrates that the information needed to carry out the data plan exists within multiple information systems and across multiple points of service that may not be readily available to the APN CM who is accountable for the evaluation plan. Because the information associated with each point of service is generally considered to be proprietary to that service, the combined efforts of the stakeholders themselves are necessary to ensure the availability of the information required to carry out the evaluation plan. Thus, the evaluation plan moves beyond a plan to measure the effectiveness of ''case management'', but rather a plan to determine the organization's clinical effectiveness, cost effectiveness and overall efficiency of managing the population for which the APN CM is responsible.

For example, one of the patient outcomes being monitored is patients' adherence to a plan to weigh themselves on a regular schedule. This self-monitoring is designed to detect an early sign of CHF so that clinicians can intervene before a clinical crisis requiring an emergency room visit or hospitalization occurs. Patient weights, collected from telephone surveys and home visits, can be linked to data from the hospital's admit-discharge-transfer and financial information systems to see whether such self-care led to less costly hospitalizations and/or fewer emergency department visits and readmissions.

To develop a conceptual data plan for another clinical problem, the APN CM must collaborate with stakeholders to set priorities for evaluation, identify the most important performance indicators that measure the evaluation targets, specify where the data exist, and establish a cooperative approach to data collection. In developing a data plan, one must consider time constraints, the human and financial resources available to collect data, and the ease with which data can be collected. The conceptual data plan for CHF is relatively complex and reflects a system-wide commitment to evaluation of care delivery. Not every health care delivery system is at this stage of development with regard to a data-based approach to evaluation. However, the approach presented here provides APN CMs with a comprehensive strategy for evaluating care. By taking a broad view at the outset, APN CMs, administrators, and clinicians can set evaluation priorities and also develop long range plans for data

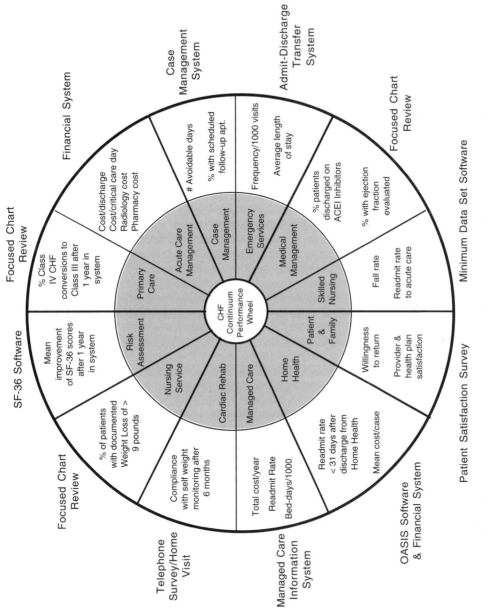

FIGURE 19–2 • Conceptual data plan for coordinating cross-continuum outcomes data for patients with congestive heart failure (CHF). (Copyright 1998 by Vicky A. Mahn, MIDS, Inc., Tucson, AZ; reprinted with permission.)

collection and management that will improve their setting's capacity to evaluate patient care.

APN CMs serve as a bridge among clinicians, administrators, and IS staff as decisions are made regarding database structures, IS, and the electronic infrastructures that support the necessary technology to monitor health care outcomes across the continuum. APN CMs must have a basic grasp of IS so that they can communicate effectively with IS staff. APN CMs often articulate and prioritize the relevant questions that need to be answered about a given population, define the data needed to answer the questions, and identify the multiple sources of required data and the methods for extracting it. APN CMs need to be able to envision the kinds of reports that will help stakeholders evaluate the processes and outcomes of care. They need to determine whether the data need to be collected in real time or whether historical data can be used. For example, if CMs are going to collect baseline health information during the case management intake process, will they, or other providers, need to have access to this information immediately after it is collected? Conversely, might the information only need to be accessed at some future point in time? This input is critical for the IS staff, who must consider the cost and complexity of implementing electronic interfaces in systems that support case management. Information that is required immediately after collection typically requires a "real-time" electronic interface. Real-time interfaces tend to be more costly to initiate and maintain than a batch interface, which brings information into the system at periodic intervals (e.g., weekly, monthly, or quarterly). The APN CM can serve as a consultant to the informatics team in setting up the IS structures that will support the evaluation plan. Ultimately, the design needs to be based on how the data will be utilized. The APN CM is in a unique position to define how the data will be used to monitor processes and measure outcomes associated with case management.

Evaluating Existing Sources of Data. Once the evaluation plan is established, a review of existing data sources needs to be conducted in order to avoid redundant data collection efforts. Typically, hospital IS contain a broad array of information that can be useful to case management evaluation. For example, the quality management or utilization management department may already collect the information required for case management performance measures. Other data sources include patient satisfaction surveys, injury claims, and infection control, financial, and cost accounting records. It is not uncommon for these data to reside within proprietary, stand-alone computer systems within individual departments. Individual departments may perceive that they "own" such information, and may require the APN CM to obtain administrative approval, computer security clearance, or consultation with those skilled at report writing in order to access the information. In addition, nursing departments may collect data on patient acuity, CQI teams, and other unit-based quality reports. Clinical documentation systems may also house data elements common to the medical record, such as patient demographics, New York Heart Association (NYHA) classification of CHF, disease history, SF-36 data, and functional independent measures.

One of the most commonly used sources of information is discharge abstract (DAB) and admissions-discharge-transfer (ADT) data. This database contains information particular to every patient encounter for hospital-based services. It usually contains registration and billing information for every inpatient, outpatient, and emergency room admission or encounter with the health care system. For inpatients and emergency patients, the record should contain one DRG and at least one diagnosis code from the International Classification of Diseases, 9th Revision (ICD-9). It is not uncommon for hospital IS departments to store as many as 15 ICD-9 codes for those patients with multiple diagnoses. The primary ICD-9 diagnosis code under which the patient was discharged is generally the first one listed in the electronic record. The record may also contain ICD-9 procedure codes if the patient underwent any procedures. Procedure codes include not only surgical procedures, but other less invasive procedures such as electrocardiographic monitoring, urinary catheter insertions, or ventilator support. Table 19–5 lists data elements that are typically found in the hospital's DAB and ADT IS that are useful to the APN CM in evaluating patterns of utilization, cost, and, to some degree, quality outcomes. Although the majority of hospital systems contain charge data, NCMs may not have access to actual cost data. In this event, APN CMs should collaborate with an expert in the financial office to determine the most accurate methodology for establishing costs of care within their organizations.

In the absence of sophisticated outcome or case management software applications, the system-savvy APN CM can request her or his IS department to prepare the data from the DAB and ADT system for a particular period of time (e.g., a month, a fiscal quarter, or even an entire year). The file that is prepared should be in a string-delimited, ASCI format with one record per encounter. In other words, all the data elements for each separate encounter are contained in one long row of data within the electronic record. In this manner, an electronic file can be easily transferred into applications such as pivot tables in Microsoft Excel for more user-friendly data analysis and query. This function is relatively easy to learn, and is an effective way to search a database and analyze common patterns of utilization. Pivot tables in Excel allow the case manager to

- Profile utilization, costs, and charges by physician or service
- Profile costs and charges by payer
- Identify common procedures for a selected case type
- Identify co-morbidities using ICD-9 diagnosis codes
- Trend cost and charges by LOS
- Explore patterns in discharge disposition
- Calculate mortality rates
- Examine utilization patterns for the emergency department, including LOS
- Calculate proxy measures of readmission

TABLE 19–5 DATA ELEMENTS TYPICALLY AVAILABLE FROM HOSPITAL INFORMATION SYSTEMS THAT ARE USEFUL FOR CASE MANAGEMENT EVALUATION			
• Facility ID	• Admission date	• Primary care	• DRG
• Account no.	• Admission time	physician	• DRG description
• Medical record no.	• Reason for admission	• Admitting physician	• Primary ICD-9
• Social Security no.	• Admit status	• Attending physician	diagnosis
• Date of birth	• Emergency admit	• Total charges	• Secondary ICD-9
• Gender	• Discharge date	• Total cost	diagnoses (15)
• Patient type	• Discharge time	• Insurance carrier	• Primary ICD-9
• Financial class	• Discharge disposition	• Insurance type	procedure
• Home zip code		• Insurance plan	• Secondary ICD-9
			procedures

For example, it would be quite possible to query the hospital database for all inpatients with a primary discharge diagnosis code of CHF. The APN CM might then wonder if there were any patterns of interest in CHF patients admitted through the emergency department. They could then "drill down" into the data, discovering findings that they never thought to ask in the beginning of their search. The data could be queried to determine patterns in admission times to the emergency department, mortality rates, most frequently performed procedures, or readmission rates of specific payer groups or physicians. Although it is not necessary for the APN CM to possess technical expertise in informatics, having skills in database querying gives the APN CM an edge in obtaining meaningful information rapidly to avoid long turnaround times traditionally associated with requests for reports from an IS department.

Utilization of Comparative Performance Data. State, national, and proprietary databases also exist, and may be excellent sources of comparative data on which to evaluate a health care organization's performance. These include

- U-92 claims data sent to state intermediaries
- HCFA Medicare claims
- Prospective payment commission reports
- Professional review organizations (PRO)
- The National Center for Health Services Research
- The JCAHO
- Milliman and Robertson, Inc. Healthcare Management Guidelines

Comparative data serve to inform an organization about how well it performs in a given area compared to other organizations. For example, an organization may track its readmission rates for patients with CHF. However, until its readmission rates are compared to other facilities, the organization will not know whether its performance falls within an acceptable range for a given population. Ideally, the comparison should be made among homogeneous subgroups that are stratified according to similar characteristics, such as bed size, geographic region, teaching status, or facilities with similar payer mixes. When clinical outcomes are being compared across facilities, it is generally expected that such data will be adjusted for clinical severity. A variety of techniques have been applied to risk-adjust clinical outcome data; however, the most accurate technique is still accumulation of patient-specific physiological and medical history data. For example, if a patient population undergoing open heart surgery was to be risk-adjusted using physiological and historical data, such information as the patients' history of diabetes, obesity, ejection fraction, location of the coronary occlusion, and smoking history would have to be collected. The collection of such information generally requires chart review and is extremely labor intensive. Furthermore, it may well be that such risk adjustment contributes very little in altering comparative performance, particularly when the database is of significant size. Health care organizations must weigh the need for risk-adjusted data against the resources required to collect the data needed to compute the risk algorithms associated with each risk factor. The use of NCM time and expertise to collect such data must be carefully considered, because it may not be the best use of case management resources. A full discussion of risk adjustment and stratification is beyond the scope of this chapter; however, the APN CM must be prepared to address the process of how risk- or severity-adjusted algorithms were applied to organization-specific data before presenting comparative data to medical staff and other stakeholders within the system (Iezzoni, 1997).

Issues Related to Common Measures of Performance: Descripton and Sources. To complement the data analyses and information management competency, it is important for APN CMs to understand specific performance measures and issues associated with their interpretation.

Bed-Days per 1,000 Covered Lives

Calculation:

$$X = \frac{\text{Sum of all inpatient days for a selected health plan}}{\text{Total count of members enrolled in the health care plan}}$$

Example:

- 182 total inpatient days during the month of January
- 12,845 members enrolled in January
  - ✔ 182 ÷ 12,845 = 0.01417
  - ✔ 0.01417 × 1,000 = 14.17 days in January per 1,000*
  - ✔ 14.17 × 12 months = 170.04 days/1,000 (annualized)

* Note: This figure is generally reported as an annualized rate.

One of the most utilized markers of utilization of hospital services in managed care is bed-days per 1,000 covered lives. This measure is widely used by executives to monitor "the big picture." As an industry standard, this measure gives health care providers and managed care organizations the ability to compare utilization of inpatient days with a common denominator.

Determination of whether bed-days are within acceptable ranges of performance may be based upon comparative data or medical management guidelines, such as Milliman and Robertson, Inc. Healthcare Management Guidelines, which lists expected bed-day ranges for a wide variety of DRG and ICD-9 diagnosis codes. Bed-day ranges are presented for three types of care environments: (1) health care systems with very little managed care, which have little incentive for adhering to the guidelines; (2) those with a moderate degree of managed care, which have more incentives to follow the guidelines; and (3) those with a high degree of managed care, which have great incentives to follow guidelines closely. Bed-day ranges are also presented for both Medicare and commercial populations. The calculation of bed-days is a function of both LOS and admission frequency. Therefore, if bed-days per 1,000 covered lives are higher than desired, the APN CM will need to ascertain whether bed-days are higher as a result of excess hospital admissions or whether they are a result of a longer average LOS. These are important data, because interventions to reduce admissions are very different from those needed to reduce LOS within the acute care environment.

Inpatient Admissions per 1,000 Covered Lives

Calculation:

$$X = \frac{\text{Total number of admissions}}{\text{Total count of members enrolled in the health care plan}}$$

Example:

- 67 patients admitted during the month of January
- 12,845 members enrolled in January
  - ✔ 67 ÷ 12,845 = 0.00522
  - ✔ 0.00522 × 1,000 = 5.22 admits per 1,000 lives*
  - ✔ 5.22 × 12 months = 62.7 per 1,000 lives per year (annualized)

* Note: This figure is generally reported as an annualized rate.

Inpatient admissions are widely used by executives to monitor overall utilization of inpatient services. Similar to admissions per 1,000 covered lives, industry standards exist for various case types for both commercial and Medicare populations (e.g., Milliman & Robertson, Inc. Health Management Guidelines). This allows APN CMs to benchmark their organization's utilization against similar markets.

Cost per Patient Day

Calculation:

$$X = \frac{\text{Total direct costs}}{\text{Total patient days}}$$

Example:

- $286,342.21 direct costs assigned to a medical unit in June
- 1908.9 patient days in June
  - ✔ $286,342.21 ÷ 1908.9 = $150.00/patient day in June

Cost per patient day is typically used to describe incremental costs of care associated with a particular unit or point of service, and helps middle-level managers make budgeting and financial projections. APN CMs can also use this calculation to report savings accrued when patients are redirected to alternative levels of care as a result of changes made in care delivery processes.

Cost per Discharge

Calculation:

$$X = \frac{\text{Sum of total costs accrued from admission to discharge}}{\text{Count of all patients discharged in the population of interest}}$$

Example:

- Total costs for patients discharged with DRG 127 (CHF) = $3,538,784
- Total number of patients discharged with DRG 127 = 914
  - ✔ $3,538,784 ÷ 914 = $3,871.75 per case

Cost per discharge is often used to evaluate cost-of-care trends for a particular case type or population over time. It is reported as an average (mean). This measure is even more meaningful when the population of interest is risk- or severity-adjusted. In this case, a more meaningful indication of cost could be achieved if costs were calculated for each of the four levels of NYHA classifications of CHF.

Mean Cost per Covered Life

Calculation:

$$X = \frac{\text{Cost of all care provided over course of year to all enrollees}}{\text{Count of all enrollees in the health plan}}$$

Example:

- Total cost of care provided by health plan = $18,487,234
- Total number of enrollees during the year = 2,421
  - ✔ $18,487,234 ÷ 2,421 = $1,488.38 per enrollee

The calculation of mean cost per covered life is a difficult measure to capture for most health care organizations because it requires claims data from the payers to determine all costs associated with care across the continuum. Ideally, this would include claims data from inpatient, emergency, outpatient, skilled nursing, rehabilitation, hospice, physician office visits, HHC, and pharmaceuticals. Despite the difficulty in gathering the data necessary to produce this measure, it is of particular interest to administrators in a capitated managed care environment, because it illustrates cost shifting that results when patients are redirected to alternative levels of service. It is an important fiscal measure to case managers who are following clients over time and across multiple points of service in their continuum.

Readmission Rates. One of the most commonly calculated indicators in case management is readmission rate. Readmission within 30 days of discharge from an acute care episode is thought to reflect the effectiveness of the treatment plan and the discharge plan. When calculating readmission rates of patients discharged with a particular diagnosis (e.g., DRG 127 [CHF]), the measure would be calculated as follows:

Calculation:

$$X = \frac{\text{Count of patients with a nonelective inpatient encounter within 30 days of discharge from a previous inpatient encounter with DRG 127 (CHF)}}{\text{Total count of all inpatients discharged with DRG 127}}$$

Example:

- Total number of patients with nonelective inpatient stay within 30 days of discharge for DRG 127 = 82
- Total number of patients discharged with DRG 127 = 914
  - ✔ 92 ÷ 914 = .10 (10% of all those discharged with DRG 127 had a nonelective readmission for the same DRG)

However, these data are difficult to obtain because the majority of hospital IS cannot "look forward" from the date of discharge of a particular DRG or ICD-9 code and track a true readmission event. In reality, the majority of hospital IS actually "look backward" from the date of discharge with a particular DRG or ICD-9 code and include those patient data with any inpatient encounter *prior* to that date. What is actually being counted is a "preadmission rate" rather than a readmission rate. To avoid this problem, many hospitals still devote time to reviewing charts and collecting readmission statistics manually. Although there are some IS that can provide "true" readmission rates by looking forward in the database, the APN CM must know how the rates are actually calculated in her or his IS, because "backward readmission rates" must be acknowledged as proxy measures of the actual readmission rate. As in the case of bed-days per 1,000 covered lives, conclusions about how well the health care facility has performed in the area of readmissions can best be drawn using comparative data.

In addition to the calculation of readmission rates, it may be quite informative to view readmission patterns sorted by elapsed days between discharge and the readmission encounters. Figure 19-3 illustrates a histogram of readmission patterns for a group of patients who were discharged with CHF and readmitted to the hospital with any nonelective diagnosis within the next 30 days. Although the overall readmission rate is reported to be 13.2%, what is most significant is that 75/164 (46%) of all readmissions occurred within the first 7 days after discharge. This information becomes a significant leverage point for APN CMs, as they discover that their case management intervention needs to occur within hours of discharge, rather than days or weeks.

Analysis of LOS Data. Traditionally, average length of stay (ALOS) has been a common performance measure believed to reflect the overall efficiency of clinical management. Recently, ALOS has come under fire as an effective performance measure. It is criticized as an arbitrary indicator of success, particularly when the focus in health care is shifting toward a population management focus. For example, the total knee replacement population in Hospital A may have an ALOS of 5.9 days.

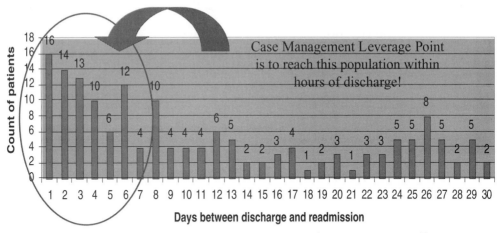

Readmission Patterns sorted by elapsed days between discharge and readmission
75/164 (46%) of all readmissions occur within 7 days of discharge

FIGURE 19–3 • Histogram of readmission rates reveals leverage points for case management. (Copyright 1998 by MIDS, Inc., Tucson, AZ; reprinted with permission.)

Typically, patients at Hospital A are discharged home with outpatient physical therapy for follow-up. In contrast, Hospital B may boast an aggressive program in which the ALOS is reported as 3.8 days. In this program, patients undergoing total knee replacement are typically transferred to either a rehabilitation program or a skilled nursing facility (SNF) for continued recuperation and therapy. Despite the reduced LOS in Hospital B, it may have cost them more in terms of total cost of care for the population than it cost Hospital A, who had the longer LOS. Until the costs of the rehab or SNF admissions can be compared to the additional costs of keeping patients in the acute care environment for several extra days, no conclusions can be made about the efficiency of Hospital A compared to Hospital B. Furthermore, quality and satisfaction outcomes must either improve or remain unchanged for the value of either strategy to be demonstrated. Finally, the payer mix of the population must also be taken into consideration when analyzing costs and reimbursements related to care resources. What may be discovered is that, despite a reported cost savings on the acute care hospital side, cost to the health care system as a whole has significantly increased without added value in terms of quality or satisfaction. Because APN CMs monitor LOS outcomes within the greater context of cost, reimbursement, utilization patterns, and quality, they are in a unique position to help their organizations avoid the trap of such "silo" thinking.

Traditional approaches to tracking ALOS data include trending ALOS in monthly or quarterly increments, and comparing performance to the previous year. In addition, the organization may compare its ALOS for a given population to the performance of other health care systems. Although these methods may be useful to describe LOS patterns, there are different approaches that may be used to examine LOS data so that potential case management leverage points can be identified. Presenting LOS in a histogram is useful because it displays the distribution patterns of various lengths of stay. At a glance, the number of encounters with very short lengths of stay can be distinguished from the number of encounters with very high lengths of stay. Figure 19–4 illustrates a population of patients with a discharge diagnosis of simple pneumonia (DRG 089). In this histogram, approximately 18% of 417 admissions had a LOS of 1 to 2 days. A review of the discharge dispositions for these patients ruled out that their short LOS was due to transfer to other levels of skilled care or death. In fact, over 95% of these patients were discharged home. One could hypothesize that these patients were not sick enough to have required hospitalization in the first place. This outcome represents a high number of unnecessary admissions with short length of stay and is not consistent with a managed care organization's goal of reducing its bed-days per 1,000 covered lives. Despite the fact that the total ALOS is lower because of the numbers of these brief stays, unnecessary resource consumption is a well-documented component of increasing costs in health care. The APN CM would then focus interventions on the preadmission phases of care decision making, implementing such tools as checklists to score the severity of illness, admission criteria, decision algorithms, or practice guidelines that may be helpful in reducing the number of unnecessary admissions.

At the other end of the LOS spectrum shown in the histogram in Figure 19–4, 24% of all encounters had lengths of stay greater than or equal to 7 days. Here it may be hypothesized that these patients developed complications or had some breach in quality that necessitated continued hospitalization. An opportunity may exist for the APN CM to ensure the delivery of timely interventions that minimize complications. Tools such as standard order sets, critical pathways, clinical protocols, or policies and procedures may be effective ways to improve the process of care for this population. A thoughtful review of LOS data by clinical experts can often identify leverage points for improvements that are not apparent to administrative experts.

Utilization of Control Charts in Interpreting Performance Trends. Skills in database query and statistical analysis are becoming increasingly important to CMs

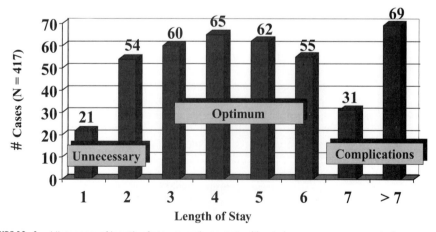

FIGURE 19–4 • Histogram of length of stay reveals opportunities to improve management of pneumonia population by decreasing unnecessary admissions and potential quality wastage days. (Copyright 1999 by MIDS, Inc., Tucson, AZ; reprinted with permission.)

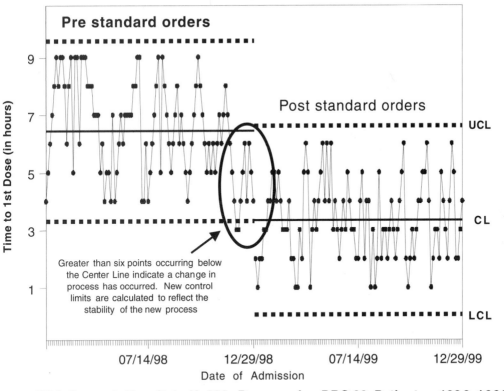

FIGURE 19–5 • Sample control chart representing statistical process control of time to delivery of antibiotics in patients admitted with pneumonia. UCL = upper control limit; CL = centerline; LCL = lower control limit. (Copyright 1999 by MIDS, Inc., Tucson, AZ; reprinted with permission.)

and the health care industry. In fact, numerous workshops, courses, and curricula are being offered that are geared solely toward health care statistics and outcome evaluation. The APN CM should also learn to analyze variations in performance data using statistical process control techniques. Statistical process control allows the data to be viewed over time in order to identify meaningful, nonrandom changes in performance (Wheeler, 1993). Through the use of control charts, the APN CM can determine whether a significant change in process has occurred as a result of an intervention to the system, or whether an intervention has failed to move the process in the desired direction. For example, an APN CM for a pulmonary population has established a standard order set, clinical guidelines, and protocols for pharmacy and nursing staff to follow in the management of patients with pneumonia. One of the goals of the program is to significantly reduce the average time from admission to the administration of the first dose of antibiotics. A control chart will serve as "the voice of the process." Figure 19-5 illustrates an Individual Control Chart which examines, in two phases, the time interval between admission and the delivery of the first antibiotic dose. The left side represents the period of time prior to the implementation of standard orders that call for rapid administration of antibiotics following admission with pneumonia. The right side reflects measurements that were taken after the implementation of standard orders. The average time interval is represented by the centerline (CL). Prior to the implementation of standard orders, the average time was approximately 6.5 hours. The upper control limit (UCL) represents the longest time interval that is statistically probable, and the lower control limit (LCL) represents the shortest time that is statistically probable. As long as the ordering and administration process remains unchanged, the time to antibiotic administration will fall between the UCL and the LCL 95% of the time (when set at two standard deviations) unless there is some alteration in the process. In this example, the healthcare team determined that the current performance was suboptimal, and decided upon standard orders as the strategy most likely to change the process and to decrease the time interval between admission and initiation of treatment. Following the implementation of standard orders, the time intervals were again measured. The right side of the graph illustrates that the mean time interval (CL) has decreased to 3.25 hours. The six data points that occur below the CL beginning in October 1998 demonstrate that this change in time interval was not random; i.e., it was not due to chance—a change known as "common cause variation." The center of the chart represents a statistically significant change that occurred because the clinicians changed the standard of care—referred to as "special cause variation." Thus, the right side of Figure 19–5 reflects the new control limits or the statistical probability that the new procedure, using standard orders, will occur within these limits 95% of the time. In this manner, an APN CM can effectively evaluate changes in health care delivery processes that drive desired cost and quality outcomes. Further evidence of the importance of the data management and information management competencies for evaluating the outcomes of advanced nursing practice are addressed in Chapter 25.

Exemplar of APN CM Practice

This exemplar illustrates the activities of the APN CM caring for a high-risk, complex client over time, and the simultaneous development of a community-wide program to manage clients in her specialty. June was a 65-year-old female with a longstanding diagnosis of MS. June lived alone in an apartment and, through Medicare and self-funding, managed her symptoms and caregiving needs independently. She attended a weekly exercise program provided by an APN CM and a physical therapist who both specialize in MS. During the announcement portion of the exercise class, June became aware of a special program funded through Medicare called the Carondelet Community Nursing Organization, a HCFA Demonstration Project. This national demonstration randomly assigned participants into a study and a control group. The purpose of the study was to demonstrate the quality and cost-effectiveness of nurse-managed community care delivery systems (Lamb & Zazworsky, 1997). Those selected into the study group were partnered with a NCM. June was randomly assigned to the study group, assessed as a high-risk participant, and partnered with an APN CM who specialized in MS. The exemplar highlights the range of APN competencies used over time with a particular patient.

DIRECT CARE

EXEMPLAR 3

On the first visit, the APN CM met June in her home and began to get acquainted. Together, they identified June's priority problems and developed a plan of care that would support June's holistic needs. The first visit is a critical step in establishing a trusting relationship. Not only are the skills of assessment and planning utilized during this first meeting, but it is also the time when the "insider-expert" role (Lamb & Stempel, 1994) of the APN CM is established. In the beginning of the relationship, June wanted an expert for her growing problems with bladder incontinence, leg spasticity, and caregiving needs. This was a delicate time to build a partnership and not foster a dependency. Therefore the APN CM helped June identify her greatest concern related to her health and well-being as being able to live in her own home. The APN CM acknowledged June's need to be in control and began to negotiate the areas in which the APN CM would offer assistance, such as patient and caregiver education and coaching, coordination of local and national resources, and being a liaison with other health care providers. At this point, emphasis was on the APN CM role as a facilitator and coach, rather than as a direct caregiver; the goal was not to take care of June, but to have June learn how to manage her own care safely and to know when to seek further assistance.

During the first month, the APN CM concentrated on the bladder and caregiver issues. Because the bladder problems depended on availability and competency of her caregivers, both were priorities. June's goal was to remain in her own home and utilize part-time caregivers to assist her with activities of daily living and mobility. June was morbidly obese and relied on a wheelchair for 100% of her mobility. She required two caregivers to transfer her from the chair to the bed in the morning, one during the day, and two in the evening. June was alone through the night. Safety became the third priority. The APN CM informed the patient about Lifeline and provided her with information regarding the installation of the service. June had the Lifeline installed within the next week.

The caregiver situation was an ongoing issue because of staff turnover and their varying skill level. Thus the APN CM identified two key caregivers who would serve as the main communicators of care. A communication book was started in which all caregivers recorded information related to patient care. The APN CM set up a checklist for daily activities such as medication times, daily exercises, deep breathing and coughing, and measuring urine output. These techniques enhanced caregiver continuity and consistency and helped the APN CM identify patterns to facilitate symptom management.

The next priority was gaining some type of control over bladder management. Prior to working with the APN CM, June's evening caregiver would insert an indwelling Foley catheter for the night, and the morning caregiver would remove and clean it. Although the caregivers were not formally trained health care technicians, they were very willing to assist June with her physical needs. Therefore, the APN CM initiated a plan of care that included educating June regarding options for treating neurogenic bladder—self-catheterization, intermittent catheterization per caregivers, or using a long-term indwelling catheter—and the pros and cons of each. June chose the long-term catheter, with a home health care (HHC) RN monitoring her for catheter problems. This was a short-term option at the time while June obtained an appointment with the urologist who specialized in MS. The APN CM coordinated the HHC orders with June's primary care physician and the home health agency. The APN CM also attended the first HHC RN visit to review the expectations of the patient and the agency regarding the indwelling Foley catheter management. The HHC RN educated the patient regarding signs and symptoms of urinary tract infection (UTI), care of the Foley catheter, and how to contact staff for other related problems.

Although HHC RNs function independently, the relationship between the HHC RN (as in any other relationship with other health care providers) and the APN CM was one of collaboration and coordination to benefit the patient. These relationships were complementary rather than competitive. The APN CM was recognized for clinical expertise, coordination of care, patient advocacy, and evaluation skills, while the HHC RN provided the specific skilled nursing care needed intermittently. Together, the APN CM and the HHC RN coached the patient and caregivers toward the patient's self-management.

The wellness plan shown in Table 19–6 reflects the initial plan that June and the APN CM negotiated. The APN CM's goal was to create a simple plan for June to follow and maintain control of during the first month. The actual patient care plan was more extensive and addressed other areas, including bladder, bowel, emotional, caregiving, respiratory, substance abuse (June was a chain smoker), physical activity, and nutrition issues.

Wellness plans are patient guides similar to a hospital discharge plan. A wellness plan is short and concise and describes realistic goals that are identified and negotiated with the patient. Typically, the patient writes two to three goals with defined time frames for each goal. The APN CM utilizes these plans based on the patient's needs. Wellness plans are helpful in long-term relationships related to behavior changes, such as building readiness in self-management skills. Wellness plans may not be pertinent when patients are in an acute episode of their disease process. In a crisis situation, patients tend to be more dependent and require specific direction and coordination.

CONSULTATION

E X E M P L A R   3 (continued)

After establishing the initial relationship with June, the APN CM began to work with the HHC RN and caregivers to build confidence in managing the Foley catheter and trouble-shoot problems. Because June was experiencing numerous problems related to bladder spasms, pain, and catheter leakage, the APN CM arranged a patient conference with June's caregivers and the HHC RN. In this conference, the APN CM served as a facilitator and educator in order to resolve commonly occurring problems and negotiate action plans. The APN CM accompanied June to her urology visit to clarify short-term and long-range plans for managing her bladder problems. Although June had an

TABLE 19–6 SAMPLE WELLNESS PLAN	
GOAL	ACTION ITEMS
1. Install Lifeline 2. Manage bladder and Foley catheter independently.	• Contact Lifeline (885-8540) and coordinate installation by next Tuesday (2/16/99) • Contact urologist (Dr. Smith, 572-7100) for appointment • Notify HHC RN(673-8731) for infection, leg spasms, bladder spasms, other Foley problems • Contact NCM (Donna, 790-3456) for other problems, questions, or concerns
Patient Signature/Date	NCM Signature/Date

Wellness Plans can include motivation scales, barriers to achieving your goal(s), and nursing recommendations.

indwelling Foley catheter, she was not ready to accept the long-term implications of a suprapubic catheter. In order to determine the extent of her bladder potential, the urologist recommended urodynamic testing to determine future treatment directions.

Over the next 2 months, June underwent testing and treatment but was unable to achieve a realistic level of independence that would accommodate her preferred living arrangement. Therefore, the APN CM and June discussed further options with her caregivers and the urologist and decided to continue with the indwelling catheter. The next step was to become independent of HHC. This meant that key caregivers would need to be trained to insert and manage the Foley catheter, as well as obtain urine samples for culture and sensitivity. The APN CM coordinated the training with the urologist and office staff. HHC was discontinued after June's caregivers were successfully trained. Over the next 3 months, the APN CM took on less of a direct care expert role and served as an occasional consultant to June and her caregivers when certain problems arose and the caregivers were unsure of whom to call. As pointed out in June's wellness plan, one of her goals was to manage her Foley catheter independently, with the assistance of her nonlicensed caregivers. Coaching by the APN CM resulted in the caregivers becoming confident in their abilities to identify and report symptoms of UTI and to collect urine samples accurately. The urologist also gained confidence in the caregivers' abilities and began to communicate directly with them as needed. At this point, the APN CM was performing reassessments at 6-month intervals to assure that the care plan was working. If the APN CM identified a decline in patient health status or the quality of caregiver interventions, the plan of care would be revised and educational needs revisited.

LEADERSHIP: DEVELOPING PARTNERSHIPS WITH PHYSICIANS AND OTHER HEALTH CARE PROVIDERS

An APN CM who specializes in a particular area must network and establish relationships with physicians and other providers who specialize in the same area. These relationships benefit the patient and create a team approach to care. It is not unusual for the APN CM to have the direct lines/extensions to physicians in order to discuss patient issues promptly when needed. APN CMs help patients build relationships with their physicians and other health care providers. As a result, patients learn how to communicate more effectively with their providers and become more confident in making health care decisions on their own. Self-care management empowers patients so that they begin to trust themselves, and the client-nurse relationship shifts from one of dependency to one of a coaching partnership.

The successful management of patients with MS requires a collaboration among physical therapists, exercise physiologists, speech therapists, occupational therapists, enterostomal therapist, nutritionists, behavioral health specialists, and social workers. The APN CM establishes relationships with June's team members to serve as the liaison and to communicate expectations among providers, caregivers, and patients.

E X E M P L A R **3** *(continued)*

Over the next 6 years, two potential hospitalizations were averted because of the collaborative relationships between June's caregiving team and her insider-expert relationship with the APN CM. Early identification of problems and prompt recognition of symptoms expedited care and insured that these complications could be managed at home.

In one instance, the APN CM received a call from the morning caregiver stating that June was not feeling well. After an in-depth telephone assessment, the APN CM identified that the primary problem was related to June's respiratory status. Having had past experiences with June's fragile respiratory status, the APN CM quickly determined that a face-to-face assessment was necessary, and revised her schedule to accommodate an immediate home visit. Within the next hour, the APN CM arrived at June's apartment and assessed the probability of early pneumonia. This diagnosis was supported by pulmonary auscultation, a decrease in the patient's pulse oximeter reading, a productive cough, and an increase in respiratory rate. The APN CM contacted June's physician, reported the findings, and requested a home chest x-ray and sputum culture and sensitivity. The x-ray was completed by noon and the physician confirmed the APN CM's diagnosis of pneumonia. By late afternoon, June was on an oral antibiotic and the HHC agency delivered oxygen and a nebulizer before the end of the day. The APN CM requested HHC nursing three times a week for closer monitoring of June's cardiopulmonary status. June's emotional status was not compromised because she was able to stay home; her caregivers could continue to meet her needs efficiently and effectively. As a result of this crisis, June decided to quit smoking. This became a permanent behavior change.

The APN CM coordinated the services of the MS network team members to achieve the most realistic outcomes for June. For example, June experienced leg spasms and required a regular regimen of daily exercises and medication management. The APN CM consulted with the neurologist to discuss medication management and the benefits of physical therapy (PT). After relaying this conversation to June and eliciting June's agreement, the APN CM called the home health agency and requested that a physical therapist experienced with MS take June's case. A joint visit to June's home with the APN CM, the physical therapist, and June's caregivers was planned. The physical therapist provided an evaluation and recommended a program. The APN CM then arranged to videotape the exercise program with the physical therapist and caregivers on the next visit so that it could be used to guide caregivers in how to conduct the exercises between visits by the physical therapist. Not only did the videotape serve as a training guide, it also served as a quality assurance mechanism to promote consistency and accuracy of the exercise regimen across caregivers.

The physical therapist continued to visit twice a week for 2 weeks while the caregivers implemented the daily program. The therapist and the APN CM discussed June's progress and her caregivers' abilities and decided to discontinue PT visits after the next visit. The APN CM discussed the plan with June and reassured her that the physical therapist would return to adjust her program as needed.

RESEARCH USE AND INTERPRETATION: EVALUATION OF INDIVIDUAL PATIENT OUTCOMES

A useful tool for evaluating changes in patient behavior and knowledge resulting from the case management intervention is the Knowledge-Behavior-Status (K-B-S) scale, which is part of the Omaha Documentation System, a problem-oriented nursing taxonomy that primarily focuses on community care issues (Martin, 1992). This system allows the APN CM to assess and communicate more objectively patients' levels of knowledge regarding their disease process, their behavior associated with managing their disease, and their health status. Using a Likert scale from 1 to 5, a number is assigned to each K-B-S problem domain identified for the patient. In this manner, changes over time can be quantified and conclusions may be drawn about the effectiveness of case management interventions. This approach may also be used to evaluate aggregate population outcomes. Mean changes in K-B-S scores over time are quantifiable measures of outcomes associated with case management intervention. In addition, a quality assurance system must be established to ensure that all clinicians using the Omaha system do so with an acceptable degree of inter-rater reliability.

EXEMPLAR 3 (*continued*)

The APN CM was accountable for evaluating outcomes of care, both for her individual MS patients and the aggregate MS population. The Omaha Documentation System was used at each visit to document June's neuromuscular status, genitourinary status, physical activity, and pain. Every 6 months, the APN CM reassessed June's knowledge, behavior, and status for each problem. On one of the reassessment visits, June complained of severe leg problems related to increased spasticity and pain. The APN CM explored the patient's patterns related to leg pain and the potential etiologies, such as UTI, medication adjustments, or exercise changes. June and her caregivers were able to describe the changes related to each of the potential etiologies. The caregivers described how they took a urine sample to the physician's office 2 days ago and a severe UTI had been ruled out. They then discussed the recent time changes of June's spasticity medication regimen as a possible reason for June's increase in night spasticity. Finally, the caregivers described the resulting decrease in June's leg exercise routine because of her onset of leg pain. The APN CM notified the neurologist and reported the leg pain assessment. Together, the neurologist, the APN CM, and June decided to change the spasticity medication regimen, add a new spasticity medication temporarily, and have the physical therapist reassess and adjust June's exercise program. When the APN CM documented the K-B-S, both knowledge (K) and behavior (B) measurements relating to the problems of neuromuscular status, physical activity, and pain remained unchanged from previous assessments; however, status (S) scores had declined from the previous visit. The APN CM recognized that June, with the help of her caregivers, was demonstrating excellent self-management skills. However, June's overall physical function had declined. Reassessments at 3 and 6 months would enable the APN CM to determine whether June's episode of leg problems was temporary or an indication of disease progression.

RESEARCH INTERPRETATION AND USE: EVALUATING POPULATION OUTCOMES

EXEMPLAR 3 (*continued*)

A more formal approach to evaluating aggregate population outcomes requires a research approach. Continuing with the MS example, Carondelet Health Network Community Case Management received a demonstration grant in 1990 from the National MS Society to provide nurse case management for patients with chronic progressive MS (Lamb, 1993). Participants were randomly assigned to a study and control group and received face-to-face interviews by trained health professionals at the beginning of the study and 6 months and 1 year later. At each interview, patients were given standardized questionnaires to evaluate quality of life, symptom management, satisfaction with health care services, caregiver burden, cost of care, empowerment, level of disability, and health service use. The following instruments were utilized:

- Index of Well Being (Campbell, Converse, & Rogers, 1976)
- General Symptom Distress Scale (LaLonde, 1987)
- Satisfaction with Health Care (Hall, Feldstein, Fretwell, Rowe, & Epstein, 1990)
- Caregiving Impact Scale (Poulshock & Deimling, 1984)
- Cost of Care Index (Kosberg & Cairl, 1986)
- Minimal Record for Disability for Multiple Sclerosis (National MS Society, 1985)
- Health Service Use (Brown, Arpin, Corey, Fitch, & Gafni, 1990; Spitzer, Roberts, & Delmore, 1976)

Quantitative research methods did not demonstrate significant differences between groups in any of the items measured. However, further exploration of the data, called a "drill down," demonstrated a significant difference in empowerment scores of those participants in the study group who reported a higher level of disability and required a more intensive level of case management interventions. During a "drill down," a qualitative approach is used. NCMs were interviewed by a doctorally prepared APN CM about the complexity of their patients and the care provided to them in order to capture the impact of the interventions on the high-risk MS patients. Outcomes were presented to administrative leaders and contracting payers to substantiate the value of case management services for high-risk populations such as patients with MS.

RESEARCH INTERPRETATION AND USE: EVIDENCE-BASED
PROGRAM DEVELOPMENT

E X E M P L A R **3** (continued)

Putting research into practice is another defining component for the APN CM. For example, an outcome of the MS research study was the identified need for exercise and the lack of community resources for the MS community with regard to exercise. The APN CM developed a group exercise program with the help of the MS study participants and a physical therapist who specialized in MS. The APN CM set up a research design to demonstrate the benefits of the exercise program. Before and after an 8-week group exercise class, the physical therapist measured functional status using the Manual Muscle Test, while the APN CM measured satisfaction, exercise compliance, and community referrals. The evaluation demonstrated positive outcomes; using these data, the APN CM was successful in obtaining funding from a local community foundation to continue the exercise program. The APN CM and the physical therapist have trained numerous RNs, physical therapists, and volunteer nursing and medical students over the 9 years since the community program started. In addition, the APN CM has networked with the local MS society to do the marketing/promotions. (See Chapter 21 for additional information on marketing.)

EDUCATION, EXPERIENCE, AND CERTIFICATION: PREPARING FOR THE APN CM ROLE

A variety of certification bodies for case management have sprung up within the past 4 to 5 years, each with its own eligibility requirements and practice standards (Table 19–7). Some certifications, such as the Commission for Case Management Certification (CCMC), The National Board of Continuity of Care, and the America Institute of Outcomes–Case Management (AIOCM), offer an interdisciplinary case management certification. Others, such as the ANA, offer case management certification and standards of practice specific to nurse case management. Still others, such as the American Board of Occupational Health Nurses and the Association for Rehabilitation Nurses, now offer case management certification and standards of practice specific to nurse case management within a particular specialty. Although there is still no certification specific to the APN CM role, the certification of CMs by specialty organizations may be the mechanism by which APN CM certification occurs. In the meantime, APN CMs are advised to maintain certification in their clinical specialty and seek a second certification in case management under the more generic certification bodies such as the CCMC or ANA. Currently, not all case management certification bodies endorse

TABLE 19-7 CASE MANAGEMENT CERTIFICATION CRITERIA

ORGANIZATION	ELIGIBILITY CRITERIA	CREDENTIAL
Commission for Case Management Certification (CCMC) *www.ccmcertification.org*	• Minimum postsecondary degree in any field that promotes the physical, psychosocial, or vocational well-being of persons served • Current licensing or certification in professional practice • Minimum of 12 months of full-time case management employment • Successful completion of exam • Recertification required every 5 years	CCM (Certified Case Manager)
American Nurses Association (ANA) *www.nursingworld.org*	• Active RN license • Baccalaureate or higher degree in nursing • Functioned within the scope of a NCM a minimum of 2,000 hours within past 2 years • Show proof of current, core specialty certification or function as a RN a minimum of 4,000 hours • Successful completion of exam • Recertification required every 5 years	RNCM (Nurse Case Manager)
American Institute of Outcomes–Case Management (AIOCM) *www.aiocm.com*	• Degree of BS, BA, MS, MA, MD, PhD, Associate Degree, or nursing diploma with professional license • Three to 5 years of professional experience • Completed required outcomes–case management education (scored on point system) • Successful completion of exam • Recertification required every 2 years	CMC (Case Management Certified)
Association for Rehabilitation Nurses (ARN) *www.rehabnurse.org*	• Current RN license • Minimum of 2 years of practice in rehab setting within past 5 years or 1 year of practice in rehab setting with 1 year of advanced study beyond baccalaureate in nursing • Successful completion of exam • Recertification required every 5 years	CRRN (Certified Registered Rehab Nurse)
American Board of Occupational Health Nurses *www.aaohn.org*	• Current RN license • Minimum of 5 years of practice in occupational health setting • Currently employed in an industry • Successful completion of exam • Recertification required every 5 years	COHN (Certified Occupational Health Nurse)
National Board of Continuity of Care *www.ptcny.com*	• Bachelor's degree or higher • Two years of full-time experience in continuity of care position within past 5 years • Successful completion of exam • Recertification required every 5 years	A-CCC (Advanced Competency Certification in Continuity of Care)

the minimal requirement of a postsecondary degree in a health care–related area; however, all require extensive experience and employment as a CM. In addition, all certifying bodies require the candidate to submit an extensive profile of her or his practice and pass a written examination.

One of the newest certifications available is the Administrative Case Management Certification offered by the Center for Case Management. This certification was developed based on the belief that there is a distinct level of knowledge and experience required by those who are responsible for the development, implementation, and evaluation of case management programs. This certification advocates a master's degree in health care–related areas but acknowledges the competencies of those individuals with baccalaureate preparation in conjunction with substantial case management experience by permitting non-master's-prepared individuals to become certified. This certification tests for competencies in management, human resources, employment issues, and budgetary issues. Although there is a small component focused on clinical competency in the management of chronic diseases such as asthma, cardiovascular disease, and diabetes, this certification is primarily geared toward those in administrative leadership positions responsible for the oversight of the business and operational management aspects of case management. APN CMs who assume such responsibilities are excellent candidates for this certification, although it does not appear to be directly relevant to the APN CM role as described in this chapter (K. Bower, personal communication, June 1999).

The AIOCM offers certification for health care professionals who have attained expertise in managing data and information used to improve the performance of case management–related processes and outcomes. This credential recognizes those individuals who are proficient in outcomes management implementation projects, data management methodologies, health care economics, statistics, quality improvement, and linking outcomes data to health care decision making. The AIOCM certification is not limited to NCMs or social workers. Medical doctors, executives, respiratory therapists, pharmacists, or any allied health professional may become certified. Certification criteria include meeting standards of general education, 3 to 5 years of health care experience, education in outcomes case management, and successful completion of the AIOCM certification examination.

The APN CM should continue to meet the requirements for APN licensure for her or his clinical specialty (e.g., gerontology, rehabilitation, oncology, adult medical-surgical, critical care) and within her or his jurisdictions of practice. If certification in a practice area or specialty is not yet a requirement for APN licensure, or is not yet available, the APN CM should be certified at a basic level in both case management and specialty nursing, in addition to having an advanced degree in nursing. Depending upon the job market and the availability of CMs, certification as a CM may or may not give the APN interested in being a CM an edge when seeking a job.

To meet the growing need for APN CMs, many schools of nursing are providing graduate curricula with a specialty in nurse case management (see Chapter 4). There is still considerable debate about whether separate case management programs are needed, or whether the CNS and NP programs should just increase their level of case management instruction (Falter et al., 1999). According to Falter and co-workers (1999), the knowledge and skills that are the foundation of case management preparation are health care economics, resource management, quality concepts applied to case management, care delivery systems, management and interpretation of outcome data, and APN role preparation. The Lienhard School of Nursing at Pace University, in Pleasantville, New York, revised its core master's curriculum in 1998 to include case management concepts, which were seen as generic to all APN roles. This program prepares APN CMs with the option of tailoring their clinical focus to one of three advanced practice nursing areas: adult CNS, psychiatric–mental health CNS, and family NP. The curriculum includes courses in economics, quality, systems, and roles. Clinical course work prepares students for certification in their APN role and prepares them to perform case management roles in a variety of health care settings. Other programs, such as the one at San Francisco State University, offer a master's degree in nursing that provides nurses with the advanced integrated knowledge and the skills cited previously to become successful APN CMs in the home care and long-term care environment.

Fralic (1992) observed that the successful NCM is able to operate in an unstructured environment and has a high tolerance for ambiguity, uncertainty, and change. The NCM is "required to bring innovation, enthusiasm, and confidence to the role" (Fralic, 1992, p. 14). APN graduate education fosters these qualities through its emphasis on role socialization, self-learning, and self-direction, as well as content on change theory. In addition, advanced clinical and leadership skills help students develop these characteristics. Master's-level course work should also include core courses in conceptual models and nursing theory, risk analysis, statistics, family and community assessment, and the conduct and use of research. Just as role socialization and mentoring are critical to the development of the CNS (Hamric & Taylor, 1989), students in APN case management curricula must experience the NCM role during clinical and mentoring experiences with practicing APNs in the case management role. Given the APN CM role's similarity to the traditional CNS role, it is reasonable to assume that a developmental process exists in which the APN CM experiences the phases of role development as described by Hamric and Taylor (1989) (see also Chapter 5). As nurse case management continues to evolve, more and more graduate programs are likely to offer courses specific to the case management role, with a dual emphasis in a specialized area of clinical practice that has been traditionally associated with APN roles.

CRITICAL ELEMENTS OF THE APN CM PRACTICE ENVIRONMENT

Whether employed in acute care, in the community, or as an independent contractor, the APN CM must address critical elements in order to achieve a successful practice. This chapter focuses primarily on the elements related to APN CM competencies. However, it would be remiss if a discussion of the business aspects of case management was not offered, because success in the business decisions associated with case management programs will determine the survival and success of APN CM clinical practice.

Business Elements

When examining the business of the APN CM, accountability from both the direct practice perspective and business perspective must be defined (Porter-O'Grady, 1996). This means demonstrating value through quality, cost, and satisfaction in terms that are meaningful to patients, providers, and payers. These processes translate into the business functions of reimbursement structuring, cost-benefit analyzing, marketing, and contracting (see Chapter 21). Therefore, the APN CM must work with the staff in finance, marketing, and contracting departments to determine how best to demonstrate that accountabilities for quality, cost, and satisfaction are being met.

ACCOUNTABILITY

Product lines, scorecards, and dashboards are all part of today's health care accountability jargon. The APN CM is a member of the teams who design and produce reports on outcomes for administrators and clinicians at the organizational, departmental, and practice levels. For example, if the organization decides to decrease bed-days per 1,000, the APN CM will work with the product line administrators to achieve related goals at the department and practice levels through data trending/analysis, guideline development, implementation, evaluation, and staff training. For example, following the implementation of a CHF admission protocol, standard orders, and a critical pathway the clinical APN CM may report to the cardiovascular product line director on the reduced numbers of unnecessary CHF admissions and critical care bed-days by payer. The community APN CM may give a report to the same cardiovascular product line director on the reduced CHF readmission rate by payer. Both clinical and community APN CMs would provide reports that translate the reductions into cost savings by payer.

PRODUCTIVITY AND ACUITY

Productivity reports should capture direct patient care (hospital, home, or provider visits; telephone contacts; etc.) and indirect care (e.g., documentation, patient conferences, and travel time). All of these items should be recorded by payer in order to calculate an average cost per case. Other time related to committee meetings or continuing education may or may not be averaged into the payer breakdown. Another method when measuring productivity is to include nurse case management intervention activities during visits. A study by Papenhausen (1996), demonstrated that community NCMs spent their visit time performing the following intervention activities: 30% assessing and monitoring, 17% teaching and informing, 7% in direct service, 23% supporting and sharing, and 11% exploring alternatives and goal setting. With this type of information, the APN CM can establish targets with NCMs, administrators, and contracted providers related to productivity and contract accountability. Productivity information and cost-benefit analyses enable the organization or private practice to negotiate better contracts for its services.

Acuity addresses level and complexity of care related to the case-managed patient. This information must be captured in order to demonstrate the costs and benefits of APN CM interventions. For example, Ward and Rieve (1997, p. 254) illustrated an acuity-based framework for CMs in a disease management/episodic-based case management model. In this model, patients who are at the lowest levels of complexity and risk, and require only 1 to 2 hours of CM intervention, are assigned an acuity level of 1. Patients requiring extensive diagnostic testing, multiple complex treatments, and over 15 hours of CM intervention, are assigned an acuity level of 5. Acuity tools that objectively quantify risk are necessary to establish valid selection criteria for triggering a case management referral. Without such criteria, other providers who initiate referrals for case management may make inappropriate referrals to case management services. As a result, undue workload on case management staff is created. Case management should not be viewed as a dumping ground for all discharge planning or continuum transition issues, but rather as a distinct level of service provided to clients who demonstrate a specific need.

INDIRECT COSTS

Other business items the APN CM must consider relate to the general business elements of daily operations, such as office telephone, beeper, cellular phone, copying, faxing, invoicing/billing abilities, procedural coding (when appropriate), support staff, and rental space. These indirect expenses need to be tracked and calculated into reimbursement structures. For APN CMs who choose to practice independently, additional considerations must be given to obtaining and maintaining a business license, Federal Identification Number, worker's compensation insurance, liability insurance, business structuring (e.g., sole proprietor, partnership, or corporation), and attorney and certified public accountant services (see Chapter 20).

REIMBURSEMENTS

Depending on the employment environment, the APN CM may receive reimbursements from a number of different sources. If the APN CM is working for a hospital or integrated delivery network (IDN), the APN CM will want to establish a mix of reimbursement vehicles. Conversely, the independent APN CM may negotiate directly with the HMO, employer, or insurance carrier for services. In this case, additional credentialing needs may be anticipated. The following business issues should be considered within the various reimbursement structures.

Fee-for-Service (Indemnity). A fee-for-service contract with insurance companies, third-party administrators, employers, and HMO is just what it means—the APN CM is paid a fee for services delivered. The appropriate hospital/IDN departments involved in contracting (e.g., legal, contracts, finance) will assist in formulating a proper contract that includes scope of services to be provided, reporting needs, reimbursements, and billing requirements. In most cases, the APN CM will receive authorization for the initial visit and then must submit an authorization request for a certain number of additional anticipated visits needed along with a plan of care.

Capitated Contract. A capitated contract is established between a HMO and the hospital or provider based on a per member per month reimbursement. In this contract, the hospital negotiates a monthly capitation payment and the APN case management cost center will be allocated a fixed payment. This type of arrangement must also be clearly defined in scope of services (i.e., hospital and home visits, service authorization capabilities) and reporting needs (outcomes of visits, service use). Another critical component in this type of arrangement is activity tracking. The APN CM must track time, broken down by payer, related to direct and indirect patient care. The APN CM can use this information to develop special services/programs such as group education for hospitalized CHF patients or a CHF clinic. Finally, through activity tracking, the APN CM can let administrators know if the capitated fee covers the cost of APN CM services being delivered.

Subcontracting ("Carve Outs"). Subcontracting or "carve outs" are another form of contract that occurs in specialized areas such as worker's compensation, behavioral health, or disease management. These contracts are set up by vendors who need an APN CM in a particular geographic area to deliver a specialized service. This type of arrangement is conducive to the APN CM in private practice. For example, the private practice APN CM will subcontract with a company to be its representative for worker's compensation cases. Depending on the needs of the patient, the private practice APN CM may need to establish special financial arrangements with local providers to deliver care on behalf of the worker's compensation company.

BILLING METHODS

Billing methods depend on the contractual arrangement between the contractor and the organization. The APN CM must collaborate with the finance department (if employed by an organization) or with a certified public accountant (if in private practice) regarding the preferred method for billing. Unfortunately, nurse case management is not recognized as a billable service under Medicare guidelines and therefore NCMs cannot bill independently as can some other APNs ("Rules and regulations," 1998). However, with the continued congressional interest in HCFA-sponsored Community Nursing Organizations, NCM services are being reimbursed through a risk-adjusted capitation model (Lamb & Zazworsky, 1997).

MARKETING

Marketing APN CM services must take place both externally and internally across the organization and to the appropriate contracted providers. Zazworsky and Hospodar (1996) demonstrated a marketing plan format that described target markets; competition analysis; strengths, weaknesses, opportunities, and threats (SWOT) analysis; and product development, pricing, and promotions applied to nurse case management. It is imperative that both internal and external markets be addressed, because success rests not only on desired outcomes but also on appropriate referrals. Internal and external marketing require assistance from the organization's public relations and/or marketing department for theme/message design, a communication plan, material development, and implementation assistance. Internally, the APN CM may spend many hours performing staff education/orientation through a customer relations framework. For example, the APN CM may communicate otherwise complex case management referral criteria in a simple, user-friendly format such as a referral form checklist or decision algorithm. Externally, the APN CM may offer the same referral form checklist to contracted providers (e.g., physicians, NPs, social workers, HMO authorization personnel). More comprehensive policies and procedures may then be developed to supplement such tools (see Chapter 21 for further discussion of marketing).

Regulatory and Credentialing Requirements

The NCM is not currently recognized by the ANA as an ANP role. However, as more and more universities offer master's programs in nurse case management, and, as national demonstration projects such as the Community Nursing Organizations verify the quality and cost-effectiveness of nurse case-managed patients, nurse case management is forging a new type of APN. This will in turn require legislation regarding Medicare billing. Therefore, current organizations such as the ANA and the Center for Case Management are taking a leadership role in establishing the standards of practice and credentialing requirements in preparation for Medicare billing by APN CMs.

Currently, health care organizations that employ NCMs establish competency-based criteria and job descriptions and NCMs are accountable to that organization. If other

CMs who are employed by physicians, HMOs, insurance companies, or independent CMs want access to a patient and his or her medical record, a process must be developed and approved through the appropriate channels within the organization, such as the medical staff office, legal department, or the medical executive committee. For HMOs or insurance companies, the provider contract may include stipulations for their CMs to have access to patients' records. Unless the NCM has a dual credential as a CNS, NP, or CNM, it may not be evident which CMs will be functioning in an APN capacity and which NCMs will be functioning at basic levels. A distinction may well be necessary if certain NCMs will be given the authority to make independent decisions about treatment plans, while others will not. In the future, APN CMs may be involved in the contracting or credentialing development and approval process for CMs.

Organizational Structures and Cultures

The APN CM typically practices in a hospital or IDN setting through an acute care clinical model and/or community-based model. Because an APN CM's practice typically crosses many units, departments, and points of service within the organization, it is important to consider carefully the reporting structures that will best support APN CMs in their role. A wide variety of administrative structures exist for CMs. NCMs may be based in the following departments or settings: quality and performance improvement, utilization resource management, medical staff office, social work, home health, nursing, or even finance or IS. Many health care systems have redesigned their organizational structures to create independent case management departments that blend the functions of quality management, utilization resource management, discharge planning, social work, and performance improvement. Still other organizations have positioned their nurse case management resources to be more closely aligned with nursing or medical services. In these structures, the APN CM may report directly to the chief nursing or medical officer, or to an administrative leader with oversight for the product line within the APN CM's clinical specialty (e.g., cardiovascular, maternal-child, medical-surgical, critical care, oncology).

Regardless of the reporting structure, the primary concern for the APN CM should be to exist within a reporting structure that supports "whole-system" thinking and places a high value on creative innovation and process improvement. APN CMs should seek to avoid reporting structures that confine or limit their practice to one unit or department's interests, or seem to place a particular emphasis on task-oriented activities. Optimally, the organization and its administrators should recognize that the APN CM is in a unique position to promote excellence in clinical practice and system performance. To achieve such outcomes, the APN CM may at times require the formal and tacit authority that comes with the position and title of those to whom the APN CM reports. Those who lead APN CMs must be prepared to "take the heat" if necessary for changes that are perceived as coming from the APN CM. Although the APN CM will not need daily, or even weekly, supervision, she or he will need to be kept abreast of organizational issues that are likely to affect the practice and business environment. The APN CM should have routine debriefing sessions scheduled with her or his immediate supervisor to clarify goals and expected outcomes, identify any resource needs, discuss any barriers, and exchange information relating to pending contracts, changes in the product line, medical practice issues, or staff education needs. Ideally, APN CMs should have representation on the hospital quality oversight committee and any high-level division meetings that are pertinent to their areas of practice. Active membership on key medical committees and direct access to administrative decision makers are imperative. This is where APN CMs have particular opportunities to integrate clinical expertise with communication, negotiation, and leadership skills to promote effective and efficient clinical processes. For those APN CMs who contract independently, being able to become familiar with the organizational structure and culture, and becoming a "trusted insider" to the organization, will be critical to successful contracting and service delivery.

CONCLUSION: LOOKING TOWARD THE FUTURE OF APN CM PRACTICE

The future of APN CM practice will parallel the fluctuations in the health care arena. As provider and health plan organizations struggle to capture market share and maintain competitive prices, the providers of value-added use and cost containment strategies may shift from a "nice to have" to a "need to have" framework. This can have positive or negative consequences on the APN CM role. On the positive side, the APN CM may be the critical link in a continuum-based organization when it makes the transition from a predominantly fee-for-service model to a shared or global risk model. On the downside, many health care organizations are currently experiencing tremendous financial losses. In fact, over 60% of hospitals in the United States failed to make a profit in 1998 (N. Hagenow, personal communication; 1999). As a result, many are returning to the "core business" of acute care delivery and dramatically reducing resources once allotted to the continuum of care model. APN CMs who work in community health, health promotion, and complication management may become expendable unless the value of their contributions is made dramatically clear to high-level decision makers and consulting teams who are so often brought in to make difficult decisions when the survival of a health care organization is at stake.

In this paradoxical environment, new opportunities for the APN CM will undoubtedly present themselves. It appears that more nursing programs are designing curricula to prepare NCMs at the graduate level. Schools with CNS and NP curricula are redesigning curricula to ensure that these APNs have some case management skills. It may be that the need for APN CMs will result in other types of blended roles in addition to the blended CNS/NP role described in Chapter 16, such as the NP/CM or the CNS/CM. As with the blended CNS/NP role, preparation for a blended role in this field will require dual preparation in case management skills as well as the skills of the additional APN role. Managed care, national initiatives to restructure health care, and the demand for chronic disease management, health prevention and promotion, and acute care complication management will create more opportunities for APN CMs to improve health care delivery processes and systems that support proactive care management.

It is also likely that private practice opportunities for APN CMs will grow significantly. As large health care insurance carriers contract with employers and individual patients all over the world, they will be faced with the need to outsource their clinical oversight at a local level. Furthermore, there is a growing desire for employer control over health care dollars. Although managed care promotes prevention, most plans fall short of providing an organized process for early risk identification and high-risk management that effectively controls costs for individual employers. The APN CM can take advantage of this shortcoming and contract directly with employers as a consultant and direct provider for health promotion and disease management services. The APN CM can design an appropriate structure with the employer to maximize outcomes for both employers and employees.

Finally, as concern for Medicare and Medicaid stability grows, the government continues to explore avenues for cost control. The HCFA-sponsored Community Nursing Organizations, for example, demonstrate the value of APN CM autonomy to order ancillary evaluations, such as physical therapy or occupational therapy, based on patient need. Acting within the scope of advanced nursing practice the APN CM can coordinate the appropriate physician and/or medical treatment follow-up based on the initial evaluation. This process expedites care, regardless of the acute or chronic nature of the disease, and accurately matches services with the right service provider. In this model, case management is reimbursed on the basis of risk. As this model continues to gain national support, the APN CM will see more opportunities for community practice and reimbursement.

ACKNOWLEDGMENTS

The authors wish to acknowledge our past patients and families for teaching us the art of caring, the Carondelet Health Care Network for instilling in us the skills of creative innovation, and Christopher J. Heller, M.D., for coaching us in the science of measuring value in health care.

R E F E R E N C E S

American Nurses Association. (1988). *Nursing case management.* Kansas City, MO: Author.

Baird, S. (1995). The impact of changing health care delivery on oncology practice. *Oncology Nursing: Patient Treatment and Support, 2*(3), 1–13.

Becker, M. H. (1974). *The health belief model and personal health behavior.* Thorofare, NJ: Charles B Slack.

Boult, C., Pacala, J. T., & Boult, L. B. (1995). Targeting elders for geriatric evaluation and management: Reliability, validity, and practicality of a questionnaire. *Aging: Clinical and Experimental Research, 7*(3), 159–164.

Brooten, D., Gennaro, S., Knapp, H., Jovene, N., Brown, L., & York, R. (1991). Functions of the CNS in early discharge and home follow-up of very low birthweight infants. *Clinical Nurse Specialist, 5*(4), 196–201.

Brown, S. (1996). Direct clinical practice. In A. B. Hamric, J. A. Spross, & C. M. Hanson (Eds.), *Advanced nursing practice: An integrative approach* (pp. 109–138). Philadelphia: W. B. Saunders.

Browne, G. B., Arpin, K., Corey, P., Fitch, M., & Gafni, A. (1990). Individual correlates of health service utilization and the cost of poor adjustment to chronic illness. *Medical Care, 28*(1), 43–58.

Bryson, K., Naqvi, A., Callahan, P., & Fontenot, D. (1990). Brief admission program: An alliance of inpatient care and outpatient case management. *Journal of Psychosocial Nursing, 28*(12), 19–23.

Bushnell, F. K. (1992, October). Self-care teaching for congestive heart failure patients. *Journal of Gerontological Nursing,* pp. 27–32.

Calkin, J. (1984). A model for advanced nursing practice. *Journal of Nursing Administration, 14*(1), 24–30.

Campbell, A., Converse, P., & Rogers, W. (1976). *The quality of American life.* New York: Russell Sage.

Case Management Society of America. (1994). CMSA proposes standards of practice. *The Case Manager, 5*(1), 59–70.

Cesta, T. (1993). The link between continuous quality improvement and case management. *Journal of Nursing Administration, 23*(6), 55–61.

Connors, H. (1993). Impact of care management modalities on curricula. In K. Kelly & M. Maas (Eds.), *Managing nursing care: Promise and pitfalls* (pp. 190–207). St. Louis: Mosby.

Cooper, D. M. (1990). Today—assessment and intuition: Tomorrow—projections. In D. M. Cooper, P. A. Minarik, & P. S. A. Sparacino (Eds.), *The clinical nurse specialist: Implementation and impact* (pp. 285–298). Norwalk, CT: Appleton & Lange.

Cronin, C., & Maklebust, J. (1989). Case-managed care: Capitalizing on the CNS. *Nursing Management, 20*(3), 38–47.

Daleiden, A. (1993). The CNS as trauma case manager. *Clinical Nurse Specialist, 7,* 295–298.

Doell Smith, L. (1994). Continuity of care through nursing case management of the chronically ill child. *Clinical Nurse Specialist, 8,* 65–68.

Eichert, J. H., & Patterson, R. B. (1997). Factors affecting the success of disease management. *Infusion, 3*(12), 31–38.

Eichert, J. H., Wong, H., & Smith, D. R. (1997). The disease management development process. In W. E. Todd & D. Nash (Eds.), *Disease management: A system approach to improving patient outcomes* (pp. 27–60). Chicago: American Hospital Publishing.

Ethridge, P. (1991). A nursing HMO: Carondelet St. Mary's experience. *Nursing Management, 22*(7), 22–27.

Ethridge, P., & Lamb, G. (1989). Professional nursing case management improves quality, access and costs. *Nursing Management, 20*(3), 30–35.

Falter, E. J., Cesta, T. G., Concert, C., & Mason, D. J. (1999). Development of a graduate nursing program in case management. *Journal of Case Management, 5*(3), 50–56.

Flynn, A., & Kilgallen, M. (1993). Case management: A multidisciplinary approach to the evaluation of cost and quality standards. *Journal of Nursing Care Quality, 8*(3), 58–66.

Fralic, M. (1992). The nurse case manager: Focus, selection, preparation, and measurement. *Journal of Nursing Administration, 22*(11), 13–14, 46.

Friedman, N. M., Gleeson, J. M., Kent, M. J., Foris, M., & Rodriguez, D. J. (1998). Management of diabetes mellitus in the Lovelace Health Systems' Episodes of Care Program. *Effective Clinical Practice, 1*(1), 5–11.

Gaedeke-Norris, M., & Hill, C. (1991). The clinical nurse specialist: Developing the case manager role. *Dimensions of Critical Care Nursing, 10,* 346–352.

Gournic, J. (1989). Clinical leadership, management, and the CNS. In A. B. Hamric & J. A. Spross (Eds.), *The clinical nurse specialist in theory and practice* (2nd ed., pp. 227–250). Philadelphia: W. B. Saunders.

Hall, J. A., Feldstein, M., Fretwell, M. D., Rowe, J. W., & Epstein, A. M. (1990). Older patients' health status and satisfaction with medical care in an HMO population. *Medical Care, 28,* 260–270.

Hamric, A. B. (1992). Creating our future: Challenges and opportunities for the clinical nurse specialist. *Oncology Nursing Forum, 19*(1, Suppl.), 11–15.

Hamric, A. B. (1989). History and overview of the CNS role. In A. B. Hamric & J. A. Spross (Eds.), *The clinical nurse specialist in theory and practice* (2nd ed., pp. 3–18). Philadelphia: W. B. Saunders.

Hamric, A. B., & Taylor, J. W. (1989). Role development of the CNS. In A. B. Hamric & J. A. Spross (Eds.), *The clinical nurse specialist in theory and practice* (2nd ed., pp. 41–82). Philadelphia: W. B. Saunders.

Hospodar, J. A., & Zazworsky, D. (1997, September/October). Population health management development through a national Medicare demonstration project. *The Alliance for Healthcare Strategy and Marketing,* pp. 9–11.

Hospodar, J. A., & Zazworsky, D. (1999, January). High-risk efforts. *The Alliance for Healthcare Strategy and Marketing,* pp. 6–7.

Iezzoni, L. I. (1997). *Risk adjustment for measuring healthcare outcomes.* Chicago: Health Administration Press.

Jenkins, M., & Sullivan-Marx, E. (1994). Nurse practitioners and community health nurses: Clinical partnerships and future visions. *Nursing Clinics of North America, 29,* 459–471.

Kolter, P., & Zaltman, G. (1971). Social marketing: An approach to planned social change. *Journal of Marketing, 35,* 3–12.

Kosberg, J. I., & Cairl, R. E. (1986). The Cost of Care Index: A case management tool for screening informal care providers. *Gerontologist, 26,* 273–278.

Ladden, M. (1991). On-site perinatal case management: An HMO model. *Journal of Perinatal-Neonatal Nursing, 5*(1), 27–32.

LaLonde, B. (1987). The General Symptom Distress Scale: A home care measure. *Quality Review Bulletin, 13*(7):243–250.

Lamb, G. (1993). *Comprehensive case management for individuals with progressive multiple sclerosis: An experimental study* (Interim Report). New York: National Multiple Sclerosis Society.

Lamb, G., Mahn, V., & Dahl, R. (1996). Goals of an effective delivery system for the chronically ill. *Managed Care Quarterly, 4*(3):46–53.

Lamb, G., & Stempel, J. (1994). Nurse case management from the client's view: Growing as insider-expert. *Nursing Outlook, 42,* 7–13.

Lamb, G., & Zazworsky, D. (1997). The Carondelet model: Case study 1. *Nursing Management, 28*(3), 27–28.

Lynn-McHale, D., Fitzpatrick, E., & Shaller, R. (1993). Case management: Development of a model. *Clinical Nurse Specialist, 7,* 299–307.

Madden, M., & Reid Ponte, P. (1994). Advanced practice roles in the managed care environment. *Journal of Nursing Administration, 24,* 56–62.

Mahn, V. (1993). Clinical nurse case management: A service line approach. *Nursing Management, 24*(9), 48–50.

Mahn, V. (1999). Use of claims data to identify the right population to case manage: Pandora's Box or the wave of the future. MIDS Monitor, July Supplement. MIDS Inc.: Tucson.

Mahn, V. A., & Spross, J. A. (1996). Nurse case management as an advanced practice role. In A. B. Hamric, J. A. Spross, & C. M. Hanson (Eds.), *Advanced nursing practice: An integrative approach* (pp. 445–465). Philadelphia: W. B. Saunders.

Martin, K. S., Scheet, N. J. (1992). The Omaha System: Applications for community health nursing. Philadelphia: W. B. Saunders.

Martin, K., Leak, G., & Aden, C. (1992). The Omaha system: A research-based model for decision making. *JONA, 22*(11), 47–52.

Milliman & Robertson (1999). Healthcare Management Guidelines. J. M. Schibanoff (ed.). San Diego, Milliman & Robertson, Inc.

National Multiple Sclerosis Society. (1985). *Minimal record of disability for multiple sclerosis.* New York: Author.

Newman, M. (1990). Toward an integrative model of professional practice. *Journal of Professional Nursing, 6,* 167–173.

Newman, M. (1994). *Health as expanding consciousness* (2nd ed.). New York: National League for Nursing Press.

Newman, M., Lamb, G., & Michaels, C. (1989). Nurse case management: The coming together of theory and practice. *Nursing & Health Care, 12,* 404–408.

Nugent, K. (1992). The clinical nurse specialist as case manager in a collaborative practice model: Bridging the gap between quality and cost of care. *Clinical Nurse Specialist, 6,* 106–111.

Office of Technology Assessment. (1986). *Nurse practitioners, physician assistants, and certified nurse midwives: A policy analysis* (Health Care Technology Study No. OTA-HCS-37). Washington, DC: Author.

Papenhausen, J. L. (1996). Discovering and achieving client outcomes. In E. L. Cohen (Ed.), *Nurse case management in the 21st century* (pp. 257–268). St. Louis: Mosby.

Parker, M., Quinn, J., Viehl, M., McKinley, A., Polich, C., Detzner, D., Hartwell, S., & Korn, K. (1990). Case management in rural areas: Definition, clients, financing, staffing, and service delivery issues. *Nursing Economics, 8*(2), 103–109.

Plocher, D. W. (1996). Disease management. In P. R. Kongstvedt (Ed.), *The managed health care services* (3rd ed.). Gaithersburg, MD: Aspen Publishers.

Porter-O'Grady, T. (1996). Nurses as advanced practitioners and primary care providers. In E. L. Cohen (Ed.), *Nurse case management in the 21st century* (pp. 10–20). St. Louis: Mosby.

Poulshock, S. W., & Deimling, G. T. (1984). Families caring for elders in residence: Issues in the measurement of burden. *Journal of Gerontology, 39*(2), 230–239.

Prochaska, J. O., DiClemente, C. C., & Norcross, J. C. (1992). In search of how people change: Applications to addictive behaviors. *American Psychologist, 47*(9), 1102–1114.

Rieve, J. A. (1999). Case identification and selection outcomes. *The Case Manager, 10*(3), 22–25.

Riley, T. (1992). HIV-infected client care: Case management and the HIV team. *Clinical Nurse Specialist, 6,* 136–140.

Rotz, N., Yates, J., & Schare, B. (1994). Application of the case management model to a trauma patient. *Clinical Nurse Specialist, 8,* 180–186.

Rules and regulations. (1998). *Federal Register, 63*(211), 58871–58874.

Schroer, K. (1991). Case management: Clinical nurse specialist and nurse practitioner, converging roles. *Clinical Nurse Specialist, 5,* 189–194.

Sherman, J., & Johnson, P. (1994). CNS as unit-based case manager. *Clinical Nurse Specialist, 8,* 76–80.

Smith, M. (1993). Case management and nursing theory-based practice. *Nursing Science Quarterly, 6*(1), 8–9.

Spitzer, W. O., Roberts, R. S., & Delmore, T. (1976). Nurse practitioners in primary care: Assessment of their deployment with the utilization and financial index. *CMAJ, 114*(12), 1099–1108, June 1976.

Stempel, J., Carlson, A., & Michaels, C. (1996). Working in partnership. In Cohen, E. L. (Ed.), *Nurse case management in the 21st century* (pp. 124–132). St. Louis: Mosby.

Strong, A. (1991). Case management of a patient with multisystem failure. *Critical Care Quarterly, 11*(6), 10–18.

Strong, A. (1992). Case management and the CNS. *Clinical Nurse Specialist, 6,* 64.

Tidwell, S. (1994). The critical care clinical nurse specialist as case manager. In A. Gawlinski & L. Kern (Eds.), *The clinical nurse specialist in critical care* (pp. 62–79). Philadelphia: W. B. Saunders.

Todd, W. E., & Nash, D. (Eds.). (1997). *Disease management: A systems approach to improving patient outcomes.* Chicago: American Hospital Publishing.

Trinidad, E. (1993). Case management: A model of case management. *Clinical Nurse Specialist, 7,* 221–223.

Wagner, J., & Menke, E. (1992). Case management of homeless families. *Clinical Nurse Specialist, 6,* 65–71.

Ward, M. D., & Rieve, J. A. (1997). The role of case management in disease management. In W. E. Todd & D. Nash (Eds.), *Disease management: A systems approach to improving patient outcomes* (pp. 235–259). Chicago: American Hospital Publishing.

Ware, J. E., Snow, K. K., Kosinski, M., & Gandek, B. (1993). *SF-36 Health Survey manual and interpretation guide.* Boston: The Health Institute, New England Medical Center.

Wedzicha, J. A., Bestall, J. C., Garrod, R., Garnham, R., Paul, E. A., & Jones, P. W. (1998). Randomized controlled trial of pulmonary rehabilitation in severe chronic obstructive pulmonary disease patients, stratified with the MRC dyspnea scale. *European Respiratory Journal, 12,* 363–369.

Wheeler, D. J. (1993). Understanding variation: The key to managing chaos. Knoxville, TN: SPC Press.

Zagorin, E. (1996). Continuum of care case study. *Rehab Management: The Interdisciplinary Journal of Rehabilitation, 9*(6), 66–67.

Zander, K. (1990). Case management: A golden opportunity for whom? In J. McCloskey & H. Grace (Eds.), *Current issues in nursing* (pp. 199–204). St. Louis: Mosby.

Zander, K. (1993). The impact of managing care on the role of a nurse. In K. Kelly & M. Maas (Eds.), *Managing nursing care: Promise and pitfalls* (pp. 65–82). St. Louis: Mosby.

Zazworsky, D. (1997). Exercise assessment for multiple sclerosis. *Home Health Focus, 4*(4), 29–30.

Zazworsky, D., & Gibson, B.(1997). Exercise program for multiple sclerosis. *Home Health Focus, 4*(5), 38–39.

Zazworsky, D., & Hospodar, J. A. (1996). Marketing nurse case management services. In E. L. Cohen (Ed.), *Nurse case management in the 21st century* (pp. 202–210). St. Louis: Mosby.

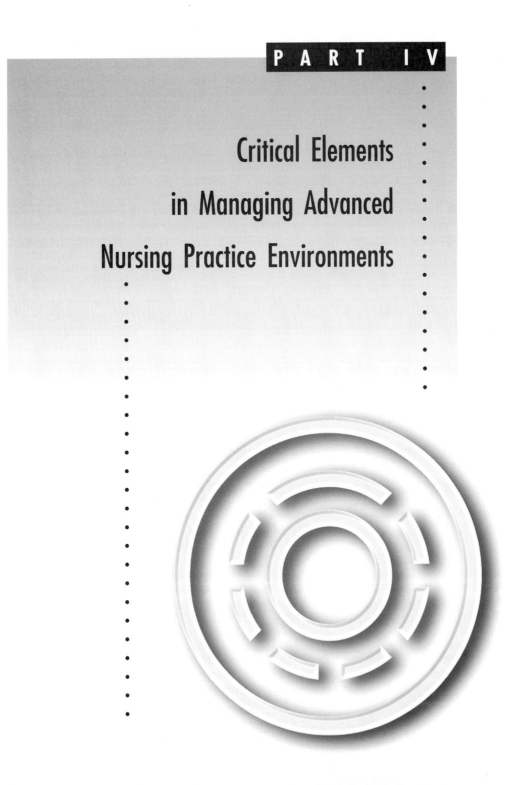

PART IV

Critical Elements
in Managing Advanced
Nursing Practice Environments

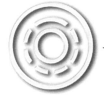

Managing Advanced Nursing Practice

BUSINESS PLANNING AND REIMBURSEMENT MECHANISMS

• C H R I S T I N A   C .   K I N G

INTRODUCTION

Today's patients need and demand health services beyond those that have been traditionally available. From the patient's perspective, services must be accessible and affordable. From the payer's perspective, they must be cost-effective. Both groups desire and demand high-quality services. The work of the health care system, and, subsequently, the advanced practice nurses (APNs) practicing within it, is to fulfill the health-related needs of the patient within an increasingly demanding and complex environment. There are many different processes that contribute to this system, most of which may be classified either as those related to direct patient care (with a clinical focus), or as those that support the patient care process indirectly (with an administrative focus). Successful APNs develop, implement, and continuously analyze the direct and indirect processes of care used to meet patient outcomes, while being cognizant of the other critical environmental elements that affect advanced nursing practice. The success of the resulting health care system is measured by the ability of the APN provider using these existing processes to attain desired patient outcomes within the constraints of available resources and reimbursement. The price of system failure is measured in terms of human suffering.

Innovation in health care often stems from the professional and ethical commitment of nurses and other health care providers to improve patient care, either directly or indirectly. Innovations in both direct patient care and the supporting indirect care infrastructure receive increasing attention from health care providers, insurers, and regulating bodies as resources decrease and need increases. One particular innovation that has been successful in patient care settings, such as hospitals and larger group practices, is the conceptualization and organization of the direct and indirect processes of patient care within the context of systems thinking (HCA Quality Resource Group, 1992a, 1992b).

According to Batalden (P. B. Batalden, personal communication, June 17, 1995), successful change leading to the continual improvement and innovation of patient care is driven by four key elements: the tension for change, the presence of actionable alternatives, the knowledge and skills to do things differently, and organizational support for the new behaviors. The current health care environment provides significant tension for change. Through the political leadership of national organizations and the active participation of nurses in the political process, nursing has the ability to influence the direction of that change (see also Chapter 10). The APN is uniquely poised as the viable alternative to the traditional physician provider, and, as such, demonstrates the expertise, knowledge, and skills to do things differently. The acceptance of the need for change by health care organizations, the commitment to nursing's professional ethics, and the covenant nurses hold with society provide support for the new behaviors.

Simply put, any system represents the flow of resources through a process that results in the desired outcomes (see Figure 20–1). The size and complexity of the developed system is dependent upon the number and complexity of processes being used to attain the desired outcome. Examination of the system includes assessment and evaluation of the resources used, the processes utilized, and the outcomes attained. The reader will recognize the similarity to Donabedian's (1966) framework of structure, process, and outcome described in Chapter 25. This chapter focuses on the process of APN business planning from a systems-thinking approach. Although the emphasis is on an APN managed practice, all APNs need to be aware that patient care delivery is conceptualized as comprising the direct and indirect patient care processes that ensure that available resources are allocated in such a manner as to meet the desired patient outcomes. Business planning is itself a process that focuses primarily upon the development, implementation, and evaluation of those indirect processes that support patient care. It stands in contrast to a business plan, which

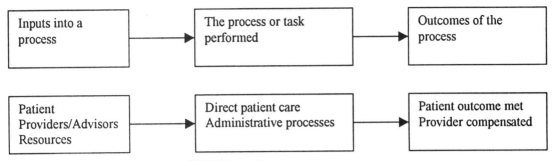

FIGURE 20–1 • Flowcharts of processes.

is a document used by legal and financial advisors to evaluate the success potential of a particular business venture, such as an individual APN practice. The business plan may be conceptualized as an outcome product of the business planning process. Reimbursement, as part of overall business planning, is another indirect process supporting patient care, and is one of the critical elements affecting the success of advanced nursing practice. Examples are provided to illustrate these important concepts.

BUSINESS PLANNING

Success in and satisfaction with one's APN role revolve around the right match between APNs and the work they do, and the ability to be flexible and innovative within the scope of that role. APNs participate in two different groups of processes within the advanced practice role. Direct care processes—hands-on patient-based processes and tasks—are evidenced by the APN's clinical practice (see Part III). Indirect processes are the administrative processes and tasks that support direct patient care. Examples of indirect processes are the steps taken to register a patient and collect demographics, the process of third-party billing, and the identification of a medical and office supplies vendor (see Table 20-1). Both direct and indirect processes are essential to the successful management of any health care system, whether it be a small, self-contained APN practice or a large, multihospital network.

Over an APN's career, the balance between direct and indirect process involvement, and the size of the system in which these processes occur, may vary. One way of characterizing the shift in this balance and size of the system is to consider that the

TABLE 20–1 EXAMPLES OF DIRECT AND INDIRECT PROCESSES AND SKILLS	
CLINICAL/DIRECT PROCESSES AND SKILLS	ADMINISTRATIVE/INDIRECT PROCESSES AND SKILLS
Wound management	Support staff supervision
Childbirth education	Presentation/teaching/precepting experience
Lactation consultation	Grant-writing capabilities
Suturing	Computer literacy
Intrauterine contraceptive device insertion	Budget development
Pain management	Medical billing
Intubation	Word processing/desktop publishing

APN adopts an entrepreneurial approach, an intrapreneurial approach, or a mixture of both at any given time. Both entrepreneurs and intrapreneurs are individuals who continually search for and who are receptive to opportunities and innovation. Innovation comes through the creation of a new process (whether direct, indirect, or both), or through radical changes to an existing process so that it seems "like new." An entrepreneur plans, organizes, finances, operates, and participates in a new health care delivery organization. Entrepreneurs have control over and responsibility for an increased proportion of indirect processes of care in their role as compared to intrapreneurs. An intrapreneur is generally an employee of an existing health care system, in which many of the indirect processes of the care delivery system may be controlled and managed by other employees or departments. The intrapreneur improves, redesigns, or augments an employer's current direct care processes, with a lesser role in the day-to-day business administrative functions of clinical practice. Entrepreneurs function within the context of the larger, societal health care system. Intrapreneurs function within an institutional health care system, a microcosm of the larger arena. When embarking on program or practice oversight, the APN needs to understand the balance between direct and indirect processes as well as the size the business will have over time (see Chapter 26 for excellent examples of both entrepreneurial and intrapreneurial practices).

The decision about the proportion of one's role to devote to direct care versus indirect processes is based upon the professional and personal values and goals of the APN. Determining one's professional values may be a complex process because these values may have been internalized and therefore may be difficult to articulate. Professional values include those tenets of nursing practice that provide significance and meaning to the APN's practice of nursing. Some sources of professional values include the various publications of the nursing profession, such as the *Code for Nurses* (American Nurses Association [ANA], 1985), writings of nursing theorists to which the APN has been exposed, and artwork depicting care and compassion (Donahue, 1985). The mission and goal statements of the APN national organizations clearly portray these values as well.

Married to one's professional values are one's personal values, especially one's comfort with risk taking, and one's preference as to the arena in which care is delivered. Risk taking is a key characteristic of the APN who is considering involvement in an entrepreneurial practice. A desire to function within an organizational setting is a key characteristic of an intrapreneurial approach. Some questions that may assist the APN in clarifying professional and personal values include the following (these sample questions are intended to be illustrative only, and are not assumed to be exhaustive):

- *To clarify one's internalized theoretical basis for practice:* What model of nursing practice, or approach to care delivery, best describes how I perceive my own nursing practice? Do the options before me favor this model, or some other approach? If they favor another approach, how compatible is it with my own beliefs? (See Chapters 2 through 5.)
- *To determine one's tolerance for being entrepreneurial (requires increased risk taking):* Do I thrive on risk taking, like some risk, or prefer situations with a conservative level of risk involved? How is a "loss" or being "unsuccessful" defined? If I like taking risks, how much of a loss can I afford to take—both professionally and personally—should my venture prove unsuccessful?

- *To determine one's preference for an intrapreneurial approach:* Do I prefer being a part of a team, or being on my own? If I like being on a team, what other team members would I like to be included on this team? How big a team am I most comfortable with? If I prefer working on my own, how will I interact with my colleagues? (See Chapters 7, 8, and 11.)

An ideal skills inventory serves as the springboard for the clarification of the APN's professional goals. The extent to which the APN balances the clinical role with administrative demands depends on the APN's skills and preferences, and begins with an inventory of those clinical skills and administrative talents that the APN would like to bring, or acquire, in an ideal advanced practice role. Table 20-1 lists examples of clinical versus administrative skills. Some questions that may refine one's ideal inventory include

- *To clearly articulate one's existing area of clinical expertise:* Do I have well-developed advanced clinical skills? If so, what are they?
- *To better articulate one's ideal role:* What tasks do I particularly enjoy, feel neutral about, and particularly dislike? Of those that I dislike, but that need to be performed, do mechanisms exist for those tasks to be performed by someone else?
- *To identify one's areas for growth:* What processes would I like to do more of, or learn more about? Does the current situation provide opportunities for me to do them?

The ability to actualize one's ideal APN role provides a strong incentive toward managing one's program or practice. However, APNs must realize that they will be the "boss" and may need to manage not only their own work, but the work of a support staff as well (Stewart, 1989). Being in charge may include attention to the rules and regulations of many different entities governing APN clinical practice, grant execution and reporting, and general business practice. Because business and managerial skills are not taught in basic nursing programs, these skills will need to be learned. Graduate nursing programs are responding to this need and to the demands of dynamic and changing practice environments by incorporating business and practice management concepts into APN education. Many APNs have sought dual degrees in nursing and business administration. Some questions related to one's ability to assume an increased managerial role in indirect processes include

- *To determine internal and external loci of support:* Do I have the unflagging support of those closest to me, both personally (significant other, children, friends, etc.) and professionally (physician collaborators, APN colleagues, financial and legal advisors, etc.)? (See Chapter 11.)
- *To determine basic management skills:* Do I have well-honed organizational skills? Do I enjoy paying attention to details? Am I comfortable in a leadership position? (See Chapter 10.)
- *To determine basic financial management skills:* Am I familiar with, or willing to learn, the budgeting cycle and processes of my employer? Have I participated in budget preparation and resource allocation in the past? Am I comfortable developing a budget for my own practice?
- *To determine external regulatory guidelines affecting practice:* Do I know where to locate copies of the applicable regulations affecting this program? Do I understand, or do I have access to advisors who understand, the specific

ramifications of state and federal laws applicable to this program, such as those pertaining to the Clinical Laboratory Improvement Amendments (CLIA) of 1988 (42 C.F.R. § 493)? Are there any institutional rules and regulations that may limit my ability to practice within the full scope of my role? What are the procedures for obtaining approval of the various institutional committees that may be involved? (See Chapter 22.)

- *To determine financial resources:* Where will funding for the program (capital for start-up expenses) come from? Do I have the financial ability to live without a steady income if the grant is not refunded, or for at least 1 year while the practice is growing?
- *To determine human resources skills and systems:* Am I willing to be responsible for the work of others? What does that entail? Are administrative systems in place for hiring, evaluating, and terminating staff for the duration of the program/ practice?

These are among the many questions to be answered by APNs prior to deciding how extensive their role will be in the management of their program or practice. Fortunately, there are several resources to help clinicians better understand the indirect processes, or "business," of clinical practice. The reader is referred to Buppert (1999) for an in-depth discussion of NP business and legal concerns. The American Medical Association (AMA 1996a, 1996b, 1996c, 1996d, 1999), in collaboration with the Coker Group, has published a series regarding independent practice management that is useful for any APN role. *Entrepreneur* and other business magazines provide useful information related to business management and administration. The Small Business Administration provides general and specific information regarding business management and referral to local supports, including the local office of the Service Corps of Retired Executives (SCORE). There are many on-line World Wide Web resources related to business management. Some specific sites that may be useful to the development of small businesses include the following:

- *www.americanexpress.com* (American Express Company, 1998)
- *www.smallbizsearch.com*
- *www.dol.gov/dol/osbp/public/sbrefa/main.htm*

DIRECT PROCESSES OF CARE

Practice environments represent small health care systems based upon a patient population with an identified need. This patient population is identified through a variety of ways, including individual APN preference based upon the role and scope of practice of the individual APN. For certified nurse-midwives (CNMs) and certified registered nurse anesthetists (CRNAs), the patient population is essentially defined by their roles with child-bearing women and their families, and with patients undergoing surgical anesthesia, respectively. Nurse practitioners (NPs) and clinical nurse specialists (CNSs) have a broader population base, although their clinical subspecialty describes their patient population (i.e., family NP, psychiatric CNS) (see Part III). Sometimes APNs identify patient populations through other modifiers, such as age, health promotion specialty, or disease state specialty—for example, CNMs who care for adolescent mothers-to-be, CNSs who have expertise in cardiac risk factor modification and rehabilitation, and adult NPs or CNSs who specialize in management of asthma or diabetes. In other instances, it is the geographical location or organizational setting that differentiates one's patient population of interest. Examples of these populations are the rural underserved populations cared for by National Health Service Corps providers, veterans cared for by the Veterans Affairs Medical Centers, and participants in Kaiser Permanente's managed care program who are cared for by their own staff of providers. APNs must be able to clearly and succinctly define the patient population being served by their clinical practice (marketing to this population is discussed in Chapter 21).

Missions, Visions, and Values

After the patient population has been identified, and the patient care processes have been outlined, the APN may choose to formalize this information in a mission and vision statement. The mission and vision statement describe the APN practice's reason for existence and future direction to the patient and to prospective funding agencies, and at times serve to remind the APN entrepreneur about where the program or practice's priorities should lie. The written summary of program or practice values may be combined with the mission and vision statements into one document, such as a brochure or program information sheet. This summary is available for review by any interested party, and should be given to every patient at the time of the first program or practice encounter.

The mission states the goal of the direct processes of care in one sentence. The vision describes the "ideal" 5-year goal, that is, what the APN envisions the direct processes of care to be 5 years from their inception. The mission and vision statements enhance interdisciplinary collaboration as APNs clearly articulate their goals and vision of patient care to existing and potential colleagues, consultants, and third-party payers. If the APN is functioning through an intrapreneurial approach, the program's mission and vision should be examined with knowledge of the organization's mission and vision to ensure that the program fits into the overall goals of the organization. If the program's mission conflicts with that of the organization, problems may take the form of delays in funding, changes to the program's direct or indirect processes of care, barriers to program implementation, and outright denial of program development. If other providers, individuals, or groups have a stake in the program, the mission and vision statement should be determined through consensus of the group.

The values of a practice, or program, describe those ethical precepts that govern relationships between the provider, the practice, the patients, and external groups. They may be related to direct care processes—patient focused, or indirect care in nature. Professional ethics are discussed in Chapters 12 and 21. Ethical precepts pertaining to patient-focused values are described briefly here.

INFORMED CONSENT

Informed consent is a legal principle that guarantees that a mentally competent adult (or a mentally competent legal guardian or parent serving as proxy for a child) has control over his or her own body. It requires that any provider, including APNs, obtain a patient's informed consent prior to any medical or nursing treatment. The

APN must describe the general nature of the treatment and any consequences involved, the normal risks and hazards inherent to the treatment, any known side effects or complications that may occur, and any alternative treatments available to the patient. The patient's understanding of this information, and the agreement to proceed with treatment based upon this understanding, comprises the patient's informed consent. Both the APN's information and the patient's agreement within the informed consent discussion must be documented as part of the patient's medical record. In many instances, a standardized form to document a patient's informed consent is used.

CONFIDENTIALITY

Confidentiality is a highly ethical issue that requires careful consideration. The balance between the patient's right to privacy and society's need to be protected is important. State laws clearly explicate those patient issues, such as sexually transmitted diseases or tuberculosis, that are reportable by law. Patient confidentiality is critical to the provider-patient relationship. It is the patient's right to decide what information the APN, and all other members of the health care team, may share with others. It extends to any communication between the APN and the patient, all personal data, information contained in the medical record, and any billing information related to the patient's care. The patient must formally give permission to the APN to release any of this information, usually in the form of a signed release of information. The release of information describes what information may be released, to whom, and for how long that particular release is allowed. Separate releases are required for any information related to mental health, substance abuse, and human immunodeficiency virus test reporting.

PRIVACY

In addition to the right to a confidential provider-patient relationship, the patient is entitled to a degree of personal privacy within the clinical encounter. Courtesy commands that the patient's dignity be maintained, including providing the patient with well-fitting patient gowns and cover sheets during the physical examination. Attention should be paid to the physical layout of the patient encounter area, ensuring that conversations cannot be overheard and that the room is secure from line of gaze through open doors and/or windows. Unless the patient agrees, or is a minor (*not* seeking certain types of reproductive health, substance abuse, or mental health care, as determined by individual states' laws), family members should not be invited into the patient encounter.

SECURITY

Both the patient and the APN should feel as if the patient care area is a safe and secure place for the encounter. Policies should clearly articulate how to maintain patient, provider, and staff safety, including provisions for securing a patient's valuables during procedures and for managing hostile persons in the area (including a policy for managing violent and armed persons). The level of security needed is dependent upon the APN's practice environment and available resources within the facility.

RESOLUTION OF COMPLAINTS

It is essential to monitor patient satisfaction with the clinical experience from the time the patient enters the waiting room through the time the final bill is paid for services. There are many patient satisfaction tools available to health care providers to measure patients' responses to the way care is delivered (see Chapter 25 on outcomes evaluation). Despite one's best efforts, however, patients may be dissatisfied with some aspect of their experience at some point during an APN's career. It is important that any sign of dissatisfaction, or patient complaint, be addressed immediately, preferably at the time of the complaint. A formal policy related to the management of patient complaints includes how patient complaints are recorded, who investigates and responds to the patient's concerns, and how quickly the complaint is addressed. Specific guidelines for managing patient complaints may be supplemented by risk management information provided by the APN's malpractice carrier.

COMMUNICATION

Ethical clinical practice demands honesty and integrity in all patient interactions. Under the best circumstances, communication lines will be open and both the APN and the patient will understand each other, and feel as if they have been understood. In circumstances in which misunderstandings occur, it behooves the APN to manage the issue as if it were a patient complaint—seeking to address the concerns in an objective and timely manner. Communications of a vital nature to patient care, such as the reporting of a critical diagnostic test result or the termination of the provider-patient relationship, demand that additional steps be taken to ensure the patient is notified, and that he or she understands the implications of the communication. In the instance of an abnormal test result, all telephone conversations should be documented with the date and time of the patient contact, along with any specific plans for treatment or follow-up testing resulting from the initial test result. Termination of the provider-patient relationship may be accomplished in a three-step process. First, a policy describing those scenarios under which the APN will terminate the relationship is clearly articulated, and made available to the patient if requested. Second, the APN speaks directly with the patient, detailing the behaviors that meet the criteria for termination. Third, a summary of the discussion is promptly sent to the patient in a certified, return receipt letter. A copy of the letter sent to the patient is kept in the patient's medical record along with the signed postal receipts. Some states have regulations regarding the termination of the provider-patient relationship. The APN is referred to individual state-specific guidelines from the board of nursing and/or boards of medicine and osteopathy for further information.

Clinical Relationships

Although the APN is assumed to be the primary care provider in this discussion, attention must be paid to the development of clinical relationships with APN, physician, pharmacist, and other allied health colleagues. (In-depth discussions related to clinical mentorship, consultation, and collaboration are found in Part II.) To be successful, the APN must maintain a collegial relationship with other health care providers (Hanson, 1993). An important legal consideration is defining the parameters of the association with a collaborating physician through the development of a collaborative practice agreement (see Chapter 22). Most state statutes for APNs require some form of medical collaboration. A strong relationship with a collaborating physician, or group of physicians, is essential to the success of APN practice.

Consultants and Referrals

APNs need to find consultants and referral sources for patients whose medical problems require additional expertise from a specialist. Locating referrals for indigent patients or the uninsured who need medical care or hospitalization may be difficult because of the lack of services for these populations. A list of consultants and referral sources, outlining the services offered and their willingness to accept referrals, should be generated. Their participation in third-party payer plans, such as health maintenance organization (HMO) networks or preferred provider organizations (PPOs), also should be noted and clearly understood by the APN entrepreneur. Consultants are identified through word-of-mouth recommendations from clinical mentors and colleagues, through the recommendation of lay public support groups who have worked with certain specialty groups, and through direct provider interviews. For example, a local chapter of the American Heart Association may be aware of the providers offering heart-healthy nutrition classes. Over time, the APN develops a referral and consultation base, and develops strong relationships with those providers who are able to assist the APN in meeting patients' needs. Once the relationship is established, acknowledging the consultant's assistance and support is equally important. This acknowledgment may be as simple as learning from the consulting registration staff what demographic information they need in order to schedule the patient, providing the most recent office notes to the consultant in time for the patient's appointment, and sending seasonal cards thanking them for their support.

INDIRECT PROCESSES OF CARE

Indirect processes support patient care and center around administrative and operational structures and functions. Although they require a different set of advisors, staff, and equipment, they are equally important in the successful APN practice. Business relationships and business structures are necessary to define the context and framework under which clinical practice is performed. Knowledge of the external regulatory bodies that impact APN practice is essential in today's complex and rapidly changing health care arena. The subsequent discussion presents an overview of these issues but in no way is intended to be comprehensive. The APN is referred to business consultants for up-to-date information reflective of the laws and guidelines within a particular state and practice setting.

Business Relationships

Separate from, but as important as, the clinical advisors and resources described earlier are the administrative advisors and resources required to develop and maintain smooth indirect processes to support patient care. An independent practice will need to contract or consult with an accountant, attorney, banker, and insurance agent for specific services (Stewart, 1989). In addition, the services of a practice management consultant with medical billing expertise should be enlisted. The accountant should assist the APN in setting up an accounting system, establishing internal controls, and preparing an operating budget (AMA, 1996d). The accountant should set up the practice to assure that the best tax advantages and flexibility are obtained (AMA, 1996d). Attorneys with expertise in health care law should establish the legal structure of the practice, and provide advice on an as-needed basis for special purposes (AMA, 1996d). The attorney and accountant should have a working relationship so that the legal structure selected provides the best legal, financial, and tax advantages for the providers involved. The banking relationship serves to establish a line of credit or business loan (if needed), and to establish business banking needs (AMA, 1996d). A business insurance agent provides expertise in the areas of health, liability, and workers' compensation insurance programs. The practice management consultant serves to develop policies and procedure manuals, billing procedures and fee schedules, and job descriptions for an entrepreneurial enterprise (AMA, 1996d). A medical billing expert provides guidance in both the efficient completion and processing of billing forms in order to receive third-party reimbursement or capitation payment for the provider's services, and the thorough and accurate completion of any third-party payer's contracting paperwork required for the APN's participation in selected contracts. The APN needs to carefully decide which of these functions can be done independently and which need to be purchased as externally contracted services. It is important for the APN entrepreneur to ask: Is this an area of strength and interest, or is this an area that I do not want to attend to? Is this an indirect process of care to which I want to devote time and energy?

The selection of day-to-day administrative support staff services (separate from the services of business advisors) revolves around the processes of care being delivered, and the environment in which services are delivered. Once the APN knows what the direct patient care process will include, and has identified those indirect processes that will support the patient encounter, additional ancillary personnel may be identified to meet process needs. In the community-based primary care setting, a practice requires someone to assist in patient registration and scheduling (the first process box in Figure 20–1), someone to assist the clinician in certain elements of patient care (the second box), and someone to collect or process patient fees (the third box). Any additional administrative roles support these primary roles, and may include someone to manage patient medical records, someone to telephone triage acutely ill patients, or someone to perform office cleaning functions. The actual individuals who fill these roles, along with their skills and qualifications, need to be matched with APN and practice goals for patient care. In hospital-based settings, CRNAs, CNSs, and CNMs often collaborate with the nurse managers of the area in which they practice to obtain the assistance of the unit's support staff and ancillary personnel. An organizational chart and job descriptions of the roles required should be developed, placed in a common personnel manual, and shared among staff members so that everyone is aware of his or her role within the successful functioning of the system. An example of an organizational chart is presented in Figure 20–2. Some payers require a copy of the organizational chart prior to enrolling the provider, as Medicaid does for APNs providing children's services. The experience, education, and other qualifications of the APN, other professionals providing services, and support staff should be described briefly and made available to interested parties.

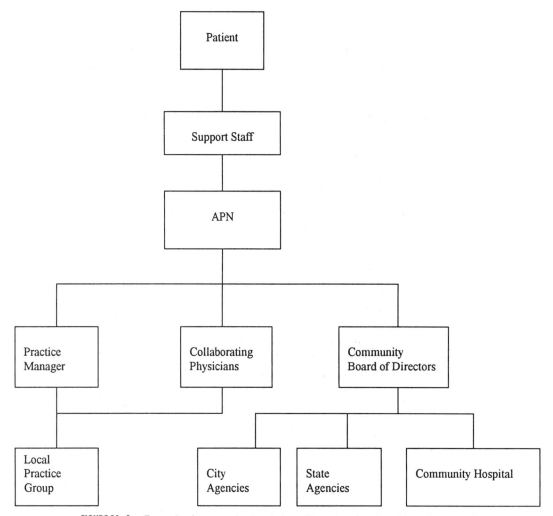

FIGURE 20–2 • Example of an organizational chart. (Based on data from Mercy Maritime Family Practice, Peaks Island, ME.)

Program and Business Structure

The structure that a particular intrapreneurial program takes is dependent upon the organization's overall guidelines for program development. An entrepreneurial program structure is often dictated by the requirements of whichever funding agency has provided the start-up and operating capital. The APN developing a program dependent upon the guidelines of other organizations is referred to the particular organization participating in program sponsorship. Many grant-funding agencies have criteria for funding and program guidelines available on the World Wide Web.

APN practice may assume one of several business structures depending upon the organizational context in which the practice is set. Practices may be hospital based or community based. Hospital-based practices may be inpatient or ambulatory in nature. Community-based practices are usually primary care settings or freestanding health centers or birthing centers, but may also be a part of a PPO, HMO, or other payer-based primary care site. Practices may be established on a for-profit or not-for-profit basis. Each business structure requires that the APN consult with business advisors to determine the best business structure to match the values and goals of the APN. It is not the intent of this chapter to provide professional legal, business, or accounting advice, only to provide basic information for the establishment of those applicable business relationships. The APN is referred to professional advisors for the clarification of specific questions or issues.

There are three basic ways to structure the practice: a sole proprietorship, a partnership, or a corporation (Vogel & Doleysh, 1994). The primary differences between these structures lie in differing tax restrictions and liability. The simplest form of business organization is a sole proprietorship, which involves one owner. It is relatively straightforward and inexpensive to establish, and control remains with the sole owner. For tax purposes, the business income is taxed at the personal tax rate. The major disadvantage of the sole proprietorship is the unlimited liability that accompanies the structure. The owner assumes all liability, including that for any negligent acts of employees.

Most medical practices are for-profit partnerships. A general partnership may be advantageous for the APN because partnering with another professional may attract venture capital. The unlimited liability for each individual partner remains, as does the personal tax rate on business income. A disadvantage of this structure is the possibility of personality conflicts and disagreements arising between the partners over control and decision making. As mentioned previously, the legality of relationships between different professionals is often dictated by state law. CRNAs can join business arrangements as consultants to hospitals and anesthesia groups. Freestanding birthing centers are a respected alternative to tertiary hospitals for uncomplicated deliveries.

A corporation is a separate legal entity for both tax and liability purposes. Incorporation protects the owners from some, though not all, liability because a corporation's liability is limited. Consequently, because the medical professional owners retain a portion of any liability incurred, it is strongly advised that APNs and other providers have an individual liability policy. A professional corporation can elect a small business (Subchapter S) status, which allows owners to retain the benefit of taxation at the personal rate or, as is sometimes said, to avoid double taxation—first on corporate income and second on shareholder dividends. Other advantages of a corporation include the ability to start pension and profit-sharing plans and the possibility of attracting venture capital investors. The main disadvantage for a corporation not electing small business status is the higher tax rate incurred by corporations. A corporation may also be more expensive to establish and operate.

Selecting a name for the practice may be an option worth considering in certain situations. Rather than using an individual's name, a specific practice name may assist in describing the services offered and reflect the business focus—for example, Women's Health Services, Access to Continence Care and Treatment (Newman, 1996), and The Family Health and Birth Center (see Chapter 17). Many professionals use their own name to connote a more personalized service, as well as to promote themselves. Most individual states regulate the selection and registration of business names as part of the registration of the business structure process. The process entails registering the business name, a formal state agency search to ensure that the name is not being used by another business, payment of a registration fee, and the issuance of a formal document confirming assignment of the business name to the APN.

External Regulatory Bodies

An interwoven fabric of regulations and guidelines serves as the basis upon which APN professional practice is built and developed. State licensure requires the fulfillment of advanced educational preparation, with the exception of those APNs licensed prior to existing regulations and "grandfathered" for the purpose of continued licensure. Educational requirements are often coupled with role-specific certification as prerequisites for licensure to practice. State practice acts clearly delineate whether the APN has prescriptive privileges within the state. Federal and state regulations determine which business structures and practice environments an APN may work within and obtain reimbursement, and whether this practice is independent, collaborative, or supervised. National and specialty nursing organizations have described and articulated both the code of nursing ethics and the scope of advanced nursing practice, to both nursing and society as a whole. Chapter 22 and the individual APN chapters in Part III present an in-depth discussion of APN credentialing and regulation.

Although APN students routinely learn about the importance of the rules and regulations established by many different stakeholders to health care systems, the impact upon daily practice may not be appreciated until the student becomes a practicing clinician. The major external regulatory vehicles affecting APN practice include

- Those state and federal statutes pertaining to the regulation and credentialing requirements for advanced practice nursing
- Guidelines for health care organizations regarding multiple facets of the management, environment, and delivery of health care established by the Joint Commission on Accreditation of Health Care Organizations (JCAHO)
- Occupational Safety and Health Administration (OSHA) regulations related to safe working conditions for employees
- CLIA regulations pertaining to laboratory services
- Additional Health Care Financing Administration (HCFA) regulations pertaining to Medicare reimbursement processes
- Those additional regulations and guidelines determined by certain funding agencies, such as grant providers

The JCAHO (1995) evaluates a health care organization's system performance in both patient-focused (direct care) and organizational (indirect care) areas in order to improve the quality of care provided to the public. Patient-focused functions include patient rights and organization ethics, assessment of patients, care of patients, education, and continuum of care. Organizational functions include improving organization performance, leadership, management of the environment of care, management of human resources, management of information, and surveillance, prevention, and control of infection. Additionally, the JCAHO examines an organization's governance, management, and functions related to medical and nursing staff. Each year, the JCAHO publishes detailed information about the performance-focused standards upon which a health care organization is evaluated. These standards are described in the first volume of the accreditation manual for the particular health care organization of interest (e.g., manual for hospitals, for ambulatory care clinics, etc.). The second volume of the manual contains the scoring guidelines used for accreditation purposes during JCAHO site surveys. Surveys are performed every 3 years by JCAHO-employed provider and nonprovider survey teams. The teams spend several days evaluating the organization using the scoring guidelines found in volume II of that year's manual. An overall score is determined along with any recommendations for improving scoring deficiencies. Accreditation is based upon the organization's compliance with JCAHO guidelines and implementation of any recommendations to resolve deficiencies (JCAHO, 1995 and *www.JCAHO.org*).

APNs are often involved in patient-focused processes of interest to the JCAHO as a result of being expert clinicians. Their level of involvement in organizational processes is dependent upon the degree of individual APN responsibility for indirect care processes. Regardless of how many standards may directly relate to an individual APN's practice, all APNs should be aware of the guidelines upon which their organization is being evaluated. On an individual level, many of the APN competencies discussed in Part II are touched upon by some or many of the JCAHO standards during the actualization of APN roles. The JCAHO standards may assist APNs in the development of their own standards of patient care and professional performance. In this manner, the JCAHO serves as a valuable resource to augment professional nursing standards and guidelines related to the delivery of clinically excellent patient care in caring, compassionate, high-quality health care organizations.

Health care safety management and hazard control are proven processes that produce results by preventing accidents, reducing injury rates, and increasing organizational efficiency (Tweedy, 1997). Areas include emergency planning and fire safety, general and physical plant safety, managing hazardous materials, managing biological waste, safety in patient care areas, and health care support area safety (Tweedy, 1997). In terms of external regulators, safety management is carefully scrutinized by both the JCAHO and the OSHA. APNs functioning as entrepreneurs or employers must be well versed in the rules, regulations, and implementation of safety programs governing these areas of safety management and hazard control. All APNs should be aware of their individual responsibilities regarding workplace safety, especially with respect to the management of biological waste and the OSHA guidelines regarding bloodborne pathogens.

Created as part of the Department of Labor, the OSHA was charged by the Occupational Safety and Health Act of 1970 to assure safe and healthful working conditions for American workers (29 C.F.R. § 1910). The general duty clause required every employer to furnish "a place of employment which is free from recognized hazards that cause or are likely to cause death or serious physical harm to employees" (29 C.F.R. § 1910). In 1991, the act was amended to include bloodborne pathogens as a specific occupational exposure to be managed (29 C.F.R. § 1910.1030). Under this amendment, occupational exposure is defined as the reasonably anticipated skin, eye, mucous membrane, or parenteral (piercing mucous membranes, or the skin barrier) contact with blood or other potentially infectious materials that may result from the performance of an employee's duties (29 C.F.R. § 1910.1030.b). In order to prevent the employee's exposure, the employer is required to develop an exposure control plan. APNs in acute care settings are usually required to attend mandatory employee training for safety management. APNs in ambulatory settings are bound by the same regulations, and need to be aware of their settings' processes for fulfilling this important OSHA mandate.

Diagnostic Services

Any provider or laboratory service planning to collect, prepare, and analyze patient specimens is bound by CLIA rules and regulations. Congress adopted the CLIA in response to published findings about the quality of laboratory testing (Hurst, Nickel, & Hilborne, 1998). Enacted to safeguard the public, the CLIA establish minimum acceptable criteria standards for all categories of laboratory testing in the United States. Providers offering laboratory services meet the criteria and apply for the appropriate level of CLIA certification. Certification is based upon the complexity of testing being performed. Fees for the certificates are based upon the test complexity, the number of specimens being processed, and the cost of surveyor inspection (Schwartz, 1996). There are four categories of laboratory testing defined by the CLIA: waived tests, provider-performed microscopy (PPM), moderate-complexity procedures, and high-complexity procedures. If laboratory specimens are going to be performed by the APN, the first two categories of CLIA testing apply to the usual level of procedures performed. Moderate- and high-complexity procedures are generally performed by independent or hospital-based laboratories.

Waived tests are simple laboratory examinations and procedures cleared by the Food and Drug Administration for home use. They are simple and accurate (making the likelihood of error minimal), and pose no significant harm to the patient. Examples of CLIA-waived tests include fecal occult blood, nonautomated dipstick or tablet urinalysis, urine pregnancy visual color comparison tests, and all qualitative color comparison pH testing of body fluids. The laboratory would apply and pay for a CLIA Certificate of Waiver, allowing the laboratory to perform only waived tests. The certificate is valid for 2 years.

PPM is a subcategory of the moderate-complexity level of testing. These examinations may be performed by physicians, by dentists, or by midlevel providers during the patient visit on a specimen obtained from the provider's patient or a patient of the group practice (American Academy of Family Practice, 1998). Other key criteria related to PPM include that the primary instrument for the test is the microscope; that the specimen must be labile or a delay in the testing could compromise test accuracy; and, that limited specimen handling is required. Examples of PPM procedures include wet mounts, including preparation of vaginal, cervical, or skin specimens; all potassium hydroxide (KOH) preparations; pinworm examinations; and nasal smears for eosinophils. The certificate for this level of laboratory service, the Certificate for Provider-Performed Microscopy Procedures, allows the provider to perform waived tests as well.

Moderate- and high-complexity laboratories are allowed to perform procedures of increasing complexity, requiring additional pieces of instrumentation, and necessitating increased amounts of specimen handling during processing. In addition to a specific listing of tests related to the appropriate level of complexity, moderate- and high-complexity laboratories are required to meet personnel and quality assurance/quality control proficiency testing and survey requirements in order to obtain a Certificate of Registration. These laboratories are also required to obtain Certificates of Compliance and Accreditation verifying compliance with all the applicable CLIA and HCFA requirements. CLIA information may be obtained via the World Wide Web at the following sites: *www.hcfa.gov/medicaid/clia* and *www.aafp.org/pt.*

If the APN does not intend to perform laboratory testing within the scope of the practice setting, the APN will need to identify providers of diagnostic testing services who will accept requisitions for diagnostic tests. In the absence of an in-house laboratory, external laboratory services basically include specimen collection, specimen processing, and reporting of results. Some APN practices choose to collect specimens themselves, then have them transported to the laboratory for processing and reporting. These practices require a separate refrigerator and/or freezer for specimen storage pending transfer to the processing area, along with the containers and media for proper specimen collection. For those practices choosing to collect and process their own specimens, additional equipment and supplies will be needed depending upon the nature of the tests being performed. Local laboratories may be identified by asking for assistance from a local hospital, or by speaking with a laboratory service representative directly. The APN should inquire about issues such as how the lab's specific requisition forms should be completed; specimen collection, pickup, and drop box availability; how results are reported (by telephone, by fax, by dedicated computer printer, or by mail); what patients should expect; and how they are billed. This information is often described in a separate manual provided to the practice by the laboratory service.

In addition to laboratory services, imaging services need to be identified. Often local hospitals will allow providers to refer patients for radiological services through the outpatient referral process. As with the laboratory services, issues related to the requisition of testing, the testing process (including any patient preparation requirements), the reporting of results, and patient billing should be discussed and recorded for future reference.

Recent revisions in Medicare regulations have resulted in the heightened enforcement of the policy of medical necessity with respect to diagnostic services. In an attempt to decrease costs related to inappropriate diagnostic testing, certain laboratory and radiological services have been identified as requiring proof of medical necessity in order for them to be covered under Medicare. In order to have these services covered, the provider must ensure that they are medically appropriate for the patient's diagnosis or symptoms. The determination of medical necessity is made by the HCFA, and codified through a listing of those *International Classification of Diseases, 9th Revision: Clinical Modification* (ICD-9-CM) (AMA, 1998) diagnoses and symptoms that will justify the diagnostic service requested. For example, in order to have a thyroid-stimulating hormone (TSH) testing paid for by Medicare, the patient must have a certain ICD-9-CM diagnosis on the listing for TSH testing, such as goiter (ICD-9-CM codes 240.0–240.9), acquired hypothyroidism (ICD-9-CM codes 244.0–244.9), or malaise and fatigue (ICD-9-CM code 780.7). (*N.B.:* Other diagnoses and symptoms are allowed for TSH testing. These diagnoses and symptoms are for use as examples only.) Those diagnostic tests for which medical necessity has been determined are listed in local Medicare medical policies found either through the laboratory service or directly from the local Medicare intermediary newsletter.

If the patient's diagnosis does not comply with HCFA guidelines but testing is determined to be necessary by the provider, the patient must be notified, in advance, that the cost of this testing may become the responsibility of the patient. This notification is formalized in the completion of an Advanced Beneficiary Notice (ABN), detailing the test requested, the symptoms or disease state necessitating the testing, and that the patient has been advised that the testing does not meet the guidelines for Medicare reimbursement. The patient signs the ABN, and the signature is witnessed by another staff person. Although on the surface this process may seem to limit provider discretion, underlying this process is a deepening of the provider's knowledge of appropriate utilization of diagnostic testing, and a recognition that diagnostic testing is an expensive and limited resource with significant financial impact on the health care system.

PROCESS RESOURCES: EQUIPMENT/SUPPLIES/ CAPITAL FUNDING

To follow in the paradigm of systems thinking, the processes of care to be delivered and the setting in which these processes occur will determine the tools needed to deliver that care. Equipment and supplies to deliver home-based primary care to an elderly population will be different from those required to implement a hospital-based wound care clinic for children who have sustained burns. The most effective way to determine what is needed for a program or practice is to flowchart all of the processes of care (both direct and indirect) with all the items needed for a particular step itemized below their respective boxes (see Figure 20–3). A secondary gain is that this process allows the APN to clearly identify the costs linked with particular services delivered (see Table 20–2 for the initial cost-based inventory of the steps illustrated in Figure 20–3). This approach is the basis for cost-based analysis. Cost-based analysis examines the actual costs of the supplies, equipment, and personnel needed to perform a particular process of care. Additional costs related to business operations overhead are calculated into the final cost, which is then used to determine the charge to the patient for that process of care. (The reader is referred to Neumann and Boles [1998] for an in-depth discussion of cost-based analysis.)

Additional methods available for identifying needed equipment and supplies include

- Relying upon clinical expertise of the APN, and her or his familiarity with the items needed to deliver the identified service
- Referring to a clinical procedures manual that lists the equipment needed
- Consulting with the collaborating physician
- Interviewing other providers who are performing the same or similar services
- Interviewing support staff to determine what they require to perform their role
- Referring to standardized equipment listings.

After determining the program/practice needs, lists or inventories are generated. These equipment and supply inventories serve to

- Establish an initial budget and time line for business planning purposes, and provide information related to budgetary requests required by lenders and grantors. (These inventories may be included in any business plan, grant application, or office procedure manual, thus eliminating the need to rewrite them for each application.)
- Create an initial ordering or shopping list
- Record business assets (For purposes of this discussion, the purchase price of the item represents its monetary equivalent. Consultation with a business advisor is required to determine actual business value and depreciation.)
- Establish minimum par levels for an inventory of disposable supplies
- Identify the locations of where items are kept in the office to facilitate inventory management

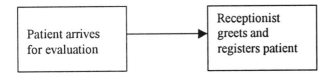

Who Performs: Patient

                        Receptionist

Related Processes: Triage

                        Scheduling

                        Registration

                        Patient confidentiality

                        Medical records

Required Resources: Office space: leased/purchased office

                        Durable equipment: desks, chairs, end tables, lamps/lights with bulbs, magazine

                        rack, patient education brochure rack, bulletin board, decorative plants, pictures,

                        curtains/draperies for the windows, rugs/carpet/floor covering, waste baskets,

                        telephone, photocopying machine, locked cash box/drawer, calculator, credit

                        card equipment and electronic transfer linkage, computer system, fax machine

                        Reuseable items: magazine subscriptions, patient education brochures,

                        tacks/fasteners for bulletin board displays, actual bulletin board displays,

                        telephone answering system/software, computer software

                        Disposable items: facial tissues, coloring books, crayons, pencils/pens, erasers,

                        business cards, appointment book, demographic/registration forms, office

                        encounter form (superbill), patient medical record folders/dividers, patient chart

                        stickers (allergy, year, alphabetical), photocopy/fax paper

FIGURE 20–3 • Itemization of a patient care process.

TABLE 20–2 COST-BASED INVENTORY OF PATIENT REGISTRATION PROCESS: DISPOSABLE ITEMS*

ITEM	VENDOR	PAR LEVEL	UNIT COST ($)[†]	TOTAL COST ($)[†]
Facial tissues	ABC Office Supply	12 boxes	0.75	9.00
Coloring books	State Children Program	36	FREE	FREE
Crayons	State Children Program	36 packs	FREE	FREE
Pencils	ABC Office Supply	5 boxes of 12	2.00	10.00
Pens: black	ABC Office Supply	10 boxes of 12	3.00	30.00
Erasers	ABC Office Supply	5	0.50	2.50
Business cards	Printing Shop	2 boxes of 1,000	40.00	80.00
Appointment book	ABC Office Supply	1	15.00	15.00
Demographic forms	Printing Shop	2 pads of 100	10.00	20.00
Superbills	Printing Shop	1 box of 2,000	275.00	275.00
Medical record folders	XYZ Forms	1 box of 100	20.00	20.00
Medical record dividers	XYZ Forms	1 box of 100 sets	20.00	20.00
Chart stickers: allergy	XYZ Forms	1 roll of 100	5.00	5.00
Chart stickers: year	XYZ Forms	1 roll of 500	5.00	5.00
Chart stickers: alpha	XYZ Forms	1 set of 20 each	15.00	15.00
Photocopy paper	ABC Office Supply	1 box of 10 reams	75.00	75.00
Fax paper	ABC Office Supply	1 box of 6 rolls	45.00	45.00

* If the APN sees 2,000 patients in a 12-month period, and the above disposable items are depleted in the same amount of time, then the cost of the disposable items used during patient registration process per year is TOTAL COST/TOTAL NUMBER OF PATIENTS = COST PER PATIENT PER YEAR (approximate), or $626.50/2000 = $0.31 (approximate).
[†] Prices are approximate and are used for illustration only.

The initial inventories for medical and office equipment and supplies follow the same template, and could be set up as comparable spreadsheets within any commercial office software package. The AMA (1996c) suggested creating three separate inventories: durable equipment, reuseable equipment/supplies, and disposable supplies. One advantage to this separation is that it enables the program administrator/practice manager to quickly assess how much money is needed to set up the program/practice, as opposed to how much will be needed on an ongoing basis for replenishment of supplies. The first lists the furniture and equipment needed to set up the office and examination room(s). This list includes durable equipment (e.g., desks, chairs, file cabinets, examination tables, autoclave, electrocardiograph, computers). The second lists the reuseable equipment needed, such as trash cans, staplers, tape dispensers, linen baskets, otoscope, stethoscope, and computer software (Rehm & Kraft, 1998). The third lists the disposable supplies needed. It will be helpful to separate the disposable supplies into two lists, one for office supplies and one for medical supplies. The office supply list includes items such as pens, pencils, tape, staples, and photocopy/printer paper. The medical supply list includes items such as alcohol swabs, gauze pads, Band-Aids, examination table paper, and syringes. For accounting and budgeting purposes, request professional advice to separate these items into capital and noncapital expenses. (See Table 20–2 for a sample listing of supplies based upon two steps in a patient care process.)

Each list includes the specific name of the equipment or supply needed and the number of units required. Quotes from potential vendors for the item should be sought. Once a vendor is identified, the price per unit (unit cost) and a total price for that item (total cost) is added to the inventory template. It is possible to obtain some disposable supplies gratuitously from other sources. For example, in primary care, often the laboratory analyzing the bloods specimens drawn at the practice will provide alcohol swabs, small gauze pads, Band-Aids, and other supplies used during venipuncture or other specimen collection as part of their service to the practice. Many pharmaceutical representatives are often willing to provide pens, note pads, and clipboards for free, although these items will have the names of their products on them as part of their marketing plan. Some larger facilities operate in-house supply "swaps" in which the excess supplies of one department are offered in trade for the excess supplies of another department. Although these sources of inexpensive disposable supplies are available, when planning an initial budget, it is essential to calculate that the program/practice is responsible for purchasing these items from traditional vendors.

Although the primary focus of APNs is direct clinical practice, the APN should also support processes that are indirect or administrative in nature with appropriate resources. Decisions related to which processes will be performed in house, as opposed to being contracted externally, will impact the types of equipment and supplies needed. Examples of indirect processes of care include

- *Creating a patient data base.* There are several medical office computerized systems available, of varying complexity and cost, for the management of patient information. Some of the processes supported by these programs are appointment scheduling, generation of patient encounter forms (superbills), and electronic claims filing.
- *Transcription services.* For intrapreneurial APNs, transcription services may be available through the larger organization's facilities. For independent APNs, the decision to contract for transcription services should include a review of the available voice-to-text computer software programs that allow the APN to directly dictate the patient's progress note (or other printed material) into a commercially available word processing or desktop publishing program. There are several voice-to-text programs available with different degrees of complexity and adaptability and varying sizes of medical vocabulary lexicons. The prices for these programs range from $99 for a basic voice-to-text program to $4,000 for a complex system that may be used by several providers at once.
- *Ensuring staff safety.* Material safety data sheets (MSDSs) are required for all items that pose a potential occupational risk to the employees working with them, such as alcohol, Betadine, or cancer chemotherapeutic agents. The MSDS information is available from the manufacturer upon request at no cost. Other OSHA regulations, such as those pertaining to biomedical waste disposal and blood-borne pathogen exposure, must also be implemented into practice, and appropriate records kept for review. As with transcription services, personnel safety systems may be available within the larger institution, or will need to be either developed or purchased for a freestanding practice.
- *Patient education materials.* Patient education materials are available in a variety of formats, including videotape, interactive computer software, and traditional written brochures or pamphlets. The APN should review the direct patient care processes for which educational materials can be anticipated. Part of the initial planning process includes reviewing available materials that can be incorporated into the APN's practice. Educational material should be evaluated for quality, readability/literacy level, availability in different languages, and cost. Oral presen-

tations to individuals or groups are also an important component of patient education.

One process of care that requires particular attention is the use of pharmaceutical agents in direct patient care by APNs with prescriptive privileges. Some of the supporting processes involved in writing a patient prescription include

- *Writing the physical prescription.* Should the APN have prescription privileges in the state in which she or he practices, the APN will need to have prescription pads available. The prescription pads will include the APN's name and credentials and the name of the APN's practice setting on the pad. In several states, the name of the collaborating physician must be on the prescription pad. Free prescription pads are available through Medi-Scripts, a prescription printing service funded by a collaboration of pharmaceutical companies. For further information, see Table 20–3.
- *Receiving drug samples.* A system to track lot numbers, expiration dates, and the patients to whom the drug was dispensed needs to be developed to address the issue of lot number recalls.
- *Including controlled substances in the course of patient care.* The APN must obtain an individual Drug Enforcement Agency (DEA) number prior to prescribing controlled substances. A completed DEA registration form will be required, with the registration fees paid, prior to the APN being able to prescribe controlled substances allowed by statute. The DEA registration is renewable every 3 years. Cost for NP registration in 1999 was $210 for the 3-year period. Forms may be requested by telephoning the DEA at 1-800-882-9539. In addition to a DEA number, a locked, secure location for storage needs to be established, and a procedure for access must be determined prior to acceptance of a supply should the APN dispense controlled substances from the office.

The use of medications within a program or practice is dependent upon the nature of the services to be delivered, but is also constrained by the scope of practice granted by individual state nurse practice acts. When the decisions regarding the use of pharmaceutical agents have been made, a listing of anticipated pharmacy supplies, along with cost, vendor, and par level information, may be generated from the same software spreadsheet as the other inventories. When preparing a pharmaceutical inventory, enrollment in the state immunization program is extremely useful for those practices providing children's services. States provide immunizations free to children who fall within certain eligibility guidelines (e.g., Medicaid recipients, uninsured, or participants in a federally funded health center). These programs involve practice enrollment, a monthly vaccine utilization report, and some record keeping regarding recipient eligibility. Some state programs have established a World Wide Web–based system, allowing practices to report monthly usage and to reorder vaccine on line. The maximum benefit of the Web-based system is that it allows confirmation of childhood vaccinations to other enrolled practices within a secure and confidential network environment (see, e.g., the ImmPact program used in Maine and New Hampshire; for more information, contact ImmPact by telephone at 1-800-867-4775, or by TTY at 1-888-706-3876).

When choosing a pharmaceutical agent for their patients, APNs are also aware of the financial impact of the drug on the patient. With the advent of managed care came the start of insurer-based drug formularies that limit the medications covered by a patient's prescription plan. Most managed care organizations have copies of their formularies available to providers so that patient needs may be matched with the insurer's cost-containment guidelines. If a patient takes a medication that is not on the formulary, possible substitutions should be evaluated. If there is no suitable alternative, all formularies have a vehicle by which a provider may appeal the formulary decision for a particular patient need.

For patients who are indigent or who meet low-income guidelines, many pharmaceutical companies offer subsidized and free prescriptions. A listing of which drugs are covered by these programs is usually available from the local sales representatives of the parent company. The process for obtaining free medications for an indigent patient entails completion of a brief form by the provider and the patient, who attest that the patient meets the income criteria for the particular program of interest. A written prescription, usually for a specific period of time as designated by the pharmaceutical program (e.g., 1 month, 3 months), accompanies the completed form. The medications are sent directly to the provider's office on behalf of the patient, who then needs to be notified that they have arrived. (A compilation of the prescription assistance programs is available from Pharmaceutical Research and Manufacturers of America [1997]. The address may be found in Table 20-3.)

It is important to note that certain companies will not accept prescriptions from APNs even though many APNs have prescription-writing privileges. The primary reason for this exclusion is that the state to which the prescription and enrollment form are sent does not permit APNs to write prescriptions. The secondary reason for this exclusion is that the parent company is unaware of revisions to the state practice act that allow APNs to write prescriptions in that particular state. The solution for the first scenario is through the development of a prescribing policy whereby the APN's collaborating physician writes the prescription for that patient's medications. The solution to the second scenario is continued efforts on the part of APNs to educate and collaborate with pharmaceutical companies to ensure that accurate, timely information is being used. Patients who mail away for their prescriptions

TABLE 20-3 USEFUL BUSINESS PLANNING RESOURCES FOR APNs

HCFA Laboratory Program
P.O. Box 849036
Dallas, TX 75284-9036
(Please contact HCFA to determine local
  intermediaries)

Medi-Scripts
Franklyn Building
5 Latour Avenue
Suite 850
Plattsburgh, NY 12901-9955
Telephone: 1-800-387-3636
Fax: 1-800-364-3209

**Pharmaceutical Research and Manufacturers
  of America**
1100 Fifteenth Street NW
Washington, DC 20005-1707

Drug Enforcement Administration
Central Station
P.O. Box 28083
Washington, DC 20038-8083
Telephone: 1-800-882-9539

**Joint Commission on Accreditation of
  Healthcare Organizations**
One Renaissance Boulevard
Oakbrook Terrace, IL 60181
Web site: *www.JCAHO.org*

through their insurance prescription plan may also suffer from the inconvenience of being told that the APN is unable to write for their prescriptions. The solutions for this group of patients are the same.

THE BUSINESS PLAN SUMMARY

Once the process of business or program planning has been accomplished, the APN should summarize the mission, vision, values, and processes of care and required resources to meet the patient's needs into one document. Traditionally this summary has taken the form of a business plan, which was then distributed to potential sources of financial backing. Even if the program is not seeking external funding, a summary is needed to describe the available services to others. One way of writing this summary is to modify the traditional business plan so that it reflects a systems-thinking approach to patient care (see Table 20–4 for an outline of a business summary). The reader is referred to Buppert (1999), the AMA (1996d), the Small Business Administration, and local business advisors for additional information and advice.

Consideration must be given to the audience for whom the summary is being prepared. As discussed earlier, grant-funding agencies have specific guidelines for the compilation of the program's operational documentation. If the summary is written for the community of patients being served, issues related to literacy, language, and emphasis need to be addressed. If the summary is written for potential investors or potential physician colleagues, issues related to capital expenditures, numbers of patients to be served, and services to be delivered need to be emphasized. Consequently, the first step in preparing the summary is to identify the anticipated audience.

The summary should start with a cover page that details the name, address, and contact telephone number of the program or practice, the name(s) and credentials of the involved APNs and collaborating physicians and any other team members, and the date that the summary is prepared. The next page of the summary should include the brief mission and vision statements written during the planning process. Any organizational values (separate from those that are patient focused and described elsewhere) should be included in the summary. Some business plan formats request that mention be given to the numbers of patients to be served and the estimated amount of capital required for start up and maintenance. A table of contents should be included for quick reference to key areas of the summary. The second section of the summary describes the direct processes of patient care to be rendered and any background information that affected the determination of these services. The third section describes the patient population to be served, and provides information about the particular marketing strategies to be employed to build the practice or program (see Chapter 21). The fourth section compiles the organizational chart and the description of the program structure and management, and provides the reader with information regarding the advisors the APN has gathered to ensure the success of the program. The fifth section focuses specifically on the monetary aspects of the program or practice. Detailed budgetary information is summarized here in a spread sheet or other accepted business accounting format. The sixth section focuses on how the program will comply with the applicable regulations and guidelines. The final section describes the performance measures against which the APN and the system will be evaluated. Parameters and timelines for internal and external review are defined.

TABLE 20-4 OUTLINE OF A PROGRAM/PRACTICE SUMMARY

I. Introductory Elements
   A. Cover page
   B. Overview/summary
      1. Mission and vision statements
      2. Overarching program/practice values
      3. Other required elements
   C. Table of contents
II. Description
   A. Background information
   B. Direct processes of care to be delivered
   C. Key factors in the delivery of patient care
III. Market
   A. Description of the patient population to be served
      1. Patient demographics
   B. Analysis of the market
   C. Marketing strategy
      1. Initial
      2. Ongoing
   D. Competition
   E. Advertising and promotion
IV. Program/Practice Structure
   A. Structure/ownership
   B. Management
   C. Clinical advisors and services offered (includes APN)
   D. Business advisors and services offered
   E. Support staff and services offered
V. Resources
   A. Budget
      1. Projected income
         a. Start-up capital: business loans, grants
         b. Ongoing capital: patient revenues, other funding
      2. Projected expenses
         a. Office space and overhead
         b. Durable equipment
         c. Reuseable equipment
         d. Disposable items
         e. Provider and staff compensation
VI. Compliance
   A. Federal and/or state regulations
      1. JCAHO
      2. OSHA
      3. HCFA
   B. Other agency regulations
   C. Provider-specific licensing, credentialing, privileging
VII. Outcome evaluation
   A. APN performance measures
   B. System performance measures
   C. Internal review parameters and timeline
   D. External review parameters and timeline

A successful system is able to describe what it does, how it does it, and how it evaluates the outcome. Using a systems-thinking approach in the actualization of their roles allows APNs to describe what they do, how they do it, and how they evaluate the outcomes of their care. A successful APN develops, implements, and evaluates both patient care and indirect processes that support it by organizing these tasks as a system. Today's health care environment demands that patient care delivery be innovative and resource efficient. Today's health care consumers demand that patient care delivery be individualized, compassionate, and effective. A sound knowledge of the system in which care is delivered continues in the spirit of the holistic approach to nursing care that will enable the APN to meet the demands of today's complex environment and the patients it serves.

REIMBURSEMENT MECHANISMS

Reimbursement refers to the monetary compensation of the clinician for services provided to patients and their families. The process of reimbursement is perhaps the most important and complex indirect process supporting patient care. Figure 20–4 provides an overview of the process of reimbursement. As with other indirect care processes, the level of APN involvement in this process is dependent upon the individual APN's role in indirect processes as a whole. All APNs are involved in the completion of the patient's clinical encounter, the documentation of the encounter in the patient's medical record, and, frequently, the completion of the patient's bill for services. Some APNs may be involved in the subsequent steps in the reimbursement process: the actual payment collection, either from the patient or from the third-party payer, and the posting of the payment to the patient's account in the provider's office. All APNs should be cognizant of the major concepts and issues related to third-party reimbursement and to APN compensation by the larger programs affecting health care economics. As illustrated in Figure 20–4, reimbursement builds bridges between the clinical encounter, the patient's medical record, the patient's bill for services, the claim submitted to the appropriate third-party payer (if any), and the payment of the APN for services delivered. In this section, an overview of documentation is presented, along with a description of the major third-party payment schemes. The patient's financial responsibility for self-pay is presented. Examples are used to illustrate steps in the reimbursement process.

Documentation

NURSING CLASSIFICATION SYSTEMS

Clinically excellent, holistic patient care delivered by APNs includes both nursing and medical diagnoses, interventions, and outcomes. Consequently, patient medical record documentation by an APN would reasonably include a combination of both nursing and medical diagnoses, interventions, and outcomes language. According to the HCFA, patient medical record documentation is required to chronologically record pertinent facts, findings, and observations as to an individual's health history, including past and present illnesses, examinations, tests, treatments, and outcomes (HCFA, 1997). The undergraduate education of nurses emphasizes the nursing process and the use of standardized languages for nursing diagnoses, interventions, and outcomes in the record keeping of nursing care. APNs, however, are not routinely prepared at the graduate level to continue the use of this nursing-sensitive language. One possible reason for this may be economically driven. In today's health care arena, APNs are unable to bill third-party payers, or obtain reimbursement, for nursing diagnoses and/or interventions unless the diagnosis or intervention is recognized as a medical one. (The reader is referred to Henry, Holzemer, Randell, Hsleh, and Miller

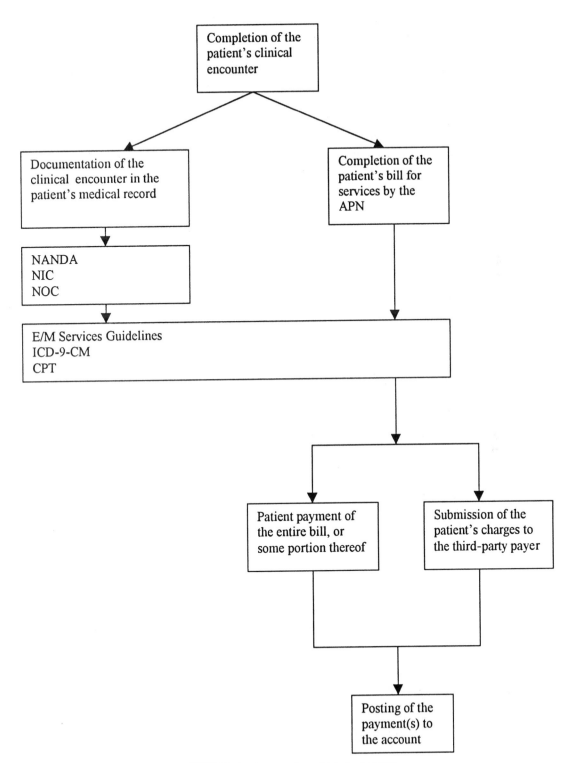

FIGURE 20-4 • An overview of reimbursement.

[1997] for a review of nursing interventions as compared to medical terminology.) The ramifications to nursing of this bias in monetary compensation are far reaching, and beyond the scope of this discussion. However, the value of nursing care and the strides being made in standardizing and codifying what nurses do is being recognized and incorporated into various elements of reimbursement strategies, such as state nursing association recommendations for standardized language and automated billing software. (The reader is referred to *www.alternativelink.com* for information related to the integration of nursing interventions into the ABC Coding Systems for Third Party Billing.) Proposals to examine the financial basis of nursing interventions, again using standardized language, are in process (B. Head, personal communication, November 5, 1999). In the future, direct financial compensation may be paid for nursing diagnoses and interventions that are independent of a medical model counterpart.

The nursing profession has organized nursing knowledge into three main areas: nursing diagnoses, nursing interventions, and nursing-sensitive patient outcomes (Bulechek & McCloskey, 1999). These areas correspond well to patient medical record documentation capturing the components of the patient's assessment, plan, and evaluation. The North American Nursing Diagnosis Association (NANDA) has worked toward the establishment and implementation of a classification system for nursing diagnoses since 1973 (Carpenito, 1999). In review, a nursing diagnosis is a clinical judgment about individual, family, or community responses to actual or potential health problems/life processes (Carpenito, 1999). The current strategic goals of NANDA include plans to include NANDA diagnoses in standardized language systems and health care databases, and to promote the use of nursing diagnoses in nursing practice, education, and research (*www.nanda.org/goals*).

Nursing diagnoses provide the basis for the selection of nursing interventions that achieve the identified patient outcomes for which the nurse is accountable. An outcome is defined as a variable concept representing a patient or family caregiver state, behavior, or perception that is measurable along a continuum and responsive to nursing interventions. Ideally, outcomes should be chosen to optimize health as well as alleviate problems (McCloskey & Bulechek, 1992). The Nursing Outcomes Classification (NOC) exists to codify a standardized language of nursing-sensitive patient outcomes (Iowa Intervention Project, 1997; *www.uiowa.edu/noc/overview.htm*). The Iowa Intervention Project developed an evolving codified taxonomy of nursing interventions, the Nursing Intervention Classification (NIC), to list the treatments that nurses perform, to assist practitioners in documenting their care, and to facilitate the evaluation of nurse-sensitive patient outcomes (McCloskey & Bulechek, 1992).

In June, 1999, the ANA passed a resolution recognizing several standardized nursing languages, including NANDA and NIC. Four state nursing associations—those in Iowa, Michigan, Minnesota, and Nebraska—endorse the use of standardized nursing languages, specifically NIC and NOC (C. M. Prophet, personal communication, October 25, 1999; B. Head, personal communication, November 5, 1999). Familiarity with these standardized languages that capture the nursing care provided by APNs, and utilizing them consistently in clinical practice and documentation, provide APNs with valuable tools in support of APN practice now and in the future.

MEDICAL CLASSIFICATION SYSTEMS

Familiarity with the medical-model guidelines and external regulations that govern reimbursement programs enables the APN to obtain health care reimbursement through compliance with existing structures, and demonstrates to third-party payers that the APN is a knowledgeable participant in health care. This degree of professional accountability may reduce barriers to full APN participation as independent providers in their own right, and expand the inclusion of nursing care within the realm of reimbursed elements of patient care. The foundation of the reimbursement process is proper patient medical record documentation of medical necessity. According to the AMA (2000), payers require the following information to determine medical necessity:

- Knowledge of the emergent nature or severity of the patient's concern or condition
- The signs, symptoms, complaints, or background facts describing the reasons for care

This information must be substantiated by the patient's medical record, and must be available to payers upon request with a signed patient authorization (AMA, 2000). Failure to document services rendered translates into the nonperformance of the service, which may leave the APN open not only to questions regarding the medical necessity of the encounter, but also to potential liability issues. Any and all services submitted for reimbursement must be evidenced by the appropriate documentation in the patient's medical record. Notation of unusual services or extenuating circumstances should leave no room for misinterpretation or assumption. From a financial standpoint, insurance carriers will frequently limit or deny reimbursement for services because of insufficient documentation. In addition, they may request refunds from the provider if audited medical records do not substantiate the reported services.

To bill for services, many insurance carriers require the use of specific medical documentation guidelines, classifications, and reimbursement codes. Documentation guidelines provide standardization and structure for the clinical encounter record. The various classifications available provide a standard language, used by both insurance carriers and health care providers, to provide a uniform interpretation of medical conditions and to identify the billable services of the provider. There are three main systems used to record and classify care delivered: the evaluation and management (E&M) services documentation guidelines (HCFA, 1997), the ICD-9-CM codes (AMA, 1998), and the Current Procedural Terminology (CPT) codes (AMA, 2000).

The *E&M Services Guidelines* (HCFA, 1997) were developed to compensate providers for clinical and cognitive effort, rather than time expended. (They are available on line at the HCFA website [*www.hcfa.gov*], or through the local Medicare intermediary.) There are seven components of E&M services:

1. *Nature of the presenting problem:* the reason or need for the client's office visit
2. *History:* the client's chief concern, a brief history of the present issue or illness, and a related systems review. A family and/or social history is included.
3. *Physical examination:* focused, addressing only the affected body area or organ system; or, comprehensive, addressing a complete examination of a single system of concern, or a multiple system physical examination
4. *Medical decision-making:* the complexity in establishing a diagnosis and selecting a certain management strategy. It includes a list of all possible medical diagnoses (the differential diagnoses) and management options, an analysis of medical records, all diagnostic tests, and other information analyzed.

5. *Counseling:* discussions or meetings with client, family, caregivers, and nursing staff (as in long-term care). Counseling can include discussions about disease process, results of diagnostic tests, prognosis, education and instructions on management, and treatment options.

6. *Coordination of care:* time spent working with other health care providers and agencies to direct care. This process must be well documented in the client's medical record if it is intended to denote the level of service, or care, delivered.

7. *Time:* In the case of encounters that predominantly consist of counseling or coordination of care, time is the key component used to determine the level of E&M services provided. Time is defined as "face-to-face" time in the office; time spent reviewing records and tests and arranging further services; or time spent with staff, such as in the nursing home. Time should be averaged in minutes and recorded in the client's medical record.

The major elements used to determine the level of service provided under the E&M system are the patient history, the physical examination, and the complexity of medical decision making required to manage the patient. Elements of at least these three components must have been performed and consequently documented in the patient's medical record. The documentation guidelines provide minimum assessment data points within each component that will support a particular level of E&M service. Each level of service is assigned a separate five-digit CPT code. The codes vary for new patients and existing patients even if the same level of service has been provided. (See Box 20–1.)

The ICD-9-CM codes are diagnostic codes that identify the diagnosis, symptom, or condition to be treated. Their purpose is to aid in standardizing coding practices across the United States (AMA, 1998) as directed by the HCFA. The HCFA has prepared guidelines for use of the ICD-9-CM codes in the area of medical billing. These guidelines are available on line at the HCFA's website (*www.hcfa.gov*) and from Medicare's local intermediaries. The codes are published each year in two volumes that are combined into one spiral-bound text for ease of use. Volume 1 contains the Tabular List of Diseases, based upon the ICD-9-CM code attached to the diagnosis, symptom, or condition of concern. Volume 2 contains the Alphabetic Index to Diseases. To identify the appropriate code for a particular symptom, a clinician would begin the search in Volume 2 under the alphabetical listing. Once the code is obtained from Volume 2, the clinician then turns to the tabular listing of the code itself to determine any additional modifiers necessary to clarify the entity being coded. For example, if the NP diagnoses otitis media, Volume 2 indicates that "Otitis" is coded as 382.9. Volume 2 also indicates that additional information is needed to determine which code best matches the type of otitis media the patient has: acute (382.9), with effusion (381.00), allergic (381.04), serous (381.01), with spontaneous rupture of ear drum (382.01), and so on. A listing of common ICD-9-CM codes used in family practice may be found at *www.aafp.org/fpm/981000fm/icd9.html.*

The primary function of the ICD-9-CM is to facilitate medical billing. Therefore, it is sometimes used at the point of care to classify the patient's diagnosis(es) on the patient's billing form, or superbill. The superbill is named such because all subsequent forms generated for that encounter are based upon this first bill completed at the time of service. The superbill may have a listing of frequently seen diagnoses or symptoms accompanied by the appropriate ICD-9-CM code for the provider to check off. This practice is discouraged by the HCFA because of a concern that diagnostic bias may be introduced by the presence of preprinted diagnoses. The HCFA would

BOX 20-1 • EXAMPLE OF IMPLEMENTING DOCUMENTATION GUIDELINES: SUBJECTIVE, OBJECTIVE, ASSESSMENT, PLAN, EVALUATION

S: R.M. is a 6-year-old boy brought to the office by his mother. He is an existing patient. She reports that R.M. has had a 24-hour history of severe sore throat, headache, and fever at home to 102°F. She states he is unable to swallow solids because of throat pain but is taking fluids well. R.M. reports that his best friend has also been ill with similar symptoms. Denies ear pain, nasal congestion, nausea, vomiting, or diarrhea. Mom has been treating his symptoms at home with over-the-counter medications for fever management, salt water gargles, rest, and increased amounts of fluids with fair symptom relief.

R.M. has been a healthy child, with no prior episodes of acute illness, injury, or hospitalization. He has no known drug or environmental allergies. His only medication is a children's multivitamin. He takes no prescription medications or alternative modality supplements.

O: *GEN:* Alert, well-developed, well-nourished, flushed child in mild distress. *VS:* T, 101.9°F oral; HR, 115; RR, 20; Wt, 35 kg. *HEAD:* NC, AT. No frontal or maxillary tenderness with palpation or percussion. *ENT:* Bilateral external auditory canals clear. Bilateral tympanic membranes pink, translucent, neutral, and freely mobile. Bony landmarks clearly visible. Nasal mucosa pink, moist, mildly edematous. Nasal passages partially obstructed by swollen turbinates. Clear rhinorrhea in the vaults. Buccal mucosa pink and moist. Tonsillar pillars, tonsils, and posterior pharynx beefy, swollen, and covered with white purulent exudate. *NECK:* Supple with significant tonsillar and anterior cervical adenopathy. *QUICK STREP TEST:* positive (CPT 87880QW Rapid antigen strep testing).

A/P:
1. Strep pharyngitis (ICD-9-CM 041.00 Streptococcus, unspecified)
2. Fever (ICD-9-CM 780.6 Fever)
   - Throat swab for culture and sensitivity (CPT 99000 Laboratory specimen handling)
   - Antibiotic regimen based upon weight
   - Supportive measures including symptomatic management of fever and throat pain with over-the-counter medications (NIC 3900 Temperature regulation)
   - Anticipatory guidance provided to mother and child regarding streptococcal infection, anticipated course of illness, and treatment implementation (NIC 5602 Teaching: Disease process; NIC 5616 Teaching: Prescribed medication; NIC 7040 Caregiver support)
3. Risk for infection transmission
   - Anticipatory guidance provided to mother and child regarding meticulous hand washing and other activities that decrease the spread of infection (NIC 7040 Caregiver support; NIC 5618 Teaching: Procedure/treatment)

E: Mother to be notified of throat culture results and any need to alter antibiotic therapy based upon sensitivities. If child not improved or worsens in next 48 hours, he is to return to clinic for re-evaluation. R.M. due for next well-child check in 7 months.

E & M: 99213 Expanded services, existing patient

prefer that the provider write the diagnosis or symptom independently, without the possible influence of the preprinted list. The billing coder for the medical practice then transcribes this code onto a uniform billing form (HCFA-1500 claim form) that is submitted for reimbursement. If the provider does not know the code assigned to her or his assessment findings, the coder assigns the code based on the diagnosis(es), sign(s), or symptom(s) written on the patient's superbill. In addition, each service or procedure performed for a client must be represented by a diagnosis that would substantiate those particular services or procedures. In other words, the procedure performed must match the diagnosis coded. For example, if a urine dipstick was performed in the office, the superbill should show diagnoses related to urinary tract infection, polyuria, dysuria, and the like. This practice has received particular attention in the realm of diagnostic testing through the use of ABNs (see earlier) for those services that may not fall within Medicare's guidelines of medical necessity. In addition to its role in reimbursement, the ICD-9-CM serves as a guide to the practicing clinician for the classifications of diseases and symptoms. It is a useful tool in the evaluation of morbidity data for indexing medical records, medical care review, ambulatory and other medical care programs, and basic health statistics (see example in Box 20-2).

Supplemental coding information is located in the ICD-9-CM to capture those patient encounters with the health care system that may not entail a disease or injury classified elsewhere in the manual. There are three main types of encounters that fall into this category, and that receive a "V code":

- When a well person encounters the health care system for some specific purpose (e.g., organ or tissue donation [V42.0 for kidney recipient], prophylactic vaccination [V04.8 for influenza vaccination])
- When a person with a known disease or illness encounters the system for a specific treatment related to that disease or illness (e.g., chemotherapy [V58.1])

BOX 20-2 • EXAMPLE OF THE DEMOGRAPHIC USE OF THE ICD-9-CM CODES

An adult NP wants to know which symptoms or diagnoses are most common in her practice. Collaborating with the medical billing administrator in her practice, the APN defines a sort of the administrative billing data base by ICD-9-CM code. The sort tallies the numbers of patient encounters associated with each code. The resulting list captures the most frequent diagnoses seen in her practice. Among the top five ICD-9-CM codes represented, hypertension, unspecified (401.9) and type 2 diabetes mellitus, uncontrolled (250.22) rank numbers 1 and 2. Based on this information, the NP commits to implementing the Sixth Report of the Joint National Committee on Prevention, Detection, Evaluation, and Treatment of High Blood Pressure guidelines (Joint National Committee, 1997) for the management of hypertension, and the American Diabetes Association (1999) guidelines for the management of diabetes. Flow sheets for blood pressure readings, urinalysis results, glycosylated hemoglobin testing, and scheduled referrals to specialists and routine follow-ups are developed. The following year, the NP commits to evaluating what percentage of patients with hypertension are reaching the goal of systolic blood pressure less than 140 mm Hg and diastolic blood pressure less than 90 mm Hg, and what percentage of patients with diabetes are reaching the goal of a glycosylated hemoglobin below 7 gm/dl.

- When some circumstance exists that influences the person's health status but is not in itself a current illness or injury (e.g., inadequate housing [V60.1], no other household member able to render care [V60.4]).

Environmental events, circumstances, and conditions that are the cause of injury, poisoning, and/or other adverse effects are assigned "E codes." Examples of E codes include those pertaining to motor vehicle traffic accidents (E810 through E819); accidental poisoning by drugs, medicinal substances, and biologicals (E850 through E858); and accidents caused by fire and flames (E890 through E898). Both V and E codes may be found in volume I of the ICD-9-CM manual. The ICD-9-CM codes, and user-friendly cross-indices, are available in paper, disc, and CD-ROM formats from the AMA.

CPT codes are those listed in the *Current Procedural Terminology* manual published annually by the AMA (2000). This text is a listing of the descriptive terms and identifying codes for reporting medical services and procedures (AMA, 2000). As with the ICD-9-CM, the CPT manual serves to provide a uniform language that accurately describes medical, surgical, and diagnostic services. The CPT codes for reimbursement should accurately reflect the services or procedures performed for those ICD-9-CM codes assigned to the patient's diagnosis(es) or symptom(s). All services or procedures are assigned a five-digit code, and represent procedures consistent with contemporary medical practice and performance by many providers in multiple locations. The CPT manual is divided into several sections: Evaluation and Management (see earlier), Anesthesiology, Surgery, Radiology, Pathology and Laboratory, and Medicine. Medicare and state Medicaid carriers are required by law to use CPT codes for the payment of health insurance claims; the majority of insurance carriers recognize and use CPT codes. Although there may be a CPT code that describes a current medical procedure, an insurance carrier is not obligated to reimburse the provider for that service.

Occasionally, modifiers are used to indicate that a service or procedure has been performed and not changed in its description or code, but altered by some specific or extenuating circumstance. The use of modifiers attached to the end of CPT codes eliminates the need for separate procedure codes in these instances. Understanding the proper use of modifiers substantially affects insurance claim reimbursement. The reader is referred to the CPT manual for an in-depth explanation of the use of modifier codes. CPT codes are also available in paper, disc, and CD-ROM formats from the AMA.

Reimbursement for APNs

At the conclusion of the patient encounter, two parallel processes occur (Figure 20–4): the APN documents the clinical encounter in the patient's record and completes the patient's superbill. Ideally, the medical record should provide data in support of the level of E&M service selected, the ICD-9-CM diagnoses used, and the CPT codes utilized. As discussed previously, it is anticipated that the record will also document nursing diagnoses and interventions appropriate to the clinical scenario. Both medical and nursing outcomes and plans for evaluating the efficacy of the plan of care are expected to be included. Viewed through the lens of process improvement and innovation, the implementation of these external resources allows APNs to improve the existing processes of patient medical record documentation. Improvement may be obtained through the use of guidelines both to support the appropriate level of third-party reimbursement and to capture key elements of patient care.

Guidelines can be adapted by individual APNs to create encounter forms incorporating the anticipated elements of the patient's history, physical examination, and diagnostic testing for any particular APN practice. Today's health care economic landscape presents several obstacles to the inclusion of APNs in reimbursement strategies, from the barriers related to scope of practice (see Chapters 22 through 24) to the lack of recognition of nursing diagnoses and interventions through monetary compensation. From a systems-thinking approach, APNs must continue efforts to rectify these inequities through an understanding of, active participation in, and knowledge-based improvement of the current processes of reimbursement. An overview of the patient payer and third-party payer reimbursement strategies is presented here. The reader is referred to the individual programs described for the most recent legislation and information affecting APN participation or enrollment.

FOSTERING PATIENT RESPONSIBILITY

Clients need to assume some level of self-care and financial responsibility for their health care. Self-care measures include active participation in the development and implementation of the plan of care for wellness maintenance and/or illness management. Financial responsibility includes recognition of the valuable services provided by the APN, and subsequent compensation of the APN for those services. Patients should be familiar with their insurance programs, particularly with regard to understanding that many programs do not provide the "blanket insurance" elements that were common in the past. Patients without insurance should expect to pay for the services rendered at the time of their delivery unless prior arrangements have been made with the APN. This policy will obviously not apply to patients being seen in free care clinics, or enrolled in Medicaid or other subsidized programs.

Financial Responsibility Statement. The billing process includes the development of clear and concise written procedures and policies that will enhance the efficiency of the practice, allow review of individual patient bills to assure accuracy, and clearly communicate to clients where their responsibilities for payment lie (AMA, 1996c). A clearly written patient financial responsibility statement, specifically describing payment expectations, should be provided to and signed by each client upon entry into the APN's practice. These expectations not only include what is expected from the patient, but also describe what the patient may expect from the APN's billing procedures and staff. It would be advantageous to include a signed statement allowing the assignment of insurance benefits directly to the APN as part of the financial responsibility statement. This release expedites the processing of insurance claims when the patient's signature is required.

Installment Plans. In the event that the uninsured, or self-pay, client is unable to pay for services at the time they are rendered, offering alternative payment plans provides financial flexibility while supporting the patient's financial responsibility to pay for the care delivered. These alternatives should be negotiated and documented prior to the patient's appointment. The agreed upon payment should then be collected at the time of service. Based upon systems developed by consumer lenders, installment payment plans enable patients to pay their bills in regularly scheduled partial payments. These plans are negotiated between the APN's practice and the patient on a case-by-case basis, according to predetermined policies established by the practice.

Interest is not added to the installment payment because the payment is not considered a financial loan per se.

Sliding Fee Scales. Sliding fee scale programs set up by the business using state and federal guidelines may be offered to eligible applicants who have been denied Medicaid because of exceeding that program's income guidelines. Often, the income guidelines for a sliding fee program allow individuals and families to earn up to 150% of the federal poverty-level income, thus enabling access to health care by the working poor, the underinsured, and the uninsured. Practices offering sliding fee scales require that the patient apply for and be refused other forms of medical financial aid prior to applying for the practice's program. From a patient's perspective, the information needed to complete the application for sliding fee scale is often identical to that used for a state Medicaid application. Consequently, it is possible for the patient to have to compile the mandatory financial information only once, while applying to two different funding programs.

Charity Care and Bartering Arrangements. Other reimbursement strategies employed by providers are charity care and barter system arrangements. Charity care is usually offered by larger practice groups or hospital facilities because they are more financially able to absorb direct reimbursement losses incurred by caring for those unable to pay for services. Hospitals, in particular, may have designated charity care as part of their mission, or may have access to foundation and trust funding designated to sponsor care for those unable to pay. Barter systems have recently been instituted in health care facilities as an innovative option for patients having difficulty paying their bills (P. Tucker, personal communication, May 1999). Issues related to potential individual income taxation need to be addressed prior to the initiation of a bartering system. APNs interested in exploring this option are advised to seek legal and taxation advice from professional advisors prior to entering into this innovative financial arrangement.

Failure to Pay. Consequences for failure to meet the agreed upon payments under practice-based aid programs may result in collection services being initiated against the patient, and/or the decision by the provider to not offer services to the patient any longer. As discussed earlier, issues related to denial of care need to be clearly documented prior to any action being taken by the provider, and need to include providing the patient with an opportunity to secure the services of another provider.

PAYMENT MECHANISMS

There are as many different payment mechanisms as there are different health insurance companies. Each company has its own process for becoming a recognized provider and obtaining reimbursement for care delivered to its beneficiaries. Because of the wide diversity of rapidly changing third-party plans and the increase in managed care entities, and because the ability for APNs to obtain reimbursement is in part dependent upon the individual state practice acts governing advanced practice, any discussion of specific third-party payer plans should be approached with caution. The information for each plan varies quickly from month to month and state to state. The need for uniformity is ever present as health care reimbursement becomes more difficult and costly to obtain. The basic process involved in reimbursement, as an independent provider, is illustrated in Figure 20–5. As discussed previously, the individual APN may not be directly involved in the daily processes related to obtaining reimbursement. Nevertheless, APNs should be familiar with and participate in the major programs and concepts that provide the mainstay of American health care.

Medicare. Medicare provides health insurance benefits for 39 million beneficiaries in the United States (*www.medicare.gov*). Since its authorization by Title XVIII of the Social Security Act in 1965, Medicare has provided access to care to individuals ages 65 years and older. In 1972, Medicare coverage was extended to include those individuals under age 65 with long-term disabilities (of at least 2 years' duration and eligible for Social Security Disability Insurance) and with end-stage renal disease. In 1982, the Tax Equity and Fiscal Responsibility Act introduced a risk-based option, facilitating the involvement of HMOs. In 1983, the inpatient hospital PPS was adopted. This system replaced cost-based payments with a plan in which a predetermined rate was paid based on patients' diagnoses. The Balanced Budget Act of 1997 includes the most extensive legislative changes for Medicare since its inception. Among these changes are the expansion of covered preventive benefits and the establishment of Part C (Medicare + Choice), which creates new managed care and other health plan choices for beneficiaries (*www.hcfa.gov/medicare*). In 1997, Medicare opened up to private company HMOs to provide beneficiaries with additional benefits at a proposed lower cost (Northeast Health Care Quality Foundation, 1999). Some of these private HMOs have already left the Medicare program because of the negative impact on their business and financial viability. (See Chapter 23 for futher discussions of the Medicare program.)

Medicare coverage consists of two parts. Hospital insurance (Part A) covers inpatient hospital services, short-term care in skilled nursing facilities, postinstitutional home health care, and hospice care. Those individuals eligible for Social Security are automatically enrolled in Part A. Other qualified beneficiaries need to initiate the enrollment process. Supplementary Medical Insurance (Part B), covers physician services, outpatient hospital services, home health care not covered by Part A, and other medical services such as diagnostic testing, durable medical equipment, and ambulance costs. Enrollment in Part B is voluntary to beneficiaries receiving Part A. Medicare Part A is funded primarily through payroll taxes, although beneficiary cost sharing in the forms of deductibles and co-insurance may apply. Beneficiaries participating in Part B pay into the system through monthly premiums that are established yearly based upon system expenses as well as through deductibles and co-insurance programs for various services. Medicare + Choice (Part C) benefits are available through participation in coordinated care or private fee-for-service plans and medical savings accounts (*www.hcfa.gov/medicare*).

Providers can either participate in Medicare or be nonparticipating providers. For participants, the Medicare fee schedule for physicians' professional services, services and supplies provided incident to physicians' professional services (e.g., certain medications and biological agents), and patient physical and occupational therapy services, diagnostic tests, and radiology services is 5% higher than for nonparticipants (National Heritage Insurance Company [NHIC], 1999). In 1999, 84.6% of all physicians, practitioners, and suppliers billed under Medicare signed participation agreements, a 2.2% increase from 1998 (NHIC, 1999). At present, only NPs and CNSs are permitted to bill Medicare. Payments are set at 85% of the physician's fee schedule.

APNs who are Medicare providers must be participating providers, which means they will accept "assignment," the allowable charge determined by Medicare. To

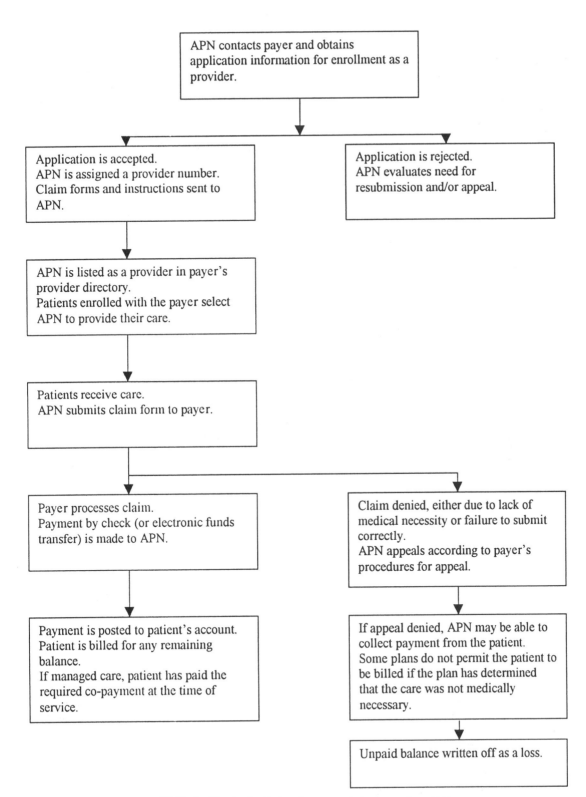

FIGURE 20–5 · The basic third-party payer reimbursement process.

become a participating provider, the APN must apply to Medicare for a Universal Provider Identification Number (UPIN). The qualifications for NPs requesting a Medicare UPIN were revised in the HCFA 2000 Physician Fee Schedule regulation as follows (NHIC, 1999):

As of January 1, 2001, the NP must possess:
- a state license
- national certification

As of January 1, 2003, the NP must possess:
- a state license
- national certification
- a master's degree.

The UPIN number is the APN's permanent identification number with the Medicare program irrespective of the practice location. In other words, even if the APN moves to another state and establishes a practice there, the UPIN number will remain the same. A local provider number is also assigned that is to be used within the local Medicare intermediary's cachement area. Applications for the UPIN may be obtained from the local Medicare intermediary. A listing of local intermediaries may be obtained from the HCFA by telephone at 1-800-MEDICARE.

Medicaid. Medicaid provides health insurance benefits as well as other assistance for eligible low-income individuals and families. Medicaid is a jointly funded state-federal insurance program. Coverage varies by state according to federal requirements that stipulate eligibility and basic services covered. Payment is usually lower than is available through other insurance groups. In 1989, Congress mandated that state Medicaid agencies provide direct reimbursement to family NPs, Pediatric NPs, and CNMs. Some states cover the services of other APNs; however, the resulting inconsistencies have caused significant confusion. APNs receive Medicaid reimbursement in 49 states, 39 of which reimburse at 80% to 100% of a physician's rate (Pearson, 2000). As with Medicare, the APN must apply for a provider number and be knowledgeable of the local state Medicaid regulations. Every state publishes a handbook of Medicaid rules complete with updates, and Medicaid payers publish newsletters periodically. A recent change in Title XXI of the Social Security Act offers services for children through the Children's Health Insurance Program (CHIP). See Chapter 23 for detailed information about this payment mechanism for APN services.

Federal Employee Health Benefit Program (FEHBP). The FEHBP is the health insurance plan for the approximately 10 million federal employees and their dependents. This is a voluntary, contributory program open to all employees of the federal government. Contracts are held with private health insurance carriers to offer health insurance plans to federal employees. Public Law 101-509, enacted in 1990, allows federal employees enrolled in the FEHBP direct access to NPs, CNSs, and CNMs, thus enabling direct reimbursement for APN services. Under this provision, insurance carriers for federal plans must make payment directly to these APNs if their services are covered under the plan. Collaboration with or supervision by a physician or any other health care provider is not needed. The payment level is determined by the individual health insurance plan. Additional information is available on the World Wide Web: *www.opm.gov/insure/*.

Private Health Insurance—Fee-for-Service Plans. Private health insurance plans include carriers such as Blue Cross/Blue Shield, Aetna, Prudential, and Metropolitan. Many of these carriers are merging into larger entities as the move to managed care demands system-wide changes and efficiencies. These traditional fee-for-service plans reimburse providers for patient charges according to the usual and customary charges for that local area. An insurance policy does not explicitly need to include the coverage of nursing services for APNs to be reimbursed for their services. APNs' direct reimbursement by private insurance carriers varies from state to state (Pearson, 2000). When considering application for third-party reimbursement, the nurse needs to be familiar with the state's nurse practice act, state insurance laws and codes (including reimbursement amendments), judicial decisions, and opinions by the attorney general. State health insurance laws do not necessarily prohibit third-party reimbursement to nurses. In Florida, for instance, direct third-party reimbursement is essentially a 1 : 1 process. The individual nurse applies to the third-party insurer and requests provider status. If reimbursement is rejected, familiarity with the state's nursing practice act and the state's health insurance laws can assist the nurse in appealing the decision.

Managed Care. Managed care denotes a spectrum of arrangements that entail some connection between financing and delivery of care, usually with cost containment (American Academy of Nursing, 1993). In managed care, the financial risk associated with health care delivery is shared between the payers, the contracted providers, and the enrolled beneficiaries. Risk is lessened for payers by the exclusive enrollment of beneficiaries with a particular health status profile. Risk is lessened for any one provider by the addition of providers to the pool of providers sharing the care for a particular population of patients. Risk is lessened for the beneficiaries through the utilization of providers who are within the contracted pool, or "network," of providers. The distribution of financial risk has received increased media coverage recently as some managed care companies face financial difficulties. Such turmoil is evidenced by the alteration of key components of typical managed care contracts. Examples include changes in patient population (e.g., the dis-enrollment of Medicare beneficiaries), pharmaceutical coverage (e.g., the increased practice of allowing a decreased supply of chronic medications to be dispensed at one time to increase collected co-payments), and departure of companies from a particular cachement location (e.g., the withdrawal of the Tufts Plan from Maine).

Managed care companies base their reimbursement to providers on a combination of historical area charge data, relative value scales, and actuarial data. Managed care entities will usually either discount a physician's fee for services or require that a predetermined fee be charged. However, the majority of managed care companies pay providers a "capitated" fee, which means the provider cares for a client population for a prearranged amount per client (per capita). Capitation amounts typically vary by member age, gender, and risk status and are negotiable. The capitated fee is paid to the provider monthly based upon the number of plan enrollees who have selected that provider as their primary care provider. Key areas of managed care contracts include practice exclusivity, sign-on bonuses to the practice for new members recruited to the HMO, and profit sharing (Jenkins & Torrisi, 1995).

Managed care programs are offered by commercial insurance carriers and include PPOs and HMOs among others. HMOs encompass any variety of prepaid group practice arrangements. These programs usually offer health care services to members enrolled in the plan for a predetermined, prepaid, or discounted fee. Prepaid means that the organization receives a fixed payment or premium to care for members of a certain population and that the organization bears the financial risk for the care that members receive. Participating providers are required to provide services for contracted reimbursement amounts. This reimbursement can range from a discounted fee for service to a lump sum for all services required. There are four main types of HMOs (Knight, 1998):

1. Staff-model HMOs employ salaried physicians who work in the HMO's own clinics.
2. Group-model HMOs contract with a large multispecialty group practice.
3. Individual practice association (IPA)–model HMOs contract with individual physicians or affiliations of independent physicians.
4. Network HMO models are similar to IPAs except that they contract with several larger physician groups. Some models are mixed combinations of group, staff, network, or IPA models.

A PPO is a network of providers, usually physicians and hospitals, that have discounted their fees for an increased volume of patients (Meazy & McGivern, 1993).

Some HMOs make extensive use of APNs in order to increase the cost-effectiveness of primary care. Jenkins and Torrisi (1995) stated that many private and public HMOs and other managed care organizations, however, have been slow to enroll primary care APNs as providers who receive direct capitation payments. California APNs have experienced "lock out" from some managed care contracts. As discussed earlier, APNs must provide the data needed by payers to demonstrate cost efficiency, and must work together at the policy-making level to eliminate these financial restraints to trade (see Chapter 23).

Reimbursement Summary

Reimbursement is an indirect process supporting patient care that provides a vehicle for APN compensation for the services rendered to patients. The process begins with the end of the patient clinical encounter, and ends with the posting of the patient's payment, either through individual accountability or through third-party reimbursement. The involvement of APNs in the reimbursement process is dependent upon whether the APN is allowed by the applicable state and federal regulations to practice independently, and is able to obtain direct reimbursement for those independently delivered services. The level to which the APN is involved in the administrative procedures is dependent upon whether the APN has chosen to practice in an entrepreneurial or intrapreneurial manner. Most times, the process of reimbursement is, and should be, delegated to an individual familiar with medical billing, and able to dedicate the time and effort required to become expert in this level of practice management. If the APN decides to become directly involved in reimbursement procedures, it is strongly urged that a professional billing advisor, similar to the attorney or accountant consulted during business planning, be contracted or hired. This advisor serves to provide the APN with the latest and most accurate information regarding this vital process in the APN's financial viability.

Some authors report that reimbursement should equal 90% of the patient's billable charges (Buppert, 1999). The reality of health care economics is that this number varies considerably over time depending upon the payer mix, specifically upon the percentage of Medicare, Medicaid, and capitated payments to be received. Medicare pays approximately 65% of the billed charges (NHIC, 1999). Medicaid pays a roughly equivalent proportion, usually based upon the local Medicare fee structure. Capitated contracts can result in financial losses if enrolled beneficiaries utilize the health care system more frequently than the anticipated risk calculation had allocated. Patients unable to pay, or who refuse to pay, create a percentage of "bad debt" that is written off as a business loss. During the business planning phase, the APN should become intimately familiar with the reimbursement rates in the local area, the anticipated payer mix of the patient population to be served, and the available resources and personnel to design and implement a reimbursement process that meets the APN's financial expectations. As with any system, the reimbursement process should undergo periodic evaluation to determine where improvements in the process may be made, including electronic claim submission, tighter internal audit controls, and efficient cross-training of staff to ensure consistency during staff absences.

EXEMPLAR: THE JAMESTOWN S'KLALLAM TRIBE

In January 1999, I was fortunate to be able to make a site visit to the Jamestown S'Klallam Tribe of Native Americans in Puget Sound. Information gathered during this visit is very instructive as APNs strive to understand business planning and opportunities for innovative ways to offer services to underserved populations.

E X E M P L A R

The Jamestown S'Klallam Tribe evolved directly from several constituent communities of S'Klallam people. The S'Klallam Tribe belongs to a Salish cultural and linguistic group related to British Columbia Tribes as well as to most Tribes in the Puget Sound area. (The history of the Tribe may be found at *http://www.olympus.net/personal/skallam/history.htm.*) In 1981, the Jamestown S'Klallam Tribe successfully obtained federal recognition to re-establish treaty rights granted in the 1855 Point No Point Treaty. As part of this recognition, the Tribe may formally maintain a government-to-government relationship with the United States within the spirit of Indian self-determination, determine its own priorities, and meet the needs of the Tribal membership in the manner it determines is most effective.

The significance of the Jamestown S'Klallam Tribe to the discussion of business planning for APNs is reflected in the Tribe's Social and Health Services Program. The mission of the program is to strengthen Tribal culture and community, promote family stability, improve the health status of Tribal people, increase opportunities, and help meet the basic needs of the membership (Jamestown S'Klallam Tribe, 1998). The goal to improve the health status of the community is specifically met through case management and the managed care program (MCP). The MCP was designed to provide the most medical services for Tribal people with the limited funds available from the Indian Health Service. From a systems standpoint, the goal to improve the health status of Tribal people is met through the provision of health care insurance coverage to all Tribal members, a local universal health care model based upon their specific community needs and resources. Every Tribal member falls into one of four medical insurance plans:

- *Medicare:* Eligible enrollees must enroll for Parts A and B. The MCP purchases supplemental policies, reimburses patients for the Part B premiums, co-payments, and deductibles; and pays for prescription drugs at authorized and participating pharmacies not covered by the other plans.

- *Medicaid:* Any one eligible for Medicaid is required to enroll. The MCP assists with Medicaid applications. Services not covered by Medicaid will be paid to the same level of benefits received under other plans by the MCP.
- *Private Insurance:* If a tribal member has private insurance through his or her own or spouse's employer, the MCP may reimburse the member for all or part of the monthly premium, or the tribe may choose to purchase the Washington State Basic Health Plan (BHP) coverage for the members. Out-of-pocket expenses, deductibles, and preauthorized preventive benefits may be reimbursed by the MCP.
- *Basic Health Plan:* If a tribal member is uninsured, the MCP purchases BHP coverage for the individual, and may reimburse the member for out-of-pocket co-payments.

Additional supplemental benefits are available through the MCP based on the availability of funding. The program successfully developed relationships with the local network of existing health care providers to obtain required health care services for their fully insured community. In addition, the program works with members to eliminate barriers related to access to these local providers by providing some transportation to appointments. Additional local services provided by the program include, but are not limited to, child care assistance, community health education and disease prevention presentations, elder services, mental health, substance abuse prevention and treatment, and a women, infants, and children's (WIC) clinic. All of these services are well within the scope of practice of APNs and offer innovative practice opportunities. Currently, there are 448 Jamestown S'Klallam members, with approximately 641 Indian people in the area successfully served by tribal programs.

CONCLUSION

Through the development of innovative programs and practices grounded in a systems-thinking approach, APNs define, demonstrate, document, and thereby claim their contributions to patient care. Business planning establishes a clear picture of how the APN will function on a daily basis, as well as how midrange and long-term goals are to be met. Knowledge of the processes involved in care delivery increases the sharing of information between APNs and their patients, other health care providers, and colleagues. Reimbursement is identified as the major indirect process of care that has a direct impact on the success of the APN's business planning efforts. Equally important to success is the APN's candid self-evaluation and determination of whether an entrepreneurial or intrapreneurial approach is the most appropriate model under which to deliver patient care. The recognition that others, such as other APNs, physicians, attorneys, and practice managers, in the greater health care system have skills and expertise to offer provides the APN with a "safety net" of advisors who should play an active role in the actualization of advanced nursing practice. Above all, the success of the APN is grounded in the professional recognition of and active participation in the larger system to ensure that the needs of patients are met through the delivery of clinically excellent, holistic health care.

ACKNOWLEDGMENTS

The author wishes to thank Collen M. Prophet, MA, RN, and Barbara Head, PhD, RN, of the Center for Nursing Classification for their guidance and input related to the potential use of nursing classifications by APNs. The author wishes to thank Cindy Lowe, Health Director, W. Ron Allen, Tribal Chairman; and the members of the Jamestown S'Klallam Tribe of Sequim, Washington, for their time and support in the preparation of the clinical exemplar.

REFERENCES

American Academy of Family Practice. (1998). ICD-9 codes for family practice: 1998–1999. Available: *http://www.aafp.org/fpm/981000fm/icd9.html*

American Academy of Nursing. (1993). *Managed care and national health care reform: Nurses can make it work.* Washington, DC: Author.

American Diabetes Association. (1999). Standards of medical care for patients with diabetes mellitus. *Diabetes Care, 22*(Suppl. 1), 532–541.

American Express Company. (1998). *Small business exchange: Creating an effective business plan.* Available: *http://www.americanexpress.com/smallbusiness/resources/starting/biz_plan/*

American Medical Association. (1996a). *Financial management of the medical practice: The physician's handbook for successful budgeting, forecasting and cost accounting.* Norcross, GA: Coker Publishing Company.

American Medical Association. (1996b). *Integration strategies for the medical practice: The physician's handbook to integration alternatives.* Norcross, GA: Coker Publishing Company.

American Medical Association. (1996c). *Managing the medical practice: The physician's handbook for successful practice administration.* Norcross, GA: Coker Publishing Company.

American Medical Association. (1996d). *Starting a medical practice: The physician's handbook for successful practice start-up.* Norcross, GA: Coker Publishing Company.

American Medical Association. (1998). *International classification of diseases. 9th revision: Clinical modification (ICD-9-CM 1999)* (Vols. 1 and 2). Dover, DE: Author.

American Medical Association. (1999). *Automating the medical record.* Norcross, GA: Coker Publishing Company.

American Medical Association. (2000). *Current procedural terminology.* Chicago: Author.

American Nurses Association. (1985). *Code for nurses with interpretive statements.* Kansas City, MO: Author.

Bulechek, G. M., & McCloskey, J. C. (1999). Nursing intervention: Effective nursing treatments (3rd ed.). Philadelphia: W. B. Saunders.

Buppert, C. (1999). *Nurse practitioner's business practice and legal guide.* Gaithersburg, MD: Aspen Publishers.

Carpenito, L. J. (1999). *Handbook of nursing diagnosis* (8th ed.). Philadelphia: J. B. Lippincott.

Donabedian, A. (1966). Evaluating the quality of medical care. *Milbank Quarterly, 44,* 166–206.

Donahue, M. P. (1985). *Nursing: The finest art.* St. Louis: C. V. Mosby Co.

Hanson, C. (1993). Our role in health care reform: Collegiality counts. *American Journal of Nursing, 93*(12), 16A–16E.

HCA Quality Resource Group. (1992a). *Organizing hospital care as a system: An annotated guide.* Nashville, TN: Author.

HCA Quality Resource Group. (1992b). *Organizing work as a system.* Nashville, TN: Author.

Health Care Financing Administration. (1997). *1997 Documentation guidelines for evaluation and management services.* Available at: *http://www.bcfa.gov/medicare/mcarpti.htm*

Henry, S. B., Holzemer, W. L., Randell, C., Hsieh, S. F., & Miller, T. J. (1997). Comparison of nursing interventions classification and current procedural terminology codes for categorizing nursing activities. *Image: The Journal of J Nursing Scholarship, 29*(2), 133–138.

Hurst, J., Nickel, K., & Hilborne, L. H. (1998). Are physician's office laboratory results of comparible quality to those produced in other laboratory settings? *JAMA, 279*(6), 468–471.

Iowa Intervention Project (Johnson, M., & Maas, M. [Eds.]). (1997). *Nursing outcomes classification.* St. Louis: C. V. Mosby.

Jamestown S'Klallam Tribe. (1998). *Jamestown S'Klallam Tribe: The "strong people".* Sequim, WA: Author.

Jenkins, M., & Torrisi, D. (1995). A nurse practitioner, community nursing centers, and contracting for managed care. *Journal of the American Academy of Nurse Practitioners, 7*(3), 119–124.

Joint Commission on Accreditation of Healthcare Organizations. (1995). *1996 Accreditation manual for hospitals, Volume II: Scoring guidelines.* Oakbrook Terrace, IL: Author.

Joint National Committee on Prevention, Detection, Evaluation, and Treatment of High Blood Pressure and the National High Blood Pressure Education Program Coordinating Committee. (1997). The sixth report of the Joint National Committee on Prevention, Detection, Evaluation, and Treatment of High Blood Pressure (JNC VI). *Archives of Internal Medicine, 157,* 2413–2446.

Keepnews, D. (1994). *The reimbursement manual: How to get paid for your advanced practice nursing services* (Supplement). Washington, DC: American Nurses Publishing.

Knight, W. (1998). *Managed care: What it is and how it works.* Gaithersburg: Aspen.

McCloskey, J. C., & Bulechek, G. M. (Eds.). (1992). *Nursing interventions classification* (2nd ed.). St. Louis: Mosby–Year Book.

Meazy, M. D., & McGivern, D. O. (Eds.). (1993). *Nurses, nurse practitioners: Evolution to advanced practice.* New York: Springer-Verlag.

National Heritage Insurance Company. (1999, November). *HCFA Medicare B bulletin.* Hingham, MA: Author.

Neumann, B. R., & Boles, K. E. (1998). *Management accounting for health care organizations* (5th ed.). Chicago: Precept Press.

Newman, D. K. (1996). Program and practice management for the advanced practice nurse. In A. B. Hamric, J. A. Spross, & C. M. Hanson (Eds.), *Advanced practice nursing: An integrative approach* (pp. 545–568). Philadelphia: W. B. Saunders.

Northeast Health Care Quality Foundation. (1999). *Health matters for Medicare consumers* (Vol. 3). Dover, NH: Author.

Pearson, J. L. (1999). Annual update of how each state stands on legislative issues affecting advanced nursing practice. *Nurse Practitioner: The American Journal of Primary Health Care, 24*(1), 11–13, 17–18, 21–22, 24–27, 31–34, 39–40, 42–44, 50.

Pharmaceutical Research and Manufacturers of America. (1997). *Directory of prescription drug patient assistance programs.* Washington, DC: Author.

Rehm, S., & Kraft, S. (1998). How to select a computer system for a family physician's office. Available: *http://www.aafp.org/fpnet/guide/*

Schwartz, I. (1996). Private office laboratories: Coping with federal guidelines. *Infections in Urology, 9*(6), 175–183.

Stewart, P. (1989). The CNS in private practice. In A. B. Hamric & J. A. Spross (Eds.), *The Clinical Nurse Specialist in Theory and Practice* (2nd. ed., pp. 435–455). Philadelphia: W. B. Saunders.

Tweedy, J. T. (1997). *Healthcare hazard control and safety management.* Bethesda, MD: Board of Certified Healthcare Safety Management; and Delray Beach, FL: GR/St. Lucie Press.

Vogel, G., & Doleysh, N. (1994). *Entrepreneuring: A nurse's guide to starting a business.* New York: National League for Nursing.

Additional Readings

American Association of Colleges of Nursing. (1999). Direct Medicare reimbursement for nurse practitioners and clinical nurse specialists. AACN Government Affairs Issue Summary, 106th Congress First Session (rev.). Available: *http://www.aacn.nche.edu/government/issues/medreimb.htm*

American College of Nurse-Midwives. (1994). Joint statement of practice relations between obstetrician/gynecologists and certified nurse midwives (reaffirmed). Available: *http://www.acnm.org/prof/jnstat.htm*

American College of Nurse-Midwives. (1997). Collaborative management in midwifery practice for medical, gynecological and obstetrical conditions (rev.). Available: *http://www.acnm.org/prof/collab.htm*

American College of Nurse-Midwives. (1997). Definitions (rev.). Available: *http://www.acnm.org/prof/defcnm.htm*

American College of Nurse-Midwives. (1997). Guidelines for the incorporation of new procedures into nurse-midwifery practice. Available: *http://www.acnm.org/prof/guide.htm*

American College of Nurse-Midwives. (1997). Independent midwifery practice (rev.). Available: *http://www.acnm.org/prof/independ.htm*

American College of Nurse-Midwives. (1997). State and federal action on primary care and direct access to obstetrical and gynecological providers. Available: *http://www.acnm.org/prof/diracces.htm*

American College of Nurse-Midwives. (1998, January). States in which certified nurse-midwives have prescriptive authority. Available: *http://www.acnm.org/prof/prescrip.htm*

American College of Nurse-Midwives. (1998, February). Third party reimbursement for CNMs; State laws. Available: *http://www.acnm.org/prof/mandate.htm*

American Nurses Association. (n.d.). States recognizing advanced practice under independent acts, separate titles of advance practice acts, or regulations. Available: *http://www.ana.org/gova/tiltrial.htm*

American Nurses Association. (1996). *Scope and standards of advanced practice registered nursing.* Washington, DC: American Nurses Publishing.

American Nurses Association. (1997). States which recognize clinical nurse specialists in advanced practice. Available: *http://www.ana.org/gova/cns.htm*

Berwick, D. M. (1998, June). *Managing for world-class improvement: Distinctive characteristics of the future outstanding health care organization.* Paper presented at Quality Day, Dartmouth Medical School, Hanover, NH.

Blair, C. (1997). Advanced practice nurses as entrepreneurs. *American Journal of Nursing, 97*(11), 16AAA–16DDD.

Blondell, R. D., Norris, T. E., & Coombs, J. B. (1992). Rural health and family medicine. *American Family Physician, 45,* 2507–2510.

Bulechek, G. M., & McCloskey, J. C. (1999). *Nursing intervention: Effective nursing treatments* (3rd ed.). Philadelphia: W. B. Saunders.

Buppert, C. K. (1995). Justifying nurse practitioner existence: Hard facts to hard figures. *Nurse Practitioner, 20*(8), 43–48.

Buppert, C. (1997). Employment agreements: Clauses that can change an NP's life. *Nurse Practitioner, 22*(8), 108–119.

Carlson, E. (1998). What's happening: Emerging roles for the gerontological nurse practitioner. *Journal of the American Academy of Nurse Practitioners, 10*(9), 403–405.

Cavanah, C. (1998, November). Entrepreneur's complete guide to software. *Entrepreneur,* pp. 129–139.

Centers for Disease Control and Prevention. (1998). New study shows lower mortality rates for infants delivered by certified nurse midwives. Available: *http://www.cdc.gov/nchs/releases/98news/98news/midwife.htm*

Covey, S. R. (1989). *The seven habits of highly effective people: Restoring the character ethic.* New York: Simon & Schuster.

Davies, A. R., Doyle, M. A. T., Lansky, D., et al. (1993, March). *Outcomes assessment: Implementation workbook.* (Functional Outcomes Program; supported by Grant 92-005 by the Henry J. Kaiser Family Foundation). Boston, MA: New England Medical Center, Inc.

DeBarth, K., & Kelly, K. (1996). Successfully sharing a private practice with MDs: Overlooked business opportunities for NPs and PAs. *The Clinicians Reference Guide: A Supplement to Clinician Reviews,* pp. 108–112.

Freedman, E. (1999, March). Your so-called life. The overachieving entrepreneur's guide to making time for a real life. *Entrepreneur,* pp. 146, 148–151.

Garr, D., Rhyne, R., & Kukulka, G. (1993). Incorporating a community-oriented approach in primary care. *American Family Physician, 47,* 1699–1702.

Health Care Financing Administration. (1999). *Medicare and you resource kit.* Baltimore, MD: Author.

Henry, P. F. (1996). Analysis of the nurse practitioner's legal relationships. *Nurse Practitioner Forum, 7*(1), 5–6.

Internal Revenue Service. (1995). *Understanding your EIN (Employer Identification Numbers)* (Publication No. 1635–Revised [Rev. 6-95]; Catalog Number 14332X). Washington, DC: U.S. Department of the Treasury.

Jones, J. E., & Bearley, W. L. (1986). *Participative management tree* [Pocket reference card]. King of Prussia, PA: Organization Design and Development, Inc.

Jones, K. R., Jennings, B. M., Moritz, P., & Moss, M. T. (1997). Policy issues associated with analyzing outcomes of care. *Image: The Journal of Nursing Scholarship, 29*(3), 261–267.

Michalek, M. R. (1994, Spring/Summer). The advanced practice job search. *Advanced Practice Nurse,* pp. 12–41.

Mohr, W. K. (1996). Dirty hands: The underside of marketplace health care. *Advances in Nursing Science, 9*(1), 28–37.

Nugent, K. E., & Lambert, V. A. (1997). Evaluating the performance of the APN. *Nurse Practitioner, 22*(4), 190–198.

Peters, S. (1998, October). States of the nation: Progress for NPs in South Carolina. *Advance for Nurse Practitioners,* p. 14.

Reid, A. H. (1999, March). *Grant writing.* Presentation provided through Maine Bureau of Health, Division of Community and Family Health, York, ME.

Richards, R. N. (1998). How to select a practice site and practice type. *Medscape Orthopedics & Sports Medicine, 2*(4). Available: *http://www.medscape.com/Medscape/OrthoSpo02.n04/mos4514.rich/pnt-mos4514.rich.html*

Rodgers, S. (1998, October). Profession's leadership needs to address NP glut. *Advance for Nurse Practitioners,* p. 93.

Rodkin, D. (1998, October). Full speed ahead: 15 shortcuts to business success. *Entrepreneur,* pp. 132–138.

Ruberry, B. (1998, November). Danger Zone: When bad things happen to good entrepreneurs: What every small business owner needs to know about crisis management. *Entrepreneur,* pp. 153–157.

Shay, L. E., Goldstein, J. T., Matthews, D., Trait, L. L., & Edmunds, M. W. (1996). Guidelines for developing a nurse practitioner practice. *Nurse Practitioner, 21*(1), 72–81.

Simpson, L., & Lee, P. R. (1993). Primary care: An idea in search of a paradigm? *American Family Physician, 47,* 323–326.

Smith, A. (1998). The job market: What does the future hold for Pas and NPs? *Clinician News, 2*(3), 1, 8.

Smith, S. S. (1999, March). Future speak: Interview with Alvin and Heidi Toffler. *Entrepreneur,* pp. 127–130.

Stodder, G. S. (1997, July). Independence days: Entrepreneurs offering a compassionate option to nursing homes are fueling the $12 billion assisted living industry. *Entrepreneur,* pp. 130, 132–133.

Stodder, G. S. (1998, July). Goodwill hunting: Who cares about socially responsible business practices? Seventy percent of consumers, that's who. *Entrepreneur,* pp. 118–125.

Taylor-Seehafer, M. (1998). Point of view: Nurse-physician collaboration. *Journal of the American Academy of Nurse Practitioners, 10*(9), 387–391.

Turner, S. O. (1996). *Transitions in healthcare: Assisting employees in transition—a manager's guide.* Aliso Viejo, CA: American Association of Critical-Care Nurses.

Turner, S. O. (1996). *Transitions in healthcare: Business skills for health professionals—instructor's guide.* Aliso Viejo, CA: American Association of Critical-Care Nurses.

Turner, S. O. (1996). *Transitions in healthcare: Career strategies in the new system—instructor's guide.* Aliso Viejo, CA: American Association of Critical-Care Nurses.

Turner, S. O. (1996). *Transitions in healthcare: Managing change and transition—instruc-tor's guide.* Aliso Viejo, CA: American Association of Critical-Care Nurses.

Turner, S. O. (1996). *Transitions in healthcare: The changing healthcare system—instructor's guide.* Aliso Viejo, CA: American Association of Critical-Care Nurses.

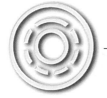

Marketing and Contracting Considerations

- S U S A N   E.   D A V I S   D O U G H T Y
- J E N N I F E R   M.   K E L L E R

HEALTH CARE AS A BUSINESS: A CALL TO ACTION FOR ADVANCED PRACTICE NURSES

Despite the fact that advanced practice nurses (APNs) have been around for decades, there is still a lack of knowledge among health care colleagues and consumers about what APNs do. In this century, certified nurse-midwives (CNMs) answered a call for safe birthing, certified registered nurse anesthetists (CRNAs) practiced long before the medical specialty of anesthesiology developed, clinical nurse specialists (CNSs) responded to a need for expert practitioners at the nurse-patient interface, and nurse practitioners (NPs) grew out of the health care crisis of the 1960s to provide increased access to patient care services. Today, health and illness care are driven by market forces, and it is a serious problem that many Americans cannot access or afford health services. APNs can help solve this problem if they understand marketing concepts and use marketing strategies. APNs who cannot get beyond an aversion toward marketing will be left behind. This chapter outlines key marketing concepts and strategies, delineates marketable properties of APNs, itemizes essentials for effective external and internal marketing, and helps both the new graduate and the experienced APN to develop a personal marketing plan. Contracting considerations including employment contracts, service contracts, and managed care contracts are also addressed.

WHAT IS MARKETING?

Marketing is anything and everything APNs do to promote their practice. It is about meeting the needs of clients and positioning services/businesses in the marketplace. Marketing consists of four key elements, popularly known as the four "Ps": product, price, place, and promotion. All of these principles can be applied to the marketing needs of APNs. Marketing differs from advertising in that advertising or promotion is a small part of marketing. In particular, advertising has a bad reputation for being focused on materialism. Almost no one believes advertising's claims, yet it persists because it works. Health care professionals are often uncomfortable with the notion of self-promotion, and some consider it unethical. Curtin (1985) stated, "Information is the coin of the realm, media its trading place, and advertising its medium." She suggested that nurses must let go of the notion that advertising is not done by respectable health care professionals and recognize that it can be done honestly if incorporated into a marketing strategy that allows both the nurse and the consumer to win. In today's health care market, which is becoming more diversified and competitive, nothing could be more important for APNs to understand.

KEY MARKETING CONCEPTS FOR APNs

Marketing is focused on satisfying the needs and desires of consumers. An important marketing concept is that of organizing information about client needs through a marketing survey using two components: service differentiation—that is, identifying aspects of a service valued by clients yet unmatched by competitiors—and market segmentation, or dividing clients into groups according to factors that influence selection and use of services (Luckacs, 1984). Service differentiation for an NP survey might include gathering data for a group of people about preferred location, hours of service, or availability of follow-up care. Market segmentation data in the survey might include individual and group characteristics such as age, gender, socioeconomic status, population density, and benefits sought.

Good marketing is designed to educate others about nursing and sell a service from a position of strength (Caveen, Cheshire, Power, & Woolley, 1992). It is important for APNs to take a position regarding marketing as it relates to the provision of health care today. APNs cannot afford to be passive. Nursing values and information oriented toward the well-being and goals of the client can support ethical marketing. Responses to competition for finite health care resources include numerous health care marketing seminars, hiring of health care marketing consultants by agencies, and the development of marketing positions by most health care organizations. In the past, nursing's values have not embraced marketing. Yet developing marketing skills and markets for advanced nursing practice could literally determine the survival of APNs. The slogans "Because I'm worth it" and "We bring good things to life" positioned L'Oreal and General Electric for success. As with the corporate world, APNs can position themselves as unique providers of certain services so that consumers automatically think of the APN when they seek that service. Examples of marketing niches for APNs can be found in Table 21-1.

Based on this overview of marketing, key marketing goals for APNs include:

- Educating consumers and colleagues about advanced nursing practice
- Generating income and obtaining funding
- Developing broad-based, interdisciplinary support for advanced nursing practice
- Being able to meet existing, but unmet, client needs
- Making health problems visible
- Creating new job opportunities and stable niches in changing systems
- Understanding how to exist within or co-exist with managed care organizations

Areas of growth in nursing are to be found at the edges of traditional practice. The evolution of health care helps APNs identify areas in which to expand. A new paradigm for care involving the APN at its core demands letting go of old paradigms in which APNs only talk to other nurses or limit professional and educational contacts to their area of specialty. It requires forging unique collaborations among disciplines to create networks and establish partnerships (Shoultz, Hatcher, & Hurrell, 1992) (see Chapter 11). It also includes reading economic, political, and marketing literature outside of nursing to learn about issues and strategies. For example, the revolutionary business concept of cooperative competition, or "co-opetition" (Brandenburger & Nalebuff, 1996) offers a way for today's competitors to find new common ground for business collaboration tomorrow. "When competitors reach a standoff in market advantage, they can switch to cooperation to increase their mutual strengths and benefits" (Coile, 1999, p. 5). Creating shared business alliances using "co-opetition" is one of many concepts advanced nursing practice can borrow from the corporate world.

Health care reform efforts should be seen as opportunities for creating new advanced nursing practice models for innovative services. An innovative role that has emerged as physician residency positions are deleted is the role of the acute care NP (see Chapter 15). There is a viable argument for "replacing" critical care residents with NPs at the same salary without costs for rotation or turnover (Edmunds, 1991; Keane, Richmond, & Kaiser, 1994). Support for institutional policies, loyalty to the institution, and continuity of care provided by the NP benefit the institution, and the NP typically enjoys the level of skill and responsibility demanded. Graduate programs in nursing to prepare critical care APNs are evolving (Clochesy, Daly,

TABLE 21-1 EXAMPLES OF ADVANCED NURSING PRACTICE MARKETING NICHES OR SERVICES

Adolescent gynecology specialist
Architectural consultant
Birthing center
Brokering services (e.g., elder care)
Chronic illness management
Correctional health care
Day care consultant
Diabetes management
Elder care
Employee programs for health care cost-containment
Ethics consultant
Family counseling
Fitness/exercise consultant
Health policy consultant
Health/wellness promotion
HIV/AIDS care
Homeless shelters
Lactation consultant & equipment rental
Mammography, breast health counseling
Medical, nursing, health care writing
Menopause center
Mobile health services (e.g., mammography van)
Multidisciplinary clinical practice
Nurse case manager
Nurse educator
Occupational health/worker's compensation consultant
Pacemaker center
Pain management
Product development (e.g., pharmaceutical, toys, personal care, therapeutic devices)
Psychiatric counseling
Radio/TV/media consultant
Retirement center
Risk management consultant
Same-day surgery center
School/college health
Special populations (e.g. lesbian/gay health, Latino health, immigrant health)
Stress management consultant
Women's health
YMCA/YWCA/Boys'/Girls' club

Idemoto, Steel, & Fitzpatrick, 1994), and the success of the role will depend on assertive APNs who insist on practicing nursing rather than simply performing medical tasks that the attending physicians do not want to do. In addition, these nurses must command a salary commensurate with their responsibilities (Dracup & Bryan-Brown, 1994; Edmunds & Ruta, 1991). An alternative way to frame this issue that would market acute care APNs is to persuade the institution to put acute care residents who remain in the intensive care unit under the auspices of the department of nursing, so that nursing would control the hospital stay. Entrepreneurial critical care APNs could gather data justifying this concept in terms of benefit to the client and the institution, and APNs could work along with residents, each providing the service that they are best prepared to provide at the same time improving interdisciplinary collaboration. Once again, maximizing friendly competition and minimizing unfriendly competition is the goal.

MARKETABLE PROPERTIES OF APNs

Realistic self-appraisal of marketable skills is essential, not only for APNs who lose jobs or move to a new area but for all APNs in the current health care environment. APNs cannot develop markets and sell themselves if they do not clearly recognize their unique skills and how these skills can meet client needs. Such an appraisal also helps APNs to determine what areas of practice need to be developed in order to better position themselves for the marketplace. Many NPs are tempted to skip this step because they do not have the time or interest; they may think that the exercise is not valuable (Fitzgerald, 1999). APN entrepreneurs have invested tremendous energy and resources in their careers and owe it to themselves to perform a self-appraisal, a key step in determining one's marketability (Fitzgerald, 1999). Questions that can help APNs make an inventory of their skills and identify opportunities for applying these unique skills might include

1. What motivates me in my practice?
2. What do I do best in my practice?
3. Where do I get the most satisfaction in my practice?
4. What am I most proud of about my practice?
5. Do I have a skill a consumer or organization would pay for?
6. How might I attract a consumer or organization to pay for my skills?

Richard Bolles (1990, 1994) has written prolifically about how an individual can determine his or her best fit in a career and then how to market oneself to attain that goal. Individuals are instructed to formulate a picture of their ideal job by identifying the specific wants and needs that allow them to flourish (Bolles, 1990). By learning how to identify strengths, such as favorite transferable skills, favorite tasks, favorite people with whom to work, and favorite kinds of information with which to work, the APN can identify the unique services she or he has to offer. The first author's experience illustrates the concept of the importance of fit.

E X E M P L A R   1

I was prepared as a CNS in critical care nursing with a master's degree in medical-surgical nursing in 1975. I found a great deal of satisfaction establishing a nurse-managed center for patients with pacemakers. I marketed the concept to the hospital administrators, and it became an excellent revenue source as well as a marketing source for the hospital (Doughty, 1989). Because work with pacemaker patients demanded more primary care skills than I had learned in my graduate program, I completed an additional year in the adult and aging NP track in graduate school. When I moved to Maine in 1983, positions for CNSs were at a minimum. I took a position as a Director of Critical Care Nursing at a tertiary center and employed a new repertoire of management skills in this position. However, I missed direct patient care, and, after 4 years as a nurse executive, I realized I was more creative and satisfied when working directly with patients. I stated an intention to return to the clinical area and started to identify what I loved to do. I saw myself listening to my pacemaker patients' stories and helping them solve problems and create a healthy lifestyle.

Within 1 month I received three job offers. One was as a NP in a holistic obstetrics-gynecology (OB-GYN) practice with another NP and three gynecologists. The notion of listening to women's stories and helping them create health appealed to me to the extent that I volunteered in a family planning clinic to reactivate my gynecology skills. I left my executive position and built a practice at the holistic center. Most of my practice involved working with perimenopausal and menopausal women, and I experienced a great deal of satisfaction from my work. I marketed myself through community lectures and groups for menopausal women as well as in newsletter articles and radio interviews, emphasizing my unique contributions to the public as alternative ways to create health through menopause. Today, I have my own interdisciplinary, holistic women's health center. (The development of this new center, which is the culmination of many dreams, is discussed later in this chapter in the section entitled "Marketing Strategies: Marketing a Service.") I continue to market myself and my new practice through public speaking, interviews, fact sheets, business cards/office stationery, legislative lobbying for increased advanced nursing practice opportunities, and networking with colleagues. I consistently educate my patients about what a NP is, and refer to myself as a NP when addressing individuals or groups.

ADVANCED NURSING PRACTICE, PUBLIC RELATIONS, AND THE MEDIA

Public relations and promotion are closely linked in that promotion incorporates a variety of public relations strategies. Certain public relations barriers need to be addressed in order for the marketing of APN services to be successful:

- *Invisibility of nursing* and a general lack of knowledge about advanced nursing practice
- *Effects of negative publicity* (e.g., inaccurate portrayals of APNs by the American Medical Association [AMA], or adverse publicity, like a nurse being arrested for murdering patients or making a medication error)
- *Traditional images of nurses* in the media

Invisibility of Nursing

Although the American Nurses Association (ANA) and other APN role-specific groups speak for APNs at the national level, APNs have the responsibility to market themselves at the state and local levels by educating legislators, physicians, and consumers about what they are equipped to do. The lack of knowledge about advanced nursing practice in medical schools was boldly illustrated as recently as January 1999 in an issue of the *Reporter,* a monthly publication of the Association of American Medical Colleges. The article was positive about what it referred to as "physician extenders," including physician assistants (PAs) and CNMs. However, any mention of NPs, CRNAs, and CNSs was glaringly absent. The reality is that advanced nursing practice invisibility is a pervasive problem not only among consumers, but among health care professionals as well.

The power of language is also an important contributor to the invisibility factor. When one says the word "doctor," everyone knows what is being talked about. The terms "nurse-midwife" and "nurse anesthetist" are also clear. However, when one says "advanced practice nurse" or "nurse practitioner" or "clinical nurse specialist," many consumers are not only unfamiliar with these terms but oftentimes uncomfortable using them. For example, a young administrator (Marie) was describing her child's health care provider to a nurse researcher who had been an APN. During the conversation, Marie said ''the doctor'' did this, then she did this and this. At the end of Marie's description of her child's visit to the provider, the nurse researcher said, ''Marie, the person you described sounds a lot like a nurse practitioner.'' Marie said with some embarrassment, ''Well . . . she is a nurse practitioner.'' When asked, her only reason for using the term ''doctor'' was that it was easier to say. She realized immediately the impact (invisibility, unintentional invalidation) of not using the appropriate term (e.g., NP, APN). A teachable moment had arisen and a collegial discussion ensued about the power of language and its role in concealing nursing's contributions to health care.

Effects of Negative Publicity

Physician dominance in the health care market and its link to adverse publicity of advanced nursing practice has also proven to be an obstacle to effective marketing for APNs. Fear of encroachment and lack of understanding about what APNs are educated to do has caused some physicians and the AMA to attempt to block legislation permitting nurses to practice within their scope. As health care reform has evolved to override state laws that prohibit APNs from practicing, the barrier of the medical profession itself has become more evident, and the American public has been exposed to ''negative marketing.''

In 1994, the AMA conducted an expensive campaign to convince the public that the quality of health care would be compromised if APNs were ''allowed'' to practice primary care. The nursing profession had a choice as to how to respond, and in the past might have ignored the smear campaign because it could only reflect on the AMA. The media, however, is powerful in presenting a position, and Virginia Trotter Betts, RN, JD (ANA president at the time), used the opportunity to market APNs' safety records. She responded to the AMA board by pointing out how their accusations against their nurse colleagues were inaccurate and ill-advised in the face of the desperate need for primary health care for all Americans. She did not confine her rebuttal to correspondence with the AMA, but also took her message to the popular press: *The Wall Street Journal* and *USA Today*.

From a public relations standpoint, it is crucial that APNs support their medical colleagues who do value and understand the role of APNs and who refuse to participate in the AMA's attempts to discredit APNs. It is important to delineate major differences in practice scope and the range of services that nurses and physicians are prepared to provide (DeAngelis, 1994). APNs also must write to their state and federal representatives and visit them, educating them about nursing's role in health care reform. The ANA and other professional organizations can assist in this process.

Traditional Images of Nurses

Traditional images of nurses in the media show that improved, widespread strategic promotion is a particularly important marketing concept for APNs to grasp. Almost 20 years ago, Kalisch and Kalisch's (1981) classic work on nurses and the media recommended that nursing specialties work with the media to improve their image, that the public be informed that the primary role of the nurse is to promote health and not serve as handmaiden to the physician, and that nurses are knowledgeable and accountable as well as sympathetic caregivers. Although the Kalisch's research was done two decades ago, an inaccurate perception of nursing still exists in many arenas. It is not as simple as blaming the media's traditionally negative images of nursing for the current paucity of nursing coverage in the media. In order to be successful in the evolving health care industry, nurses must be active in promoting positive images of nursing in the mass media. "Without counterbalancing examples of nursing reality in the serious and influential media, the power of trivialized or negative images is enhanced" (Buresh, 1998, p. 72).

Newer research suggests that Americans use the media as their primary source of information about health. "This finding is enormously important to nursing. It means that nursing cannot ignore or underestimate the power of the media to influence nursing's public credibility and prestige both now and well into the 21st century" (Buresh, 1998, p. 69). The public needs to be constantly oriented toward several functions that nurses serve in many settings: nurses promote health, teach prevention, and diagnose and treat common illnesses; specially prepared APNs deliver anesthesia and provide pain management, and provide safe prenatal, intrapartum, and postpartum care, and, finally, nurses broker services for the elderly or chronically ill. To change public perceptions of nursing, APNs must make themselves available to consult with health policy writers, health care journalists, and architects/planning boards and must create more nurse-run health centers.

In April 1998, the CBS network's "60 Minutes" aired a segment entitled "The Nurse Will See You Now." The feature was about CAPNA, the Columbia Advanced Practice Nurses primary care practice in Manhattan. Throughout the segment, the featured APNs answered all of Morley Safer's questions positively, a fine example of avoiding negative marketing techniques. For example, when asked "Why aren't you a doctor?", Edwige Thomas, NP, replied: "I chose to be a nurse. As medicine has progressed, nursing has progressed." APNs were often referred to as "prevention specialists." The focus was on nurses' abilities to engage people, to know their patients well and, as a result, know when things are not normal. Using Columbia University affiliations and fund-raising, Mary Mundinger, dean of the College of Nursing, raised money from various foundations to pay for a $1 million advertising campaign to get the word out about CAPNA. The television commercial featured a voice over with the slogan "Gotta go to CAPNA: Columbia Advanced Practice Nurses . . . Primary Care Specialists." The video footage featured a montage of images including fit, healthy bodies interspersed with the NPs at work. Superimposed words that kept repeating over the images included: "Choices," "Experienced," and "Responsible." Morley Safer concluded the segment citing the results of a 1993 Gallup poll that suggested that 86% of Americans would be willing to have an NP for primary care. (See Table 21-2 for other public relations strategies.)

As health care evolves and comes under scrutiny, more barriers to effective marketing for APNs will arise. Every profession is requiring creative courage directly proportional to the degree of change the profession is experiencing (Baker & Pulcini, 1990). This implies a willingness to go beyond conventional thinking and to perceive barriers as opportunities to rise to the challenge of placing APNs exactly where the client needs their services.

MARKETING STRATEGIES FOR THE NEW GRADUATE

Marketing oneself as a new graduate is one of the most challenging tasks for APNs. The transition period from student to APN provides many exciting new opportunities

TABLE 21–2 MEDIA AND PUBLIC RELATIONS STRATEGIES

Network with health journalists
Gain television news show exposure
Write magazine and journal articles
Send out press releases
Produce public service announcements
Publish research reports
Write for daily newspapers and news magazines
Give radio news interviews
Open a site on the Internet/World Wide Web
Volunteer to give community presentations
Volunteer to work in a free clinic and/or provide free services (e.g., homeless shelter)
Join community organizations
Get involved with politics (e.g., run for public office)

but can also be the source of much anxiety. Helping students through the transition is essential to the success of future marketing ventures.

Brown and Olshansky's (1998) research-based model "Limbo to Legitimacy" takes into account the experiences of the new NP during the first year in primary care practice (see Chapter 4). Stage 1 of this developmental, nonlinear model is relevant to all APNs in the first year of practice and raises important marketing considerations. This stage is characterized by recovering from school, negotiating bureaucracies, looking for a job, and worrying. Maintaining positive self-esteem is key to successful completion of this transition. Bolles (1994) suggested teaching graduates five approaches to sustaining a positive outlook during transitions such as prolonged job searches:

- Keep physically fit by developing an action plan that makes time for positive self-care.
- Deal with emotions by building an effective support network.
- Monitor mental stamina and focus on positive views.
- Build spirituality as a form of support in difficult times.
- Remain active by using time and talents within the community.

According to Payne (1997), the job of executives, recruiters, and faculty is to help new graduates stay open to alternatives in health care. Key elements include helping them to remain enthusiastic, market their unique skills, and understand the need for flexibility. Examples would be encouraging new graduates to view part-time positions as pathways to full-time employment, view cross-training as a challenge, and consider new or unusual job opportunities as pathways to a rewarding professional nursing career.

Developing a Personal Marketing Plan

Accurate self-assessment of strengths as well as conceptualizing a desired practice area are essential first steps in developing a personal marketing plan. Developing a professional marketing portfolio is a useful strategy to aid in this process. A professional portfolio is defined as a representative sample, a collection of documents about who you are professionally and what you have to offer (Vallano, 1999). A portfolio differs from a résumé or curriculum vitae in that, in addition to a listing of all previous positions and educational background, it contains examples of one's work. Professional portfolios contain a description of skills and provide a profile of the applicant and his or her major accomplishments and contributions (see Table 21–3). When a specific position arises that an APN desires, the APN chooses from the portfolio those promotional tools that best relate to that position, such as a résumé listing previous positions and responsibilities, a curriculum vitae listing academic experience and achievements, publications authored by the APN, project results, letters of recommendation from former employers, client and colleague recommendations, honors, awards, and/or ideas for research projects. Restifo (1999) recommends using the portfolio for communicating personal strengths in situations such as performance appraisals, job and return-to-school interviews, presentations, job fairs, and networking sessions. In addition, an APN who is a preceptor to a new graduate can use the portfolio to show career development in her or his specialty.

Scanland (1990) described an excellent example of marketing oneself. She sought a new work environment that provided more flexibility, learning, and growth opportunities and a setting in which she could use both her expertise in geriatrics and her NP skills. She targeted a family practice residency program in the area and gathered data on the gap between the needs of the elderly in that area and the supply of physician services. She contacted the program director and convinced him to hire her to conduct both a clinical practice and resident geriatric education program by matching information from her survey with that from her portfolio.

An APN might also find it useful to include information that helps differentiate between what physicians do and what APNs do. Many studies have been published that describe role differentiation and how primary care, for example, differs when provided by an APN (Kassirer, 1994; Safreit, 1992; Scanland, 1990; Mundinger et al., 2000). Professional organizations such as the ANA, the American Academy of Nurse Practitioners, the American College of Nurse Practitioners, the Oncology Nursing Society, the American College of Nurse-Midwives, and the American Association of Nurse Anesthetists distribute fact sheets or brochures describing the advantages of working with particular APNs. Thus, the portfolio serves as a data bank from which the APN can construct a position-specific marketing tool.

TABLE 21–3 COMPONENTS OF A PROFESSIONAL PORTFOLIO FOR APNs

- Business documents like your resume or curriculum vitae (CV), letters of recommendation, list of references
- Nursing documents such as license, professional certificates, malpractice insurance information, NCLEX results, diplomas and grade transcripts, contact-hour certificates, and continuing-education course information (course descriptions, outlines)
- Identification such as a driver's license, birth certificate, Social Security card, passport, and work visa
- Health information such as PPD or chest x-ray results, immunization record and titers

- Items showing special recognition you've received like honors and awards, newspaper clippings and photos
- Evidence of your teaching including programs, presentation evaluations, lesson plans, and handouts
- Items from your on-the-job work such as performance appraisals, thank-you letters, reports, papers, research findings
- Professional activities including articles or a list of publications, photos (e.g., of posters, exhibits)

From Restifo V. (1999, February 8). Your professional portfolio. *Nursing Spectrum*, p. 17; reprinted with permission.

Contracting Considerations

Obtaining a working knowledge of negotiation skills is the foundation for handling contract considerations. Negotiating and advocating for patients comes much easier than negotiating a new contract, salary, and/or benefits package. Coming from a largely female profession, nurses may be inexperienced negotiators when it comes to self-promotion. Gender differences can play a significant role in negotiating contracts that help APNs achieve their goals (Wyatt, 1999). Nurses need to avoid the "burnt toast" syndrome. In the second author's experience, this syndrome is characterized by maternal, self-effacing behaviors. When mothers in traditional roles prepare breakfast and make the toast, many will keep the burnt piece for themselves and give the nicely done pieces to their family members. Nurses can no longer afford to eat "burnt toast." Robbins' (1998) Negotiation Framework can help nurses become more comfortable with negotiating:

- Step 1: Prepare and plan
- Step 2: Define the ground rules
- Step 3: Clarify and justify
- Step 4: Bargain and problem solve
- Step 5: Close and implement

Learning to negotiate well can mean the avoidance of agreeing to mediocrity and can ensure achieving desired outcomes.

Negotiating a contract is an important marketing skill. Historically, nurses have also been inexperienced with establishing contractual and legal relationships. However, a political and economic reality of the current health care environment is that there is resistance to recognizing APNs as legitimate providers of care. Therefore, the ability to negotiate some type of contract is another skill APNs need to acquire. The three most common contracts for APNs are employment contracts, service contracts, and managed care contracts.

An employment contract (Table 21–4) helps the APN to clarify all parameters of a new position, including clause(s) that outline requirements for ending the professional relationship. The value of an employment contract is still being debated, but, at the very least, some type of written agreement should be drafted. APNs should avoid "non-compete" clauses, which may affect geographic location, patient referrals, and future employment opportunities. In addition, they should be alert to "gag" clauses that might constrain clinical practice or interactions with patients. When contracting with a health care institution, APNs should ensure that practice privileges are clearly outlined to protect the APN-patient relationship if a patient needs to be admitted. The contract will vary according to the nature of individual APN practice, but the goal of negotiating a contract is always to protect the APN through outlining expectations, objectives, and the nature of relationships with those with whom the contract is being formed. APNs must always attend to the certification/licensing requirements in states where they will practice (see Chapter 2).

When negotiating an employment contract/agreement, it is important to know what one wants and needs ahead of time. That might seem obvious, but nurses often do not anticipate and negotiate for important personal and professional benefits. In addition to salary, some suggested items to negotiate include

- Employer-paid malpractice insurance
- Medical, dental, and vision benefits

TABLE 21–4 TERMS OF EMPLOYMENT	

Your contract should include:

1. Official relationship with physician partnership, medical group, or corporation
2. Terms of employment
   Start date
   Probation period
   Criteria for probationary review
   Duration of contract
   Annual review
   Salary increases
3. Clinical responsibilities and supervision
   Supervising/consulting MD
     responsibilities
   Job description or expected duties
   Work hours
   Call hours
   PA/NP cross-coverage
   Work sites
4. Compensation
   Salary and method of calculation
   Bonuses and/or incentives
5. Benefits
   Insurance for self and family
     –Medical
     –Dental
     –Vision
     –Disability
     –Life
     –Automobile
   Medical malpractice coverage
   Retirement plan
6. Business expenses
   State licensure and supervisory fees
   Hospital medical staff fees
   Automobile costs and insurance
   Association dues
   Books and professional journals

7. Vacation and sick time
   Vacation conditions
   Sick leave and limits
   Maternity leave
8. Continuing education
   Conditions and amounts
   Listed separately from vacation
9. Contract renewals and terminations
   Option to renew
   Clinician evaluation criteria
   Termination "for cause" specifics
   Termination "without cause"
     –Notice period
     –Compensation/benefit buyout
10. Other standard clauses
    Contract is total agreement (no verbal agreements accepted—neither contract negotiations nor contract changes)
    Contract modifications must be signed by both parties
    Conduct differing from the contract does not waive the right to uphold all contract clauses
11. Proper signatures with names and title typed below
12. Date of signing

From Woomer, S. (1994). Negotiating an employment contract. *The Clinician's Reference Guide 1994, (a supplement to Clinician Reviews),* pp. 21–28; reprinted with permission.

- Short- and long-term disability
- Life insurance
- Liability insurance
- Vacation
- Continuing education time and funds
- Licensure and certification fees
- Journal subscriptions and textbooks
- Profit sharing, bonuses, and/or incentives
- Retirement vesting
- Practice management issues such as administrative time, call responsibilities, and prescription privileges
- Creative scheduling, such as flex-time and job sharing

In terms of vacation, APNs should aim for the physician standard in the setting/ practice. For continuing education time, they should aim for at least 4 to 5 paid days per year and a minimum of $1,000 for continuing education expenses (Fitzgerald, 1999).

The goal of managed care is to decrease overall health costs and to provide more services for less reimbursement (Levin, 1993). When participating in managed care, a contract is essential to clarify commitments of a position. Table 21-5 lists the key components of a managed care contract. Managed care contracts with providers include an agreement for the APN to provide certain kinds of services for a company,

TABLE 21-5 KEY COMPONENTS OF A MANAGED CARE CONTRACT

Negotiating a contract with a managed care organization (MCO) will demand the assistance of an attorney experienced in negotiating these contracts, since the contract will cover much more than just compensation.

- What is included? What is excluded?
- Requirements for:
  - Utilization management
  - Quality assurance
  - Credentialing
  - Member grievance
  - Recordkeeping
  - Claims submission
  - Hours of operation
  - Appointment response times
  - On-call coverage
  - Employing other providers
  - Arranging backup with other groups
  - Maximum/minimum number of patients
  - Antidisparagement
  - Business confidentiality
- Fee (capitation) schedule
- Special needs programs (carve outs): criteria, process for transfer of care for those eligible
- Stop-loss provisions
- Referral pools
- Withholds
- Level of distribution from withhold/referral pools over prior five years
- Bonus system
- Provisions for closing the practice to additional practice from the MCO
- Claims processing: in-house or contracted out?
- Who does lab work?
- Renewal of contract: based upon? Renewal rate with provider
- MCO's review of office practices
- Directory listing: how will it read?
- Any prohibition on joining other MCOs?
- Definitions of "experimental emergency" and "preexisting condition"
- Who bears the brunt of a mistake in eligibility or coverage determination?
- Can preadmission or referral approval be rescinded retroactively?
- Formulary contents
- System for verifying member eligibility
- Routine for notification of members selecting practice
- Provisions for dispute resolution
- Marketing provided
- Who owns the records/data?

Adapted from Buppert, C. (1999). *Nurse practitioner's business practice and legal guide.* (pp. 259–261, 341–344). Gaithersburg, MD: Aspen Publishers, Inc.; reprinted with permission.

such as pre-employment histories and physical examinations. Provision of health education to employees of a company may or may not include the employee's family members, and this should be clarified by the contract. APNs who work in a health maintenance organization (HMO) have been eliminated by the HMO simply because a large managed care contract refused to recognize the NP as a legitimate provider of care (Baker & Pulcini, 1990). A well-written contract that addressed such contingencies would have protected the APN and prevented the elimination of the role. Newer legislation is continuing to open doors for APNs to ensure they are included in the primary care medical provider panels so that they will be reimbursed.

An important aspect of professional development also includes making an informal contract with oneself to re-evaluate short-term and long-term goals. It is to the APN's advantage to review objectives at least quarterly to determine if she or he is moving along the career path as anticipated and to recommit to the most important criterion for personal satisfaction in a position. A critical component of this contract includes the balance of the physical, intellectual, emotional, and spiritual dimensions and reviewing whether the position is consuming an unbalanced amount of energy. In that case, neither the APN nor the client benefits.

MARKETING CONSIDERATIONS FOR EXPERIENCED APNs

External and Internal Marketing

Two facets of marketing that are useful ways to clarify the role(s) of APNs in every setting include external and internal marketing. *External marketing* refers to all the techniques that APNs might use to promote themselves or their practices to their consumers or the public at large. Suggestions include speaking at community meetings, circulating business cards, writing a column in the newspaper, advertising in the yellow pages, or sending out fliers or brochures about the practice. *Internal marketing* involves differentiating the unique capabilities of APNs in their practice environment and showing how what they have to offer is different from the care provided by anyone else, whether it is of higher quality, more complex, more accessible, or less expensive (Brunk, 1992). Referring to it as a holistic management process, Hallums (1994) described internal marketing as the important work undertaken by an organization to motivate and train its "internal customers" (employees) to work as a unified group to deliver customer service and satisfaction. Grasping the importance of internal marketing is crucial for APNs. Internal marketing strategies are often central to establishing credibility and developing collaborative, interdisciplinary relationships. They can also help to encourage and promote the adoption of evidence-based practice.

In order to research the marketing activities of APNs, the American Academy of Nurse Practitioners surveyed 12,000 NPs (Towers, 1990). A total of 5,964 NPs responded to the survey. Less than half of those responding reported that they marketed themselves; those in rural areas marketed themselves most, those in inner city areas the least. Of those who did market themselves, over 50% used pamphlets. Yellow pages and newspaper advertising were used by less than half of all respondents. A third of the respondents, the highest percentage, reported using special referral arrangements as a marketing strategy. As the results of this survey indicate, APNs may not be using external marketing as effectively as possible.

Capitalizing on creativity is the hallmark of both external and internal marketing for APNs. Tapping into one's creativity often gets overlooked when doing routine care and management of patients. For example, in settings where protocols are standard, it is difficult to "creatively" manage a urinary tract infection. Generally the choices are limited, and in health care it is easy to get stuck in these narrow ways of thinking. The second author used a unique, creative internal marketing strategy that was very successful.

E X E M P L A R   2

While working in a multispecialty group practice in the Southwest several years ago, my NP/PA colleagues and I met regularly to discuss practice issues. As a group, we decided it was necessary to educate physicians, administrators, and clinical and clerical support staff about the role of NPs/PAs in our organization. We put together a presentation called "A Day in the Life of an NP and a PA." With a total of 85 physicians and 13 NPS/PAs in the practice, we felt it was very important for the entire medical staff and top administration to be in attendance. The best forum for our program was at our health center's monthly medical and administrative staff meeting. This presentation was a first within the organization. We knew two things: first, this might be our *only* chance to capture the attention of our physician and administrative colleagues, and second, the presentation had to be extremely well done in order to enhance our credibility.

After much brainstorming, we came up with a creative, humorous, and informative program. We made a list of the most memorable questions we had been asked in our careers as NPs/PAs, such as "What do all those letters after your name mean?", "When are you going to become a doctor?", "Do I have to pay the full $5.00 co-pay to see you instead of a doctor?", "I am so confused . . . what is the difference between an NP and a PA?", and "As an NP, are you the one who stands in the room with the doctor when he does a Pap smear?" We then enlisted the help of our collaborative physicians to serve as "plants" in our audience. Each collaborating physician was provided with the question that was to be addressed by the NP/PA in her or his dyad. "Dyad" was the term we had mutually chosen with our medical director to define the relationship between each NP or PA provider and her or his collaborating physician in our practice. We felt this dyad recognition in our presentation was important because some of the physicians had historically been uncomfortable referring patients to NPs and PAs if they were not aware of the dyad arrangement. The overall mood was humorous and informal. On cue during the program, each physician "plant" stood up and asked the question assigned to her or him. The corresponding NP or PA would then answer the question with factual information illustrating the role of the NP or PA. For example, in response to the question "When are you going to become a doctor?", a NP replied with enthusiasm about positive reasons for choosing to be an APN instead of a physician. In response to "As an NP, are you the one who stands in the room with the doctor when he does a Pap smear?", I addressed the need for consumer education and widespread external and internal marketing of APNs. Other issues that were addressed in our question-answer format were the educational requirements for NPs and PAs, quality-of-service issues, and the role of NPs and PAs as primary care providers.

Prior to the start of the program, the NPs and PAs were seated in front of the audience with large name tags and each was given the opportunity to introduce herself or himself in a brief biographical format (e.g., name, department, site, collaborating physician name, education, related work/volunteer background, and special interests clinically and personally). Many of the staff members had never met each other, so this was a great opportunity for recognition and networking. The feedback we received was tremendous. Many physicians, administrators, and human resources representatives made a special point to thank us for a most informative and interesting program. Overall, internal referrals to NPs and PAs increased and further marketing projects were launched. As an outgrowth of this program, we did a training for receptionists and medical assistants about the role of NPs and PAs in health care. The result was more appropriately scheduled appointments and no more overhearing receptionists saying, "You can't see the doctor today, *just* the NP or PA. Sorry!" The most important outcome of this marketing effort of all was my appointment as the first APN on the medical center's new board of directors. In this setting, we needed to start with aggressive internal marketing strategies before branching out to external strategies. Do not assume that your administrators and physician colleagues have any idea what you do!

MARKETING STRATEGIES: MARKETING A SERVICE

Eighty percent of all new products fail in the open market (Gardner & Weinrauch, 1988). Survival of small businesses depends on several critical factors (Gardner & Weinrauch, 1988):

- Accurate identification of consumer needs
- Financial resources
- Timing of entry into the workplace
- Planning for growth to meet further demands

Accentuation of how a proposed service differs from that provided by others is important. These services may include such things as higher quality, more accessibility, or different hours of service. Services targeted toward specific market segmentation data, such as retirement centers, hospital staff, individuals living with chronic pain, or new mothers needing breast-feeding counseling, help the APN to tailor marketing plans for success based on client needs. The first author offers the following experience of identifying and marketing a service to a targeted population.

E X E M P L A R   3

As a NP in a holistic OB-GYN practice, I recognized a need in the community for midlife women to have access to information about whether to take hormones or herbs, how to improve quality of life, and how to prevent problems of aging that start in midlife. Certain obstacles prevented universal access in that practice, and I dreamed of an interdisciplinary holistic center on a bus line with a fund for indigent women and handicapped accessibility. Intrinsic to my dream was the concept of circle leadership among the disciplines without a medical hierarchy, consistent with the work of Christina Baldwin (1994). According to Baldwin, "The circle is an organizational structure that locates leadership along the rim and provides an inclusive means for consultation. Circling is a useful structure for learning, governance, creating community, providing services, and observing ritual" (1994, p. 34).

After a year of planning with a nurse massage therapist and a highly skilled medical receptionist, I completed the business plan and went to the bank. I hoped to get partial funding as a business loan and to secure a personal loan for the remainder of the start-up costs. The bank was so impressed with the marketing projections and data in the business plan that they funded the entire start-up cost.

Critical to the success of the women's center was the agreement of a close friend and colleague, another experienced women's health NP with a background in business and a master's degree in business administration, to buy in as a partner. Many of the business decisions that had to be made in the infancy of the practice were tempered with expertise and practical orientation. She believed in the vision, and she and I remained connected to the constant question, "How will this decision affect the women who want our services?"

Initially, the other disciplines included massage, mental health, movement, and nutrition. We recruited a physical therapist and a gynecologist. We sat in "circle" weekly to discuss how the center was doing and how we were doing with the center. We held retreats quarterly to bond as a team. A naturopath also joined our group. Our marketing efforts are detailed in Table 21–6.

Obstacles to third-party reimbursement for APN autonomous practice in Maine precipitated legislation to ensure reimbursement. The state NP group hired a lobbyist and forged this legislation. My business partner was extremely active in this effort, gathering data and testimonials. Prior data that had been generated on cost and efficacy influenced the banking and insurance committee, who first heard the bills. Patient testimonials were what convinced all involved that APNs made a difference and needed to have separate identification numbers and reimbursement. A unanimous vote for eligibility for reimbursement for certified NPs and CNMs went from the committee to both houses, where it passed without debate.

Marketing a service effectively depends on making others aware of its unique features. It is helpful to gather data on how clients discovered a service so that future energy and resources can be channeled into what is known to be successful.

TABLE 21–6 MARKETING EFFORTS FOR HOLISTIC OB-GYN PRACTICE

Marketing the concept to the bank for start-up costs
The business plan included detailed data based on experience as well as income projections.
Marketing to the community
1. Other providers
   • Contracts with three gynecologists to provide backup care on an urgent basis
   • Community letters and meetings with internists and gynecologists about the niche our service provided to help women with complex midlife needs or hormone therapy that was not working
   • Meetings with a community breast surgeon, oncologist, and nurse practitioners about complex menopausal symptom relief for women who could not take estrogen
2. Potential women clients
   • Open houses highlighting the services of the center
   • Day-long workshops presented by the team about midlife issues. Topics included
     –Osteoporosis: Reframing Your Frame
     –Heart Disease: Finding Your Heart's Desire
     –Mental Clarity: Mysteries of the Menopausal Mind
     –The Joy of Soy: Cooking with Soy Made Easy
   • Free monthly menopause support group supported by the American Menopause Foundation, which helped market to area media
   • Multiple community education workshops and lectures to YWCA, women in business, insurance executives
   • Lunch meetings and tours through center
   • Newspaper stories featuring third-party reimbursement hassles for an APN practice
   • Newspaper columns about women's health
   • Newspaper advertisement
   • Yellow pages advertisement
   • Promotional Fact Sheet about center (see Figure 21–1)
3. Other APNS who wanted to start similar practices
   • Reprints about the practice
   • Panel discussions with slide show at state APN meetings
   • Meetings, tours, and opportunities for shadowing in the practice (professional fee charged for time spent with us)
   • Lectures to the university NP programs in the city
   • Preceptor to one ANP graduate student each semester

Brochures, articles in the newspaper, newsletters, letterhead stationery, business cards, flyers, personal interviews with the media, and group community classes all help promote a unique service (Figure 21-1). Yellow pages advertising is expensive, so it is wise to routinely audit how often clients use the yellow pages to initiate contact. Groups such as Rotary, American Association of Retired Persons, American Association of University Women, Junior League, and Kiwanis often invite speakers to address health topics. These opportunities allow the APN not only to promote a service but to clarify misinformation about APNs. Joining professional and civic organizations is an important part of marketing a service as well, and the opportunity to sit on a board of directors or a health-related committee does much to enhance one's professional reputation.

Writing a Successful Business Plan

Although writing a successful business plan is not usually a component of traditional advanced nursing practice curricula, it is a vital aspect of the entrepreneurial move-

---

NEW ENGLAND WOMENCENTER
FACT SHEET

WHAT?
New England Womencenter is an interdisciplinary women's health center offering nurse practitioner, medical doctor, and naturopathic doctor services, massage, psychotherapy, movement, exercise, and yoga. We are dedicated to meeting the needs of women of all ages and specialize in midlife and menopausal issues.

FOR WHOM?
Women of all ages with varied needs come to New England Womencenter.

- Women who want to develop their own plan of wellness with the help of our center's practitioners and therapists.
- Women who want to explore their options for health. Many women come to the center because of our specialty in menopausal issues and expertise in prescribing plant-based hormones.
- Women who are having their first gyn exam or have been hesitant to have this exam due to past experiences.
- Women who are interested in either beginning psychotherapy or continuing their exposure to therapy.
- Women who are interested in movement, self-defense, yoga, or exercise.
- Women who are having their first massage or who enjoy regular massage.

WHO ARE WE?
   SUSAN DOUGHTY, RN, CS, MSN, NP
   KATHLEEN COLEMAN, RNC, MSN, ANP
   JEAN CURRAN, MD, PA
   PRISCILLA SKERRY, ND
   ALLISON BASILE, LCPC, MMT
   JERI LYNN SCHROEDER, MS, MA, LCPC
   LENORA TRUSSELL, RN, CPK

Location in the Old Port ● 66 Pearl Street. Portland, Maine. Free & covered parking in the area . . . We have luncheon and evening hours . . . Workshops, classes, newsletter appointments, support groups. Office or telephone consultations . . . Accepting BCBS & other.

CALL 207-761-4700 (761-4744 fax)

FIGURE 21-1 • Promotional fact sheet for New England Womencenter.

ment in advanced nursing practice. According to Haag (1997), approximately 1 million new businesses are started each year in the United States alone. Of those 1 million new businesses, only about one in five will survive to see their fifth anniversary. "A business owner who fails to plan, plans to fail" (Covello & Hazelgren, 1995). The process of writing a business plan includes the following steps (Haag, 1997, p. 26):

• Define the business concept.
• Gather data on the feasibility and specifics of the concept.
• Focus and refine the concept.
• Outline the specifics of the business.
• Put the plan in compelling form.

Many "how-to" guides exist on what critical elements to include in a business plan (see Table 21–7 for more information).

It is helpful for the APN to remember that people usually will not appreciate what a professional does unless they are educated to the facts (Abraham, 1994). People want to know more about unique services, yet potential employers may have no concept of the expertise APNs could bring to their businesses or practices and would never advertise for one (Weill et al., 1989). In fact, once employers work with APNs, they often wonder how they ever got along without one. APNs have many strengths that increase their marketability, and these strengths are rooted in basic nursing practice.

Presenting oneself to the medical community is an important marketing strategy in promoting a service. Having self-confidence about one's skills and knowing one's particular areas of expertise and limits help to communicate a willingness for collaboration. Establishing credibility with regard to one's competency and abilities is essential. Inaccurate reports about NPs taking away paying patients as well as the less insured are common, as are unsupported accounts of practice errors and poor management of client problems. Successful APN-physician collaboration helps alleviate such fears (see Chapter 11). When one is outlining possible benefits to physicians for including an APN in their referral network, it is important to stress unique areas of expertise: prevention, counseling, education, and the ability to see patients with special, time-consuming needs.

In her quest for "the best fit," Levin (1993) developed a solo practice born out of the idea that what was needed was not more health care but an alternative type of health care for women that was different from the existing medical model in her

TABLE 21–7 BUSINESS PLAN COMPONENTS
Cover/Title Page
Executive Summary
Table of Contents
Business Description and History
Business Structure
Product/Service Description
Market Analysis and Strategy (Plan)
Operations
Management Team
Financial Data/Projections
Appendix

From Haag, A. B. (1997). Writing a successful business plan. *AAOHN Journral, 45*(1), 27; reprinted with permission.

community. She identified the specific strengths she possessed that would enable her to succeed. These strengths included self-confidence, comfort in dealing with other health care providers as colleagues, accountability, enjoyment in marketing herself to the lay and medical communities, flexibility, and patience. She attributed her success to her business plan, which included advantages over the competition, and the uniqueness of her nursing-based practice.

Consumer Marketing

It is important to use every opportunity to remind clients that they are receiving good care because APNs are specially prepared to provide this care. Also, the office staff has a role in helping APNs in this process by having a critical understanding of the APN's uniqueness and skills and sharing that knowledge with the public. Being able to describe the differences and complementary aspects of APNs in comparison to other providers is essential. When APNs deal with pharmaceutical reps, it is important to educate the sales representative about the difference between what an APN does and what a physician does. Reps should be asked to have APNs included as providers in their patient-oriented product brochures. To constantly see the word "doctor," such as "see your doctor with any questions," sends a distinct message to potential clients, health policy decision makers, and legislators (Smithing & Wiley, 1990). Finally, a critically important endorsement for the nursing profession is for the APN to be sure to use an APN for personal as well as for family care.

Avoiding Common Marketing Mistakes

In 1989, Weill and colleagues projected that the biggest obstacle to future viability of the APN's role was lack of consumer awareness and minimal demand for preventive services as a result of inadequate marketing by APNs. Today, we are experiencing a greater demand for preventive services and yet a lack of consumer awareness about the APN role remains. An understanding of this notion, a strong belief in oneself and in the APN role, and a strong understanding of one's own APN philosophy are critical to reversing this trend and enhancing marketing time and energy. When marketing a service, it is important to avoid the common marketing mistakes noted by Abraham (1994) by doing the following:

1. Be sure to audit which particular strategies provide the best return (Calmelat, 1993).
2. Continuously ascertain and develop unique services.
3. Be sure to differentiate from the competition.
4. Always give clients a reason to return for repeat services.
5. Address clients' needs as a priority.
6. Educate and inform clients about any changes made in the practice, such as an increase in prices.
7. Maintain enjoyment in providing the service. Avoid burnout.

CONCLUSION

Marketing oneself and one's services is critical to the survival of APNs and might well influence the future of the nursing profession itself. As the health care environment changes, clients are becoming sophisticated about what they want as well as about what they need. APNs must become familiar enough with marketing concepts and be flexible enough so that they can position themselves to meet client needs. As a result of successful marketing strategies, clients will not only request APNs, they will demand their services, recognizing the value they provide in the ever-expanding and complex world of health care.

REFERENCES

Abraham, J. (1994). *The Abraham experience.* Rolling Hills Estates, CA: Citation Publishing Group, Inc.

Baker, M. M., & Pulcini, J. A. (1990). Innovation: Nurse practitioners as entrepreneurs. *Nurse Practitioner Forum, 1*(3), 169–174.

Baldwin, C. (1994). *Calling the circle.* Newburgh, OR: Swan-Raven & Company.

Bolles, R. N. (1990). *How to create a picture of your ideal job or next career.* Berkeley, CA: Ten Speed Press.

Bolles, R. N. (1994). *What color is your parachute?* Walnut Creek, CA: Ten Speed Press.

Brandenburger, A. M., & Nalebuff, B. J. (1996). *Co-Opetition.* New York: Doubleday.

Brown, M., & Olshansky, E. (1998). Becoming a primary care nurse practitioner: Challenges of the initial year of practice. *Nurse Practitioner, 23*(7), 46, 52–66.

Brunk, Q. (1992). The clinical nurse specialist as an external consultant: A framework for practice. *Clinical Nurse Specialist, 6*(1), 2–4.

Buresh B. (1998, Spring). Extra!: Healthcare forms new media partnership—nursing must participate. *Revolution—The Journal of Nurse Empowerment,* pp. 68–75.

Calmelat, A. (1993). Tips for starting your own nurse practitioner practice. *Nurse Practitioner, 18*(4), 58, 61, 64, 67–68.

Caveen, W., Cheshire, L., Power, B., & Woolley, D. (1992). Grasping the marketing nettle: A professional development course for nurse practitioners in stoma care. *Professional Nurse, 7,* 580, 582, 584–585.

Clochesy, J. M., Daly, B. J., Idemoto, B. K., Steel, J., & Fitzpatrick, J. J. (1994). Preparing advanced practice nurses for acute care. *American Journal of Critical Care, 3*(4), 255–259.

Coile, R. C. (1999). The Three C's: Consumerism, Cyberhealth, and Co-Opetition. In R. Gilkey (Ed.), *The 21st century health care leader* (pp. 3–21). San Francisco: Jossey-Bass.

Covello, J., & Hazelgren, B. (1995). *Your first business plan.* Naperville, IL: Sourcebooks, Inc.

Curtin, L. (1985). Survival of the slickest. *Nursing Management, 16*(2), 7–8.

DeAngelis, C. D. (1994). Nurse practitioner redux. *JAMA, 271,* 868–871.

Doughty, S. (1989). The CNS in a nurse managed center. In A. Hamric & J. Spross (Eds.), *The clinical nurse specialist in theory and practice* (pp. 415–434). Philadelphia: W. B. Saunders.

Dracup, K., & Bryan-Brown, C. (1994). The advanced practice nurse in critical care: Yes or no? *American Journal of Critical Care, 3*(31), 163.

Edmunds, M. W. (1991). After 26 years, it's time for "NP" to be a household name. *Nurse Practitioner, 16*(11), 59.

Edmunds, M. W., & Ruta, M. V. (1991). NPS who replace physicians: Role expansion or exploitation? *Nurse Practitioner, 16*(9), 46, 49.

Fitzgerald, M. A. (1999). Negotiating your future: Employment, contract and practice issues for the nurse practitioner. *Clinical Letter for Nurse Practitioners, 3*(3), 1–11.

Gardner, K., & Weinrauch, D. (1988). Marketing strategies for nurse entrepreneurs. *Nurse Practitioner, 13*(5), 46, 48–49.

Haag, A. B. (1997). Writing a successful business plan. *AAOHN Journal, 45*(1), 25–32.

Hallums, A. (1994). Internal marketing within a health care organization: Developing an implementation plan. *Journal of Nursing Managmeent, 2,* 135–142.

James, J. (1994). *Building a twenty-first century mind.* Speech before the American Association of Colleges of Nursing NTI. Atlanta, GA.

Kalisch, P. A., & Kalisch, B. J. (1981). Communicating clinical nursing issues through the newspaper. *Nursing Research, 30*(3), 132–138.

Kassirer, J. P. (1994). What role for nurse practitioners in primary care? *New England Journal of Medicine, 330*(3), 204–205.

Keane, A., Richmond, T., & Kaiser, L. (1994). Critical care nurse practitioner: Evolutions of the advanced practice role. *American Journal of Critical Care, 3*(3), 232–237.

Levin, T. E. (1993). The solo nurse practitioner: A private practice model. *Nurse Practitioner Forum, 4*(3), 158–164.

Luckacs, J. L. (1984). Marketing strategies for competitive advantage. *Nurse Practitioner, 9*(9), 37, 38, 40.

Payne, M. E. (1997, July/August). Counselling new graduates to find jobs. *Recruitment, Retention & Restructuring Report,* pp. 4–7.

Restifo, V. (1999, February 8). Your professional portfolio. *Nursing Spectrum,* p. 17.

Robbins, S. (1998). *Organizational Behavior* (8th ed.). Englewood Cliffs, NJ: Prentice-Hall.

Safreit, B. J. (1992). Health care dollars and regulatory sense: The role of advanced practice nursing. *Yale Journal on Regulation, 9*(2), 417–487.

Scanland, S. (1990). What's happening: The nurse teaches the doc. *Journal of the American Academy of Nurse Practitioners, 2*(4), 174–177.

Shoultz, J., Hatcher, P. A., & Hurrell, M. (1992). Growing edges of a new paradigm: The future of nursing in the health of the nation. *Nursing Outlook, 40*(2), 57–61.

Smithing, R. T., & Wiley, M. D. (1990). Marketing and management. See your physician. *Journal of the American Academy of Nurse Practitioners, 2*(1), 38.

Towers, J. (1990). Report of the national survey of the American Academy of Nurse Practitioners, Part IV: Practice characteristics and marketing activities of nurse practitioners. *Journal of the American Academy of Nurse Practitioners, 2*(4), 164–167.

Vallano, A. (1999). *Kaplan careers in nursing: Managing your future in the changing world of healthcare.* (pp. 153–154). New York: Kaplan Educational Center and Simon & Schuster.

Weill, J. A., Love, M. G., Pron, A. L., Tesoro, T. A., Grey, M., Hickel, M., Teti, B. S., & Serota, J. (1989). Future potential, phase I: Nurse practitioners look at themselves. *Journal of Pediatric Health Care, 3*(2), 76–82.

Wyatt, D. (1999, January). Negotiation strategies for men and women. *Nursing Management,* 22–25.

Additional Readings

Ball, G. B. (1990). Perspectives on developing, marketing, and implementing a new clinical specialist position. *Clinical Nurse Specialist, 4*(1), 33–36.

Boccuzzi, N. K. (1998). CAPNA: A new development to increase quality in primary care. *Nursing Administration Quarterly, 22*(4), 11–19.

Buppert, C. (1999, February 8). Malpractice insurance: To have or to have not? *Nursing Spectrum (New England Edition),* pp. 13–14.

Burgess, S. E., & Misener, T. R. (1997). The professional portfolio: An advanced practice nurse job search marketing tool. *Clinical Excellence for Nurse Practitioners, 1,* 468–471.

Cawley, J. F. (1998). Whither independence? *Clinician News, 2*(1), 40.

Crow, G. (1998). The entrepreneurial personality: Building a sustainable future for self and the profession. *Nursing Administration Quarterly, 22*(2), 30–35.

Curtin, L. (1993). Barbarians at the gate. *Nursing Management, 24*(12), 9–10.

Gelman, E. (1999, January 5). Be prepared—with a master's degree [editorial]. *Patient Care for the Nurse Practitioner,* p. 5.

Giordano, B. P. (1994). Watch out for "friendly fire" from our medical allies! *AORN Journal, 59*(2), 360, 362.

Hau, M. L. (1997). Ten common mistakes to avoid as an independent consultant. *AAOHN Journal, 45*(1), 17–22.

Henry, P. F. (1996). Analysis of the nurse practitioner's legal relationships. *Nurse Practitioner Forum, 7*(1), 5–6.

Hodges, L. C., Satkowski, T. C., & Ganchorre, C. (1998). Career opportunities for doctoral-prepared nurses. *MEDSURG Nursing, 7*(2), 114–120.

Kowal, N. (1998). Specialty practice entrepreneur: The advanced practice nurse. *Nursing Economics, 16*(5), 277–278.

Leccese, C. (1998, January). Who's making what—and where? *Advance for Nurse Practitioners,* pp. 30–35.

MacDonahue, D. (1997). Interviewing hints. *Massachusetts Nurse, 67*(9), 9, 14.

Manthey, M., & Avery, M. D. (1996). Remembering the nurse in the business of advanced practice. *Advanced Practice Nursing Quarterly, 2*(1), 49–54.

Monahan, B. B. (1996). The nurses media handbook: A reference for nurses planning to meet the media . . . first in a two part series. *Massachusetts Nurse, 66*(5), 2, 6, 12.

Niederlitz, P. (1997). Laid off? What's next? The job search process. *AORN Journal, 66*(3), 502–503.

Nolan, C. M., Conway, L. G., Litteer, T. B., Peterson–Sweeney, K., Richardson, K., Smith, S. W., & Stoler, P. M. (1988). Marketing strategies of nurse practitioners in New York State. *Nurse Practitioner, 13*(8), 37, 41–42.

Pearson, L. J. (1999). Stands on legislative issues affecting advanced nursing practice. *Nurse Practitioner, 24*(1), 18–24.

Porter-O'Grady, T. (1998). The private practice of nursing: The gift of entrepreneurialism. *Nursing Administration Quarterly, 22*(2), 23–29.

Price, J. L. (1998). A reflective approach to career trajectory in advanced practice nursing. *Advanced Practice Nursing Quarterly, 3*(4), 35–39.

Scarano, R. M. (1998). PA/NP practice and contract law: Avoiding pitfalls of managed care. *Clinician Reviews, 2*(1), 33.

Schaffner, R. J., & Bohomey, J. (1998). Demonstrating APN value in a capitated market. *Nursing Economics, 16*(2), 69–74.

Schneider, B. (1997). Have you thought of entering business as an entrepreneur or intrapreneur, a satisfying alternative career in nursing? *Washington Nurse, 27*(2), 45.

Sebas, M. B. (1994). Developing a collaborative practice agreement for the primary care setting. *Nurse Practitioner, 19*(3), 49-51.

Selph, A. K. (1998). Negotiating an acute care nurse practitioner position. *AACN Clinical Issues, 9*(2), 269-276.

Shamansky, S. L., Schilling, L. S., & Holbrook, T. L. (1985). Determining the market for nurse practitioner services: The New Haven experience. *Nursing Research, 34*(4), 242-247.

Shepard, P. M. (1997). Medicine and the Internet. *Clinician News, 1*(2), 12, 14-15.

Sherrod, D. R. (1997). Advising nursing students in a tightened job market. *Journal of Nursing Education, 36*(7), 344-346.

Simpson, R. L. (1998). From nursing to nursing informatics consultant: A lesson in entrepreneurship. *Nursing Administration Quarterly, 22*(2), 87-90.

Sloan, A. J. (1995). Employment contracts—who needs them? (Parts I and II). *Virginia Nurses Today, 3*(4), 28, 30; *3*(5), 20-21.

Smithing, R. T., & Wiley, M. D. (1989). Marketing and management. Marketing: An issue of particular relevance to nurse practitioners. *Journal of the American Academy of Nurse Practitioners, 1*(1), 33.

Smithing, R. T., & Wiley, M. D. (1989). Marketing and management. Marketing techniques in print. *Journal of the American Academy of Nurse Practitioners, 1*(3), 103-104.

Smithing, R. T., & Wiley, M. D. (1990). Marketing and management. Marketing techniques in person. *Journal of the American Academy of Nurse Practitioners, 2*(2), 88-89.

Stahler-Miller, K. (1987). *Marketing yourself: How to make your excellence visible.* Workshop held at the Maine Medical Center, Portland, August.

Steiger, N., Hagenstad, R., & Anderson, A. (1996). Budget development and implementation for the APN in independent practice. *Advanced Practice Nursing Quarterly, 2*(1), 41-48.

Straka, D. A. (1996). Are you your resume? *Advanced Practice Nursing Quarterly, 2*(1), 75-77.

Thomas, B. (1997). A successful job search begins with a realistic resume and a positive approach to the market. *AORN Journal, 66*(4), 702-703.

Waldrop, J. B. (1999, April). Getting the word out. *The Clinical Advisor,* p. 84.

Ward, R. (1998). Public relations for advanced practice nurses. *AWHONN Lifelines, 2*(5), 47-48.

Waxman, K. T. (1998, August). Marketing your skills outside the hospital walls. *Nursing Management,* pp. 48-51.

White, K. R., & Begun, J. W. (1998). Nursing entrepreneurship in an era of chaos and complexity. *Nursing Administration Quarterly, 22*(2), 40-47.

Woomer, S. (1994). Negotiating an employment contract. *The Clinician's Reference Guide 1994 (a supplement to Clinician Reviews),* 21-28.

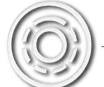

Understanding the Regulatory and Credentialing Requirements for Advanced Practice Nursing

• C H A R L E N E   M .   H A N S O N

INTRODUCTION

Impressive strides have been made over time in the areas of credentialing and regulation of advanced practice nurses (APNs). The health care provided by APNs has had far-reaching effects on members of society, and thus the evolution of advanced nursing practice in the United States is a source of pride to nurses. However, with success comes ever higher accountability and the need for more standardized ways to credential, certify, regulate, and sanction competent practice for a growing number of APNs. At both federal and state levels, this is a time of shifting priorities and changing models for nursing practice in all settings. It is an environment in which any discussion of regulatory issues is, by definition, fluid, dynamic, and subject to rapid change. APNs must influence health policy at both national and grassroots levels to assure regulatory configurations that allow for successful APN practice and reimbursement. It may be as simple as interpreting health policy decisions to patients and co-workers locally, or as complex as hammering out equitable regulatory decisions about reimbursement with the Health Care Financing Administration (HCFA) in Washington, DC.

The challenge to provide standards of quality upon which advanced nursing practice can be framed, defended, and regulated is a serious one that requires constant attention. Issues involving education, scope of practice, specialty practice, reimbursement, and prescriptive authority are all embedded in regulatory language. To make the problem more difficult, regulatory issues are governed by multiple federal, state, educational, and professional entities whose work occurs in different venues complicating efforts to collaborate (Hanson, 1998). The complexity of regulatory issues and the multiplicity of stakeholders are the bases for recommendations by the Pew Health Professions Commission that national policy initiatives are urgently needed to research, develop, and publish national scopes of practice and continuing competency standards for state legislatures to implement (O'Neil et al., 1998).

This chapter describes basic national and state credentialing and regulatory realities and provides a discussion of the critical elements of health policy and regulation that currently face APNs. (Chapter 23 deals with major health policy issues confronting health care providers and consumers nationally.) In reading this chapter, it is important to understand that, for specific questions about up-to-the-minute, current APN rules and regulations, especially those that pertain to specific state statutes regarding ANP prescriptive authority and reimbursement, the reader is referred to individual local and state regulatory bodies for practice requirements.

Finally, the skills required for successful policy activism and advocacy, which are crucial to negotiating regulatory mechanisms, are part of the APN core competency of clinical and professional leadership. The concepts and skills outlined in Chapters 10 and 11 are crucial to the role APNs play in setting credentialing and regulation policy mechanisms and should be considered when reading this chapter.

CURRENT PRACTICE CLIMATE FOR APNs

The appropriate use of APNs during an era of unsettled health care change is an important issue that needs serious and thoughtful deliberation about practice and education as we move into the new century. This fit requires an in-depth study of the entire milieu that affects APNs. The differences in education, certification, and individual scope of practice regulations from one advanced nursing specialty to another complicate issues for policy makers and regulators. The climate within nursing practice is also greatly affected by what is happening in other health care disciplines. For example, the move toward managed care and away from solo specialty medical practice continues to have implications for APNs (Rentmeester & Kindig, 1994). Currently, the combined health care needs of an aging population, a period of economic retrenchment in health care, and the movement of both the public and private sectors of health care to a managed care environment have fostered a positive trend for advanced nursing practice. Community-based health care systems that rely on interdisciplinary health care team approaches have positively affected APN specialties but in some instances have heightened tensions between the disciplines of medicine and nursing. Health policy issues surrounding practice parameters, reimbursement, and choice of provider require careful consideration. All of these environmental phenomena have an impact, either directly, or indirectly, on the credentialing and regulatory policies that govern APN practice. Therefore, it is incumbent upon individual APNs to understand and practice within the parameters of these mechanisms.

Nursing's earliest efforts to establish professional identity for APNs focused on advancing APN education as well as gaining independence over nursing practice and autonomy from the medical community. These efforts were critical to the evolution of advanced practice in nursing, and great strides have been made over the years. The reality of the complex health care system and the needs of a patient population that requires a multifaceted approach to multiple problems stress interdisciplinary team-building. This does not imply "parallel play" or working side by side, but requires a true blending of nursing and medical models to offer a comprehensive health care approach. Larger teams of health care providers need to collaborate to provide comprehensive care to families and whole communities. However, to be able to move forward as full-fledged team members in cooperation with other interdisciplinary health care providers, APNs need to shift their practice ideal from one of complete autonomy to a truly collegial interdisciplinary paradigm. This change in practice stance is necessary. Does any health care professional, including the most renowned vascular surgeon, practice with full independence? Or does this surgeon call upon the internist, the clinical nurse specialist (CNS), and the physical therapist to assist with providing competent and expert care? Will APNs do themselves a disservice if they maintain an isolationist stance based on barriers and past professional turf issues? Have APNs reached a point in their evolution at which they can feel comfortable as peers and colleagues with providers in other disciplines?

When APNs seek to change statutes and regulations it is not because they see themselves as needing to practice in a vacuum of independence apart from the rest of the health care team. It is a hard fact that APNs must have authority over their own practices and the decisions they make about patient care. Only in this way can APNs move out of the darkness of being, as Wilcox (1995) stated, a "shadow provider." This is the challenge for APNs across the nation who are working to clarify statutory policies within state boards of nursing. It may be that APNs will feel comfortable only when their position within the health care community is fully secure in all states, and this will require serious political and legislative work related to credentialing and regulatory issues.

SCOPE OF PRACTICE FOR APNs

By definition, scope of practice describes practice limits and sets the parameters within which nurses in the various APN specialties may practice. Scope statements define what APNs can do for/with patients, what they can delegate, and when collaboration with others is required. Scope of practice statements tell APNs de facto what is beyond the limits of their nursing practice. The scope of practice for each APN specialty group is explicated in Chapters 13 through 19. Scope-of-practice statements are key to the debate about how the U.S. health care system uses APNs as health care providers; scope is inextricably linked with barriers to advanced nursing practice. The ability to diagnose and manage clients that is inherent to the role of the APN is fluid and evolving, and is in many instances tied to the collaborative relationships that APNs have with physician colleagues. Certified registered nurse anesthetists (CRNAs), who administer general anesthesia, have a markedly different scope of practice from that of the primary care nurse practitioner (NP), for example, although both have their roots in generic nursing. In addition, it is important to understand that scope of practice differs from state to state and is based on state statutes promulgated by the various state nurse practice acts and the rules and regulations for APN practice. On the Internet, scope-of-practice statements can be found by searching state government Web pages in the areas of licensing boards, nursing, and APN rules and regulations.

Accountability becomes a crucial factor as APNs move toward authority over their own practices. First, it is important that scope-of-practice statements identify the scope of each APN role. Furthermore, it is crucial that scope-of-practice statements that are presented by national certifying entities are carried through in scope-of-practice language in state statutes. APNs must recognize state variances to scope of practice in a highly mobile society. This factor is discussed more fully later in this chapter in the section "A Wave of the Future: Telehealth/Telepractice."

APNs owe Barbara Safriet, Associate Dean at Yale Law School, a debt of gratitude for her clear vision and clarity in helping APNs understand and think strategically about scope-of-practice and regulatory issues. In her landmark 1992 monograph, Safriet noted that APNs are unique in that there is a multiprofessional approach to their regulation based on ignorance and the fallacy that medicine is all-knowing and knows all about advanced nursing practice. Restraints result from ignorance about APN abilities, rigid notions about professional roles, and turf protection.

> *States have used a variety of approaches to extend the scope of practice of nursing. Some have revised their Nurse Practice Acts (NPAs) to delete the absolute prohibition on diagnosis and treatment, or to add "nursing diagnosis." Some have added an "additional acts" clause to the NPA, authorizing some specially trained nurses to "perform acts of medical diagnosis and treatment" as specified by rules of the state nursing and/or medical boards or as "agreed upon by the professions of nursing and medicine." Some have added a generic category, or specific categories, of advanced practice nurses and have either defined their scope of practice or have authorized state nursing and/or medical boards to promulgate rules that do so. Some have revised their Medical Practice Acts (MPAs) to authorize physicians to "delegate" diagnosis and treatment tasks to nurses who have the necessary additional training."*

(Safriet, 1992, pp. 445–446)

APN Titling

The American Nurses Association's (ANA's) definition of an APN requires that the role be clinically focused and that the APN give direct clinical care to patients. As described in Chapter 3, there are four groups of APNs: NPs in primary and acute care, certified nurse-midwives (CNMs), CRNAs, and CNSs. In addition, emerging APN case manager roles can be included in these groups (see Chapters 16 and 19). This designation of what constitutes an APN is primarily driven by two factors: the ability for APNs to be directly reimbursed and the degree to which nurses desire prescriptive and admitting privileges. The reason for this clear definition is that there must be an efficacious way for state boards, insurers, prescribing entities, and the like to monitor the scope of practice, prescribing, and reimbursement patterns of APNs. There must be a "count" that can be validated in order to assure patient safety and to monitor proper certification and credentialing. The issues surrounding the titling and credentialing of APNs have been difficult since the inception of the role. There is an ongoing dialogue between national certifying bodies and state regulators, as well as among bodies who accredit educational programs, to bring standardization to the multiple APN specialties. CRNA and CNM certification and credentialing are the most clearly uniform and standardized based on their longevity and singleness of purpose and specialty. The credentialing and oversight of NPs and CNSs is more clouded based on the multiplicity of programs and specialties and the continuing need to develop certification in some areas. The advent of new national practice standards for the CNS is a clear move in the right direction (see Chapter 13).

IMPLICATIONS OF STANDARDS OF PRACTICE AND STANDARDS OF CARE FOR APNs

Standards of practice for nursing are defined by the profession nationally and help to further explicate and delineate scope of practice. Standards are overarching, authoritative statements that the nursing profession uses to describe the responsibilities for which its members are accountable (ANA, 1996). APNs are held to both the standards of practice promulgated by the nursing profession and to standards of the various APN specialties. At both levels, standards of practice describe the basic competency levels for safe and competent practice (e.g., see Chapters 17 and 18 for the standards of practice for CNMs and CRNAs, respectively). Professional standards of practice match closely with the core competencies for APNs outlined in Chapter 3, which undergird advanced nursing practice.

Standards of care differ from the standards of practice set forth by the nursing profession described previously. These standards are often termed "practice guidelines." Practice guidelines provide a foundation by which health care providers administer care to patients. These guidelines crosscut the health professions disciplines and are the frameworks/standards by which basic safety and competent care are measured. For APNs this means that the standard used to evaluate APN practice is often the same as the standard used to review medical practice. Standards of care are derived from evidence-based practice and are evolving over time. The Agency for Healthcare Research and Quality (AHRQ, formerly AHCPR), at the federal policy level, has taken on the responsibility to conduct the research needed to provide clinical practice guidelines that define a standard of appropriate care in some specific areas (Buppert, 1999). It is very important that APNs are part of interdisciplinary teams that develop and test practice guidelines for care. Much work needs to be done in this area. AHCPR guidelines are currently available in areas such as depression, otitis media with effusion, sickle cell disease, pain management, low back pain, and smoking cessation. AHCPR guidelines can be accessed on line at *http://www.ahrq.gov* (Buppert, 1999).

LEGAL CONCERNS SURROUNDING ADVANCED NURSING PRACTICE

There are several reasons why the multiplicity of titles and roles for APNs is a problem from a policy viewpoint. The first and foremost reason is that it is confusing to policy makers and regulators. It is especially a problem at agencies such as the Health Care Financing Agency, where major designations for Medicare and Medicaid reimbursement set the standard for all reimbursement across the country. In addition, discrepancies among states make mobility difficult for APNs in terms of prescriptive authority and reimbursement.

APNs are primarily responsible to and are disciplined by individual state boards of nursing. One of the licensing and credentialing difficulties faced by APNs is the variance in board regulations from state to state. In some states APN practice is governed solely by the board of nursing; in others it is jointly administered by the boards of nursing and medicine; and in still others it is governed by the boards of nursing and pharmacy. In many states CNMs are answerable to nurse-midwifery boards that are attached to boards of medicine. CNSs who are not in prescribing roles may be governed solely by the board of nursing. Although written prescriptive statements delegating medical acts to the APN that are co-signed by a physician preceptor are not as prevalent as they were in the 1980s, they are still the norm in some states, predominantly in the South.

As APNs move in and out of what is considered the domain of medicine, serious thought must be given to the standard by which APNs will be judged if they are deemed to have made an error. Although there are not many documented cases citing APNs who have injured patients by wrongful actions, the question about whether APNs should be tried by the courts using medical standards or nursing standards is important and needs to be clarified. It is incumbent upon APNs to set clear standards for practice that are based on clinical competency. CNMs and CRNAs are currently furthest along in this process.

APN CREDENTIALING AND REGULATION

Several important definitions and concepts are central to the discussion of credentialing and regulation of APNs in the United States. As APNs become more mobile across state and international boundaries, and as communications allow for increased interaction, it is important that credentialing and regulatory parameters are well understood.

"Credentialing" is an umbrella term that refers to the regulatory mechanisms that can be applied to individuals, programs, or organizations (Styles, 1998). Credentialing can be defined as "getting your ducks in a row" for the purpose of meeting standards, protecting the public, and improving quality. As an example, for the individual APN, credentialing may include, but is not limited to, the following:

- Graduation from an approved graduate nursing program
- Attainment of national certification
- State licensure/recognition as a registered nurse (RN) and APN
- Approval as a nurse prescriber
- Medicare/Medicaid provider numbers
- Approval of hospital privileges

For a graduate nursing program preparing APNs, credentialing may include accreditation by the Commission on Collegiate Nursing Education (CCNE) or the National League for Nursing Accreditation Center (NLNAC); regional and state university boards and commissions; or groups such as the American College of Nurse-Midwives or the American Association of Nurse Anesthetists (Faut-Callahan & Caulk, 1998). For an institution, credentialing may include adhering to Joint Commission on Accreditation of Healthcare Organizations or Occupational Safety and Health Administration guidelines.

Credentialing may be mandatory, as in state licensure, or voluntary, as with some national certification processes. In some instances, bodies that regulate APNs to assure public safety may recognize voluntary credentialing bodies, such as national nursing certification organizations, as a part of the mandatory state credentialing mechanism.

APN program accreditation and approval, scope of practice, standards of practice, practice guidelines, and collaborative practice agreements all have important implications for APNs in terms of proper credentialing and interactions with the court system. These documents create the standard by which APN practice is monitored and regulated, deemed safe or unsafe, and by which APNs are disciplined from state to state. These components of APN education and practice are described in the following sections.

Master's Education as a Component of APN Credentialing

The first credential that the new APN has to satisfy is successful graduation from an approved APN nursing program. Over time most educational programs have moved the curriculum to the graduate nursing level. For example, the year 2007 is the projected time by which all NPs who use the title APN are to be prepared in master's of nursing programs (Buppert, 1999). In many states, both eligibility to sit for national certification and the ability to obtain APN licensure/recognition by the state require a transcript of successful completion of a master's degree in the designated nursing specialty from an approved university; this is rapidly becoming the norm in all states.

APN PROGRAM ACCREDITATION

Graduate programs in nursing and related fields that prepare APNs must be accredited as educationally sound, with appropriate content for the specialty and adequate clinical hours of supervised experience. The NLNAC and the CCNE accredit graduate programs in the nursing major (Commission on Collegiate Nursing Education, 1998). The accreditation process provides an overall evaluation of the graduate program for the most part, but currently does not deal with the specifics of approval of specialty NP and CNS content. The American College of Nurse-Midwives and the American Association of Nurse Anesthetists oversee and review CNM and CRNA education within the framework of designated graduate programs. The National Organization of Nurse Practitioner Faculties (NONPF), the National Certification Board of Pediatric Nurse Practitioners and Nurses (NCBPNP/N), and other like bodies provide curriculum guidelines, program standards, and competencies to assist NP programs in this task. Currently there is strong momentum toward collaborative relationships between nursing accreditors, APN certifiers, and APN specialty organizations such as the NONPF to provide specialty review within the overarching accreditation process. Furthermore, the certifying bodies review programs, to some degree, to sanction eligibility to sit for national APN certification exams, but many educators feel that this process comes too late. There is a need to be proactive and oversee program appropriateness and strength before students graduate and are ready for credentialing. Given the increased numbers of APN programs in a variety of nursing specialties, the work being done to standardize education for APNs is of major importance. The proposed standardization of the approval process for NP educational programs would greatly assist state boards of nursing in their role of recognizing and regulating APNs for practice.

SPECIALTY PROGRAM REVIEW FOR NEW AND EXISTING PROGRAMS

Oversight of specialty education for APNs occurs using several different models. The clearest models are those that are administered by the American Association of Nurse Anesthetists and the American College of Nurse-Midwives. These bodies provide a process to review and regulate CRNA and CNM programs across the country that is separate from but feeds into the overall graduate nursing accreditation process. The review and monitoring of NP education at the specialty level is much more complex because of the multiplicity of specialties. The most clearly established review processes for NP programs are those administered by the NCBPNP/N, which approves pediatric NP programs, and the National Association of Women's Health, which accredits women's health programs (Association of Women's Health, Obstetric, Neonatal Nurses, 1996). In 1997, the National Task Force on Quality Nurse Practitioner Education established national criteria by which to monitor and approve NP programs using six broad-based criteria (Table 22–1).

TABLE 22–1 NATIONAL TASK FORCE CRITERIA FOR NURSE PRACTITIONER PROGRAM EVALUATION

Criterion I—Organization and administration of NP programs
   Institutional support
Criterion II—Students
   Student admission and progression
Criterion III—Curriculum
   Content areas, competencies, basic course work
Criterion IV—Resources, facilities, and services
   Physical resources, clinical site and preceptorship resources
Criterion V—Faculty and faculty organization
   Faculty preparation, credentialing, and clinical practice
Criterion VI—Evaluation
   Program, students, faculty, clinical sites

Data from the National Task Force on Quality Nurse Practitioner Education (1997).

The National Task Force Criteria for Evaluation of Nurse Practitioner Programs were developed and endorsed by a consortium of NP education and practice associations, NP regulators, and NP national certifiers and accreditors. These criteria, in conjunction with the American Association of Colleges of Nursing's (AACN's) *Essentials of Master's Education for Advanced Practice Nursing* (1995), which define graduate nursing core and APN core (pathophysiology, physical assessment, and pharmacology) curriculum requirements provide the needed structure and guidance for APN nursing education. There has been good progress by NP educators in the late 1990s to bring the multiplicity of NP educational programs into a standardized approval process for NP education (National Association of Neonatal Nurses, 1995). Although CNS education is embedded fully within the nursing paradigm, the CNS community is working toward clear structure and progression of CNS specialty education to assure compliance with credentialing and regulation as APN providers.

POSTGRADUATE EDUCATION

The number of postgraduate APN programs that are targeted to students who have already attained a graduate degree in nursing but who wish to become APNs or want to work in a different APN role is markedly increasing (AACN and NONPF, 1999; NONPF, 1996). Post-master's APN education is often tailored to meet the individual needs of post-master's students. Standardization of post-master's advanced practice nursing programs is needed because many of these programs, depending on the specialty, currently do not fall within the purview of formal graduate nursing accreditation. Additional education to meet requirements of a new specialty advanced area of practice need to be met from both a didactic and a clinical standpoint. It is important that master's-prepared nurses who aspire to do post-master's work to acquire an APN credential identify programs that offer curricula that meet the standards of eligibility for national certification and state licensure for the particular APN role.

DUAL AND BLENDED ROLE EDUCATION

New configurations of programs and tracks for specialty APNs that are dual or blended (see Chapters 3 and 16 for clarification of these roles) are widespead. These programs require careful consideration of content and clinical experiences to assure mastery of basic APN competencies and clinical experiences in both areas. New certification examinations and program review processes are being developed to meet the quality assurance and regulatory needs of these new specialties. Many APNs are dually prepared and are thus able to sit for more than one national certification. Today's complex health care system, fostered by managed care, makes this a viable option for many APNs who are functioning in diverse settings.

State Licensure/Recognition as a Component of APN Credentialing

State law that provides oversight to APN practice is divided into two forms: statutes as defined by the nurse practice act enacted by the state legislature, and rules and regulations explicated by state agencies under the jurisdiction of the executive branch of state government (Buppert, 1999). Licensure is the authority delegated to the individual states by the federal Constitution, which provides standards to assure basic levels of public safety. In most states, the board of nursing has sole authority over APN practice; however, in 11 states there is joint authority with the board of medicine (Buppert, 1999). The states require that all APNs carry current licensure as an RN. Advanced nursing practice status is achieved through rules and regulations that are part of the individual state nurse practice act. Authority to practice is tied to scope of practice and varies from state to state depending on the degree of practice auton-omy the APN is granted. Most states require national certification and proof of completion of an approved APN program. Pharmacology requirements vary from state to state, although currently most states require a graduate core pharmacotherapeutics course during the APN educational program and yearly continuing education (CE) credits thereafter to maintain prescriptive privileges. Current status of APN licensure and scope of practice and application information is best found by accessing the desired state government Web page.

Most states require a temporary permit for new APN graduates to practice as an APN while awaiting national certification results. New graduates should contact the board of nursing and submit the required application for a temporary APN permit if the state allows such practice.

PRESCRIPTIVE AUTHORITY

Credentialing/licensure for prescriptive authority occurs at the state level. The process varies from state to state depending on how the statute is written. Prescribing author-ity may be regulated solely by the board of nursing, as it is in several states; jointly by the board of nursing and the board of pharmacy, as it is in several others; or by a triad of boards of nursing, medicine, and pharmacy. It is incumbent upon the APN to clearly understand the mechanism whereby prescriptive authority is regulated in a given state.

As prescriptive authority has evolved over the past several years, certain basic requirements have become fairly standard (although not entirely) for APN prescribers. They are as follows:

1. Graduation from an approved master's-level APN program
2. Licensure/recognition in good standing as an APN
3. National certification in an APN specialty
4. A recent pharmacotherapeutics course of at least 3 credit hours (45 contact hours)
5. Evidence of a collaborative practice arrangement (in some states)
6. Ongoing CE hours in pharmacotherapeutics to maintain prescribing status
7. State prescribing and national Drug Enforcement Administration numbers in some instances
8. A pharmacy formulary (in some states)

These requirements vary from state to state but provide a core regulatory process for prescriptive authority (Buppert, 1999; Hanson, 1996). A good resource for under-standing differences in prescriptive practice from state to state is the yearly update provided by Pearson each January in the *Nurse Practitioner Journal,* which provides a chart describing prescribing regulations in all 50 states (Pearson, 2000).

State boards of nursing need to clearly document the numbers of hours of pharma-cology required for an APN to receive and maintain prescriptive privileges in terms of both educational program and year-to-year continuing education. Advanced nursing programs, which previously integrated pharmacological content within clinical management courses, have moved toward separately defined pharmacology courses in order to comply with recent state requirements for a designated amount of pharmacology in advanced nursing education. Pharmacology content should be taught by faculty pharmacists or a nurse-pharmacist faculty team who have an in-depth knowledge of therapeutic prescribing. Some states are currently requiring that specific course and content hours be verifiable in order to be used in an application for prescriptive authority. Furthermore, several states require documentation of the number of hours of CE for pharmacology per year or per cycle. The direction is clearly to require APNs to attend ongoing CE in pharmacology in order to maintain prescriptive privileges. Therefore, states need to move toward contracting with universities or other educational providers to offer timely CE offerings and distance learning modalities (e.g., interactive television or Web-based offerings) in order to meet the needs of isolated rural clinicians. Over time, the states will most likely move in the direction of interdisciplinary pharmacology education for both nurses and physicians.

National Certification as a Component of APN Credentialing

NATIONAL CERTIFICATION

National certification for APNs, over time, has served several purposes, including regulation and licensure, entry into practice, validation of competence, and a way to recognize expert practice (Lewis, Camp, & Rothrock, 1996). Multiple bodies for certification have surfaced to fill the need for APN certification, which has resulted in varying certification requirements (Hodnicki, 1998). APN certification is national in scope and is a mandatory requirement for APNs to obtain and maintain credentialing in most but not all states (Pearson, 2000). More and more state regulatory bodies are currently using national certification examinations as a component of the credentialing mechanism. CRNAs are credited with the first national certification in 1945, with other APN specialties following suit, although there were few standards for certification in place (Hodnicki, 1998). A perceived weakness of APN certification is the multiplicity of certification configurations for APN practice. Table 22–2 provides a comparison of certification requirements for CRNAs, CNMs, NPs, and CNSs.

RECERTIFICATION

Overall, APNs must fulfill CE and practice requirements to successfully maintain their national certification, although differences in requirements exist from specialty to specialty. Each APN certification entity clearly lays out the requirements and time frame for recertification. Generally, national certification for most specialties lasts from 5 to 8 years and requires that the candidate retest unless the established parameters are met. Table 22–3 provides a comparison of recertification requirements for APN specialty groups.

MANDATORY CONTINUING EDUCATION REQUIREMENTS

CE requirements differ from specialty to specialty as to the type and amount of CE needed to maintain current national certification. Instruction should be in the area of APN specialty, although it may be interdisciplinary. For example, CRNAs may

TABLE 22–2 COMPARISON OF CERTIFICATION REQUIREMENTS FOR APNs

CRITERIA	ANCC (NP)	ANCC (CNS)	NCC (WHNP or NNP)	ACC (CNM)	DOA (CRNA)
Education	Master's	Master's	Post-basic RN or master's (req. 2000 A.D.)	Certificate, master's, doctoral	Certificate (those already admitted Master's for all entering as of 1998
RN licensure in U.S. or its territories	Yes	Yes	Yes	Yes	Yes
Program length	12 months with 1/3 didactic, 2/3 clinical		9 months min. with 200 hrs didactic and 600 hrs clinical		24 months minimum
Practice requirements	No	Per specialty	No	No	No
Curriculum outline	Yes	Yes	Yes	Yes	Yes
Clinical hours mandated	2/3 total program length	1,000–1,500 per specialty	600 hours	Not stated	450 cases and 800 clinical hours
Program accreditation or pre-accreditation required	No	No	No	Yes	Yes

* ANCC = American Nurses Credentialing Center; NP = nurse practitioner; CNS = clinical nurse specialist; NCC = National Certification Corporation; WHNP = women's health nurse practitioner; NNP = neonatal nurse practitioner; ACC = ACNM Certification Council Inc.; DOA = Division of Accreditation; CRNA = certified registered nurse anesthetist.
From Hodnicki, D. R. (1998). Advanced practice nursing certification: Where do we go from here? *Advanced Practice Nursing Quarterly*, *4*(3), 34–43, © Aspen Publishers, Inc; reprinted with permission.

choose to attend a conference with collaborating anesthesiologists, or family NPs (FNPs) may attend a conference with family practice physicians. It is encouraging to note that more and more conferences are offering interdisciplinary speakers and panels at discipline-specific conferences. APN expert clinicians are serving as conference faculty for medical CE and vice versa. Ongoing CE hours can be met by attending CE courses and workshops, working toward degree requirements, completing journal CE offerings, writing for publication, completing on-line offerings, simulations, audiotape and CD-ROM materials, and the like. There are a wide variety of nursing and medical materials that offer CE credit to subscribers. The move to interdisciplinary offerings has broadened the scope of information available. Each APN specialty determines the number of hours required for successful recertification.

MANDATORY PRACTICE REQUIREMENTS

Most, but not all, APN specialties have built in specific requirements for an adequate number of clinical practice hours between the years of recertification to assure that APNs are maintaining currency and competence through regular practice as an APN. Each certification process clearly spells out the clinical hour practice requirement for the specialty. Some APN specialties accept clinical teaching and other modalities

TABLE 22–3 COMPARISON OF RECERTIFICATION REQUIREMENTS FOR APNs

CRITERIA	ANCC (NP)	ANCC (CNS)	NCC (WHNP or NNP)	ACC (CNM)	DOA (CRNA)
Due date	5 years	5 years	3 years	8 years	2 years
RN licensure	Yes	Yes	Yes	Yes	Yes
Retest option	Yes	Yes	Yes—must take prior to recert expiration date	Yes or complete 3 modules†	Yes but provisional recertification available
Practice hours	1,500	1,000–1,500	None	None	850 hours over 2 years recommended
Continuing education from accredited provider	37.5–150 contact hours plus other categories	75 contact hours plus other categories	45 contact hours	20 contact hours†	40 contact hours
Random audit performed	20%	20%	20–30%		All applications reviewed
Lapsed recertification option	Appeal process or retest	Appeal process or retest	Retest only		May be granted late start on recertification

* ANCC = American Nurses Credentialing Center; NP = nurse practitioner; CNS = clinical nurse specialist; NCC = National Certification Corporation; WHNP = women's health nurse practitioner; NNP = neonatal nurse practitioner; ACC = ACNM Certification Council Inc.; DOA = Division of Accreditation; CRNA = certified registered nurse anesthetist.
† Currently under discussion. From Hodnicki, D. R. (1998). Advanced practice nursing certification: Where do we go from here? *Advanced Practice Nursing Quarterly, 4*(3), 34–43, © Aspen Publishers, Inc; reprinted with permission.

as part of the practice requirement. APNs who do not meet stipulated CE and practice requirements must retake the national certifying exam to continue to practice.

National certification assures national consistency of professional standards and helps the public to understand scope of practice (AACN, 1995). It is one way to assure that competent APNs provide needed health care to patients and families. Therefore, standardization of APN certification and recertification processes is critical in order to assure the credibility of APN specialties (Hodnicki, 1998). Table 22–4 presents Internet website addresses for major APN accreditation, regulatory, and certification bodies.

TABLE 22–4 INTERNET ADDRESSES TO NATIONAL APN ACCREDITATION, REGULATION, AND CERTIFICATION WEBSITES

American Academy of Nurse Practitioners (AANP)	www.aanp.org
American Association of Colleges of Nurses & Commission on Collegiate Nursing Education (AACN and CCNE)	www.aacn.nche.edu (links to CCNE)
American Association of Nurse Anesthetists (AANA)	www.aana.com.index.htm
American College of Nurse-Midwives (ACNM)	www.acnm.org
American Nurses Credentialing Center ANCC)	www.nursingworld.org/ancc
National Certification Board of Pediatric Nurse Practitioners and Nurses (NCBPNP/N)	www.pnpcert.org
National Certification Corporation for Obstetrical, Gynecologic And Neonatal Nursing Specialties (NCC)	www.nccnet.org
National Council of State Boards of Nursing (NCSBN)	www.ncsbn.org
National League for Nursing and National League for Nursing Accreditation Corporation (NLNAC)	www.nln.org/nlnac

Collaborative Practice Arrangements

The general term "practice guidelines" can be confusing to the APN in that it is used in several different contexts. First, as defined earlier, it is an evidence-based standard of care. However, it is also used to refer to a collegial agreement between the APN and the physician to define parameters of practice for the APN. Collegial practice agreements take many forms, from a one-page written agreement defining consultation and referral patterns to a more specific prescribed "protocol" for specific functions. The term "protocol" in relation to advanced nursing practice was common several years ago as a directed, specified guideline for practice that defined each patient problem and the care directive. Some states used this "cookbook" approach to NP practice as a way to oversee prescriptive and other treatment modalities. For the most part, specific protocols for care are no longer used in most settings because it is difficult to maintain currency and to adhere to the given individuality of patients and practices. As APNs have proven their ability to provide competent care with positive outcomes, protocols have been replaced by overall practice guidelines and collaborative practice agreements. However, it is important to note that the specificity of the collaborative arrangement is most often based on trust and respect between the collaborating APN and physician colleague. APNs must often "earn their stripes" as competent health care providers in the medical world before they are granted more autonomous practice.

The norm today in APN regulation is shifting toward loosely configured collaborative relationships that offer support to all parties and protect the safety of patients. In any case, to achieve compliance with state regulations for practice, the collaborative agreement, if required in a given state, must have a current signature and provide relevant and up-to-date information. Collaborative relationships vary widely from APN specialty to specialty. The chapters in Part III of this text help to explain the differences in collaborative structures for APNs.

Institutional Credentialing

The need for hospital privileges for APNs varies according to the nurse's practice. For example, CNMs and many rural NPs cannot properly care for patients without the ability to admit to the hospital should the need arise. Conversely, many CNSs are employed by hospitals and have no need for admitting privileges. CRNAs and some NPs have not needed to admit patients to the hospital independently in order to give comprehensive care, but may need to see patients in the emergency room.

The rules for practice as part of the hospital staff are even more specific and variable than those for prescriptive authority and are bound to the local hospital or medical facility and the medical staff of the granting institution. Unfortunately, most of the criteria and guidelines are written exclusively for medical practitioners and therefore are not compatible with the APN's education and supporting credentials. In many hospitals, professional privileges are granted by a committee made up of physicians and administrators. The first step for APNs seeking hospital privileges is to seek out the nurse administrators and find out how the credentials committee is organized, who makes up the membership, and what support there is for nonphysician applicants. Is there even a process for nurses or others to petition for privileges?

Nursing administrators are often members of these committees, and the APN should meet with nurse colleagues for advice and support prior to the application process.

A second step is to obtain the application package and begin to collect the necessary documents, which include licenses and certifications, transcripts, letters of support, provider numbers, and so on. Support from collaborating physicians is key; in some committee structures, a collaborating physician may serve as the petitioner for a nurse colleague. Dialogue between the hospital administration, physician staff, and other stakeholders such as APN colleagues and other team members is necessary if admitting privileges are required for the desired practice role. Alliances with consumers often add support to the application. Some hospitals have specific guides and protocols for all nonphysician providers; others do not.

The determination of the specific privileges desired is critical to the process. For example, is it necessary to be able to admit or discharge patients; write orders; do particular procedures; visit in-hospital patients; or take an emergency room call? Many hospitals have different levels of hospital privilege, ranging from ''full'' to modified privileges, for specific functions. Asking for full privileges may not be prudent or useful in a particular setting. A good rule is to ask for what is needed, establish a solid track record, and expand privileges later as the need arises. It is important to remember that the attainment of hospital privileges is often a professional turf issue and fraught with political overtones. The task of overcoming this barrier to practice requires astute planning, negotiating, and careful attention to the ''cast of characters'' and set policies of the institution.

EXEMPLAR 1: MEETING THE REQUIREMENTS FOR CREDENTIALING AND REGULATION

Jeni is in the final semester of her FNP program at a state university. She is in the process of negotiating a contract with a provider network of physicians and APNs in a satellite health maintenance organization (HMO) practice. Jeni knows that she must begin the process of acquiring the necessary credentials in order to be able to practice in her state. When she applied to take her FNP program, she made sure that the university and graduate program were accredited in good standing. Now that she is ready to leave, she must prepare for a new and challenging professional life.

In her seminar class, Jeni received the application to sit for national certification the month after she graduates from her master's program and has sent the application forward to assure her seat at the examination. Her next step is to access the Internet and download the APN rules and regulations for her state as well the application for a temporary permit to practice as an APN for the interim between graduation and the time that she gets the results from her national certifying exam. Jeni reviews both of these documents carefully so that she fully understands the application process and the materials and fee that she will need to submit.

Jeni carefully notes in the APN rules and regulations that, to be able to prescribe in her state, she must show proof that she has completed a 45-contact-hour approved course in pharmacotherapeutics and that she must complete 6 hours of CE in pharmacotherapeutics each year to maintain her status as a prescriber. She makes a note to request the transcript for her pharmacotherapeutics course to attach to her application for her APN license.

The HMO that Jeni plans to practice with has sent her several documents that she must complete in order to be able to practice. First, upon signing her contract, she will need to negotiate a written collaborative arrangement with her precepting physician, who will see the patients who are beyond her scope of practice. Second, she needs a Medicaid provider number in order to see children in the Medicaid program and a

Medicare number in order to see elders. In addition, this managed care system requires that Jeni apply to the local hospital privileging committee so that she can see patients on rounds, do admitting and discharge planning, and follow nursing home patients on a regular basis.

As part of her "package," Jeni has negotiated for the employer to pay the premium on her malpractice insurance as an APN. She needs to call her insurance carrier to discuss the transfer of her student policy to a full policy to cover her as a certified APN with the appropriate scope of practice that she will need in her new position. Jeni uses the support of her colleagues and mentors as she works though this important process of preparing her credentials to practice as an APN.

ISSUES THAT AFFECT APN CREDENTIALING AND REGULATION

Reimbursement

On a par with the need to be able to prescribe medications for patients is the need to be appropriately reimbursed for care. Clearly, APNs must be paid for services rendered for health care whether they work independently, share a joint practice with a physician colleague, or are employed within a managed care system or provider network. Although the individual states regulate the insurance industry, many of the private-pay insurance standards that are used to set payment mechanisms are modeled after federal Medicaid and Medicare policy. Federal mandates that encourage direct payment of nonphysician health care providers are often blocked at the state level by discriminating rules and regulations. Many third-party reimbursers, including some major insurance companies, are now reimbursing NPs directly; others are not. As states move more directly into managed care models, both in the private and public sectors, and into large purchasing groups in which APNs are providing care as part of interdisciplinary teams, reimbursement is becoming more readily available. However, tensions persist with regard to provider status and membership on patient panels. From a credentialing standpoint, attention to HCFA rules, Medicare and Medicaid provider numbers, Cinical Laboratories Improvement Act regulations, and managed care provider requirements are extremely important. For a detailed description of specific reimbursement mechanisms and issues for APNs, see Chapters 20 and 23 as well as the role-specific chapters in Part III.

Payment for APN services has long been controversial. The argument continues about whether nurses should be paid the same fee for service as a physician or be paid only a percentage of the physician payment. This is always a negotiable issue, and there is disagreement within medicine and nursing alike. It is difficult for nurse lobbyists who represent many types of APNs from several specialties to negotiate fair and equitable reimbursement that meets the needs of everyone.

Payment by private insurers is contract specific and varies with each state's insurance commission. The current climate of large-scale mergers between major private insurance companies to accommodate complex managed care structures has important relevance for APN reimbursement. It is critical that APNs position themselves to sit on policy-making boards for private enterprise. A prime example comes from the 1980s, a time when NPs lost their liability coverage nationally. NPs worked with the National Alliance of Nurse Practitioners, and through negotiation and education, gained access to the executive board at Cotterell, Mitchell, and Fifer as part of an advisement group. This activity cemented a long-term relationship that has brought a clear understanding about the practice of NPs and a newsletter for risk management with this major liability carrier (Hanson, 1985).

There is another key issue with regard to reimbursement for APNs. It should be noted that in managed care contracts the level of reimbursement is immaterial. APNs and all other providers must deliver care at a fixed, preset price; this can be an advantage if APNs are less costly to employ. Thus, it becomes critical for APNs to fully understand how much it costs them to provide care for patients with a variety of preventive, episodic, and chronic health problems and to be able to articulate to contractors that they are competitive in the marketplace.

Policy issues surrounding the reimbursement of APNs require careful reflection before strategies to remove constraints to payment are undertaken. Several important questions should be considered when shaping policy. For example, what services do APNs want to be paid for? Are they different from physician services or the same? Are there specific nursing services that need to be reimbursed? Is direct payment the issue, or does it matter who gets the payment? Will the payment level be the same as or lower than what physicians receive for equivalent service? These are important questions because, in most states, APNs historically have been reimbursed indirectly, "incident to" physicians and at a considerably lower rate. It is advantageous for APNs who are planning to practice clinically, no matter what the setting or physician relationship, to seek counsel about the reimbursement realities in their state before beginning to care for patients. Only then are APNs in an appropriate position to seek status as reimbursable providers with Medicare, Medicaid, and the many private payers.

A Wave of the Future: Telehealth/Telepractice

Regulatory issues surrounding the changes in the way health care providers practice based on electronic capabilities will challenge policy makers and APNs well into the new millenium. A model described as "mutual recognition" refers to the use of a system much like that used for driver's licenses, whereby states share the jurisdiction, discipline, and information sharing to regulate practice based on an interstate compact (National Council of State Boards of Nursing [NCSBN], 1998; Williamson & Hutcherson, 1998). An APN is licensed in a home state but other states recognize the licensure. The mutual recognition model would hold the APN accountable for the laws and regulations in the state where the APN provides the health care but would rely on the licensure from the home state (Williamson & Hutcherson, 1998). The following example illustrates this practice model.

EXEMPLAR 2

As a pediatric NP in a pediatric HMO practice, you have been co-managing the health care of 4-year-old David in North Carolina since he was born. David has insulin-dependent diabetes mellitus. The child and his mother have grown to trust and depend on your care for David over time. While at Disneyland in Florida, David develops diarrhea and vomiting. His mom chooses to e-mail you for advice rather than take David to an unfamiliar emergency room and provider. You respond back to the mother with directions about management of the gastroenteritis and potential changes in David's insulin dosage if needed. In doing so, you have cared for David in a state other than the one in which you are licensed and recognized as an APN. However, a system of regulatory mutual recognition between states would allow for you to care for David using your North Carolina APN credentials.

Interestingly, new technologies and a system of "virtual practice" as described in the previous example focuses attention on old pervasive barriers that have plagued APNs for many years (Safriet, 1998). Although implementation of a mutual recognition system is well underway for RNs, the same type of recognition is lagging behind for APNs because of the lack of stability and standardization of regulatory schemes from state to state with regard to scope of practice, prescriptive authority, and reimbursement. Although the dysfunctional aspects of this current regulatory regime for APN providers are problematic, it may provide a basis for positive change. Based on the Comprehensive Telehealth Act of 1997 (Senate Bill 385), physicians and other health care providers, including nurses, fall within the boundaries of electronic practice and all require regulation. Therefore, the potential for policy makers to focus on "what is being done" rather than on "who is doing it" is positive for APNs (Safriet, 1998). Telehealth legislation could provide the catalyst needed to ensure that all states recognize and authorize key elements or APN scopes of practice (e.g., prescriptive authority). Since some states are lagging behind, national strategy such as this could bring these states into alignment with the rest of the country. It will be important for APNs to carefully monitor the development of practice beyond state boundaries and work closely with the APN nursing associations to effect regulatory change that removes barriers and augments practice.

From a legal and regulatory standpoint, clear statutes are needed that offer broad practice standards to allow for mobility across state lines. This change will require national standards of practice as well as certification and credentialing requirements that can satisfy many different jurisdictions—not an easy task! These standards will require diligent collaboration between educators, state boards of nursing, the specialty professional associations, and all practicing APNs (Hanson, 1998). Part of the professional agenda that APNs need to address is the need for accountability and responsibility for competence in practice. As a professional group, APNs must build strong national standards of practice, scope, and skills. Experienced practitioners need to help peers gain greater competence and new skills. It is important that APNs not lose sight of the need to support each other and to mentor colleagues as the practice arena broadens.

The Influence of the Managed Care System

The national health care reform debate that began with the Clinton administration has served as a catalyst for change at both the state and the local levels as well as in Congress. There has been a definite movement toward a myriad of configurations for capitated systems of care (providers are prepaid for caring for a population of patients) that requires nurses to understand, to a much higher degree, how much it costs to manage patients as well as how to interface with new systems as providers. There are several areas in which managed care directly affects the regulation of APN practice.

Managed care organizations build networks of providers by hiring, purchasing services from, or contracting with physicians and APNs, hospitals, and others to provide services to patient members. When APNs join a provider network, they must meet all of the requirements, regulations, and standards of care established by the plan (Knight, 1999). For example, a primary care NP applying for a position would need to meet all of the state APN licensure criteria, including the credentials to prescribe medications, appropriate Medicare and Medicaid provider status, malpractice history and coverage, national certification status, and hospital admitting status. Some managed care groups choose to hire credential verification organizations that are far distant from the practice, or conduct searches of national databases to verify credentials (Knight, 1999). It is incumbent upon the APN to have all credentials and regulatory documentation in good and accessible order when preparing to practice in a managed care environment that may be governed by managed care administrators in a distant state.

In 1994, Peter Buerhaus, Director of the Harvard Nursing Research Institute, outlined four critical issues that nurses facing managed care competition need to address. First, APNs must realize the range of opportunities for APNs in fee-for-service, prepaid markets and proceed appropriately into these markets. Second, as part of that effort, APNs must ensure that the minimum package of benefits includes APN services. Third, any managed care system must meet both the clinical and economic interests of APNs. Fourth, nurses must make sure that the turmoil does not detract from the value of nursing services (Buerhaus, 1994).

How APNs fit into managed care systems is a critical issue for nurses. It is important for APNs to know how to contract for their services at the individual level as they negotiate an employment package, but, even more importantly, they need to be present at the negotiating table where the rules for managed care systems are made (see Chapter 21). This means that APNs must position themselves visibly on executive boards and committees and be included as members of management teams who are setting the policies for managed care provider services.

Research has shown that APNs are viable alternatives to physician-based health care. This increased visibility makes it imperative that APNs monitor the competencies of their own practices. Recent acts of Congress that have cut federal programs for the poor will augment the need for APNs while they reduce funds for health care and increase the stress placed on the health problems of the underserved. The ANA's *Nursing's Agenda for Health Care Reform* (1991) has lasted well in these unsettled times for health care and continues to be an important reference for APNs who want to better understand how to improve access and reduce cost. Nursing's agenda is a prevention-driven, managed care approach that conserves resources. It includes several themes: universal access to health care, emphasis on primary and preventive care, shared consumer and provider accountability for health care decision making, and holistic health care services that emphasize affordable quality.

INFLUENCING THE REGULATORY PROCESS

APNs can directly influence the regulatory process in several ways in addition to using political strategies. At all levels, regulators are keen to find practicing APNs and APN educators who will take an active role in assisting them to develop and implement sound regulatory policies and procedures. Chapter 10 provides an in-depth discussion of skills needed for leadership and political advocacy. Following are some additional ways that APNs can actively engage in the regulatory process that affects their practice.

- Seek out gubernatorial appointment to the board of nursing or to the advanced practice committee that advises the board of nursing in your state.
- Seek membership as the APN member of the advisory council for either the state medical board or the state board of pharmacy.
- Seek appointment to the board of accreditation or the test-writing committees for national certification examinations.
- Seek appointment to HCFA panels where Medicare and Medicaid provider issues are decided.
- Seek appointment to hospital privileging committees and assure that privileging materials are appropriate for APNs.
- Seek appointment on advisory committees and task forces that are advising the NCSBN.
- Offer testimony at state and national hearings where proposed regulatory changes in APN regulation, prescriptive authority, and reimbursement schemes will be aired.
- Respond to offers to review/edit/provide feedback on circulated draft regulatory polices that directly affect APN education and practice.

In order to accomplish these activities, APNs need to use research data, a powerful tool for shaping health policies (Hamric, 1998). By actively participating in the regulatory process, APNs assure themselves of a strong voice in regulatory and credentialing processes. At the very least, it is incumbent upon the practicing APN to carefully monitor the process through websites and newsletters to stay informed.

CONCLUSION: FUTURE REGULATORY CHALLENGES FACING APNs

"Certification is a form of credentialing and credentialing is a form of regulation" (M. Styles, 1998). At no time has it been more important that APNs understand and value the important relationships that underpin the complex processes and systems that regulate practice. New models of health care and varying configurations of how APNs practice in interdisciplinary teams escalates the importance of regulatory considerations to new levels. The growth of telehealth and telepractice modalities makes the picture even more complex. APNs will need to provide leadership and clear direction for the development of broad-based practice standards that will satisfy state statutes and "fit" all of the APN specialties.

Both of the recent health professions reports disseminated by the Pew Health Professions Commission have been very clear about the fact that there is a need for generic benchmarks and standards for health care education and practice (Gelmon et al., 1999; O'Neil et al., 1998). Furthermore, the Pew Commission recommended interdisciplinary competence for all health care professionals. More specifically, advanced nursing practice leaders were charged to "develop standard guidelines for advanced nursing practice and reinforce them with curriculum guidelines, examination requirements, and accreditation regulations" (O'Neil et al., 1998).

The future requires that APNs promulgate clear, competency-based standards for both education and practice that will allow for growth and movement across state lines. It is important that APNs accomplish this work in preparation for the next trajectory–interdisciplinary credentialing and regulation based on defined patient outcomes–because this phenomenon will become a reality in the not too distant future. The wave of the future is to move to interdisciplinary regulation–whereby, for example, family practice physicians, FNPs, and CNMs caring for menopausal women would all be held to a like standard of education and practice. Porter-O'Grady (1998) suggested that regulation for the health professions will require a new approach that dispels notions of exclusivity, exclusion, or independence from other disciplines. This move toward overarching regulation for the health professions, when and if it comes to pass, will require much higher levels of collaboration among the disciplines and specialties than we now enjoy and, most importantly, broad-based standards and regulations for APN practice.

REFERENCES

American Association of Colleges of Nursing. (1995). *Essentials of master's education for advanced practice nursing.* Washington, DC: Author.

American Association of Colleges of Nursing and National Organization of Nurse Practitioner Faculties. (1999). *1998–1999 enrollment and graduations in baccalaureate and graduate programs in nursing* (Publication no. 98-99-1). Washington, DC: American Association of Colleges of Nursing.

American Nurses Association. (1991). *Nursing's agenda for health care reform.* Washington, DC: Author.

American Nurses Association. (1996). *Scope of practice and standards of advanced nursing practice.* Washington, DC: Author.

Association of Women's Health, Obstetric and Neonatal Nurses and the National Association of Nurse Practitioners in Reproductive Health. (1996). *The women's health nurse practitioner: Guidelines for practice and education.* Washington, DC: Authors.

Buerhaus, P. I. (1994). Managed competition and critical issues facing nurses. *Nursing and Health Care, 15,* 22–26.

Buppert, C. (1999). *Nurse practitioner's business practice and legal guide.* Gaithersburg, MD: Aspen Publishers.

Commission on Collegiate Nursing Education. (1998). *Procedures for accreditation of baccalaureate and graduate nursing education programs.* Washington, DC: Author.

Comprehensive Telehealth Act of (1997), S. 385, 105th Congress (1997).

Faut-Callahan, M. F., & Caulk, S. S. (1998). Credentialing of certified registered nurse anesthetists. *Advanced Practice Nursing Quarterly, 4*(3), 54–62.

Gelmon, S. B., O'Neil, E. H., Kimmey, J. R., and the Task Force on Accreditation of Health Professions Education. (1999). *Strategies for change and improvement: The report of the Task Force on Accreditation of Health Professions Education.* San Francisco: Center for the Health Professions, University of California at San Francisco.

Hamric, A. B. (1998). Using research to influence the regulatory process. *Advanced Practice Nursing Quarterly, 4*(3), 44–50.

Hanson, C. M. (1985). Statesboro, GA: *Personal archives.* National Alliance of Nurse Practitioners.

Hanson C. M. (1996). Health policy issues: Dealing with the realities and constraints of advanced practice nursing. In A. B. Hamric, J. A. Spross, & C. M. Hanson (Eds.), *Advanced nursing practice: An integrative approach* (pp. 496–515). Philadelphia: W. B. Saunders.

Hanson, C. M. (1998). Regulatory issues will lead advanced practice nursing challenges into the new millennium. *Advanced Practice Nursing Quarterly, 4*(3), v–vi.

Hodnicki, D. R. (1998). Advanced practice nursing certification: Where do we go from here? *Advanced Practice Nursing Quarterly, 4*(3), 34–43.

Knight, W. (1999). *Managed care: What it is and how it works.* Gaithersburg, MD: Aspen Publishers.

Lewis, C. K., Camp, J., & Rothrock, J. (1996). *The Trilateral Initiative for North American Nursing: Nursing specialty certification in the United States. An assessment of North American nursing.* Philadelphia: Commission on Graduates of Foreign Nursing Schools.

National Association of Neonatal Nurses. (1995). *Report of NANN neonatal nurse practitio-*

ner program accreditation. Washington, DC: Author.

National Council of State Boards of Nursing, Inc. (1998). *APRN licensure: Draft uniform requirements.* Chicago: Author.

National Organization of Nurse Practitioner Faculties. (1995). *Advanced nursing practice: Curriculum guidelines and program standards for nurse practitioner education.* Washington, DC: Author.

National Organization of Nurse Practitioner Faculties. (1996). *Workforce policy project technical report for nurse practitioner educational programs 1988-1995* (pp. 7-41). Washington, DC.

National Task Force on Quality Nurse Practitioner Education. (1997). *Criteria for evaluation of nurse practitioner programs.* Washington, DC: National Organization of Nurse Practitioner Faculties.

O'Neil, E. H., and the Pew Health Professions Commission. (1998). *Recreating health professional practice for a new century.* San Francisco: Pew Health Professions Commission.

Pearson, L. (2000). Annual update of how each state stands on legislative issues affecting advanced nursing practice. *The Nurse Practitioner: The American Journal of Primary Health Care, 25*(1), 16-68.

Porter-O'Grady, T. (1998). A new age for regulation. *Advanced Practice Nursing Quarterly, 4,*(3), 94-95.

Rentmeester, K., & Kindig, D. A. (1994). *Physician supply by specialty in managed care organizations.* Madison: School of Medicine, University of Wisconsin.

Safriet, B. (1992). Health care dollars and regulatory sense: The role of advanced practice nursing. *Yale Journal of Regulation, 9,* 417-487.

Safriet, B. (1998). Still spending dollars, still searching for sense: Advanced practice nursing in an era of regulatory and economic turmoil. *Advanced Practice Nursing Quarterly, 4*(3), 24-33.

Styles, M. M. (1998). An international perspective: APN credentialing. *Advanced Practice Nursing Quarterly, 4*(3), 1-5.

Wilcox, P. (1995, April). *Advanced practice model response to needs of women at risk for female malignancies.* Abstract presented at the Oncology Nurses Society national conference, Anaheim, CA.

Williamson, S. H., & Hutcherson, C. (1998). Mutual recognition: Response to the regulatory implications of a changing health care environment. *Advanced Practice Nursing Quarterly, 4*(3), 86-93.

Additional Readings

Antrobus, S., & Brown, S. (1997). The impact of the commissioning agenda upon nursing practice: A pro-active approach to influencing health policy. *Journal of Advanced Nursing, 25*(2), 309-315.

Brent, N. J. (1997). *Nurses and the law: A guide to principles and applications.* Philadelphia: W. B. Saunders.

Gorenberg, B. D., Alderman, M. C., & Cruise, M. J. (1991). Social policy statements: Guidelines for decision making. *International Nursing Review, 38*(1), 11-13.

Hebda, T., Czar, P. & Mascara, C. (1998). *Handbook of informatics for nurses and health care professionals.* New York: Addison-Wesley.

Koerner, J. (1998). Tapping into uncommon wisdom through mentorship. In C. Vance and R. K. Olson (Eds.), *The mentor connection in nursing* (pp. 7-233) New York: Springer-Verlag.

Mason, D. J., & Leavitt, J. K. (1998). *Policy and politics in nursing and health care* (3rd ed.). Philadelphia: W. B. Saunders.

Milstead, J. A. (1997). A social mandate: APN leadership for the whole policy process. *Advanced Practice Nursing Quarterly, 3*(3), 1-8.

Milstead, J. A. (1998). *Health policy and politics: A nurses guide.* Gaithersburg, MD: Aspen Publishers.

Mundt, M. H. (1997). Books on health policy and health reform: How is nursing represented? *Journal of Professional Nursing, 13*(1), 19-27.

Penney, N. E., Campbell-Heider, N., Miller, B. K., Carter, E., & Bidwell-Cerone, S. (1996). Influencing health care policy: Nursing research and the ANA social policy statement. *Journal of the New York State Nurses Association, 27*(3), 15-19.

Pew Health Professions Commission. (1995). *Critical challenges: Revitalizing the health professions for the twenty-first century, third report.* San Francisco: Center for the Health Professions, University of California at San Francisco.

Starfield, B. (1997). Primary care and health policy. The future of primary care in a managed care era. *International Journal of Health Services, 27*(4), 687-696.

Sullivan, T. J. (1998). *Collaboration: A health care imperative. Part III, intraorganizational collaboration.* New York: McGraw-Hill.

Whitman, M. (1998). Nurses can influence public health policy. *Advanced Practice Nursing Quarterly, 3*(4), 67-71.

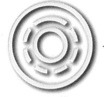

Health Policy Issues in a Changing Environment

AN INTERDISCIPLINARY PERSPECTIVE

• J E A N   J O H N S O N
• L.   G R E G O R Y   P A W L S O N

INTRODUCTION

Although clinical practice is the hallmark of advanced practice nurses (APNs), health policy issues influence virtually all aspects of clinical practice. Policies established at the federal, state, and corporate levels influence, for example, which patients are seen by APNs, what services are reimbursed, what and how APNs are paid, and the scope of APN practice. Health policy also defines issues of concern to APNs beyond direct clinical practice, including the financing of health care in general and the overall tax burden resulting from health care expenditures. This chapter discusses health policy in a broad perspective, including (1) the definition of health policy, (2) financing and cost of health care, (3) access to health care, and (4) quality. Specific issues related to APN practice are integrated into these general topics.

While recognizing that there are areas of conflict between nursing and medicine, this chapter is written by an APN and a physician in the hope that we can convey the possibility and desirability of collaboration. Given the extraordinary pressures on health care providers from purchasers, government, corporations, and others, it is important to try to find the common concerns among health professionals, particularly medicine and nursing, rather than automatically taking adversarial positions based on discipline. When the well-being of individual patients and the health of our nation is at stake, we firmly believe in the importance of working together. However, we also have not omitted or underestimated those areas in which conflict is present or likely.

This chapter also complements several other chapters in the book, specifically Chapters 10, 20, and 22. No single chapter can cover all the topics relevant to practice issues, and many issues can be more fully understood when viewed from a different perspective. For these reasons, the reader is strongly encouraged to refer to the other chapters noted.

WHAT IS HEALTH POLICY AND WHY IS IT IMPORTANT?

Health policy in its broadest sense can be taken to mean any decision that affects health care at a group or macro level, including access, finance, reimbursement, delivery, quality, and cost. Longest (1998) stated that policy decisions are intended to direct or influence the actions, behaviors, or decisions of others. In a more limited sense, health policy is often used to mean public policy related to health care delivery, specifically decisions regarding health care that are made in a public forum, mostly through local, state, or federal government actions by their legislative, judicial, or executive branches. However, this latter definition leaves out the increasing number of decisions about health care that are made by insurers, providers, purchasers, or others outside of government who nonetheless form and shape health care systems.

The importance of health policy stems from a number of factors. The most obvious factor is that health care has become a major economic activity in the United States. The health care industry is one of the top three employers in this country, and health care expenditures represent 16% of our gross domestic product (GDP) which is the value of all goods and services produced in the United States, at a cost of more than $1 trillion for 1998 alone (Smith, Freeland, Heiffler, & McKusick, 1998). In order to understand the magnitude of public interest in health care spending, it is important to know the amount of public funds used. In 1998, total health care expenditures amounted to $1.3 trillion. Public funds accounted for just over 46% ($610 billion) of this spending. Public funds paid for 20% ($270 billion) of Medicare costs, 15% ($200 billion) of Medicaid costs, and 11% ($140 billion) of military, veterans, and state and local governments costs. Private funding accounted for the other 54% ($690 billion). The majority of private funding was from employer-sponsored insurance at 32% ($415 billion), self-pay at 17% ($220 billion), and other private funding at 5% ($55 billion).

The portion of total health care spending in the United States financed directly by government is the lowest among developed countries; however, state, federal, and local tax dollars still account for 45% of all health care expenditures (Braden et al., 1998). Although the United States spends more on health care, measured either per capita or as a percentage of GDP, than any other developed country in the world, the United States has the highest proportion of its citizens with no insurance and ranks near the bottom of this group of developed nations in a number of key health indicators, such as perinatal and maternal mortality, and life expectancy.

The Basis of Health Policy in the United States: Health Care as a Right Versus the Free Market

Although there is no legal or statutory "right" to health care in the United States, most of the public sees health care as a "right" (Curran, 1989). One of the main arguments for health care being a "right" is that, like other basic rights, health care and health are a prerequisite to allow citizens some equitable chance at "life, liberty and the pursuit of happiness" (Daniels, 1985). If health care is a basic human right, like freedom of religion or speech, it can be argued that the public (government) should have a primary role in ensuring that everyone has some measure of equitable access to health care. In this formulation, a key role of government would be to ensure that health care is equitably distributed among its citizens.

Much of the history of health policy in the United States can be seen as a struggle between those who see health care as a right and government as the guarantor of that right, and those who hold that health care is best handled in the "free market" and therefore see most government intervention as either undesirable or actually harmful. Both traditions have a strong place in U.S. history. Those who hold to the idea of the free market believe that the best means to distribute goods and services (except perhaps defense, fire, and police services) is by an open and direct transaction between those who desire a good or service and those who wish to sell a good or service. Inherent in this belief is that goods and services should be distributed on the basis of willingness and ability to pay a negotiated price. In a market-based economy, government interventions are usually seen as distorting the free market. The most prominent example of the failure to come to a resolution of these opposing forces is the patchwork health care systems created for different groups in the United States. There are systems fully financed and delivered by the federal government (veterans and active-duty military), a system that is federally financed and privately delivered (Medicare), a system financed by federal and state revenues and privately delivered (Medicaid), systems in which care is largely financed and provided by local government (public and county hospitals and clinics), and, finally, our largest sector with private financing and delivery (private insurance purchased individually or through an employer) (see Table 23–1 for a summary).

TABLE 23–1	PROGRAMS, FINANCING, AND DELIVERY BASED ON PUBLIC AND PRIVATE BASES		
PROGRAM		FINANCING	SERVICE DELIVERY
Veterans Administration, military health care, county hospitals		Public	Public
Medicare, Medicaid		Public	Private
Employer or individually purchased insurance		Private	Private

The origins of this patchwork can be traced to public support for legislation covering specific groups who were felt at the time to be especially needy or deserving or for whom the free market did not seem to work well. These groups include the aged, blind, or disabled (Medicare), veterans (Veterans Affairs [VA] health care); active-duty military (Department of Defense); children living in low-income, single-parent families (Medicaid); and Native Americans (Indian Health Service). Although there have been repeated attempts in virtually every decade of this century (most recently in 1994–1995) to enact some level of government-sponsored or mandated health insurance for all citizens, in the end, the fear of federal government control and the tax burden of the very large dollar amounts created by pooling current health expenditures into one program have resulted in a failure to enact universal coverage (Heclo, 1995).

Public distrust of government, especially at the federal level, has a long history. Indeed, the Constitution includes the phrase "all powers not herein specified are reserved to the states." This distrust has recently led to the "new federalism" movement of some health policy decisions (and other public services) to the state level. A number of states (Hawaii, Minnesota, Washington, and Vermont among others) have tried to set up state-based programs that would provide insurance coverage to most people who are uninsured. However, these attempts have not been fully successful (Holahan, Weiner, & Wallin, 1998). Thus the United States remains the only economically developed nation that does not have government-financed or mandated health insurance available to all, or nearly all, its citizens (Anderson & Poullier, 1999).

Organizations and Institutions Shaping Health Policy

Formulation of most health policy through law and regulation lies with the executive, legislative, and judicial branches of government at the federal, state, and local levels. Traditionally the initial formulation of health care law lies with the legislative branch, while the role of the executive branch is to implement those laws through regulation and program development. The judicial branch ensures that laws enacted by the legislative branch are consistent with state or federal constitutions, and that the executive branch follows the wishes of the legislature. Given that the executive and legislative branches can be, and often are, controlled by different parties, health policy reform has often been a major point of conflict between the executive and legislative branches. At the federal level, jurisdiction over health care in Congress is highly fragmented among different committees that oversee the various systems of publicly financed health care. For example, health-related committees in the U.S. Senate include Veterans Affairs (VA program), Armed Services (military), Labor and

Human Resources (Public Health Service), and Finance (Medicare and Medicaid) (Iglehart, 1993).

There are also a large number of nongovernmental groups that attempt to influence health policy. These can be classified as follows (examples in parentheses); provider groups (American Nurses Association), suppliers (Pharmaceutical Research and Manufacturers Association), insurers (Health Insurance Association of America), disease-related interest groups (American Cancer Society), purchasers (National Association of Manufacturers), "the public" (American Association of Retired Persons), and groups purporting to represent payers (American Taxpayers Union). Most major health policy issues call forth a remarkable number of these special interest groups into direct advertising, and mobilizing their memberships to do "grassroots" lobbying. The influence they have is determined by many factors, including the size of campaign contributions, their ability to influence elections by "getting out the vote" and mobilizing public opinion, and their capacity to provide critical information to legislators or regulators.

For policies promulgated through laws, the focus of intervention by such groups may come at any point in the process. The intervention may be exerted during the legislative process when the Senate or House writes a bill, as a bill is amended in committee, on the floor, or in House-Senate conference committee meetings. In addition, lobbying groups have an opportunity to influence how legislation is operationalized during the writing of regulations. The regulatory system establishes the rules and guidelines for the implementation of policies. Finally, the judicial system offers another road for influence through a court challenge to some aspect of the law or regulations (Feldstein, 1988).

Examples of APN Involvement in Health Policy

APN influence during the legislative phase of policy development is exemplified in the success of achieving Medicare payment to APNs in 1997. Nursing organizations coalesced to influence key senators and representatives to insert language into the Medicare bill that allowed for direct reimbursement without physician supervision or constraints on type of visit. Considerable grassroots efforts in which nursing organizations reached out to members to call and write their Congressional representatives were highly effective. APNs tracked the legislation throughout the regulatory process to ensure that the intent of Congress was upheld in the regulations. Without careful monitoring of the regulatory phase, gains that were achieved in the legislation phase could potentially be greatly reduced.

APNs have become politically sophisticated over the past several decades and have exerted considerable influence over health legislation. Although APN organizations have limited funds to invest in lobbying as compared to some other organizations, APN groups have developed the ability to form coalitions to work together targeting specific issues that have a high benefit for practice and patients, rather than having limited input in a broad set of issues. Results of this strategy can be seen in certified nurse-midwives (CNMs) obtaining Medicaid reimbursement in the 1970s, and nurse practitioners (NPs), clinical nurse specialists (CNSs), and CNMs expanding Medicare reimbursement in 1997.

Nursing has often been accused of not speaking with a unified voice. As APN groups have become more politically adept, the level of comfort and trust has increased in working as a coalition of groups for a common interest and remaining silent, if possible, when there is not a common interest. During the Clinton Health Reform era, nursing groups of all types came together and developed a strategy to make nursing's agenda integral to the reform plan. Even though the reform act was eventually defeated, the nursing profession proved it could be an important and unified force in the policy arena.

Professional Practice and Health Policy

Laws and regulations governing who can provide health care have their origins in the early 1900s with the rise of "professionalism." A profession is usually defined by a set of knowledge and skills acquired through training and education coupled with a self-generated set of standards and values. The public has been willing to allow individuals from most professions to have a strong influence in promulgating laws that define the level of education required as well as the scope of activities provided within the profession. These laws usually restrict others not educated in a similar manner from practicing that profession.

There is clearly a large degree of trust required between professionals and society to allow this model to flourish. It is helpful to remember that, prior to these laws being established, there were no barriers to anyone in the field of health care. For example, anyone could designate herself or himself a physician or nurse. Over time, each state passed laws that defined and regulated what constitutes the practice of medicine and nursing as well as other professions and who can engage in practice of these professions. In many states the oversight of these laws, including administrative enforcement, is given over to publicly appointed bodies (such as state nursing or medical boards) whose members are drawn largely from the profession.

Even though barriers to entry into a profession and restrictions as to who may engage in some set of services may protect the public from harm, they also clearly restrict competition and the free market. Although professionalism is still flourishing, there is growing evidence of greater distrust of professionals as self-defining entities, particularly when self-regulation leads to economic advantages at the expense of the public.

Over the opposition of some medical groups, APNs have taken on responsibilities that had previously been the sole prerogative of medicine. APNs and physicians have worked together effectively in the clinical area for decades, and some of the strongest supporters of APNs have been physician colleagues. However, economic pressures in the health system together with expanding numbers of physicians and APNs have created tensions, particularly at the level of national organizations. These economic tensions will likely intensify as physician salary and employment choices decrease. The American Medical Association has taken a strong stand and established guidelines for members to facilitate physicians controlling patient care (AMA, 1995). The paradox about the current context of interprofessional politics is that economic territorialism is occurring simultaneously with the need to develop efficient and effective health care teams. The renewed impetus to develop health care teams has been spurred by population-based health care as well as an increased chronic illness burden, each requiring varied expertise in order to deliver effective and efficient care.

THE HEALTH CARE MARKET AND FINANCE ISSUES

Fundamentally, the health care market is, like all markets, the interaction among those who use and purchase health care and those who provide health care services.

However, it is a very "distorted" market because of the complexity of financing and the presence of "third parties" in the form of insurers, purchasers, and payers other than the patient. Economists describe a "free" or perfect competitive market by four major characteristics: (1) the presence of a large number of buyers and sellers, (2) the unrestricted mobility of resources that allows easy exit and entry of both suppliers and buyers to the market, (3) a homogeneous (standard) product, and (4) possession of all relevant information by both supplier and buyers. The further a market is from these characteristics, the more imperfect the market, which for some may indicate a greater need for governmental intervention. In considering the health care market, none of the four characteristics noted is even close to optimal. Although there would seem to be a large number of buyers and suppliers, the fact that health care is now purchased by an ever-shrinking number of insurance companies and government agencies from ever larger health care provider groups is of concern. Furthermore, in many emergent situations, the patient may be able to exercise little or no choice of provider. Professionalism and training, the life-or-death needs for health care in some situations, and the high cost of hospital technology all mitigate against easy entry and exit. Finally, health care is far from a "standard" product. Large variation is seen throughout the United States in basic procedures such as the rate of cesarean sections, the rate of bypass surgeries, and so on. Most would argue that consumers are not particularly well informed about health care services. Although there is agreement that the health care market is far from perfect, there is still a great deal of disagreement as to how much regulation or government intervention is needed to improve the system (Feldstein, 1988).

Health Care Finance

Health care finance can be best understood as the flow of money from the source of funds to those providing services. In health care, the proximate source of the funds for the provider is often an insurer, or other entity, that collects the dollars and pools the risk for health care costs. The ultimate source of financing is individuals who earn money, who purchase health care or private insurance directly, pay taxes that are earmarked for health care, or forgo some of their earnings/wages in the form of fringe benefits that allow employers to purchase health care on their behalf. An important point is that neither government nor employers are really the source of the funds. The real source of funds is employees who forgo wages and pay taxes.

In most developed countries there is a dominant system of financing using tax funds with the government acting as insurer and purchaser. In a few instances, such as in Great Britain, the government serves as provider as well. A few other countries, including Germany and the Netherlands, rely primarily on employer-based insurance, but these countries mandate coverage by all employers and provide government-financed insurance for nearly all those not employed. As noted, the financing of health care in the United States is more complex than that in most other countries and uses a combination of direct payment and purchase of insurance, insurance purchased through fringe benefits by employers, multiple forms of public (government) insurance, and multiple forms of provider reimbursement in many of these programs.

The most direct means of health care financing is direct purchasing and payment by private citizens, as occurs with cosmetic plastic surgery. This type of payment is the norm with non-health-care goods and services. However, as health care technology evolved, it became obvious that some health care services were beyond the means of most people to pay directly out of pocket. As a result, private insurance developed. Private insurance is a means by which a group of people can pool funds to protect those who pay into that pool from "catastrophic" expenses for rare events.

TRADITIONAL INSURANCE

Private health care insurance was developed in the 1930s with the creation of Blue Cross. The first Blue Cross plan was started to enable a group of teachers in Texas to pool funds to pay for hospital care. Health insurance expanded during and after World War II. During World War II there was both a shortage of workers and a government freeze on wages. To retain or attract employees, companies began to offer health insurance as a fringe benefit. Health care benefits were not only exempt from the wage freeze but, through legislation passed by Congress, were exempt from federal taxes as well. Economic studies show that most workers, except those at very low pay levels, are often willing to trade off some portion of wages for fringe benefits. Their tendency to do so is greatly enhanced by the favorable tax treatment of health insurance. This tax exemption accounts for more than $100 billion per year in forgone taxes (Reinhardt, 1993). This tax benefit is most realized by those with higher incomes and is another factor that reduces the apparent cost of health care for most employed people.

The concept of health care insurance to protect against catastrophic events has become distorted by the inclusion of coverage for expenses that are neither rare nor particularly expensive. Insurance coverage for common and relatively inexpensive events like office visits to a physician or APN do not fit the definition of insurance (rare and costly events), but instead are a form of prepayment of expenses that are likely to be incurred. The distortion of the health care market created by insurance, and even more by prepayment, is termed "the moral hazard" of insurance. This is simply the tendency to overuse (or undervalue) services for which the person consuming the service does not have to pay the full cost. It is helpful in understanding "moral hazard" to consider how consumers would behave if they "insured" themselves or, more accurately, prepaid and pooled funds for groceries. If groceries were paid for by insurance, most people would probably choose to shop at a high-quality, expensive gourmet grocery store. Both insurance and tax subsidies (discussed later) introduce moral hazard by lowering (sometimes to zero) the direct cost of health care services to the consumer.

Until recently, the most common form of health insurance in the United States was "indemnity" insurance purchased by an employee through his or her employer. The concept of indemnity is that the insurer agrees to "indemnify" (protect) those who are insured from losses sustained up to some set amount. In classic indemnity insurance, the person goes to a health care provider of choice, pays the provider for the service, and then files a claim with the insurance company for reimbursement at a preset level. An early modification to indemnity insurance, which was quickly adapted by most insurers, was the imposition of the insurer as the direct payer of the service provider. This protected the insured individual from having to come up with funds to pay the provider first, and allowed the insurance company to negotiate with providers for lower rates based on volume purchasing. Note that this introduced a fundamental change in the health care market. While the consumer of health care services (the patient) remains the same, the entity that actually purchases and pays for the service is now an insurance company. This shift, accelerated by the growing consolidation of insurers and the rise of large, often for-profit provider entities (hospitals, physician groups, home care providers, nursing home chains) has been termed by Starr (1982) the "corporatization" of American health care.

Many small to moderate-sized employers offer employees one or more insurance plans that can be purchased as an employment-related fringe benefit, usually along with some additional direct payment by the employee. In this case, the insurance company becomes the "at risk" entity, which means that the insurance company agrees to pay the cost of all covered health care benefits for enrolled employees. The "risk" is that the premiums paid by the employee and employer may not be sufficient to cover the costs. A growing number of larger employers are "self-insured." This means the company accepts the risk for paying the costs of health care services covered by the health care benefits provided by the company. Most self-insured companies use insurance companies to perform such tasks as estimating the probable cost of health benefits (actuarial or risk analysis), overseeing eligibility and enrollment, and management of claims made by providers.

HEALTH MAINTENANCE ORGANIZATIONS

With their roots in traditional indemnity insurance, most health insurance companies did not see themselves as the actual purchasers of care, and had no interest in providing health care services themselves. A few industries, such as railroads and timber, provided health care for their workers as long ago as the late 19th century. These companies hired and paid for their own health care providers and in some cases built their own hospitals. During World War II, the Kaiser Aluminum Corporation created a company-sponsored health care plan for its employees. After the war, Kaiser began to offer membership in their plan to other employers and individuals for a set yearly payment. Prior to the war, consumer groups in Washington, DC, and Seattle, Washington, started "group health cooperatives." Like the Kaiser plan, these health plans acted as risk pool manager, payer, and provider of health care for people who joined the health plan. Membership was defined by a yearly "membership" payment. Kaiser and the two group health plans were termed "prepaid health plans" and later named "health maintenance organizations" (HMOs), which evolved to managed care organizations. The basic concept was that, for some predetermined "prepaid" premium, the health plan would provide all needed care either directly, through employing health care staff (thus the designation staff-model HMO), or indirectly, by contracting with providers. The critical difference compared to traditional indemnity health insurance is that HMOs tend to act more as direct providers or active purchasers of health care in addition to their actuarial and risk pool management functions. HMOs were much more aggressive than traditional insurers in competitive contracting with a limited group of providers, lowering prices paid for services, and intervening in the process of health care to try to reduce utilization. As HMOs evolve from staff and group models to individual practice associations and point of service plans and traditional insurers begin to implement fee schedules and utilization management, the distinction between HMOs and other insurers is becoming less. In many regards, all care is now "managed care."

PUBLIC FINANCING

A final form of health care financing that is dominant in all other developed countries is publicly financed health care through taxation by government. Unlike private insurance, public funding for health care nearly always involves coverage for some people who cannot afford to purchase private health care insurance on their own. For public (government-financed) programs, the source of funds is taxpayers, with the government serving as funds collector, manager, and payer (as in the traditional Medicare and Medicaid programs). The government may also serve as purchaser (as with the Medicare + Choice program) or as funds collector, manager, and provider, as for active-duty military through the Department of Defense, for military veterans through the VA, or for Native Americans through the Indian Health Service. The advantages of public financing include lower administrative costs, creation of the largest possible risk pool, and maximal equity in the quality and accessibility of health care. Finally, as noted earlier, one of the largest and often least noted sectors of public financing of health care is the tax subsidy provided by the tax-exempt status of private health care insurance that is purchased directly or provided as a fringe benefit of employment.

Reimbursement

Reimbursement is simply the way those who purchase health care services pay those who provide services. Payment in health care is complicated by the fact that, presently, the payer is most often not the person who receives the services, but rather an insurance company. Historically, indemnity insurers reimbursed the insured individual a set amount for any service that was covered by the insurance plan. The patient could go to any provider who was defined in the insurance contract as qualified to deliver the service. Qualification was usually defined as anyone licensed as a specific type of provider. The patient, not the insurance company, paid the provider the amount charged, and then would file a claim with the insurer and receive the amount defined in the insurance contract. The amount received by the patient could be more or less than the amount charged by the provider.

With the emergence of the insurer as active purchaser rather than as passive payer, insurers began to restrict reimbursement to those providers who signed an agreement or contract with the insurer. These contracts defined the terms and often the level of reimbursement provided by the insurer. This trend was greatly accelerated by the emergence of HMOs and "managed care." In addition to limits on who they would pay, insurers moved to directly pay providers based on one of the following: the amount charged by the provider (fee for service [FFS]), a set level of reimbursement set by the insurer (fee schedule), or a capitation payment (per member per month payment regardless of the services provided). It is vital for APNs to understand reimbursement, particularly because of their ability to be directly reimbursed by Medicare and Medicaid (for some APNs). It is also critical to understand payment as APNs become recognized providers and contract effectively with managed care organizations.

CHARGE OR COST-BASED FEE FOR SERVICE

In the simplest form of FFS reimbursement, the provider sets a price (charge) for a defined service provided to a patient, and the patient pays that amount. This is the way that most goods and services are paid for. As insurers began to control costs and pay providers directly, more complex variations of FFS arrangements were developed. The most common of these arrangements bases the amount that the insurer reimburses either the patient or the provider for a given service on the lesser of the "actual, customary, prevailing, or reasonable" charge. The actual charge is the amount on the bill from the provider; the customary charge is the average charge that the same provider charged for the same service in the past (usually over a 1-year period); the prevailing charge is some percentage of the average charge for all providers in a given area for the specific service; and reasonable charge is the amount determined by the insurer to be "reasonable" for the service.

The proportion of reimbursement based on FFS has been steadily declining, especially with the enactment of the Medicare fee schedule for physicians. Some large insurers, and by definition preferred provider organizations, negotiate a discount on what the provider usually charges. This is termed "discounted FFS" and can take the form of a fixed percentage reduction of the charges.

APNs have had limited success in gaining access to FFS reimbursement. Much of the reason for this was timing. Just as APNs gained enough influence and political strength to be recognized by insurers, there was a shift away from the traditional FFS reimbursement.

A variation of charge-based reimbursement is cost-based reimbursement, which has been used for payment to hospitals. In cost-based reimbursement, the provider and insurer negotiate a contract in which the provider is reimbursed the "allowable costs" of producing a service. The contract defines what costs are "allowable" or considered to be legitimate costs of producing the service. Until recently, cost-based reimbursement was used extensively by Medicare and some private insurers to pay hospitals, nursing homes and home care providers. Very few insurers now pay on the basis of cost-based reimbursement.

FEE SCHEDULES

In this case the price paid for a service or group of services, often called "bundled services," is determined by the insurer. The critical difference from charge or FFS reimbursement is that the insurer, not the provider, has final say in setting the reimbursement. The fee schedule may be developed based on some percentage of historical charges or costs, or on an analysis of the work and expenses that go into producing a given service, as with the Medicare resource-based relative value scale. In the case of Medicare and most other insurers at this time, providers must sign an agreement to accept the fee schedule, in most cases as full payment, if they want to be reimbursed by Medicare for seeing the patient. Patients who obtain services from providers who are not under contact with the insurer will usually have to pay for those services themselves. Most health plans, and most notably Medicare, either limit or altogether forbid (through contract or, in Medicare, through statutory law) the provider from charging the patient the difference between what the provider "charges" to patients paying FFS and the fee schedule amount. Payments under Medicare's various "prospective payment" programs (hospitals, skilled nursing facilities, and most recently home care services) are basically variants of a fee schedule developed using a fraction of historical costs as the basis of paying for the service. A per diem payment—that is, a set amount per day of services—is also in effect a type of fee schedule.

APNs have gained considerable inroads into reimbursement under fee schedules. Like that for physicians, APN reimbursement under Medicare and Medicaid is through a fee schedule. APNs are paid a set percentage of the fee that a physician receives. For instance, CNSs and NPs eligible for Medicare reimbursement receive 85% of the physician rate if billing independently, or 100% if the billing is "incident to" a physician visit. The policy dilemma for APNs is whether to politically position themselves as "cost-effective" providers and continue to accept 85% of an already low reimbursement rate, or push to get 100% of the physician rate based on the premise that the same or very comparable service is provided.

CAPITATION

As a fee schedule changes the control of reimbursement from the provider to the insurer, capitation changes the locus of financial risk from the insurance company to the provider entity that accepts capitation. With capitation, providers are paid a negotiated amount per member per month or per year. For that fixed amount, the provider agrees to provide all necessary health care services that are covered by the insurance benefit and specified in the provider's capitation contract. Capitation can cover a total (for all services) or be limited (as for primary care, specialty care, or hospital care only). Because of the risk of adverse selection (i.e., getting patients who require more services than average), providers can afford to accept full risk only if they are part of a large group.

The fundamental challenge to APNs under the capitation reimbursement mechanism is to be a recognized provider who can contract with a managed care entity or be accepted as part of a group practice. In either situation, APNs need to fully assess the financial risk associated with capitation. For primary-care-only capitation, there is a lesser risk of financial losses from adverse selection, and it may be possible for individual or groups of APNs to negotiate capitation contracts with HMOs.

SALARY

In addition to these three mechanisms of reimbursement, providers may be salaried. Although this is a relatively new phenomenon for physicians, this has been the standard form of payment for most APNs. Thus, while a provider or provider group may be reimbursed via a mix of capitation, FFS, and fee schedule, the individual providers may pay themselves or be paid a salary, or a salary plus incentive based on charges or resource-based relative value units (RBRVUs) generated. If providers are in unincorporated private practices, they may receive whatever revenues remain after practice expenses are paid.

ETHICAL ISSUES RELATED TO REIMBURSEMENT

Each form of reimbursement introduces certain economic and ethical issues. In FFS or charge-based reimbursement, providers can set prices at whatever level they choose, which is the way most businesses operate. Although this is the way most non-health-care markets operate, FFS tends to result in overuse of health care services and high costs. Like FFS, cost-based reimbursement results in high costs because there is no incentive for the provider to keep costs down. In these modes of reimbursement, the economic interest of the provider is to maximize the price, or allowed cost, and the number of services provided.

With a fee schedule, salary with incentives, billings, RBRVUs, or net revenues, there are economic incentives for providers to minimize the costs of producing the service but still provide as much as possible. This method of payment may encourage providers to supply services that are of small or no benefit to the patient. With capitation, or a salary plus incentives based on controlled utilization of services by patients, providers have an incentive to minimize both the cost of producing a given service and the number of services. This creates the pressure for providers to withhold services that may be of substantial benefit to the patient. Finally, when providers are paid a salary, there is no direct incentive related to the number or price of services provided to a given patient. Salary also removes any incentive for increased productivity or to provide services quickly and efficiently. However, in practices dependent on practice revenues (like private group practice as opposed to physicians employed by a government agency), the provider's salary is ultimately affected by practice revenues and practice expenses.

From the patient's perspective, it would be most desirable to get the maximum number of useful services at the lowest cost. If the patient is only paying through an insurance premium with no out-of-pocket payments, there is a strong incentive to use services that may be of very small benefit. For the taxpayer in public programs or the insurer and employees who pay for private insurance, the goal is to try to pay for only those services that are essential and at the lowest possible overall cost. The ethical dilemmas raised by different types of reimbursement arise where the interests of the provider, the patient, the insurer, and those who pay for insurance are in conflict. Thus each mode of reimbursement presents the patient, provider, and insurer-financier with ethical dilemmas. In FFS the challenge is for the provider and patient not to oversupply and overuse services; in capitation, it is for the provider not to withhold needed services.

Cost and Cost Containment

The total expenditures on health care as a percentage of all goods and services (the GDP) have been growing in the United States throughout the 20th century. Since the 1950s, with the widespread introduction of insurance for most Americans and the acceleration of health care technology development, health care cost increases have pushed the proportion of GDP devoted to health care to over 16%.

Most studies of health care cost increases have found that there are three major factors driving the rise in health care costs relative to GDP or general inflation (Newhouse, 1993). These factors are technology, demographics (growth and aging of the population), and health care price inflation. The most powerful factor, accounting for well over half of the cost increase, is the ever-growing use of health care technology. In U.S. society there is a very high value placed on the individual and an imperative in health care to do everything possible. In addition, the use of insurance and tax exemptions means that the person receiving the services does not see the total cost of the service.

Furthermore, with more effective and lower risk treatments, problems like hypertension, hypercholesterolemia, impotence, and infertility are being constantly redefined to include everyone with a less than ideal level of risk or function, rather than just those at very high risk or with markedly impaired function. Artificial joints, laser eye surgery, laparoscopic surgery, and virtually risk-free diagnostic procedures, such as magnetic resonance imaging, constantly lower the risk-benefit barriers of diagnostic and therapeutic interventions. This removal of patient risk as a barrier to technology, along with insurance and tax exemptions, gives rise to increased use of technology, including procedures that are very expensive and provide limited benefit in prolonging life or enhancing the quality of life. Moreover, most technologies do not totally replace existing ones but are simply added to existing procedures, and thus increase total cost.

Those interventions that do prolong life exacerbate another major factor leading to higher health care costs, namely population growth and the aging of the population. Between 1900 and 1960, average life expectancy rose from 45 years to nearly 70 years, and between 1960 and the present life expectancy has risen from 70 to 78 years. The most rapidly growing portion of the population is people over 85. In addition to longer survival, people are also living longer with major disease and disability.

The other major factor that has affected health care costs is that price increases for health care have in most years exceeded price increases in other sectors of the economy. Prices charged for a defined service like an office visit rose faster than GDP or general inflation, especially in the period from 1950 to 1975. The spread of insurance and the enactment of Medicare, with their use of FFS and cost-based reimbursement, contributed to the rise in inflation. Again however, technology played a role because what was being delivered as part of a unit of service (e.g., an emergency room visit for a person with a myocardial infarction) was modified by new technologies. Many of these new technologies, such as the use of tissue plasminogen activators, not only add costs directly but may require the use of more highly trained, and often more costly, personnel to deliver the technology. Thus the cost of producing, and the price charged for a "standard" unit of service such as the emergency room visit, is increased.

There have been numerous attempts to try to reduce the rate of rise of health care costs, most of which have totally failed. Even those that appear to have had some impact have only provided a brief, usually one-time reduction. The reasons why health care costs are so difficult to control include the moral hazard of insurance, with its disconnect between the benefits received by the patient and the perceived cost; our society's drive to prolong life regardless of the cost (the rescue mentality); ample public financing of basic research and technology development (most notably through the National Institutes of Health); our fascination with technology; a strong history of focus on the individual; and, until recently, a relative undersupply of providers in the face of failure of market forces to control prices (Aaron & Schwartz, 1984).

Some of the mechanisms by which government and private insurers attempt to control costs have included payment and market reforms, utilization management strategies, and shifting costs to reduce demand (Table 23–2). All of these interventions have been present in the health care market for the past decade or more, many of them under the general title of "managed care." Although medical sector cost inflation has been affected at times, especially by some of the payment and market reforms, health care costs have, in most years, continued to rise 1% to 3% per year faster than either general inflation or the GDP. The various pronouncements that "health care inflation has been tamed" have proven to be untrue. In 1996–1997, health care costs actually rose less rapidly than other costs or GDP (Health Care Financing Administration [HCFA], 1998b). However, in 1998 and even more in 1999, it appeared that health care costs had again begun to outpace inflation and growth in the GDP (Crippen, 1999). Short of a major depression or a change in our attempts to extend life and use technology, health care costs will continue to rise faster than inflation or GDP for the foreseeable future. However, the rate of relative increase in the future is likely to be lower because of the increasing market power of insurers and the relative oversupply of providers, which will mitigate or even reduce the prices

TABLE 23–2 SUMMARY OF COST CONTROL STRATEGIES

Payment Reforms
- Imposition of fee schedules instead of cost-based reimbursement (Medicare's Prospective Payment System [PPS] for hospitals and Resource Based Relative Value System [RBRVS] fee schedule for doctors)
- Limiting total increases in PPS and RBRVS to some index of inflation or GDP and reducing the fee schedule rates if volume increases occur
- Use of capitation payments to give providers incentive to reduce both costs and volume of services as well as to cap total expenditures

Market Reforms
- Mergers that increase the relative economic power of insurers to set price
- Contracting only with selected providers who agree to lower fees
- Competitive contracting (bidding out services to the lowest bidder)
- Profiling providers on the basis of utilization and price (total cost) and eliminating the high-cost providers from the plan
- Use of a specific group rating instead of community rating (charging an enrolled group a premium based on that specific group's risks and utilization, rather than on the average risk and utilization in the community as a whole)

Utilization Management
- Requiring second opinions for expensive services such as surgery
- Concurrent and retrospective reviews resulting in denial of payments
- Guidelines, case management, disease management, and other attempts to change the way medicine is practiced

Reducing Demand by Shifting Costs to Consumers
- Higher co-pays
- Higher deductibles
- Higher self-pay premiums
- Excluding services (contraception, transplants, infertility services)

charged per unit of services. Taming the increase in health care technology is much more problematic. The double-digit rise in the cost of pharmaceuticals in the past 2 years is just one manifestation of this seemingly uncontrollable sector.

ACCESS

Access to care has been a major policy issue for many years. It is of growing concern and was one of the factors (as well as concern about rising costs) that drove the health care reform initiative during the early years of the Clinton administration. The issue of access has become more prominent as a result of the unrelenting increase in the number of uninsured individuals, especially during a time of economic prosperity. The estimated number of uninsured people is now 44.6 million, representing an increase of 2.7 million just from 1996 (U. S. Census Bureau, 1998).

Access to health care is a complicated issue. Barriers to access are related to a number of factors, including inability to pay for health care as well as lack of availability of specific types of health care providers or institutions. It can be argued that health care is not accessible if care is not available within a geographically reasonable area for a specific type of provider, such as a CNM or NP, or if cultural background, values, and language are disparate between patient and provider.

APNs have been a forceful voice to ensure access to care in its most comprehensive aspects. Access concerns by APNs are linked to APN roots. APNs largely developed as a result of a policy response to access problems. Much of the focus of the HHS Division of Nursing, which implements the funds appropriated by Congress to support nursing education and special projects through Title VIII of the Nurse Practice Act, has been to support programs that enhance access.

AFFORDABILITY

The rise in health care costs, coupled with a growing number of people with no or inadequate insurance, has created significant problems in the affordability of health care for many people in the United States. Public perception has been that the uninsured are mostly individuals who are unemployed. That perception has changed over the past several years with the recognition that the majority of uninsured individuals work either full or part time, and often in multiple jobs. A recent report on the decline in health insurance coverage of workers indicates that, whereas 15% of workers were uninsured in 1979, approximately 23.3% of workers were uninsured in 1995. This number is even higher among those who work for small employers and especially those in the service sector (Kronick & Gilmore, 1999).

Several reasons have been advanced for the increased numbers of uninsured people, including a change in immigration patterns, a shift in employment to small firms or self-employment, and, most importantly, the growing cost of health care. Kronick and Gilmore (1999) proposed that the rise in the uninsured is more related to rising health care expenditures making insurance unaffordable for increasing numbers of workers even when it is offered by their employer, and the shift to group rating from community rating by insurance companies. This latter factor results in insurance premiums for employees in some firms being double or triple the rates in other similar companies. Thorpe and Florence (1999) found that a growing number of workers cite the high cost of insurance as their reason for refusing coverage. As a result of this, and reductions in Medicaid and other safety net programs, the number of people with no health insurance has been steadily growing, reaching 44 million, or 16% of the total population, in 1999. The Institute for the Future (2000) anticipates that this trend will continue, with an increase of uninsured occurring at a rate of about 750,000 people per year. This estimate would increase if there were an economic recession.

It is important to understand the profile of individuals who are uninsured. Because Medicare covers nearly all Americans 65 years and older, most uninsured are under 65. The likelihood of being uninsured increases if one works for a small business (less than 100 employees), is self-employed or a temporary worker, or is an employee in a low-wage firm (Gabel, Hurst, Whitmore, & Hoffman, 1999). Not all uninsured are poor, but they are not well off. Seventy-two percent of the nonelderly uninsured have incomes above the poverty line (Rowland, Feder, & Keenan, 1998). More than 50% of the uninsured are in families in which the head of the household works full time for the entire year, and 32% are in families in which the head of the household works part time for the year or full time for part of the year (Kaiser Family Foundation, 1994).

Having no insurance is a major factor limiting access to and use of health services. However, there is substantial reason to be concerned also about the population who are "underinsured." Although there is no clear definition of what "underinsured" is, being underinsured relates to the degree of financial exposure for the care of illness. One measure of underinsured is out-of-pocket expenses exceeding 10% of family income for a serious illness. Using this measure, Short and Banthin (1995) estimated that 18.5% of the population, or nearly 40 million people, was underinsured.

Lack of access has been operationally defined by several measures. The most traditional measure is the number of uninsured individuals. Individuals are considered uninsured if they have no insurance coverage either through employer-sponsored insurance or public safety net programs such as Medicare or Medicaid. It is important to note that some uninsured may be eligible for coverage through a safety net program, yet for many reasons do not apply. Additional measures include the number of individuals unable to obtain care, the number of emergency room visits for nonemergent care, and reports of fair or poor health with no physician visits in the past year (Berk & Schur, 1998). Berk and Schur (1998) compared six different surveys related to inability to obtain care during the period of 1982 through 1995. In all cases uninsured individuals reported inability to obtain care more frequently than those who were insured. The consequences of not having access to health care include hospitalization for otherwise avoidable health problems and a greater disease burden (Weissman, Gastonis, & Epstein, 1992; Syrne, 1998).

State and federal government-sponsored programs have been the backbone of providing access to care for those who otherwise could not financially afford insurance. The federal programs include Medicare and the V.A. Federal-state programs include Medicaid and the Child Health Initiative Program.

Medicare

PROGRAM DESCRIPTION

Medicare was enacted in 1965 to provide health coverage to individuals over 65 years of age, and to those who are blind or disabled. Many at the time considered Medicare as the first step to providing universal health insurance coverage, starting with a specific group (the elderly, blind, and disabled) of whom many were poor (nearly 20% under the poverty level at the time) and who had relatively high health care costs. Although the expansion to other groups (with the exception of those with kidney failure) has not occurred, Medicare now covers approximately 37 million Americans. Medicare Part A, funded from a special part of the Social Security Tax, covers hospital stays, skilled nursing facilities, home health care, hospice care, and certain products. Part B, funded from general tax revenues (75%) and premiums paid by enrollees (25%), covers most costs of physician and APN visits; outpatient medical and surgical services; supplies; physical, occupational, and speech therapies; diagnostic tests; and durable medical equipment. Part B also covers outpatient clinical laboratory services, home health care (if the individual is not covered by Part A), and outpatient hospital services and blood products (as an outpatient) (see Table 23–3).

Even though Medicare provides coverage for a broad array of services, individuals with Medicare coverage can experience considerable out-of-pocket expenses as a result of co-payment and deductible costs and the costs of noncovered services such as long-term care and pharmaceuticals. Other products and services not included are eyeglasses, most dental care, hearing aids, and routine eye exams.

Although nearly 80% of Medicare recipients have additional coverage through private Medicare supplemental insurance or Medicaid, few of the private insurers

TABLE 23-3 MEDICARE COVERED SERVICES

PART A	PART B
Hospitalization, including semiprivate room, meals, and general nursing	Medical expenses, including physician and APN services; inpatient and outpatient medical and surgical services; occupational, physical, and speech therapy; diagnostic tests; and durable medical equipment
Skilled nursing facility, including semiprivate room, meals, skilled nursing and rehabilitative services	Clinical laboratory services, including blood tests, VA and others
Home health care, including intermittent skilled nursing, physical therapy, speech-language services, home health aide services, and durable medical equipment	Home health care (if patient does not have Part A)
Hospice (including pain) and support relief, home care, inpatient care	Outpatient hospital services for diagnosis or treatment of an illness or injury
Blood during a hospital or skilled nursing facility stay	Blood as an outpatient

cover long-term care or pharmaceuticals. Thus a substantial number of Medicare enrollees are underinsured relative to their risks of health care costs and personal resources. These uncovered costs can be catastrophic for elderly individuals and couples. The cost of a hospital stay followed by a period of rehabilitation, along with home care costs and drug costs, can be financially devastating. For instance, the out-of-pocket expenses related to stroke may easily exceed $10,000 in the first year. These costs would include the hospital co-pay, the co-pay on the first 100 days of skilled nursing care and the full costs (often more than $300 per day) for each skilled nursing home day thereafter, the full costs of drugs outside the hospital, and the 20% co-pay for all outpatient physician or APN care and durable medical equipment, such as a wheelchair, that may be needed. Individuals experiencing prolonged stays in skilled nursing facilities with recurrent hospitalizations can also exhaust their Medicare hospital benefits, resulting in expenses that can overwhelm all but the very wealthy.

As noted many older persons purchase supplemental private insurance. These policies are designed to pay primarily for the deductibles, co-pays, and long hospital stays not covered by Medicare. Policies that are labeled "Medicare Supplemental Insurance" are regulated by the federal government and grouped into 10 "standard" policies each offering a slightly different combination of benefits (HCFA, 1998d). Most of these policies cost $3,000 or more a year, and individuals must purchase them from personal funds. Elderly and disabled individuals with severe illness and low incomes cannot afford this expense, and, as noted, few of these policies cover long-term care or pharmaceuticals.

Medicare coverage for pharmaceuticals has been frequently considered and debated since the program's inception in 1965. A Medicare drug benefit was actually enacted as part of the "Catastrophic Coverage Act of 1987," but was repealed the following year largely because of fears of its impact on higher taxes and of government control of pharmaceuticals. The issue was once again before Congress in 1999, but was tabled. This issue will continue to be raised. The cost of a Medicare drug benefit is estimated to be $118 billion over the next decade. Critics of Medicare's failure to provide a drug benefit cite numerous anecdotes of individuals who experience acute illness because they were not able to pay for the prescriptions that would prevent or treat the illness. The politics surrounding this issue are complex and involve potential conflict with the pharmaceutical companies. The policy options considered by Congress include using a portion of the budget surplus to fund a drug benefit with a cap on the amount covered. Another option that the pharmaceutical companies strongly oppose is to limit the prices pharmaceutical companies could charge.

MEDICARE FINANCING

Much of the current policy debate about Medicare centers on the viability of Medicare Part A, which is funded through the Medicare Trust Fund. The Trust Fund receives revenues from the Medicare part of the Social Security Tax, which are then used to pay expenses of Medicare Part A. Projections of the viability of Part A of Medicare are based on the balance between the rate of future expenditures and anticipated revenues. The projections are very dependent on both the anticipated rate of growth of health care expenditures and on employment, which determines income and thus Social Security Tax revenues. Prior to 1997, even the most optimistic projections predicted that the Trust Fund would be depleted in the early years of the 21st century. In addition, expenditures in Part B of Medicare, which as noted gets most of its funding from the general tax fund (mostly from the Federal Income Tax) have become one of the largest single tax expenditures. Concerns about the viability of the Part A Trust Fund, and the drain on general revenues by Part B, have led Congress to enact a steady stream of cost control measures, including most recently the Medicare provisions that were included in the Balanced Budget Amendment of 1997 (BBA).

The political pressures surrounding changes in the Medicare program are considerable, with the more than 37 million persons who benefit from the program pushing for benefit expansion, and those who pay Social Security and income taxes in favor of holding costs down. Given this political pressure and the lack of effective ways of controlling costs, policy makers have focused most of the changes on trying to control expenditures by changing reimbursement procedures from cost or FFS to fees that can be controlled by Medicare. The evolution of hospital payments from cost-based reimbursement to prospective payment using diagnosis-related groups (DRGs) and of physician payments from FFS to a fee schedule based on RBRVUs are two changes enacted in the 1980s and early 1990s that illustrate this trend. The 1997 BBA removes the remaining cost-based reimbursements and extends prospective payment to skilled nursing facilities, hospital outpatient settings, home care, and rehabilitation hospitals, as well as reducing the rate of increase of prospective payment and RBRVU-based payments to physicians and hospitals. The current Medicare fee schedule payment to APNs represents an example of how pressure to allow APNs to bill directly was combined with a cost control measure.

Attempts to control expenditures through limiting Medicare benefits to low-income elderly, requiring higher income elderly to pay higher premiums for Part B, or any other measures directed at recipients have met strong opposition from politically active elders. As recently as 1999, President Clinton floated an option for "means testing" enrollees' benefits but withdrew this option because of immediate opposition (Goldstein, 1999). However, some measures, including linking the Part B premium paid by recipients to 25% of total program costs, and limiting skilled nursing and home care benefits with restrictions on prior hospital stays, are a few of the measures that have been enacted to control costs on the recipient side.

The decision to cut provider rates has had significant consequences. Many hospitals, particularly academic health centers, and hospitals providing care to uninsured populations are experiencing severe financial difficulty. Health plans are choosing to scale back or eliminate their Medicare choice options. APNs need to be knowledgeable about changes in Medicare in order to know how efforts to control costs may affect the financial viability of practice. Updates on changes in Medicare can be obtained at *www.hcfa.gov/medicare/medicare.htm.*

Medicaid

The Medicaid program was enacted in 1965 as Title XIX (along with Medicare, which is Title XVIII) of the Social Security Act. In 1996, 36.1 million individuals were covered by Medicaid (HCFA, 1998a). A major revision of the Medicaid program occurred in 1996 with the enactment of the Welfare Reform Act. Prior to enactment of this bill, enrollment in Medicaid was automatic for persons receiving cash assistance under a number of federal low-income assistance programs, most notably Aid to Families with Dependent Children (AFDC, which was abolished by the Welfare Reform Act). The de-linking of Medicaid enrollment from cash assistance programs such as AFDC has resulted in substantial decreases in the number of low-income non-elderly enrolled in Medicaid. In addition, the Welfare Reform Act prohibited states from enrolling non-citizens in Medicaid other than in very limited situations.

Medicaid provides health insurance coverage for certain groups of individuals and families with specified levels of low income and assets. It is a program funded jointly by the states and the federal government. The formula used to determine the state contribution is based on the average per capita income of the state. Thus, states with low per capita income contribute less than the 50% maximal match required of wealthier states.

Although the federal government through intermediaries, carriers, and other contractors administers Medicare, Medicaid is administered by individual states, with substantial latitude in terms of eligibility standards, scope of service, payment rates, and the administering entities. States have some discretion in determining eligibility requirements, but there are some groups that states must offer coverage to in order to get federal matching dollars. These mandated groups include U.S. citizens who are

- In families who meet requirements that previously applied to the AFDC program
- Recipients of Supplemental Security Income (SSI)
- Infants born to Medicaid-eligible mothers
- Children below the age of 6 and pregnant women who meet the state's earlier AFDC financial requirements or whose family income is at or below 133% of the federal poverty level
- All children up to age 19 born after September 30, 1983, in families with incomes at or below the federal poverty level
- Medicare beneficiaries who meet Medicaid income and asset restrictions

Note that people eligible for Medicaid must *both* meet the income/asset tests *and* be a member of one of the defined groups. In addition, with the loss of automatic enrollment linked to cash assistance programs like ADFC, many low-income people do not apply for Medicaid coverage until they are hospitalized or have some other major health need.

States have the option of providing Medicaid coverage to other "categorically needy" groups. Eligibility criteria applicable to all states for these groups are more flexible than the mandatory groups—for example, infants up to 1 year and pregnant women whose family income is up to 185% of the poverty level are eligible. In addition, states have the option to have a "medically needy" program to extend coverage to individuals who have too much income to qualify under the mandatory or optional categorically needy groups but who have high medical care costs. This medically needy option allows individuals to "spend down" to Medicaid eligibility by incurring medical care expenses to offset their excess income. An example is an individual entering a nursing facility with income and assets in excess of Medicaid limits, but who, after paying for nursing home care for a period of time, depletes his or her assets and has an income that is less than the cost of the nursing home plus the Medicaid income limit. If the state offers a "medically needy" program under Medicaid (and 38 states do so), the remainder of the nursing home stay may be covered under Medicaid. (See Table 23-4 for a summary of Medicaid services.)

The Medicaid program is often thought to cover poor children. In fact, attempts to cut Medicaid costs have often been based on reducing "abuse" in the system by welfare mothers. However, two thirds of Medicaid enrollees, who were AFDC recipients, get one third of the benefits. Although elderly and disabled individuals represent only one third of the enrollees, they receive two thirds of the benefits, largely for long-term stays in nursing homes. A 1996 comparison of Medicaid payment

TABLE 23-4 MEDICAID SERVICES

REQUIRED FOR CATEGORICALLY NEEDY	REQUIRED FOR MEDICALLY NEEDY	FEDERALLY FUNDED COMMON OPTIONAL SERVICES
Inpatient hospital	Prenatal care and delivery services	Clinic services
Outpatient hospital	Ambulatory services to individuals under age 18	Nursing facility services for under 21
Physician services	Home health services to individuals entitled to nursing facility services	Intermediate care facility/ mental retardation services
Medical and surgical dental services		Optometrist services and eyeglasses
Nursing facility for individuals age 21 and over		Prescribed drugs
Home health care for those eligible for nursing facility		Tuberculosis (TB)-related services for TB-infected individuals
Family planning services and supplies		Prosthetic devices
Rural health clinic services		Dental services
Laboratory and x-ray		
Pediatric and family NP services		
Federally qualified health center services		
Nurse-midwifery services		
Early and periodic screening, diagnosis, and treatment for individuals under age 21		

by age of recipients show that those 85+ years received $12,169 per year while those 0 to 5 years received services valued at $1,406 per year (HCFA, 1999).

Policy makers have pursued a variety of strategies to contain the cost of Medicaid, mostly focused on the nonelderly portion of the program. Because of the federal match, many states have tried to expand Medicaid programs, which can substitute for programs that are fully state funded. This tendency has been a factor that has increased the cost of Medicaid at the federal level. One result of the increases at the federal level is the previously discussed changes enacted in the 1996 Welfare Reform Act. Another major strategy for cost control has been to move Medicaid recipients into managed care plans. In 1991, 9.5% of Medicaid enrollees were in a managed care plan. The percentage of Medicaid recipients enrolled in managed care has now increased to 40%, but virtually all these are the nonelderly Medicaid enrollees. In a number of states, movement of Medicaid enrollees to managed care has been beset by problems of disenrollment, loss of Medicaid eligibility, and failure of those enrolled to understand HMO restrictions on use of non-HMO resources, such as the continued use of emergency rooms in public hospitals. In this situation, the HMO receives the payment for providing care but the public hospital provides the care with no HMO reimbursement.

Currently, only specific groups of APNs are eligible for Medicaid reimbursement. These groups include pediatric NPs, family NPs, and CNMs. A major policy agenda of NPs is to extend Medicaid reimbursement to all NPs.

Children's Health Insurance Program

The Children's Health Insurance Program (CHIP) was passed as a part of the BBA as Title XXI of the Social Security Act. Congress and the Clinton administration agreed to set aside $24 billion from general tax revenues over a 5-year period to create this program to expand health care insurance coverage for low-income children. CHIP is intended to extend insurance to children in low-income families who are not eligible for Medicaid but who do not have or cannot afford private health care insurance. Like Medicaid, CHIP is a program in which federal funds must be matched by a set proportion of state funds.

CHIP represents the largest investment in children's health since the enactment of Medicaid in 1965. The impetus for CHIP was the recognition of the growing number of uninsured children in low-income families. Over 11 million children in 1996 were uninsured, a number that had grown by nearly 800,000 in just 1 year (Congressional Budget Office, 1998). Projections when the program was enacted indicated that 3.8 million uninsured children would be eligible for CHIP, or about 1 in 4 uninsured children in this county (Selden, Banthin, & Cohen, 1999).

To date, all states and territories have approved CHIP plans. However, some states were slow to implement CHIP because of the requirement for matching funds and the provisions requiring active enrollment efforts for both CHIP- and Medicaid-eligible children. It is of interest to note that Congress anticipated that federal funding for the CHIP program would come from the federal tobacco settlement. As events unrolled, the federal settlement was scuttled but most states participated in an agreement with the tobacco companies. However, the income from the settlement was not earmarked for CHIP or any other health program. A major battle has developed in many states over the use of the tobacco settlement funds, including their use for the CHIP program.

There were three alternative forms for implementation of the CHIP program. Twenty-six states have implemented CHIP as part of the Medicaid program; 16 states developed a separate child health insurance plan; and 12 states have a combination plan (see Figure 23–1). States also have several benefits plan options. One benchmark plan is the standard Blue Cross/Blue Shield preferred provider option offered under the Federal Employees Health Benefits Program. Another is a benefit plan generally available to state employees, and the third uses the benefit plan of the HMO with the largest commercial enrollment in the state (HCFA, 1997a).

Policy makers are concerned that parents or employers might see CHIP as a substitute for offering private insurance coverage to employees. In a survey of low-wage employers, nearly one fifth said they would stop paying premiums if CHIP was available (Aston, 1999). However, most employers stated they would not drop their contributions if there was a waiting period for eligibility. Numerous states have

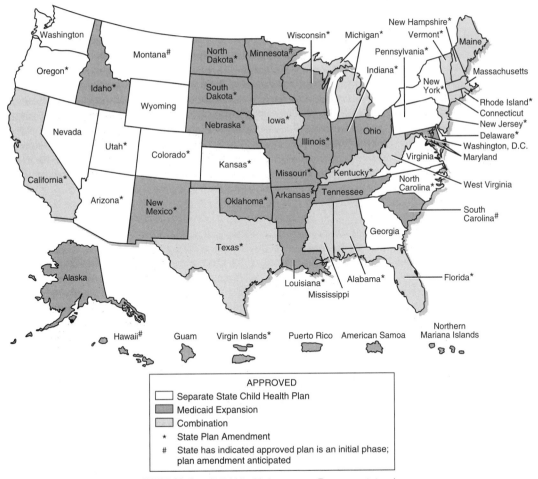

FIGURE 23–1 • Child Health Insurance Program state plans.

established waiting periods as a disincentive for employers to opt out of offering health insurance.

A greater concern related to the program is enrollment of uninsured children (Rosenbaum, Johnson, Sonosky, Marcus, & DeGraw, 1998). Efforts are currently underway to reach out to families and communities through schools, churches, and day care centers to let parents know about the availability of coverage (HCFA, 2000). APNs need to be part of the effort to identify children who are eligible for CHIP. (Information about outreach for the CHIP is provided in Table 23–5.) There is currently concern about children with special needs accessing the program. For example, there is evidence that states have not incorporated elements into the program that provide for children with optical needs (Fox Health Consultants, 1998). One million children are now enrolled in CHIP, with the expectation of covering 2.3 million by September 2000 (DeParle, 1998).

CHIP payment to APNs has presented some challenges. Although states recognize payment to family NPs, pediatric NPs, and CNMs through Medicaid, it has been difficult in some states, such as New York, for eligible APNs to get payment if the program was implemented under a separate state health plan and not through Medicaid. State and national organizations representing APNs have been active in working with these states to ensure access to APN care.

TABLE 23–5	REGIONAL INFORMATION FOR CHIP OUTREACH		
REGION	STATE	REGION	STATE
Boston—I	Connecticut	Dallas—VI	Arkansas
	Maine		Louisiana
	Massachusetts		Oklahoma
	New Hampshire		New Mexico
	Rhode Island		Texas
	Vermont	Kansas City—VII	Iowa
New York—II	New Jersey		Kansas
	New York		Missouri
	Puerto Rico		Nebraska
	Virgin Islands	Denver—VIII	Colorado
Philadelphia—III	Delaware		Montana
	Dist. of Columbia		North Dakota
	Maryland		South Dakota
	Pennsylvania		Utah
	Virginia		Wyoming
	West Virginia	San Francisco—IX	American Samoa
Atlanta—IV	Alabama		Arizona
	Florida		California
	Georgia		Guam
	Kentucky		Hawaii
	Mississippi		Nevada
	North Carolina		Northern Mariana Islands
	South Carolina	Seattle—X	Alaska
	Tennessee		Idaho
Chicago—V	Indiana		Oregon
	Michigan		Washington
	Minnesota		
	Ohio		
	Wisconsin		

For further information and direct contact go to: *www.hcfa.gov* or *www.insurekids.now.gov/childhealth/states.asp*.

AVAILABILITY

In addition to affordability, availability is an important dimension of access. Availability can be viewed as geographic access, access to providers with specific expertise such as midwifery or cardiology, and access to providers who understand or share cultural values of their patients.

APNs have their policy roots in enhancing geographic access. CNMs have a long history of providing services to traditionally underserved populations. They secured Medicaid reimbursement in the 1970s, enabling them to deliver services to poor women living in areas with no accessible providers. A demonstration of the commitment by CNMs to providing services to underserved women is the Frontier Nursing Service support of the first distance education program designed to increase the number of midwives in underserved areas. Governmental concern in the 1960s about substantially unmet health care needs of society, particularly individuals in rural and poor urban areas, strengthened the growth of NP roles. The Rural Health Clinics Act of 1979 implemented Medicaid and Medicare reimbursement to APNs to address availability issues.

Although there is a growing indication that a more than adequate supply of health professionals exists, as of June 1997, there were 2,597 designated primary medical care, health professional shortage areas (HPSAs). Of these areas, 1,742 (67%) were in nonmetropolitan areas. More than 20 million people live in a HPSA (Federal Office of Rural Health Policy, 1997). Federal policies that have attempted to address geographic accessibility have had limited success. The policies have focused on two main strategies: recruitment of individuals from underserved areas in the hope they will come to educational programs and then return to their home communities, or transplantation of graduates of programs into underserved areas in the hope that they will remain in these communities. Through the use of distance learning, a new approach is being used to take educational programs to qualified individuals already living in underserved areas.

The National Health Service Corps (NHSC) is a federal agency within the Department of Health and Human Services charged with addressing the problem of geographic access. The NHSC has a scholarship and loan repayment program for health professionals who agree to work in underserved areas for a specific period of time. By law, the NHSC has had to use 10% of its total funding to support APNs, dentists, and others. This requirement is currently being renegotiated. The NHSC has proposed to use funds to support the type of health professional that communities want. APNs are not usually requested first, mainly because communities do not fully understand the benefits of having an APN. This could jeopardize the funding available to APNs. However, the NHSC is exploring the idea of a partnership approach with APN organizations to work with communities to enable them to better understand the advantages of having services provided by APNs.

Availability of specific services is a problem. An example of limited availability is that of mental health services, which directly affects mental health APNs. Physical health needs have always taken priority in the eyes of most policy makers. Mental health needs have not had equal parity with physical health. The Mental Health Parity Act (MHPA) of 1996 (P.L. 104–204) requires insurers to offer the same benefits for mental health care as for other health benefits. All employers with more than 50 employees must offer mental health insurance benefits, but, because of the Employee Retirement Income Security Act, employers that self-insure are exempt. In effect, access to mental health continues to be problematic, mainly because of limited reimbursement through the many exclusions and limits on the MHPA.

Fourteen states have passed more stringent mental health laws than the federal law. Even with this legislation addressing mental health issues, the Washington Haye Group (1998) reported that behavioral health care benefits as a percentage of total benefits costs decreased from 6.1% in 1988 to 3.7% in 1997. Although insurance plans offer mental health and substance abuse coverage, mental health benefits usually carry substantial limits for inpatient stays and substance abuse counseling and may carry higher co-pays and deductible than coverage for physical health (Buck, Teich, Umland, & Stein, 1999). Attempts to expand mental health services have fallen short mainly because of concerns about the costs of mental health parity. Psychiatric/mental health APNs have a significant challenge. Even though their services can be reimbursed, significant problems continue to exist with regard to access because of the constraints noted here.

QUALITY

The federal government has a major interest in quality of care. As the largest purchaser of health care in the country, ensuring the adequacy of care that is purchased or provided is a critical government role. In addition, changes in the health system with the rapid move to managed care and, heightened competition, and, in some cases, extreme pressure to reduce costs, have created congressional interest because of concerns of constituents. The federal government has also become active within the quality-of-care context in ensuring that public funds are effectively and efficiently used. Efforts focused on fraud and abuse are intended to ensure that the government gets the care it is paying for.

Consumer Protection in Managed Care

Consumer protection issues have become the focus of major debate in Congress for the past two congressional sessions. Consumer concerns about managed care have been the engine that has propelled this issue into mainstream politics. Although there is substantially conflicting evidence on how well managed care entities provide care, there have been numerous complaints from consumers about the difficulties related to managed care. The media have broadcast the personal stories related to problems faced by consumers in terms of denial of payment for emergency room visits, difficulty getting access to subspecialists, and denial of certain types of treatments. One of the most visible consumer issues in the past 2 years has been the "drive-by deliveries," in which women were being discharged within 24 hours after delivery based on managed care payment constraints. Congress passed a law requiring managed care organizations to provide coverage for at least 2 days unless complications warranted a longer stay.

Dissatisfaction with managed care plans seems to be increasing (Allen & Rogers, 1997). One factor noted for the increase in dissatisfaction is related to patients not having a choice in selecting their health insurance plan. A study by Gawande and colleagues (1998) found that individuals having no choice about the health plan in which they are enrolled were more dissatisfied with the plan. Those individuals who had a choice about health plans were as satisfied as individuals with traditional health insurance. The impact of limited choice was seen during the Clinton health care reform debate when advertisements with "Harry and Louise" focused on the lack of choice available to consumers if the Clinton plan were approved. Many analysts attributed the failure of the reform to the power and simplicity of the issue of choice.

In response to concerns about managed care, a number of highly visible policy activities have taken place. In 1996, President Clinton convened the President's Advisory Commission on Consumer Protection and Quality in the Health Care Industry to focus attention on quality of care issues (President's Advisory Commission, 1998). This commission's report has led to several initiatives. One was the recommendation for a patient's bill of rights (discussed later). Another was the formation of the Forum for Health Care Quality and Reporting, composed of public and private parties, to focus on further development of performance measures and quality improvement processes. Another outcome was the establishment of the Quality Interagency Coordination Task Force (QuIC) to ensure that all federal agencies involved in purchasing, providing, studying, or regulating health care services are working in a coordinated way to improve quality of care (Agency for Health Care Policy and Research, 1999). The major goals of QuIC are

- Improving patient and consumer information
- Identifying key opportunities for improving clinical care
- Improving efforts to measure quality of care
- Developing the health care work force
- Improving information systems

What Is Quality of Care?

Quality of care has been defined by the Institute of Medicine (1990, p. 4) as "the degrees to which health services for individuals and populations increase the likelihood of desired health outcomes and are consistent with current professional knowledge."

Quality of care issues have been conceptualized as problems related to overuse, underuse, or poor delivery of health services. The U.S. health system has been criticized for providing too little health care to some (underuse), too much care to others (overuse), and inappropriate care to still others (misuse). Underuse occurs when services known to be effective are not used. An example is the National Committee on Quality Assurance (NCQA) (1999) findings that 30% of women ages 52 to 69 in surveyed managed care plans had not received a mammogram in the past 2 years. Another example is the failure to use beta-blocker medications after heart attack in light of evidence that mortality can be reduced by 43% when they are used. Soumerai and colleagues (1997) found that only 21% of eligible Medicare patients in New Jersey received beta-blockers.

Overuse is characterized by providing excessive and unnecessary services that do not contribute to improving health. Use of antibiotics to treat colds and acute bronchitis is an example of overuse. Gonzales, Steiner, and Sande (1997) found that nearly half of all patients diagnosed with acute bronchitis received antibiotics. Another example is that Bernstein and colleagues (1993) found that 16% of hysterectomies in seven health plans were unnecessary.

Misuse of services results in missed diagnoses, injury to patients, high costs, and sometimes death or major disability. Use of more expensive antibiotics to treat ear infections was associated with more adverse effects and worse outcomes than use of less expensive antibiotics (Brennen et al., 1991). Medication errors also constitute misuse of services and can be prevented (Bates et al., 1995).

In the 1998 Congress, in spite of this new concern about quality, purchasers and managed care organizations successfully defeated attempts to pass a patient's bill of rights. The argument against passage was based on a concern that the legislation, particularly legislation that would allow patients to sue their health plans, would raise the cost of health care and thus create more uninsured people who could not afford health insurance premiums. The Patient's Bill of Rights resurfaced in the 1999 session and, to the surprise of many, the Republican-controlled House passed a bill that established a review system for patients' complaints, enhanced access to subspecialists, and allowed patients to sue their HMO, whereas only providers could be sued previously.

The House vote was significant in that Republican members broke with their party leadership. The public let their members know that this was an important grassroots issue. Constituent pressure, coupled with all-out lobbying efforts by the AMA, American Nurses Association, and others, defeated a well-financed opposition. House members face election in November, and those wanting to be elected listened to voters. As of this writing, the House and Senate versions of a patient bill of rights need to be reconciled because the Senate passed a more conservative version that did not include allowing lawsuits to be brought against health plans.

Quality-of-Care Monitoring Activities

Several major national initiatives focusing on quality of care have emerged during the 1990s. The NCQA, an entity that has had major policy influence, is a private, not-for-profit organization that has done seminal work to measure and report the quality of managed care plans. The NCQA board of directors includes employers, consumers, health plans, policy experts, and physicians. However, there are no APNs on this board. The mission of the NCQA is to produce information to guide purchasers and consumers in their choice of high-quality and higher value health plans. The major functions include collection of performance data and accreditation of health plans. Currently nearly half of all health plans covering three quarters of all enrollees are involved in NCQA accreditation. Increasing numbers of large corporations such as Ameritech, Ford, Federal Express, and Xerox require the health plans they contract with to be NCQA accredited (NCQA, 1999). Plans are evaluated on five different categories: access and services, qualified providers, enrollees' health status, improved health status, and living with illness. As part of accreditation, plans have a site visit by teams of physicians. At present, no APNs are included as site visitors.

The Health Plan Employer Data and Information Set (HEDIS) is a data set developed by the NCQA and composed of more than 50 standardized measures of health plan performance. HEDIS is consistently updated by the NCQA. HEDIS 2000 was released in February 1999 and includes new measures related to women's health and chronic illness. The most recent NCQA report, *State of Managed Care Quality,* was released in July 1999 (NCQA, 1999). Although managed care is vilified nationwide, the NCQA findings shed light on important findings relevant to policy. Health plans that report their HEDIS findings provide better quality of care than those that do not, and patient satisfaction is greater in plans with better clinical performance measures (NCQA, 1999). Another important finding is that health plans make substantial improvement following the incorporation of a new HEDIS measure, indicating there is room for continued improvement and that plans are responsive. The NCQA also developed *Quality Compass,* which incorporates data from HEDIS and accreditation visits (Thompson, Best, Ahmed, Ingalls, & Sennett, 1998). This database provides information to employers, consumers, and others that forms the basis for report cards on plans.

In addition to the NCQA, the AHRQ, formerly AHCPR, has done significant work to inform policy decisions. The AHRQ funded a project to create a quality improvement software tool called the Computerized Needs-Oriented Quality Measurement Evaluation System (CONQUEST). This software product assists users to collect and evaluate health care quality measures suited to and adaptable to their needs. The intent of this package is to assist individual providers, groups, or institutions to have a flexible tool for internal quality monitoring.

The AHRQ also supported the development of the Healthcare Cost and Utilization Project (HCUP), a set of 33 clinical indicators of performance measures used primarily to assess hospital systems (AHCPR, 1999). The Joint Commission for Accreditation of Healthcare Organizations has approved use of HCUP quality indicators for several hospital systems as part of their performance management initiative.

The latest version of the Consumer Assessment of Health Plans Study (CAHPS) was developed by the NCQA with help from the AHRQ. This instrument combines elements of the 1998 HEDIS Member Satisfaction Survey and the past version of CAHPS. This tool now allows consumers to compare plans, both Medicaid and commercial, in ways not previously available.

Businesses, because of their role in purchasing health care on behalf of employees, have also gotten involved in quality activities. For instance, the Pacific Business Group on Health (PBGH) has been a leader in establishing performance measures for more than a dozen of the largest health plans in California. The PBGH negotiated on behalf of health purchasers who put $8 million at risk if the plans did not meet their performance measures (Schauffler, Brown, & Milstein, 1999). The purpose of building a financial incentive for meeting specific targets based on information (including consumer satisfaction as well as a number of specific clinical measures such as immunization rates) is to provide a monetary reason for plans to provide quality care.

APNs need to be involved in quality improvement activities at all levels. Mary Wakefield, Ph.D., a faculty member at George Mason University, was on the President's Advisory Commission, but there has been very limited participation by APNs with the NCQA or QuIC. One result of not being included in quality measurement and reporting activities is that performance measures important to APN practice and patient outcomes are not being captured. Another is that APNs will remain invisible in the health system if they are not included as a category of providers on whom data are collected.

Fraud and Abuse

The policy issue related to the efficient use of taxpayer dollars is reflected in the commitment of the current administration to detecting fraud and abuse in billing. Fraud and abuse detection initiated by the HCFA is one method being used to ensure appropriate use of Medicare and Medicaid dollars. Fraud is defined by the HCFA as "the intentional deception or misrepresentation that an individual knows to be false or does not believe to be true and makes, knowing that the deception could result in some unauthorized benefit to himself/herself or some other person" (HCFA, 1998c). Abuse is defined as "actions that are inconsistent with accepted, sound, medical, business or fiscal practices. Abuse directly or indirectly results in unnecessary costs to the program through improper payments" (HCFA, 1997b). Each Medicare contractor, whether an intermediary or carrier, has a Medicare Fraud Unit in place. Once an investigation takes place and there is sufficient evidence to warrant potential prosecution, the case goes to the U.S. Department of Health and Human Services Office of the Inspector General (OIG). The OIG's office then prepares the case for referral to the Department of Justice for criminal and or civil prosecution. If a provider or institution is found guilty of committing fraud or abuse, penalties can range from a civil penalty of $5,000 to $10,000 per false claim and treble damages under the False Claims Act to imprisonment up to 10 years. The penalties associated with fraud or abuse can clearly be substantial.

Every APN needs to be familiar with the laws regarding fraud and abuse. There are a number of potential pitfalls that could be construed as fraud or abuse. Examples of billing fraud and abuse that APNs need to be careful about are "incident to" billing as well as kickback issues. The Medicare legislation enabling billing under Medicare creates opportunities as well as cautions. Ignorance of billing requirements will not be a justification for billing practices that could be construed as fraud or abuse. Confusion about "incident to" has been based in the limited guidelines from the HCFA about the requirements governing this billing. Johnson and Torras (1999) have provided a number of criteria that must be met for "incident to" billing for supplies or services; they must be

- An integral, although incidental, part of the physician's services
- Commonly rendered without charge or included in the physician's bill
- Of the type that is commonly furnished in an office or clinic
- Furnished under the physician's direct supervision
- Furnished by an individual who qualifies as an employee of the physician or clinic

All of these criteria must be met in order to comply with the requirements for "incident to" billing. It is important for APNs to note that services "incident to" APN services can be billed. That stipulation as part of the BBA provides an avenue for billing that has previously not been open to APNs.

The anti-kickback statute could also be inadvertently abused by APNs if there are grounds for the APN to get a financial benefit from a particular arrangement—for instance, with a pharmaceutical company. APNs need to be careful about what can be construed as an arrangement for financial enhancement for the clinician. It is difficult to identify specific examples of problems related to "incident to" billing or kickback schemes because there have been no reported incidents involving APNs as of this writing.

APNs and Physicians

At the beginning of the chapter, the importance of nursing and medicine working together for the welfare of patients and the health of the nation was recognized. The policy arena, although it provides the opportunity for important collaboration, has frequently created an adversarial forum for both disciplines to engage in economic competition. Because the basis for nearly all policy decisions rests on economics, many national organizations have staked out policy positions that maintain or enhance the economic position of their respective discipline. The current context of health systems change is rooted in cost containment that has led to the threat of lower physician salaries and potential job loss. Within this context, physicians have experienced significant loss of control over how they practice medicine as well as loss of income. The actual or potential losses make it difficult for physicians to embrace expanded practice for APNs, who may be seen as competitors for jobs and income.

Understanding this economic and policy landscape allows physicians and APNs to recognize the factors that may create an adversarial relationship in order to look for common ground in the pursuit of better patient care. The past few years have been spent by each discipline trying to strengthen its own position. It is time to work together in addressing the very critical issues facing our country, including access to basic health care for all and fair payment for services delivered, and ensuring valid methods of assessing quality of care.

Specific examples of how physicians and APNs could collaborate include defining practice models to efficiently and effectively care for elderly, disabled populations. Working through options regarding this issue requires crafting an interdisciplinary model of care that recognizes the strengths of each discipline. There are many geriatrics practices in which NPs and physicians work together and care for this very challenging population. Neither nursing nor medicine alone can care for individual patients with multiple interacting health and social problems. For instance, in a nursing home practice a core team of providers, including an NP, a physician, a CNS who may be a head nurse on a nursing unit, and a psychiatric nurse specialist, could form a professional team. The team could meet regularly for case conferences, and share accountability and responsibility for frequent and effective communication. There would be overlapping yet distinctive areas of expertise among team members.

Another example of a policy problem for which physicians and APNs have a shared concern is the growing number of uninsured individuals. National attention could effectively be focused on this issue and solutions identified with medicine and nursing working together. A model of interdisciplinary collaboration is demonstrated by a recently developed initiative entitled Primary Care Action. Numerous nursing and medical professionals representing major organizations have joined together to identify a common set of policy goals and to develop a plan for attaining those goals that includes enhancing the quality of primary care and providing universal coverage.

CONCLUSION

Policy advocacy needs to be a part of every APN's professional role. It is important to be a member of a professional organization that advances issues critical to APN practice and the health of the nation. The first step to being involved in policy formulation is to be knowledgeable about the policy process and issues. In order to be involved, APNs need to understand the details related to funding issues, measures of quality and how they reflect NP practice, and specific programs designed to improve access. Websites have been identified in Table 23–6 that can provide APNs with current and comprehensive information about important policy issues. The important lesson in policy is that, after understanding an issue, a single person can make a difference. An individual backed by organizational strength, particularly by coalitions of organizations, can make an even more significant difference.

TABLE 23-6	URL ADDRESSES TO NATIONAL APN ACCREDITATION REGULATION AND CERTIFICATION WEB SITES
American Association of Nurse Practitioners (AANP)	*www.aanp.org*
American Association of Colleges of Nurses and Commission on Collegiate Nursing Education (AACN and CCNE)	*www.aacn.nche.edu* (links to CCNE)
American Association of Nurse Anesthetics (AANA)	*www.aana.com.index.htm*
American Association of Nurse-Midwives (ACNM)	*www.acnm.org*
American Nurses Credential Center (ANCC)	*www.nursingworld.org/ancc*
National Corporation Pediatric Nurse Practitioners and Nurses (NCBPNP/N)	*www.pnpcert.org*
National Certification Corporation for Obstetrical, Gynecologic and Neonatal Nursing Specialists (NCC)	*www.nccnet.org*
National Council State Boards of Nursing (NCSBN)	*www.ncsbn.org*
National League for Nursing Accreditation Corporation (NLNAC)	*www.nln.org/nlnac*

REFERENCES

Aaron, H. T., & Schwartz, W. B. (1984). *The painful prescription.* Washington, DC: Brookings Institute.

Agency for Health Care Policy and Research. (1999). Quality Interagency Coordination Task Force (QuIC): Fact Sheet (Publication No. 99-P031). Available: *http://www.ahcpr.gov/qual/quicfat.htm*

Allen, H. M., & Rogers, W. H. (1997). The consumer health plan value survey: Round two. *Health Affairs, 16*(4), 156.

American Medical Association. (1995). *Physicians assisstants and nurse practitioners.* Chicago, American Medical Association.

Anderson, G. F., & Poullier, J. P. (1999). Health spending, access and outcomes: Trends in industrialized countries. *Health Affairs, 18*(3), 178.

Aston, G. (1999). States act to reserve CHIP funds to cover uninsured children. *American Medical News, 42*(23), 1.

Bates, D., Cullen, D., Laird, N., Petersen, L. A., Small, S. D., Servi, D., Laffel, G., Sweitzer, B. I., Shea, B. F., Hallisey, R., et al. (1995). Incidence of adverse durg events and potential adverse drug events: Implications for prevention. *JAMA, 274,* 29-34.

Berk, M. L., & Schur, C. L. (1998). Measuring access to care: Improving information for policy-makers. *Health Affairs, 19*(1), 180.

Bernstein, S. J., McGlynn, E. A., Siu, A. L., Roth, C. P., Sherwood, M. J., Keesey, J. W., Kosecoff, J., Hicks, N. R., & Brook, R. H. (1993). The appropriateness of hysterectomy: A comparison of care in seven health plans. Health Maintenance Organization Quality of Care Consortium. *JAMA, 269,* 2398-2402.

Braden, B. R., Cowan, C. A., Lasjenby, H. C., Martin, A. B., McDonnell, P. A., Sensenig, A. L., Stiller, J. M., Whittle, L. S., Donham, C. S., Long, A. M., & Stewart, M. W. (1998). National health care expenditures, 1997. *Health Care Financing Review, 19*(20), 83-126.

Brennan, T. A., Leape, L. L., Laird, N. M., Hebert, L., Localio, A. R., Lawthers, A. G., Newhouse, J. P., Weiler, P. C., & Hiatt, H. H. (1991). Incidence of adverse events and negligence in hospitalized patients: Results of the Harvard Medical Practice Study I. *New England Journal of Medicine, 324,* 370-376.

Buck, J. A., Teich, J. L., Umland, B., & Stein, M. (1999). Behavioral health benefits in employer-sponsored health plans, 1997. *Health Affairs, 18*(2), 67-78.

Congressional Budget Office. (1999). Expanding health insurance coverage for children under Title XXI of the Social Security Act 1998. Available: *www.cbo.gov/byclasscat.cfm?class-0&cat-9*

Crippen, D. (1999). Health care costs and insurance coverage: Congressional Budget Office testimony before the Subcommittee on Employer-Employee Relations, Committee on Education and the Workforce, U.S. House of Representatives, June 11, 1999. Available: *www.cbo.gov/showdoc.cfm?index-1324&from-3&sequence-0*

Curran, W. J. (1989). The constitutional right to health care: Denial in the court. *New England Journal of Medicine, 320,* 788-789.

Daniels, N. (1985). *Just health care.* Cambridge, England: Cambridge University Press.

DeParle, N.-A. (1998). Statement on the State Children's Health Insurance Program before the House Commerce Committee, Subcommittee on Health & Environment, September 18, 1998. Available: *www.hcfa.gov/init/testim918.htm*

Federal Office of Rural Health Policy. (1997). *Facts about rural physicians.* Washington, DC: Health Resources and Services Administration.

Feldstein, P. (1988). *The politics of health legislation.* Ann Arbor, MI: Health Administration Press.

Fox Health Consultants. (1998). *States' CHIP policies and children with special care needs.* Washington, DC: Author.

Gabel, J., Hurst, K., Whitmore, H., & Hoffman, C. (1999). Class and benefits at the workplace. *Health Affairs, 18*(3), 144–150.

Gawande, A. A., Blendon, R., Brodie, M., Benson, J. M., Levitt, L., & Hugick, L. (1998). Does dissatisfaction with health plans stem from having no choices? *Health Affairs, 17*(5), 184–194.

Goldstein, A. (1999, June 30). Clinton details overhaul plan for Medicare. *The Washington Post,* p. 1A.

Gonzales, R., Steiner, J., & Sande, M. (1997). Antibiotic prescribing for adults with colds, upper respiratory tract infections, and bronchitis by ambulatory care physicians. *JAMA, 278,* 901–904.

Health Care Financing Administration. (1997a). Children's Health Insurance Program Answers to frequently asked questions—released September 11, 1997 (first set). Available: *www.hcfa.gov/init/qa/q&a9-11.htm*

Health Care Financing Administration. (1997b). Frequently asked questions: Fraud and abuse, 1) Q. What is the difference between fraud and abuse. Available: *www.hcfa.gov/webfaq3.htm#fraud1*

Health Care Financing Administration. (1998a). Medicaid national summary statistics, Table 1: Medicaid recipients, vendor, medical assistance and administrative payments. Available: *www.hcfa.gov/medicaid/2082-1.htm*

Health Care Financing Administration. (1998b). *Medicare and Medicaid Statistical Supplement: HealthCare Financing Review OHHs.* Washington, DC: Author.

Health Care Financing Administration. (1998c). Medicare definition of fraud. Available: *http://www.hcfa.gov/medicare/fraud/DEFINI2.HTM*

Health Care Financing Administration. (1998d). What is Medicare: Medigap and Medicare select Medicare supplemental insurance. Available: *www.medicare.gov/additional.html*

Health Care Financing Administration. (2000). Children's Health Insurance Program HCFA outreach contacts. Available: *http://www.hcfa.gov/init/outreach/rocontct.htm*

Heclo, H. (1995). The Clinton health plan: Historical perspective. *Health Affairs, 14,* 86–98.

Holahan, J., Weiner, J., & Wallin, S. (1998). Health policy for the low income population: Major findings from the Accessing the New Federalism. (Occasional Paper #18). Washington, DC: Urban Institute.

Iglehart, J. K. (1993). Health care reform: The labyrinth of Congress. *New England Journal of Medicine, 329,* 1593–1596.

Institute for the Future. (2000). *A forecast of health and health care in America: The future beyond 2005.* San Francisco, Jossey-Bass Publishers.

Institute of Medicine. (1990). Medicare: *A strategy for quality assurance.* K. N. Lohr (Ed.). Washington, D.C., National Academy Press.

Johnson, D., & Torras, H. (1999). NP billing and coding tips. *Washington Word.*

Kaiser Family Foundation. (1994). *Uninsured in America: Straight facts on health reform.* Menlo Park, CA: Author.

Kronick, R., & Gilmore, T. (1999). Exploring the decline in health insurance coverage, 1979–1995. *Health Affairs, 18*(2), 30.

Longest, B. B. (1998). *Health policy in the United States* (2nd ed.). Chicago: Health Administration Press.

National Committee on Quality Assurance. (1999). NCQA's *State of Managed Care Quality Report,* QUALITY COMPASS 99 Show Simple Formula for Health Care Quality: Accountability: Available: *www.ncqa.org/pages/communications/news/somcgrel.html*

Newhouse, J. P. (1993). An iconoclastic view of health care cost containment. *Health Affairs, 12*(suppl), 152–171.

President's Advisory Commission on Consumer Protection and Quality in the Health Care Industry. (1998). *Quality first: Better health care for all Americans—final report to the President of the United States.* Washington, DC: Author.

Reinhardt, U. E. (1993). Recognizing the financial flaws in American healthcare. *Health Affairs, 12*(Suppl), 172–193.

Rosenbaum, S., Johnson, K., Sonosky, C., Markus, A., & DeGraw, S. (1998). The children's hour: The State Children's Health Insurance Program. *Health Affairs, 17*(1): 75–89.

Rowland, D., Feder, J., & Keenan, P. S. (1998). Uninsured in America: The causes and consequences. In S. H. Altman, U. E. Reinhardt, & A. E. Shields (Eds.), *The future United States health care system: Who will care for the poor and uninsured?* (pp. 25–44). Chicago: Health Administration Press.

Schauffler, H. H., Brown, C., & Milstein, A. (1999). Raising the bar: The use of performance guarantees by the Pacific Business Group on Health. *Health Affairs, 18*(2), 134.

Schwartz, W. B., & Aaron, H. J. (1984). *The painful prescription: Rationing hospital care.* Washington, DC: Brookings Institute.

Selden, T. M., Banthin, J. S., & Cohen, J. W. (1999). Waiting in the wings: Eligibility and enrollment in the State Children's Health Insurance Program. *Health Affairs, 18*(2), 126.

Sheils, J., & Alecxih, L. (1996, October 21). *Recent trends in employer health insurance coverage and health.* Paper for American Hospital Association.

Short, P., & Bathin, J. (1995) Caring for the uninsured and underinsured. *JAMA, 274,* 1302.

Smith, S. S., Freeland, M., Heffler, S., & McKusick, D. (1998). The next ten years of health spending: What does the future hold? *Health Affairs, 17*,(5)128–140.

Soumerai, S. B., McLaughlin, T. J., Spiegelman, D., Hertzmark, E., Thibault, G., & Goldman, L. (1997). Adverse outcomes of underuse of beta-blockers in elderly survivors of acute myocardial infarction. *JAMA 277,* 115–121.

Starr, P. (1982). *The social transformation of American medicine.* New York: Basic Books.

Syrne, S. L. (1998). Social and economic disparities in health: Thoughts about intervention. *Milbank Quarterly, 76,* 493–503.

Thompson, J. W., Bost, J., Ahmed, F., Ingalls, C. E., & Sennett, C. (1998).The NCQA's quality compass: Evaluating managed care in the United States. *Health Affairs, 17*(1), 152–158.

Thorpe, K. E., & Florence, C. S., (1999). Why are workers uninsured? Employer-sponsored health insurance in 1997. *Health Affairs, 18*(2), 213–218.

U.S. Census Bureau. (1998). Health insurance coverage 1997. Available: *www.census.gov/hhes/www/hlthin97.html*

Washington Haye Group. (1998). *Health care plan design and cost trends—1988-1997.* Washington, DC: Author.

Weissman, J. S., Gastonis, C., & Epstein, A. M. (1992). Rates of avoidable hospitalization by insurance statistics in Massachusetts and Maryland. *JAMA, 268,* 2388.

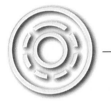

Strengthening Advanced Nursing Practice in Organizational Structures and Cultures

ADMINISTRATIVE CONSIDERATIONS

• B R E N D A M. N E V I D J O N

INTRODUCTION

In the last decade of the millennium, the future of advanced practice nurses (APNs) seemed to change every 2 to 3 years. With the increase in managed care, futurists predicted that more nurse practitioners (NPs) would be needed to provide primary care. As schools of nursing ramped up to prepare more NPs, physicians responded by questioning the competencies of lesser prepared professionals and increased their interest in primary care. An idea that has gained interest is the use of acute care NPs (ACNPs) to replace decreasing numbers of residents in teaching hospitals. The continuation of the clinical nurse specialist (CNS) role, especially in acute care settings, was uncertain given the financial challenges faced by hospital administrators. Many CNSs quickly returned to school to prepare as NPs because nurse executives, often on the advice of consultants, eliminated CNS positions in the early cycles of budget reductions. Then, a few years later, nurse executives who eliminated CNS positions reintroduced them because they understood the negative impact on basic nursing care that resulted from lack of CNS practice. Certified registered nurse anesthetists (CRNAs) found their job security challenged by an abundance of anesthesiologists. Birthing centers gained a foothold as certified nurse-midwives (CNMs) offered women a choice in birthing experience. The blended role of CNS and NP has gained in popularity, and the evolving nurse case manager role is being discussed in the literature as a potential advanced practice role. As the millennium closed, other roles, such as practice-based educators or clinical consultants, were starting to appear in the literature and job title nomenclature as potential advanced practice roles, continuing the confusion for the many audiences that interact with nurses about what advanced practice nursing means.

While the roles of CRNAs and CNMs have a century-long history, the other roles evolved much later and have constantly undergone change and challenges (Bear, 1995; Lyon, 1996; see Chapter 1). Lack of consensus about the definition of roles, need for second licensure, reimbursement, prescriptive privileges, and scope of authority are a few of the external, national environment issues that compound the internal issues about how to use APNs. Nurse administrators who consider using APNs in their health care organizations must deal with internal organizational issues also, such as how to define the value an APN will bring or identifying what groups APNs might threaten. As changes continue to occur in where and how health care is delivered, traditional and often inflexible organizational boundaries are disappearing. Opportunities exist to create responsive organizations by building strong alliances among the health care professions to meet society's needs for accessible and affordable health care. Numerous internal and external factors influence how nursing is practiced and how care is delivered in all health care settings, whether office based, home health, or acute care institutions.

The literature on advanced nursing practice indicates that administrative support is an important variable in the success of APN practice (Hamric & Taylor, 1989). The purpose of this chapter is to outline the factors that contribute to the justification and use of APNs now and for the future. It provides information to help nurse administrators be champions of APNs in their organizations, whether introducing a new position or advocating to continue current ones. The chapter also helps APNs understand the needs of administrators and how organizational culture, policy, and finance affect them. Recent history has shown that, without an appreciation for and documentation of the contributions of APNs, administrators will eliminate financial support for them. Administrators, particularly nurses in administration, have a responsibility to remain knowledgeable about APN roles and what these roles can accomplish for patient care and thus for an organization. A clearly articulated vision of advanced nursing practice by the nursing leadership of an organization will sustain commitment to the roles through difficult times. Collaboration is essential between APNs and nurse administrators to define the expected contributions of the APN, including patient outcomes, cost savings, and revenue generation. Without a commitment from the most senior nursing voices in an organization, individual APNs are without a critical ally.

FACTORS AFFECTING ADMINISTRATIVE COMMITMENT TO APNs

The Changing Health Care Environment

Although access to and quality of care are concerns, economics continues to be the driving force behind changes in the health care environment. Both private and governmental payers led initiatives aimed at reducing the cost of health care. Their key issues included cost containment, new forms of payment, consumer preferences, health reform efforts, and technological developments (Shortell, Gillies, & Devers, 1995). Managed care was embraced in the 1990s as the way to save money. However, health care as a percentage of the U.S. gross national product has continued to rise. The uninsured now number more than 43 million people.

As seen in Table 24-1, there are many internal and external factors that create opportunities for or impediments to the practice of nursing and the delivery of patient care. The external factors drive many of the internal factors. For example, the external payer environment has frequently led to reactive decisions about services and the future of specific disciplines in hospitals. However, the predicted restructuring of care delivery has not occurred as uniformly and quickly throughout the country as one might think from media coverage. Nonetheless, administrators have been challenged by decreasing reimbursement as managed care is increasing, thus increasing regulatory controls, increasing cost of technology, and increasing acuity of care. Nurse administrators have responded by changing the skill mix of staff, developing cross-training programs, eliminating types of positions, and expanding the scope of

TABLE 24-1 PRESSURES ON HEALTH CARE ADMINISTRATORS	
EXTERNAL FACTORS	INTERNAL FACTORS
Managed care	Diminishing resources
Rise in integrated delivery networks (IDNs)— consolidation	Restructuring work processes
Competition—market shifts	Changes in skill mix
Global pricing	Creation of new types of workers
Emphasis on costs	Reduction in acute care beds
Demand for outcomes data	Increased acuity in all settings
Interest in patient satisfaction	Need for standard outcomes data
Insurers as driving forces regarding clinical decisions	Enhanced training needs
Emphasis on primary care	Fewer workers through retirement, buy-out, terminations
Technological advances	Application of technology/automation
Increased Internet usage	Emphasis on interdisciplinary efforts
Changing demographics	Changing organizational structures
Shift to less acute/ambulatory/home care	Expanded scope of nurse executives
Regulatory requirements	Job/career insecurity
Licensing/credentialing requirements	New reporting relationships
Changes in the medical profession	Pressure to constrain wages
Better informed consumers	Multisite practices, affiliations, networks
Federal and state health care initiatives	Administration-physician relationships
	Nurse-physician relationships

middle managers. Commitment to APNs has varied throughout this time because these roles can be seen as expensive, fixed costs in a nursing department's budget.

Radical health care reform did not occur under the Clinton administration, but two key pieces of federal legislation left their mark on the health care industry. The 1996 Health Insurance Portability and Accountability Act increased flexibility in coverage, and the 1997 Balanced Budget Act (BBA) affected reimbursement. The BBA also created the State Children's Health Insurance Program (SCHIP). The nursing community heralded the BBA as a victory for their lobbying efforts because it contains a provision to extend Medicare reimbursement for APNs to all geographic areas and clinical settings (Haber, 1997; Minarik, 1997). Prior to this legislation, reimbursement was limited to APNs in rural areas and NPs only in nursing homes. Interestingly, Wilken (1995) found that the more rural states had fewer NPs available than the need would require. She also noted that increased NP numbers in urban areas occurring simultaneously with declining numbers in rural areas was important to health care policy. Her research showed that the availability of NPs is influenced by state-level initiatives such as support of educational programs, recruitment and retention efforts, and the presence of direct third-party reimbursement. The long-term impact of the 1997 BBA, although not yet known, may also directly help increase availability of NPs. The January issue of *Nurse Practitioner* provides an annual update on each state's legislative issues regarding NPs and is a useful reference when considering employment opportunities (Pearson, 2000).

APNs are eligible to receive direct reimbursement in the majority of states. However, obtaining reimbursement privileges from managed care and insurance organizations has been difficult. With the increase in integrated delivery networks (IDNs), APNs may find that they are not recognized as primary care providers and thus are ineligible for reimbursement because they are not included on the provider list. However, state laws and private insurance companies tend to follow federal legislation, so gains at the national level will have a broader influence in time. Not only professional organizations of APNs, such as the American Association of Nurse Anesthetists, but also nursing specialty organizations, such as the Oncology Nursing Society, are vital links to influencing federal legislation (Camp-Sorrell & Spencer-Cisek, 1995; see also Chapter 23).

States are experimenting with modifications to their Medicaid plans to improve access for their citizens. Although Medicaid enrollees are predominantly women and children, a disproportionate share of the funds covers services for people with chronic diseases and disabilities (Licking & Sampson, 1995). SCHIP is expected to reach an additional 5 million children without health care coverage (Lowe & Havens, 1998). Family and pediatric NPs are recognized as primary care providers and, thus, there is an opportunity to integrate APNs into delivery systems designed to meet the needs of these additional 5 million children. Nurse administrators can and should advocate for APNs as programs and services are designed.

As a result of turbulent health care reimbursement changes, the momentum of moving care to the outpatient arena accelerated and the role of "gatekeeper" emerged. Managed care organizations (MCOs) are focused on reducing the cost of care by controlling utilization of services through greater control of their approval. Physicians have experienced increased workloads with flat or decreased income. The Health Care Advisory Board (1999) found that, across the United States, relationships between physicians and hospital administrators are seriously strained. Academic organizations have not been immune to the changes. Johnson (1994) suggested that, if the medical profession did not increase the supply of primary care physicians, the government should redirect graduate medical education funds to schools of nursing for NP education. The BBA decreased funding for graduate medical education, which is creating pressures on the competing missions of teaching hospitals. Faculty are faced with conflict from the competing demands to see more patients while maintaining the teaching and research activities required for academic advancement. The decline in the number of residents is causing teaching hospitals to consider APNs or "house" physicians as alternatives. The dilemma for administrators is that an APN's or house physician's salary is more expensive than that of a resident physician. However, if the cost of educating and supervising the resident is factored in, the difference in cost may be slight.

Nurse administrators have created opportunities for APNs by developing new roles in acute care settings. Rather than eliminate the CNS role completely, some hospitals converted their master's-prepared nurses to case managers or care coordinators. APNs have been used extensively to facilitate development of critical pathways and multidisciplinary guidelines. These guidelines have successfully decreased costs by eliminating duplication and providing closer monitoring of the processes of care. In academic medical institutions and teaching hospitals, as noted previously, there are fewer house staff and fellows to provide medical care on inpatient units, and the focus of their clinical education includes more ambulatory clinic time. Thus APNs are being used to cover many functions previously performed by physician learners.

Technology and advances in the understanding of disease, especially through genetics, have affected the cost of care and led to changes in the care environment. The rate of discovery in the last two decades has been incredible. Translation of new knowledge into clinical treatment has become more rapid. Advances in electronic communication, in particular access to the Internet, have meant immediate worldwide information distribution. Patients and their families can gain in-depth details of their disease in a matter of minutes and come to their provider with greater information than the provider may have. With a more informed public, providers encounter patients who expect more time to discuss their disease and treatment options. At the same time, payers may be restricting access to certain technologies and pressuring providers to see more patients. There is opportunity for APNs to develop collaborative practices to maximize the use of each discipline.

Regulatory agencies, such as the Joint Commission on Accreditation of Healthcare Organizations (JCAHO), recognize the changing health care environment. JCAHO has revised its standards to reflect the dynamic nature of health care and reflect the shift in the locus of care. The Joint Commission requires consistent standards of care across an organization's care delivery sites (i.e., inpatient units, ambulatory clinics, and hospital-affiliated physicians' practices or offices). These requirements become especially important as regional and national networks of health care providers form.

Care Delivery Systems

The changing health care environment has led to a change in the structure of the care delivery system. Loose alliances of former competing organizations or formal contractual arrangements, such as IDNs, have increased throughout the country. IDNs can be developed horizontally or vertically and be for profit or not for profit. In a horizontally integrated delivery network, a group of like organizations form a legal entity. One example is an IDN of several hospitals, with one usually being the tertiary/quaternary site. A vertically integrated delivery network, in contrast, brings together organizations from along the continuum of care. This network would include primary care, an acute care hospital, home health, a skilled nursing home, and perhaps even an insurance product. IDNs can cover a wide geographic area or consolidate care options in one city. It is more common to see one or two IDNs be the option in a community as opposed to the several hospitals that once existed. Ownership of the system may also be distant as regional consolidation occurs. In the case of national for-profit systems, such as Columbia HCA or Tenet, centralized administration exerts significant control over local operations. For-profit niche players, such as heart hospitals and cancer treatment facilities, have competed effectively against full-service institutions in many communities. Their strategy of having a joint venture with the specialty physicians provides what physicians want: control and enhanced income.

Although the reorganization that is occurring should provide opportunities for APNs, support for their use varies widely among MCOs and IDNs. Some of the reasons for this are that physicians do not want the competition, executives who set policy do not appreciate the benefits of APNs, and the managers who do know the benefits usually are not in positions of influence within the organization (Sinclair, 1997). Mason, Cohen, O'Donnell, Baxter, and Chase (1997) researched how 67 MCOs used NPs as primary care providers in New York and Connecticut. They found that the MCO executives who used NPs were highly satisfied with them. Their data indicate the need for intensive efforts to educate MCO leaders as well as the public about the role, scope, and strengths of NPs. The most effective way to use APNs in IDNs is undetermined, but some characteristics of IDNs would indicate possibilities for APNs, particularly the blended CNS/NP role (see Chapter 16). These APNs are able to cross settings to follow specialty patients and are able to work with nurses in those multiple settings regarding the needs of these patients. Systematic planning and coordination of care across settings are necessary to ensure desired outcomes, patient satisfaction, and financial performance. APNs can meet gaps in services and cross boundaries. They can facilitate the integration of nursing into the overall mission of the organization and devise cost-effective and quality clinical program innovations. System-wide chief nurse executives, in particular, should find the APN an excellent candidate for ensuring the standard of nursing practice across all sites.

Barger (1997) outlined some of the ways in which an APN could be better prepared to be effective in managed care delivery systems. She cited an example of time management in which a director of a primary care network found APNs to be less efficient in using their time than physician assistants (PAs). APNs spent an average of 45 minutes with patients, more than the practice could afford. She attributed this difference to the educational preparation of NPs, which encourages spending more time with the patient than does traditional medical training. However, she sees APNs as being in the best position to bridge managed care and community partnerships because of their skills in networking, coordinating, and integrating tasks.

As the organizational structures for care delivery have been reshaped, the work and structures inside have been reshaped too. Some organizations have introduced a product line structure in which nursing is often decentralized. The structure may result in a marginalized nursing leadership that cannot advocate for appropriate patient care delivery models. However, a product line or decentralized structure does not necessarily indicate a lack of senior nursing voices; in fact, many product line administrators are nurses. It can mean variability in the advanced practice role with each product line defining the position.

Changes to reduce cost have resulted in fewer resources for patient care units, reductions in the overall number and changes in the skill mix of hospital employees, and the introduction of new kinds of workers to provide direct and indirect patient care. An APN role that suffered through these changes is that of the CNS. Because the CNS was too often "all things to all people," the actual contributions made by the CNS to patient care have been underestimated. One of the more frequent administrative responses was to eliminate the position as a cost-containment initiative. However, the literature reveals that new and reconfigured roles for the CNS and other APNs emerged from the chaotic inpatient environment (Fitzpatrick, 1998; Genet et al., 1995; Goksel, Harrison, Morrison, & Miller, 1993; Spisso, O'Callaghan, McKennan, & Holcroft, 1990; Payne & Baumgartner, 1996). Early in the development of case management, many CNSs were asked to lead the role definition. These positions build on the CNS's expertise in patient care and corporate financial management. The evolution of the role of APN case manager in hospitals is one example of how organizations are responding to the need to ensure effective and efficient care across traditional institutional boundaries in order to remain competitive (see Chapter 19).

Another role that is emerging in hospital settings is that of the ACNP (see Chapter 15). Although somewhat present in pediatric acute care settings, NPs have not been widely used with other inpatient populations. Today, in contrast, NPs have roles with trauma services, chronic medical services, and perioperative services.

The prediction that hospitals in the future will be purely intensive care facilities may create a justification for nurse administrators who are considering reintroducing the CNS role. Having a CNS available to consult with staff about complex patient care situations will be increasingly necessary to support the staff at the bedside. Subacute, transitional, or skilled nursing and hospice units exist today as freestanding organizations or within hospitals. The goal of these units is to provide care in the most appropriate setting to meet the patient's needs. In the process, it is expected that the cost of care will be reduced by enhancing efficiency, eliminating unnecessary activities, and reducing overhead costs. Nurse administrators face daily pressure to have models of care that will achieve those goals and help the organization be attractive to managed care business. They need clinical leaders who understand the continuum of the patient's needs and develop appropriate services. APNs will fulfill that need.

Regardless of the care environment, APNs and administrators must work together to be successful in designing new nurse roles and to preserve and enrich nursing's values and heritage within current and emerging systems.

Professional Tensions

Whatever the specific role in advanced nursing practice, APNs have experienced tensions with other professions and within nursing. Those tensions can influence the commitment of nurse administrators to the APN roles. At the same time that organizations need to be creative and take risks in developing new ways of delivering care, increasing financial constraints may be creating a conservative, risk-averse atmosphere. For instance, although CNMs and CRNAs have worked for many years with their physician colleagues, there have been many occasions of conflict. In organizations in which there is dispute about these roles, chief nursing officers (CNOs) can help mediate the disagreement—or could risk their own survival if they alienate physicians.

When the NP role was introduced, there was mixed reaction by physicians and nurses alike. Physicians reacted to the thought that someone with less preparation was taking over their medical functions. Members of the nursing community, then and today, questioned whether the NP is a "mini-doctor" or an APN (Sinclair, 1997). Cultivating collaborative partnerships with physicians reduces the fear factor. Clearly demonstrating APN competencies (see Chapter 3) eliminates concerns about whether these positions are truly nursing. The CNO can help shape collaborative APN-physician relationships by modeling collaboration with medical leadership and taking a lead in educating the organization about APNs.

Tensions can and do occur among various APN specialty organizations when they have different political agendas, such as the issue of medical supervision versus collaboration. They occur between administrators who want to use APNs and insurers who do not want to reimburse for the services. They occur between APNs and other health care professionals, such as PAs.

When there is conflict and lack of clarity about a role, administrators may shy away from introducing the role into an organization even if there is a good business case. The CNO should be the voice to influence decisions, but may also be one who does not understand the value of the various APN roles. Thus APNs must build meaningful working relationships with key administrators, beginning with the CNO. This includes assessing the CNO's understanding of the APN's potential contributions and undertaking sustained efforts to educate and inform the CNO about advanced practice if necessary. If the CNO is knowledgeable and committed to advanced practice, the partnership between CNO and APN can lead to innovative solutions to the stresses felt in health care organizations.

ASSESSING THE POTENTIAL FOR SUCCESS WITHIN ORGANIZATIONAL CULTURES

There are compelling reasons for CNOs and other administrators to consider APN roles as the answers to many of the important challenges of today's health care environment. Table 24-2 lists some of the attributes that provide justification for

---

TABLE 24-2 JUSTIFICATION FOR APN ROLES

- Use of theory-based and evidence-based clinical care
- Knowledge of clinical practice, including both medical and nursing perspectives
- Knowledge of health care systems
- Ability to develop and integrate practice within organizations, communities, and systems
- Ability to make independent judgments and ethical decisions
- Ability to practice in multiple care settings, such as tertiary, hospice, and home care
- Flexibility
- Ability to identify the nature and costs of nursing interventions and their effects on patient outcomes
- Expertise in specific areas of advanced nursing practice within the domain of nursing, such as pain management and women's health
- Ability to translate research into practice
- Ability to analyze care for a population, not only an individual
- Skill in educating staff

APN roles. Descriptions of the core competencies of APNs and other attributes that make them invaluable to nurse executives can be found in Chapter 3 and in the role chapters in Part II. Many of the variables that contribute to the success of the APN role are within the control of the CNO, so the needs and concerns of the CNO are important. Likewise, those variables that are within the control of the APN need to be acknowledged. The next sections are considerations for both CNO and APN.

Facilitators and Inhibitors for Role Success

Abdellah (1997) gave examples of APNs worldwide and noted that frustrations experienced by APNs included balancing components of blended roles, defending the role, lack of involvement in decision making, and lack of authority to make change. The last two are an alert to nurse administrators. They indicate that nurse administrators may be missing an opportunity to position APNs effectively within the nursing organization. However, they may also indicate that APNs have not been assertive in taking a leadership role. Given today's health care climate, clinical leadership is essential for redesigning care delivery (see Chapter 10). APNs should be the CNO's designees to lead redesign efforts because they are the experts in direct patient care and interact with the patient's needs along the continuum of care. They are also ideal candidates to lead a multidisciplinary team in performance improvement initiatives.

CNOs want APNs who are able to build partnerships and work comfortably in interdisciplinary teams. Support from physician and nurse colleagues tops the list of factors that help or hinder an APN (Hupcey, 1993). Acceptance by colleagues creates a successful environment in which to develop a practice. The opposite holds if support and acceptance are absent. Resistance to the role may be due to beliefs about APN roles (whether they are part of nursing or not) or to concerns about reimbursement. Sometimes it is simply a lack of understanding of a particular role by colleagues that raises a barrier to successful implementation. Woods (1998) presented preliminary findings of a longitudinal study of factors facilitating or inhibiting implementation of advanced practitioner roles in the United Kingdom. In addition to the support of colleagues, Woods found that other key factors for success were the APN's own confidence in her or his ability, having increased autonomy, being valued as a resource by staff, and good staffing levels. Inhibiting factors included lack of resources, lack of understanding/unrealistic expectations of the role, poor staffing levels, nurse colleagues feeling threatened, and inadequate compensation for the role.

Confusion among physicians about the specific nature of APN roles may stop them from giving support. CNOs and APNs can alleviate this confusion in a number of ways. These include providing information regarding the attributes of APN roles and the relationship of these roles to enhancing physician practice, the benefits of sharing and collaborating in research activities, and freeing up physician time for teaching responsibilities. The CNO needs to be able to show the positive influence on patient satisfaction and the value added by APNs to patient care. She or he can share information informally through distributing relevant literature or having discussions at clinical and administrative meetings or formally when presenting a budget request for a position. The importance of using appropriate data to support one's point of view cannot be overemphasized. The demonstration of successful role implementation is the most powerful force for CNOs and APNs to garner organizational support. Building institutional success stories, the folklore about the roles, can be most helpful to CNOs.

Considerations When Applying for a Position

There are many factors for the APN to consider when applying for a position in an organization or practice (Table 24–3). Although it may seem that many of these factors relate to larger organizations, they can be equally important when considering entering a primary care practice or physician group. Being knowledgeable of the regulatory conditions in a particular state is important if the APN is considering relocation. Some states are more supportive of APN practice than others. Once there is an understanding about the state's regulatory environment, conditions specific to a position are critical. There are specific factors to consider when evaluating the likelihood for success of a position.

MISSION AND VISION OF THE ORGANIZATION

The organization's mission and vision can orient an APN candidate to the potential support for the role. Organizations with a strong community focus may be seeking to develop APN-run clinics. Academic organizations, with their triple mission of patient care, teaching, and research, may seek doctorally prepared CNSs to influence the advancement of all nursing practice. IDNs may create an APN role that crosses boundaries of the discrete entities within the network to ensure a consistent standard of care for patients.

A candidate should assess how members of the organization understand the mission and vision and an APN's contributions to achieving them. Likewise, the nurse administrator will evaluate the APN candidate as to her or his interpretation and understanding of the organization and its goals. The nurse administrator will look for the fit between the mission and vision of the organization and the APN's personal abilities and reasons for seeking the position. In the interview process, the selection committee and hiring administrator will also evaluate the political abilities of the candidates, particularly if the position is new.

PHILOSOPHY AND SUPPORT OF THE NURSE EXECUTIVE TEAM

CNOs provide the vision and shape the culture for nursing practice within an organization. This vision is derived from the organization's mission and goals and reflects the CNO's beliefs about nursing. For APN roles to be firmly established, CNOs must promote a nursing philosophy that recognizes advanced nursing practice as central to the quality of and access to care and to the advancement of the profession. However, CNOs are also faced with pressures of balancing cost and quality and a

---

TABLE 24–3 ORGANIZATIONAL CONSIDERATIONS FOR APNs WHEN APPLYING FOR A POSITION

- Organization's mission, structure, strategic priorities, culture
- Nursing philosophy, share of organizational power, definition of APN roles
- Commitment to interdisciplinary care and continuous improvement principles
- Expected outcomes, financial objectives
- Reporting relationship, credentialing requirements, reimbursement potential
- Resources, other APNs
- Models of care delivery, clinical programs, patient populations
- State regulations for APNs

workforce shortage. APNs are the clinical surveillance within the organization. They are able to see patterns of care as well as assess and meet the individual needs of patients. Because APNs are able to move throughout the care continuum, they can manage resource utilization effectively. Also, they are able to address development needs among the nursing staff. When CNOs understand this, it is easy to maintain a commitment to advanced practice even in difficult times. For example, the author refused to eliminate the CNS role in her organization even though consultants were suggesting to administration that this was an easy budget cut.

Whether the APN is aligned within the nursing structure or not, the nurse executive is influential in preparing the organization for the successful implementation of the role. The CNO can broker relationships, making sure the APN is introduced effectively in the organization by using formal communication tools such as newsletters as well as setting meetings with key individuals during the APN's orientation. The CNO can align resources that help an APN achieve the expected outcomes, such as arranging access to current technology versus "hand-me-downs." CNOs need to ensure that there is a voice for nursing in the credentialing and privileging process. If not the CNO, then another nurse administrator should be a member of the organization's credentialing committee. The author has seen credentialing delegated to a nurse executive review committee, with the organization's credentialing committee simply accepting the nursing committee's approval. In an organization with well-established acceptance of APN roles, this works. Where there is ambivalence or unfamiliarity with the roles, the CNO needs to be in a position to clarify a particular role and advocate for APN privileges. APNs can assist the CNO by having timely and well-prepared application packets that do not omit information.

A collaborative effort between the nurse executive team and APNs ensures integration of administrative and advanced clinical thinking. This greatly enhances the potential for successful implementation of advanced nursing practice and sustaining the role during difficult periods.

COLLABORATIVE, INTERDISCIPLINARY RELATIONSHIPS

When considering a position, evaluating the collaborative atmosphere is essential. The advertising of a position does not necessarily mean that the people within the organization embrace an APN role. Learning about the partnerships that exist and seeking examples of past successes can be helpful in understanding who may be champions of the role. These champions are not just found in the physician or nursing arenas. Any of the organization's formal and informal leaders can be supporters more readily if they understand the purpose of the position and, as appropriate, participate in the interviewing process.

The CNO should help identify these leaders and then anticipate and respond to their needs for specific information. Existing APNs in the organization are sources of information about key supporters and detractors and should communicate that information to the CNO. Being aware of these leaders and partnering with the supporters builds a strong network that can prevent an APN from being seen as an intruder. Chapter 11 describes the importance of collaboration in detail.

EXPECTED OUTCOMES

Without clear expectations, an APN may find it difficult to be successful. In setting the expectations for a particular position, a nurse administrator can shape an understanding of what defines success. Assessing the need for an APN can determine which advanced practice role will fulfill the need. Involving stakeholders in planning for the new position ensures commitment to the person who is hired. A well-developed position description and agreed-upon reporting relationships establish the foundation for the APN and facilitate entry to the organization. The process of recruiting the best APN includes a comprehensive interview process to ensure that all stakeholders have an opportunity for input about their expectations. Finally, an orientation to the organization, including communication about the expectations of the APN, is necessary to foster success.

The requirements of the position will determine the educational preparation and previous professional experiences needed by the APN. For example, an organization seeking ways to maximize its reimbursement potential may develop APN positions such as NPs and CNMs to achieve this goal. If APN positions are needed to provide services 24 hours a day, 7 days a week, the decision about the type of position may differ from what it would be were APN services needed during limited times of the week. An academic organization faced with declining availability of residents may want to use NPs to cover medical functions, such as ACNPs in a critical care unit or neonatal NPs in an intensive care nursery.

The goals and objectives of the position determine the nature of the practice requirements, such as primary care delivery, consultation, program planning, and expansion of physician practices. The nature of the clinical program will determine the selection of the appropriate APN role—whether a CNS is needed, or someone who can blend the roles of CNS and NP, or a nurse case manager with CNS expertise. The number and type of other disciplines and professionals within the practice setting is another consideration. A CNS position may be selected to enhance staff nurses' clinical and communication skills within a clinical program that includes physicians, PAs, and ACNPs. A blended role CNS/NP may be desired if the purpose is to manage the care of a group of patients across multiple settings in an IDN. The purpose of a position will also determine the licensure and credentialing requirements (see Chapter 22).

Nuccio and colleagues (1993) suggested that role expectations solicited from staff nurses can be useful in developing supportive relationships. Paul (in Paladichuk, 1998) also spoke to the importance of the APN–staff nurse partnership. Delineation of roles and clear-cut communicating and reporting structures strengthen these relationships. APNs potentially affect the practice of clinical administrators, pharmacists, and nonprofessional direct and indirect care providers. The broadest interpretation of these advanced nursing roles to other staff, well before their introduction, helps ensure their success. The emerging focus on advanced nursing practice, especially within the context of work redesign, affects other care providers in different ways. In some organizations, APNs assume functions previously performed by other professionals, including physicians, social workers, and clinical dietitians. ''Territorial disputes'' may arise. The CNO can minimize the potential for these disputes by maintaining the focus of decision making on patient care requirements and how to address them in the most cost-effective and efficient manner with the best possible outcomes. Sincerely expressed respect for the work of other professionals, coupled with sensitivity and diplomacy, modulates the potentially negative effects of these negotiations.

REPORTING RELATIONSHIPS

There is no singular reporting structure for APNs. Rarely will an APN report directly to a CNO unless the organization is small. Instead, specific roles, legal requirements, and other variables in the organization will shape the reporting relationship. For instance, NPs, CNMs, and CRNAs who practice in hospital settings must obtain privileges through the credentialing committee and have a designated physician supervisor/collaborator. They may have accountability to a nurse supervisor as well. The CNS most likely will not go through this same process and usually does not have a physician supervisor. The individual to whom the APN reports can indicate the importance of the position, but this should not be overvalued. Depending on the organization, where an APN is listed on an organizational chart may be much less important than what access the APN has to key leaders.

All APNs should carefully examine a potential practice setting before accepting a job offer. Consideration should be given to how the job is positioned in the organization and to the position or individual to whom the APN is accountable. Parrinello (1995) described three models of practice: the physician practice model, the nursing model, and the joint practice model. In the physician practice model, the APN typically joins a group practice and reports to a physician. In the nursing model, the APN reports to a nursing director and is assigned to work with physicians. This is the traditional CNS structure, but it is also how nurse case managers may be assigned and it is often used with ACNPs, such as those in intensive care units. The joint practice model is a cohesive physician and nurse care delivery model in which the funding for the APN is a combination of nursing/hospital and professional revenue funds. Each has advantages and disadvantages that the APN needs to understand. Table 24-4 outlines some of these advantages and disadvantages. Regardless of the model, both APNs and nurse administrators should align their efforts to ensure the best clinical care.

Nurse executives are instrumental in creating an environment in which any of the models are accepted. By thinking broadly about the needs of the patients and the organization, the nurse executive is the champion of all nursing. She or he sets the tone of acceptance for other nurses in the work setting regardless of what practice model exists. To do so, the nurse executive must ensure that clear expectations of APNs are established and communicated. Nurse executives who have system-wide responsibilities in IDNs have an additional opportunity to create APN roles that cross organizational boundaries and extend their capability as clinical surveyors for the system.

TABLE 24-4 MODELS OF PRACTICE IN ORGANIZATIONS		
MODEL	ADVANTAGES	DISADVANTAGES
Physician Practice Model	Funding linked to the success of the group practice, not nursing budget; clinical work closely linked with physicians and clearly defined	Potential conflict in definition of collaboration versus supervision, isolation from nursing colleagues
Nursing Model	Clear identification with nursing, credibility with staff, focus on broader APN skills	Potential for decreased collaboration with physicians, risk for losing continued funding within the large nursing budget
Joint Practice Model	Captures the best of physician and nursing-based models, interdependency recognized	Complexity of a matrix structure and potential to be caught between two supervisors

RESOURCES

To succeed, APNs need resources. Some are as simplistic as adequate space for direct and indirect patient care activities. The organization needs to assure the APN of appropriate salary support and opportunities for raises or sufficient opportunities to generate income through professional fees. Assistive staff, such as clinical assistants, secretarial support, and data entry personnel, may be required. Access to automated systems is essential in today's environment. Continuing education opportunities in both academic and nonacademic programs are essential for maintaining one's skills. The organization's support of these activities can be seen in the financial support dedicated to the role and service. Asking to see a budget for the APN position is an easy way to evaluate whether the organization has planned for the needed resources. Finally, contact with the CNO and other nursing leaders will ensure synchrony between the APN and the organization.

Creating New Roles

The chaos in the health care system, as traditional care delivery systems are failing, creates significant opportunities for APNs to develop new roles. For example, the ACNP has evolved partially as a result of the challenges being faced in academic medical centers as resident and fellow numbers are declining and training is changing. Although the basis of NP role development and education has been primary care in the ambulatory setting, the question of how to provide medical coverage for hospitalized patients has generated a new role for NPs and a new curriculum for NP preparation. Whether this role will thrive is uncertain. The medical community has responded to that same question of how to provide coverage for hospitalized patients by promoting the role of the hospitalist, a physician dedicated full time to managing the care of hospitalized patients. Blended roles are also evolving, such as CNS/NP, NP case manager, and CNS case manager (see Chapters 16 and 19). Regardless of whether an APN or a nurse executive is proposing a new advanced practice role, several factors should be considered.

Justification for the Role. With passage of the BBA, restrictions on NP and CNS billing were removed. Increased managed care penetration has resulted in a greater need for primary care providers and specialists to work harder to maintain their revenue stream. The changes in resident programs have left inpatient care management uncovered. All are reasons that APN roles have been and can be created with new emphasis. Beginning with the needs of patients establishes a justification for the new role, and the CNO is the likely leader for starting this process.

Identifying Stakeholders. With any new initiative, understanding who the stakeholders are and what their expectations might be is important. For a new APN role, determining who will be affected by the role means assessing who might gain or lose something if the role is created. Physicians who are experiencing increased workloads may welcome the addition of a NP to the care team. Conversely, staff nurses may respond to a case manager negatively because they see that some of their responsibilities are being reassigned. The nurse executive can be helpful in identifying the stakeholders. As noted earlier, the presence or absence of support from co-workers or superiors has been shown to be the major factor in influencing NP role success (Hupcey, 1993).

Laying the Groundwork. Once a justification is developed and the stakeholders are known, it is time to lay the groundwork for introducing the role in the organization. A thorough communication plan will ensure that all audiences are informed about the role and the expectations of the person in the role. In determining who initiates the communication plan, understanding the politics of the organization is important. In some circumstances, having the nurse executive introduce the role may be the most effective; in others, a physician leader may be the most appropriate (see Chapter 10).

Marketing the Role Within the Organization. Once the position has been established and the person hired, ongoing promotion of the APN's services may be needed. This is particularly key with roles such as CNS and nurse case manager, the first because it is vulnerable to elimination and the second because it is new and variably defined. NPs, CRNAs, and CNMs in nontraditional roles will also benefit from ongoing education about their roles within the organization. APN roles based in a physician practice tend to be clearly defined by the physician group and usually have activities extending from the medical model, such as doing histories and physicals on patients. However, that does not eliminate the need for the APNs to explain their role and services to other staff.

MEASURING AND MONITORING THE VALUE OF APN ROLES

During the turmoil of the changing health care payer environment, much has been written about the value of NPs to provide primary care. The lay media as well as the professional literature have viewed the use of APNs as a way to increase access to care and to control cost. However, the literature also reinforces the necessity of measuring the impact of advanced practice roles on the cost and quality of care (Byers & Brunell, 1998; Carroll & Fay, 1997; Fitzpatrick, 1998; Mundinger, 1999; Schaffner & Bohomey, 1998). By demonstrating their ability to deliver high-quality, cost-effective care, APNs show their value and secure a position in the health care marketplace. Table 24–5 lists resources APNs and CNOs can use for developing measurement and monitoring strategies (see also Chapters 20 and 25).

Carroll and Fay (1997) reviewed the challenges APNs and administrators face in measuring the impact of APN practice. They discussed several considerations: defining the scope of practice of the APN; building consensus about the definition and the relationship of structure, process, and outcomes variables; designating the settings and systems of practice; influencing stakeholders; and assuring the scientific rigor of a study. In making informed decisions about the utilization of APNs in an organization, the CNO is often the administrator who will research the literature for studies that document cost and quality outcomes of using APNs. CNOs are inundated with a tremendous amount of information, so it is helpful to the CNO when APNs forward articles to them, particularly reports about outcomes and cost savings attributed to APNs.

Byers and Brunell (1998) described a comprehensive model for evaluating the impact of an APN. As they noted, evaluation strategies have typically focused on

TABLE 24-5 RESOURCES FOR APN IMPACT MEASUREMENT INFORMATION

RESOURCE	MEASURES
Joint Commission on Accreditation of Healthcare Organizations 708-916-5950 Website: *www.jcaho.org*	Standards, indicators
National Committee for Quality Assurance 202-955-5697 Website: *www.ncqa.org*	HEDIS
Medical Outcomes Trust 617-426-4046 Website: *www.outcomes-trust.org*	SF-36, SF-12
Health Outcomes Institute 612-858-9188	Health Status Questionnaires
Foundation for Accountability 503-223-2228	FAACT tools

specific components of an APN's role. They proposed measurement of structure, process, and outcomes to assess quality and the use of benchmarks or demonstrated best practices for comparison. They recognized the limitations of accomplishing comprehensive evaluation, such as lack of consolidated data sources, difficulty in longitudinal data collection, and limited resources. Nurse executives need to consider allocation of resources to support APNs in practice evaluation beyond the basics required by regulatory agencies or performance management systems. Byers and Brunell advocated the development of a statewide or national database of APN-dependent measures, such as rate of complications following an APN-provided procedure, that would provide critical information for APNs.

Two studies have demonstrated the value of APN models of care in the managed care environment. Mundinger (1999) described the experience of the Columbia University School of Nursing in implementing an APN-run primary care clinic. In the evaluation phase of this clinic, patients were randomized from the Presbyterian Hospital Emergency Room and Urgicenter to either the APN clinic or a physician primary care practice. To reduce variability in the practices, the APNs were given admitting privileges to the hospital. Additionally, the APNs became full members of the Columbia-Presbyterian Physicians Network, the centralized operations unit for contracting, and had fee equity with their physician colleagues. With the success of this first effort in extending primary care to an underserved community and subsequent to the completion of the trial period, the School of Nursing introduced two other practices. Using their experience with APNs on the Nutritional Support Team at the University of Rochester Medical Center, Schaffner and Bohomey (1998) described how APNs could demonstrate their value to institutions by cost reduction. They used a simple documentation of activities to capture savings and show the value of APNs in a capitated market.

As previously noted, the CNS role has been more vulnerable than other APN roles to elimination when budget cuts are made. In the 1980s, many articles were written about measurement of CNS activities and the importance of the role to inpatient care. However, in the 1990s, CNOs often eliminated the positions, an indication that the value of the role was not tangible. In the past few years, the CNS role has begun to be reintroduced and its value in managed care is being noted (Bakker & Vincensi, 1995; Rago, 1997; Vollman & Stewart, 1996).

In any organization, to measure and monitor the contributions of any APN, there must be a clear definition of the role and of the role objectives and time frame for achieving them. These must be understood by the APN and the person or persons to whom the APN is accountable. Consensus about the scope of practice, definitions of outcomes, and practice settings are a few of the variables to consider. Ongoing communication about performance and achievement of objectives is one step in measuring the value of the role. Formally setting annual goals and reviewing performance using the organization's performance management system should be done annually.

Deciding the appropriate number of patients for whom the APN is responsible is based on the context and nature of the clinical practice and forms the basis for one measure: productivity. In Frampton and Wall's study (1994), NPs and PAs believed that 81% to 91% of the patients they saw were appropriately cared for and did not require the services of a physician. Other factors that influence this number include the organization's standards of practice and the number and diversity of other staff members within the clinical practice. For example, Dang and Haller (1995) found a range of 7 to 16 patients per case manager in the academic hospitals surveyed. MCOs often have established targets for the numbers of patients seen by NPs or CNMs. Hummel and Pirzada (1994) noted that teams of "non-physician providers" (NPs or PAs) and physicians were extremely cost-effective when the number of patients cared for expanded.

CONSIDERATIONS FOR THE FUTURE

The turmoil of the current health care environment is expected to continue for the next couple of decades. This holds both opportunity and threat for APNs. The passage of the BBA offers opportunity for expanding practice options for NPs and CNSs in the near future (Keepnews, 1998). Direct billing by APNs will answer some of the questions about their practice, such as what types of patients they see. The BBA also defines CNS for the first time in Medicare law, which gives CNSs the opportunity to serve Medicare beneficiaries. APNs need to view the development of IDNs or community-based programs as realms in which they can advance their services and create new opportunities. However, the BBA is also affecting physicians and, in a few years, APNs may find increased competition with physicians who are struggling to maintain their practices and their income. It is therefore essential that nursing organizations be united in their efforts to shape policy.

Berger and colleagues (1996) defined several future advanced practice roles to promote the optimal use of knowledge, skills, and abilities of APNs. They do not all fit the APN definition in this book, but do represent the reality of the marketplace in which new titles and role definitions continue to arise. Although these authors acknowledge the confusion that has existed in defining advanced practice roles and functions, they propose the following roles: case manager, clinical educator, clinical researcher, clinical consultant, NP, corporate/community NP, and patient care manager. These roles take into account the need to serve patients with increasingly complex health care concerns while being cost conscious, and some of them incorporate the unique skills of APNs. No doubt, there will be debate about whether nursing needs more titles within the area of advanced practice, but during a state of major change more roles and titles are likely to develop. Nurse executives in particular, but all executives, could assist in reducing the confusion about APN roles by not introducing more nomenclature into the job lexicon. Increasing clarity about the APN roles described in this text is an important responsibility of nurse executives as well as other nursing leaders.

Hester and White (1996) examined CNSs' perceptions of their future. They found that CNSs perceived that their roles were changing to meet the challenges of the changing delivery system. An area in which APNs can take a lead is the research of patient outcomes, particularly related to quality and cost. This means that APNs must become more knowledgeable about the "business" of health care and learn to speak the language of administrators. As early as 1989, Brown described the need for CNSs to serve as "shuttle diplomats" who interpret economic realities and administrative decisions to nursing staff and clinical realities to administrative staff. Brown (1989) described the CNS as able to be "the person in the middle, a person expected and required to speak the language of both subcultures, understand the issues and dilemmas of each, and participate in the problem-solving of both arenas" (p. 285). The need for shuttle diplomacy by all APNs, particularly those working in large, complex organizations, has never been more critical, especially in relating clinical activities to institutional costs. Nurse executives must help APNs with this development. The era of APNs being able to self-define their positions and be vaguely accountable within an organization is over.

The APN's direct clinical practice is the foundation for APN success in the 21st century. As noted throughout this book, clinical care is increasingly complex; the aging population is living longer with multisystem chronic illnesses, increases in technology continue, and burgeoning research findings, particularly in genetics research, need to be incorporated into clinical care. Having a strong expert clinical practice base is critical for APNs to enact the clinical leadership and critical thinking skills so valued by administrators. The characteristics of APN direct practice noted in Chapter 6 (use of a holistic perspective, formation of partnerships with patients, expert clinical thinking and skillful performance, use of research evidence, and diverse health and illness management approaches) are the sources of the APN's value-added contributions to patient care, and their other competencies (see Chapter 3) emanate from this practice expertise. Nurse executives must be careful not to overload APNs with committee and project work to the extent that they lose these skills or become less visible in key practice arenas. Although this is tempting in the short term, weakening an APN's practice strength compromises the reason the positions were established and can diminish the APN's effectiveness in the long term. APNs must also be vigilant in communicating with their administrators when nonclinical activities are requiring them to compromise their practice expertise.

According to Milstead (1997), the role of political activist is one that APNs should embrace. Certainly, APNs need to follow national and state legislation closely and make their views known. They can also be valuable educators of politicians and their staffs about the issues faced by patients and by nurses in advanced practice. Many of the APN's clinical skills, such as communication, conflict resolution, and critical thinking, transfer well into the political arena. Nurse executives can be allies to APNs in the political arena and present a strong voice for nursing (see Chapters 22 and 23).

SUMMARY

APNs and CNOs should think in terms of the skills that APNs bring to an organization, especially as changes continue in the provision and the location of care delivery within an organization and within the community. APNs should promote their skills as new opportunities and new relationships emerge, and nurse executives should assist them in doing so. Furthermore, the community's and the organization's needs and strategic imperatives are the context for current and future job-related opportunities of APNs. By committing to the mission and objectives of the organization and consistently developing and expanding their skills, APNs ensure their place in the future of health care delivery.

REFERENCES

Abdellah, F. G. (1997). Managing the challenges of role diversification in an interdisciplinary environment. *Military Medicine, 162*(7), 453–458.

Bakker, D. J., & Vincensi, B. B. (1995). Economic impact of the CNS: Practitioner role. *Clinical Nurse Specialist, 9*(1), 50–53.

Barger, S. E. (1997). Building healthier communities in a managed care environment: Opportunities for advanced practice nurses. *Advanced Practice Nursing Quarterly, 2*(4), 9–14.

Bear, E. M. (1995). Advanced practice nurses: How did we get here anyway? *Advanced Practice Nursing Quarterly, 1*(1), 10–14.

Berger, A. M., Eilers, J. G., Pattrin, L., Rolf-Fixley, M., Pfeifer, B. A., Rogge, J. A., Wheeler, L. M., Bergstrom, N. I., & Heck, C. S. (1996). Advanced practice roles for nurses in tomorrow's healthcare systems. *Clinical Nurse Specialist, 10*(5), 250–255.

Brown, S. J. (1989). Supportive supervision of the CNS. In A. B. Hamric & J. A. Spross (Eds.), *The clinical nurse specialist in theory and practice* (2nd ed., pp. 285–298). Philadelphia: W. B. Saunders.

Byers, J. F., & Brunell, M. L. (1998). Demonstrating the value of the advanced practice nurse: An evaluation model. *AACN Clinical Nurses, 9*(2), 296–305.

Camp-Sorrell, D., & Spencer-Cisek, P. (1995). Reimbursement issues for advanced practice. *Oncology Nursing Forum, 22*(8, Suppl.), 31–34.

Carroll, T. L., & Fay, V. P. (1997). Measuring the impact of advanced practice nursing on achieving cost-quality outcomes: Issues and challenges. *Nursing Administration Quarterly, 21*(4), 32–40.

Dang, D., & Haller, K. (1995). *Analysis of nonphysician provider roles.* Unpublished manuscript, The Johns Hopkins Hospital, Baltimore.

Fitzpatrick, E. R. (1998). Analysis and synthesis of the role of the advanced practice nurse. *Clinical Nurse Specialist, 12*(3), 106–107.

Frampton, J., & Wall, S. (1994). Exploring the use of NPs and PAs in primary care. *HMO Practice, 4,* 165–170.

Genet, C. A., Brennan, P. F., Ibbotson-Wolff, S., Phelps, C., Rosenthal, G., Landefeld, C. S., &

Daly, B. (1995). Nurse practitioners in a teaching hospital. *Nurse Practitioner, 20*(9), 47–54.

Goksel, D., Harrison, C. J., Morrison, R. E., & Miller, S. T. (1993). Description of a nurse practitioner inpatient service in a public teaching hospital. *Journal of General Internal Medicine, 8,* 29–30.

Haber, J. (1997). Medicare reimbursement: A victory for APRNs. *American Journal of Nursing, 97*(11), 84.

Hamric, A. B., & Taylor, J. W. (1989). Role development of the CNS. In A. B. Hamric & J. A. Spross (Eds.), *The clinical nurse specialist in theory and practice* (2nd ed., pp. 41–82). Philadelphia: W. B. Saunders.

Health Care Advisory Board. (1999). *The physician perspective: Key drivers of physician loyalty.* Washington, DC: The Advisory Board Company.

Hester, L. E., & White, M. J. (1996). Perceptions of practicing CNSs about their future role. *Clinical Nurse Specialist. 10*(4), 190–193.

Hummel, J., & Pirzada, S. (1994). Estimating the cost-effectiveness of nurse practitioner/physician team in long-term care facilities. *HMO Practice, 8*(4), 162–164.

Hupcey, J. E. (1993). Factors and work settings that may influence nurse practitioner practice. *Nursing Outlook, 41*(4), 181–185.

Johnson, S. J. (1994). GME financing: A well-kept secret. *Nursing Management, 25*(4), 43–46.

Keepnews, D. (1998). New opportunities and challenges for APRNS. *American Journal of Nursing, 98*(1), 62–64.

Licking, M., & Sampson, D. (1995). HCFA regulations and financing. *Short Communications, 20*(12), 6–9.

Lowe, M., & Havens, D. H. (1998). Hot issues for NPs in 1998. *Journal of Pediatric Health Care, 12*(3), 161–163.

Lyon, B. L. (1996). Defining advanced practice nursing role diversity is essential in meeting nursing's social mandate. *Clinical Nurse Specialist, 10*(6), 263–264.

Mason, D. J., Cohen, S. S., O'Donnell, J. P., Baxter, K., & Chase, A. B. (1997). Managed care organizations' arrangements with nurse practitioners. *Nursing Economics, 15*(6), 306–314.

Milstead, J. (1997). Using advanced practice to shape public policy: Agenda setting. *Nursing Administration Quarterly, 21*(4), 12–18.

Minarik, P. (1997). Medicare reimbursement for nurse practitioners and clinical nurse specialists passes; states' legislative and regulatory forum II. *Clinical Nurse Specialist, 11*(6), 274–275.

Mundinger, M. O. (1999). Can advanced practice nurses succeed in the primary care market? *Nursing Economics, 17*(1), 7–14.

Nuccio, S., Costa-Lieberthal, K. M., Gunta, K. E., Mackus, M. L., Riesch, S. K., Schmanski, K. M., & Westen, B. A. (1993). A survey of 636 staff nurses' perceptions and factors influencing the CNS role. *Clinical Nurse Specialist, 7*(3), 122–128.

Paladichuk, A. (1998). Interview. Sara Paul, RN, MSN, FNPC. The advanced practice/staff nurse partnership: Building a winning team. *Critical Care Nurse, 18*(2), 92–97.

Parrinello, K. M. (1995). Advanced practice nursing: An administrative perspective. *Critical Care Nursing Clinics of North America, 7*(1), 9–16.

Payne, J. L. (1996). CNS role evolution. *Clinical Nurse Specialist, 10*(1), 46–48.

Pearson, L. J. (2000). Annual update of how each state stands on legislative issues affecting advanced nursing practice. *Nurse Practitioner, 25*(1), 16–83.

Rago, K. A. (1997). Clinical nurse specialist: A cost-effective role in the managed care environment. *Progress in Cardiovascular Nursing, 12*(4), 38–39.

Schaffner, R. J., Jr., & Bohomey, J. (1998). Demonstrating APN value in a capitated market. *Nursing Economics, 16*(2), 69–74.

Shortell, S. M., Gillies, R. R., & Devers, K. J. (1995). Reinventing the American hospital. *Millbank Quarterly, 73*(2), 131–158.

Sinclair, B. P. (1997). Advanced practice nurses in integrated health care systems. *Journal of Obstetric, Gynecologic, and Neonatal Nursing, 26*(2), 217–223.

Spisso, J., O'Callaghan, C., McKennan, M., & Holcroft, J. W. (1990). Improved quality of care and reduction of housestaff workload using trauma nurse practitioners. *Journal of Trauma, 30*(6), 660–665.

Vollman, K. M., & Stewart, K. H. (1996). Can we afford not to have clinical nurse specialists? *AACN Clinical Issues, 7*(2), 315–323.

Wilken, M. (1995). State regulatory board structure, regulations, and nurse practitioner availability. *Nurse Practitioner, 20*(10), 68–74.

Woods, L. P. (1998). Implementing advanced practice: Identifying the factors that facilitate and inhibit the process. *Journal of Clinical Nursing, 7,* 265–273.

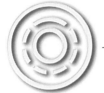

New Directions for the Advanced Practice Nurse in Health Care Quality

PERFORMANCE AND OUTCOME IMPROVEMENT

• S H I R L E Y   A.   G I R O U A R D

INTRODUCTION

Changes in the organization, delivery, and financing of health care during the past decade and the continued pressure on the health care system to be more accountable to policy makers, consumers, and the general public have made evaluation a critical issue for advanced practice nurses (APNs). By virtue of their educational and practice competencies, APNs must be able to provide society with evidence of their contributions to health care. Employers, consumers, insurers, competing providers, and others are calling on APNs to justify their contributions to health care outcomes and the health care system. In particular, attention needs to be given to establishing the "value" of advanced nursing practice, where value = quality/cost.

The evaluation of advanced practice nursing is an important and timely component of the present quality of health care agenda discussed in Chapter 23. The assessment of APNs' contributions has implications beyond that of determining the impact of APN practice on individuals or groups of patients. The APN has a social responsibility to promote the optimal health of individuals, families, and communities. This responsibility to the public includes contributing to the resolution of problems that limit the health care system's ability to achieve optimal health for individuals. These issues include problems of access to services and concerns about the quality, effectiveness, and cost of interventions. Verification of nursing's contributions to improved health requires the assessment of the structures, processes, and outcomes related to nursing practice. The knowledge gained from these efforts can be used to improve the health of the public by improving the organization, delivery, and financing of health care services and enhancing the practice, education, and research activities of nurses.

The Institute of Medicine (IOM) (Lohr, 1990) defined quality of care as "the degree to which health services for individuals and populations increase the likelihood of desired health outcomes and are consistent with professional knowledge" (p. 3). Given the APN's focus on expert clinical practice to achieve desired health outcomes, this definition is consistent with APN roles and with nursing and other health care knowledge. McGlynn (1997) identified five characteristics of quality, derived from the IOM definition, that suggest considerations for the APN to use to evaluate the quality of health care services:

1. Quality performance occurs on a continuum (ranging from unacceptable to excellent).
2. Quality assessment is focused on services provided.
3. Quality can be evaluated from the individual or population perspective.
4. Evidence is needed to identify which interventions/services improve outcomes.
5. Professional consensus regarding effectiveness is needed when scientific evidence is lacking.

This definition and these characteristics have been widely accepted by a variety of stakeholders in health care and emphasize the need for the APN to be diligent in determining the outcomes of advanced practice. The APN may be involved in research to measure and improve outcomes, apply existing knowledge, educate from this perspective, or engage in other activities related to assuring and improving the quality of health care. From these activities, APNs will be better able to strengthen their awareness of and justify their contributions to health care quality. The contributions of APNs' performance in other health care system components, such as health care plans or public health agencies, also need to be evaluated. In addition, the importance of measuring APN performance is consistent with current accountability concerns.

This chapter discusses why greater attention needs to be given to evaluating the quality and quantity of APN practice, and provides a framework for understanding the quality movement. Challenges associated with meaningful evaluation are reviewed and the content and relevance of Donabedian's model for evaluation activities are described. The chapter also reviews related literature and proposes an approach to improve evaluation activities. Finally, possible activities for APNs in evaluation and quality assessment processes are identified.

THE NEED FOR EVALUATION AND ASSESSMENT

The purpose of the health care system must be to continuously reduce the impact and burden of illness, injury and disability, and to improve the health and functioning of the people of the United States.

(President's Advisory Commission, 1998, p. 2)

This statement of purpose for the health care system by the President's Advisory Commission on Consumer Protection and Quality in the Health Care System reflects the focus of the "quality movement." As discussed in Chapter 23, quality of care is a major policy issue for the nation. Health care providers, payers, and consumers are all concerned about issues related to the quality of care. Although different stakeholders may emphasize different issues, all need information. For example, health care plans may focus on assuring their ability to rank well on performance measures reported to an accrediting body and to delivering care at the lowest possible cost; consumers are interested in their ability to access care when they need it; and payers are interested in evidence to support their payment of health care services. Obviously, the APN must be involved in providing such information. Also, APNs need quality-related information to be able to assess their performance.

The Quality Movement

The current quality movement emphasizes the demand for information about whether or not the health care system is meeting its purpose: Are consumers and society getting what they need, want, and pay for? The resulting emphasis on quality measurement was fostered by theories and practices from private industry and business, evidence of quality problems identified by research, concerns about managed care's impact on quality, and the growing consumer movement in health care. The importance of health care, the traditional values of the nursing profession, and the professional and social responsibilities of the APN are all consistent with the aims of the quality movement. None of these concepts should be alien to the APN because they are clearly the core of nursing. The conceptualizations of advanced practice nursing (Chapter 2) and the definition of advanced nursing practice (Chapter 3) support a primary role for the APN in the quality movement. The President's Advisory Commission's statement of purpose is also congruent with the traditional values of the nursing profession. Nurses, especially those engaged in advanced practice, have always been involved in assessing and improving the quality of nursing care, have long recognized the need for an evidence (research) base for practice, and believe they are accountable for their practice.

Girouard (1996) identified the need for APN evaluation and how this need was derived from the existing environment of health care. These issues remain and are perhaps even more critical. Changes in the organization and delivery of nursing and health care that have taken place in the last 5 years have resulted in an even greater emphasis on quality and accountability. APNs have the opportunity to operationalize their roles in a context that is consistent with their values about patient care. The challenge facing the APN is to increase efforts to become more involved in the quality movement at every level—from the bedside to the side of the policy maker. As Urden (1999) suggested, APNs have a major role to play in outcome evaluation given their knowledge and skills in evaluating care.

Assessing the quality of the health care system includes the identification, specification, and measurement of the structures and processes that produce positive outcomes for individuals and groups of patients. Issues related to access to health care insurance and the costs and efficacy of health care services are also fundamental concepts for understanding the current health care quality climate. Given the extensive literature related to quality, the APN needs to become familiar with the definitions and conceptual frameworks used to address quality concerns. In addition, the APN should be familiar with quality-related activities taking place at the national level, within states, within the practice setting, and within the APN's area of specialization. The discussion that follows provides some basic information about the frameworks, concepts, and definitions being used by individuals and organizations leading the quality movement.

Outcomes of health care services have traditionally been measured by assessing health status indicators such as survival and morbidity, functional level, comfort and well-being, and consumer/patient satisfaction. Outcomes are dependent on the structures and processes of providing the service. Thus defining the structural components of a service—the characteristics of system resources such as numbers of health care providers, facilities, technological support, financing, and organization of care delivery—is necessary to understand how outcomes are achieved. Similarly, processes, such as the elements of nursing interventions (assessments, treatments, etc.) used to achieve specific outcomes, must be identified. It may be helpful to consider outcomes as the dependent variables and structures and processes as the independent variables of a research equation where outcomes = structures + processes. Measurement of structures, processes, and outcomes using this definition can take place at a number of levels: the consumer or individual patient, the organization, the health plan or payer source, the community, the state, or the nation.

Key Concepts and Terms

The term "performance measurement" has become widely used by those involved in measuring health care quality. Simply stated, it refers to assessing how well a provider, health care organization, or health plan does in relation to a given measure of performance. Performance measures include those developed by the Foundation for Accountability (FACCT) to assess whether or not the needs of patients are being met and by the National Committee for Quality Assurance's (NCQA's) Health Plan Employer Data and Information Set (HEDIS) to assess, for example, immunization rates and the care provided to plan members. Performance measures are tools to assess whether or not a health care provider is delivering health care services that are appropriate, safe, competent, and timely to achieve desired outcomes (Palmer et al., 1995).

The language of the quality movement has its own vocabulary. The use of terms and concepts is not always clear, especially since different individuals and groups may use them in different ways. Some of the additional concepts/terms related to quality of care include quality assessment, quality assurance, quality improvement (often modified by "total" or "continuous"), total quality management, core measure sets, quality indicators, and report cards. Although it is beyond the scope of this chapter to discuss these in depth, the APN should be familiar with how these terms are generally used and clarify their use in discussions with providers and others. "Quality assessment" refers to the process of determining whether the processes of care achieve good outcomes or meet processes believed to be associated with positive health care outcomes. "Quality assurance" generally refers to a process that includes assessment, problem identification, application of improvements, and an evaluation of whether or not the "corrective" action resulted in the desired changes in outcomes or processes of care. Related to this are the terms "quality improvement," "total quality management," and "continuous quality improvement." They reflect procedures/actions taken to improve the quality of processes or outcomes of care.

As the demand for accountability and the assessment of quality has increased, there is a need for health care quality measures that can serve the informational needs of the wide variety of users of health quality information. Core measure sets, some of which are being developed by accrediting bodies such as the NCQA and the Joint Commission on Accreditation of Healthcare Organizations (JCAHO), are those measures that address national goals for health care quality. In addition, their measurement is standardized so the information gained can be used for allocating resources, tracking improvements in health care across patient populations and institutions, and directing quality improvement activities. The term "quality indicators" is often used synonymously with performance indicators. In an effort to report to others on the quality of care, report cards may be used to provide the results of measuring health care performance (often for a health plan). They employ standardized measures of performance.

Stakeholders

The quality movement involves many stakeholders: consumers/patients; providers, including the APN; professional organizations; purchasers of health care services; accrediting bodies; state and federal agencies; others who assess health care quality; policy makers; and researchers. During the past 5 years, the depth and breadth of quality-related efforts by these stakeholders has increased significantly. The following discussion provides an overview of these efforts.

Consumers, primarily through the efforts of advocacy organizations, are a major force in the demand for health care quality information. For example, New England

SERVE, an advocacy organization for children and families with special health care needs, conducted research to identify core measures and assess the quality of health care for its constituents. Numerous other advocacy organizations have collaborated with other stakeholders to develop and implement measures to assess quality of care. One of the most important collaborations is FACCT, created in 1995. With trustees from consumer organizations, corporate and government purchasers, health plans, and others, it is dedicated to helping consumers make better health care decisions. FACCT does this by engaging all stakeholders in the development of tools to assess and use information about health care quality. Sets of health care quality measures have been developed for both children and adults focusing on consumer concerns related to diabetes care, depression, asthma, breast cancer, health risk behaviors, satisfaction with care, and the health status of the elderly (see the Foundation for Accountability website at *www.facct.org*).

Through their participation in the work of FACCT and other quality-related organizations, providers have contributed to the development of quality measures and their application and evaluation. Nurses serve on committees and work with many groups, such as accrediting organizations, to further efforts to improve health quality measurement and reporting. National efforts to improve quality measurement and reporting are enhanced by sets of measures promulgated by many professional associations, such as the American Nurses Association's *Nursing Report Card for Acute Care* (1995). Specialty nursing organizations have also become more involved in these and related activities. For example, the American Academy of Nursing recently brought together child/family health care nursing specialty associations to determine current activities with the aim of developing a core set of quality principles for child/family nursing.

Purchasers of care—both private and public—are concerned about how well their health care premium money is spent. They, like providers, are involved in many of the ongoing initiatives to measure quality of care. In addition, purchasers influence health care quality through their negotiations with health plans, decisions about benefits, and the incentives they use to influence the health behavior of their employees or those covered by the health insurance they purchase on behalf of their constituents. Purchasers can require insurers and providers to assess and report on specific quality-related structures, processes, or outcomes. For example, some purchasers require the health plans they contract with to provide HEDIS information for their employees to use in making decisions about their choice of health plans (see the NCQA's website at *www.ncqa.org*).

Accrediting organizations are also contributing to improving quality through their quality measurement activities. For example, the JCAHO has developed quality measures for use by the health care organizations it accredits and, through the ORYX initiative, is promoting the development and use of measures developed by others (see the JCAHO website at *www.jcaho.org*). One of the more influential organizations in the quality movement is the NCQA, a not-for-profit organization that assesses and reports on the quality of managed care plans. The NCQA accredits managed care organizations and is responsible for the development and revision of HEDIS. It includes more than 75 performance measures to assess quality, including patient satisfaction.

There are a number of reasons state governments are involved in the quality movement: they are major purchasers of health care for state employees and others; they have responsibility for Medicaid; they provide health care services in public institutions such as nursing homes, hospitals, and prisons; they have regulatory responsibility for protecting the health and safety of the public; and they are consumers. States vary considerably in how they carry out their quality-related roles. Through their public health agencies, states are more likely to monitor structural components than outcomes. Some states and localities have created agencies that collect data to measure health care quality. For example, the Maryland Health Care Access and Cost Commission uses data from surveys and health plans to provide reports comparing health plan performance. Medicaid agencies are becoming increasingly involved in quality measurement as the federal government moves forward in quality monitoring for Medicaid, as it has done for Medicare.

A number of federal agencies play significant roles in the quality movement. The Agency for Healthcare Research and Quality (AHRQ; formerly the Agency for Health Care Policy and Research [AHCPR]) supports research in quality measurement, including the measurement of consumer satisfaction through the Consumer Assessment of Health Plans Study (CAHPS) initiative. The AHRQ has also sponsored the development of an inventory of measures and measurement sets being used to assess quality, the Computerized Needs-Oriented Quality Measurement Evaluation System (CONQUEST). Another major player is the Health Care Financing Administration (HCFA), with responsibility for the Medicare and Medicaid programs. In 1997, legislation mandated that the HCFA establish quality requirements for health plans that enroll Medicaid and Medicare beneficiaries. In addition, the agency will have similar requirements for fee-for-service care. One example of the HCFA's quality-related activities is the new requirement that home health care agencies use the Outcomes and Assessment Information Set (OASIS) to measure quality and patient satisfaction. OASIS is a standardized system for the collection and analysis of quality-related data. There are numerous other efforts underway to address quality concerns. The HCFA has been involved in the development of HEDIS, CAHPS, and FACCT measures for holding Medicare and Medicaid providers accountable for the health care they provide. Among the many other federal agencies involved in the quality movement are the Maternal Child Health Bureau and the Centers for Disease Control and Prevention.

The contributions of nurses and other researchers to the quality movement are important to nursing's ability to gain new knowledge about quality issues. As is discussed later in this chapter, progress continues to be made in the development and standardization of quality measures and data collection and analysis. Researchers provide much needed information about how to improve quality assessment, the relationship of structures and processes to outcomes, the impact of quality improvement efforts on improving practice, and the development and testing of analytical and statistical tools to enhance assessment.

This discussion of stakeholders would not be complete without mentioning the significant contributions health care philanthropies make directly and by funding important quality-related efforts throughout the country. Among the many foundations supporting work in quality are the Robert Wood Johnson Foundation, the David and Lucile Packard Foundation and the Commonwealth Fund, to name just a few.

Accompanying the increase in the amount of work being done in the quality movement is greater collaboration among stakeholders. This provides opportunities to enhance the use of resources to increase the nation's capacity to address health care quality issues. The synergy that comes from using the collective knowledge and expertise of all stakeholders will do much to accelerate the positive outcomes that can be achieved by the quality movement. The APN is an important player and, as discussed later in this chapter, has many opportunities for participation and much to offer.

AN APPROACH TO EVALUATION

Evaluation research uses the methodological approaches inherent in any research effort. As a form of applied rather than basic research, it focuses on findings that have practical application. Evaluation research is the application of social science research methods involving collecting, analyzing, and interpreting data to determine the implementation, effectiveness, and efficiency of interventions in order to evaluate and improve practice. The formulation of hypotheses, the manipulation of variables, and the study of relationships characterize evaluation research, which uses both quantitative and qualitative methods. APNs should be involved with this type of research for a number of reasons: to assess their role, to determine the effectiveness and efficacy of the interventions they directly or indirectly provide, to measure program or organizational quality, to meet accountability standards, or to identify the inputs—structure and processes—related to particular outcomes.

Because the APN's role in the quality movement is critical, fulfilling this role requires a framework for organizing thinking and developing approaches. This is particularly important given the complexity of evaluating quality in a rapidly changing healthcare system.

Donabedian's Framework

Donabedian's (1966) model for patient care evaluation was one of the earliest frameworks, and is among the best known and most used by nurses as well as other health care providers and researchers. Donabedian's model has been applied to nursing by Bloch (1975) and to the clinical nurse specialist (CNS) by Hamric (1983, 1989). It provides an excellent framework for evaluating the impact of all categories of APNs (Table 25-1). Structural variables relate to the components of a system of care or intervention and would include such elements as numbers and types of providers, agency policies and procedures, characteristics of clients served, practice regulations, and payment sources. Process variables relate to the behavior or actions of the APN. The end result of the interaction among structural and process variables is the outcome, the impact of advanced nursing practice on access, quality, or costs. Structure, process, and outcome variables can be studied as independent or dependent variables. Specific examples of the types of variables that the APN might study are listed in Table 25-2.

A number of nursing leaders provide suggestions for approaching outcomes assessment in relation to structures and processes (Aiken, Sochalski, & Lake, 1997; Henry & Holzmer, 1997; Hester, Miller, Foster, & Vojir, 1977; Mitchell & Shortell, 1997; Murdaugh, 1997; Rosenthal & Shannon, 1997). The importance of assessing the impact of changes in organizational factors on the quality of care is identified and discussed. Knowledge about these factors is necessary to design delivery systems to meet patient care needs and improve the performance of the health care system.

National Frameworks/Approaches

The President's Advisory Commission (1998) called for a national framework for quality measurement and reporting to

TABLE 25-1 A MODEL FOR PATIENT CARE EVALUATION			
	STRUCTURE	PROCESS	OUTCOMES
Donabedian & Bloch	Characteristics of: • Setting • System • Care providers	Care processes Appropriateness and completeness of care delivery Coordination of care For nursing, the quality of nursing process	Care recipient End result of care in terms of change in patient's: • Physical health state • Cognitive state • Psychosocial state • Behavioral state
Hamric & Girouard	APN characteristics: • Education • Certification Institutional characteristics: • APN impact on institutional practices • APN professional activities • APN time documentation	APN role component performance: • Direct practice • Education • Consultation • Research • Collaboration • Leadership APN impact on staff performance APN evaluation of performance growth Acceptance of APN role Satisfaction with APN: • Staff • Administrators • Non-nurse providers • Clients	APN impact on patient-related outcomes: • Health status • Knowledge • Psychosocial • Behavioral • Resource utilization • Costs • Client satisfaction

Adapted from Hamric, A. B. (1989). A model for CNS evaluation. In A. B. Hamric & J. A. Spross (Eds.), *The clinical nurse specialist in theory and practice* (2nd ed., pp. 83–104). Philadelphia: W. B. Saunders; reprinted with permission.

- Evaluate quality at multiple levels: patient, provider, health care organization, or population group (a heath plan or community)
- Create synergy among efforts: use of core or common measures by those involved in measuring quality
- Serve the needs of consumers/patients: determine their needs and concerns
- Focus on vulnerable populations
- Encourage innovations and their assessment
- Improve data collection and reporting

TABLE 25-2 STRUCTURE, PROCESS, AND OUTCOME VARIABLES—EXAMPLES		
STRUCTURE	PROCESS	OUTCOME
• Educational level of APN • Time spent in role components • Level of third-party reimbursement • Organizational characteristics • Mission, goals of organization • Staffing patterns • Certification • Physical environment • Regulations, policies	• Patient education procedures • Referral patterns • Prescriptive practice behavior • APN behavior • Nurse/APN satisfaction • Collaboration • Staff nurse practices • Nursing processes	• Mortality • Morbidity • Utilization of services • Quality of life • Social functioning • Costs of care • Client satisfaction • Health status • Activities of daily living • Client knowledge

McGlynn (1997) stressed the importance of identifying the level of evaluation to determine accountability. For example, the APN needs to identify the level being assessed: Is the focus of the evaluation on the APN's direct interventions or the assessment of an innovation led on a nursing unit or part of a team approach?

The use of core or common measures in the evaluation of quality is a key component of the current quality movement. Whatever the purpose of the APN's evaluation activities, attention needs to be given to support the concept of synergy suggested by the President's Advisory Commission. The use of common measures is obvious when the purpose of the evaluation is external—to compare the performance of one organization to another using performance measures such as those used in HEDIS to evaluate health plans. Relevance, scientific soundness, and feasibility all need to be addressed. This approach is also important for internal uses, as when APNs are evaluating impact on their patients. Synergy is necessary, in part, to be able to justify the APN's role in comparison to those of other providers. In addition, contributions to the development and testing of core measures useful in evaluating APN practice and assessing outcomes will assure that issues of importance to the APN are included in core measure sets.

Traditionally, the nursing profession has focused on the needs of patients in practice, education, and research. Thus the call to use evaluation approaches that serve consumers should be easy for the APN to address. FACCT (see the FACCT website at *www.facct.org*) provides a framework for evaluating quality from the consumer/patient perspective that reflects the tradition of nursing practice. The measures it has developed and is developing are organized into five domains:

1. The Basics—access to services and qualified caregivers
2. Staying Healthy—services to promote health and prevent illness and disability
3. Getting Better—helping patients get better after an illness or injury
4. Living with Illness—supporting and helping chronically ill patients and their families achieve the best possible outcomes
5. Changing Needs—helping patients adjust to and cope with a chronic condition or with the end of life

This framework, with its focus on the patient/consumer, suggests the need for the evaluator to attend to health status, risk factors, and problems of an individual patient or group of patients.

The President's Advisory Commission called for additional attention to the needs of vulnerable populations. As reflected in the literature, APNs have consistently served the chronically ill, children, the elderly, and other persons with special needs or those who have difficulties accessing the health care system. This is reflected in the missions and goals of nurse practitioner (NP) primary care practices and school-based health clinics, nurse-led geriatric care programs, and certified nurse-midwife (CNM) practices. Because APNs are already involved in serving vulnerable populations in a systematic way, opportunities for evaluating outcomes abound.

APNs are also well known for their development, application, and assessment of innovations in the delivery of health care services, another component of the President's Advisory Commission's framework. For example, CNSs' programs to improve the recovery of cardiac surgery patients, the NP's role in primary care for schoolchildren, the CNM's promotion of improvements in perinatal care sensitive to the needs of consumers, and the pediatric NP's leadership in asthma care for children all represent innovations in care delivery. Further development of consistent and comparable evaluation of these and similar programs is well within the scope of the APN's role.

Finally, the President's Advisory Commission's framework includes improving quality-related data and reporting. As Starr (1997) noted, improvements in this area through the development and application of computer information systems can lower the costs of "quality." Health care, and certainly nursing, lags behind other sectors of society in the use of information systems. APNs can be helpful in identifying the types of data to be collected and in assuring that data are relevant to their practice. In addition, the APN needs to be involved at all levels to address issues such as confidentiality, data quality, relevance of data, and reliability and validity of data.

Frameworks from the Nursing Literature

In addition to the frameworks discussed previously, APNs have identified a number of ways to organize an approach to quality assurance and outcomes measurement. Chance (1997) provided a brief overview of many of the conceptual frameworks and models used to assess the quality of nursing care, including behavioral, economic, systems, and self-care theory. The processes used in nursing outcomes research (Broome, 1999) include four steps: (1) identify the intervention to be addressed and the target population; (2) develop an infrastructure for data collection; (3) identify and analyze relevant structural, process, and outcome variables; and (4) make changes (and re-evaluate) related to the findings of the evaluation.

Curley (1998) described a "synergy model" developed by the American Association of Critical-Care Nurses Certification Corporation to link practice by certified nurses to outcomes. The model is based on the premise that nursing competencies are driven by the needs of patients. When matched, outcomes for patients are improved. An important consideration for the APN is the measurement of outcomes that are nursing sensitive (Brooten & Naylor, 1995; Hamric, 1989; Oermann & Huber, 1999). Do APN practices make a difference? Cassidy (1999) illustrated this in a model for assessing the care of patients with Type II diabetes. At the University of Pennsylvania School of Nursing, a community-based practice uses a model of socially acceptable care to meet the needs of the frail elderly (Naylor & Buhler-Wilkerson, 1999). Future evaluation will focus on the measurement of quality and costs of a program developed using this model.

Ventura, Crosby, and Feldman (1991) developed a model for assessing NP effectiveness that can be applied to the evaluation of nurses in other advanced practice roles. They created the model with the assistance of a consultant and advisory committee to provide a framework for evaluation and for their review of the evaluation literature. As shown in Figure 25–1, they include preliminary conditions (predisposing, preparation and enabling) that influence the APN's ability to perform in the role. These can be considered structural variables and include regulations, educational background, acceptance of the role, and reimbursement issues. In the model, utilization also includes structural variables for evaluation. Delivery of care in this model represents many of the process variables discussed in this chapter. Short-term outcomes, such as patient knowledge at time of hospital discharge and freedom from pain, are those assessed in a time frame close to the delivery of care. Long-term outcomes are those that would be measured longitudinally and might include the patient's ability to return to work, life span, and long-term costs related to what was influenced over time by the delivery of care. This model is essentially a recasting of Donabedian's

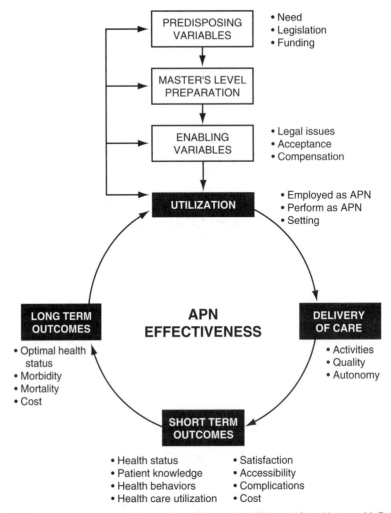

FIGURE 25–1 • Model for evaluating advanced practice nursing. (Adapted from Ventura, M. R., Crosby, F., & Feldman, M. J. [1991]. An information synthesis to evaluate nurse practitioner effectiveness. *Military Medicine, 156,* 286–291; reprinted with permission.)

framework. It is useful in contemporary measurement for the identification of indicators and the specification of their interrelationships.

Discussion

Evaluation is the systematic application of research procedures to assess the conceptualization, design, implementation, and utility of health care interventions. Evaluation procedures make it possible to determine what APN structural and process elements improve access, promote the best quality, contribute to patient outcomes, and provide cost-effective services. The definitions and frameworks discussed earlier can be used as a guide to the development of measures to assess structures and processes and their relationship to outcomes. In addition, they are helpful in approaching the assessment of innovations and in identifying data needed to understand quality. When there is confidence in the measurement of quality, the findings of evaluations can be used as a guide for quality improvement activities. For example, if APNs identify immunization rates that vary among public health clinics, they can compare the structures and processes used to achieve good performance, and they can promote and implement system changes that will attain the best rates.

Where research has been conducted, the findings can be used to guide future research efforts (see Chapter 9). Clarity about the questions to be asked will serve to ameliorate many of the problems and issues inherent in the complex evaluation process and practice context. In addition, there are research design and methodological questions to be addressed. Suggestions from critiques of the literature include using multiple sites, using longer time frames, using comparison groups, focusing on nurse-dependent outcomes, and developing reliable and valid methods to assess outcomes.

CHALLENGES IN EVALUATING QUALITY AND ADVANCED NURSING PRACTICE

Although the quality of health care can be defined and measured, the science to support quality assurance is in its infancy. This state of the science results because, until recently, this issue was not a national priority. Thus sufficient resources to move the science forward did not exist. In addition, methodological and technical issues made it difficult to achieve the goal of systematic quality assurance. The recent changes described previously and improvements in the science of quality assurance suggest that there will be rapid development in this area. The promise does not come without many challenges to improving quality measurement, assurance, and improvement (Lohr, 1990). In addition to the general challenges, there are issues specific to the APN's role and work. Given their knowledge and expertise, APNs can help to address the challenges both for themselves and for the nation.

Lohr (1997) identified a number of continuing challenges to quality assurance (including measurement and improvement):

* The types and numbers of services that affect both physical and mental health and the artificial separation of these services
* The need for and difficulties with measuring continuity of care
* The need to focus on both individuals and populations
* Problems with access to and availability of care/services
* The numbers and types of outcomes—clinical, biological, health, and functional status—that need to be assessed
* The need to examine processes, especially when outcomes cannot be practically measured
* The need for providers to remain current about the rapidly growing knowledge base required to practice well

Other challenges identified in the literature (AHCPR, 1995; Champagne, Tornquist, & Funk, 1997; Eddy, 1998; McGlynn, 1997; O'Leary, 1998; President's Advisory

Commission, 1998) include those related to multiple uses and users of quality information, the need for clarity in all aspects of the process, methodological and technical issues, and barriers to the application of research findings in practice. By becoming familiar with these challenges, APNs can consider these issues as they become more involved in all levels of the quality movement.

The President's Advisory Commission (1998) engaged in public hearings and an extensive review of available data and information about the climate surrounding health care quality. They reported that the health care system continues to undergo rapid and complex change, including the growth of managed care, changes in technology and new innovations, and increased demand for health care quality information by a wide variety of stakeholders. Characteristics of the health care system, such as pluralistic insurance practices, increasing numbers of uninsured, concerns about costs, the growth of self-funded insurance (where federal and state governments do not have oversight authority), and the impact the system has on consumers (e.g., confusion and dissatisfaction), add to the problems associated with the development and implementation of a standardized system for measuring and assuring quality health care services. Other system changes that add to the difficulty of achieving quality assurance goals are the complexity and numbers of health plans, the development of complex provider networks, the changing roles of primary care providers, changes in health care financing, changes in the way health care services are delivered, and the explosion in health care knowledge and technology.

Establishing Criteria

The difficulties in measuring quality (Eddy, 1998) include the probability factor—that is, the probability that an outcome will occur despite certain interventions. For example, a person may have a heart attack although she or he has reduced the risk factors. Low occurrences of health outcomes make this problem even more difficult to address. For example, measuring death rates for cancer as an outcome measure is problematic because the incidence of death is low. Similarly, it takes many years to determine survival rates, and this long delay between interventions and outcomes makes it difficult to determine the relationship of the intervention to the outcome. Also problematic are the clinical details needed to assess outcomes and the ability to measure and communicate clinical details to consumers and other stakeholders. Eddy regarded these elements as "natural" factors that cannot be changed but need to be "worked around" to improve quality assessment. He identified four "man-made" factors—inadequate information systems, the multiplicity of measures that have been developed, the complexity of health plans, and needed cost/funding of quality assurance activities, including the burden on providers and health care plans to provide data.

O'Leary (1998), McGlynn (1997), and the AHCPR (1995) provided further clarification of the issues facing the quality movement, which are similar to those identified by Eddy. These include (1) establishing explicit clinical criteria and developing related measures to meet the needs of the many users and the uses they make of data and information about health care quality; and (2) identifying measures that offer significant opportunities for improvement and are relevant, scientifically sound, and feasible. Compounding the problems in quality measurement are existing variations in practice and practice settings, variations in the quantity and type of health care services, variations in data and documentation, and provider differences in education and training.

APN Role

The problems inherent in the role of the APN conducting effective evaluation were identified by Hamric (1989) and others. Hamric discussed how the independent role of the APN makes it difficult to develop uniform performance criteria for evaluation. In addition, the time and other resources needed to conduct meaningful evaluation may not be available to the APN. The complexity and difficulties in conducting outcome evaluation often result in conceptually and methodologically flawed evaluation that contributes little to accountability. Evaluation approaches are more difficult than simply exploring or describing a phenomenon, and require advanced levels of knowledge and skill—as well as time—representing a greater challenge for the APN. In addition, to be successful, such approaches often require collaboration with other researchers within and outside the profession. Similarly, evaluating outcomes is complex because, in assessing the APN's contribution to patient outcomes, one must account for intervening variables, such as the effects of changes in health care reimbursement that limit services, and the impact of other providers on outcomes.

The methodological problems associated with evaluating the impact of the APN, although not unique, are compounded by the fact that the focus of the research is on the APN's contribution to patient care. As Jennings (1991) suggested, defining process, structure, and outcome variables is a demanding task. For example, determining who should identify the outcomes, what the outcomes should be, and the magnitude of these outcomes requires careful attention and is likely to involve a number of stakeholders if the evaluation is to be recognized and appreciated. Evaluation of advanced nursing practice is also more challenging because traditional measures of quality, such as mortality, morbidity, and length of stay, are not always sensitive indicators of nursing interventions. Thus the APN must develop methods for assessing more nursing-sensitive patient outcomes such as functional status, mental status, satisfaction, and burden of care (Brooten & Naylor, 1995; Naylor, Munro, & Brooten, 1991).

Additional issues to be considered when evaluating the impact of advanced nursing practice include the requirement to focus primarily on the patient's needs. This focus on patient's needs may preclude thinking about planning an evaluation when a program or intervention is being introduced. It is also difficult to understand the impact of a structure or process of care when baseline data with which to compare the results of the evaluation are not available. For example, assessing the costs of APNs is often difficult because costing-out nursing interventions and nursing's relative contribution to patient outcomes is complex and data are often not available. Useful and generalizable evaluation results also require a larger sample and more than one location—often difficult methodological problems for the APN.

Discussion

Although these challenges may at first appear overwhelming to the APN, a careful review should make them less daunting. As an expert clinician, the APN is continuously faced with the need to provide research evidence for practice. As Champagne and colleagues (1997) noted, APNs must provide leadership to achieve this goal. Thus APNs have dealt with the challenges of providing a scientific basis for practice when information and knowledge are increasing rapidly. When involved in research, the APN will need to clarify the reason for the research and identify the stakeholders who will benefit from the knowledge gained. The APN also must be concerned about the unit of analysis—are individual patients, nursing units, or patient populations the appropriate focus of research? To assure the use of sound scientific methods, the APN may need to collaborate with experienced researchers. Certainly APNs are acutely aware of the climate surrounding health care quality, because it is the climate within which their roles are operationalized. For example, a NP evaluating the effect of the NP role on adolescent pregnancy may experience significant problems when a public health department is no longer available to refer patients for pregnancy prevention services. Similarly, the introduction of other programs in a community, such as new home care services, may make it difficult for the pediatric CNS to assess the impact of care on hospital length of stay.

The complexities of assuring that individuals and populations are receiving the best possible care should not deter the APN from developing evaluation strategies. The stewardship of quality of care cannot be the domain of other health care providers or other stakeholders without the involvement and leadership of the APN. To achieve the purpose of the health care system and to enhance the role of the APN and the nursing profession in achieving positive health outcomes for the nation, APNs, in partnership with others, must participate at all levels. The following discussion of the literature provides examples of the types of activities and research that illustrate the importance of the APN in the quality process and provides guidance for the identification of strategies.

REVIEW OF LITERATURE

Since the publication of the last edition of this book (Hamric, Spross, & Hanson, 1996), significant progress has been made by APNs and researchers. The quality and quantity of the information available in the literature and in the public domain reflect the growing sophistication of APNs and a greater recognition of the contributions of advanced practice. For example, in 1996 the American Academy of Nursing sponsored an invitational conference to discuss issues related to care delivery systems and outcome measures. Aiken and colleagues (1997) discussed the effects of organizational change on patient outcomes. They provided a theoretical framework for studying the impact of organizational changes on outcomes and discussed methodological issues. In addition, they presented an argument for increasing knowledge, especially in a rapidly changing health care environment, about the impact of structural changes, such as nurse staffing and changes in payment mechanisms, on patient care outcomes. In a review of acute care studies, Mitchell and Shortell (1997) concluded that, although there is not conclusive evidence about the impact of organizational issues on mortality, adverse events appear to be related to organizational factors. They encouraged further research focused on these and other outcomes. Patient satisfaction and experience with care and structures and processes of care, as reported by Rosenthal and Shannon (1997), appeared to be related. Because the evidence is not conclusive, they identified the need for standardization of measures and additional research. Similarly, Hester and associates (1997), in their review of studies of the relationship between pain management and delivery system factors, did not find significant evidence of the relationship among structures, processes, and outcomes. They also called for additional work to assess these relationships.

The review of the literature in the first edition of this book (Girouard, 1996) is not repeated here, but APNs, particularly students and those new to the evaluation process, are encouraged to review that discussion for examples of classic and important studies. The "Additional Readings" section at the end of this chapter lists many of these classic works. The review that follows includes some of the more recent literature related to evaluation and quality that focuses on advanced practice nursing. It also includes studies conducted by APNs or those of particular interest. As the APN seeks information and research findings related to evaluation and quality, the quest should extend beyond the nursing literature. Much can be learned and adopted from the contributions of others in the health care community.

Structural Evaluation

Structural variables related to the APN provide information about the role, factors relating to performance, and what structures influence particular outcomes. As Hamric (1989) discussed, structural evaluation can provide a starting point for evaluation of the APN. Structural analysis can describe staffing patterns, indirect patient care actions such as committee and consultative activities of the APN, and characteristics of the APN or the practice setting. These data are relatively easy to obtain and analyze and can provide important information for evaluating the impact of the APN. APNs should examine and analyze existing data and research findings to determine both substantive and methodological approaches to define relevant structural variables and to clarify structural variables as inputs for outcome measurement.

Structural variables that have received a good deal of attention in the literature relate to amount of time spent on various APN roles, acceptance of the role, and characteristics of the APN. Other approaches to evaluating the structure of advanced nursing practice include measuring performance in relation to structural standards, such as numbers of meetings and workshops attended and given, numbers of requests for consultation, and numbers and types of clients served. Organizational characteristics, such as staffing patterns, agency mission, and governance, are also important variables. These types of indicators may be useful for internal purposes but are not likely to provide the type of information needed regarding the impact of the APN on access, quality, or cost unless they can be identified as having a relationship to outcomes. For example, if the outcomes of the APN's practice are better in settings where more registered nurses (RNs) are employed, this would provide clear guidance for employers seeking to set high standards of quality.

Practice setting provider structures such as collaborative practice models illustrate how structural variables can be assessed. Physician attitudes toward NPs are important in collaborative models. Aquilino, Damiano, Willard, Momony and Levy (1999) found that primary care physicians who previously worked with NPs and general practice physicians had more favorable attitudes toward NPs than did other primary care physicians. Posner and Freund (1998) found that productivity and outcomes were not significantly different when the composition of anesthesia teams included certified registered nurse anesthetists (CRNAs). McMullen (1998) examined the satisfaction of patients, physicians and staff nurses with the performance of NPs in an NP-physician collaborative service. All were satisfied with the role of the NP. Patients reported that NPs, in comparison to the traditional physician service, communicated better with other nurses and other APNs and did not talk inappropriately in front of them. Staff nurses rated the NP as good to excellent in relation to patient courtesy, quality of care, respect for staff nurses, staff teaching, and patient teaching. In a study of patient satisfaction with CNS care in a breast cancer clinic, Garvican, Grimsey, Littlejohns, Lownes, and Sacks (1998) reported that patients were more satisfied with the CNS's care than with other aspects of their hospital care. Johnson (1998) surveyed women regarding their perceptions of the terms "midwife" and "nurse-midwife" and knowledge about the services and confidence in each. A significant relationship between familiarity with terms and knowledge about scope of services and confidence in the two types of providers was found.

Job satisfaction is an important issue for the APN and the supervisor, because performance and outcomes are likely to be linked to job satisfaction. Numerous studies assess the job satisfaction of the APN. Although it is unlikely that measuring job satisfaction alone will contribute much to understanding the effect of the APN on patient care, the information may be useful for developing and structuring positions within an agency and thus may reduce the costly effects of recruitment, retention, and performance related to dissatisfaction. Beal and Philips (1999) examined turnover rates among NPs in neonatal intensive care units (ICUs) and found that role dissatisfaction with limitations of the role or with management were the most common dissatisfiers.

APNs also have much to contribute to understanding changes in health care delivery structures. Harrison (1999) studied nurses' perceptions of the impact of managed care on advanced practice nursing in one state. She found that NPs believed managed care would foster exploration of new approaches to quality and cost-effectiveness, expansion of the NP role in primary care, and greater partnering with clients in self-responsibility for care. Perceived threats to practice included preauthorization difficulties, payment denials, a tenuous job market, and encroachment on nursing roles by others. Mason and colleagues (1999) found that more than half of NPs in New York and Connecticut had never applied to be credentialed by a managed care organization (MCO). As a result, they were not listed on MCO panels, and their services were billed at the physician rate and under the physician's name. Work environment is also of interest to the APN. Otto and Davidson (1999) found that levels of CRNA exposure to radiation during fluoroscopic procedures were above recommended levels, thus exposing the CRNA's unprotected thyroid to risk.

One can also study the extent to which a target population is being reached to address access issues. Paine and colleagues (1999) studied the characteristics of patients served by CNMs and the numbers and reasons for visits. They found that 70% of visits were made by women and infants vulnerable to access or outcome problems, refuting the belief of some that CNMs only provided services for pregnant women who could afford childbirth alternatives. Hamric, Worley, Lindebak, and Jaubert (1998) found that 71% of patients seen by APNs in their study were either Medicare/Medicaid (40%), were self-pay (18%), or received care through a state-funded (other than Medicaid) program (13%). Only 18% had commercial insurance. These studies demonstrate that APNs often provide services for underserved populations; further evaluation of APNs' relationship to access strengthens justification of their roles. In a study of the care delivery changes related to telemedicine, Borchers and Kee (1999) examined the use of a telemedicine system to conduct family and home assessments and to identify the issues of concern to APNs using this system. They found that this innovation was an inexpensive approach to early intervention and identified the advantages and disadvantages of an image video technology. Further support for the role of APNs employing remote video technology in the home health care setting was demonstrated by Johnston, Wheeler, Deuser and Sousa (2000). They found significant improvements in access, cost savings, and patient satisfaction among patients using the technology when compared to those who did not use the video technology. In a study of ethnicity and sources of prenatal care, Gardner, Cliver, McNeal, and Goldenberg (1996) found that more white women (73%) received care from a private CNM, physician, or HMO than did Mexican-Americans (51%), African Americans (44%), or Puerto Ricans (37%). Recognizing issues associated with multicultural patient care, Peterson and Smith (1996) reported how an interdisciplinary, multicultural patient care team could increase cultural awareness and sensitivity.

Process Evaluation

Process evaluation focuses on what the APN does or on programmatic components—that is, the nature of an intervention. As with structural characteristics, process variables can be examined independently of outcomes to describe what the APN or a program does. Strategies APNs may use to evaluate their care-giving process include assessments by those supervised directly, such as unit leaders, or indirectly, such as staff nurses; evaluation by other health care providers or clients; reviews of improvements in various components of the nursing process; and peer review (Hamric, 1989). Administrative assessment of the APN's performance based on goals or job description criteria is another useful method for evaluation of APN processes. Numerous instruments have been developed to facilitate such evaluation (Girouard & Spross, 1983; Hamric, Gresham, & Eccard, 1978; Houston & Luquire, 1991; Ingersoll, 1998; Kearnes, 1992; Tierney, Grant, & Mazique, 1990). The most effective way to conduct this type of evaluation is to base it on mutual goals and objectives that are used as an ongoing management tool.

The effective APN engages in processes to assure patient care quality for both the care delivered by the APN and the care provided by others. Evaluation of these processes is important to strengthen and justify the role of the APN and her or his contributions. Pelletier-Hibbert (1998) found that the coping strategies of nurses dealing with the care of organ donation patients and families were enhanced when they had access to a CNS, received education related to grieving, and had opportunities to discuss their feelings. East and Colditz (1996) found that women's experiences with childbirth were enhanced by the extra attention they received when included in a fetal intrapartum oxygen saturation monitoring study. Innovative approaches to assessing the use of clinical and cost information to explain trends and assess variances have been proposed (Bozzo, Carlson, & Diers, 1998; Diers & Bozzo, 1997; Diers, Bozzo, Blatt, & Roussel, 1998). These models could be used by the APN to operationalize process variables to study independently, or to assess their relationship to outcomes.

One of the major tools used to improve quality of care and reduce costs is the development, implementation, and evaluation of clinical guidelines for patient care. This issue has received much attention from a variety of researchers within and outside nursing. These types of evaluations, especially when linked to outcomes, provide an important opportunity to document APN contributions to quality and cost-effectiveness. Jacavone, Daniels, and Tyner (1999) described the CNS role in facilitating improvements in the processes used to provide care for cardiac surgery patients. The importance of translating evidence-based practice guidelines into clinical practice is well known (see Chapter 9) but rarely studied. Strohschein, Schaffer, and Lia-Hoagberg (1999) developed, implemented, and assessed a process to promote the use of practice guidelines by nurses. They found that more than 90% of public health nurses participating in the project felt that clinical practice guideline manuals would be useful in their practice. McDaniel (1999) assessed the feasibility of implementing an inpatient smoking cessation program by measuring the time and costs associated with conducting the intervention using AHRQ guidelines. In a study of an implementation of pain management guidelines promulgated by the AHRQ, White (1999) found that, following an educational program and the introduction of new routes for administering postoperative analgesia, nursing documentation of pain assessment improved.

Outcome Evaluation

Clearly, the most important issue in evaluation is the evaluation of outcomes—measuring the effects of structures and processes on patients and the health of population groups. Outcomes reflect the end result of a treatment or intervention. Given the social responsibility of the nursing profession, improvement in patient outcomes is the reason for nursing's existence. Strickland (1997) suggested that nursing outcome studies should begin with the selection of an appropriate design, with randomized clinical trials most likely to result in changes in outcomes and careful operationalization of the intervention. She also supported the need for improved measures. Lang and Marek (1992) identified the outcome indicators used by nurses in quality assurance and research activities. As shown in Table 25-3, they encompass physiological, psychosocial, functional, quality-of-life, service utilization, and patient satisfaction/experience with care indicators. In addition, costs of care are important considerations in the present health care climate. As reported by Girouard (1996) and Urden (1999), there have been numerous studies to support the impact of the APN on outcomes both directly and through the APN's role providing leadership in quality assurance activities. The following review provides a few examples of the growing number of outcome studies by and about APNs. The reader is also referred to each of the role chapters in Part II of this book for reports of numerous outcome studies specific to individual APN roles.

York and colleagues (1997), using a randomized clinical trial, assessed the outcomes associated with the use of a CNS providing follow-up for early discharge of high-risk childbearing women. Outcomes for the women and infants followed by the CNS were more positive than those for women not receiving the CNS intervention. During the course of their pregnancy, women at high risk for complications had fewer rehospitalizations than the control group. Low birth weight births for women with diabetes were three times higher in the control group than in the group followed by the CNS. Aikins and Feinland (1998) reported that CNMs achieved high rates of intact perineum and low episiotomy rates in home birth settings. In a study of comprehensive discharge planning for elderly, hospitalized patients by APNs, Naylor and associates (1999) found that patients in the experimental group who received the APN intervention had fewer hospitalizations and a longer interval between discharge and rehospitalization when compared to patients who did not receive the APN intervention. These outcomes reflected their improved health status.

Tilly, Garvey, Gold, Powell, and Proudlock (1996) found that hospital admissions and emergency room visits were decreased and patient well-being was improved

| TABLE 25-3 | TYPES OF OUTCOME INDICATORS AND EXAMPLES |

Physiological status
- Vital signs
- Laboratory values
- Skin integrity
- Wound healing
- Weight
- Symptom control—fatigue, nausea, incontinence

Behavior
- Application of knowledge and skills
- Problem-solving, compliance
- Motivation
- Therapeutic competence
- Self-care

Home/Family
- Family living patterns
- Home environment
- Support
- Role function
- Family strain
- Financial

Psychosocial
- Patterns of behavior
- Communications
- Relationships
- Mentation
- Emotion
- Attitude
- Mood
- Affect
- Coping
- Social contact
- Social functioning
- Occupational functioning
- Spiritual

Knowledge (Client)
- Cognitive understanding:
  - Of nursing problems
  - Of diet, medications, treatment

Utilization of Services
- Length of stay
- Number of clinic visits
- Telephone contacts
- Rehospitalization
- Unnecessary admission/tests
- Financial costs

Functional Status
- Activities of daily living
- Mobility
- Communications
- Self-care

Quality of Life
- Life satisfaction
- Well-being
- Symptom control
- Standard of living
- Functional capacity
- Safety

Patient Satisfaction
- With care
- With care provider
- Care process
- Scheduling
- Access

From Lang, N. M., & Marek, K. D. (1991). Outcomes that reflect clinical practice. In *Patient outcomes research: Examining the effectiveness of nursing practice* (Proceedings of a conference sponsored by the National Center for Nursing Research) (Publication No. 93-3411). Washington, DC: U.S. Department of Health and Human Services.

for adults and children with the introduction of an asthma education program. In McDaniel's (1999) study of the feasibility of clinical practice guidelines in smoking cessation, 70% of the participants in the program continued to abstain from smoking at 1 month postdischarge. Using a multidisciplinary intervention, Blondin and associates (1996) developed and implemented a program for earlier extubation of cardiac surgery patients. The intervention significantly reduced the numbers of hours patients were intubated postoperatively. Aiken, Smith, and Lake (1994) found lower mortality rates among Medicare patients in hospitals known to have good-quality nursing care.

Patient's experience or satisfaction with care is an additional outcome of interest to APNs and to the quality movement. The APN is certainly interested in the impact of her or his practice on how patients feel about their care and their experience with the health care system. The demands of consumers, as reflected in the earlier discussion of the quality movement and the interest in evaluation, are being used by a variety of stakeholders to assess the performance of health care providers. APNs have recognized this demand and are responding in a variety of ways. As Barnason, Merboth, Pozehl, and Tietjen (1998) reported, when CNSs developed and implemented a structured intervention for pain management, patients reported greater satisfaction with their pain management and the ability to better assess what level of pain was acceptable to them. Nine CNM practices studied pain management of women in labor (CNM Data Group, 1998). They found use of a wide variety of techniques, with paced breathing (55%), activity and position change (42%), narcotics

(30%), and epidurals (19%) the most frequently used. Coward (1998) showed that a support group for cancer patients improved their satisfaction with life. In a study of the bereaved, McCorkle, Robinson, Nuamah, Lev, and Benoliel (1998) found less psychological distress among those who received a CNS home-based intervention.

Indication of greater attention to nursing issues in outcomes research is reflected in the development of tools to measure outcomes and the funding of research in this area. As reflected in the literature, the APN has an important role to play in this process. For example, Lauver (1996) described a clinical benchmarking process to improve outcomes. Benchmarking—identifying and establishing acceptable parameters for outcomes—was used to provide direction for improving practice and, thus, outcomes. Kilpack, Campion, Stover, Wood, and Cocke (1996) described a collaborative effort of a hospital and vendor to develop outcome indicators and use benchmarking data to guide the evaluation and planning of interventions to reduce pressure ulcers. Recent grants awarded by the AHRQ to nurse researchers (AHCPR, 1999b) suggest the importance of outcomes measurement, recognition of the nursing component of outcomes and the growing sophistication of the nursing community in this area. Mion is the principal investigator for a grant to study the effects of nursing interventions based in emergency departments to maintain the frail elderly in community settings (AHCPR, 1999a). As the principal investigator for a study of nurse staffing and quality of care, Buerhaus will be looking at adverse nurse-sensitive events in the hospital setting (AHCPR, 1999a).

Cost as an Outcome Measure

The costs of care are a major concern of stakeholders and often drive policy and care decisions. They are also an important component of accountability. The APN needs to know the costs associated with interventions and the impact of system structures and processes in the value equation. Whenever appropriate and feasible, outcome studies should include the dimension of cost. As APNs seek to justify their roles and assure that advanced practice nursing remains viable, the cost component of health care cannot be overlooked. There are a number of possible approaches to assessing costs: directly, by using length of stay, numbers of emergency room visits, and other utilization data as proxies for costs; or indirectly, by modeling the cost savings associated with reducing the health care costs associated with preventable diseases and disability. Kee and Borchers (1998) discussed the nursing literature related to CNS discharge planning interventions in the hospital and through the use of telemedicine to achieve positive outcomes such as reduction in hospital readmissions. Some studies examined cost issues directly, and in others cost issues were assumed, (e.g., if a hospital or emergency room visit could be avoided through the use of an APN intervention).

There is a growing literature that directly measures costs. Naylor and associates (1999), in the randomized clinical trial described previously, reported that the costs for patients who did not receive the CNS discharge planning and follow-up were $1.2 million as compared to the experimental group's costs of $0.6 million—a real and statistical difference. York and colleagues (1997) found that total hospital charges for postpartum patients in the experimental group that received CNS discharge planning and follow-up were 44% less than for the control group. There was a net savings of $13,327 for the mother and infant discharged early with the intervention. The mean cost of CNS follow-up care was 2% of total hospital charges for the control group, representing a small additional expense that reduced total care costs. Blondin and colleagues (1996) estimated that early intubation intervention resulted in total cost reductions of more than $5 million by reducing length of ICU stay. The costs of care for stroke patients were reduced with implementation of clinical pathways in a program coordinated by a CNS (Summers & Soper, 1998). Wammack and Mabrey (1998) found reductions in lengths of stay for orthopedic patients when clinical pathways were introduced. Topp, Tucker, and Weber (1998) reported that patients in an experimental group that received a CNS case management intervention had shorter lengths of stay and reduced hospital costs when compared to patients in the control group that did not have case management.

Burns, Lamb, and Wholey (1996) found that patients in a health maintenance organization (HMO) receiving integrated HMO and community services had lower utilization rates and costs. Although this finding has implications for all APNs, it is particularly important for blended role APNs and APN case managers. In a study of specialization of staff nurses, Czaplinski and Diers (1998) reported shorter lengths of stay for patients who received specialty staff nursing care than for those not receiving such care. This suggests that APN support of specialty patient care can reduce length of stay and thus total costs. At a meeting of the Eastern Nursing Research Society, a promising methodology was reported by Diers, Karlsen, and Allegretto (1999) to identify high-cost users of hospital services. Using this methodology, the APN could identify patient populations with the highest total hospital costs. By focusing on high-cost patient populations, the APN has a unique opportunity to assess patient needs related to high costs and design, implement, and evaluate interventions. Rudy and associates (1995) focused on a group of high-cost patients, those with long ICU stays. They found significant cost savings in a nurse-managed special care unit for the chronically critically ill when compared to similar patients in ICUs. Critical care CNSs and acute care NPs could introduce this care delivery innovation and be responsible for its implementation and evaluation.

Linking Structures, Processes, and Outcomes

One of the more exciting developments in the outcomes arena is the investigation of the relationship between structures, processes, and outcomes. It is interesting to note that Bloch called for this approach in 1975, but specific examples have been rare in the literature until recently. A number of the studies described earlier have investigated the relationships. For example, White (1999) introduced and evaluated the impact of an interdisciplinary team and staff education (structures and processes) to improve pain management outcomes. Studies of the use of clinical pathways (Jacavone et al., 1999; Sagehorn, Russel, & Ganong, 1999) have evaluated the relationship between processes of care and outcomes. Although they did not examine outcomes, Morin and colleagues (1999) examined issues in the use of research to establish practice protocols for acute care agencies to better understand how evidence-based practice could be improved. Milbrath (1996) demonstrated the impact of changes in structures to improve a care process—preparing children for surgery. Additional work in this area includes studies by Sovie (1999), who is examining the relationship of hospital restructuring of nursing services to patient outcomes.

Rudy and colleagues (1998) looked at the relationship between structural factors (acute care NPs, physician assistants, and resident physicians), processes (activities of caregiving), and patient outcomes. Processes of care and outcomes were similar for NPs, physician assistants, and residents; residents were less likely than the other providers to include patients' social histories in their admission notes. A study of trainee NPs in the United Kingdom (Bond et al., 1999) found that students made good diagnostic and treatment decisions (as judged by their physician mentors) and were rated well by patients. The relationship of structure and outcomes was studied by Aiken, Sloane, Lake, Sochalski, and Weber (1999). They found that dedicated acquired immunodeficiency syndrome (AIDS) units and magnet hospitals, most if not all employing APNs, were related to better processes and outcomes (delayed death and patient satisfaction) than other units and hospitals. This supports an earlier study (Aiken et al., 1993) that found NPs' AIDS clinic patients had outcomes comparable to those of patients cared for by physicians despite their poorer health status, and that patients cared for by NPs had 45% fewer problems with care. Cost savings were associated with free standing birth centers (Walker & Stone, 1996). Johnson-Pawlson and Infeld (1996) found that having more RNs in nursing homes was related to higher levels of quality care.

Mundinger and colleagues (2000) compared the primary care practices of NPs and physicians to determine whether or not there were differences in patient outcomes, utilization of services, or patient satisfaction with care. Patients referred to a primary care practice from an urgent care center and two emergency rooms were randomly assigned to a NP or physician primary care practice. The health status of patients assigned to the two groups was comparable as measured by the Medical Outcomes Study Short Form (SF-36) at the initiation of the study and after 6 months. Physiological testing of patients showed comparability between NP and physician groups except for lower diastolic blood pressure values for patients assigned to the NP practice. Utilization of health care services did not differ. Patient satisfaction scores on provider communication and overall satisfaction with care were not significantly different. Patients reported a somewhat higher rating for physicians in ''provider attributes.'' This study provides an excellent example of how to compare structures (service delivery practices), the processes of selected caregivers, and outcomes.

Discussion

The challenges put to APNs in the previous edition of this book—for the next generation of research to focus on access, quality, and costs—are beginning to be addressed through the research and dissemination of findings related to structures and processes of APN practice and their impact on outcomes. Also of importance, especially for accountability and evidence supporting the contributions of the APN, is the fact that findings related to the evaluation of quality are increasingly appearing in the public domain. For example, Licht (1999) reported in the *Washington Post* on Naylor and colleagues' (1999) study. The headline read "Getting Patients Back on Their Feet Faster: Study Says Care Before and After Discharge from the Hospital Saves Money, Spurs Recovery." The care was provided by APNs. *The New York Times* quoted an oncology CNS, Marnie McHale, in an article about the issue of cancer patient fatigue and the goal of nursing to have patients recognize that this problem can often be addressed ("Cancer Specialists Turn," 1999). In a *New York Times* article discussing hand washing in hospitals (Yoffee, 1999), the research of Elaine Larson was featured. In a press release, the AHCPR (1999a) reported the results of a study by Harrington and colleagues (1999) to identify categories for measuring the quality of care in nursing homes.

The evaluation literature discussed has contributed a great deal to the understanding of the structures, processes, and outcomes associated with advanced nursing practice. These studies provide information to identify APN roles in meeting organizational needs and articulating position expectations, and they serve as a basis for developing job descriptions and performance standards for further evaluation. Clearly, there is a strong tradition of evaluation on which to base future study of the important role of APNs in the health care system. This information can be used for planning and implementing APN programs, for educating policy makers on the merits of investing in such programs, and for "selling" APN services to managed care organizations. The approaches being used represent significant movement toward addressing the needs for evaluation put forth earlier in this chapter. Studies that address outcomes document how well the nursing profession is doing toward meeting the purpose of the health care system to reduce the impact of illness, injury, and disability and to improve the health of those it serves.

The momentum to evaluate advanced nursing practice and the study of outcomes and how to achieve them needs to continue, because, of course, much remains to be done. As Hogan (1997) stated at an invitational conference on outcome measures and care delivery systems, many nursing studies of outcomes could have obtained cost data and linked these data to outcomes. He also described the limitations of many nursing-focused studies in not assessing the structures and processes of care provided by other disciplines and their impact on outcomes. At the same conference, Brooten (1997), from a review of the literature, described research issues in linking costs and outcomes to structures and processes that will require additional research to better understand their interrelationships.

In planning future efforts, APNs should consider the limitations of reported studies in order to improve the design and implementation of evaluations of the APN's impact. The literature provides good information about the roles, activities, and perceived barriers to practice, especially for CNSs. Similar information about NPs and CNMs is also available, but there is little research related to these issues for the CRNA. Although it might be assumed that all APN role activities and barriers are similar, research to confirm this assumption is desirable. Also desirable are data about the potential of the APN to increase access to services, especially for underserved groups. To identify measures and outcomes, Wong (1998) advised APNs to use the array of "ways of knowing" to develop nurse-sensitive patient outcomes. As suggested, the quality and quantity of evaluation research is improving, but problems continue to exist in terms of conceptualization of evaluation research and the methods used to assess advanced nursing practice.

Rossi and Freeman (1989) identified the types of questions that are typically asked in evaluation research:

- What is the nature and scope of the problem requiring a new, expanded, or modified intervention?
- Where is the intervention provided and whom does it affect?
- What feasible interventions are likely to ameliorate the problem significantly?
- What are the appropriate targets for the intervention?
- Is the intervention reaching the target population?
- Is the intervention being implemented as envisioned?
- Is the intervention effective?
- How much does the intervention cost?
- What are the intervention's costs relative to its effectiveness and benefits?

These and similar questions should guide the APN engaged as a primary evaluator or in working with others to evaluate practice and assess the quality of health care. By focusing on practice, the APN uses an understanding of patient issues (Hamric, 1983) to make evaluation meaningful and relevant. The systematic evaluation of APN interventions will contribute to knowledge of nursing practice, and the knowledge thus gained can be interpreted for others to substantiate APNs' contributions to the health care system. Whether the purpose of the evaluation is to assess individual performance, job satisfaction, a programmatic change, the impact of an institutional or governmental policy, or patient care outcomes, the evaluation must address what difference advanced nursing practice makes in relation to access, quality, or cost if the evaluation results are to have value beyond the individual and the immediate work setting. The underlying question is: What difference does the APN make in the health care system? Are the APN's contributions unique and valuable, and can this be shown to others? For example,

- In assessing individual performance in a hospital setting, the CNS must be able to identify how performance contributes to the patient-focused mission and goals of the organization. Does the CNS's practice reduce length of stay, improve patient outcomes, or enhance the efficiency of staff nurses?
- The CNM concerned about job satisfaction needs to link this concept to the practice setting's ability to better meet patient needs or to provide services to groups of clients at a lower cost than those provided by physician specialists.
- A NP's evaluation of contracted services to a group of chronically ill patients in a managed care organization would need to document both the quantity and quality of services provided and the NP's ability to reduce hospitalization rates among clients.
- A CRNA evaluating anesthesia services in a chronic low back pain clinic would want to clearly document quality of service and patient outcomes.

ROLE OF THE APN IN EVALUATION AND QUALITY ASSURANCE

In an article to promote outcomes research in home care agencies, Peters (1994) offered some helpful suggestions for selecting a problem for study and initiating an evaluation effort. The problem should be one

- About which there is considerable interest or expertise
- For which baseline data exist
- Of high volume, high risk, or high cost
- With which a problem or deficiency has been identified
- That relates to the mission and goals of the agency

Peters also suggested that the nurse go slowly, select a manageable area to evaluate, involve all levels of personnel, and be creative in searching for standardized measures and approaches that can be used in the APN's practice setting.

Hamric (1989) had similar recommendations for initiating evaluation that can be used to improve APN practice and demonstrate outcomes to improve patient care. The APN is advised to discuss with the administrator the components critical to evaluation of the role, to emphasize the importance of collaboration with other nurses and disciplines, to identify the need for planning the evaluation, and to consider the desirability of working with other APNs, faculty, and researchers to implement evaluation efforts. Approaches to continuous quality improvement and community assessment are also available in the nursing literature. For example, Hawkins, Thibodeau, Utley-Smith, Igou, and Johnson (1993) discussed the role of the APN in accountability and in assuring health in communities.

Although this chapter has focused on evaluating advanced nursing practice and its impact, APNs also need to conduct individual performance evaluations of their specific activities, competencies, and setting-specific goals. The framework for individual evaluation of performance is comparable to that used for more broadly conceived evaluation but focuses on job expectations. The APN's position description can be used as a starting point for structuring the performance evaluation. In collaboration with the immediate supervisor and staff with whom the APN works and with other appropriate colleagues, the APN should identify role expectations and the purpose of the evaluation procedures. For example, the evaluation may be used as a component of annual performance reviews (Girouard & Spross, 1983), to develop annual goals and measure progress in achieving them, or to justify the contributions of the role in a setting (Hamric, 1989).

The steps in the process of individual evaluation (Hamric, 1989) include the following:

- *Selecting a focus or foci for the evaluation.* For example, the CNS may wish to assess a teaching program developed for preoperative patients (single focus) or may evaluate practice changes associated with the provision of staff in-service education programs on a surgical unit (multiple foci). The CRNA may wish to evaluate the impact of preoperative patient assessment on the perioperative experience of patients (single focus) or assess the volume and effectiveness of services provided (multiple foci). A primary care NP and her physician colleagues may decide to determine the volume of laboratory tests that the NP orders for patients with peripheral vascular disease (single focus) or the number and effects of referrals to specialty care by the NP (multiple foci).
- *Determining goals for the evaluation.* The APN would establish the specific outcomes for the activity to be assessed. The goals for the CNS's preoperative patient teaching program might include improvements in postoperative compliance with respiratory regimens and self-care activities. The staff education goal would include participation by 80% of staff in in-service education programs and measures of changes in staff behavior following participation in the programs. The CRNA or the NP in the examples given would identify similar goals.
- *Identify the components of the evaluation.* The APN would determine which structure, process, or outcomes variables, or which combination of these variables, is to be used for the evaluation. Structural variables might include the determination of resources to meet the goal. Process variables, such as participant evaluations of educational programs for patients or staff, are also to be considered if they are relevant to measuring goal achievement. Outcome variables, such as the quantity of services as a cost indicator or patient outcomes, may also be considered in relation to measuring specific goals.
- *Determine the methodology for assessing goal achievement.* Attendance at in-service education classes, record review, questionnaires and pre- and post-testing of variables are possible approaches to measuring the APN's performance. The

methodology should also include consideration of who will be doing the assessment. Staff, patients, or the APN may provide data for the evaluation. For example, patient and staff satisfaction with educational programs may be assessed through interviews or written questionnaires; the APN may collect data from records or from aggregated data available in reports prepared by medical records. Attention must also be given to the time frame for data collection in relation to the goals and intervention. Whether daily, weekly, monthly, or annual data collection is used depends on the nature of the goals to be evaluated and the resources available to the APN for evaluation activities.

- *Data analysis, interpretation, and reporting.* In planning an individual performance evaluation, the APN should decide how data will be analyzed and interpreted. The APN, the supervisor, or others may be engaged in the process. It is also important to determine how the findings of the performance evaluation will be shared. The APN and others may wish to share evaluation findings with administrative personnel, clients, and others within the setting. Whatever the decision, it should be made prior to the evaluation effort so as to provide the APN and others with access to appropriate and useful information. Attention should be given to the use of performance evaluation results for developing future goals and enhancing APNs' growth in the role within the setting and the profession.

The process of evaluation has been identified as a continuum from episodic, activity-specific assessment and feedback to periodic assessments that contribute to a broader understanding of the contributions of the APN (Hamric, 1985). Regardless of the knowledge, experience, and resources available for evaluation, the APN should be involved in a thoughtful and meaningful assessment of the role and its contributions to patient care.

There are many activities for APNs to operationalize their roles in the quality movement. Many resources are available to make the task less daunting. This section provides some suggested activities for the APN in practice, research, and education. Given the importance of evaluation and the APN's focus on practice, evaluation activities should be integrated in all APN competencies. When engaging in evaluation activities, either individually or with a team, the APN should address the following: the measure should be related to an important health concern that is meaningful to a variety of stakeholders; the measure needs to be sensitive to APN practice and able to be measured in the short term; the intervention and related factors need to be clearly defined; and, sound scientific approaches should be used.

There are a variety of possible actions to take in evaluation, which will be operationalized at different times and to varying degrees. APNs can be involved with quality assurance activities within their employment settings and with their professional organizations, consult with others and participate in conducting evaluations of their practice or patient care, and disseminate and use study findings to influence institutional and public policy that will affect patient care.

Practice

Riccardi and Kuck (1992) identified functions for the APN in quality assurance programs: developing and implementing standards of care; anticipating, identifying, and prioritizing issues related to practice and the context of care; collaborating in the development of criteria; participating in the design of studies and the analysis of data; facilitating changes in nursing practice based on findings; acting as a liaison to quality-focused and practice committees; and participating in multidisciplinary studies.

The use of quality assurance approaches was illustrated by Haase and Miller (1999). Having determined that smoking cessation counseling was not consistent in their private practice setting, they developed and implemented a strategy to use national smoking cessation counseling guidelines. All APNs should be involved in performance measurement activities in their practice settings. For example, in the hospital setting, APNs can participate in performance measurement activities required by the JCAHO (Pasero, Gordon, & McCaffery, 1999). APNs in managed care organizations can become more involved in performance measurement—using HEDIS, for example—within the primary care setting. To prepare future APNs, Noll and Girard (1993) developed a typology of quality assurance activities that relate to the competencies of the APN. For example, in the direct practice competency, APNs establish and promote standards of care, assess practice, identify problems and strategies to address them, and evaluate the effectiveness of interventions.

Education

APN curricula should include learning about the quality movement, strategies for outcome evaluation, and maintaining a current knowledge base in evaluation research. Students should integrate the elements of quality assurance into their practice experience so they can gain the knowledge and skills needed to fulfill this aspect of their roles. Course work should provide opportunities for students to identify and evaluate patient outcomes.

The APN has a major role to play through role modeling and teaching nurses and others about all components of the quality process. APNs should provide leadership for the measurement and assessment of quality in their practice setting, especially with staff nurses. In addition, the APN can assist patients and other consumers in interpreting and using performance and other quality information in their choice of health plans and providers and in knowing what they should expect from the health care system.

Research

As discussed in Chapter 9, the research competency is a critical element of advanced practice, including evaluating and conducting research to establish nursing knowledge and promote an evidence base for practice. The current quality movement demands that APNs increase their involvement in the assessment of outcomes and the improvement of quality. The APN should conduct or be involved with research at the patient, organizational, and population levels. APNs should also collaborate with researchers to seek and secure financial and other resources needed to conduct evaluations. This is particularly important in order to execute the large-scale studies needed to build a more scientific and relevant database about the impact of the APN on patient care outcomes.

Advocacy

Two other activities deserve special attention because they are critical to the ability of APNs to fulfill their social responsibility to promote optimal health and assure their place in the health care system. Given the amount of evaluation activity going on in the health care system and the attention being given to patient outcomes, APNs must be advocates for state and national government and private-sector policy efforts that foster quality assurance activities. For example, they can advocate for and support the adoption of performance measures as criteria for assessing managed care organizations through policy initiatives and within the workplace.

Successful advocacy requires both political and policy involvement (see Chapter 10)—the APN must seek these opportunities, because they will not come without effort. Related to this is the importance of disseminating findings (and having high-quality findings to disseminate) to inform policy makers, consumers, and other stakeholders about advanced practice nursing's contributions. Publications in prestigious national and international health care journals—not just nursing journals—and the use of the media to share findings with the public are two important activities. Brooten and colleagues (1999) emphasized the importance of diffusion and adoption of innovations. They described a strategy for disseminating information by identifying target audiences and sharing results through publications and presentations. Hamric (1998) discussed two examples of the influence of research findings on state regulatory policy decisions.

Resources

Fortunately, there are a number of resources available to the APN for evaluation activities. Data sources for population-based studies, frameworks for approaching quality issues, performance measures, guidelines, and other tools have grown significantly during the past 5 years. Before embarking on a quality-related activity, the APN should explore what currently exists. Much of this information, including public data sets, is available from the Internet (see Table 25-4). Although a number of resources are discussed here, the list is neither exhaustive nor reflective of all that will take place in the months and years that follow the publication of this book.

Data are available from a variety of national and state government sources and from the private sector. The federal government is an excellent source for national survey data. For example, the Healthcare Cost and Utilization Project Quality Indicators (HCUP QIs) are a set of 33 clinical performance measures for hospitals. Many states have data collected from hospitals and other health care organizations. All health care organizations collect data about their performance that can be useful to the APN to assess organizational effectiveness in achieving health outcomes.

Nursing intervention classification systems (Bowles & Naylor, 1996), although they require further testing and evaluation, can be used by the APN as a framework for describing nursing interventions and developing data sets for practice evaluation. Similarly, existing classifications of nursing-sensitive patient outcomes (Bulechek & McCloskey, 1999; Maas, Johnson, & Moorhead, 1996; Johnson, Maas, Moorhead et al., 2000) can be used to define desired outcomes and data relevant to APN practice.

The AHRQ is an excellent resource. In collaboration with the American Medical Association and the American Association of Health Plans, the National Guideline Clearinghouse database of evidence-based clinical practice guidelines and related

TABLE 25-4 WEBSITE QUALITY EVALUATION RESOURCES

These resources can be located using most search engines. In additon, most search engine sites have a button labeled "health," which can be a starting point for general searches. The sites mentioned here are those that are mentioned in the text or thought to be of particular interest to the APN. Most health care associations and organizations also have websites, and many journals can be found on line.

Agency for Healthcare Research and Quality (including CONQUEST and CAHPS)	www.ahrq.gov
American Health Care Information Management Association	www.ahima.org
American Journal of Public Health	www.apha.org
Center for Evaluative Clinical Sciences, Dartmouth College	www.dartmouth.edu/dms/cecs
Centers for Disease Control and Prevention (including Office of Disease Prevention and Health Promotion)	www.cdc.gov
Foundation for Accountability	www.facct.org
Health Care Financing Administration (including OASIS)	www.hcfa.gov/quality
The Joint Commission for the Accreditation of Healthcare Organizations (including ORYX)	www.jcaho.org
Maternal Child Health Bureau	www.mchb.hrsa.gov
MedWeb Site Directory	www.MedWeb.Emory.Edu/MedWeb
The National Committee for Quality Assurance (including HEDIS)	www.ncqa.org
National Guideline Clearinghouse	www.guideline.gov
National Institutes of Health	www.nih.gov
National Library of Medicine	www.nlm.nih.gov

documents was developed. Guidelines for pain management, low back pain, incontinence, and asthma care are among the many publicly available guidelines the APN can use as the basis for assessing conformance within her or his practice setting. Also of interest is CONQUEST, which links clinical performance measures and medical condition databases. It contains over 1,000 performance measures. The AHRQ has also been instrumental in the development and testing of a national initiative to assess health plans (CAHPS). Because this agency of the federal government has a major role in the quality movement, the APN has an excellent resource to track activities. To assess the literature associated with quality, the APN can also access the resources of the National Library of Medicine through the Internet (Humphreys, Ruffin, Cahn, & Rambo, 1999). Other government resources include the Centers for Disease Control and Prevention, the HCFA, the National Institutes of Health, and the Office of Disease Prevention and Health Promotion.

Accrediting organizations are also valuable sources. The JCAHO, the NCQA, and others can provide the APN with information about their quality-related activities. The NCQA, for example, has a national report card comparing managed care plans of HEDIS measures related to preventive care, care of the chronically ill, and patient satisfaction/experience with care. Other sources for outcome measures include FACCT and the Center for Evaluative Clinical Sciences at Dartmouth College.

Information about quality issues can also be found through professional associations, including the American Nurses' Association. The *Nursing Report Card for Acute Care* (American Nurses Association, 1995) is one example of its work in the quality area. Specialty nursing organizations are excellent resources as well, and APNs should be familiar with the quality work of other disciplines. For example, the American Medical Association and the American Academy of Pediatrics conduct major quality and quality-related research initiatives.

CONCLUSION

This chapter has presented a number of compelling arguments to motivate APNs to increase and improve efforts to evaluate the impact of advanced nursing practice in the health care system. The existing literature has been reviewed and, although it strongly suggests that APNs make a demonstrable difference in the lives of patients, the body and quality of the evidence is by no means definitive. The problems associated with evaluating the impact of the APN and the strengths and weakness of past efforts should help future evaluators improve conceptualization and methodologies for evaluation. Finally, the frameworks presented can guide the beginning and more experienced evaluator to make greater contributions to assessing the impact of the APN.

These are challenging times for advanced practice. There are many exciting opportunities to improve access, enhance quality, and control costs. The data and knowledge gained from evaluation efforts can play a major role in shaping the organization, delivery, and financing of the future health care system. True today is Hamric's statement made in 1989:

In the current health care climate, demonstrating positive changes in patients and nursing behavior attributable to [the interventions of APNs] is not only desirable, it is a necessity for survival.

(p. 103)

Not only will the APN lose, but the nursing profession and consumers will lose a great deal if the knowledge, skills, and leadership of APNs are not fully utilized in the evolving health care system. Evaluation activities are an opportunity for the APN to provide leadership within the quality movement, advance the science of caregiving, and document the important role APNs play in meeting the purpose of the health care system. APNs must continue to demonstrate their important roles in reducing the impact and burden of illness, injury, and disability and thus improve the health and functioning of individual patients and the larger population.

REFERENCES

Agency for Health Care Policy and Research. (1995). *Using clinical practice guidelines to evaluate quality of care, Vol. 1: Issues* (AHCPR Publication No. 95-0045). Washington, DC: Author.

Agency for Health Care Policy and Research. (1999a, June 7). Quality of care most important nursing home measure (AHCPR Press Release). Washington, DC: Author.

Agency for Health Care Policy and Research. (1999b, June 28). AHCPR Awards 10 large grants in areas of emphasis (AHCPR Press Release). Washington, DC: Author.

Aiken, L. H., Lake, E. T., Semaan, S., Lehman, H. P., O'Hare, P. A., Cole, C. S., Dunbar, D., & Frank, I. (1993). Nurse practitioner managed care for persons with HIV infection. *Image: The Journal of Nursing Scholarship, 25*(3), 172–177.

Aiken, L. H., Sloane, D. M., Lake, E. T., Sochalski, J., & Weber, A. L. (1999). Organization and outcomes of inpatient AIDS care. *Medical Care, 37,* 760–772.

Aiken, L. H., Smith, H. L., & Lake, E. T. (1994). Lower Medicare mortality among a set of hospitals known for good nursing care. *Medical Care, 32,* 771–787.

Aiken, L. H., Sochalski, J., & Lake, E. T. (1997). Studying outcomes of organizational change in health services. *Medical Care, 35,* NS6–NS18.

Aikins, M. P., & Feinland, J. B. (1998). Perinatal outcomes in home birth setting. *Birth, 25*(4), 226–234.

Aquilino, M. L., Damiano, P. C., Willard, J. C., Momony, E. T., & Levy, B. T. (1999). Primary care physician perceptions of the nurse practitioner in the 1990s. *Archives of Family Medicine 8,* 224–227.

American Nurses Association. (1995). *Nursing report card for acute care.* Washington, DC: American Nurses Publishing.

Barnason, S., Merboth, M., Pozehl, B., & Tietjen, M. J. (1998). Utilizing an outcome approach to improve pain management by nurses: A pilot study. *Clinical Nurse Specialist, 12*(1), 28–36.

Beal, J. A., & Philips, M. (1999). *The nurse practitioner role in the NICU: A study of role turnover.* Paper presented at the Eastern Nursing Research Society meeting, New York.

Bloch, D. (1975). Evaluation of nursing care in terms of process and outcomes: Issues in research and quality assurance. *Nursing Research, 24*(4), 256–263.

Blondin, J., Schriefer, J., Shinozaki, T., Calhoun, B., Leavitt, B., Deane, R., & LaChaunce, W. (1996). The quality cup winner: Fletcher Allen Health Care's Early Extubation Team. *Quality Management in Health Care, 4*(2), 42–54.

Bond, S., Beck, S., Dernck, S., Sargeant, J., Cunningham, W. F., Healy, B., Rawes, G., Holdsworth, S., & Lawson, J. (1999). Training nurse practitioners for general practice. *British Journal of General Pracice 49*(7), 531–535.

Borchers, L., & Kee, C. C. (1999). An experience in telenursing. *Clinical Nurse Specialist, 13*(3), 115–118.

Bowles, K. H., & Naylor, M. D. (1996). Nursing intervention classification systems. *Image: The Journal of Nursing Scholarship, 28*(4), 303–308.

Bozzo, J., Carlson, B., & Diers, D. (1998). Using hospital data systems to find target populations: New tools for clinical nurse specialists. *Clinical Nurse Specialist, 12*(2), 86–91.

Broome, M. E. (1999). Outcomes research: Practice counts! *Journal of the Society of Pediatric Nursing, 4*(2), 83–85.

Brooten, D. (1997). Methodological issues linking costs and outcomes. *Medical Care, 35,* NS87–NS95.

Brooten, D., & Naylor, M. D. (1995). Nurses' effect on changing patient outcomes. *Image: The Journal of Nursing Scholarship, 27*(2), 95–99.

Brooten, D., Youngblut, J. M., Roberts, B. L., Montgomery, K., Standing, T., Hemstrom, M., Suresky, J., & Polis, N. (1999). Disseminating breakthroughs: Enacting a strategic framework. *Nursing Outlook, 47*(3), 133–138.

Bulechek, G. M., & McCloskey, J. C. (1999). *Nursing interventions: Effective nursing treatments* (3rd ed.). Philadelphia: W. B. Saunders.

Burns, L. R., Lamb, G. S., & Wholey, D. R. (1996). Impact of integrated community nursing services on hospital utilization and costs in a Medicare risk plan. *Inquiry, 33*(1), 30–41.

Cancer specialists turn to a long-ignored side effect: Fatigue. (1999, April 10). *The New York Times,* p. A-16.

Cassidy, C. A. (1999). Want to know how you are doing? *American Journal of Nursing, 99*(9), 51–57.

Champagne, M., Tornquist, M. A., & Funk, S. G. (1997). Achieving research-based practice. *American Journal of Nursing, 97*(5), 16AAA–16DDD.

Chance, K. S., (1997). The quest for quality: An exploration of attempts to define and measure quality nursing care. *Image: The Journal of Nursing Scholarship, 29*(4), 326–331.

CNM Data Group. (1998). Midwifery management of pain in labor. *Journal of Nurse Midwifery, 43*(2), 77–82.

Coward, D. D. (1998). Facilitation of self-transcendence in a breast cancer support group. *Oncology Nursing Forum, 25*(1), 75–84.

Curley, M. A. (1998). Patient-nurse synergy: Optimizing patients' outcomes. *Journal of Critical Care, 7*(1), 64–72.

Czaplinski, C., & Diers, D. (1998). The effect of staff nursing on length of stay and mortality. *Medical Care, 36,* 1626–1638.

Diers, D., & Bozzo, J. (1997). Nursing resource definition in DRGs: RIMS/Nursing Acuity Project. *Nursing Economics, 15*(3), 124–137.

Diers, D., Bozzo, J., Blatt, L., & Roussel, M. (1998). Understanding nursing resources in intensive care: A case study. *American Journal of Critical Care, 7,* 143–148.

Diers, D., Karlsen, B., & Allegretto, S. (1999). *A method for studying high cost users.* Paper presented at the 11th Annual Scientific Sessions Eastern Nursing Research Society meeting, New York.

Donabedian, A. (1966). Evaluating the quality of medical care. *Milbank Quarterly, 44,* 166–206.

East, C. E. & Colditz, P. B. (1996). Women's evaluations of their experiences with fetal intrapartum oxygen saturation monitoring and participation in a research project. *Midwifery, 12*(2), 93–97.

Eddy, D. M. (1998). Performance measurement: Problems and solutions. *Health Affairs, 17*(4), 7–25.

Gardner, M. O., Cliver, S. P., McNeal, S. F., & Goldenberg, R. L. (1996). Ethnicity and sources of prenatal care: Findings from a national survey. *Birth, 23*(2), 84–87.

Garvican, L., Grimsey, E., Littlejohns, P., Lownes, S., & Sacks, N. (1998). Satisfaction with clinical nurse specialists in a breast care clinic: Questionnaire survey. *BMJ, 316,* 976–977.

Girouard, S. A. (1996). Evaluating advanced nursing practice. In A. B. Hamric, J. A. Spross, & C. M. Hanson (Eds.), *Advanced practice nursing: An integrative approach* (pp. 569–600). Philadelphia: W. B. Saunders.

Girouard, S. A., & Spross, J. A. (1983). Evaluation of the CNS: Using an evaluation tool. In A. B. Hamric & J. Spross (Eds.), *The clinical nurse specialist in theory and practice* (pp. 207–218). New York: Grune & Stratton.

Haase, R., & Miller, K. (1999). Performance improvement in everyday clinical practice. *American Journal of Nursing, 99*(5), 52–54.

Hamric, A. B. (1983). A model for developing evaluation strategies. In A. B. Hamric & J. Spross (Eds.), *The clinical nurse specialist in theory and practice* (pp. 187–206). New York: Grune & Stratton.

Hamric, A. B. (1985). Clinical nurse specialist role evaluation. *Oncology Nursing Forum, 12*(2), 62–66.

Hamric, A. B. (1989). A model for CNS evaluation. In A. B. Hamric & J. A. Spross (Eds.), *The clinical nurse specialist in theory and practice* (2nd ed., pp. 83–104). Philadelphia: W. B. Saunders.

Hamric, A. B. (1998). Using research to influence the regulatory process. *Advanced Practice Nursing Quarterly, 4*(3), 44–50.

Hamric, A. B., Gresham, M. L., & Eccard, M. (1978). Staff evaluation of clinical leaders. *Journal of Nursing Administration, 8*(1), 18–26.

Hamric, A. B., Spross, J. A., & Hanson, C. M. (Eds.). (1996). *Advanced nursing practice: An integrative approach.* Philadelphia: W. B. Saunders.

Hamric, A. B., Worley, D., Lindeback, S., & Jaubert, S. (1998). Outcomes associated with advanced nursing practice prescriptive authority. *Journal of the American Academy of Nurse Practitioners, 10*(3), 113–118.

Harrington, C., Mullan, J., Woodruff, L. C., Burger, S. G., Carillo, H., & Bedney, B. (1999). Stakeholders' opinions regarding important measures of nursing home quality for consumers. *American Journal of Medical Quality, 14*(3), 124–132.

Harrison, J. K. (1999). Influence of managed care on professional nursing practice. *Image: The Journal of Nursing Scholarship, 31*(2), 161–166.

Hawkins, J. W., Thibodeau, J. A., Utley-Smith, Q. E., Igou, J. F., & Johnson, E. E. (1993). Using a conceptual model for practice in a nursing wellness center for seniors. *Perspectives, 17*(4), 11–16.

Henry, S. B., & Holzmer, W. L. (1997). Achievement of appropriate self-care: Does care delivery system make a difference? *Medical Care, 35*(11), NS33–NS40.

Hester, N. O., Miller, K. L., Foster, R. L., & Vojir, C. P. (1997). Symptom management outcomes—do they reflect variations in care delivery systems? *Medical Care, 35,* NS69–NS83.

Hogan, A. J. (1997). Methodological issues in linking costs and health outcomes in research on differing care delivery systems. *Clinical Nurse Specialist, 13*(5), 228–235.

Houston, S., & Luquire, R. (1991). Measuring success: CNS performance appraisal. *Clinical Nurse Specialist, 5*(4), 204–209.

Humphreys, B. L., Ruffin, A. B., Cahn, M. A., & Rambo, N. (1999). Powerful connections for public health: The National Library of Medicine and the National Network of Libraries of Medicine. *American Journal of Public Health, 89,* 1633–1636.

Ingersoll, G. L. (1988). Evaluating the impact of the clinical nurse specialist. *Clinical Nurse Specialist, 2*(3), 150–155.

Jacavone, J. B., Daniels, R. D., & Tyner, I. (1999). CNS facilitation of a cardiac surgery clinical pathway program. *Clinical Nurse Specialist, 13*(3), 126–132.

Jennings, B. M. (1991). Patient outcomes research: Seizing the opportunity. *Advances in Nursing Science, 14*(2), 59–72.

Johnson, M., Maas, M., Moorhead, S., et al. (Eds.). *Nursing outcomes classification (NOC)* (2nd ed.). St. Louis: Mosby–Year Book.

Johnson, P. G. (1998). Midwife and nurse-midwife: The effects of title on perception and confidence in services provided by professional midwives. *Journal of Nurse Midwifery, 43*(4), 296–304.

Johnson-Pawlson, J., & Infeld, D. L. (1996). Nurse staffing and quality of care in nursing facilities. *Journal of Gerontological Nursing, 22*(8), 36–46.

Johnston, B., Wheeler, L., Deuser, J., & Sousa, K. H. (2000). Outcomes of the Kaiser Permanente Tele-Home Health Research Project. *Archives of Family Medicine, 9*(1), 40–45.

Kearnes, D. R. (1992). A productivity tool to evaluate NP practice: Monitoring clinical time spent in reimbursable, patient-related activities. *Nurse Practitioner, 17*(4), 50–52, 55.

Kee, C. C., & Borchers, L. (1998). Reducing readmission rates through discharge interventions. *Clinical Nurse Specialist, 12*(5), 206–209.

Kilpack, V., Campion, P., Stover, P., Wood, M. E., & Cocke, M. W. (1996). Tracking skin integrity: A template for hospital and vendor collaboration. *Journal of Nursing Care Quality, 10*(3), 18–27.

Lang, N. M., & Marek, K. D. (1992). Outcomes that reflect clinical practice. In *Patient outcomes research: Examining the effectiveness of nursing practice* (pp. 27–38) (Proceedings of a conference sponsored by the National Center for Nursing Research), (Publication No. 93-3411). Washington, DC: U.S. Department of Health and Human Services.

Lauver, L. S. (1996). Benchmarking: Improving outcomes for the congestive heart failure population. *Journal of Nursing Care Quality, 10*(3), 7–17.

Licht, J. (1999, July 20). Getting patients back on their feet faster: Study says care before and after discharge from the hospital saves money, spurs recovery. The *Washington Post,* p. Z15.

Lohr, K. N. (Ed.). (1990). *A strategy for quality assurance* (Vol. 1). Washington, DC: National Academy Press.

Lohr, K. N. (1997). How do we measure quality? *Health Affairs, 16*(3), 22-25.

Maas, M. L., Johnson, M., & Moorhead, S. (1996). Classifying nurse-sensitive patient outcomes. *Image: The Journal of Nursing Scholarship, 28*(4), 295-301.

Mason, D. J., Alexander, J. M., Huffaker, J., Reilly, P. A., Sigmund, E. C., & Cohen, S. S. (1999). Nurse practitioners' experiences with managed care organizations in New York and Connecticut. *Nursing Outlook, 47*(5), 201-208.

McCorkle, R., Robinson, L., Nuamah, I., Lev, E., & Benoliel, J. Q. (1998). The effects of home nursing care for patients during terminal illness on the bereaved's psychological distress. *Nursing Research, 47*(1), 2-10.

McDaniel, A. M. (1999). Assessing the feasibility of a clinical practice guideline for inpatient smoking cessation intervention. *Clinical Nurse Specialist, 13*(5), 228-235.

McGlynn, E. A. (1997). Six challenges in measuring the quality of health care. *Health Affairs, 16*(3), 7-21.

McMullen, M. (1998). *Satisfaction of patients, physicians and staff nurses with the care provided by a nurse practitioner/attending collaborative service.* Paper presented at the 11th Annual Scientific Sessions Eastern Nursing Research Society meeting, New-York.

Milbrath, C. D. (1996). Improving surgical preparedness. *Eye on Improvement, 3*(6), 6-8.

Mitchell, P. H., & Shortell, S. M. (1997). Adverse outcomes and variations in organization care delivery. *Medical Care, 35,* NS19-NS32.

Morin, K. H., Bucher, L., Plowfield, L., Hayes, E., Mahoney, P., & Armiger, L. (1999). Using research to establish protocols for practice: A statewide study of acute care agencies. *Clinical Nurse Specialist, 13*(2), 77-84.

Mundinger, M. O., Kane, R. L., Lenz, E. R., Totten, A. M., Tsai, W. Y., Cleary, P. D., Friedewald, W. T., Siu, A. L., & Shelanski, M. L. (2000). Primary care outcomes in patients treated by nurse practitioners or physicians: A randomized trial. *JAMA, 283,* 59-68.

Murdaugh, C. (1997). Health-related quality of life as an outcome in organizational research. *Medical Care, 35,* NS41-NS57.

Naylor, M. D., Brooten, D., Campbell, R., Jacobsen, B. S., Mezey, M. D., Pauly, M. V., & Schwartz, J. S. (1999). Comprehensive discharge planning and home follow-up of hospitalized elders: A randomized clinical trial. *JAMA, 281,* 613-657.

Naylor, M. D., & Buhler-Wilkerson, K. (1999). Creating community-based care for the new millennium. *Nursing Outlook, 47*(3), 120-127.

Naylor, M. D., Munro, B. H., & Brooten, D. A. (1991). Measuring the effectiveness of nursing practice. *Clinical Nurse Specialist, 5*(4), 210-215.

Noll, M. L., & Girard, N. (1993). Preparing the CNS for participation in quality assurance activities. *Clinical Nurse Specialist, 7*(2), 81-84.

Oermann, M. H., & Huber, D. (1999). Patient outcomes—a measure of nursing's value. *American Journal of Nursing, 99*(9), 40-48.

O'Leary, D. S. (1998). Reordering performance measurement priorities. *Health Affairs, 17*(4), 38-39.

Otto, L. K., & Davidson, S. (1999). Radiation exposure of CRNAs during uteroscopic procedures using fluoroscopy. *American Association of Nurse Anesthetists Journal, 67*(1), 53-58.

Paine, L. L., Lange, J. M., Strobino, D. M., Johnson, T. R., DeJoseph, J. F., Declereq, E. R., Gagnon, D. R., Scupholme, A., & Ross, A. (1999). Characteristics of nurse-midwife patients and visits. *American Journal of Public Health, 89,* 906-909.

Palmer, R. H., Duggar, B., DeLozier, J., Goldenberg, D., Lawthers, A. J., Banks, N. J., Kurkland, D., Hargraves, J. L., & Peterson, L. (1995). *Understanding and choosing clinical performance measures: Development of a typology* (Publication No. 95-N001). Washington, DC: Agency for Health Care Policy and Research.

Pasero, C., Gordon, D. B., & McCaffery, M. (1999). Pain control: JCAHO on assessing and managing pain. *American Journal of Nursing, 99*(7), 22.

Pelletier-Hibbert, M. (1998). Coping strategies used by nurses to deal with the care of organ donors and their families. *Heart and Lung, 27,* 230-237.

Peters, D. (1994, June/July). Strategic directions for using outcomes. *The Remington Report,* pp. 9-13.

Peterson, R., & Smith, J. (1996). A patient care team approach to multicultural patient care issues. *Journal of Nursing Care Quality, 10*(3), 75-79.

Posner, K. L., & Freund, P. R. (1998). Trends in quality of anesthesia care associated with changing staffing patterns, productivity and concurrency of case supervision in a teaching hospital. *Anesthesiology, 91,* 839-847.

President's Advisory Commission on Consumer Protection and Quality in the Health Care Industry. (1998). *Quality first: Better health care for all Americans.* Washington, DC: Author.

Riccardi, E., & Kuck, A. W. (1992). Improving patient outcomes: The role of the clinical nurse specialist in quality assurance. *Journal of Nursing Care Quality, 6*(2), 46-50.

Rosenthal, G. E., & Shannon, S. E. (1997). The use of patient perceptions in the evaluation of health care delivery systems. *Medical Care, 35,* NS58-NS68.

Rossi, P. H., & Freeman, H. E. (1989). *Evaluation: A systematic approach* (4th ed.). Newbury Park, CA: Sage Publications.

Rudy, E. B., Daly, B. J., Douglas, S., Montenegro, H. D., Song, R., & Dyer, M. A. (1995). Patient outcomes for the chronically critically ill: Special care unit versus intensive care unit. *Nursing Research, 44*(6), 324–331.

Rudy, E. B., Davidson, L. J., Daly, B., Clochesy, J. M., Sereika, S., Baldisseri, M., Hravnak, M., Ross, T., & Ryan, C. (1998). Care activities and outcomes of patients cared for by acute care nurse practitioners, physician assistants and resident physicians: A comparison. *American Journal of Critical Care, 7,* 267–281.

Sagehorn, K. K., Russell, C. L., & Ganong, L.H. (1999). Implementation of a patient-family pathway: Effects on patients and families. *Clinical Nurse Specialist, 13*(3), 119–122.

Sovie, M. (1999). *Hospital restructuring's impact on outcomes.* Paper presented at the 11th Annual Scientific Sessions Eastern Nursing Research Society meeting, New York.

Starr, P. (1997). Smart technology, stunted policy: Developing health information networks. *Health Affairs, 16*(3), 95–105.

Strickland, O. L. (1997, First Quarter). Outcomes research: Are we rigorous enough? *Reflections,* pp. 8–10.

Strohschein, S., Schaffer, M. A., & Lia-Hoagberg, B. (1999). Evidence-based guidelines for public health nursing practice. *Nursing Outlook, 47*(2), 84–90.

Summers, D., & Soper, P. A. (1998). Implementation and evaluation of stroke clinical pathways and impact on cost of stroke care. *Journal of Cardiovascular Nursing, 13*(1), 69–87.

Tierney, M. J., Grant, L. M., & Mazique, S. I. (1990). Cost accountability and clinical nurse specialist evaluation. *Nursing Management, 21*(5), 26–28, 30–31.

Tilly, K. F., Garvey, N. J., Gold, M., Powell, E., & Proudlock, M. L. (1996). Outcomes management and asthma education in a community hospital: Ongoing monitoring of health status. *Quality Management in Health Care, 4*(3), 67–78.

Topp, R., Tucker, D., & Weber, C. (1998). Effect of a clinical case manager/clinical nurse specialist on patients hospitalized with congestive heart failure. *Nursing Case Management, 3*(4), 140–147.

Urden, L. D. (1999). Outcome evaluation: An essential component for CNS practice. *Clinical Nurse Specialist, 13*(1), 39–46.

Ventura, M. R., Crosby, F., & Feldman, M. J. (1991). An information synthesis to evaluate nurse practitioner effectiveness. *Military Medicine, 156,* 286–291.

Walker, P. H., & Stone, P. W. (1996). Exploring cost and quality: Community-based versus traditional hospital delivery systems. *Journal of Health Care Finance, 23*(1), 23–47.

Wammack, L., & Mabrey, J. D. (1998). Outcomes assessment of total hip and total knee arthroplasty: Critical pathways, variance analysis and continuous quality improvement. *Clinical Nurse Specialist, 12*(3), 122–131.

White, C. L. (1999). Changing pain management practice and impacting on outcomes. *Clinical Nurse Specialist, 13*(4), 166–172.

Wong, S. T. (1998). Outcomes of nursing care: How do we know? *Clinical Nurse Specialist, 12*(4), 147–151.

Yoffee, E. (1999, November 9). Doctors are reminded, "wash up!" *The New York Times,* pp. D-1, D-3.

York, R., Brown, L. P., Samuels, P., Finkler, S. A., Jacobsen, B., Persely, C. A., Swank, A., & Robbins, D. (1997). A randomized clinical trial of early discharge and nurse specialist transitional follow-up care of high-risk childbearing women. *Nursing Research, 46*(5), 254–261.

Additional Readings

Abraham, I. L., Chalifoux, Z. L., & Evers, G. C. (1992). Conditions, interventions, & outcomes: A quantitative analysis of nursing research (1981–1990). In *Patient outcomes research: Examining the effectiveness of nursing practice* (Proceedings of a conference sponsored by the National Center for Nursing Research), (Publication No. 93-3411). Washington, DC: U.S. Department of Health and Human Services.

Alexander, J. S., Younger, R. E., Cohen, R. M., & Crawford, L. V. (1988). Effectiveness of a nurse managed program for children with chronic asthma. *Journal of Pediatric Nursing, 3*(5), 312–317.

Baradell, J. G. (1994). Cost-effectiveness and quality of care provided by clinical nurse specialists. *Journal of Psychosocial Nursing and Mental Health Services, 32*(3), 21–24.

Bartucci, M. R. (1985). A comparative study of outpatient care as perceived by renal transplant patients. *Journal of the American Association of Nephrology Nurses, 12*(2), 119–124.

Batey, M. V., & Holland, J. M. (1985). Prescribing practices among nurse practitioners in adult and family health. *American Journal of Public Health, 75,* 258–262.

Baughan, D. M., White-Baughan, J., Pickwell, S., Bartlome, J., & Wong, S. (1990). Primary care needs of Cambodian refugees. *Journal of Family Practice, 30,* 565–568.

Boyd, N. J., Stasiowski, S. A., Catoe, P. T., Wells, P. R., Stahl, B. M., Judson, E., Hartman, A. L., & Lander, J. H. (1991). The merit and significance of clinical nurse specialists. *Journal of Nursing Administration, 21*(9), 35–43.

Brooten, D., Kumar, S., Brown, L. P., Butts, D., Finkler, S. A., Bakewell-Sachs, S., Gibbons, A., & Delivoria-Papadopoulos, M. (1986). A randomized clinical trial of early hospital discharge and home follow-up of very low birth weight infants. *New England Journal of Medicine, 315,* 934–939.

Brooten, D., Roncoli, M., Finkler, S., Arnold, L., Cohen, A., & Mennuti, M. (1994). A randomized trial of early hospital discharge and home follow-up of women having cesarean birth. *Obstetrics and Gynecology, 84*(5), 832–838.

Buchanan, J. L., Bell, R. M., Arnold, S. B., Witsberger, C., Kane, R. L., & Garrard, J. (1990). Assessing cost effects of nursing-home-based geriatric nurse practitioners. *Health Care Financing Review, 11*(3), 67–78.

Burge, S., Crigler, L., Hurth, L., Kelly, G., & Sanborn, C. (1989). Clinical nurse specialist role development: Quantifying actual practice over three years. *Clinical Nurse Specialist, 3*(1), 33–36.

Burgess, A. W., Lerner, D. J., D'Agostino, R. B., Vokonas, P. S., Hartman, C. R., & Gaccione, P. (1987). A randomized control trial of cardiac rehabilitation. *Social Science and Medicine, 24,* 359–370.

Capan, P., Beard, M., & Mashburn, M. (1993). Nurse-managed clinics provide access and improved health care. *Nurse Practitioner, 18*(5), 50, 53–55.

Cavero, C. M., Fullerton, J. T., & Bartlome, J. A. (1991). Assessment of the process and outcomes of the first 1,000 births of a nurse midwifery service. *Journal of Nurse-Midwifery, 36*(2), 104–110.

Chambers, L., & West, A. (1978). Assessment of the role of the family nurse practitioner in urban medical practices. *Canadian Journal of Public Health, 609,* 459–468.

Cherry, J., & Foster, J. C. (1982). Comparison of hospital charges generated by certified nurse-midwives' and physicians' clients. *Journal of Nurse-Midwifery, 27*(1), 7–11.

Cox, K., Bergen, A., & Norman, I. J. (1993). Exploring consumer views of care provided by the Macmillan nurse using critical incident technique. *Journal of Advanced Nursing, 18*(3), 408–415.

Cromwell, J., & Rosenbach, M. (1988). The economics of anesthesia delivery. *Health Affairs, 10*(1), 17–26.

Crosby, F., Ventura, M. R., & Feldman, M. J. (1987). Future research recommendations for establishing NP effectiveness. *Nurse Practitioner, 12*(1), 75–76, 78–79.

Damato, E. G., Dill, P. Z., Gennaro, S., Brown, L. P., York, L. P., & Brooten, D. (1993). The association between CNS direct care time and total time and very low birth weight infant outcomes. *Clinical Nurse Specialist, 7*(2), 75–79.

Davis, L. G., Riedman, G. L., Sapiro, M., Minogue, J. P., & Kozer, R. R. (1994). Cesarean section rates in low-risk private patients managed by certified nurse-midwives and obstetricians. *Journal of Nurse-Midwifery, 39*(2), 91–97.

Dixon, B. A. (1993). Institutional survey of nurse anesthesia practice in patients receiving opioids via patient-controlled analgesia. *Nurse Anesthetist, 4*(3), 112–117.

Doblin, B. H., Gelberg, L., & Freeman, H. E. (1992). Patient care and professional staffing patterns in McKinney Act clinics providing primary care to the homeless. *JAMA, 267,* 698–701.

Draye, M. A., & Pesznecker, B. L. (1979). Diagnostic scope and certainty: An analysis of FNP practice. *Nurse Practitioner, 4*(1), 42–43.

Ellings, J. M., Newman, B. B., Hulser, T. C., Bivins, H. A., Jr., & Keenan, A. (1993). Reduction in very low birth weight deliveries and perinatal mortality in a specialized, multidisciplinary twin clinic. *Obstetrics and Gynecology, 81*(3), 387–391.

Fenton, M. V. (1985). Identifying competencies of clinical nurse specialists. *Journal of Nursing Administration, 15*(12), 31–37.

Ferguson, L. A., & Sapelli, D. M. (1992). Nurse practitioner sutured wounds: A quality assurance review. *American Association of Occupational Health Nursing Journal, 40*(12), 577–580.

Fleming, S. T. (1992). Outcomes of care for anesthesia services: A pilot study. *Quality Assurance in Health Care, 4*(4), 289–303.

Garrard, J., Kane, R. L., Radosevich, D. M., Skay, C. L., Arnold, S., Kepferle, L., McDermott, S., & Buchanan, J. L. (1990). Impact of geriatric nurse practitioners on nursing-home residents' functional status, satisfaction and discharge outcomes. *Medical Care, 28*(3), 271–283.

Georgopoulos, B. S., & Jackson, M. M. (1970). Nursing Kardex behavior in an experimental study of patient units with and without clinical nurse specialists. *Nursing Research, 19*(3), 196–218.

Georgopoulos, B. S., & Sana, J. M. (1971). Clinical nursing specialization and intershift report behavior. *American Journal of Nursing, 71*(3), 538–545.

Gifford, M. S., & Stone, I. K. (1993). Quality, access and clinical issues in a nurse practitioner colposcopy outreach program. *Nurse Practitioner, 18*(10), 33–36.

Girouard, S. (1978). The role of the clinical specialist as change agent: An experiment in preoperative teaching. *International Journal of Nursing Studies, 15*(2), 57–65.

Graveley, E. A., & Littlefield, J. H. (1992). A cost-effectiveness analysis of three staffing models for the delivery of low-risk prenatal care. *American Journal of Public Health, 82,* 180–184.

Hag, M. B. (1993). Understanding older adult satisfaction with primary health care services in a nursing center. *Applied Nursing Research,* 6(3), 125–131.

Hanneman, S. G., Bines, A. S., & Sajtar, W. S. (1993). The indirect patient care effect of a unit-based clinical nurse specialist on preventable pulmonary complications. *American Journal of Critical Care,* 2(4), 331–338.

Hastings, G. E., Vick, L., Lee, G., Sasmor, L., Natiello, T. A., & Sanders, J. H. (1980). Nurse practitioners in a jailhouse clinic. *Medical Care,* 18, 731–744.

Hill, J., Bird, H. A., Harmer, R., Wright, V., & Lawton, C. (1994). An evaluation of the effectiveness, safety and acceptability of a nurse practitioner in a rheumatology outpatient clinic. *British Journal of Rheumatology, 33,* 283–288.

Hill, K. M., Ellsworth-Wolk, J., & DeBlase, R. (1993). Capturing the multiple contribution of the CNS role: A criterion-based evaluation tool. *Clinical Nurse Specialist, 7*(5), 267–273.

Hinshaw, A. S. (1992). Welcome: The patient outcomes research conference. In *Patient outcomes research: Examining the effectiveness of nursing practice.* (Proceedings of a conference sponsored by the National Center for Nursing Research). (Publication No. 93-3411). Washington, DC: U.S. Department of Health and Human Services.

Holmes, G., Livingston, G., & Mills, E. (1976). Contribution of a nurse clinician to office practice productivity: Comparison of two solo primary care practices. *Health Services Research, 11*(1), 21–33.

Kane, R. L., Garrard, J., Skay, C. L., Radosevich, D. M., Buchanan, J. L., McDermott, S. M., Arnold, S. B., & Kepferle, L. (1989). Effects of a geriatric nurse practitioner on process and outcome of nursing home care. *American Journal of Public Health, 79,* 1271–1277.

Kasch, C. R., & Knutson, K. (1986). The functional message behavior inventory: Linking nursing action with health care outcomes. *Nurse Practitioner, 11*(6), 61–67.

Kearnes, D. R. (1994). Impact of a nurse practitioner and physician collaborative practice on older adults admitted to a large urban hospital: Differences in treatment and outcome. *Nurse Practitioner, 19*(8), 32, 34–36.

Knaus, W. A., Draper, E. A., Wagner, D. P., & Zimmerman, J. E. (1986). An evaluation of outcome from intensive care in major medical centers. *Annals of Internal Medicine, 104,* 410–418.

Knickman, J. R., Lipkin, M., Jr., Finkler, S. A., Thompson, W. G., & Kiel, J. (1992). The potential for using non-physicians to compensate for the reduced availability of residents. *Academic Medicine, 67,* 429–438.

Koelbel, P. W., Fuller, S. G., & Misener, T. R. (1991). An explanatory model of nurse practitioner job satisfaction. *Journal of the American Academy of Nurse Practitioners, 3*(1), 17–24.

Koelbel, P. W., Fuller, S. G., & Misener, T. R. (1991). Job satisfaction of nurse practitioners: An analysis using Herzberg's theory. *Nurse Practitioner, 16*(4), 43, 46–52, 55–56.

Komaroff, A. L., Sawayer, K., Flatly, M., & Browne, C. (1976). Nurse practitioner management of common respiratory and genitourinary infections, using protocols. *Nursing Research, 25*(2), 84–89.

Kurz-Cringle, R., Blake, L. A., Dunham, D., Miller, M. J., & Annecillo, C. (1994). A nurse-managed inpatient program for patients with chronic mental disorders. *Archives of Psychiatric Nursing, 8*(1), 14–21.

Lemley, K. B., O'Grady, E. T., Rouckhorst, L., Russel, D. D., & Small, N. (1994). Baseline data on the delivery of clinical preventive services provided by nurse practitioners. *Nurse Practitioner, 19*(5), 57–63.

Levy, B. S., Wilkinson, F. S., & Marine, W. M. (1971). Reducing neonatal mortality rate with nurse-midwives. *American Journal of Obstetrics and Gynecology, 109,* 50–58.

Linde, B. J., & Janz, N. M. (1979). Effect of a teaching program on knowledge and compliance of cardiac patients. *Nursing Research, 28*(5), 282–286.

Lipman, T. H. (1988). Length of hospitalization of children with diabetes: Effect of a clinical nurse specialist. *Diabetes Education, 14*(1), 41–43.

Little, D. E., & Carnevali, D. (1967). Nurse specialists effect on tuberculosis. *Nursing Research, 16*(4), 321–326.

Martin, J. P. (1989). From implication to reality through a unit-based quality assurance program. *Clinical Nurse Specialist, 3*(4), 192–196.

McBride, A. B., Austin, J. K., Chestnut, E. E., Main, C. S., Richards, B. S., & Roy, B. A. (1987). Evaluation of the impact of the clinical nurse specialist in a state psychiatric hospital. *Archives of Psychiatric Nursing, 1*(1), 55–61.

McCorkle, R., Benoliel, J. Q., Donaldson, G., Georgiadou, F., Moinpour, C., & Goodell, B. (1989). A randomized clinical trial of home nursing care for lung cancer patients. *Cancer, 64,* 1375–1382.

Melillo, K. D. (1993). Utilizing nurse practitioners to provide health care for elderly patients in Massachusetts's nursing homes. *Journal of the American Academy of Nurse Practitioners, 5*(1), 19–26.

Molde, S., & Diers, D. (1985). Nurse practitioner research: Selected literature review and research agenda. *Nursing Research, 34*(6), 362–367.

Neidlinger, S. H., Scroggins, K., & Kennedy, L. M. (1987). Cost evaluation of discharge planning for hospitalized elderly. *Nursing Economics, 5*(5), 225-230.

Nemes, J., Barnaby, K., & Shamberger, R. C. (1992). Experience with a nurse practitioner program in the surgical department of a children's hospital. *Journal of Pediatric Surgery, 27,* 1038-1040.

Nevidjon, B., & Warren, B. (1984). Documenting the activities of the oncology clinical nurse specialist. *Oncology Nursing Forum, 11*(3), 54-55.

Nuccio, S. A., Costa-Lieberthal, K. M., Gunta, K. E., Mackus, M. L., Riesch, S. K., Schmanski, K. M., & Westen, B. A. (1993). A survey of 636 staff nurses: Perceptions and factors influencing the CNS role. *Clinical Nurse Specialist, 7*(3), 122-128.

Office of Technology Assessment. (1986). *Nurse practitioners, physicians' assistants and certified nurse midwives: A policy analysis* (HCS 37). Washington, DC: U.S. Congress.

Oleske, D. M., & Hauck, W. W. (1988). A population based evaluation of the impact of interventions for improving care to cancer patients in home settings. *Home Health Services Quarterly, 9,* 45-61.

Orient, J. M., Kettel, L. J., Sox, H. C., Jr., Sox, C. H., Berggren, H. J., Woods, A. H., Brown, B. W., & Lebowitz, M. (1983). The effect of algorithms on the cost and quality of patient care. *Medical Care, 21,* 157-167.

Pickwell, S. M. (1989). The incorporation of family primary care for southeast Asian refugees in a community-based mental health facility. *Archives of Psychiatric Nursing, 3*(3), 173-177.

Powers, M. J., Jalowiec, A., & Reichelt, P. A. (1984). Nurse practitioner and physician care compared for nonurgent emergency room patients. *Nurse Practitioner, 9*(2), 39, 42, 44-45.

Pozen, M. W., Stechmiller, J. A., Harris, W., Smith, S., Fried, D. D., & Voigt, G. C. (1977). A nurse rehabilitator's impact on patients with myocardial infarction. *Medical Care, 15,* 830-837.

Ramsey, P., Edwards, J., Lenz, C., Odom, J. E., & Brown, B. (1993). Types of health problems and satisfaction with services in a rural nurse-managed clinic. *Journal of Community Health Nursing, 10*(3), 161-170.

Reid, M. L., & Morris, J. B. (1979). Prenatal care and cost effectiveness: Changes in health care expenditures and birth outcome following the establishment of a nurse-midwifery program. *Medical Care, 17,* 491-500.

Repicky, P. A., Mendenhall, R. C., & Neville, R. E. (1980). Professional activities of nurse practitioners in adult ambulatory care settings. *Nurse Practitioner, 5*(2), 27, 31, 33-34.

Robichaud, A. M., & Hamric, A. B. (1986). Time documentation of clinical nurse specialist activi-

ties. *Journal of Nursing Administration, 16*(1), 31-36.

Rogers, T., Metzger, L., & Bauman, L. (1984). Common concern. Geriatric nurse practitioners: How are they doing? *Geriatric Nursing, 5*(1), 51-54.

Salkever, D. S., Skinner, E. A., Steinwachs, D. M., & Katz, H. (1982). Episode based efficiency comparisons for physicians and nurse practitioners. *Medical Care, 20,* 143-153.

Sampselle, C. M., Peterson, B. A., Murtland, T. L., & Oakley, D. J. (1992). Prevalence of abuse among pregnant women choosing certified nurse-midwife or physician providers. *Journal of Nurse-Midwifery, 37*(4), 269-273.

Schultz, J. M., Liptak, G. S., & Fioravanti, J. (1994). Nurse practitioners' effectiveness in NICU. *Nursing Management, 25*(10), 50-53.

Scupholme, A., DeJoseph, J., Strobino, D. M., & Paine, L. L. (1992). Nurse-midwifery care to vulnerable populations, Phase I: Demographic characteristics of the national CNM sample. *Journal of Nurse-Midwifery, 37*(5), 341-348.

Scupholme, A., Paine, L. L., Lang, J. M., Kumar, S., & DeJoseph, J. (1994). Time associated with components of clinical services rendered by nurse-midwives: Sample data from Phase II of nurse-midwifery care to vulnerable populations in the United States. *Journal of Nurse-Midwifery, 39*(1), 5-12.

Shamansky, S. L. (1985). Nurse practitioners and primary care research: Promises and pitfalls. *Annual Review of Nursing Research, 3,* 107-125.

Shaughnessy, P., Kramer, A., & Little, D. (1990). *The teaching nursing home experiment: Its effects and limitations* (Study Paper 6). Boulder: Center for Health Services Research, University of Colorado.

Smith, J. E., & Waltman, N. L. (1994). Oncology clinical nurse specialists' perceptions of their influence on patient outcomes. *Oncology Nurse Forum, 21*(5), 887-893.

Spisso, J., O'Callaghan, C., McKennan, M., & Holcroft, J. W. (1990). Improved quality of care and reduction of house staff workload using trauma nurse practitioners. *Journal of Trauma, 30,* 660-663.

Spitzer, W. O., Sackett, D. L., Sibley, J. C., Roberts, R. S., Gent, M., Kergin, D. L., Hackett, B. C., Olynich, A., Hay, W. I., & Lefroy, J., et al. (1990). 1965-1990: 25th anniversary of nurse practitioners. A classic manuscript reprinted in celebration of 25 years of progress: The Burlington randomized trial of the nurse practitioner, 1971-1972. *Journal of the American Academy of Nurse Practitioners, 2*(3), 93-99.

Sterling, Y. M., Noto, E. C., & Bowen, M. R. (1994). Case management roles of clinicians: A research case study. *Clinical Nurse Specialist, 8*(4), 195-207.

Tri, D. L. (1991). The relationship between primary health care practitioners' job satisfaction and characteristics of their practice settings. *Nurse Practitioner, 16*(5), 46, 49-52, 55.

Trotter, C., & Danaher, R. (1994). Neonatal nurse practitioners: A descriptive evaluation of an advanced practice role. *Neonatal Network, 13*(1), 39-47.

Van Cott, M. L., Tittle, M. B., Moody, L. E., & Wilson, M. E. (1991). Analysis of a decade of critical care nursing practice research: 1979 to 1988. *Heart and Lung, 20,* 394-397.

Ward, C., & Dracup, K. (1995). Identifying patients appropriate for nurse-managed ICUs. *American Journal of Critical Care, 4,* 255.

Weilitz, P. B., & Potter, P. A. (1993). A managed care system: Financial and clinical evaluation. *Journal of Nursing Administration, 23*(11), 51-57.

Weinberg, R. M., Liljestrand, J. S., & Moore, S. (1983). Inpatient management by a nurse practitioner: Effectiveness in a rehabilitation setting. *Archives of Physical Medicine and Rehabilitation, 64,* 588-590.

Wright, S. W., Erwin, T. L., Blanton, D. M., & Covington, C. M. (1992). Fast track in the emergency department: A one-year experience with nurse practitioners. *Journal of Emergency Medical Care, 10,* 367-373.

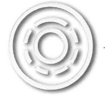

C H A P T E R   2 6

Innovative Practice Models

UNITING ADVANCED NURSING PRACTICE AND EDUCATION

· D I A N A   T A Y L O R
· L U C Y   M A R I O N

INTRODUCTION

From the time that nursing education transitioned to the university setting, there has
been a concern that education must be clearly linked with practice. Faculty practice,
as a component of advanced nursing practice, has developed as a link between

795

education and practice. The challenge for advanced practice nurse (APN) faculty has been and continues to be finding ways to link scholarship with expert clinical practice. In the rapidly changing health care environment, practice-education partnerships may provide advanced nursing practice with the best approach to solutions for both practice and education. Faculty practice may reverse the trend of moving the most knowledgeable APNs away from the patient or the practice setting while providing opportunities for testing nursing theory, developing innovative practices, and exploring research questions.

This chapter summarizes the historical development of practice-education partnerships, provides a definition of faculty practice based on existing research and practice, describes the current state of practice by APN faculties, describes existing practice-education models, and proposes future directions, challenges, and strategies for partnerships between advanced nursing practice and education. Although this chapter is limited to the discussion of "practice" by APN faculty, the domain of faculty practice is clearly more than clinical practice by nurse educators. This chapter focuses on the multiple components of faculty practice by APNs—education, research, administration, and clinical practice—and the collaborative models between APN faculty and practicing APNs that strengthens practice, integrates clinical scholarship, and improves the education of future APNs.

THE PAST: HISTORICAL PERSPECTIVES ON DEVELOPING PRACTICE IN NURSING EDUCATION

Faculty practice was a non-issue in the early days of nursing education because the educator was the practitioner. During the era of diploma schools, nurse training was conducted in the hospital. Although theory classes may have been taught by nurses with specialized knowledge, most clinical expertise was gained from nurses who cared for patients. The head nurse usually functioned as the main source of clinical teaching.

Over time, nurse "training" transitioned into nursing "education" where the teaching center shifted from the hospital to educational institutions (Christy, 1980; Mauksch, 1980b). With the growth of baccalaureate programs, nursing faculty became increasingly focused on education for themselves and their students. Practice, although important, played a secondary role. In the world of academia, advanced degrees and research, not clinical proficiency, were of primary importance. Although educators were concerned about the declining influence of practice on nursing education and vice versa, the distance between education and service widened.

The expansion of clinical nurse specialist (CNS) roles in the 1960s and the advent of nurse practitioner (NP) roles in the 1970s may have stimulated nursing educators to re-examine more seriously the significance of practice. Much of the early clinical education for certified registered nurse anesthetists (CRNAs), certified nurse-midwives (CNMs), and NPs was supervised by physicians. As ANP education moved to the graduate level, there was a need for nurse educators to become expert practitioners. Advanced practice certification required a practice component, which also established practice as a legitimate faculty role. However, this clinical role developed slowly within graduate education (Table 26–1).

The first attempt to unite nursing service and nursing education, which provided the basis for the early faculty practice models, occurred in 1956. Dorothy Smith,

TABLE 26-1	HISTORY OF FACULTY PRACTICE DEVELOPMENT
YEAR	**HISTORICAL EVENT**
1956	First nursing education/service unification model at University of Florida
1961	Academic-Service Collaboration model at Case Western Reserve University
1970	Unification model expansion at Rush University and University of Rochester
1979	American Academy of Nursing (AAN) Resolution in support of faculty practice
1985	AAN/Robert Wood Johnson Foundation–supported faculty practice symposium
1993	National Organization of Nurse Practitioner Faculties publication: *Nursing Faculty Practice—Models and Methods* (Potash & Taylor, 1993)
1993–1995	American Association of Colleges of Nursing symposia on advancing faculty practice
1997	National Organization of Nurse Practitioner Faculties publication: *Nursing Faculty Practice: Applying the Models* (Marion, 1997)

Dean of the School of Nursing at the University of Florida and the Director of Nursing Service at the University Hospital, envisioned an education-service structure that would provide a demonstration of the intellectual nature of clinical nursing, support nursing education within nursing service, develop nursing systems that crossed education and service, and guarantee faculty practice (Fagin, 1986). With Dorothy Smith as the administrator of both nursing education and nursing service, the faculty taught students and provided patient care within their faculty role.

In 1961, Rozella Schlotfeldt, using a different model at Case Western Reserve University, developed an "academic-service collaboration" system for uniting education and service. This collaborative model formalized collaboration between faculty and clinicians through joint appointments. Instead of one person simultaneously holding positions at both the school and the clinical agency, a faculty member's prime responsibilities were with the school, along with an appointment within the clinical area. Although the administrations of the school and the clinical area were separate, some of the salary costs were shared. Case Western Reserve University's standards of academic leadership and practice collaboration have influenced many current methods for faculty clinician appointments (Fagin, 1985).

In the early 1970s, Luther Christman, Dean of the College of Nursing at Rush-Presbyterian University, and Loretta Ford, Dean of the School of Nursing at the University of Rochester, developed an organizational structure, generally known as the "unification" model, that unified administration of the clinical agency and the school of nursing (Christman, 1982). The unification model of faculty practice was an organizational innovation whose primary purpose was to improve the relationship between nursing service and nursing education. In the unification model, all levels of faculty served jointly as clinicians and educators, and the Dean of the School of Nursing assumed authority and accountability in nursing education, nursing practice, and nursing research, demonstrating that clinical expertise by nursing faculty members can unite nursing service and nursing education (Grace, 1981).

These two examples of nursing education-service unification were important for providing legitimacy to faculty practice, demonstrating nursing autonomy as well as interdisciplinary collaboration, and attaining national and political support for nursing services (DeLeon, 1994; Fagin, 1986). Data show that, although these models have not been widely replicated because of an overemphasis on merger and unification and too little focus on the practice partnerships, they have reduced the existing education-practice gap (Andreoli, 1993; Gresham-Kenton, 1989). More importantly, these early models provided the impetus for the development of a wide variety of practice-education endeavors. Throughout the 1970s, nursing faculties attempted to institutionalize practice within the academic system using a variety of organizational structures (Barnard, 1983; Barnard & Smith, 1985).

In 1979, the American Academy of Nursing supported faculty practice through the passage of a resolution (American Academy of Nursing, 1980). With support from the Robert Wood Johnson Foundation, the Academy sponsored four symposia that have continued to provide the knowledge base for the development and implementation of faculty practice. In these symposia on faculty practice, nursing leaders provided important perspectives on the role of faculty practice in nursing education. Mauksch (1980b) proposed that nursing practice is an essential component of the role of the nurse educator if one is to keep the respect of other health professionals, improve communication with students, and increase realism in the classroom. According to Mauksch, nursing service also accrues benefits from faculty practice. Students are prepared to enter institutional practice, nursing staff profit from increased exposure to new knowledge and new ideas for patient care, educators have increased knowledge of the nursing care delivery system, and the potential exists for greater mutual respect between clinicians and educators. All of these factors contribute to the advancement of the nursing profession.

During the 1980s, nursing faculty experimented with multiple strategies for integrating practice and education roles. Collaborative arrangements developed between individual faculty and practitioners independent of structural or organizational changes (Fagin, 1986; Mauksch, 1980a). An "integrated model" in which faculty and graduate students shared patient care responsibilities was developed at Pennsylvania State University and the University of Wisconsin–Milwaukee (Stainton, 1989). At multiple locations nationwide, CNS faculty were influential in the development of "collaborative models" in which CNSs provided the links between hospital-based nursing service and nursing education. The focus was on collaboration at the level of the APN (communication, consultation) and at the level of the organization (organizational consent and policy) (Styles, 1984). Another example, a "partnership model" of faculty practice, was implemented at the University of Pennsylvania, incorporating clinical and educational excellence, research and scholarship, and professional empowerment as broadly defined faculty practice goals (Fagin, 1986). Structural changes within the School of Nursing allowed clinicians (CNM, CNS, and NP roles) to advance within the academic system. The addition of a formalized academic appointment track for the clinical professor allowed for promotion and advancement for the clinically expert nurse educator. Common to these integrated or partnership models is the focus on redesigning faculty roles rather than redesigning the organization in order to link advanced nursing practice and education.

Also in the 1980s, the federal government, through the funding programs administered by the Division of Nursing in the Health Resources Services Administration (HRSA), supported faculty practice projects. The "Special Projects" program allowed the Division of Nursing to support the development and implementation of clinical practice innovations that were linked with the nurse practitioner/nurse-midwifery training and advanced nursing practice training programs (HRSA, Division of Nursing, 1998).

By the early 1990s, descriptions of faculty practice models, issues, and debates were published widely. In spite of a lack of consensus about its definition, purposes, or implementation, faculty practice remains the prevailing method for uniting practice and education. ANP educators were searching for ways to integrate practice into their teaching and research roles because of ethical, professional, regulatory, and academic requirements. New partnerships and links with community agencies, church groups, school-based clinics, and health care delivery systems have been formed for APN faculty research and practice. One approach, called "reintegration," was proposed by a group of clinician-educators (Langford et al., 1987). An expansion of the "unification model" of nursing education and nursing practice, "reintegration" was the predecessor for new practice-education partnerships. Moving away from the earlier structural changes proposed by unification model approaches, reintegration focused on the processes of practice-education integration through synthesis of clinical practice, educative function, scholarly activity, and community and institutional service.

Another model for linking practice and education was described as an "entrepreneurial model" (Potash & Taylor, 1993) in which faculty design their practice, determine their goals and objectives, and provide client services as part of their faculty duties. In the entrepreneurial model, faculty may utilize the practice as a teaching site, a research site, or both; frequently they are paid for their services for direct patient care, consultancy, or technical assistance. These arrangements permit many variations in services, client population, setting, business arrangements, and outcomes. A few schools of nursing have emerged as leaders in promoting this entrepreneurial model of faculty practice and are described later in this chapter. An entrepreneurial approach to faculty practice shifts the focus from an education-service orientation to a business model in which resources are assessed, resources are matched to goals, and outcomes are evaluated (Walker, 1993). Business principles combined with educational goals can be directed toward advancing nursing education, nursing practice, and nursing research, especially those involved with health-related interventions, costs, and patient outcomes. Currently, the American Association of Colleges of Nursing (AACN) continues to support the development of practice-education activities and innovations through annual symposia for faculty development.

By the year 2000, almost 50 years after Dean Dorothy Smith pioneered the first model to link nursing practice with nursing education, integration may occur through flexible partnerships that are based on population needs and health professional education planning. During the next decade, nursing education will continue to develop or expand faculty practice as an important component of both education and research missions. ANP faculty, in collaboration with their practice partners, will continue to provide the leadership.

THE PRESENT: EVOLUTION OF FACULTY PRACTICE AND ADVANCED NURSING PRACTICE-EDUCATION MODELS

Academic nursing became three dimensional, with important substance, where instruction and research were joined by a third peer—faculty practice.

Mary Mundinger (1997, p. 63)

Current Status and Definitions of Faculty Practice

In an applied discipline, faculty practice consists of faculty "doing" what the teacher-practitioner teaches others to do. In the context of nursing, practice connotes the focus and intent to study, improve, and master both the substance and the process of delivering nursing care (McClure, 1987). Historically, definitions of faculty practice have been numerous and diverse. Durand (1985) claimed, "faculty practice means the practice of nursing as performed by faculty in the context of being faculty" (p. 38). Joel (1983) defined faculty practice as "direct or indirect involvement in provision of service [by nursing faculty] to the consumer" (p. 49) and believed that faculty practice must be scholarly and result in publication. Although provision of care to clients is often the central focus of faculty practice, "moonlighting," defined as working after hours for pay, is not considered faculty practice by most schools of nursing (Nugent, Barger, & Bridges, 1993). In contrast, Anderson and Pierson (1983) maintained that faculty practice should be an addition to the expected teaching role accomplished through joint appointment, moonlighting, or summer employment (p. 9). A 1993 survey of selected members of the National Organization of Nurse Practitioner Faculties (NONPF) (Potash & Taylor, 1993) concluded that the definition of faculty practice should include multiple roles (consultant, researcher, administrator, and clinician), in multiple settings (clinics, hospitals, home care), and using multiple structural and economic models (entrepreneurial, volunteer, joint practice).

Faculty practice by APNs is scholarly-based professional activity: the provision or facilitation of the delivery of nursing care through advanced behaviors of research, mentoring, leadership, collaboration, and direct patient care that encompasses patient outcomes as well as scholarship and student learning. On one level, faculty practice has the good of the faculty and its students as its prime concern, offering an area in which faculty members can maintain their clinical expertise and identity as nurses. On another level, faculty practice functions primarily for the good of the profession and of the recipients of nursing care; furthermore, activities resulting in research and publication both enhance the profession and ultimately improve patient care.

A review of faculty practice definitions from five schools of nursing (Oregon Health Sciences University, the University of California–San Francisco, the University of Colorado Health Sciences Center, the University of Oklahoma, and the University of Texas–Houston) at which most faculty practitioners function as APNs, yields the following composite definition of faculty practice:

> Faculty practice includes all aspects of the delivery of health care through the roles of clinician, educator, researcher, consultant, and administrator. Faculty practice activities within this framework encompass direct nursing services to individuals and groups, as well as technical assistance and consultation to individuals, families, groups, and communities. In addition to the provision of service, practice provides opportunities for promotion, tenure, merit, and revenue generation. A distinguishing characteristic of faculty practice within the School of Nursing is the belief that teaching, research, practice, and service must be closely integrated to achieve excellence. Faculty practice provides the vehicle through which faculty implement these missions. There is an assumption that student practica and residencies as well as research opportunities for faculty and students are an established component of faculty practice.

Clinical faculty practice by the APN is the direct (or indirect) nursing of individuals, groups, and families. Direct clinical practice includes services directed toward individuals, families, and groups whether in primary, secondary, or tertiary settings. Indirect clinical practice includes the provision of consultation services or technical assistance (e.g., a geriatric consultation service for elderly clients and their families, consultation for a pediatric pain management clinic, or a diabetes consultation service). The general faculty practice definition extends beyond APN practices. It encompasses other specialized roles as well (e.g., educator, administrator, or researcher). The practice role of the educator (other than student teaching) may be in curriculum consultation, program development and evaluation, or provision of continuing education activities (e.g., summer institutes, professional training). Administrative faculty practice may include the formation of a consultation practice in which faculty provide technical assistance to health care organizations. The practice role of the nurse researcher, aside from direct scientific investigation, might include consultation to health care organizations for the supervision of clinical nursing research projects. It is important to understand that these roles are not advanced nursing practice as defined in Chapter 3.

Research on Faculty Practice

Regardless of how narrow or broad the definition of faculty practice, many schools of nursing have institutionalized some form of practice in education. Generally, studies of faculty practice by university nursing faculty suggest that practice is an important component of their educator role. Various authors discuss benefits assumed to be associated with faculty practice (Herr, 1989; Just, Adams, & DeYoung, 1989; Kramer, Polifroni, & Organek, 1986; Millonig, 1986; Pohl, 1999). A study of 55 schools of nursing with active faculty practice programs described four major benefits of faculty practice. For the schools surveyed, faculty practice benefits included (1) enhanced learning experiences for students, (2) initiation of clinical research projects, (3) higher faculty satisfaction, and (4) a solution for clinical learning site shortages (Maurin, 1986).

In a 1989 survey of 909 nursing educators (about half were APNs), 94% reported "skill maintenance" as the primary reason for faculty practice; they also reported personal satisfaction, improved credibility, and financial reasons for developing practice as part of their educator role (Just et al., 1989). In a 1999 survey of 453 APN faculty (70% doctorally prepared) conducted by the NONPF, 50% ranked maintaining clinical skills as the most important reason for faculty practice, followed by personal/pleasure (37%), student education (28%), and maintaining certification (32%). Only 18% ranked promotion and 23% ranked salary supplementation as the most important reason for practice (Pohl, 1999).

Specific practice competencies identified as important by university-level faculty include demonstration of expertise in a specialized area of clinical nursing, use of research findings in the practice of nursing to improve client health, and provision of theory-based nursing practice.

In general, faculty practice has been thought to enhance teaching, improve the quality of patient care, improve the credibility of nursing education, maintain clinical skills, and generate research opportunities. Although most descriptive surveys report the benefits of faculty practice, little objective evidence exists about patient, professional, or organizational outcomes related to faculty practice. More recently, research has focused on client/patient outcomes. Frenn, Lundeen, Martin, Riesch, and Wilson (1996) summarized the positive outcomes from nursing centers, such as improved client health behaviors, improved health status, client satisfaction, cost-effectiveness, and quality of care. At the level of the organization, faculty practice appears to improve the relationship between nursing service and nursing education. As collaborative models of interdisciplinary practice develop within practice-education partnerships, it is assumed that benefits of team practice will extend to both patients and clinicians (Henry, 1997). Extending these benefits to the nursing profession, faculty practice also appears to contribute to the advancement of the profession by ensuring that highly prepared graduates enter the workforce, by improving nursing practice through research, and by increasing mutual respect between educators and clinicians that contributes to the advancement of the profession. When data from large samples demonstrate that measurable outcomes, such as improved curricula development, enhanced patient outcomes, or increased clinical research, are strongly correlated with practice, much of the current ambiguity surrounding benefits will be resolved.

Current Advanced Nursing Practice-Education Models

Since the inception of the "unification" model of faculty practice, in which nursing educators linked with hospital-based nurses, new models of linking nursing practice and nursing education have been developed. Most of these faculty practice models have been developed by APN faculty and are vital to the education of APNs. Faculty practice models can be described by *structural types* (nursing centers, joint appointments, faculty development), by *faculty roles* (teacher, practitioner, administrator, consultant roles), by *specialty practice* (community health, elder care, primary care, school health, midwifery services, anesthesia services, symptom management), or by *administrative aspects* of faculty practice (volunteer model, collaborative arrangements, revenue generating, contractual model) (Table 26–2). Certainly, some of these typologies will overlap in any one faculty practice. For example, midwifery faculty may implement a birth center using a revenue-generating reimbursement system in their role of practitioner-educator. CNS faculty may collaborate or contract with an oncology service to provide cancer treatment symptom management. Community health faculty and NP faculty may collaborate to provide health services to a homeless shelter on a contractual or volunteer basis.

This section describes a variety of different types of faculty practices. All of these faculty practices are implemented by APNs (CNMs, CNSs, CRNAs, and NPs). Although the following examples represent multiple roles, types of practice arrangements, and practice specialties, there are similarities among all of them that demonstrate the importance of faculty practice in the development and education of APNs. Discussion is limited to direct and indirect clinical practice by APN faculty, although faculty practice roles of educator, researcher, and administrator are also outlined in Table 26–2. Examples of a faculty development model have been described by Wandel (1991) and Turner and Pearson (1989). Faculty practice by researchers and administrators has been commonly implemented as technical assistance to health care organizations (Campbell & King, 1992; Donnelly, Warfel, & Wolf, 1994; Potash & Taylor, 1993).

UNIFICATION MODEL OF FACULTY PRACTICE: IMPLEMENTING THE
PRACTITIONER-TEACHER ROLE

Luther Christman's unification model of faculty practice has been modified (Andreoli, 1993) at Rush-Presbyterian University (Chicago), where one of the first models of merging service and education was implemented. Faculty are involved in patient care activities, staff development, consultation, patient education, hospital committees, clinical management, and clinical research. In this modified unification model, teacher-practitioners provide indirect patient care for 40 weeks of each year while

TABLE 26-2 FACULTY PRACTICE MODELS FOR ADVANCED NURSING PRACTICE

STRUCTURAL TYPES	APN FACULTY ROLES	SPECIALTY PRACTICE	ADMINISTRATIVE TYPE
Faculty development	Clinician, researcher, administrator	All specialties; all APN roles	Volunteer, contracts, joint appointments
Technical assistance & consultation	Administrator, researcher	Hospital, long-term care, community institutions; outcome research, research utilization; CNS, nurse administrators	Contracts, joint appointments, joint ventures, volunteer
Clinical consultancy	Clinician, educator	All specialties—usually hospital or institution based; CNS, CRNA	Joint appointments, contracts
Clinical/summer camp health services	Clinician, educator, administrator, researcher	Child/adolescent health, rehabilitation, chronic disease; CNS, NP	Contracts, research grant support
Institution-based services • Hospital • Long-term care	Clinician, administrator, researcher	Midwifery, oncology, ambulatory care, anesthesia, child/adult chronic disease management; CNS, CNM, CRNA, some NPs	Contracts, joint appointments, other collaborative arrangements
Case management services	Clinician	Home health, community health, oncology, symptom management, perinatal, neonatal; CNS, some NPs	Contracts, nursing centers, joint ventures, joint appointments
Community-based services • Wellness • Mental health • Homeless clinics	Clinician, administrator, researcher	Community health, primary care, underserved populations, homeless health clinics; CNS, CNM, NP	Grant supported, contracts, volunteer
Nursing centers	Clinician, administrator, researcher	Wellness, geriatric, rural, student health, midwifery, community health; all APN roles	Contracts, school owned, joint ventures, grant supported

supervising undergraduate students and provide direct care during school breaks, on holidays, and during nursing shortage periods. Faculty are active in patient-related clinical conferences and participate in team decision making about patient care. In the consultant role, the teacher-practitioner consults with staff nurses and physicians in an area of expertise (e.g., skin problems, incontinence, pain, ethical decision making, acquired immunodeficiency syndrome [AIDS] complications). Other consultation activities include the development of patient teaching aids; development of a new patient-centered model of care with associated technology and reorganization; and creation of clinical pathways for decreasing length of stay, decreasing costs, and improving quality of care. The practitioner-teacher is also involved with management activities, such as working with unit leadership in staff meetings, chart audits, new staff orientation, and staff performance appraisals. Committee membership for the practitioner-teacher might also include review of accreditation criteria, standards of practice, nursing care evaluation, new products, and discharge planning procedures.

The multiple roles of the teacher-practitioner in the unification model suggests a high workload, no matter how integrated these roles. In addition, the nonclinical activities of the teacher-practitioner emphasize institutional service unrelated to education (staff development, medical center committees). It is unclear how educational issues, such as curriculum development, are managed by the teacher-practitioner in this unification model. However, this faculty practice model can inform education about ways to reduce unnecessary workload on the education side of the teacher-practitioner responsibility. Although an early model of faculty practice, the unification model may provide a model for faculty practice implementation in an integrated managed care environment of the future.

CONSULTANCY AS FACULTY PRACTICE—CLINICAL AND EDUCATIONAL

This model of faculty practice is most often implemented by CNS faculty through contractual arrangements or joint appointments to nursing staff or health care agencies. CRNAs often assume the role of consultant to nursing staff for pain management support. Polifroni and Schmalenberg (1985) described activities of faculty clinical consultants as *direct patient care* (assumes responsibility for specific aspects of patient care), *role modeling* (paired with staff nurses to assess difficulties or demonstrate new or different ways of proceeding with care), *staff development* (patient assessment, problem-oriented records, peer review, teaching and learning projects), *administrative projects* (new forms, standards of care, flow sheets in critical care units), *information resource* (source of current information for staff), and *nurse manager support* (managerial and clinical matters). The faculty member functions as a resource person on the average of 1 day per week in giving nursing care and consulting with nursing staff or working collaboratively with nursing administration.

A faculty practice program at the Texas Tech University Health Sciences Center School of Nursing includes the provision of nursing continuing education and staff development (Miller, 1997). In 1982, the School of Nursing faculty initiated the "Personal Order Service" whereby, through contractual agreements, courses were specifically designed and taught on-site for hospitals and other health care agencies in rural Texas. The educational offerings reflect varied needs. Some relate to issues of leadership and management; others are more clinically focused. In some cases, a faculty member provides ongoing consultation to staff and administrators. Fees are negotiated on a total cost recovery basis through individualized contracts.

CLINICAL CAMPS OR SUMMER CAMP HEALTH SERVICES

Both NP and CNS-prepared faculty have developed faculty practices at clinical and summer camps for healthy children and adolescents, adolescents with chronic diseases, and adults with developmental disabilities and mental illness (Aroian & Rauckhorst, 1985; Arthur & Usher, 1994). The primary purpose of these faculty practices is the maintenance of clinical skills. These faculty practices are often developed using contractual arrangements for summer funding for faculty on 9-month appointments. In addition to salary augmentation, these summer faculty practices provide autonomy, time flexibility, and the ability to develop nurse-initiated interventions. Some faculties have also included student participation and the development of research projects.

INSTITUTION-BASED FACULTY PRACTICE IN HOSPITALS

Faculty at the University of Virginia School of Nursing developed an inpatient oncology and geriatric rehabilitation unit where they provided direct patient care as part of their faculty role (Lee, Levy, Dix, & Tatum, 1987). Noted benefits of this faculty practice to advanced nursing practice were described in a number of ways. First, this faculty practice served as an experimental model in an inpatient hospital. Second, it provided clinical experience for APN students in a nurse-directed environment. Third, the faculty practice provided an opportunity for collaborative clinical research between faculty and staff nurses. Administratively, this project was a joint venture between the school of nursing and nursing service. Faculty practitioners were in nontenure track, 12-month positions that were funded jointly by the two institutions.

Gresham-Kenton (1989) described collaborative models of CNS practice that implemented a variety of collaborative methods between hospital-based nursing service and nursing education. These models illustrate a corporate approach in which initial decision making occurs at the level of nursing dean, director, or vice president. Successful implementation depends on the CNS in a practitioner-teacher role. Some of these arrangements have included an exchange of resources or shared funding. Examples of successful collaborative models include an inpatient and home-care pediatric service in Colorado and a Teaching Nursing Home Project in New Jersey.

Many nurse anesthesia faculty practices are integrated into hospital-based anesthesiology departments in which CRNA faculty contract to provide a portion of the anesthesia services along with supervision of students. Some CRNA faculties have joined as small faculty practice groups and contract as a group; other CRNA faculty act as independent contractors in a part-time faculty-practitioner role. At the University of Tennessee–Memphis School of Nursing, CRNA faculties have full-time faculty appointments in the School of Nursing but the hospital reimburses the school for the CRNA faculty clinical services (R. Lester, personal communication, 1995). Because most CRNA training programs are situated in schools of medicine or schools of allied health, CRNA faculty practice development has been limited. However, a few CRNA faculties have included practice as a part of their faculty appointment. For example, at the University of Alabama–Birmingham, CRNA faculty practice in hospital sites for at least 1 day each week, and the hospital reimburses the CRNA program, which supplements the CRNA faculty salary (J. Williams, personal communication, May, 1995).

Most CRNA faculties have part-time academic appointments and part-time clinical appointments, which allow CRNAs to supplement their academic salaries and combine their teaching role with their practice role. At Rush University in Chicago, where Luther Christman pioneered the "unification" model of practice-education, the roles of the chief nurse anesthetist and nurse anesthesia program director have been merged to create the role of the practitioner-teacher (M. Faut-Callahan & M. Kremer, personal communication, September, 1999). Over time, both of these leadership roles have become complex and demanding, with unique requirements that make role combination difficult. However, the faculty practice plans developed by CRNA practitioner-teachers have provided a model for delineating new role requirements to assist both the institution and the CRNA in balancing their workloads.

The CRNA faculty at the University of Alabama School of Health Related Professions has developed a salary supplement arrangement that allows CRNA faculty to supplement salaries with clinical revenues in the same way that nonclinical faculty supplement salaries with research grants (J. Williams, personal communication, May 1995). CRNA faculty have full-time appointments in the university and, as part of their academic contract, are allowed 52 days per year for clinical practice. In addition, liberal vacation policies allow for additional clinical practice and approximately $20,000 per year of salary supplementation.

Nurse-midwifery faculties have developed multiple arrangements within hospital settings. Some CNM faculties have developed independent birth centers or birth centers associated with medical centers (see the later section, "Nursing Centers"). Other examples of CNM faculty practices include contractual arrangements between the school of nursing and a hospital for specific nurse-midwifery services (intrapartum services, resident/medical student teaching, pregnancy/postpartum care services). Joint appointments of CNM faculty shared between schools of medicine and nursing provide another alternative to the contractual arrangements, but the nurse faculty may have dual institutional requirements (see the discussion of the Yale University model under "The Business of Education-Practice Partnerships"). Still another arrangement used by CNM faculty involves the CNM being employed by (or contracting with) an obstetrics-gynecology faculty practice within a school of medicine but providing education primarily to medical students and residents and secondarily to nurses (Davis & Zatuchni, 1993).

INSTITUTION-BASED FACULTY PRACTICE IN LONG-TERM CARE FACILITIES

The teaching nursing home model of community-based practice, developed in the 1980s in response to the historical lack of research and training in long-term care, offers a synergy between education, research, and clinical care. With shifts of emphasis away from long-stay hospitalization for elderly people, the availability of clinical training for APNs to gain experience in caring for elderly people or those with chronic conditions has been reduced. The teaching nursing home as an academic-service partnership involving nursing and/or medicine in collaboration with a long-term care facility has been found to raise the profile of care of the elderly through a structure of joint appointments or contractual arrangements. A study undertaken to determine the enduring impact of the Teaching Nursing Home Project between 1982 and 1987 revealed that a structured school of nursing–nursing home affiliation could be a cost-effective association to improve the quality of resident care in nursing homes (Mezey, Mitty, & Bottrell, 1997). Research into the chronic disorders and specialist needs of the elderly has been found to increase through joint appointment arrangements in teaching nursing homes (Aiken, 1988). However, ethical issues must be considered in relation to the possibility of over-researching or overpracticing with a group of vulnerable individuals who may not be able to give adequate informed consent. The contractual model of faculty-service partnership in the teaching nursing home is similar to a consultation, where the faculty might identify and research practice problems and subsequently feed back new knowledge into both the service and educational system to improve teaching and promote better patient care. Secondary effects of a teaching nursing home model have been to raise the profile of the long-term care facility and to attract qualified and motivated staff who are interested in being part of an innovative project (Chilvers & Jones, 1997).

CASE MANAGEMENT AS FACULTY PRACTICE

The Loyola University Niehoff School of Nursing, in association with a university-affiliated home health agency, provides joint appointments to agency administrators and CNSs in the School of Nursing. APN students are assigned to the home health agency for learning experiences (Murray, Hackbarth, Sojka, & Swanston, 1987). In this joint venture, two faculty share a half-time CNS position at the home health agency, where 75% of their practice time is delegated for patient case management and 25% is delegated for administration, research, and fund-raising.

Stark, Walker, and Bohannan (1991) described an oncology case management example of faculty practice at The University of Texas Health Science Center–Houston School of Nursing. Doctorally-prepared faculties with specialization in clinical oncology nursing provide case management for a group of hospitalized cancer patients in a large teaching/research oncology center. Graduate nursing students work in collaboration with a faculty member who provides case management services, including symptom management during cancer treatments. Networking by the faculty member helps facilitate opportunities for student and staff nursing research. The School of Nursing provides administrative and contracting services for the individual faculty member, in this case a contract with oncology medical faculty for 50% of the nurse faculty's salary.

There are few examples of case management as faculty practice in the current literature; this area of advanced nursing practice is one of future development for nursing educators as well as an area that needs the attention of nursing centers operated by schools of nursing.

COMMUNITY-BASED FACULTY PRACTICES

Health Promotion and Wellness Services. As the changing focus of health care and nursing moves from the hospital to the community, nursing faculty are active in developing community-based health promotion programs in a variety of settings. These settings include work sites, senior centers, apartment complexes for elderly and handicapped individuals, and homes of individual clients and families. The role of the APN is that of educator, counselor, and coach. Nurses assist with realistic and priority goal setting, but responsibility and accountability for change remains with the clients. One innovative model combines community health APN faculty with health professions students to provide health promotion to employees on a university campus (White, 1999). The program, called Wellness Wednesdays, provides individualized health promotion assessment, guidance in goal setting and establishment of personal health promotion plans, follow-up, and community service coordination.

Another wellness-oriented faculty practice evolved from student intervention with small industries as part of their undergraduate community health nursing clinical experience (Wold & Williams, 1997). Advanced practice community health nursing faculty combine prevention-based clinical practice, professional training, and outcomes evaluation with APN-student teams. Students consistently rate this experience as very important to their "real-life" learning and application of health promotion principles and strategies. Research from this faculty practice has shown that previous student interventions had been statistically significant in reducing cardiovascular risk in employee groups. This faculty from Georgia State University in Atlanta is now marketing this concept to small industries as a cost-saving strategy for rural health services as well as clinical placement sites for students (Wold & Williams, 1997).

Mental Health Services. Psychiatric nursing faculty have a rich history of engaging in various community-based practice activities such as consultation, crisis intervention, psychosocial rehabilitation planning, case management, individual/group/family therapy, medication management, community outreach, and client-consumer advocacy (Richie et al., 1996). The mental health nursing faculty at Vanderbilt University School of Nursing offer a wide spectrum of mental health services and psychosocial rehabilitation in collaboration with primary care nursing faculty within a larger nurse-managed community clinic (Adams & Partee, 1998).

Homeless Shelter Clinics. Nursing has been in the forefront in the development of health service delivery within homeless shelters. Two examples of community-based APN faculty practice within homeless shelters are highlighted here. Kean College of New Jersey Department of Nursing developed a partnership with a homeless shelter in which faculty and students provide direct health and nursing services to homeless families (Campbell, 1993). The partnership allowed establishment of a site for interdisciplinary student learning and multidisciplinary faculty practice and research. Nursing faculty coordinated with other disciplines from Kean College, such as medical record administration, social work, sociology, psychology, public administration, and early childhood education faculty. Specific services that faculty and students provide to homeless families include family assessment, planning, and implementation of interventions, such as traditional health care services, parenting skills, how to access social service agencies, counseling to assist families in coping during the homeless crisis, and remediation or assistance with learning for children whose education has been interrupted. Unique to this faculty practice is the interdisciplinary student learning, in which students help organize and administer the shelter, set up and maintain records, locate and obtain funds, or train personnel to work with shelter residents alongside other professional graduate students. Benefits of this faculty practice are not limited to student experiences. Nursing faculty and students have access to actual service situations that future APNs must be able to manage, and opportunities to study and learn from actual service situations in order to remain current in practice. The faculty practice also benefits the homeless shelter by enabling the shelter to negotiate access to experts without incurring the expenses that usually accompany consultation. Collaboration in grant writing and access to the College Grants Office is another benefit.

Although the previous faculty practice was implemented by community health CNS faculty, two other faculty practices in homeless shelters have been implemented by NP faculty at State University of New York–Buffalo and the University of California–Los Angeles Schools of Nursing. In both of these settings, faculty and students provide primary care to homeless shelter residents. Funding for homeless shelter health services in these (and other) faculty practices is through public health contracts, university or federal grants, and faculty volunteers.

NURSING CENTERS

The previous examples of faculty practices were primarily models involving one to several faculties who have developed individual arrangements with an organization or agency external to the school of nursing. The nursing center owned or operated by a school of nursing is a more recent development of group faculty practice. Nursing centers are characterized by nurse management; nursing control of practice; direct access to nursing services; holistic, client-centered services; and reimbursement for services rendered (Riesch, 1992a, 1992b). Nursing centers may be community based, affiliated with hospitals or schools of nursing, or freestanding entrepreneurial centers; most are sponsored by nursing schools. According to a 1991 study by Barger, 51 nursing centers have been developed since 1985 and provide a wide variety of health-related services. Nursing centers have had a significant impact on the development of practice models in nursing. They have created opportunities for faculty to design nursing models of care that transcend the biomedical model of care to provide services to underserved groups (Norbeck & Taylor, 1998).

Phillips and Steele (1994) described the roles of APN faculty in nursing centers. CNS faculty have developed nursing centers focused on specialty care, such as cardiac care, oncology, premature birth prevention, and primary care or case management of people with chronic diseases (multiple sclerosis, AIDS). Nursing services by CNS faculty include symptom and treatment management, prevention of complications, and disability limitation. CNSs have expanded both the boundary and the dimension of their scope of practice in nursing centers (Davis-Doughty, 1989). NP faculty in nursing centers also deliver a wide variety of primary and specialty care services. Many of the services developed by NP faculty overlap with those of primary care physicians, such as primary care services to adolescents in group homes or acute and chronic disease management in ambulatory clinics. However, other NP faculty practices in nursing centers involve independent nursing interventions such as school health educational services, spiritual counseling services, and health promotion interventions. Nurse-midwifery faculties have developed freestanding birth centers or midwifery services as part of an existing faculty group practice. A few examples of nursing centers established by nursing faculty follow; they represent specialty or role-specific practice ventures as well as examples of innovative models of the integration of advanced nursing practice and education.

Nursing Centers for Older Adults. Hawkins, Igou, Johnson, and Utley (1984) described the development of the Wellness Center located in a senior center building, a joint venture of the Boston College School of Nursing and a small local township. The nursing center provided preventive health maintenance, early detection of disease, health maintenance for chronic conditions, and coordination of care with other professionals. The School of Nursing originally provided a full-time NP (or a full-time equivalent) and established a community advisory board. Multiple research projects were generated from the center, such as measurement of the cost-effectiveness of care, measurement of outcomes from interventions, description of clinical phenomena (incontinence), and the study of interdisciplinary team function. A federal grant funded by the Division of Nursing to expand services combined with Medicare reimbursement supported additional faculty.

At the University of Washington School of Nursing, a joint venture with a local developer resulted in the establishment of a faculty-operated long-term care facility, the Ida Culver House. A local developer, working with the School of Nursing, built a state-of-the-art senior living center and health care center. Faculty operate the health care facility, which provides a living laboratory for nursing research and student education experiences (H. Young, personal communication, 1998).

Rural Nursing Centers. Nursing faculty have developed nursing centers in rural communities that are directed to special populations such as migrant health outreach services, multiphase health screening for the elderly, and long-term care for people with hypertension. Many of these faculty practices are nursing centers without walls; faculty locate the centers in unique places such as grocery stores, laundromats, gas stations, cafes, churches, local school events, schools, and day care centers.

Faculty at the University of Texas–Galveston (Fenton, Rounds & Iha, 1988) developed a Community Nursing Center in a rural community. Community health nursing faculty and NP faculty jointly provide primary care and community nursing services in a rural Texas community. In addition to disease management and health promotion services, nursing faculty assess community needs, identify necessary resources, gain support of the community, and increase access to health care services. Services are provided in nontraditional ways through outreach activities. The nursing center is also used as a clearinghouse for government and private health organizations that can provide financial aid, assistance with disabilities and daily living, and transportation and case management. Faculty are also involved in fund-raising activities. Funds come from a combination of state and federal grants, insurance reimbursement, private foundation support, community resources, and local fund-raising.

Student Health Centers and School-Based Nursing Centers. NP-managed clinics have been particularly effective in providing cost-effective, quality primary care services, especially in college health settings, where NPs serve a dual role as providers and clinic managers (Hale, Harper, & Dawson, 1996). A few nursing schools have begun operating student health services using a nursing center model.

Since 1991, the George Mason University Student Health Center (SHC) has been a primary health care center directed by nursing faculty. The focus of care goes beyond simply managing current health care needs by emphasizing prevention of future health problems, wellness, and quality of life. In addition, this NP faculty-directed SHC offers a cost-effective, consumer-responsive alternative for delivering primary care services to the members of the university community.

Negotiations with surrounding specialists have resulted in a prompt and cost-effective referral system as needed by patients with conditions exceeding the capabilities of the SHC providers. Responses to student surveys regarding the quality, availability, and cost of care, as well as the process involved in receiving that care, indicate the highest level of satisfaction among students using these services. The SHC has a fertile, convenient faculty practice site as well as several clinical placements for NPs as well as undergraduate students.

The faculty at the University of Tennessee–Memphis operate the campus student health service, where students pay an annual fee at the time of registration and receive all of their primary care from nursing faculty. In addition to providing health services for students at the Memphis campus, the faculty contract with other schools for student care. The student health center is used by other APN faculty to evaluate nursing therapeutics and nursing practice models (examples are also found at the Pace University and California State University–Sonoma Schools of Nursing).

Many faculties are establishing nursing centers in elementary and high schools, especially in rural and inner-city schools, where children and adolescents have special health care needs. Similar to community nursing centers, these faculty practices are developed in collaboration with teachers and parents to meet the primary health care needs of the school-age child and adolescent. Most of these school-based nursing centers are funded by state or federal grants and staffed by CNS and NP faculty. Two nursing schools have developed school-based services administered by faculty traveling to various sites in a mobile van. CNS and NP faculty from San Francisco State University School of Nursing provide primary health care to inner-city high school students. In rural Mississippi, CNS and NP faculties from Alcorn State University provide similar services modified for school-age children and adolescents in rural communities. Gladstone School Center, a primary care clinic operated by Xavier University School of Nursing faculty, is located in an inner-city Chicago elementary school. All of these faculty practices provide nursing services to ethnic populations who are traditionally medically underserved.

Midwifery/Birthing Centers. Rather than focusing on the boundaries of obstetrical nursing practice within the medical model, CNMs have successfully built on a core of practice established through a long tradition and distinct philosophy that characterizes the dimensions of CNM practice. Many of these CNM faculty practices provide an interdisciplinary focus in which midwifery students are taught alongside medical and nursing students.

Most CNM faculty are involved in clinical practice as part of their faculty role. Administrative arrangements are usually contractual between the CNM faculty and a clinical agency external to the school of nursing, or through a primary appointment with a school of medicine. Although many midwifery/birth centers are in operation, only a few are functioning as faculty practices. A notable exception is the University of Utah School of Nursing, where CNM faculty own and operate a Family Birth Center (Amos, 1995; see also Chapter 17).

Community Nursing Centers. Community nursing centers are the outgrowth of public health nursing and are considered the contemporary version of 19th-century settlement houses (Henry, 1997). Although community nursing centers take many forms, their common mission is to expand access to nursing care to vulnerable and underserved populations. They may be freestanding clinics, institutionally based centers that draw their mission from their parent organization, wellness and health promotion centers, or centers founded for specific target populations (Dunn & Graves, 1996; Lockhart, 1995).

Hampton University School of Nursing in Virginia has operated a community health nursing center since 1984, providing primary care, health promotion, and family-centered care to a racially diverse patient population. Health promotion and wellness programs are provided at the nursing center and in the community. Faculty at the center integrate practice, teaching, and research. Undergraduate students are involved in community health projects, and NP students provide care under the supervision of faculty practitioners. Other nursing schools contract with the center to provide clinical experience for their graduate students. Clinical research conducted at the center includes description of cardiac risk factors for African American men and the impact of clinical interventions on patient outcomes. The center contracts with physicians and local laboratories for consultation and diagnostic services. The center provides health care to homeless shelter residents as well as family planning services through contractual arrangements with the local health department. Employee health services are provided to Hampton University employees through informal agreements established with university administration. Approximately 20% of the center budget is funded by patient revenues, with the remainder funded through grants and university resources (Potash & Taylor, 1993).

The Community Nursing Organization (CNO) of the School of Nursing at Virginia Commonwealth University, established in 1992 as a center without walls, implements faculty-student practice through a partnership with 16 community-based organizations. The CNO provides health care for partner agencies whose emphasis would otherwise be education and social services. The Homeless & At-Risk Project, one community-based partnership of the CNO, provides women and families with temporary care as they establish stability in their lives. Faculty and students provide primary health care, health promotion, screening, and education to homeless and at-risk women and children. Services are provided in shelters, day care settings, soup kitchens, and a free clinic (Henry, 1997).

One nursing center that combines primary care and mental health service, the Vine Hill Community Clinic of Vanderbilt University School of Nursing, is accepting third-party reimbursements, managed care capitation contracts, and sliding-scale self-pay after 8 years of grant funding (Adams & Partee, 1998). The primary care clinicians (NPs and students) are responsible for 4,000 capitated clients and serve an additional 1,000 clients as primary care providers. Chronic conditions (diabetes, hypertension, and depression) were found to be the most common primary diagnoses, followed by acute infections and gynecological problems. Primary mental health diagnoses include affective and anxiety disorders followed by schizophrenia. The mental health clinicians and students provide services to an active caseload of 250 clients, with students offering the benefit of extended, no-cost therapy. Educational outcomes are also linked with patient outcomes in this nurse-managed primary care practice. For example, increased APN student sensitivity to the stigma of mental illness through clinical learning activities was related to client's recovery.

THE FUTURE: NEW PRACTICE-EDUCATION MODELS

The growth of nursing centers, the necessary testing of outcomes of nurse-managed care in community-based settings, and the education of future APNs depend largely on collaborative efforts across education, practice, and research. Developing nursing centers as interdisciplinary and self-sustaining clinical, educational, and research service and training programs builds on Ernest Boyer's (1990) notions of academia as an interactive community that links education and service with common purposes and shared concerns. As integrated health service systems become the norm, academic nursing and nursing centers must consider partnerships that allow them to retain their unique characteristics. Academic nursing provides the structure for faculty with diverse interests to practice; it provides innovative learning experiences for students; and research models can be developed through active participation of community and clinical partners. With the dramatic changes in health care, models that are innovative and successful today may be inappropriate tomorrow. To effectively educate future practitioners, educators, and researchers, academic nursing in collaboration with clinical partners must continue to produce new models for nursing care.

New models of care delivery provide practice opportunities for APNs to provide community-based care as hospitals assume a smaller role in the delivery of care. Although education for community-based care traditionally has been at the baccalaureate level, all levels of nursing education must prepare graduates for out-of-hospital care. Increased emphasis on content related to the health of communities is essential for all APNs (Hall & Stevens, 1995; National Organization of Nurse Practitioner Faculties, 2000). Community assessment and education for health promotion and disease prevention will emerge as vital to reducing the long-term costs of health care. APNs will require knowledge of systems of care, finance, budgeting, and reimbursement. The legal parameters of practice are changing, with greater emphasis on practice guidelines and standards of care. These changes require greater skill in informatics and evaluation methods. Nursing centers can provide a setting for educating nurses in emerging models of community-based care and where students can acquire skills needed for leadership in community-based care.

Successful education-practice ventures are promoting nursing practice in the form of new, complementary, community-based alternatives that are responsive to patient needs. This care by nurses is based on measured outcomes and not simply used as a substitute for care by other providers. Differentiating a distinct scope of nursing practice that is separate but complementary to medicine will establish nursing centers as critical to a reformed health care system. These new models assume partnerships between education and service. New forms of research are being integrated into faculty practices, for the development of health policy research and for measurement of cost/quality outcomes. More importantly, new practice-education partnerships are being created to link socially responsible health care with institutional and professional goals.

Partnership Models—Linking Practice and Education Across Institutions and Communities

Partnerships, alliances, and coalitions, whether formal joint ventures or one-time collaborations, are forming worldwide among diverse organizations and constituencies. Partnerships, traditionally a corporate model, allow organizations to remain current as markets, technologies, resources, research, and information move quickly. However, participating groups can maintain their independence and identity and often gain wider acceptance and credibility than they can through isolated efforts. As collaborative education-practice models foster multidisciplinary approaches to the delivery of health care and health professional education, coalitions, alliances, and partnerships can provide new models of curricula for proactive, APN roles. Furthermore, they offer nurses the opportunity to establish partnerships with professionals from other disciplines, with community leaders, and with health care consumers.

Health coalitions are emerging as a force for change in many communities to promote more universal access to health care and to reflect the values of self-help, citizen participation, and community control (Gale, 1998). Faculty practice in the form of partnership with a community coalition can be a dynamic strategy for uniting nursing practice, education, and community. The Escalante ElderCARE Coalition was formed in 1991, with the Community Health Division of the Arizona State College of Nursing taking a leadership role. Since that time, more than 50 elder/senior networks and community agencies have become involved. More than $300,000 in grant funding has been awarded for Healthy WAY services with low-income seniors as health care and program partners. The conceptual model, Health WAY (*Wellness Activities with You*, not to you or for you), includes health promotion services, participation of community elders in program planning and evaluation, and education of health professionals. Participation theory is the basis for the conceptual model. A large number of undergraduate and graduate nursing students have been involved in the nontraditional delivery of services provided by the coalition. Both health status outcome measures and process indicators (elder satisfaction, coalition effectiveness, and cost-savings measures) provide the basis for evaluating the effectiveness of the coalition model.

The Linkages program, an expansion of the Community Nursing Organization (CNO) of the School of Nursing at Virginia Commonwealth University (described in the previous section), links service and learning for students in nursing, medicine, and the master's of public health (MPH) program (Henry, 1997). Faculty, students, community partners, and clients work and learn together to meet the needs of a particular community. All participants are involved in planning, implementation, and evaluation of the program. For example, nursing and MPH students work with a community agency providing case management services for high-risk women and their families. The nursing students provide direct care and coordinate their case management support with the nurses and lay workers of the agency. The MPH students complete their research courses in the agency working on evaluation of the outcomes of coordinated care. Everyone participates in reflection sessions, in which they discuss their experiences toward broader understanding of the differing contributions of each person. Expansion of this program now includes collaboration with the local Area Health Education Center (AHEC, a federally funded project) and extends health services available to vulnerable women and children as well as providing experienced clinical preceptors for student supervision.

At Columbia University in 1994, a partnership between the School of Nursing and the Columbia-Presbyterian Medical Center Ambulatory Care Network Corporation resulted in the establishment of an innovative model of practice-education collaboration. Called a cross-site model, NP faculty provide care for patients in both ambulatory and inpatient areas. This is the nation's first NP faculty practice with full hospital privileges in a major teaching hospital (Auerhahn, 1997). Two practice sites have been established: the Center for Advanced Practice, staffed by adult and pediatric NP faculty in an independent nurse-run clinic; and the Urban Family Practice Group, which uses a team approach with family NP faculty and family medicine physicians. Both sites provide all ages with 24-hour comprehensive primary care, such as screening, preventive services, counseling, and diagnosis and management of episodic and chronic health problems. These practices are unique in that the NP manages hospitalized patients, which provides continuity of care across sites. This practice-education partnership has extended the current faculty practice models in four directions: (1) the creation of a model that emphasizes continuity of care before, during, and after hospitalization; (2) cost containment through improved access to early preventive care, resulting in fewer hospitalizations and emergency room visits; (3) increased multidisciplinary practice, education, and research between the physician and nursing faculties; and (4) a greater emphasis on health promotion and education activities for patients (Mundinger, 1997). A study in JAMA that compared APN and physician care providers in this clinic showed comparable health status in patients with asthma, diabetes and hypertension and comparable patient satisfaction in patients cared for by NP faculty providers. (Mundinger, 2000).

An alliance for academic home care, a partnership between the University of Pennsylvania School of Nursing and the Visiting Nurse Association of Greater Philadelphia, is an innovative development in the emergence of academic-practice partnerships (Buhler-Wilkerson, Naylor, Holt & Rinke, 1998; Naylor & Buhler-Wilkerson, 1999). Their mission is to develop nurse-led, interdisciplinary, integrated, community-based delivery systems that are cost-effective, accessible, socially responsible, and reimbursable, and that provide quality care to vulnerable high-risk populations of all ages. Adapting the PACE program (Program for All-inclusive Care for the Elderly), an existing government-supported program for frail elders who wish to continue to live in their communities, the Penn Nursing Network home care alliance has implemented LIFE (Living Independently for Elders). When fully operational, the LIFE program will deliver a comprehensive and integrated health and social service package to approximately 250 frail elders living in West Philadelphia, consisting of two adult day health centers with 25 full- and part-time staff. The LIFE alliance goals include responsibility and accountability for health care quality, the assumption of full risk for both clinical and economic outcomes for the most vulnerable older adults within an identified community, and a commitment to social change. Unique to most health care systems, the LIFE program has proposed a set of educational and practice goals that clearly fit with community needs and values (Naylor & Buhler-Wilkerson, 1999). For example, it proposes to offer a mix of programs and services that match community need, respect local customs, are culturally relevant, and link effectively with mainstream health care. Furthermore, the program has attempted to link educational and research agendas to both partnership and community needs by proposing a research agenda characterized by rigorous measurement of individual, family, and societal benefits and costs as well as responsiveness to sponsors' pluralistic agendas. The program has been designed to support the education of student teams in the management of the complexities of community-based care. Goals are also directed to the health of the community by the development of a community-wide data networking and sharing initiative for the elder patient population.

Consultation and policy development are also extensions of community nursing center partnerships. Community nursing center staff and students can provide in-service education for the staff and volunteers of community partners, serve on advisory committees and boards, and participate in writing grant applications with partners. Such collaboration will reduce the competition that might arise if each agency were writing independent grants. Henry (1997) described examples of community nursing center consultation to community agencies. Faculty-student teams educate lay health workers and mothers receiving Medicaid assistance about the impact of managed cared on their health care practices, or provide education to uninsured children and their parents in health promotion skills to increase self-care capacity. Such collaboration enhances the projects of the partners, provides sites for faculty practice and research, and provides students with clinical experiences in innovative programs.

In addition, partnerships in clinical practice policy development can be an extension of community nursing centers. For example, in collaboration with state health departments and school divisions, faculty-student teams developed practice guidelines for school-age children with specialized health care needs (Henry, 1997). Through such collaboration, students develop skills at developing policy and procedure manuals that outline the legal parameters of practice. More than traditional clinical practice protocols, these collaborative practice policies can be used at the local school level to assure safe care for children with chronic health problems.

The Business of Education-Practice Partnerships

New and future education-practice models will depend on partnerships that link practice and research interests for faculty and enhance education of students while attending to the "business" of providing professional nursing services. Faculty practitioners need to be able to provide health care services in the same way that APNs outside the university milieu engage in fiscally sound practice. University-community health care partnerships that allow for billable services are necessary to provide funds for salaries and day-to-day operating costs. Both entrepreneurial and intrepreneurial models can be used to unite education, service, and research. It is clear that entrepreneurial arrangements permit many variations in services, client population, locale of care, business arrangements, and outcomes. Chapter 20 describes entrepreneurial and intrepreneurial opportunities for practice arrangements that support APN practice.

To be successful clinicians in the rapidly changing health care system, APNs will be required to have an understanding of basic business functions, including accounting, finance, economics, marketing, and reimbursement practices. The University of Indianapolis School of Nursing offers a business preceptorship to all NP students through a collaborative arrangement with community-based primary care nurse managers. NP student outcomes include knowledge and skills for service expansion, case load assignment and management, profitability analysis, and grant writing. Students came to realize the importance of an integrated NP role with an understanding of how business knowledge can make them proactive rather than reactive to change (Wing, 1998).

One of the many benefits of faculty practice contracts has been the formalization and visibility of nursing services through business and organizational procedures. Prior to the development of faculty practice contracts, nursing educators would "moonlight" or volunteer their services. Informal arrangements, without reimbursement, kept these valuable nursing services unstructured, invisible, and outside of the organizational mainstream. Other positive results include the empowerment of nursing faculty as they negotiate intrainstitutional policies and develop business plans. A description of some of these faculty practices, along with the "how-to" of establishing a business plan, can be found in *Nursing Faculty Practice: Models and Methods* by Potash and Taylor (1993). Some newer examples of faculty practices that use contracting can be found at the University of South Carolina, Vanderbilt University, and the University of Texas–Houston schools of nursing. The University of Tennessee College of Nursing in Memphis has widely instituted an entrepreneurial practice model using contracting and nursing center structures. All faculty, including the dean, are encouraged to have a faculty practice. One provides primary care and screening to residents of the Memphis Jewish Home. The college has an annual contract with the Memphis Jewish Home that reimburses the college on a per capita basis. As noted previously, the School of Nursing also operates the university's Student Health Center, combining a managed care and a nursing center approach.

A Community Nursing Center established at the University of Rochester School of Nursing is now a professional corporation providing women's health, adolescent and child care, school health, care of the elderly, care of the disabled, wellness programs, and consultation (Walker, 1993). Operating as an entrepreneurial faculty practice, clusters of service exist under a Community Nursing Center corporate umbrella (center without walls). Future plans will facilitate collaboration among nursing professionals for group practice and research. Additional plans for this innovative faculty practice include marketing NP services across the age span, consultation services, education services, and research services for proposal writing and program evaluation. Future innovations for ensuring the economic stability of these faculty practices include gaining market position in the business and health care community via new contracts for health promotion in the workplace, interdisciplinary collaborative practice, co-managed care agreements, and health maintenance organization care contracts.

A joint practice model at Yale University School of Nursing exemplifies another way to implement an entrepreneurial faculty practice structure in which the School of Nursing generates over $1 million in clinical revenues through joint appointments. Although a joint practice model of faculty practice has been in effect for over 30 years at Yale, the current faculty practices are now poised to take advantage of managed care as it emerges in Connecticut. The Yale Midwifery Center has reorganized under a subcontract with the Yale–New Haven Hospital, and faculty members are providing care at the Community Mental Health Center through joint funding from Yale–New Haven Hospital, the State, and the School of Nursing. The faculty maintain a full-time appointment in the School of Nursing, conduct research at their practice sites, and maintain administrative and academic assignments at both institutions (Krauss, 1995).

The University of Utah School of Nursing, like the University of Rochester, is realigning its faculty practices with managed care. The challenge is to create faculty practices within an integrated system. The school has had faculty practices since 1986, and for the past 3 years has functioned under a faculty practice plan that rewards teaching, research, and practice activities. The faculty practice program includes a birth center and a symptom management clinic and will soon add a family primary care center. Although the faculty practice programs are not capitated, the school has contracts with managed care systems, and the faculty clinicians are designated providers under those contracts (Amos, 1995).

As market forces drive the health care system, nursing faculty practices are attending to the business aspects of health care delivery. As illustrated, business arrangements may be simple or complex and involve contracts with a variety of health care systems; partnership arrangements with physicians, nurses, or other health care personnel; and joint practice arrangements with agencies or groups. Some faculty practices are broad enough to include other faculty, nurses, or health personnel within one structural arrangement. Evaluation of faculty practice structures and implementation issues are beyond the scope of this chapter; the reader is referred to Potash and Taylor (1993) for a complete discussion of these issues. This publication, supported and published by the NONPF, presents a framework for starting a faculty practice and describes procedures for structuring, planning, and evaluating a practice at different stages of its development. The challenge of sustaining these practice-education partnerships is addressed in the next section.

NOW AND AGAIN: CONTINUING CHALLENGES AND PROSPECTIVE OPPORTUNITIES FOR PRACTICE-EDUCATION MODEL PARTNERSHIPS

In APN education-practice partnerships, the integration of teaching, research, and practice/service missions has led to innovative practice and teaching opportunities (Marion, 1997). These innovations have also resulted in exceptional faculty and organizational challenges, including perceptions of (1) a greater demand for quality (Taylor, 1997), (2) increased workload for the participants (Burns, 1997; Mirr, 1997), and (3) higher costs (AACN, 1998; Pew Health Professions Commission, 1998). Students, teachers, researchers, and practitioners from nursing and other health professions, business, information science, and other disciplines bring diverse perspectives on service delivery. In addition to the usual quality surveillance, the workload of academic health systems and their providers includes the additional rigors of scientific inquiry. Professionals with extraordinary standards for quality, innovation, and productivity usually will experience increases in their workloads, at least temporarily. However, their efforts may not lead to the traditional academic reward of tenure. Finally, integrating three missions within an academic practice model costs more than achieving a single mission, but the actual costs of teaching and research (or potential for savings) within a clinical partnership are unknown (AACN, 1999). Furthermore, in addition to the same stresses encountered by academic medical practices (Griner & Blumenthal, 1998; Van der Werf, 1999), advanced nursing practices face unique political, legal, financial, and bureaucratic barriers.

Of the numerous challenges to successful education-practice partnerships, four issues seem to confront most academic APN practices: achieving and maintaining quality of health services; acknowledging and balancing faculty workloads and roles; attaining sustainability in the face of barriers to academic nursing practice; and, finally, fulfilling the profession's social responsibility in a market-driven world.

Quality and Accountability for APN Practice-Education

CHALLENGES OF PRACTICE-EDUCATION EVALUATION

Generally, all strategies that are used to evaluate APN education and practice apply to APN faculty practice (see Chapter 25). More specifically, for practice-education entities, Edwards (1997) proposed a new, comprehensive model for quality evaluation in academic nursing centers. Five evaluative categories include physical and environmental facilities, organizational structure and governance, client outcomes, human resources, and financial processes. For partnerships, expanded evaluations are necessary to meet the planning and decision-making needs of sponsoring organizations and institutions; third-party payers; local, state, and national statutes; professional standards; the people who choose their services; and the profession as a whole. Evaluation data for practice-education partnerships can be used to increase accountability to constituents, to position APN centers in the mainstream of providers, and to maintain their unique services and a community focus.

If the APN practice operates as a nursing center, an evaluation of structural components will be necessary. *Structure evaluation* should include a determination of the extent to which the center and related organizations meet the standards for environmental and occupational safety, provide access to the services by individuals with disabilities, perform laboratory procedures, and store and safely dispose of medicines, materials, and equipment. Policy and procedures manuals for standards maintenance and human resource documents must comply with all governmental and affiliate organizational regulations (Edwards, 1997).

Process evaluation overlaps with structure and outcome evaluation, especially in relation to access issues and utilization of services (Patrick, 1997). The process of APN care can be evaluated for meeting the standard for "best practice," or integration of evidence-based practice, clinician judgment (including utilization management), and client preferences (Hayne, Sacket, Gray, Cook, & Guyato, 1996). Evaluation methods for the care process include chart audits, which reveal not only evidence-based practice but also APN tailoring to the client and mutual planning for care (Marion, 1997). An analysis of APN charge data (International Classification of Diseases, 9th Revision codes for diagnosis and Current Procedural Terminology codes for treatments) can effectively reveal use of evidence-based practice (Horn, 1998) as well as cost and health care utilization outcomes.

To capture what is unique in APN practice, health information systems (HIS) must be designed for more than standard medical records and physician charge data. The flexible HIS has the capability to reflect standard, nonbillable APN practices such as contracting with the client for behavior change and care in health fairs and other nontraditional settings. Also, APNs are learning how to use standard medical coding to reflect more of the processes used most frequently by nurse clinicians.

Credentialing for entry into practice and maintenance of clinical competency will likely be a requirement for APN faculty practitioners to maintain excellence in health care and to meet requirements of managed care and other payers. For APNs, this may include documentation of national certification, continuing education, demonstration of skill with new procedures, chart audits, and some diagnostic and procedure coding review (Marion, 1999). Although the reliability and validity of many of the usual measures for continuing competence have not been determined (Kane, 1992), there is increased national professional and regulatory interest in assuring continuing competence of all health professionals (Pew Health Professions Commission, 1998). Also, the American Nurses Credentialing Center, through its Continued Competency Task Force (Pulcini, 1999), is evaluating the new designs and methods for recertification, such as re-examination and simulated clinical performance by APNs in the future.

Quality in financial processes must be carefully evaluated in relation to cost outcomes (Edwards, 1997; Patrick, 1997). These processes include business planning and budget development and procedures for coding, charging, billing, collections, productivity of providers, cash flow management, and cost-effectiveness analysis. The partners' institutional requirements usually shape the center's financial methods, and reaching agreement on a financial model is a major hurdle in many instances. All providers of care have a responsibility in assuring quality financial practices, which ultimately determine the long-term sustainability of the health care center.

The evaluation of *patient/client outcomes,* according to the Cox APN model of care (Carter & Kulbock, 1995) includes assessment of the client's adherence to health prescriptions; health status, including perceived status and quality of life; utilization of health services; and satisfaction with care. Also, the APN is accountable for costs of health care and expected to be proficient in utilization management to reduce costs as part of professional services. Byers and Brunell (1998) described short- and long-term health status (clinical) outcomes as well as functional status as APN outcomes.

Faculty scholarship and student activity and learning outcomes are unique to education-practice partnerships (Edwards, 1997; Fontana, Kelber, & Devine, 1998). Each partnership must be evaluated for the potential to create knowledge and to prepare practitioners who will promote excellence in health care and nursing. Clinical scholarship by faculty includes development of clinical knowledge, professional competency development, application of technical or research skills to promote clinical practice, and service (AACN, 1999). Examples of such scholarship are peer-reviewed presentations and publications for clinician audiences, consultation reports, peer reviews of practice, state or higher recognition as a master practitioner, and establishment of practice partnerships. Student activities and learning can be measured with APN process and outcome indicators, such as diagnostic and treatment codes, charges, productivity, and satisfaction with teaching and learning experiences. Also, students may have scholarly activities leading to funded projects and poster and paper presentations. Finally, student participation may also be analyzed relative to the APN supervisor's productivity to indicate costs or benefits of that instruction. Estimation of these costs is the target of a study by the AACN and the NONPF (AACN, 1999).

OPPORTUNITIES TO IMPROVE QUALITY

Opportunities to improve the quality of health care seem to burgeon when faculty develop and/or implement nursing models. Well-prepared faculty can and do collaborate with colleagues from nursing and other disciplines to achieve and monitor the quality of academic nursing practice. Students bring their energy, creativity, and sense of inquiry into the partnerships and become a force for change. All partnership professionals can nurture students' learning. Additionally, nurses in academic practice have the occasion and responsibility to question old models and to test innovative, leading-edge health care models in search of improvement. In the centers of excellence, a "culture of competence" can emerge, and faculty, students, and respective peers can support one another to meet exemplary standards. Relevant, highly effective financial and information management processes can be developed to increase the potential for economic success in academic practices. Finally, as the source of new, quality, cost-effective health care models, nursing programs readily prepare APN students to be innovative in achieving and maintaining outstanding quality in nursing practices.

APN Faculty Practice

CHALLENGES OF BALANCING WORKLOAD AND REWARDS

The question of how extensively nursing faculty should be expected to participate in practice includes university, college, and faculty issues (Kraft, 1998; Norbeck, 1997). The external environment is increasingly hostile to university systems that award lifetime tenure to professors after a few years of employment, without requiring continuing scholarship or other productivity (Trower, 1999). The expectations of scholarship relative to tenure differ among universities according to the priority of missions. Sherwen (1998) noted that, with faculty practice, teaching faculty are invigorated, they are better able to describe aspects of nursing practice to students, they create wide networks of professionals who strengthen their teaching foundations, they utilize theory and empirical knowledge that are naturally embedded in practice, and they produce scholarly "products" such as clinically based research projects and publications. Within these universities, nurse faculty and others focus on new knowledge dissemination through peer-reviewed, data-based publications and presentations as well as teaching students at all levels. As nurses become ready to test nursing interventions with the scientific rigor required by the National Institute of Nursing Research and other institutes (Chang, 1999; McCorkle, Robinson, Nuamah, Lev, & Benoliel, 1998), there will be more practice-based questions that can be answered in academic nursing practices.

Mirr (1997) and Burns (1997) credited much of the interest in academic practice to Boyer (1990), who proposed a broader definition of university scholarship to include practice. Specifically, Boyer proposed four domains: the scholarship of discovery, teaching, application, and integration. Nursing faculty practices are a source and support of each domain. Often modeled after medical practice plans, which set forth methods for distributing practice income, nursing faculty practice plans have created a circumstance by which faculty can receive monetary and other incentives for their contributions to the organization.

OPPORTUNITIES TO RESOLVE WORKLOAD ISSUES

Opportunities related to resolving workload issues include further delineating the amount of work (costing) relative to process and outcomes of integrative faculty practice. The effect of role merger on the faculty member's energy and morale over time are not fully understood. Understanding and preventing burnout by academic clinicians can be a major focus for an interdisciplinary workforce research team. Fortunately, national discussions about faculty practice issues have resulted in clarity about practice scholarship. As with all employment, matching the person with the faculty practice expectation and environment is critical to the success of faculty practice.

Sustainability of Advanced Nursing Practice-Education Innovations

CHALLENGES TO PARTNERSHIP SUSTAINABILITY

Education-practice partnerships with APNs as providers face many challenges to sustainability. Academic nursing centers generally began as nurse-managed clinics when and where the need arose. This opportunistic approach, rather than strategic planning, provided excellent care to many underserved populations, but once the foundation or governmental funding ended, many centers closed their doors or severely limited their scope of services because of lack of funds. Such outcomes are entirely unsatisfactory for the partners—the community organizations and residents who had grown to depend on APN services and the APNs who had invested considerable time and energy in integrating the college missions. One example is an academic nursing center tailored to a high-risk population on Chicago's West Side. After 6 years of intense effort, the academic and community partners closed the center when the cost of facility repairs became too burdensome and grant funding ended before APNs could be reimbursed in Illinois (L. Marion, personal communication, September, 1999).

APN practice barriers have been external or environmental (Sekscenski, Sansom, Bazell, Salmon, & Mullan, 1994), including restrictive practice and insurance laws and regulations, limited or nonexistent liability insurance, and lack of reimbursement for traditional nursing services (Edwards, Kaplan, Barnett, & Logan, 1998). Most recently, the expansion of managed care without a concomitant recognition of APNs as providers and the lack of APN business skills have been major threats to existing practice (Norbeck & Taylor, 1998).

Just as the scope of faculty practice has developed, the need for a diversity of business and analytical skills expanded as well. In the past, skills were needed to negotiate salary reimbursement for clinical hours at the individual level or joint appointments at the institutional level. As colleges and schools of nursing embarked on establishing autonomous practices, administrators needed skills to create comprehensive business plans, develop faculty practice plans for revenue sharing, and negotiate an ever-changing set of arrangements to gain reimbursement for clinical services (Norbeck & Taylor, 1998). Sophisticated faculty and administrators have developed their own entrepreneurial infrastructure or have managed to adapt that of their parent organization or other partner to nursing practice (Mundinger, 1997; Norbeck, 1997). Increasingly, academic nursing programs now have an academic administrator or a business manager with advanced preparation in business and experience in managed care, health services delivery, and/or other aspects of practice management. Newer financial techniques, such as activity-based costing, are being used by financial officers to very accurately determine the costs of nursing services and the costs of specific work activities, including educational and research costs (Storfjell, 1997). The administrators, with the faculty, periodically assess the extent and sustainability of present practices, identify potential markets and assets for providing service, and set a strategic plan for practice that is congruous with the teaching and research mission (Potash, 1997).

Although the ability to sustain a faculty practice has improved considerably as APN entrepreneurs learn from one another (Barger, 1995), in truth many nursing practices are struggling. Medicine-nursing partnerships are strained as academic physician colleagues have revolutionized their methods of practice management and health care delivery. As academic health centers launch physician groups that must achieve sustainability, the cost of nursing enterprise support is questioned by all involved. Unfortunately, the information management industry together with nursing faculty have not developed an HIS that captures the usual health care practice management activities plus the process and outcomes of nursing practice (Palladino & Dower, 1997). This lack of definitive data is one of the greatest challenges facing nursing practice today. The use of existing codes designed for physicians is a stopgap tracking and evaluation method that will continue to be refined as better qualified nurses enter the business management arena.

OPPORTUNITIES FOR SUSTAINABILITY

Opportunities arising from the challenge of achieving sustainability can be expanded through partnerships with nursing service administrators who have the administrative and analytical knowledge and experience in sustaining health care delivery systems. These nursing service colleagues may assist with the development of an organizational strategic plan and the establishment of a practice management team that develops a business plan for each project (Potash, 1997; Rudy, Anderson, Dudjak, Kobert, & Miller, 1995). The practice team includes at least a business manager/director, the clinical faculty, and perhaps a person skilled in fund-raising (development). Faculty members who write training and/or research grants may be a part of the team from time to time. If there are community partners, their clinical, business, and development representatives become members of the team. With new projects, the team usually writes grants or otherwise solicits funds for start up and commits to a projected date for sustainability. Staffing is determined by anticipating the demand for type and amount/frequency of services. As grant funding and reimbursement become available, services can be increased accordingly. The business director usually develops templates for each type of agreement to specify the contributions of all partners and guide the various forms of contracting. For example, a nursing program may agree to provide primary care services if the community-based organization will contribute space that meets safety and access standards for a health care clinic. Also, a community agency may pay consulting fees to the faculty or nursing program until they become sustainable through third-party reimbursement.

Opportunities for sustainability will depend on business decisions and the development of HIS that support educational missions and clinical practice goals. A collaborative venture for nurses and HIS vendors is to create (1) a system that captures APN process and outcome and (2) a system of networking these data. As nursing practice leaders identify successful business models and methods, the nursing curricula can reflect this new knowledge, and students can learn in this culture of quality and innovation through experiences and observation as well as traditional study.

Balancing the Business of Practice-Education Partnerships with Social Responsibility

CHALLENGES OF MEETING THE PROFESSION'S
SOCIAL RESPONSIBILITY

Throughout nursing history, practice has evolved in response to the needs of the public. In the United States, nurses have been providing community-based primary care and medical coordination services since Lillian Wald began the Visiting Nurses Association clinic in the early 1800s in New York City and the first midwifery service began serving the rural poor in Kentucky. These pioneering health care systems were more than acute care or disease-related services and were based upon a broad definition of personal and community health. New practice-education partnerships must continue their investment in ethical health care practices in spite of the system focus on cost controls. Ethical practice should address issues of health service rationing based on culture, race, class, or age in addition to sociopolitical issues of access and reproductive choice. Successful practice-education innovations must continue the tradition of being at the forefront of health advocacy, health protection, health promotion, and community empowerment as vehicles for improving the health care delivery system (Taylor, 1998).

OPPORTUNITIES TO FULFILL NURSING'S SOCIAL RESPONSIBILITY

More diverse health providers, researchers, and policy makers can create new ways of interacting and setting priorities to address both the particular and common needs of clients. Health care partnerships can shape clinical services to fit particular sociocultural needs. Nurses and nursing organizations will more likely be involved with ethnic organizations, disability rights groups, senior health advocacy groups, and other identity movement groups in setting local and national research and service policies. Working with a diverse community also extends to the community of health care workers. APNs will collaborate with a variety of health care providers and workers who represent the diversity of patient populations.

Socially responsible care partnerships require that health professionals participate in advocating for healthy environments. Without attention to the material conditions in which clients live, including their income disparity, poor housing conditions, and threats to their personal safety, personal health services can have only limited effects. Community health partnerships address the broader circumstances of people's lives, encompassing sanitation, environmental health, housing, infectious disease surveillance and control, and programs for community-based health systems, such as child care facilities, violence prevention, and protection of reproductive freedoms (American Academy of Nursing Expert Panel on Women's Health Writing Group, 1996). Advanced nursing practice-education partnerships of the future will need to bring forward past traditions of nursing activism to balance the innovation costs and economic constraints.

Inherent in APN activism is the formation of community partnerships and empowerment that enables the opportunity for healthier lifestyles. An empowering health promotion practice holds that certain community processes (organization, mobilization, education) are necessary to enhance personal health and to create environments that are simultaneously more protective of health and more supportive of healthy personal behaviors (Labonte, 1993). Empowerment of people, so they can leave overwhelmingly unhealthy communities and start new lives with more opportunity, may be an answer that partnerships can offer. For example, an important step in helping low-income individuals and families to earn sufficient income is to identify and treat the multiple health problems so common in this group. The comprehensive health assessment, health promotion, and early detection of health problems characteristic of APN practice brings added value to a nursing partnership with social service agencies devoted to improving the quality of life among disadvantaged people.

CONCLUSION

Faculty practice, which became an important issue in nursing education during the 1980s, may be one way to unify the profession for the future. APN educators have demonstrated that they can be role models in innovative nursing practices. Faculty practice can provide revenue for an institution as well as establish models of nursing care based on research and advanced practice.

APNs, nursing administrators, and nursing educators have demonstrated that the whole is greater than the sum of the parts through their efforts at unifying education, practice, and, now, health care delivery systems through practice-education innovations. Future development of advanced nursing practice-education programs will include integrating practice into traditional academic missions of teaching and research, attention to practice-education quality and accountability, the development of stable funding and resources, workload considerations, and academic advancement standards. Although challenges continue for advanced nursing practice-education innovations, numerous opportunities exist to benefit the public by influencing policy and improving health care delivery as well as maintaining nursing social responsibilities. Within this practice environment, it will be important for APN faculty and clinicians to look for ways to structure practice opportunities that provide a balance between paying patients and those who cannot pay. Only then can future practice-education innovations offer advanced practice nursing the opportunity to address unmet health care needs, to test specific interventions, to role model effective care, and to integrate practice with education and research.

REFERENCES

Adams, S. M., & Partee, D. J. (1998). Integrating psychosocial rehabilitation in a community-based faculty nursing practice. *Journal of Psychosocial Nursing and Mental Health Services, 36*(4), 24-28, 47-48.

Aiken, L. (1988). The Robert Wood Johnson Foundation TNHP. In N. Small & P. Wilhere (Eds.), *Teaching nursing homes: The nursing perspective* (pp. 56-59). Owings Mills, MD: National Health Publication.

American Academy of Nursing. (1980). Resolution on unification of nursing service and nursing education. *American Academy of Nursing Newsletter, 1*(4).

American Academy of Nursing Expert Panel on Women's Health Writing Group. (1996). *Women's health and women's health care: Recommendations for transformative changes in health care services, nursing education and practice.* Washington, DC: American Academy of Nursing.

American Association of Colleges of Nursing. (1998). *Managed care constraints stir debate on preceptor reimbursement.* Washington, DC: Author.

American Association of Colleges of Nursing. (1999). AACN to study costs of advanced practice nurse training in outpatient settings. *Syllabus, 25*(1), 12-15.

Amos, L. (1995). A school of nursing–owned family nursing center. In *Faculty practice in a managed care environment* (Proceedings of the Second Annual Faculty Practice Conference, Tucson, AZ) (pp. 22-27). Washington, DC: American Association of Colleges of Nursing.

Anderson, E. R., & Pierson, P. (1983). An exploratory study of faculty practice: Views of those faculty engaged in practice who teach in an NLN accredited baccalaureate program. *Western Journal of Nursing Research, 5,* 129–143.

Andreoli, K. G. (1993). Faculty improve clinical operations. *Journal of Professional Nursing, 9*(4), 194.

Aroian, J. F., & Rauckhorst, L. M. (1985). Summer camp: An overlooked site for faculty clinical practice? *Nurse Educator, 10*(1), 32–35.

Arthur, D., & Usher, K. (1994). An application of nursing faculty practice: Clinical camps. *Journal of Advanced Nursing, 19,* 680–684.

Auerhahn, C. (1997). Columbia University School of Nursing faculty practice: A cross-site model. In L. Marion (Ed.), *Nursing faculty practice: Applying the models* (pp. 65–69). Washington, DC: National Organization of Nurse Practitioner Faculties.

Barger, S. E. (1991). The nursing center: A model for rural nursing practice. *Nursing and Health Care, 12*(6), 290–294.

Barger, S. E. (1995). Establishing a nursing center: Learning from the literature and experiences of others. *Journal of Professional Nursing, 11*(4), 203–212.

Barnard, K. E. (Ed.). (1983). *Structure to outcome: Making it work.* Kansas City, MO: American Academy of Nursing.

Barnard, K. E., & Smith, G. R. (1985). *Faculty practice in action.* Kansas City, MO: American Academy of Nursing.

Boyer, E. (1990). *Scholarship reconsidered: Priorities for the professoriate.* Princeton, NJ: The Carnegie Foundation for the Advancement of Teaching.

Buhler-Wilkerson, K., Naylor, M., Holt, S., & Rinke, L. (1998). An alliance for academic home care: Integrating research, education and practice. *Nursing Outlook, 46*(2), 77–80.

Burns, C. (1997). Faculty clinical practice as a tenurable activity. In L. Marion (Ed.), *Nursing faculty practice: Applying the models* (pp. 41–50). Washington, DC: National Organization of Nurse Practitioner Faculties.

Byers, J., & Brunell, M. (1998). Demonstrating the value of the advanced practice nurse: An evaluation model. *AACN Clinical Issues, 9*(2), 296–305.

Campbell, B. F., & King, J. B. (1992). Public health service administration and academia. *Journal of Nursing Administration, 22*(12), 23–27.

Campbell, M. (1993). Multidisciplinary faculty practice and community partnership. *Holistic Nursing Practice, 7*(4), 20–27.

Carter, C., & Kulbok, P. (1995). Evaluation of the Interaction Model of Client Health Behavior through the first decade of research. *Advances in Nursing Science, 18*(1), 62–73.

Chang, B. (1999). Cognitive-behavioral intervention for homebound caregivers of persons with dementia. *Nursing Research, 48*(3), 173–182.

Chilvers, J. R., & Jones, D. (1997). The teaching nursing homes innovation: A literature review. *Journal of Advanced Nursing, 26*(3), 463–469.

Christman, L. (1982). The unification model. In A. Marriner (Ed.), *Contemporary nursing management* (pp. 88–91). St. Louis: C. V. Mosby.

Christy, T. E. (1980). Clinical practice as a function of nursing education: A historical analysis. *Nursing Outlook, 28,* 492–496.

Davis, L., & Zatuchni, G. I. (1993). Nurse-midwifery within a faculty group practice. *Nurse Practitioner Journal, 18*(10), 14–15.

Davis-Doughty, S. E. (1989). The CNS in a nurse-managed center. In A. B. Hamric & J. A. Spross (Eds.), *The clinical nurse specialist in theory and practice* (2nd ed., pp. 415–434). Philadelphia: W. B. Saunders.

DeLeon, P. (1994). Nursing school administered clinics: An important policy agenda for the future. *Nursing Economics, 10,* 137–158.

Donnelly, G. F., Warfel, W., & Wolf, Z. R. (1994). A faculty-practice program: Three perspectives. *Holistic Nursing Practice, 8*(3), 71–80.

Dunn, B. H., & Graves, L. (1996). Community outreach model of faculty practice. In Hickey, J. V., Oimette, R. M., & Venegoni, S. L. (Eds.). *Advanced practice nursing: Changing roles and clinical applications* (pp. 257–269). Philadelphia: Lippincott-Raven.

Durand, B. A. (1985). Defining faculty practice: A look at theory-practice relationships. In K. E. Barnard & G. R. Smith (Eds.), *Faculty practice in action* (pp. 38–40). Kansas City, MO: American Academy of Nursing.

Edwards, J. (1997). Evaluating practice in nurse-managed centers. In L. Marion (Ed.), *Faculty practice: Applying the models* (pp. 73–83). Washington, DC: National Organization of Nurse Practitioner Faculties.

Edwards, J., Kaplan, A., Barnett, J., & Logan, C. (1998). Nurse-managed primary care in a rural community: Outcomes of five years of practice. *Nursing and Health Care Perspectives, 19*(1), 20–25.

Fagin, C. M. (1985). Institutionalizing practice: Historical and future perspectives. In K. E. Barnard & G. R. Smith (Eds.), *Faculty practice in action* (pp. 1–17). Kansas City, MO: American Academy of Nursing.

Fagin, C. M. (1986). Institutionalizing faculty practice. *Nursing Outlook, 34*(3), 140–144.

Fenton, M. V., Rounds, L., & Iha, S. (1988). The nursing center in a rural community: The promotion of family and community health. *Family and Community Health, 11*(2), 14–24.

Fontana, S., Kelber, S., & Devine, E. (1998). *Design of a computerized database for tracking prescribing patterns of FNP students.* Paper presented at the National Organization of Nurse Practitioner Faculties meeting, Savannah, GA.

Frenn, M., Lundeen, S. P., Martin, K. S., Riesch, S. K., & Wilson, S. A. (1996). Symposium on nursing centers: Past, present and future. *Journal of Nursing Education, 35*(2), 54–62.

Gale, B. J. (1998). Faculty practice as partnership with a community coalition. *Journal of Professional Nursing, 14*(5), 267–271.

Grace, H. K. (1981). Unification, re-unification: Reconciliation or collaboration—bridging the education-service gap. In J. C. McCloskey & H. K. Grace (Eds.), *Current issues in nursing* (pp. 625–643). Boston: Blackwell Scientific.

Gresham-Kenton, M. L. (1989). The CNS in collaborative relationships between nursing service and nursing education. In A. B. Hamric & J. A. Spross (Eds.), *The clinical nurse specialist in theory and practice* (pp. 343–362). Philadelphia: W. B. Saunders.

Griner, P., & Blumenthal, D. (1998). Reforming the structure and management of academic medical centers: Case studies of ten institutions. *Academic Medicine, 73*(7), 818–825.

Hale, J. F., Harper D. C., & Dawson, E. M. (1996). Partnership for a nurse practitioner-directed student health primary care center. *Journal of Professional Nursing, 12*(6), 365–372.

Hall, J. M., & Stevens, P. E. (1995). The future of graduate education in nursing: Scholarship, the health of communities, and health care reform. *Journal of Professional Nursing, 11*(6), 332–338.

Hawkins, J. W., Igou, J. F., Johnson, E. E., & Utley, Q. E. (1984). A nursing center for ambulatory, well, older adults. *Nursing and Health Care, 5*(4), 209–212.

Hayne R., Sacket, D., Gray, J., Cook, D., & Guyato, G. (1996). Transferring evidence from research to practice: 1. The role of clinical care research evidence in clinical decisions. *ACP Journal Club, 125,* A14–A15.

Health Resources Service Administration, Division of Nursing. (1998). *Special projects funding program.* Rockville, MD: Author.

Henry, J. K. (1997). Community nursing centers: Models of nurse managed care. *Journal of Obstetric, Gynecologic, and Neonatal Nursing, 26*(2), 224–228.

Herr, K. A. (1989). Faculty practice as a requirement for promotion and tenure: Receptivity, risk and threats perceived. *Journal of Nursing Education, 28*(8), 347–353.

Horn, S. D., Sharkey, P. D., & Gassaway, J. (1996). Intended and unintended consequences or HMO cost containment strateiges: Results from the managed care outcomes project. *The American Journal of Managed Care, 2*(3), 233–247.

Joel, L. A. (1983). Stepchildren in the family: Aiming toward synergy between nursing education and service from the faculty perspective. In

K. E. Barnard (Ed.), *Structure to outcome: Making it work* (pp. 43–57). Kansas City, MO: American Academy of Nursing.

Just, G., Adams, E., & DeYoung, S. (1989). Faculty practice: Nurse educators' views and proposed models. *Journal of Nursing Education, 28*(4), 161–168.

Kane, M. (1992). The assessment of professional competence. *Evaluation and The Health Professions, 15*(2), 163–182.

Kraft, S. K. (1998). Faculty practice: Why and how. *Nurse Educator, 23*(4), 45–48.

Kramer, M., Polifroni, E. C., & Organek, N. (1986). Effects of faculty practice on student learning outcomes. *Journal of Professional Nursing, 2*(5), 289–301.

Krauss, J. (1995). Joint appointments for faculty practice. In *Faculty practice in a managed care environment* (Proceedings of the Second Annual Faculty Practice Conference, Tucson, AZ) (pp. 37–45) Washington, DC: American Association of Colleges of Nursing.

Labonte, R. (1993). *Community health responses to health inequalities.* New York: New York Community Health Promotion Research Unit.

Langford, T., Ridenour, N., Dadich, K., Yoder, P., Cox, H., Axton, S., Harsanyi, B., & Cooke, S. (1987). Past unification to reintegration: One school's effort to emphasize wholeness in professional nursing. *Journal of Professional Nursing, 3,* 362–371.

Lee, V. K., Levy, E. Y., Dix, P. E., & Tatum, M. F. (1987). Faculty as primary nurses on a model inpatient unit. *Nurse Educator, 12*(5), 16–19.

Lockhart, C. (1995). Community nursing centers: An analysis of status and needs. In B. Murphy (Ed.), *Nursing centers: The time is now* (pp. 1–18). New York: National League for Nursing.

Marion, L. (Ed.). (1997). *Nursing faculty practice: Applying the models.* Washington, DC: National Organization of Nurse Practitioner Faculties.

Marion, L. (1999, April 22). *Links between faculty competence and quality of master's programs: How do you ensure competency?* Speech delivered to the American Association of Colleges of Nursing Master's Education Conference, Orlando, FL.

Mauksch, I. (1980a). Faculty practice: A professional imperative. *Nurse Educator, 5,* 21–24.

Mauksch, I. (1980b). A rationale for the reunification of nursing service and nursing education. In L. Aiken (Ed.), *Health policy and nursing practice* (pp. 211–217). New York: McGraw-Hill.

Maurin, J. T. (1986). An exploratory study of nursing services provided by schools of nursing. *Journal of Professional Nursing, 2,* 277–281.

McClure, M. (1987). Faculty practice: New definitions, new opportunities. *Nursing Outlook, 35,* 162–166.

McCorkle, R., Robinson, L., Nuamah, I., Lev, E., & Benoliel, J. (1998). The effects of home nursing care for patients during terminal illness on the bereaved's psychological distress. *Nursing Research, 47*(1), 2–10.

Mezey, M. E., Mitty, E. L., & Bottrell, M. (1997). The teaching nurse home program: Enduring educational outcomes. *Nursing Outlook, 45*(3), 133–140.

Miller, V. G. (1997). Coproviding continuing education through faculty practice: A win-win opportunity. *Journal of Continuing Education in Nursing, 28*(1), 10–13.

Millonig, V. L. (1986). Faculty practice: A view of its development, current benefits, and barriers. *Journal of Professional Nursing, 2*(3), 166–172.

Mirr, M. (1997). Initiating, negotiating, and maintaining a faculty practice. In L. Marion (Ed.), *Nursing faculty practice: Applying the models* (pp. 33–39). Washington, DC: National Organization of Nurse Practitioner Faculties.

Mundinger, M., Kane, R., Lenz, E., Totten, A., Tsai, WY., Cleary, P., Friedewald, W., Siu, A., & Shelenski, M. (2000). Primary care outcomes in patients treated by nurse practitioners or physicians. *JAMA, 283*(1), 59–68.

Mundinger, M. (1997). A philosophy of scholarly faculty practice. In L. Marion (Ed.), *Nursing faculty practice: Applying the models* (pp. 63–64). Washington, DC: National Organization of Nurse Practitioner Faculties.

Murray, K. M., Hackbarth, D. P., Sojka, S. A., & Swanston, L. J. (1987). Faculty practice in home health care: A new education and service relationship in process. *QRB, 13*(2), 42–44.

National Organization of Nurse Practitioner Faculties. (2000). *NONPF faculty-to-faculty mentoring program in community health.* Washington, DC: NONPF.

Naylor, M., & Buhler-Wilkerson, K. (1999). Creating community-based care for a new millenium. *Nursing Outlook, 47*(3), 120–127.

Norbeck, J., & Taylor, D. (1998). Faculty practice: Nursing in the 21st century. In E. Sullivan (Ed.), *Creating nursing's feature: Issues, opportunities and challenges* (pp.125–136). St. Louis: Mosby.

Norbeck, J. S. (1997). The value of faculty practice: A dean's perspective. In L. Marion (Ed.), *Nursing faculty practice: Applying the models* (pp. 103–106). Washington, DC: National Organization of Nurse Practitioner Faculties.

Nugent, K. E., Barger, S. E., & Bridges, W. C. (1993). Facilitators and inhibitors of practice: A faculty perspective. *Journal of Nursing Education, 32*(7), 293–300.

Palladino, M., & Dower, D. (1997). Nursing faculty practice: A collaborative model for information management. In L. Marion (Ed.), *Nursing faculty practice: Applying the models* (pp. 85–93).

Washington, DC: National Organization of Nurse Practitioner Faculties.

Patrick, D. (1997). Finding health-related quality of life outcomes sensitive to health-care organization and delivery. *Medical Care, 35*(11), 49–68.

Pew Health Professions Commission. (1998). Academic health centers in danger of losing sight of their academic missions. *Front & Center, 3*(1), 1–4.

Phillips, D. L., & Steel, J. E. (1994). Factors influencing scope of practice in nursing centers. *Journal of Professional Nursing, 10*(2), 84–90.

Pohl, J. (1999). NONPF 1999 faculty practice survey results. In *Proceedings of the 1999 NONPF Annual Conference, San Francisco.* Washington, DC: National Organization of Nurse Practitioner Faculties.

Polifroni, E. C., & Schmalenberg, C. (1985). Faculty practice that works: Two examples. *Nursing Outlook, 33*(5), 226–228.

Potash, M. (1997). A guide to faculty practice. In L. Marion (Ed.), *Nursing faculty practice: Applying the models* (pp. 107–130). Washington, DC: National Organization of Nurse Practitioner Faculties.

Potash, M., & Taylor, D. (1993). *Nursing faculty practice: Models and methods.* Washington, DC: National Organization of Nurse Practitioner Faculties.

Pulcini, J. (1999, March 24). American Nurses Credentialing Center: The second Continued Competency Task Force. In *National Organization of Nurse Practitioner Faculties board report* (pp. 1–8). Washington, DC: National Organization of Nurse Practitioner Faculties.

Richie, M. F., Adams, S. M., Blackburn, P. E., Cone, C. P., Dwyer, K. A., Laben, J. K., & Seidel, S. S. (1996). Psychiatric nursing faculty practice care within the community context. *Nursing and Health Care Perspectives on Community, 17*(6), 317–321.

Riesch, S. K. (1992a). Nursing centers. *Annual Review of Nursing Research, 10,* 145–161.

Riesch, S. K. (1992b). Nursing centers: An analysis of the anecdotal literature. *Journal of Professional Nursing, 8*(1), 16–25.

Rudy, E., Anderson, N., Dudjak, L., Kobert, S., & Miller, R. (1995). Faculty practice: Creating a new culture. *Journal of Professional Nursing, 11*(2), 78–83.

Sekscenski, E., Sansom, S., Bazell, C., Salmon, M., & Mullan, F. (1994). State practice environments and the supply of physician assistants, nurse practitioners, and certified nurse-midwives. *New England Journal of Medicine, 331,* 1266–1271.

Sherwen, L. N. (1998). When the mission is teaching: Does nursing faculty practice fit? *Journal of Professional Nursing, 14*(3), 137–143.

Stainton, M. C. (1989). The development of a practicing nursing faculty. *Journal of Advanced Nursing, 14,* 20–26.

Stark, P. L., Walker, G. C., & Bohannan, P. A. (1991). Nursing faculty practice in the Houston linkage model: Administrative and faculty perspectives. *Nurse Educator, 16*(5), 23–28.

Storfjell, J. (1997). The cost of faculty practice: The missing link. In L. Marion (Ed.), *Nursing faculty practice: Applying the models* (pp. 95–102). Washington, DC: National Organization of Nurse Practitioner Faculties.

Styles, M. M. (1984). Reflections on collaboration and unification. *Image: The Journal of Nursing Scholarship, 16,* 21–23.

Taylor, D. (1997). Perspectives on nursing faculty practice: The next steps. In L. Marion (Ed.), *Nursing faculty practice: Applying the models* (pp. 3–8). Washington, DC: National Organization of Nurse Practitioner Faculties.

Taylor, D. (1998). Crystal ball gazing: Back to the future. *Advanced Practice Nursing Quarterly, 3*(4), 44–51.

Turner, D. M., & Pearson, L. M. (1989). The faculty fellowship program: Uniting service and education. *Journal of Nursing Administration, 19*(10), 18–22.

Trower, C. (1999). The trouble with tenure. *National Forum: The Phi Kappa Phi Journal, 79*(1), 24–29.

Van der Werf, M. (1999, May 21). Changing economics of health care are devastating academic medical centers. *Chronicle of Higher Education,* pp. A38–A39.

Walker, P. H. (1993). A comprehensive community nursing center model: Maximizing practice income: A challenge to educators. *Journal of Professional Nursing, 10*(3), 131–139.

Wandel, J. C. (1991). Education-practice partnerships: Faculty practice as faculty development. *Journal of Professional Nursing, 7*(5), 310–318.

White, J. L. (1999). Wellness Wednesdays: Health promotion and service learning on campus. *Journal of Nursing Education, 38*(2), 69–71.

Wing, D. M. (1998). The business management preceptorship within the nurse practitioner program. *Journal of Professional Nursing, 14*(3), 150–156.

Wold, J. L., & Williams, A. M. (1997). Student/faculty practice and research in occupational health: Health promotion and outcome evaluation. *Journal of Nursing Education, 35*(6), 252–257.

Additional Readings

American Association of Colleges of Nursing. (1996). *The power of faculty practice: Proceedings of the AACN's 1995 and 1996 Faculty Practice Conferences.* Washington, DC: Author.

American Association of Colleges of Nursing. (1998). *Position statement on nursing research.* Washington, DC: Author.

American Association of Colleges of Nursing. (1999). *Position statement on defining scholarship for the discipline of nursing.* Washington, DC: Author.

American Nurses Association. (1987). *The nursing center: Concept and design.* Kansas City, MO: Author.

Baillie, L. (1994). Nurse teachers' feelings about participating in clinical practice: An exploratory study. *Journal of Advanced Nursing, 20,* 150–159.

Barger, S., & Bridges, W. C. (1987). Nursing faculty practice: Institutional and individual facilitators and inhibitors. *Journal of Professional Nursing, 3,* 338–346.

Barger, S. E., Nugent, K. E., & Bridges, W. C. (1992). Nursing faculty practice: An organizational perspective. *Journal of Professional Nursing, 8*(5), 263–270.

Barger, S. E., Nugent, K. E., & Bridges, W. C. (1993). Schools with nursing centers: A 5-year follow-up study. *Journal of Professional Nursing, 9*(1), 7–13.

Barnes, N., Duldt, B., & Green, P. (1994). Perspectives of faculty practice and clinical competence. *Nurse Educator, 19*(3), 13–17.

Batey, M. V. (1983). Structural consideration for the social integration of nursing. In K. E. Barnard, (Ed.), *Structure to outcome: Making it work.* (pp. 39–46). Kansas City, MO: American Academy of Nursing.

Berlin, L. E., Bednash, G. D., Stanley, J. M., & Scott, D. L. (1994). *1994–1995 special report on master's and post-master's nurse practitioner programs, faculty clinical practice, faculty age profiles, undergraduate curriculum expansion in baccalaureate and graduate programs in nursing.* (Publication no. 94-95-4). Washington, DC: American Association of Colleges of Nursing.

Bickel, J. (1991). The changing faces of promotion and tenure at U. S. medical schools. *Academic Medicine, 66*(5), 249–256.

Boyer, E. (1995, January 26). *Scholarship for the professional professionate.* Speech delivered to the American Association of Colleges of Nursing Doctoral Education Conference, Sanibel Island, FL.

Broussard, A. B., Delahoussaye, C. P., & Poirrier, G. P. (1996). The practice role in the academic nursing community. *Journal of Nursing Education, 35*(2), 82–87.

Budden, L. (1994). Nursing faculty practice: Benefits vs costs. *Journal of Advanced Nursing, 19,* 1241–1246.

Burke, L. M. (1997). Teachers of nursing presenting a new model practice. *Journal of Nursing Management, 5*(5), 295–300.

Busby, L. C., Moore, A., Bradley, R., Covington, C., Daddario, J., Howard, E., McIntosh, E., Taylor, C., & Welch, L. (1996). Practical aspects of faculty practice: A model for excellence. *Nursing and Health Care Perspectives on Community, 17*(6), 313–316.

Carter, B., & McGuiness, B. (1997). Expanding nursing informatics knowledge through curriculum development: A collaborative faculty practice model. In Nursing Informatics of the International Medical Association (Ed.), *Nursing informatics: The impact of nursing knowledge on health care informatics* (Proceedings of Sixth Triennial International Congress of IMIA-NI, Vol. 46). (pp. 431–436). Amsterdam: IOS Press.

Carter, B. E. L., & McGuiness, B. (1996). Developing nursing informatics through a collaborative faculty practice model. In McGuiness, B., et al. (Eds.), *Making IT happen* (HIC '96: Proceedings of the Fourth National Health Informatics Conference, Melbourne, Australia) (pp. 111–114). Melbourne: Health Information Society of Australia.

Chickadonz, G. H. (1987). Faculty practice. *Annual Review of Nursing Research, 5,* 137–151.

Choudry, U. K. (1992). Faculty practice competencies: Nurse educators' perceptions. *Canadian Journal of Nursing Research, 24*(3), 5–17.

Collison, C. R., & Parsons, M. A. (1980). Is practice a viable faculty role? *Nursing Outlook, 28,* 677–679.

Conine, T. A., Shilling, L. M., & Pierce, E. R. (1985). The relative importance of supportive data for promotion and tenure reviews. *Journal of Allied Health, 14*(2), 183–190.

Conway-Welch, C. (1995). Integration of faculty practice into a state managed care setting. In *Faculty practice in a managed care environment* (Proceedings of the Second Annual Faculty Practice Conference, Tucson, AZ) (pp. 10–15). Washington, DC: American Association of Colleges of Nursing.

Cook, J., & Wilby, L. (1998). The role of the lecturer practitioner in midwifery. *Midwifery Digest, 8*(4), 414–417.

Corless, I. B., & Nokes, K. M. (1996). Professional nursing education's response to the HIV/AIDS pandemic. *Journal of the Association of Nurses in AIDS Care, 7*(1), 15–22.

Council of the American Association of University Professors. (1984). *The standards for notice of non-reappointment: Policy documents and reports.* Washington, DC: American Association of University Professors.

Council on Medical Education. (1990). Principles for graduate medical education. *JAMA, 263,* 2917–2931.

Culbertson, R. A. (1997). Academic faculty practices: Issues for viability in competitive managed care markets. *Journal of Health Politics, Policy and Law, 22*(6), 1359–1383.

Declercq, E., Paine, L., Simmes, D., & DeJoseph, J. (1998). State regulation, payment policies, and nurse-midwife services. *Health Affairs, 17*(2), 190–200.

De Tornyay, R. (1988). What constitutes scholarly activities? *Journal of Nursing Education, 27*(6), 245.

Dickens, M. R. (1983). Faculty practice and social support. *Nursing Leadership, 6,* 121–127.

Donabedian, A. (1966). Evaluating the quality of medical care. *Milbank Memorial Fund Quarterly, 44*(3), 166–206.

Donabedian, A. (1996). The effectiveness of quality assurance. *International Journal for Quality in Health Care, 8*(4), 401–407.

Duga, A. B. (1985). Expanding nursing's practice terrain: Imperatives for future viability. *Public Health Nursing, 2*(1), 23–32.

Elcock, K. (1998). Lecturer practitioner: A concept analysis. *Journal of Advanced Nursing, 28*(5), 1092–1098.

Eng, E., Salmon, M. E., & Mullan, F. (1992). Community empowerment: The critical basis for primary health care. *Family and Community Health, 15*(1), 1–12.

Fairbrother, P., & Ford, S. (1997). Education. It's a dual not a duel . . . the role of lecturer/practitioner. *Nursing Times, 93*(16), 32–34.

Fairbrother, P., & Ford, S. (1998). Lecturer practitioners: A literature review. *Journal of Advanced Nursing, 27*(2), 274–279.

Fiandt, K. (1997). Strategies for overcoming barriers to faculty practice. In L. Marion (Ed.), *Nursing faculty practice: Applying the models* (pp. 23–32). Washington, DC: National Organization of Nurse Practitioner Faculties.

Ford, L., & Kitzman, H. (1983). Organization perspectives on faculty and practice: Issues and challenges. In K. E. Barnard (Ed.), *Structure to outcome: Making it work* (pp. 13–30). Kansas City, MO: American Academy of Nursing.

Forni, P. R., & Welch, M. J. (1987). The professional versus the academic model: A dilemma for nursing education. *Journal of Nursing Education, 3*(5), 291–297.

Gersten-Rothenberg, K. (1998). Graduate student scholarship. Should schools of nursing develop nursing centers? *Clinical Nurse Specialist, 12*(2), 59–63.

Gilson-Parkevich, T. (1983). Stepchildren in the family: Aiming toward synergy between nursing education and service from the nursing service perspective. In K. E. Barnard (Ed.), *Structure to outcome: Making it work* (pp. 51–58). Kansas City, MO: American Academy of Nursing.

Hunter, J. K., Crosby, F. E., Ventura, M. R., & Warkentin, L. (1991). National survey to identify evaluation criteria for programs of health care for homeless. *Nursing and Health Care, 12*(10), 536–542.

Hutelmyer, C. M., & Donnelly, G. F. (1996). Joint appointments in practice positions. *Nursing Administration Quarterly, 20*(4), 71–79.

Jacobson, S. F., MacRobert, M., Leon, C., & McKennon, E. (1998). A faculty case management practice: Integrating teaching, service, and research. *Nursing and Health Care Perspectives, 19*(5), 220–223.

Kean College of New Jersey Department of Nursing. (1990). *Learning Center for Health guidelines.* Union: Kean College of New Jersey.

Labonte, R. (1989). Community health promotion strategies. In C. J. Martin & D. V. McQueen (Eds.), *Readings for a new public health.* Edinburgh: Edinburgh University Press.

Lambert, C., & Lambert, V. A. (1993). Relationships among faculty practice involvement, perception of role stress, and psychological hardiness of nurse educators. *Journal of Nursing Education, 32*(4), 171–179.

Lassan, R. (1994). Nursing faculty practice: A valid sabbatical request? *Nursing Forum, 29*(2), 10–14.

LeMone, P., McDaniel, R., & Sullivan, T. (1998). Partnership for health care: An academic nursing center in a rural community college. *Nursing and Health Care Perspectives, 19*(2), 80–85.

Lessing-Turner, G. (1997). The role of joint appointments in midwifery . . . lecturer-practitioner roles. *Midwifery Digest, 7*(2), 154–156.

Lindsay, A. M. (1989). Health care for the homeless. *Nursing Outlook, 37*(2), 78–81.

Maggs, C. (1996). Debate. Professor of nursing as clinicians and academics: Is this the way forward? *NT Research, 1*(2), 157–158.

Mallik, M. (1998). The role of nurse educators in the development of reflective practitioners: A selective case study of the Australian and UK experience. *Nurse Education Today, 18*(1), 52–63.

McClure, M. (1981). Promoting practice-based research: A critical need. *Journal of Nursing Administration, 7,* 66–70.

Messmer, P. R. (1989). Academic tenure in schools of nursing. *Journal of Professional Nursing, 5*(1), 39–48.

Mezey, M. D., Lynaugh, J. E., & Cartier, M. M. (1988). The teaching nursing home program, 1982–87: A report card. *Nursing Outlook, 36*(6), 285–288.

Napholz, L. (1993). An academic nursing center integrating education, role modeling, and research. *Nurse Educator, 18*(4), 3–5.

National Council of State Boards of Nursing. (1984). *Continued competence* [Online]. Available: *http://www.ncsbn.org/files/publications/papers.asp.* Updated on July 15, 1999.

National Council of State Boards of Nursing. (1986). *Continued nursing competence* [Online]. Available: *http://www.ncsbn.org/files/publications/papers.asp.* Updated on July 15, 1999.

National Council of State Boards of Nursing. (1991). *Conceptual framework for continued competence* [Online]. Available: *http://www.ncsbn.org/files/publications/papers.asp.* Updated on July 15, 1999.

National Council of State Boards of Nursing. (1996). *Assuring competence: A regulatory responsibility* [Online]. Available: *http://www.ncsbn.org/files/publications/papers.asp.* Updated on July 15, 1999.

National Council of State Boards of Nursing. (1999). *Continued competence (1987–1992)* [Online]. Available: *http://www.ncsbn.org/files/publications/papers.asp.* Updated on July 15, 1999.

National League for Nursing Accrediting Commission. (1996). *Criteria and guidelines for the evaluation of baccalaureate and higher degree programs in nursing.* New York: NLN Press.

Nichols, C. (1985). Faculty practice: Something for everyone. *Nursing Outlook, 33*(2), 85–90.

Nichols, L. (1992). Estimating costs of underusing advanced practice nurses. *Nursing Economics, 10*(5), 343–351.

Parsons, M. A., Felton, G. M., & Chassie, M. B. (1996). Success stories: Faculty practice plan entrance strategy for nursing. *Nursing Economics, 14*(6), 372–382.

Pesut, D., & Misner, T. (1997). Decision guide for prospective faculty practitioners. In L. Marion (Ed.), *Nursing faculty practice: Applying the models* (pp. 13–22). Washington, DC: National Organization of Nurse Practitioner Faculties.

Rodgers, M. W. (1986). Implementing faculty practice: A question of human and financial resources. *Journal of Advanced Nursing, 11,* 687–696.

Rosswurm, M. A. (1981). Characteristics of 23 faculty group practices. *Nursing and Health Care, 2*(6), 327–330.

Ryan, M. C. (1997). Integrating practice, education, and research: Killing three birds with one stone. *Clinical Excellence for Nurse Practitioners, 1*(4), 244–249.

Shah, H. S., & Pennypacker, D. R. (1992). The clinical teaching partnership. *Nurse Educator, 17*(2), 10–12.

Spero, J. (1980). Nursing: A professional practice discipline in academia. *Nursing and Health Care, 1,* 22–25.

Spitzer, R., Bandy, C., Bumbalough, M., Frederiksen, D., Gibson, G., Howard, E., McIntosh, E., Pitts, V. N., & Reeves, G. (1996). Marketing and reimbursement of faculty-based practice. *Nursing and Health Care Perspectives on Community, 17*(6), 308–311.

Starck, P. (1996). Boyer's multidimensional nature of scholarship: A new framework for schools of nursing. *Journal of Professional Nursing, 12*(5), 268–276.

Steele, R. L. (1991). Attitudes about faculty practice, perceptions of role, and role strain. *Journal of Nursing Education, 30*(1), 15–22.

Walker, P. H. (1995). Faculty practice: Interest, issues, and impact. *Annual Review of Nursing Research, 13,* 217–236.

Walker, P. H., Bowallan, N., Chevalier, N., Gulio, S., & Lawrence, L. (1996). School-based care: Clinical challenges and research opportunities. *Journal of the Society of Pediatric Nurses, 1*(2), 64–74.

Wardle, M. G., & Boutin, C. (1997). Researching nurses as educators. *Nursing Connections, 10*(2), 47–52.

Watson, J. (1996). Service and education: We are all in it together. *Image: The Journal of Nursing Scholarship, 28*(4), 290–291.

White, B. J., Jarrett, S. L., & Tolve, C. J. (1997). A model of collaboration: The Academic Practice Council. *Nursing Connections, 10*(1), 5–12.

Williamson, N., McDonough, J. E., & Boettcher, J. H. (1990). Nurse faculty practice: From theory to reality. *Journal of Professional Nursing, 6*(1), 11–20.

Woodcock, E. (1999). Assessing primary care's contribution to academic health centers. *Medical Group Management Journal, 46*(2), 14–18, 20–22.

Woodcock, E. (1999, February). *Financing primary care.* Speech delivered to the Association of Departments of Family Medicine 1999 Spring Meeting, Tucson, AZ.

Wright, D. J. (1993). Faculty practice: Criterion for academic advancement. *Nursing and Health Care, 14*(1), 18–21.

Yarcheski, A., & Mahon, N. E. (1985). The unification model in nursing: A study of receptivity among nurse educators in the United States. *Nursing Research, 34,* 120–125.

Zenas, C. S. (1988). Achieving promotion and tenure: A strategic perspective. *Nurse Educator, 13*(1), 8–13.

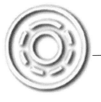

Index

Note: Page numbers in *italics* indicate figures; page numbers followed by t indicate tables.

ISBN 0-7216-8632-X

90016

9 780721 686325